a LANGE medical book

Basic and Clinical Immunology

Seventh Edition

Edited by

Daniel P. Stites, MD
Professor and Vice Chairman
Department of Laboratory Medicine
Director, Immunology Laboratory
University of California, San Francisco

Abba I. Terr, MD
Clinical Professor of Medicine
Stanford University School of Medicine
Stanford, California

APPLETON & LANGE
Norwalk, Connecticut/San Mateo, California

0-8385-0544-9

Copyright © 1991 by Appleton & Lange
A Publishing Division of Prentice Hall
Copyright © 1987, 1984, 1982, 1980, 1978, 1976 by Lange Medical Publications

91 92 93 94 95 / 10 9 8 7 6 5 4 3 2 1

Prentice Hall International (UK) Limited, *London*
Prentice Hall of Australia Pty. Limited, *Sydney*
Prentice Hall Canada, Inc., *Toronto*
Prentice Hall Hispanoamericana, S.A., *Mexico*
Prentice Hall of India Private Limited, *New Delhi*
Prentice Hall of Japan, Inc., *Tokyo*
Simon & Schuster Asia Pte. Ltd., *Singapore*
Editora Prentice Hall do Brasil Ltda., *Rio de Janeiro*
Prentice Hall, *Englewood Cliffs, New Jersey*

ISBN: 0-8385-0544-9
ISSN: 0891-2076

PRINTED IN THE UNITED STATES OF AMERICA

Table of Contents

iii

SECTION IV. IMMUNOLOGIC THERAPY

APPENDIX

Preface

This, the 7th edition of *Basic and Clinical Immunology,* is a major revision of a popular textbook for health care students and practitioners. The tradition of a comprehensive and comprehensible treatise on immunology, which began with the first edition in 1974, is maintained.

The application of new techniques in molecular biology and genetics to basic and clinical research in recent years has brought new insights into the immune response and its consequences for diseases in ways that were difficult to imagine in 1974. The editors have endeavored to make the ''new'' immunology more understandable through several features unique to this edition.

- The subject matter of the book is restricted to human immunology. The contribution of animal research to the study of the human immune response is overwhelming and essential. However, differences in anatomy, function, and nomenclature of the immune systems of each animal species can be a source of confusion in an introductory textbook of immunology. The results of critical experiments with certain animal models are nevertheless included when these help to explain human diseases.
- The use of illustrations has been greatly expanded over that in previous editions. To simplify the identification of cells and their chemical products and receptors, a uniform set of symbols is used throughout the book. A glossary of these symbols is provided at the end of the book for easy reference.
- The sections and chapters of the book have been reorganized for better understanding of normal immunologic function and disease processes.
- It is recognized that immunology is not an easy subject, both because of its intrinsic complexity and because of the vast array of information currently available. The authors—all experts in their particular fields—have made every effort to write in a readable style without sacrificing essential details.

The book is divided into 4 sections, including Basic, Laboratory, and Clinical Immunology, as in previous editions, and a fourth new section, Immuno-therapy. This section describes the drugs and other forms of therapy used to treat immunologic diseases. It also deals with the ways in which the immune system is manipulated for treatment of other diseases, through immunization, immune suppression, and immune modulation.

The Basic Immunology section has been reorganized to reflect the immune response as primarily a cellular phenomenon with secondary generation of cell products—cytokines, immunoglobulins, and mediators—that subserve immune cell function. One chapter is devoted to an overall summary of the integrated function of the immune system. The mucosal immune system is described in a separate chapter. A new chapter on physiologic and environmental effects on the immune system has been added to include material not usually covered in immunology textbooks. Each chapter has a brief introduction, a body, and a thorough summary.

The Immunologic Laboratory Tests section is extensively updated with new methods and techniques that are rapidly being added to aid in clinical diagnosis. Histocompatibility testing is treated in a separate chapter. A new chapter on the assessment of immune competence through laboratory testing provides a critical overview of the efficient use and avoidance of misuse of the enormous number and variety of tests now available.

The Clinical Immunology section is subdivided into 5 categories in this edition. Two of these—immunodeficiency diseases and allergic diseases—expand these important subjects, which were treated as individual chapters in previous editions. The large number of diseases characterized by a variety of immunologic abnormalities, autoimmunity, and disordered immune regulation in which the underlying cause is unknown are again grouped together. As in previous editions, these fascinating diseases are discussed in separate chapters based on the involved organ or body system. A fourth category covers neoplasms of the immune system and neoplasms that arise in patients with diseased immune systems. The fifth category, on infections, makes a full circle from the origin of immunology, which concerned protection against infectious diseases to the newest concern, viral infections of the immune system itself, including acquired immunodeficiency syndrome (AIDS).

Each of the book's 4 sections and each of the Clinical Immunology subsections begins with a brief introductory chapter that is both an overview and an essay on the subject of the chapters that follow. The editors hope that this feature of the seventh edition will serve as a conceptual framework for the details that must be learned by beginning and advanced students of immunology.

ACKNOWLEDGMENTS

The editors are deeply grateful to Jack Lange for his continuing encouragement and wise counsel during the preparation of this major revision. We also acknowledge the expertise and advice of Alex Kugushev during the crucial planning stages. The meticulous editing skills of Yvonne Strong and the artistic drawings of Linda Harris helped to make this an informative and understandable text of a difficult subject. Finally, the authors and editors are indebted to the editorial staff of Appleton & Lange, particularly Nancy Evans, for their efforts and patience.

Recommendations about diagnosis and treatment of disease are based on the best scientific and clinical information currently available. They are intended, however, as guidance to the clinician and not necessarily as recommendations for specific cases. Furthermore, we recognize that we may have overlooked errors despite our best efforts. We would be grateful if our readers would point these out so that they may be corrected in the next edition.

San Francisco
November 1990

Daniel P. Stites, MD
Abba I. Terr, MD

The Authors

Arthur J. Ammann, MD
Director of Clinical Research, Genentech, Inc., South San Francisco.

Nancy Ascher, MD, PhD
Professor of Surgery, Chief of Liver Transplantation, University of California School of Medicine, San Francisco.

James R. Baker, Jr, MD
Associate Professor of Medicine, Division of Allergy, Department of Medicine, University of Michigan Medical Center, Ann Arbor.

Edith L. Bossom, SBB
Supervisor, Blood Bank, University of California, San Francisco.

Marek Bozdech, MD
Head, Department of Oncology and Hematology, Kaiser Permanente at Santa Rosa, Santa Rosa, CA.

David H. Broide, MB, ChB
Assistant Professor of Medicine, University of California School of Medicine, San Diego.

Richard A. Bronson, MD
Associate Professor, Obstetrics and Gynecology and Pathology, State University of New York, Stony Brook.

Stephen N. Cohen, MD
Clinical Professor of Laboratory Medicine, Medicine, and Microbiology and Director of Clinical Laboratories, University of California School of Medicine, San Francisco.

Beth W. Colombe, PhD
Associate Research Immunologist and Associate Director, Immunogenetics and Transplantation Laboratory, University of California School of Medicine, San Francisco.

Suzanne Crowe, MBBS
Head, AIDS Research Unit, MacFarlane Burnet Centre for Medical Research, Fairfield Hospital, Melbourne, Australia.

Thomas R. Cupps, MD
Associate Professor of Medicine, Georgetown University Medical Center, Department of Medicine, Division of Rheumatology, Immunology and Allergy, Washington, D.C.

Elizabeth Donegan, MD
Associate Professor of Clinical Laboratory Medicine, Pathology, and Microbiology and Immunology, University of California School of Medicine, San Francisco.

Steven D. Douglas, MD
Section Chief for Immunology, Professor of Pediatrics and Microbiology, Children's Hospital of Philadelphia.

David J. Drutz, MD
Vice President, Medical Affairs, Daiichi Pharmaceutical Corp., Fort Lee, NJ; Adjunct Professor of Medicine, University of Pennsylvania.

Devendra P. Dubey, PhD
Assistant Professor, Dana Farber Cancer Institute and Harvard Medical School, Boston.

Connie Faltynek, PhD
Scientist, Program Resources, Inc., NCI-FCRF, Frederick, MD; Senior Research Scientist, Sterling Research Group, Sterling Drug Inc., Malvern, PA.

Paul S. Fishman, MD, PhD
Assistant Professor, Department of Neurology, University of Maryland School of Medicine, Baltimore.

Alessandro Fornasieri, MD
Research Associate, Department of Immunology, Scripps Clinic and Research Foundation, La Jolla, CA.

Michael M. Frank, MD
Clinical Director, NIAID, and Chief, Laboratory of Clinical Investigation, Bethesda, MD.

Mitchell H. Friedlaender, MD
Adjunct Associate Member, Department of Molecular and Experimental Medicine, Scripps Clinic and Research Foundation, La Jolla, CA.

Kenneth H. Fye, MD
Clinical Professor of Medicine, University of California School of Medicine, San Francisco.

Marvin R. Garovoy, MD
Professor of Surgery and Medicine, and Director, Immunogenetics and Transplantation Laboratory, University of California School of Medicine, San Francisco.

Sanford M. Goldstein, MD
Assistant Clinical Professor, Department of Dermatology, University of California School of Medicine, San Francisco.

Joel W. Goodman, PhD
Professor and Vice Chairman, Department of Microbiology and Immunology, University of California, San Francisco.

James S. Goodwin, MD
Professor of Medicine, Head, Section of Geriatrics, University of Wisconsin Medical School, Milwaukee.

Joan Goverman, PhD
Senior Research Fellow, Division of Biology, California Institute of Technology, Pasadena.

Philip D. Greenberg, MD
Professor of Medicine and Immunology, University of Washington; Member, Fred Hutchinson Cancer Research Center, Seattle, WA.

John S. Greenspan, BDS, PhD, FRCPath
Professor of Oral Pathology and Chair, Department of Stomatology, University of California, San Francisco.

Moses Grossman, MD
Professor and Vice Chairman, Department of Pediatrics, San Francisco General Hospital.

Donald Heyneman, PhD
Professor of Parasitology, University of California, San Francisco; Chair, UC Berkeley-UCSF Joint Medical Program and Associate Dean for Health Sciences, School of Public Health, University of California, Berkeley.

Gary W. Hunninghake, MD
Professor and Division Director, Pulmonary Disease Division, Department of Internal Medicine, University of Iowa Hospital, Iowa City, IA.

James P. Isbister, FRACP, FRCPA
Head, Department of Haematology, Royal North Shore Hospital of Sydney, St. Leonards, New South Wales, Australia.

Howard S. Jaffe, MD
Attending Physician, San Francisco General Hospital; Director of Clinical Research, Genentech, Inc., South San Francisco.

Stephen P. James, MD
Senior Investigator, Mucosal Immunity Section, National Institute of Allergy and Infectious Diseases, Bethesda, MD.

Naynesh R. Kamani, MD
Assistant Professor of Pediatrics, University of Pennsylvania School of Medicine, Philadelphia.

Daniel V. Landers, MD
Assistant Professor, Obstetrics & Gynecology, San Francisco General Hospital, San Francisco.

Lewis Lanier, PhD
Associate Research Director, Immunobiology, Becton Dickinson Monoclonal Center, Inc., San Jose, CA.

Robert J. Lukes, MD
Professor Emeritus, Pathology, University of Southern California School of Medicine, Los Angeles.

Donald J. Magilligan, Jr, MD†
Formerly Professor of Surgery and Chief of Cardiac Surgery, University of California, San Francisco.

James H. McKerrow, MD, PhD
Associate Professor of Pathology, Department of Pathology, University of California School of Medicine, San Francisco.

Juliet S. Melzer, MD
Associate Professor of Surgery, Transplant Service, University of California School of Medicine, San Francisco.

John Mills, MD
Professor of Medicine, Microbiology and Laboratory Medicine, University of California School of Medicine, San Francisco.

Phillippe Moullier, MD, PhD
Research Associate, Department of Immunology, Scripps Clinic and Research Foundation, La Jolla, CA.

†Deceased

G. Richard O'Connor, MD
Professor Emeritus, Ophthalmology, University of California School of Medicine, and Director, Francis I. Proctor Foundation for Research in Ophthalmology, San Francisco.

Joost J. Oppenheim, MD
Chief, Laboratory of Molecular Immunoregulation, National Cancer Institute, Frederick, MD.

Hillel S. Panitch, MD
Professor of Neurology, University of Maryland, and Clinical Investigator, Department of Veterans Affairs Medical Center, Baltimore.

John W. Parker, MD
Professor of Pathology and Vice Chairman, Department of Pathology, University of Southern California School of Medicine, Los Angeles.

Jane R. Parnes, MD
Associate Professor of Medicine, Stanford University, Stanford, CA.

Tristram G. Parslow, MD, PhD
Assistant Professor of Pathology and Microbiology and Immunology, University of California School of Medicine, San Francisco.

Charles S. Pavia, PhD
Associate Professor of Medicine, Microbiology and Immunology, and Director of the Spirochete Research Laboratory, New York Medical College, Valhalla.

R.P. Channing Rodgers, MD
Assistant Professor, Laboratory Medicine, Assistant Research Chemist, Department of Pharmaceutical Chemistry, University of California School of Medicine, San Francisco.

Francis W. Ruscetti, PhD
Head, Lymphokine Section, National Cancer Institute, Frederick, MD.

John L. Ryan, PhD, MD
Executive Director, Infectious Disease, Clinical Research, Merck, Sharp, & Dohme, Philadelphia.

Kenneth E. Sack, MD
Associate Clinical Professor of Medicine, Director of Clinical Programs in Rheumatology, University of California School of Medicine, San Francisco.

Benjamin D. Schwartz, MD, PhD
Professor of Medicine and Molecular Microbiology, Washington University School of Medicine, and Chief, Division of Rheumatology, Jewish Hospital at Washington University Medical Center, St. Louis.

William Seaman, MD
Professor of Medicine, University of California School of Medicine, San Francisco, and Chief, Arthritis/Immunology Section, Veterans Administration Medical Center, San Francisco.

Steven A. Sherwin, MD
President and Chief Executive Officer, Cell Genesys Inc., Foster City, CA.

Raymond G. Slavin, MD
Professor of Internal Medicine and Microbiology, and Director, Division of Allergy and Immunology, St. Louis University School of Medicine, St. Louis.

Alfred D. Steinberg, MD
Chief, Cellular Immunology, ARB, NIAMS, National Institute of Health, Bethesda, MD.

Daniel P. Stites, MD
Professor and Vice Chairman, Department of Laboratory Medicine, University of California School of Medicine, San Francisco.

Warren Strober, MD
Head, Mucosal Immunity Section, Laboratory of Clinical Investigation, NIAID, Bethesda, MD.

David W. Talmage, MD
Distinguished Professor, University of Colorado, Denver.

Winson Tang, MD
Research Associate, Department of Immunology, Scripps Clinic and Research Foundation, La Jolla, CA.

Abba I. Terr, MD
Clinical Professor of Medicine, Stanford University School of Medicine, Stanford, CA.

Francine L. Vriesendorp, MD
Assistant Professor of Neurology, University of Maryland Medical School, Baltimore.

Robert H. Waldman, MD
Dean, College of Medicine, and Professor, Department of Internal Medicine, University of Nebraska Medical Center, Omaha.

David M. Ward, MB, ChB, MRCP (UK)
Professor of Clinical Medicine, University of California School of Medicine, San Diego; Director of Clinical Nephrology, University of California Medical Center, San Diego.

Stephen I. Wasserman, MD
Professor and Chairman, Department of Medicine, University of California School of Medicine, San Diego.

H. James Wedner, MD
Associate Professor of Medicine, and Chief, Clinical Allergy and Immunology, Washington University School of Medicine, St. Louis.

J. Vivian Wells, MD, FRACP, FRCPA
Senior Staff Specialist in Clinical Immunology, Kolling Institute of Medical Research, Royal North Shore Hospital of Sydney, St. Leonards, New South Wales, Australia.

Curtis B. Wilson, MD
Member, Department of Immunology, Scripps Clinic and Research Foundation, La Jolla, CA.

Alan Winkelstein, MD
Professor of Medicine, University of Pittsburgh School of Medicine, and Head, Clinical Immunology Unit, Montefiore Hospital, Pittsburgh.

Bruce U. Wintroub, MD
Professor and Chairman, Department of Dermatology, University of California School of Medicine, San Francisco.

Lowell S. Young, MD
Director, Kuzell Institute for Arthritis and Infectious Diseases, Medical Research Institute, San Francisco.

Edmond J. Yunis, MD
Professor of Pathology, Harvard Medical School, and Chief, Division of Immunogenetics, Dana-Farber Cancer Institute, Boston.

Brian P. Zehr, MD
Pulmonary Medicine, Ft. Wayne, IN.

John L. Ziegler, MD
Professor of Medicine, University of California School of Medicine, and Associate Chief of Staff for Education, Veterans Administration Medical Center, San Francisco.

Section I. Basic Immunology

History of Immunology

1

David W. Talmage, MD

THE ORIGIN OF IMMUNOLOGY

Immunology began as a branch of microbiology; it grew out of the study of infectious diseases and the body's responses to them. The concepts of contagion and the germ theory of disease are attributed to Girolamo Fracastoro, a colleague of Copernicus at the University of Padua, who wrote in 1546 that "Contagion is an infection that passes from one thing to another . . . The infection is precisely similar in both the carrier and the receiver of the contagion . . . The term is more correctly used when infection originates in very small imperceptible particles." Fracastoro's conclusions were remarkable because they were contrary to the philosophy of his time in that he postulated the existence of germs that were too small to be seen. He was a practical physician who gave more credence to his own observations than to traditional beliefs.

It was more than 2 centuries later that another physician, Edward Jenner, extended the concept of contagion to a study of the immunity produced in the host. This was the beginning of immunology. Jenner, a country doctor in Gloucestershire, England, noted in 1798 that a pustular disease of the hooves of horses called "the grease" was frequently carried by farm workers to the nipples of cows, where it was picked up by milkmaids. "Inflamed spots now begin to appear on the hands of the domestics employed in milking, and sometimes on the wrists . . . but what renders the Cowpox virus so extremely singular, is, that the person who has been thus affected is for ever after secure from the infection of Small Pox; neither exposure to the variolous effluvia, nor the insertion of the matter into the skin, producing this distemper."

Jenner was unclear about the nature of the infectious agent of cowpox and its relation to smallpox, but he reported 16 cases of resistance to smallpox in farm workers who had recovered from cowpox. He described how he deliberately inserted matter "taken from a sore on the hand of a dairymaid, on the 14th of May, 1796, into the arm of the boy by means of two superficial incisions, barely penetrating the cutis, each about half an inch long." Two months later, Jenner inoculated the same 8-year-old boy with matter from a smallpox patient, a dangerous but accepted procedure called **variolation.** However, the boy developed only a small sore at the site of inoculation. His exposure to the mild disease cowpox had made him immune to the deadly disease smallpox. In this manner Jenner began the science of immunology, the study of the body's response to foreign substances.

Immunology has always been dependent upon technology, particularly lens-making and the microscopy. Eyeglasses were introduced into Europe in the 14th century, (perhaps by Marco Polo), and telescopes were used by Galileo in 1609 to discover the moons of Jupiter. However, useful microscopes were not available until the middle of the 19th century. After that, progress in microbiology was rapid. In 1850, Davaine reported that he could see anthrax bacilli in the blood of infected sheep. In 1858, Wallace and Darwin jointly submitted reports proposing evolution through natural selection, and in the same year, Pasteur demonstrated to the French wine industry that fermentation was due to a living microorganism. In 1864, Pasteur disproved the theory of spontaneous generation; in 1867, Lister introduced aseptic surgery; and in 1871, DNA was discovered by Miescher. Anthrax was first transmitted from in vitro culture to animals by Koch in 1876, thus fulfilling **Koch's postulates,** which he had said were required to prove that the bacteria caused the disease. Between 1879 and 1881, Pasteur developed the first 3 attenuated vaccines (after cowpox); these were for chicken cholera, anthrax, and rabies.

Bacteriology and histology were recognized as established scientific fields during this period. The gonococcus, the first human pathogen, was isolated in 1879 by Neisser, and 10 other pathogens were isolated in the next decade. Of particular importance to immunology was the isolation of the diphtheria bacillus by Klebs and Loeffler in 1883; this led to the production of the first defined antigen, diphtheria toxin, by Roux and Yersin in 1888. In that same year, the first antibodies, serum bactericidins, were reported by Nuttall, and Pasteur recognized that nonliving substances as well as living organisms could induce immunity. This led to the discovery of antitoxins by von Behring and Kitasato in 1890 and later to the development of toxoids for diphtheria and tetanus.

CELLULAR VERSUS HUMORAL IMMUNITY

In 1883, Metchnikoff observed the phagocytosis of fungal spores by leukocytes and advanced the idea that immunity was primarily due to white blood cells. This provoked an intense controversy with the advocates of **humoral immunity.** The discovery of complement in 1894 by Bordet and **precipitins** in 1897 by Kraus appeared to favor the humoral side of the controversy. Ehrlich's side chain theory, proposed in 1898, was an attempt to harmonize the 2 views. According to Ehrlich, cells possessed on their surfaces a wide variety of side chains (we would call them antigen receptors) that were used to bring nutrients into the cell. When toxic substances blocked one of these side chains through an accidental affinity, the cell responded by making large numbers of that particular side chain, some of which spilled out into the blood and functioned as circulating antibodies.

In 1903, Sir Almoth Wright reported that antibodies could aid in the process of phagocytosis, thus effectively settling the controversy over cellular versus humoral community. Wright called these antibodies "opsonins." This followed the practice of labeling antibodies according to their observed action, eg, agglutinins, precipitins, hemolysins, and bactericidins.

It was gradually realized that antibodies could have deleterious as well as beneficial effects and could produce hypersensitivity. The term "anaphylaxis" was coined by Richet and Portier in 1902 to denote the frequently lethal state of shock induced by a second injection of antigen. The term "allergy" was introduced by von Pirquet in 1906 to denote the positive reaction to a scratch test with tuberculin in individuals infected with tuberculosis.

THE PERIOD OF SEROLOGY

Blood group antigens and their corresponding agglutinins were discovered by Landsteiner in 1900. This led to the ability to give blood transfusions without provoking reactions. Landsteiner was a dominant figure in immunology for 40 years, developing the concept of the antigenic determinant and demonstrating the exquisite specificity of antibodies for chemically defined hap-

tens, a term he applied to simple chemicals that could bind to antibodies but were by themselves incapable of stimulating antibody formation. Landsteiner rejected Ehrlich's side chain theory because he was able to make antibodies against a seemingly infinite number of different substances, synthetic as well as natural.

In 1901, Bordet and Gengou introduced the complement fixation test, which became a standard diagnostic test in the hospital laboratory. The word "immunology" first appeared in the *Index Medicus* in 1910, and the *Journal of Immunology* began publication in 1916. The first 30 years of the Journal were devoted almost exclusively to a study of serologic reactions.

Landsteiner's book, *The Specificity of Serological Reactions,* was published in German in 1933 and in English in 1936. Marrack's text, *The Chemistry of Antigens and Antibodies,* was published in 1935. Antibodies were viewed as being formed directly on antigens, which functioned as templates, in a theory published by Breinl and Haurowitz in 1930. In 1939, Tiselius and Kabat showed that antibodies were gamma globulins, and in 1940, Pauling proposed the variable-folding theory of antibody formation. According to Pauling's theory, gamma globulin peptides are folded into a complementary configuration in the presence of antigen. This fit the "Unitarian" view of antibodies generally accepted at that time, which held that all antibodies were the same except for their specificity.

Immunochemistry was a natural outgrowth of this chemical approach to immunology. The quantitative precipitin test was developed by Heidelberger, Kendall, and Kabat and was used to study the structure of polysaccharide antigens.

THE REBIRTH OF CELLULAR IMMUNOLOGY

Two events of 1941–1942 heralded the rediscovery of the cell by immunologists. Coons demonstrated the presence of antigens and antibodies inside cells by the new technique of **immunofluorescence,** and Chase and Landsteiner reported that delayed hypersensitivity could be transferred by cells but not by serum. The very next year (1943), Avery, MacCleod, and McCarty reported that DNA was responsible for the transfer of hereditary traits in bacteria.

In 1945, Owen discovered blood chimeras in cattle twins, and in 1948, Fagraeus showed that antibodies were made in plasma cells. In 1949, Burnet and Fenner published their adaptive enzyme theory of antibody formation, which again established immunology as a biologic science. They also proposed the "self-marker" concept, which was the first formal explanation of self tolerance.

In 1953, Billingham, Brent, and Medawar demonstrated acquired immunologic tolerance in bone marrow chimeras in mice injected with allogeneic bone marrow at or before birth. In that same year, Watson and Crick described the double helix of DNA. The close association in the development of immunology and molecular biology is illustrated by these two discoveries. Two years later, Jerne proposed his natural selection theory of antibody formation, in which randomly diversified gamma globulin molecules were thought to replicate after binding to injected antigen. Jerne's theory explained the known facts of immunology of that time, such as immunologic memory and the logarithmic rate of rise of antibody. However, this theory was incompatible with the new concepts of cellular and molecular biology. Within 2 years, 2 new theories of antibody production were proposed, the first by Talmage and the second by Burnet. Both theories substituted randomly diversified cells for randomly diversified gamma globulin molecules and proposed that the interaction of antigen with receptors on the cell surface stimulated antibody production and the replication of the selected cell.

After more than 30 years, the cell selection theory and the name given to it by Burnet—**clonal selection**—have become part of the established dogma of immunology. This theory has been confirmed by numerous experiments and was popularized in 1975 by the development by Köhler and Milstein of the technique of producing monoclonal antibodies.

Cellular immunology reached its zenith in 1966 with the discovery by Claman, Chaperon, and Triplett of the presence and cooperation of **B cells** and **T cells.** Since that time, the study of the development, specificity, and activation of B cells and T cells has occupied the energy of a great many immunologists.

THE ADVENT OF MOLECULAR IMMUNOLOGY

By 1959, the field of protein chemistry had reached the point at which it was possible to analyze the structure of the antibody molecule in detail. In that same year, the 3 fragments of immunoglobulins, 2 Fab's and one Fc, were separated by Porter, and the heavy and light chains were separated by Edelman. The discovery of common and variable regions by Putnam and by Hilschmann and Craig came in 1965. Edelman et al reported the first complete amino acid sequence of an immunoglobulin molecule in 1969.

The 1960s and 1970s saw similar advances in the identification, separation, and structure of other molecules important to the immune system, such as complement components, interleukins, and cell receptors. These studies were greatly enhanced by the application of monoclonal antibody technology, which allowed sensitive and specific identification and isolation of many such molecules.

The elusive T cell receptor was finally isolated in 1982–1983 by Allison et al and Haskins et al. The steps required for antigen processing and presentation and the chemical reactions required for lymphocyte activation by antigen were also elucidated.

IMMUNOGENETICS & GENETIC ENGINEERING

The major histocompatibility antigens were discovered by Gorer in 1936, but it was not until 1968 that McDevitt and Tyan showed that immune response genes were linked to the genes of the major histocompatibility complex. Six years later, Doherty and Zinkernagel reported that the recognition of antigen by T cells was restricted by major histocompatibility complex molecules. During this time, the technology of recombinant DNA was developed. This led to the demonstration of immunoglobulin gene rearrangement by Tonegawa et al in 1978 and the production of transgenic mice by Gordon et al in 1980. The identification of genes for the T cell receptor by Davis et al came in 1984.

IMMUNOLOGY TIME LINE

1798   Edward Jenner
        Cowpox vaccination.

1880   Louis Pasteur
        Attenuated vaccines.

1883   Elie I. I. Metchnikoff
        Phagocytic theory.

1888   P. P. Emile Roux and A. E. J. Yersin
        Bacterial toxins.

1888   George H. F. Nuttall
        Bactericidal antibodies.

1890   Robert Koch
        Hypersensitivity.

1890   Emil A. von Behring and Shibasaburo Kitasato
        Diphtheria antitoxin.

1894   Jules J. B. V. Bordet
        Complement.

1897   Rudolf Kraus
        Precipitins.

1898   Paul Ehrlich
        Side chain theory.

1900   Karl Landsteiner
        Blood group antigens and antibodies.

1902   Charles R. Richet and Paul J. Portier
        Anaphylaxis.

1903   Almoth E. Wright
        Opsonins.

1905   Clemens P. von Pirquet and Bela Schick
        Serum sickness.

1906   Clemens P. von Pirquet
        Allergy.

1930   Friedrich Breinl and Felix Haurowitz
        Template theory.

1939   Arne Wilhelm Tiselius and Elvin A. Kabat
        Identity of antibodies with gamma globulins.

1941   Albert H. Coons et al
        Immunofluorescence.

1942   Karl Landsteiner and Merrill W. Chase
        Transfer of delayed-type hypersensitivity with cells.

1945   Ray D. Owen
        Chimeras in bovine twins.

1948   Astrid E. Fagraeus
        Antibodies in plasma cells.

1949   F. Macfarlane Burnet and Frank Fenner
        Adaptive enzyme theory.

1953   Rupert E. Billingham, Leslie Brent, and Peter B. Medawar
        Bone marrow chimeras in mice.

1955   Niels K. Jerne
        Natural selection theory.

1957   David W. Talmage and F. Macfarlane Burnet
        Cell selection theories.

1959   Rodney R. Porter and Gerald M. Edelman
        Structure of antibodies.

1966   Henry N. Claman et al
        Cooperation of T and B cells.

1968   Hugh O. McDevitt and Marvin L. Tyan
        Linkage of immune response genes to major histocompatibility complex genes.

1974   Peter C. Doherty and Rolf M. Zinkernagel
        T cell restriction.

1975   Cesar Milstein and Georges J. F. Kohler
        Monoclonal antibodies.

1978   Susumu Tonegawa
        Immunoglobulin gene rearrangement.

1980   Jon W. Gordon et al
        Transgenic mice.

1983   Kathryn Haskins et al
        T cell receptor isolation.

1984   Mark Davis et al
        T cell receptor genes.

NOBEL PRIZE WINNERS IN IMMUNOLOGY

1901   EMIL ADOLF von BEHRING for his work on serum therapy, especially application against diphtheria.

1905   ROBERT KOCH for his investigations and discoveries in relation to tuberculosis.

1908   PAUL EHRLICH and ELIE METCHNIKOFF for their work on immunity.

1913   CHARLES ROBERT RICHET for his work on anaphylaxis.

1919   JULES BORDET for his discoveries relating to immunity, particularly complement.

1928   CHARLES JULES HENRI NICOLLE for his work on typhus.

1930   KARL LANDSTEINER for his discovery of human blood groups.

1960   FRANK MACFARLANE BURNET and
        PETER BRIAN MEDAWAR for their
        discovery of acquired immunologic toler-
        ance.

1972   GERALD MAURICE EDELMAN and
        RODNEY ROBERT PORTER for their
        discoveries concerning the chemical
        structure of antibodies.

1977   ROSALYN YALOW for the develop-
        ment of radioimmunoassays of peptide
        hormones.

1980   BARUJ BENACERRAF, JEAN DAUS-
        SET, and GEORGE DAVIS SNELL for
        their discoveries concerning genetically
        determined structures on the cell surface
        that regulate immunologic reactions.

1984   NIELS K. JERNE, GEORGES F.
        KÖHLER, and CESAR MILSTEIN for
        theories concerning the specificity in de-
        velopment and control of the immune
        system and the discovery of the principle
        for production of monoclonal anti-
        bodies.

1987   SUSUMU TONEGAWA for his discov-
        ery of the genetic principle for genera-
        tion of antibody diversity.

SUMMARY

Immunology began as a study of the response of the whole animal to infection. Over the years, it has become progressively more basic, passing through phases of emphasis on serology, cellular immunology, molecular immunology, and immunogenetics. At the same time, immunology has grown to encompass many fields such as allergy, clinical immunology, immunochemistry, immunopathology, immunopharmacology, tumor immunology, and transplantation. Thus, it has always provided an excellent mix of fundamental and applied science.

Immunology has always depended upon and stimulated the application of technology, such as the use of microscopy, electrophoresis, radiolabeling, immunofluorescence, recombinant DNA, and transgenic mice. In general, immunology has not become an inbred discipline but has maintained close associations with many other fields of medical science. From a base in microbiology, immunologists have spread out into all of the basic and clinical departments.

REFERENCES

Alexander HL: The History of allergy. In: *Immunological Diseases.* Samter M (editor). Little Brown, 1965.

Allison JP, McIntyre BW, Bloch D: Tumor specific antigen of murine T-lymphoma defined with monoclonal antibody. *J Immunol* 1982;**129**:2293.

Billingham RE, Brent L, Medawar PB: Actively acquired tolerance of foreign cells. *Nature* 1953; 172:603.

Bordet J: *Traite de L'Immunité dans les Maladies infectieuses,* 2nd ed. Masson, 1937.

Brack C, et al: A complete immunoglobulin gene is created by somatic recombination. *Cell* 1978;**15**:1.

Burnet FM: A modification of Jerne's theory of antibody production using the concept of clonal selection. *Aust J Sci* 1957;**20**:67.

Burnet FM, Fenner F: *The Production of Antibodies.* Macmillan (Melbourne), 1949.

Claman HN, Chaperon EA, Triplett RF: Thymus-marrow cell combination. Synergism in antibody production. *Proc Soc Exp Biol Med* 1966;**122**:1167.

Coons AH, et al: Immunological properties of an antibody containing a fluorescent group. *Proc Soc Exp Biol Med* 1941;47:200.

Doherty PC, Zinkernagel RM: T-cell mediated immunopathology in viral infections. *Transplant Rev* 1974;**19**:89.

Dubos R: *The Unseen World.* Rockefeller Univ Press, 1962.

Edelman GM: Dissociation of gamma globulin. *J Am Chem Soc* 1959;**81**:3155.

Ehrlich P: On immunity with special reference to cell life. *Proc R Soc London Ser B* 1900;**66**:424.

Fagraeus A: The plasma cellular reaction and its relation to the formation of antibodies in vitro. *J Immunol* 1948;**58**:1.

Foster WD: *A History of Medical Bacteriology and Immunology.* William Heineman Medical Books, 1970.

Gay FP: Immunology, a medical science developed through animal experimentation. *J Am Med Assoc* 1911;**56**:578.

Gordon JW, et al: Genetic transformation of mouse embryos by microinjection of purified DNA. *Proc Natl Acad Sci USA* 1980;**77**:7380.

Haskins K, et al: The major histocompatibility complex restricted antigen receptor on T cells. I. Isolation with a monoclonal antibody. *J Exp Med* 1983; **157**:1149.

Hedrick SM, et al: Isolation of cDNA clones encoding T cell-specific membrane-associated proteins. *Nature* 1984;**308**:149.

Jerne NK: The natural selection theory of antibody formation. *Proc Natl Acad Sci USA* 1955;**41**:849.

Köhler G, Milstein C: Continuous culture of fused cells secreting antibody of predefined specificity. *Nature* 1975;**256**:495.

Landsteiner K: *The Specificity of Serological Reactions.* Thomas, 1936; reissued by Dover, 1962.

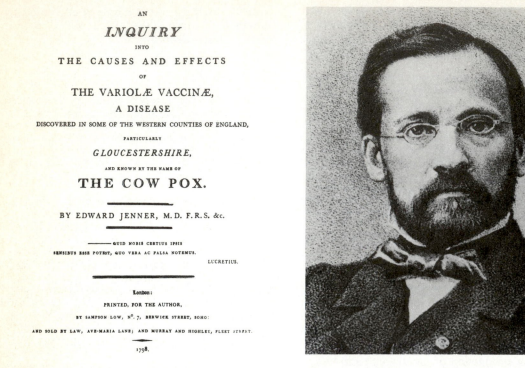

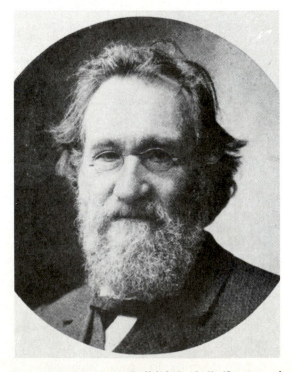

Figure 1-1. Face plate from first edition (1798) of Jenner's inquiry into the Causes and Effects of . . . the Cow Pox

Figure 1-2. Louis Pasteur (1822–1895). (Courtesy of the Museum of the Pasteur Institute, Paris.)

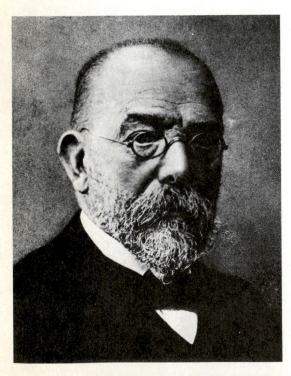

Figure 1-3. Robert Koch (1843–1910). (Courtesy of the Museum of the Pasteur Institute, Paris.)

Figure 1-4. Elie Metchnikoff (1845–1916). (Courtesy of the Rare Book Library, the University of Texas Medical Branch, Galveston.)

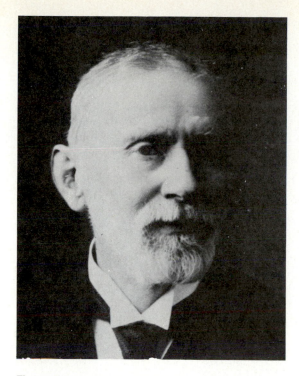

Figure 1-5. Paul Ehrlich (1854–1915). (Courtesy of the Museum of the Pasteur Institute, Paris.)

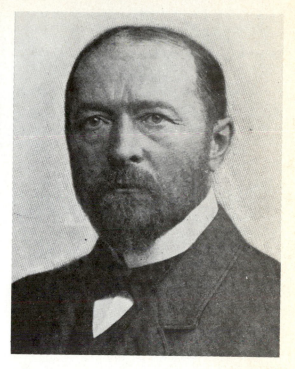

Figure 1-6. Emil von Behring (1854–1917). (Courtesy of the Museum of the Pasteur Institute, Paris.)

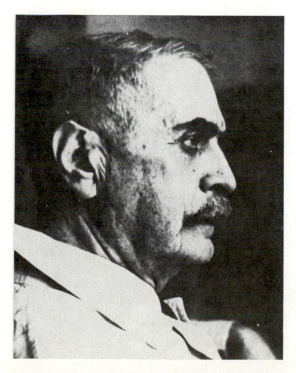

Figure 1-7. Karl Landsteiner (1868–1943). (Courtesy of the Museum of the Pasteur Institute, Paris.)

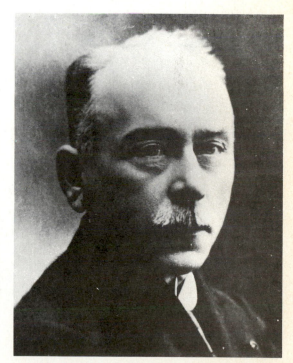

Figure 1-8. Jules Bordet (1870–1961). (Courtesy of the Museum of the Pasteur Institute, Paris.)

Landsteiner K, Chase MW: Experiments on transfer of cutaneous sensitivity to simple compounds. *Proc Soc Exp Biol Med* 1942;**49**:688.

McDevitt HO, Tyan ML: Transfer of response by spleen cells and linkage to the major histocompatibility (H-2) locus. *J Exp Med* 1968;**128**:1.

Parrish HJ: *A History of Immunization*. E & S Livingstone, 1965.

Parrish HJ: *Victory with Vaccines*. E & S Livingstone, 1968.

Pauling L: A theory of the structure and process of formation of antibodies. *J Am Chem Soc* 1940;**62**:2643.

Porter RR: The hydrolysis of rabbit gamma globulin and antibodies with crystalline papain. *Biochem J* 1959;**73**:119.

Talmage DW: Allergy and immunology. *Annu Rev Med* 1957;**8**:239.

Talmage DW: A century of progress: Beyond molecular immunology. *J Immunol* 1988;**141(Suppl)**:S5.

Structure & Development of the Immune System

2

Naynesh R. Kamani, MD, and Steven D. Douglas, MD

The cells that make up the immune system are distributed throughout the body but occur predominantly in the lymphoreticular organs, such as the lymph nodes, spleen, bone marrow, thymus, and the mucosa-associated lymphoid tissues of the gastrointestinal and respiratory tracts. In the extravascular tissues, these immune cells occupy the interstices of a network of interlocking reticular cells and fibers with a supporting framework of reticular cells. The lymphocytes are the predominant immunocytes, but monocyte-macrophages, endothelial cells, and rare eosinophils and mast cells also play roles in the immune system. All the cells of the immune system arise from pluripotent, self-renewing stem cells in the bone marrow.

Most lymphocytes are found in the spleen, lymph nodes, and Peyer's patches of the ileum. In mammals, the aggregate of lymphocytes constitutes about 1% of total body weight; the human body contains about 10^{12} lymphocytes. Approximately 10^9 lymphocytes are produced daily. Lymphocytes in the tissues are in dynamic equilibrium with those in the circulating blood and continuously recirculate through the vascular and lymphatic channels from one lymphoid organ to another.

Macrophages are found in connective tissues, lungs, liver, nervous system, serous cavities, bones and joints, and lymphoid organs. The lymphoid tissues of the body may be divided into primary or central lymphoid organs, ie, the thymus and bone marrow, and secondary or peripheral organs, eg, the lymph nodes, spleen, and Peyer's patches.

ORGANIZATION OF THE IMMUNE SYSTEM

LYMPHOID ORGANS

Thymus

The **thymus** is derived embryologically from the third and fourth branchial pouches and differenti-ates as ventral outpocketings from these pouches during the sixth week of embryonic life. During vertebrate embryogenesis, the thymus is the first organ to begin the production of lymphocytes. It is central to the development and function of the immune system; however, it is generally protected from exposure to antigen, partly by means of a barrier created by an epithelial membrane that surrounds thymic cortical blood vessels. The thymus does not directly participate in immune reactions but, rather, provides the microenvironment necessary for the maturation of T cells.

The thymus consists of 2 lobes, each of which is divided by septae into several lobules. Each lobule contains a cortex and medulla (Fig 2–1). It is believed that a humoral factor is produced by thymic epithelium that attracts stem cells to the thymus. Whether these cells are already committed to the T lymphoid lineage is unknown. Incoming cells migrate from the cortex to the medulla and in the process differentiate, acquire newer functions and surface antigens, and then emigrate from the thymus to peripheral tissues.

The most rapidly dividing cells in the thymus are large, blastlike lymphoid cells found in the subcapsular cortex. These cells contain terminal deoxynucleotidyl transferase (TdT) and express the early thymocyte T10 antigen. Approximately three-quarters of the lymphocytes within the thymus are located in the deeper cortex. These express the T6 or CD1 marker as well as both the helper-inducer CD4 and suppressor-cytotoxic CD8 markers. The medullary thymocytes are corticosteroid-resistant mature cells that express high levels of class I **major histocompatibility complex** (MHC) antigens and either the CD4 or the CD8 antigens. They constitute about 20% of the thymic lymphocytes. The medulla also contains thymic (Hassall's) corpuscles, composed of layers of epithelial cells, some macrophages, and cell debris. The function of thymic corpuscles is not known, but these structures may be the sites where lymphocyte cells die inside the thymus. The thymus has the highest rate of cell production of any tissue of the body, but the vast majority of cells produced in the thymus die there. This remark-

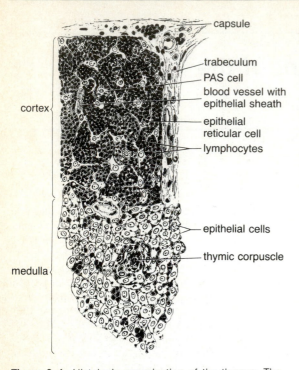

Figure 2–1. Histologic organization of the thymus. The cortex is heavily infiltrated with lymphocytes. As a result, the epithelial cells become stellate and remain attached to one another by desmosomes. The medulla is closer to a pure epithelium, although it too is commonly infiltrated by lymphocytes. A large thymic corpuscle consisting of concentrically arranged epithelial cells is seen. The capsule and trabeculae are rich in connective tissue fibers (mainly collagen) and contain blood vessels and variable numbers of plasma cells, granulocytes, and lymphocytes. (Reproduced, with permission, from Weiss L: *The Cells and Tissues of the Immune System: Structure, Functions, Interactions.* Copyright © 1972. Reprinted by permission of Prentice-Hall, Inc., Englewood Cliffs, NJ.)

able degree of cell wastage most probably results from abortive rearrangements of genetic material that occur during the generation of T cell receptor diversity (see Chapter 6).

Lymphoid cells in the thymus are surrounded by epithelial cells and other supporting cells, including interdigitating reticular cells and macrophages. The cortical and medullary thymic epithelial cells differ in their embryologic derivation and hence also in their morphologic features. A number of thymic hormones, including thymulin, thymosin $\alpha1$, thymosin $\beta4$, and thymopoietin, are produced by thymic epithelial cells. These hormones are necessary for differentiation of stem cell precursors in the thymus into mature cells.

The thymus reaches its maximum size (as a percentage of body weight) in most vertebrates either at birth or shortly thereafter. The human thymus grows until puberty and then begins a gradual process of involution. It decreases from 0.27% to 0.02% of total body weight between the ages of 5 and 15 years.

Neonatal removal of the thymus has profound effects on the immune system in many species of animals. In certain strains of mice, removal of the thymus leads to "wasting disease" (runting), with marked lymphoid atrophy and death. In other strains of mice, severe lymphopenia occurs, with depletion of cells from the paracortical areas of lymph nodes and periarteriolar regions of the spleen. Since cellular immunocompetence occurs early in human fetal development, there are few significant sequelae to neonatal thymectomy in humans. Long-term follow-up studies of individuals who received thymic radiation in early infancy have revealed decreases in the numbers of T and B lymphocytes and reduction in in vitro proliferative responses of lymphocytes to mitogens.

Impaired thymic development may be associated with immunologic deficiency disorders. The classic example of this is the DiGeorge syndrome, which results from an embryologic maldevelopment of the pharyngeal pouches, leading to various degrees of thymic hypoplasia and cellular immunodeficiency, congenital cardiac defects, an abnormal facies, and hypoparathyroidism (see Chapter 25). Abnormalities of the thymus, including both lymphoid hyperplasia and the development of thymomas, frequently occur in patients with certain autoimmune diseases, particularly systemic lupus erythematosus and myasthenia gravis.

Bursa of Fabricius & Mammalian "Bursa Equivalents"

The bursa of Fabricius, which is present in birds, is a lymphoepithelial organ located near the cloaca. The bursa is lined with pseudostratified epithelium and contains lymphoid follicles divided into cortex and medulla. In chickens, removal of the bursa of Fabricius leads to marked deficiency in immunoglobulins, impairment in development of germinal centers, and absence of plasma cells. The "bursa-dependent" lymphoid system is independent of the thymus. The mammalian equivalent of the bursa of Fabricius has not yet been definitively identified, although the mammalian gut-associated lymphoid tissues, including the appendix and Peyer's patches, histologically most closely resemble avian bursal tissues. Nevertheless, the primary site for B cell differentiation in mammals is most probably the fetal liver and, following birth, the bone marrow (Fig 2–2).

Pluripotent hematolymphoid stem cells, which have as yet not been morphologically or immunophenotypically identified with certainty in hu-

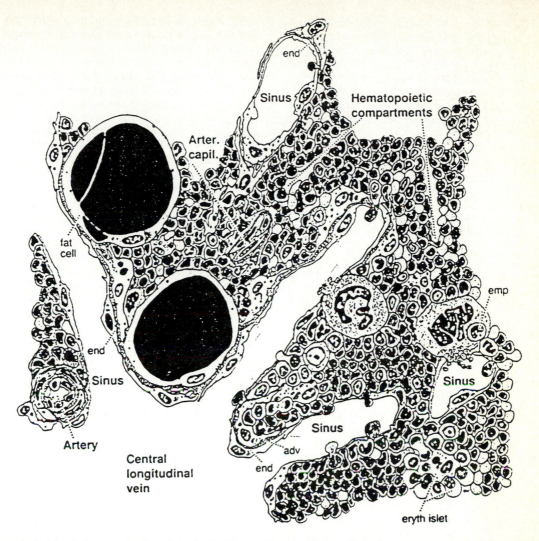

Figure 2-2. Histologic organization of the bone marrow. Hematopoietic cells lie between sinuses that drain into the central longitudinal vein. The wall of the sinus and the vein is trilaminar consisting of endothelium (end), a basement membrane, and adventitial cell (adv). With fatty change, the adventitial cells become voluminous fat cells and encroach on the hematopoietic space, whereas with active hematopoiesis, these cells become flat with the sinus wall reduced to a single endothelial cell layer. Megakaryocytes (meg) characteristically lie against the outside of the sinus wall, discharging platelets into the lumen through an aperture. Occasionally, other cell types enter megakaryocyte cytoplasm by a phenomenon known as emperipolesis (emp).

mans, are found in the fetal liver and adult bone marrow. These common progenitors give rise to lymphoid stem cells that eventually differentiate into mature lymphocytes and to hematopoietic progenitors that divide and differentiate into phagocytic cells (neutrophils and monocytes), erythrocytes, platelets, and eosinophils. Growth factors (called "cytokines"; see Chapter 7) that induce differentiation and maturation of hematopoietic cells in the bone marrow have been isolated and cloned. One of these, interleukin-4

(IL-4), previously known as B cell growth factor 1 (BCGF-1), is produced by T cells and serves as a proliferation factor not only for B cells but also for a number of other hematolymphoid progenitors, including T cells and megakaryocytic, myelomonocytic, and erythrocytic precursors.

Pre-B cells arise from lymphoid stem cells in the bone marrow and are the earliest identifiable cells of the B cell lineage. These are large lymphoid cells that express cytoplasmic μ chains but no light chains or surface immunoglobulin and are identified in fetal liver and adult bone marrow. During early B cell differentiation independent of antigen, stem cells and pre-B cells differentiate into immature and then mature B cells that express surface immunoglobulin and acquire Fc receptors for IgG. Following antigenic stimulation, B cells differentiate into immunoglobulin-secreting plasma cells or return to small, resting memory cells.

Lymph Nodes

The lymph nodes are encapsulated, bean-shaped or round structures usually located at the junction of major lymphatic tracts. In the resting state they range from 1 to 25 mm in diameter, and during states of infection or malignancy they enlarge significantly. Afferent lymphatics enter the nodes at the subcapsular sinus, from which there is centripetal flow toward the major efferent lymphatic duct, located in the hilus. Lymphocytes leave the circulation and enter the node via the **high endothelial venules (HEV)** in the paracortex, migrate toward the medulla, and eventually return to the circulation via efferent lymphatic channels that ultimately drain into the thoracic or right lymphatic duct (Fig 2–3). Lymph nodes serve as a filter for particulate foreign matter and tissue debris and participate as the central organs in lymphocyte circulation.

The histologic appearance of a lymph node depends on the state of activity of the node. The resting lymph node, which has not received recent antigenic stimulation, is morphologically divided into cortex, paracortical areas, and medulla. The margin between the cortex and paracortex may be obscure and may contain many resting lymphocytes. Within the cortex, there are a few aggregates of predominantly B lymphocytes called **primary follicles.** The paracortical areas contain postcapillary venules lined by cuboid epithelium, through which passes the blood supply to the node (Fig 2–4). The paracortex consists mostly of T lymphocytes that are situated in close proximity to interdigitating antigen-presenting cells (see the section on mononuclear phagocytes). In the resting node, the medulla is composed mostly of connective tissue surrounding the hilum. The antigen-stimulated lymph node shows an increased turnover of lymphocytes. Following antigenic stimulation, the paracortical area is hypertrophied, contains large lymphocytes and blastlike cells, and is easily distinguished from the cortex. The cortex contains germinal centers composed of metabolically active and mitotic cells, and the medulla contains numerous plasma cells, which actively secrete antibody.

Spleen

The spleen is a secondary lymphoid organ and performs a number of nonimmunologic functions, including filtration of blood and conversion of hemoglobin to bilirubin. Like the lymph nodes, it has a collagenous tissue capsule with trabeculae that penetrate the splenic parenchyma. The white and the red pulp constitute the 2 major types of splenic tissue. They are supported by a dense, close-meshed reticular network. The lymphoid

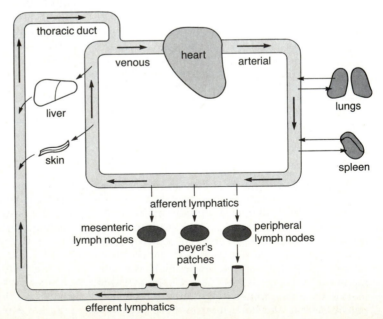

Figure 2–3. Lymphatic recirculation (Adapted from Duijvestijn A, Hamann A: Mechanisms and regulation of lymphocyte migration. *Immunol Today* 1989; **10**:23.)

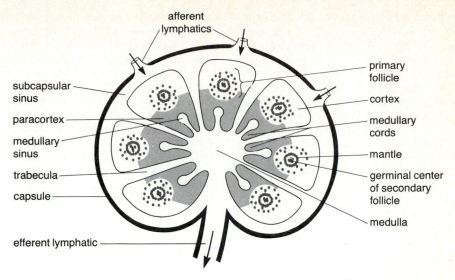

Figure 2–4. Schematic diagram of an immunologically active lymph node.

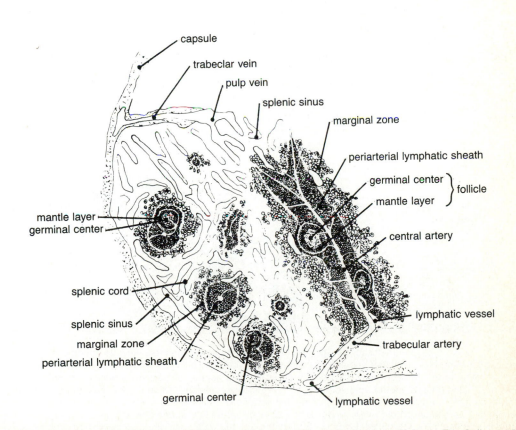

Figure 2–5. Histologic organization of the spleen. (Reproduced, with permission, from Weiss L: *The Cells and Tissues of the Immune System: Structure, Function, Interactions.* Copyright © 1972. Reprinted by permission of Prentice-Hall, Inc., Englewood, Cliffs, NJ.)

white pulp has central lymphoid follicles consisting mostly of B cells surrounded by thymus-dependent T lymphocytic regions (Fig 2–5). The erythroid red pulp serves as a filter for damaged or aged red cells and as a reserve site for extramedullary hematopoiesis (Fig 2–6). Unlike lymph nodes, lymphocytes enter and leave the spleen predominantly via the bloodstream.

Mucosa-Associated Lymphoid Tissue

The diffusely distributed, nonencapsulated lymphoid tissues of mucosal surfaces of the gastrointestinal, respiratory, and urogenital tracts are collectively referred to as the **mucosa-associated lymphoid tissues (MALT)**. Of all these tissues, the **gut-associated lymphoid tissue (GALT)** and the **bronchus-associated lymphoid tissue (BALT)** are the best-characterized. The lymphoid aggregates within these tissues are strategically located so that they are directly exposed to the external environment.

A. GALT: GALT is made up of Peyer's patches and isolated lymphoid follicles that are found predominantly in the colonic submucosa. Lymphoid cells are also scattered widely through the lamina propria, among the absorptive intestinal epithelial cells, and in small numbers in the lumen of the intestine. Peyer's patches consist of lymphoid aggregates with a central B cell–dependent follicle and surrounding T cell–dependent regions and macrophages that serve as antigen-

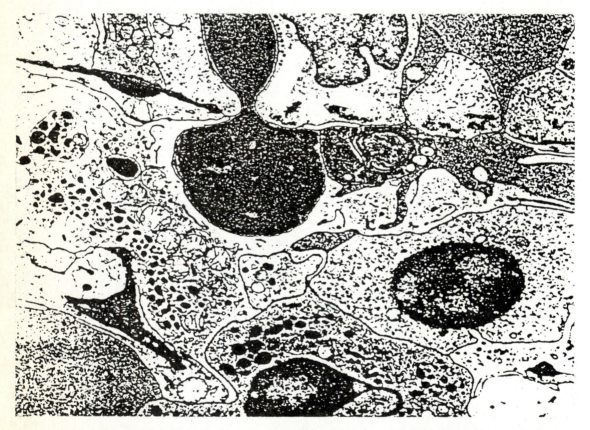

Figure 2-6. Human spleen in thalassemia. The wall of a splenic sinus crosses this field, its endothelial cells (End) cut in cross section. The base of these endothelial cells is rich in intermediate filaments and microfilaments that tend to run longitudinally. In this section, most filaments are cut in cross section and impart a stippled effect. In places the filaments are folded on one another and appear as relatively dense plaques (pl). Sinus and endothelial cells lie upon a fenestrated basement membrane (Bas Mb), represented here as short linear segments. Portions of reticular fibers (RF) branch into the perisinusal cord. Several erythrocytes (Ery), disparate in size and content, lie in interendothelial slits of the sinus. In addition, an erythroblast (Eb) is in passage through the wall, quite markedly pinched by the basal portions of the separated endothelial cells. The portion of its nuclear pole in the cord is surrounded by a macrophage (Mp), which also reaches to the cordal portion of a vesiculated, lamellated erythrocyte (Ery2) in the contiguous interendothelial slit. These slits impose a test on erythrocytes and other cells during passage through the human spleen.

presenting cells. The B cells are heterogeneous and may express any of the immunoglobulin isotypes. The T cells are predominantly regulatory and cytotoxic. These patches have efferent lymphatics that drain into mesenteric lymph nodes, but they have no afferent lymphatics. They are covered by a specialized lymphoepithelium consisting of microfold of M cells, which can be distinguished from surrounding epithelium by electron microscopy. They have short, wide, and irregular microvilli containing conspicuous axial filaments; an apical cytoplasm that has very few lysosomelike structures; and a basally situated nucleus (Fig 2–7). Luminal antigens can enter the Peyer's patches via the M cells after these cells selectively pinocytose and phagocytose particles. It is not known whether the antigens that eventually reach MALT are processed within the M cells or whether the M cells merely act as passive conduits for these antigens.

B. BALT: BALT is structurally and probably functionally quite similar to Peyer's patches and other lymphoid tissues that constitute the GALT of the intestines. It consists of large collections of lymphocytes organized into lymphoid aggregates and follicles. These are found primarily along the main bronchi in all lobes of the lungs and are situated prominently at the bifurcations of bronchi and bronchioles. The epithelium convering BALT follicles is devoid of goblet cells and cilia. In some species, BALT follicles seem to protrude into the lumen of the larger bronchi and trachea. The follicles invariably lie between branches from the pulmonary artery and the bronchial epithelium. BALT contains an elaborate network of capillaries, arterioles and venules, and efferent lymphatics; this suggests that BALT may play a role in sampling antigen not only from the lumen but also from the systemic circulation.

The M cells overlying the BALT follicles are

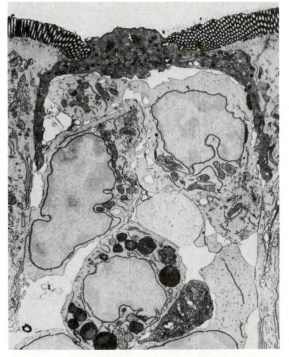

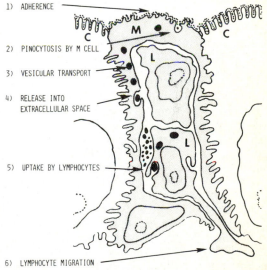

HORSERADISH PEROXIDASE TRANSPORT ACROSS LYMPHOID FOLLICLE EPITHELIUM

1) ADHERENCE

2) PINOCYTOSIS BY M CELL

3) VESICULAR TRANSPORT

4) RELEASE INTO EXTRACELLULAR SPACE

5) UPTAKE BY LYMPHOCYTES

6) LYMPHOCYTE MIGRATION

Figure 2–7. (*A*) Schematic diagram summarizing the transport of exogenous horseradish peroxidase observed by Owen and Jones. They hypothesize that the M cell transports intact macromolecules from the lumen to allow efficient "sampling" of luminal antigens by lymphocytes. L, Lymphocytes; C, columnar absorptive cells. (Reproduced with permission, from Owen RL: Sequential uptake of horseradish peroxidase by lymphoid follicle epithelium of Peyer's patches in the normal unobstructed mouse intestine: An ultrastructural study. *Gastroenterology* 1977;**72:**440.) (*B*) Electron micrograph showing the attenuated apical cytoplasm of an M cell over a cluster of intraepithelial lymphocyte (L). The protein tracer horseradish peroxidase (HRP) was introduced into the lumen 1 hour before fixation. The dense reaction product reveals the presence of HRP on the microvillous border of two adjacent absorptive cells and within small vesicles in the M cell cytoplasm. (Reproduced, with permission, from Owen RL, Nemanic P: Page 367, in: *Scanning Electron Microscopy.* Vol. II. SEM, Inc., 1978.)

structurally similar to intestinal M cells covering GALT. BALT consists mostly of collections of lymphocytes organized into follicles with infrequent germinal centers. The majority of lymphocytes in BALT are B cells.

Tonsils

By virtue of their strategic location, the palatine and nasopharyngeal **tonsils** are directly exposed to both airborne and alimentary antigens. Their architecture is similar to that of the lymph nodes. The deep crypts in tonsillar epithelium facilitate the trapping of antigens and foreign particles and greatly augment the area of contact between lymphoid tissue and airborne environmental antigens. Antigen is transported from the crypts to well-organized lymphoid follicles via the reticular epithelium. B cells predominate in these follicles, accounting for 40–50% of all lymphocytes. As in lymph nodes, the germinal centers within the follicles are antigen-dependent B cell areas, where memory clones expand and differentiate into plasma cells.

IMMUNOLOGIC CELLS

1. LYMPHOID CELLS

Morphology

The **lymphocyte** is a cell defined by certain morphologic features. Visualized by light microscopy, lymphocytes are ovoid cells 8–12 μm in diameter. They contain densely packed nuclear chromatin and a small rim of cytoplasm that stains pale blue with Romanovsky stains. The cytoplasm contains a number of azurophilic granules and a few vacuoles. In the area where most of the cytoplasmic organelles are present, the cytoplasmic rim is thickened. Phase contrast microscopy of living lymphocytes reveals a characteristic slow ameboid movement with a "hand-mirror" contour. Histochemical studies have demonstrated nucleolar and cytoplasmic ribonucleoprotein. The cytoplasm contains some glycogen. The lymphocyte contains a number of lysosomal hydrolases and mitochondrial enzymes. T and B cells are indistinguishable by conventional light microscopy.

Ultrastructure

Electron-microscopic examination of the resting circulating lymphocyte (Fig 2–8) reveals a dense heterochromatic nucleus, which contains some less electron-dense areas referred to as **euchromatin.** The nucleolus contains agranular, fibrillar, and granular zones. The nucleus is surrounded by the **nuclear membrane complex.** The cytoplasm of the resting lymphocyte contains or-

ganelle systems characteristic of eukaryotic cells (Golgi zone, mitochondria, ribosomes, and lysosomes). Many of these organelle systems, however, are poorly developed. There are many free ribosomes, a few ribosome clusters, and strands of granular endoplasmic reticulum. A small Golgi zone is present, which contains vacuoles, vesicles, and a few lysosomes. Microtubules are often present, and there are frequent mitochondria. The cytoplasm usually contains several lysosomes. The plasma membrane of the lymphocyte is a typical unit membrane, which may show small projections and, under some circumstances, longer pseudopodia or uropods. When platinum-carbon replicas of the plasma membranes of these cells are visualized by the freeze-fracture technique, they are shown to contain intramembrane particles in all membrane systems examined. Plasma membrane specialization may be related either to cell attachment to surfaces or to cell-cell interaction. By transmission electron microscopy, the cells of the plasma cell series are distinguishable from lymphocytes by the extensive development and dilation of granular endoplasmic reticulum and a well-developed Golgi zone in plasma cells (Fig 2–9). Monocular phagocytes (monocyte-macrophages) possess larger Golgi zones and more lysosomes than lymphocytes do.

The **blast cell,** in contrast to the small lymphocyte, has a nucleus characterized by loosely packed euchromatin, a large nucleolus, and a large cytoplasmic volume containing numerous polyribosomes and an extensively developed Golgi zone. It is easily identified by light microscopy and measures 15–30 μm in diameter. Blast cells are present in lymph nodes in vivo following antigenic stimulation or in cultures of lymphocytes stimulated in vitro with phytomitogens.

B & T Lymphocytes

The general features of these cell types are considered in order to provide a basic and more detailed understanding of their interactions in immune responses, their function, and their alterations in immunologic deficiency and autoimmune diseases.

A. Surface Markers: Numerous **monoclonal antibodies** have been developed that define leukocyte differentiation and cell surface molecules. As of 1989, the International Workshop on Human Leukocyte Differentiation Antigens has agreed on many clusters of differentiation (CD; see Chapter 5) groups or subgroups of distinct antigens on leukocyte cell surfaces that are recognized by the various available monoclonal antibodies. There is an important distinction between a plasma membrane **determinant,** which is a macromolecule present on the cell membrane, detected by labeled antibody methods and identifying particular cell

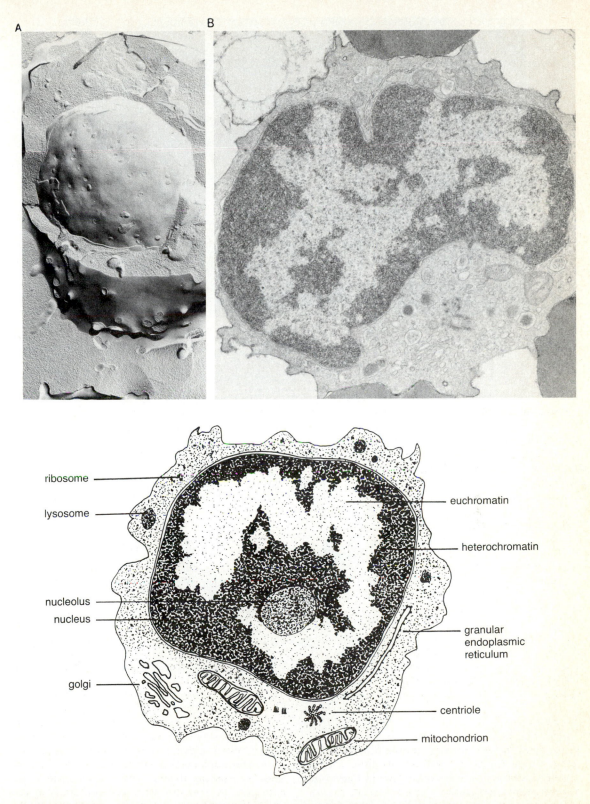

Figure 2–8. *Top:* (*A*) Freeze-fracture electron micrograph of normal human circulating lymphocyte. (Original magnification × 25,000.) (*B*) Transmission electron micrograph of normal circulating human lymphocyte. (Original magnification × 33,000.) ***Bottom:*** Diagrammatic representation of the micrograph shown at top right.

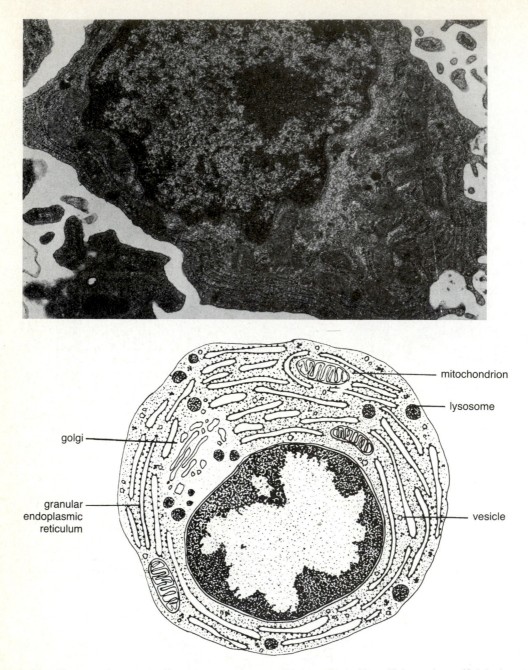

Figure 2–9. **Top:** Electron micrograph of bone marrow plasma cell from patient with multiple myeloma. (Original magnification × 19,000.) **Bottom:** Diagrammatic representation of cell shown at top.

types or subpopulations, and a **receptor,** which is a functional macromolecule characteristic of a specific cell type but with a known binding affinity for a specific ligand.

A property of most membrane determinants and receptors that is related to membrane fluidity is their ability to undergo redistribution and "cap-

ping." When a membrane component combines with its complementary molecule, it first undergoes a metabolically independent reorganization into patches over the entire cell surface ("patching") It may then undergo a metabolically dependent process by which the marker is topographically redistributed from dispersed patches to localization at one pole of the cell (capping). This capping event is usually followed by internalization of the components via membrane vesicles.

B. B Lymphocytes: The B lymphocyte in humans and most mammalian species is characterized by the presence of readily detectable surface immunoglobulin (Fig 2–10). The major immunoglobulin class on circulating B lymphocytes is IgM, which is present in monomeric form. IgD, IgG, IgA, and IgE may also be present on B lymphocyte membranes. In addition, most of the B lymphocytes have a receptor for antigen-antibody complexes, or aggregated immunoglobulin. This receptor is specific for a site on the Fc portion of the immunoglobulin molecule and is known as the **Fc receptor.** A receptor for the complement component C3d and for Epstein-Barr virus has been demonstrated on B cells (CD21 or B2). This complement receptor is distinct from the Fc receptor. A number of other B cell lineage–restricted differentiation antigens have been characterized. These include CD19 (B4) and CD20 (B1). B cells also possess other cell surface antigens not restricted to cells of the B lineage. These include CD10 (CALLA), CD9 (BA-2), and CD23, which appears to serve as the Fc receptor for IgE. B cells also express class II MHC antigens and the transferrin receptor.

C. T Lymphocytes: T lymphocytes form rosettes with sheep erythrocytes via the sheep erythrocyte receptor (CD2 or T11), and this marker is used to identify human T cells. A series of monoclonal antibodies to T cell membrane markers are used for the delineation of functional subsets of T cells. Anti-CD5 (anti-T1) is a monoclonal antibody reactive with 100% of peripheral T cells but only 10% of thymocytes. The CD5 thymocytes are the only thymocytes capable of reactivity in mixed lymphocyte culture. Anti-CD3 has essentially identical reactivity. Anti-CD4 reacts with 75% of thymocytes and 60% of peripheral T cells; it appears to identify a helper or inducer subset of peripheral blood T cells, which also are the only peripheral T cells that show a proliferative response to soluble antigens. This CD4+ subset is roughly equivalent to the $Th_1^+(Th_2^-)$ subset defined by heteroantisera. Anti-CD8 (anti-T5 and anti-T8) reacts with about 80% of thymocytes and 20–30% of peripheral T cells; anti-75 identifies a subset with both suppressor and cytotoxic capacity, similar to the Th_2^+ subset. Anti-CD1 (anti-T6), anti-T9, and anti-T10 react almost exclusively with thymocytes and not with peripheral T cells. The earliest thymocytes bear T9 and T10 markers or T10 alone; the T10 antigen is apparently lost when the cells leave the thymus for the peripheral compartment. The CD8+ subset in humans is analogous to the murine Lyt-2,3 subset, which mediates both cytotoxic and suppressor functions, and the human CD4 subset is analogous to the murine Lyt-1 subset, which has helper functions.

CD4 cells of the inducer type predominate in the thymic medulla, blood, and T cell traffic areas, including tonsillar paracortex and intestinal lamina propria. Cells of the suppressor-cytotoxic type, CD8, constitute the major T cell population in normal human bone marrow and gut epithelium. In lymph node microenvironments, there is close anatomic proximity between CD4 cells and cells expressing large amounts of Ia antigens, interdigitating cells, and macrophages (Table 2–1).

Natural Killer (NK) Cells

Functional studies have identified lymphocyte populations that serve as **natural killer (NK) cells** and antibody-dependent killer cells in the surveillance of certain tumors and virus-infected cells. The NK cell is defined as an effector cell that has the capacity for spontaneous cytotoxicity toward

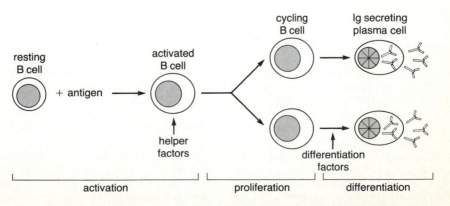

Figure 2–10. Model of B cell activation, proliferation, and differentiation.

Table 2-1. Lymphocyte distribution in various tissues in humans.[1]

Tissue	Approximate %		
	T cells		B cells
	CD4+	CD8+	
Peripheral blood	35–60	20–30	15–30
Lymph nodes and Tonsils			
Paracortex & interfollicular areas	60	20–40	Rare
Germinal centers	5–30	Rare	70–95
Lymphoid follicles (mantle zone)	Few	Few	>95
Spleen			
Periarteriolar sheath	70–90	10–30	Rare
Marginal zone–white pulp	40–55	5–20	40
Red pulp	20–40	60–80	Few
Thymus			
Cortex	>90	>90	Rare
Medulla	60–80	20–40	5–10

[1]Adapted from Hsu, S, Cossman, J, Jaffee, ES: Lymphocyte subsets in normal lymphoid tissues. *Am J Clin Pathol* 1983;**80**:21.

various target cells and is not MHC restricted. The precursor cells of these effector cells are unknown, but they lack major functional, genotypic, and phenotypic features of T cells, B cells, and monocyte-macrophages. NK cells, many of which appear as **large granular lymphocytes (LGL),** have unique morphologic features and typically possess round or indented nuclei with abundant pale cytoplasm containing azurophilic granules (Fig 2–11). LGL contain membrane-bound granules that stain for acid hydrolases, including acid phosphatase, α-naphthyl acetate esterase, and β-glucuronidase. These granules may be related to the cytolytic capacity of the LGL. LGL lack surface immunoglobulins, are nonadherent and nonphagocytic, frequently form rosettes with sheep erythrocytes, and express IgG Fc receptors (CD16). Thus, LGL exhibit morphologic and membrane characteristics intermediate between those of lymphocytes and monocytes.

Large Granular Lymphocytes (LGL)

LGL characteristically bear the cell surface antigens CD16, CD3, and Leu 7 (HNK-1). Blood LGL with NK activity have been subdivided into a majority population of CD16+ CD3− and a minority population of CD16− CD3+. Approximately 10% of peripheral blood lymphocytes are CD16+ CD3−. Following exposure to interleukin-2 (IL-2), these cells can efficiently kill targets that are otherwise NK insensitive (ie, solid tumor cells). The CD16+ CD3+ cell type is a non-MHC-restricted cytotoxic lymphocyte. These cells may recognize their targets through the CD3-Ti receptor. A distinguishing feature of the CD16− CD3+ cells is the expression of NKH-I (Leu 19), an anti-

gen not present on the majority of T cells. These CD3+ Leu 19+ cells make up 5% or less of peripheral blood lymphocytes.

Since LGL form rosettes with sheep erythrocytes and a subset does express CD3-Ti receptors, there is debate about whether NK cells are T cells or represent a distinct (third) lineage of lymphoid cells. The study of genotypic alteration, unique to human T cells (rearrangement of α, β, and γ genes) has helped to resolve this controversy. Human CD16+ CD3− cells neither rearrange α or β genes nor produce functional mRNA for these genes. The non-MHC-restricted cytotoxic cells do, however, rearrange Ti genes and produce functional Ti mRNA. Thus, this LGL subpopulation may be from the T cell lineage.

Lymphokine-Activated Killer (LAK) Cells

Lymphokine-activated killer (LAK) cells are generated when fresh lymphoid cells from the blood or spleen are incubated in IL-2. They differ from NK cells in that they have cytotoxic activity against a broader range of target cells, including freshly isolated autologous and allogeneic tumor cells and cell lines. Characterization of LAK cells shows that they are mostly negative for CD3 and positive for the CD16 and NKH 1 markers. These phenotypic characteristics and other experimental data on the augmentation of NK activity by IL-2 suggest that most of the LAK activity can be attributed to NK cells activated by IL-2. However, LAK cell activity can also be generated from thymocytes. LAK cells have shown promise against a number of metastatic cancers in clinical studies. Recently, another population of lymphocytes that are cytotoxic to specific human tumors has been

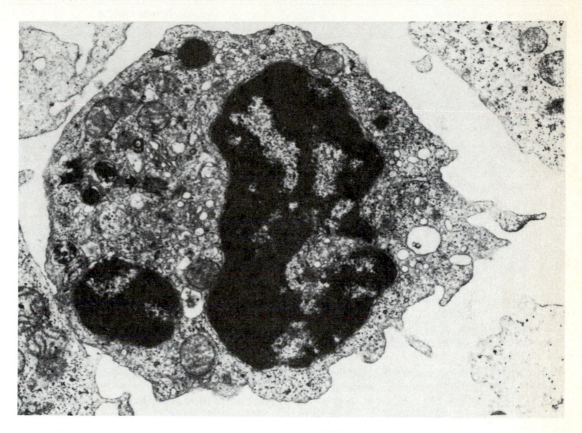

Figure 2–11. Morphology of the human NK cell. The nucleus is indented and rich in chromatin. The cytoplasm is abundant, and characteristic osmiophilic granules (spearheads) numerous mitochondria, centrioles (arrow), and the Golgi apparatus (g) are visible. (Original magnification × 17,000.) (Reproduced, with permission, from Carpen O, Virtanen I, Saksela E: *J Immunol* 1982;**126**:2692.)

identified within these solid tumors. These cells are known as **tumor-infiltrating lymphocytes (TIL).**

Dendritic Cells

Human **dendritic cells** have been identified in the peripheral blood and various peripheral lymphoid organs; they have similar cytologic features to rodent dendritic cells. They are bone marrow derived but belong to a distinct hematopoietic cell lineage, and they constitute less than 1% of peripheral blood mononuclear cells. They are potent stimulators of mixed-leukocyte reactions and are capable of presenting antigen for primary immune responses. They differ from other immunocytes in that they are Ia positive but lack Fc and sheep erythrocyte receptors, surface immunoglobulin, and other lymphocyte and monocyte markers. They have an irregular nucleus, small

nucleoli, and pale blue-gray cytoplasm. They bear many mitochondria but few lysosomes and ribosomes and have scanty rough endoplasmic reticulum. Their surfaces lack ruffles and microvilli.

Functional Properties

The functions of various subpopulations of lymphocytes are discussed in Chapters 3, 5, and 6. Several reagents stimulate lymphocytes in vitro; these include plant lectins, bacterial products, polymeric substances, and enzymes. Morphologic transformation occurs following stimulation, with the formation of blast cells or, in some instances, plasma cells. Lymphocyte transformation may also be assessed biochemically by the measurement of RNA, DNA, or protein synthesis. The detailed functional aspects of B and T lymphocytes, their interaction, and their alteration in disease are discussed in subsequent chapters.

Table 2-2. Cells belonging to the mononuclear phagocytic system.[1]

Bone marrow	Tissues	Body Cavities
Monoblasts	Macrophages occurring in:	Pleural macrophages
Promonocytes	Connective tissue (histiocytes)	Peritoneal macrophages
Monocytes	Skin (histiocytes; Langerhans cells?)	
	Liver (Kupffer cells)	**Inflammation**
Blood	Spleen (red pulp macrophages)	Exudate macrophages
Monocytes	Lymph nodes (free and fixed-macrophages; interdigitating cells?)	Epithelioid cells
	Thymus	Multinucleated giant cells
	Bone marrow (resident macrophages)	
	Bone (osteoclasts)	
	Synovia (type A cell)	
	Lung (alveolar and tissue macrophages)	
	MALT	
	Gastrointestinal tract	
	Genitourinary tract	
	Endocrine organs	
	Central nervous system (macrophages, [reactive] microglia, CSF macrophages)	

[1]Reproduced, with permission, from Van Furth R: Development and distribution of mononuclear phagocytes in the normal steady state and inflammation. In: *Inflammation: Basic Principles and Clinical Correlates.* Gallin JI, Goldstein IM, Snyderman, R (editors). Raven Press, 1988.

2. MONONUCLEAR PHAGOCYTES (MONOCYTE-MACROPHAGES)

The mononuclear phagocytes include circulating pheripheral blood monocytes, promonocytes, precursor cells in the bone marrow, and tissue macrophages. Tissue macrophages are present in several tissues, organs, and serous cavities. The organization of the mononuclear phagocyte system is shown in Table 2-2. The precursor cell in the mononuclear phagocyte lineage is the **monoblast,** which is present in the bone marrow and is morphologically similar to the myeloblast. The monoblast gives rise to the **promonocyte,** a bone marrow cell that is phagocytic and adherent and contains nonspecific esterase (Fig 2-12). Circulating monocytes are heterogeneous in size, receptor expression, and phagocytic function. There is a wide spectrum of morphologic features in the various types of mononuclear phagocytes. Their surface membranes are characterized by prominent microvilli and ruffles (Fig 2-13).

Functions of Macrophages

The major functional properties of monocyte-macrophages are ingestion of particles smaller than 0.1 μm by pinocytosis and engulfment of particles larger than 0.1 μm by phagocytosis. During engulfment, the particle first adheres to the plasma membrane of the cell and is then ingested. The monocyte-macrophage is capable of both nonimmunologic and immunologic phagocytosis. It has a plasma membrane receptor that recognizes 2 of the 4 subclasses of human IgG (IgG1 and IgG3); this binding site on the IgG molecule has been localized to the C_H3 domain of the im-

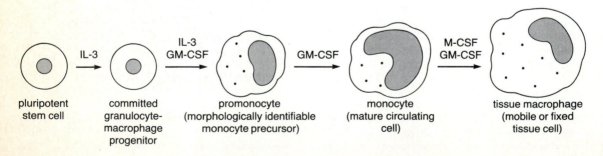

pluripotent stem cell   IL-3   committed granulocyte-macrophage progenitor   IL-3 GM-CSF   promonocyte (morphologically identifiable monocyte precursor)   GM-CSF   monocyte (mature circulating cell)   M-CSF GM-CSF   tissue macrophage (mobile or fixed tissue cell)

Figure 2-12. Cells of mononuclear phagocyte lineage.

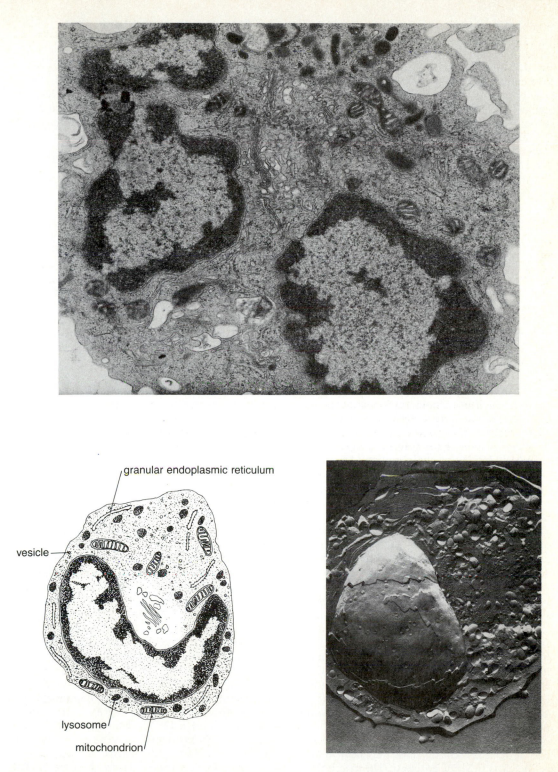

Figure 2–13. *Top:* Electron micrograph of normal human blood monocyte. (Original magnification × 34,500.) *Bottom left:* Diagrammatic representation of the monocyte. *Bottom right:* Freeze-fracture micrograph of normal human blood monocyte. (Original magnification × 10,000.)

munoglobulin molecule. Three types of human receptors for the Fc region of IgG (FcγR) have been identified. These are referred to as HuFcγRI, HuFcγRII, and HuFcγRIII. HuFcγRI is found predominantly on monocytes and macrophages, is a heavily glycosylated protein with molecular weight of 72,000, and plays a role in antibody-dependent cellular cytotoxicity reactions. HuFc-γRII (CDw32) is an MW 40,000 protein found on monocytes, platelets, eosinophils, neutrophils, and B cells; its most important role may be in initiating the oxidative burst. HuFcγRIII (CD16) is expressed on tissue macrophages but not on monocytes and is also expressed on neutrophils, NK cells, and eosinophils. Its abundant presence on tissue macrophages in the liver and spleen suggests that it plays a vital role in clearance of autologous erythrocytes and other immune complexes.

Monocyte Receptors

Monocyte-macrophages also have an independent receptor system, which recognizes the activated third component of complement. Three major types of surface receptors for C3 have been identified on immunocytes. Of these, CR1 and CR3 are expressed on monocytes. CR1 is a single-chain molecule that demonstrates polymorphism, with a molecular weight (MW) ranging from 160,000 to 250,000 depending on the allotype. CR3, which is specific for C3bi, is a heterodimer with an MW 165,000 α chain and an MW 95,000 β chain. A monoclonal antibody, anti-CD11 (anti-Mac-1), recognizes this determinant on more than 95% of fresh human monocytes and macrophages. Mac-1(CR3) is a member of an interrelated family of different cell surface adhesion molecules, including LFA-1 and p150,95, that share identical 95 K β chains. CR2 is the Epstein-Barr virus receptor found on B lymphocytes.

The monoclonal MO2 antibody (anti-CDw14) appears to be specific for peripheral blood monocytes. There are a number of other monoclonal antibodies that react with monocytes and other nonmonocyte blood elements. CD4 molecules and their corresponding mRNA have been demonstrated on monocytes, macrophages, and monocytelike cell lines. This CD4 receptor on monocytes serves as the principal site of entry for the human immunodeficiency virus (HIV) into mononuclear phagocytes.

Mononuclear phagocytes play an important role as antigen-presenting cells; they bear Ia antigens, the class II MHC antigens. The macrophage receptors for the Fc portion of IgG and C3b are the principal modes of antigen binding and recognition of appropriately opsonized antigen. Cells of the monocyte-macrophage series are active in killing bacteria, fungi, and tumor cells.

3. CELL TYPES INVOLVED IN THE INFLAMMATORY PHASE OF THE IMMUNE RESPONSE

Leukocytes consisting of neutrophils, eosinophils, basophils, and mast cells all participate in inflammatory reactions. For a description of their structure and functions, refer to Chapter 12.

HEMATOLYMPHOPOIESIS

Lymphocyte Recirculation & High Endothelial Venules (HEV)

The distribution of lymphocytes in various body tissues is determined by a number of factors, including lymphocyte class, stage of differentiation, and antigenic specificity. Thus, T cells predominate in the peripheral lymph nodes, whereas B cells migrate to MALT. Studies with animals show that antigen-specific T and B cells predominate in tissues that have been challenged with antigen. After their generation and maturation in the thymus and bone marrow, lymphocytes migrate to the secondary lymphoid organs, ie, the lymph nodes, MALT, and spleen. After traversing these tissues, lymphocytes that constitute the recirculating pool reenter the circulation via the efferent lymphatics and major lymphatic channels and repeatedly travel through the secondary lymphoid tissues via the blood and lymphatics (Fig 2–3). Approximately 10^9 lymphocytes are produced per day in the primary lymphoid organs. The average lymphocyte completes a cycle of recirculation in about 1–2 days. A small fraction of lymphocytes travel through nonlymphoid tissues such as the skin and gut (intestinal lamina propria). The mechanisms that govern their migration through these tissues parallel those relevant for traffic through secondary lymphoid organs. Labeling experiments have shown that thymic lymphocytes can be seen in peripheral lymph node high endothelial venules (HEV) within 30 minutes of being labeled in the thymus. Lymphocytes take more than 6 hours to travel from an afferent lymphatic vessel to the efferent lymphatic vessel draining the lymph node.

Approximately 1% of total body lymphocytes are present in the blood. During lymphocyte trafficking and recirculation, migrating lymphocytes leave the blood at HEV, which are specialized segments of the postcapillary venules. These HEV are characterized by distinctive, cuboidal, plump endothelial cells (Fig 2–14). In the white pulp of the spleen, lymphocytes leave the circulation via capillaries in the marginal zone of the periarteriolar lymphoid sheath. Since there are no HEV in the spleen, it is unknown how this occurs. The selective nature of the interaction between

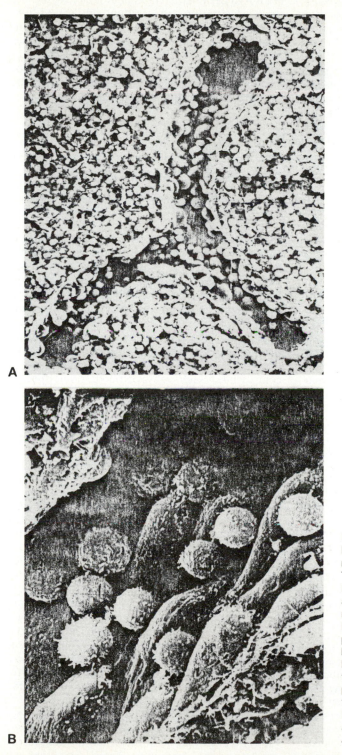

Figure 2–14. Scanning electron micrographs illustrating high endothelial venules (HEV) in mouse lymph nodes. **A:** Inverted Y-shaped HEV. The high endothelial cells bulge into the lumen. Individual small round lymphocytes can be seen attached to the endothelium, some apparently migrating between endothelial cells on their way into the lymph node parenchyma. **B:** Higher power showing numerous lymphocytes tightly bound to the high endothelial cells. Nonadherent blood elements were washed out by perfusion of the vasculature with medium prior to fixation by perfusion with glutaraldehyde in phosphate-buffered saline. (Reproduced, with permission, from Butcher EC et al: *The Pathology of the Endothelial Cell*, pp 409–424. Nossel H, Vogel H [editors]. Academic Press, 1982.)

lymphocytes and HEV and lymphocyte extravasation is mediated by organ-specific receptors, whereby lymphocytes have the capacity to distinguish between HEV in lymph nodes, mucosal tissues, and possibly other lymphoid organs.

Homing Receptors

A number of "homing" receptors have now been identified on lymphocyte surface membranes. At least 3 distinct types of homing receptors exist: one that mediates the binding of lymphocytes to peripheral lymph node HEV, one for Peyer's patch HEV, and one that mediates lymphocyte adhesion to endothelium in inflamed synovia. These receptors constitute a closely related family of MW 90,000 glycoprotein molecules. Their basic structure consists of a constant backbone region and a variable region that confers tissue specificity. This HEV-recognizing property of lymphocytes is developmentally acquired and appears to be based on lymphocyte class. Thus, "virgin" or non-antigen-exposed surface IgA-bearing B cells preferentially bind to HEV of and localize better to the mucosal lymphoid tissues such as Peyer's patches, whereas virgin regulatory T cells bind better to peripheral lymph node HEV.

The lymphocyte function-associated antigen LFA-1 is a non-tissue-specific surface molecule on lymphocytes that may play an accessory role in lymphocyte interaction with HEV. The intercellular adhesion molecule ICAM-1 has recently been identified as a ligand for LFA-1 on HEV cells, but its definitive role in HEV endothelial cell-lymphocyte interaction is unknown. Molecules on HEV endothelial cell surfaces that serve as recognition and binding sites for lymphocyte homing receptors have been identified by using monoclonal antibodies. These tissue-specific glycoproteins are referred to as "vascular addressins."

Upon exposure to antigen and following lymphocyte activation, there is a rapid increase in the blood supply to the stimulated lymphoid organ. Concurrently, a transient arrest of lymphocyte egress from these tissues occurs, allowing lymphocytes to accumulate, proliferate, and differentiate within these sites.

Common Mucosal Immune System

Support for the concept of a common mucosal immune system comes from studies showing that lymphocytes can selectively migrate between various mucosal surfaces in the body that produce secretory immunoglobulins at sites of antigen exposure. These sites include the intestines, lungs, breasts, and the female genital tract. The lymphoid tissues in these sites are all structurally similar and have plasma cells that produce secretory IgA.

For example, gut lymphoid tissue-derived cells can home to several different types of mucosal tissues but not to peripheral lymph nodes. During the late stages of gestation and lactation, gut-derived IgA-bearing plasma cells are diverted to breast connective tissue, where they secrete IgA antibodies specific for antigens to which these B cells were exposed in the gut. This results in the transfer of passive immunity to the intestinal tract of the suckling newborn (see Chapter 15).

PHYLOGENY OF IMMUNITY

The immune response originated in organisms with a nucleus (eukaryotic organisms), probably in response to a need to distinguish self from nonself. Unicellular organisms (protozoa) have undergone evolutionary changes that allow them to differentiate food or invading microorganisms from autologous cell components. Multicellular organisms (metazoa) have also evolved highly complex and functionally integrated cells and tissues that exhibit various degrees of immunologic competence. Such cell-specific or tissue-specific antigens arise from a restricted phenotypic expression of the genome (see Chapter 4). In such organisms, specialized cells or immunocytes have developed that protect the entire body from microbial invaders, from incursions of foreign tissue, and from diseases that may be caused by altered or neoplastic cells. This phemonemon is known as **immune surveillance**

From an evolutionary standpoint, cellular immunity and, particularly, phagocytosis preceded the development of antibody production in animals. Invertebrates characteristically demonstrate primitive forms of graft rejection and phagocytosis, but in no invertebrate species have molecules been identified that have a functional or physicochemical structure analogous to that of vertebrate immunoglobulins. On the other hand, all vertebrate species synthesize antibody, reject grafts, and exhibit **immunologic memory.** Thus, there is a relatively sharp delineation between the complexity of immunity in invertebrates and vertebrates; no clearly transitional forms have so far been identified.

The fully developed immune response is characterized by **specificity** and **anamnesis.** These essential criteria should be borne in mind when distinguishing true immunity from primitive or paraimmunologic phenomena in the phylogenetic analysis that follows.

IMMUNITY IN INVERTEBRATES

Unicellular invertebrate species have survived largely as a result of their remarkable reproductive capacity rather than the development of specific immune responses to environmental challenges. Perhaps the most primitive self-recognition mechanism is the ability of certain protozoa to reject transplantation of foreign nuclei. However, this phenomenon is really quasi-immunologic and probably depends on enzymatic rather than specific antigenic differences among various species.

All invertebrate species exhibit some form of self-versus-nonself recognition. However, true cellular immunity, with specific graft rejection and anamnesis, has been conclusively demonstrated only in certain earthworms (annelids) and corals (coelenterates) (Table 2–3). Although invertebrates with coelomic cavities possess a variety of humoral substances such as bacteriolysins, hemolysins, and opsonins, none of these have been specifically induced by immunization, nor do these rather ill-defined substances have any known physicochemical similarities with vertebrate antibodies. A fascinating array of primitive or quasi-immunologic phenomena, including self-recognition, phagocytosis, encapsulation, allograft and xenograft rejection, humoral defenses, and leukocyte differentiation, have been identified in invertebrates.

IMMUNITY IN VERTEBRATES

The most advanced invertebrates, the protochordates, are probably the ancestors of the true chordates, from which all higher vertebrates are descended. However, at the level of the most primitive extant vertebrate class, the agnathae, an entirely new component in the immune system is apparent, ie, **antibody.** Specific antibody synthesis is a property of all vertebrates. Cellular immunity, present in a primitive form in invertebrates, is highly developed and immunologically specific in all vertebrates. Graft rejection is accelerated after primary sensitization, and a true second-set rejection phenomenon occurs. However, some difference in the expression of immunologic functions is evident between warm-blooded and cold-blooded animals.

The hallmark of vertebrate immunity is the presence of a truly 2-component immune system; this is best demonstrated in birds, in which 2 independent central lymphoid organs exist: the thymus, which controls cellular immunity, and the bursa, which determines antibody-producing capacity. The immunologic repertoire of the various vertebrate classes is shown in Table 2–4.

Several generalizations regarding the phylogenetic emergence of immunity are possible. First, primitive and quasi-immunologic phenomena are present in the simplest forms of extant animal species. Second, T cell immunity precedes antibody immunity in evolution. Third, a truly bifunctional immune system with dual central lymphoid organs in a highly differentiated form is the most recent immunologic evolutionary development.

THE IMMUNOGLOBULIN GENE SUPERFAMILY

The immunoglobulin gene superfamily consists of a series of genes that share an evolutionary homology but do not necessarily share function, genetic linkage, or coordinate regulation. The members of this superfamily are defined by the presence of one or more structural regions homologous to the basic structural unit of the immunoglobulin molecule. This unit (the immunoglobulin homology unit) is characterized by a primary sequence of 70–110 amino acids with an essentially invariant disulfide bridge and several relatively conserved residues. The unique ability of the immunoglobulin homology unit to accommodate diversity has made possible the evolution of the complex phenotypic traits of the immunoglobulin gene superfamily. Comparisons of these sequences reveal that the similarity score between proteins that make up this superfamily is greater than 2–3 standard deviations above what would be expected between 2 random sequences.

The molecules that mediate the specific recognition of antigen, ie, the immunoglobulin molecule, the T cell receptor, and the class I and II MHC molecules, are the most significant products of this gene superfamily. However, a wide variety of gene products ranging from the above-named molecules to receptors of cartilage formation and nervous system-associated molecules are represented in this superfamily. These include (1) non-antigen-presenting β_2-microglobulin, (2) T cell-associated molecules, (3) molecules expressed on both T cells and neural cells, (4) nervous system–associated molecules, (5) immunoglobulin-binding molecules, and (6) growth factor/kinase receptors (Table 2–5).

The diversity inherent in the genes of the immunoglobulin homology unit appears to have driven the evolution of this superfamily of gene products. New functional structures have arisen during evolutionary development through the duplication of nucleotides, exons, genes, and entire families of genes. It is most likely that this superfamily arose from structures that first evolved to mediate cellular interactions and that the immune system in vertebrates developed from this group of structures.

Table 2-3. Evolution of immunity in invertebrates.[1]

Phylum or Subphylum	Graft Rejection	Immunologic Specificity of Graft Rejection	Immunologic Memory	Phagocytosis	Encapsulation	Nonspecific Humoral Factors	Phagocytic Ameboid Coelomocytes	Leukocyte Differentiation	Inducible Specific Antibodies
Protozoa	Yes. Enzyme incompatibility.	No	No	Yes; whole organism	No	No	No	No	No
Porifera (sponges)	Yes. Aggregation inhibition; species-specific glycoprotein.	Yes	Yes	No	Yes	No	No	No	No
Coelenterata (corals, jellyfish, sea anemones)	Yes; with graft necrosis.	Yes	Yes, short term	No	Hyperplastic growth around graft.	No	No	No	No
Annelida (earthworms)	Yes	Yes. First and second set graft rejection.	Short term, either positive or negative.	Yes	Yes	Yes. Nonspecific hemagglutinins, ciliate lysins, bacteriocidins.	Yes. Chemotaxis to bacteria.	Probable phytohemagglutinin response in coelomocyte.	No
Mollusca	Yes	?	?	Yes	Yes	Yes. Hemagglutinins act as opsonins.	Yes	No	No
Arthropoda	Yes	?	?	Yes	Yes	Yes	Yes	No	No
Echinodermata	Yes. Prolonged 4–6 months.	Yes. Specific second set graft rejection.	Short term only.	Yes	Yes	Yes. Hemolysins.	Yes	Yes. Cellular infiltrate in graft injection.	No
Protochordata (tunicates)	Yes. Genetically determined alloimmunity.	Probable. Tolerance possible.	Yes	Yes	Yes	Yes	Yes. Macrophage, lymphocyte, and eosinophil.	Yes. Lymphocytes present which form E rosettes and respond to phytohemagglutinin.	No

[1]Modified from Hildemann WH, Reddy AL: *Fed Proc* 1973;**322**:2188.

Table 2-4. Immunologic features exhibited by various vertebrate classes.

Class	Lymphocytes	Plasma Cells	Thymus	Spleen	Lymph Nodes	Bursa	Antibodies	Allograft Rejection
Agnatha (jawless fish)	+	−	PRIM[1]	PRIM	−	−	+	+
Chondrichthyes (cartilaginous fish)								
Primitive	+	−	+	+	−	−	+	+
Advanced	+	+	+	+	−	−	+	+
Osteichthyes (bony fish)	+	+	+	+	−	−	+	+
Amphibia	+	+	+	+	+	−	+	+
Reptilia	+	+	+	+	+ (?)[2]	−	+	+
Aves	+	+	+	+	+ (?)	+	+	+
Mammalia	+	+	+	+	+	−	+	+

[1]PRIM = primitive.

[2]? = some question regarding the presence of lymphoid structures under consideration, although such structures or their functional counterparts may have been described.

ONTOGENY

In the fetus, hematopoiesis—predominantly erythropoiesis—begins in the blood islands of the yolk sac in the second week of gestation. By about the sixth week of embryonic life, foci of hematopoiesis can be seen in the liver. During the second month, the bone marrow assumes an increasing role in this process and becomes the predominant site for hematopoiesis by the second half of gestation. The fetal spleen transiently serves as a hematopoietic organ between the third and fifth months of gestation. After birth, the bone marrow is normally the only hematopoietic organ, although both the liver and the spleen can serve as sites for extramedullary hematopoiesis if the bone marrow fails for any reason.

BLOOD CELLS

All circulating peripheral blood cells, including the lymphocytes, are derived from the pluripotent stem cells. These stem cells have the ability to self-replicate and eventually differentiate into mature blood cells. It is estimated that one of every 10,000 nucleated marrow cells in adult mouse bone marrow is a stem cell. As few as 30 pluripotent stem cells in the mouse can hematopoietically reconstitute lethally irradiated mice. These cells are lymphoid-appearing cells intermediate in size between bone marrow lymphocytes and large myeloid cells. Similar cells probably also exist in humans.

T Cells

Entry into the human thymus of blood-borne stem cells derived from sites of fetal hematopoiesis and their subsequent differentiation into lymphoid cells starts around the seventh week of gestation. Contact with the thymic epithelium, the presence of which is demonstrable by the seventh week of gestation, appears to be necessary for the maturation and differentiation of T cells in the thymus. The exact role of the thymic peptide hormones in the induction of these changes is unclear.

Important insights into murine thymocyte ontogeny have been obtained from studies of developmentally regulated expression of lymphocyte cell surface molecules involved in antigen recognition, including the T cell receptor (TCR). The first stage of T cell development from a molecular standpoint involves the rearrangement of TCR gene segments and the cell surface expression of the TCR. After surface TCR expression, cellular selection can occur. Cells that express self-reactive TCRs are eliminated, whereas those expressing TCRs that can recognize foreign antigens in the context of self-MHC molecules are positively selected. Following cell selection, thymocytes progressively acquire effector functions.

The order of appearance of critical ontogenetic events in humans is believed to be very similar to that in mice. The majority of TCR gene rearrangements occur at the stage of the earliest CD4⁻ CD8⁻ CD3⁻ fetal thymocytes. The T cell γδ re-

Table 2–5. Members of the immunoglobulin gene superfamily.

Molecules of immune recognition Immunoglobulin molecule T cell receptor MHC class I and II molecules	**T cell–associated molecules** CD7, CD28 CD2, CD3, CD4, CD8
β2-Microglobulin-associated molecules Qa and Tla CD1	**Immunoglobulin-binding molecules** Mouse Fc receptor Polyimmunoglobulin receptor (p-IgR)
T cell nervous system–associated molecules THY-1 antigen Rat Ox-2 cell surface antigen	**Nervous system molecules** Neural cell adhesion molecule (N-CAM) Rat myelin-associated glycoprotein (MAG) Peripheral myelin glycoprotein (Po)
Growth factor receptors Platelet-derived growth factor (PDGFR) Receptor for macrophage colony-stimulating factor (CSF-1R)	
Other molecules Carcinoembryonic antigen (CEA) 1B-glycoprotein (1B) Link glycoprotein (cartilage)	

ceptor ($TCR_{\gamma\delta}$) is the first CD3-associated receptor to appear during ontogeny. This is closely followed by the expression of $TCR\alpha\beta$. In humans, thymocytes from 9.5-week-old fetuses can be shown to express the $TCR_{\gamma\delta}$, and by 10 weeks, expression of $TCR_{\alpha\beta}$ is demonstrable, followed by a progressive decrease in the number of thymocytes expressing $TCR_{\gamma\delta}$. T cells acquire maturational surface markers during corticomedullary differentiation by about 14 weeks of gestation. Although fetal thymocytes can be shown to possess several functional capabilities, detectable T cell functions appear in peripheral blood lymphocytes around birth. Responsiveness to phytohemagglutinin can be shown as early as 10–12 weeks; responses to allogeneic cells and cell-mediated lympholysis occur by 12 and 16 weeks, respectively.

Studies of neonatal immune function shows that the magnitude of the responses of neonatal lymphocytes is generally comparable to that of adult lymphocytes. When deficiencies of function are demonstrable, they are secondary both to lower levels of precursors of effector T cells and to deficiencies of accessory or antigen-presenting cells.

B Cells

B lymphocytes arise from a common lymphoid stem cell derived from the pluripotent stem cells, although some studies have suggested a closer relationship of B cell precursors to myeloid precursors than to T cell progenitors. In early fetal life, the liver is the major repository of B cell progenitors. During mammalian embryogenesis, the bone marrow becomes the primary hematopoietic organ and, with it, becomes the significant source of B cell precursors.

Pre-B cells are the earliest identifiable B cell lineage progenitors. They are large, rapidly dividing cells that contain cytoplasmic μ chains but no light chains or surface immunoglobulin. They can be detected in human fetal liver by the seventh or eighth week of gestation. With proliferation, smaller pre-B cells arise; these express first cytoplasmic light chains and then surface immunoglobulin. B cells can be detected in fetal liver by about the ninth week of gestation. At this stage, they have surface complement receptors and IgM. Between the tenth and twelfth weeks, lymphocytes expressing other classes of immunoglobulin appear. By the fifteenth, the proportions of mature surface immunoglobulin-bearing B cells in the blood, spleen, and lymph nodes and the distribution of B cells expressing different immunoglobulin classes are comparable to those found in adults. If the emerging clones of B cells that express only surface IgM are exposed to antigen, they become tolerant to that antigen, a phenomenon referred to as clonal anergy. This mechanism is important in the development of B cell tolerance to high concentrations of self-antigens.

During B cell ontogeny, all B cell clones arise from surface IgM (sIgM)-expressing progenitors. Immature sIgA- or sIgG-bearing B cells also coexpress sIgM and sIgD, whereas coexpression of both sIgA and sIgG is extremely rare. IgM synthesis can be detected as early as the tenth to twelfth weeks of gestation. IgG synthesis is demonstrable somewhat later, and synthesis of serum IgA and secretory IgA cannot be detected until about the thirtieth week of gestation. At birth, the neonatal serum contains almost no IgA, small amounts of IgM, and adult levels of IgG, most of which is passively transferred maternal IgG. The rapidity with which serum immunoglobulin levels rise from neonatal levels to normal adult levels varies according to the isotype. Functionally, the neonatal immune response is qualitatively and quantitatively different from that of the adult. The neonatal IgM response is prolonged and prominent, whereas the IgG and IgA responses are relatively deficient. This defect appears to be related to lack of T cell help rather than to a lack of B cell precursors. Neonates also appear to have a relative inability of mounting an IgG2 subclass response; this may correspond to their inability to respond to carbohydrate antigens.

Monocyte-Macrophages

The mononuclear phagocyte cell lineage arises from a committed progenitor that itself is derived from the pluripotent stem cell. Differentiation of the progenitor into monocytes is probably a random event, but the differentiation and subsequent maturation of this progenitor into mature monocytes is facilitated by a number of **colony-stimulating factors (CSF)** including granulocyte-macrophage CSF (GM-CSF), interleukin-3 (Il-3), and macrophage CSF (M-CSF). Following commitment, the first identifiable cell of this lineage in the bone marrow is the promonocyte, which constitutes approximately 3–5% of the bone marrow. Although monoblasts can be seen in bone marrow during leukemic states, they cannot routinely be differentiated from myeloblasts in normal bone marrow. Each promonocyte divides in the bone marrow, giving rise to 2 daughter monocytes, which subsequently enter the peripheral circulation, circulate for about 3 days, and then migrate to different tissues. Tissue macrophages are derived from precursors in the bone marrow. Once in the tissues, local proliferation may contribute to the tissue macrophage pool although this pool is regularly replenished from the blood monocyte pool.

Embryonic macrophages can be found in the hematopoietic tissues of the yolk sac around the third to fourth week of gestation. When hematopoiesis moves to the liver, more than half of the free intravascular hematopoietic cells in the human fetal liver are of the mononuclear phagocyte lineage. Between the eighth and twenty-second weeks of gestation, high levels of colony forming units for granulocytes and monocytes (CFU-GM) can be identified in fetal liver and peripheral blood. These CFU-GM are different from those derived from adult bone marrow in that they are more actively proliferating and give rise more consistently to pure macrophage colonies in vitro. Mature monocytes do not appear in the fetal circulation until about the fifth month of fetal life. Beyond 30 weeks, monocytes constitute about 3–7% of all hematopoietic cells. The exact kinetics of monocyte production and tissue distribution during fetal life are unknown. There is a relative monocytosis during the perinatal period, with peripheral blood monocyte counts returning to normal levels by about 1 month of age. Histologic studies of the lungs of stillborn infants and neonates have suggested that very few alveolar macrophages are present in fetal lungs prior to birth but there is a significant influx of macrophages into the lungs soon after birth.

MALT

MALT cannot be identified in animal or human tissues at birth. Mononuclear cell aggregates which may be the forerunners of MALT have been identified in the intestines and less so in the lungs of the human fetus as early as 14 weeks of gestation. This assumption is supported by studies demonstrating the development of BALT follicles in fetal lungs transplanted from 18-day-old mouse fetuses into syngeneic animals. In humans, lymphoid aggregates representative of MALT are absent at birth but appear at the end of the first week of life and subsequently increase in number with age during childhood and adolescence.

Complement

Synthesis of some of the components of **complement** starts in the human fetal liver during the first trimester of gestation. Specifically, synthesis of C3 and C1 inhibitor protein have been documented as early as the 29th day of gestation, C4 and C2 by the 8th week and C5 by the 9th week of gestation. Throughout fetal life, the liver and other tissues continue to produce complement components at varying rates. Transplacental passage of complement proteins does not occur. The levels of immunochemically and hemolytically detectable complement components in newborn sera range between 60 and 90% of adult levels. They rise steadily in the first few years of life to reach normal adult levels.

SUMMARY

The immune system is composed of cells within the lymphoreticular organs, which include the primary lymphoid organs (the bone marrow and thymus) and the secondary organs such as the spleen, lymph nodes, and the MALT. Thymus-derived (T) lymphocytes and bone marrow-derived (B) lymphocytes are the predominant immunocytes. The structural architecture of lymphoid organs is generally characterized by discrete T and B cell areas interspersed with endothelial, stromal, and reticuloendothelial cells. The peripheral lymphoid tissues, ie, the tonsils, lymph nodes, and MALT, are situated in strategic areas where they are intimately and continuously exposed to antigens.

T lymphocyte precursors arise in the bone marrow, migrate to the thymus, and undergo maturation and differentiation within the thymic microenvironment. A number of differentiational and functional cell surface markers are acquired during this process. These immunocompetent T lymphocytes then emigrate from the thymus and populate the T cell areas of peripheral lymphoid organs. Postnatally, maturation of B lymphocytes occurs exclusively in the bone marrow. These short-lived B lymphocytes then travel to B cell areas of peripheral lymphoid tissues, where they can differentiate into long-lived B cells upon antigenic stimulation.

All lymphocytes continuously recirculate throughout the lymphoid tissues of the body. They leave the blood circulation via the HEV in the peripheral lymphoid tissues and eventually return to the venous circulation after traversing afferent lymphatics, lymph nodes, and the efferent lymphatics, which ultimately empty into the thoracic duct. There is preferential migration of B lymphocytes to MALT, whereas T cells migrate to peripheral lymph nodes. This selective migration is mediated via lymphocyte-endothelial interaction involving receptors on lymphocyte cell surfaces and ligands on specialized vascular endothelium.

Teleologically, the immune response arose to meet a need for organisms to distinguish self components from foreign or nonself components. Primitive forms of graft rejection and phagocytosis are present in invertebrates, but truly immunologic responses, with specificity and anamnesis, are present only in vertebrates. Ontogenetic studies of the human immune system show that although hematopoiesis begins in the fetal yolk sac in the second week of gestation, the earliest T and B cell functional characteristics cannot be demonstrated until the seventh or eighth week of gestation. The neonatal immune response is immature in comparison with the fully developed response in the immunocompetent adult.

REFERENCES

LYMPHOID ORGANS

Bienenstock J: The mucosal immunologic network. *Ann Allergy* 1984;**53**:535.

Hsu S, Cossman J, Jaffe, ES: Lymphocyte subsets in normal lymphoid tissues. *Am J Clin Pathol* 1983;**80**:21.

Janossy G et al: Cellular differentiation of lymphoid subpopulations and their microenvironments in the human thymus. *Curr Top Pathol* 1986;**75**:89.

Weiss L: The blood cells and hematopoietic tissues. Page 423 in: *Cell and Tissue Biology. A Textbook of Histology,* 6th ed. Weiss L (editor). Urban & Schwarzenberg, 1988.

Immunologic Cells

Douglas SD, Hassan NF: Morphology of monocytes and macrophages. Chapter 93 in: *Hematology,* 4th ed. Williams WJ (editor). McGraw-Hill, 1989.

Douglas SD, Hassan, NF, Blaese, RM: The mononuclear phagocyte system. Page 81 in: *Immunologic Disorders in Infants and Children,* 3rd ed. Stiehm ER (editor). Saunders, 1988.

Douglas SD, Kay NE: Morphology of plasma cells. Chapter 101 in: *Hematology,* 4th ed. Williams WJ (editor). McGraw-Hill, 1989.

Herberman RB et al: Lymphokine-activated killer cell activity. Characteristics of effector cells and their progenitors in blood and spleen. *Immunol Today* 1987;**8**:178.

Hersey P, Bolhuis R: "Nonspecific" MHC-unrestricted killer cells and their receptors. *Immunol Today* 1987;**8**:233.

Kay NE, Douglas SD: Antigenic phenotype and morphology of human blood lymphocytes. Chapter 100 in: *Hematology,* 4th ed. Williams WJ (editor). McGraw-Hill, 1989.

Sprangrude GJ, Heimfeld S, Weissman IL: Purification and characterization of mouse hematopoietic stem cells. *Science* 1988;**241**:58.

Steinman RM, Nussenzweig MC: Dendritic cells: Features and functions. *Immunol Rev* 1980;**53**:127.

Trinchieri, G: Biology of natural killer cells. *Adv Immunol* 1989;**47**:187.

Voorhis WC et al: Human dendritic cells. Enrichment and characterization from peripheral blood. *J Exp Med* 1982;**155**:1172.

Zola H: The surface antigens of human B lymphocytes. *Immunol Today* 1987;**8**:308.

Hematolymphopoiesis

Butcher EC: The regulation of lymphocyte traffic. *Curr Top Microbiol Immunol* 1986;**128**:85.

Duijvestijn A, Hamman A: Mechanisms and regulation of lymphocyte migration. *Immunol Today* 1989;**10**:23.

Yednock TA, Rosen SD: Lymphocyte homing. *Adv Immunol* 1989;**44**:313.

Phylogeny

Cohen N: Phylogeny of lymphocyte structure and function. *Am Zool* 1975;**15**:119.

Goetz D (editor): *Evolution and Function of the Major Histocompatibility System.* Springer-Verlag, 1977.

Hildemann WH, Clark EA, Raison RL: *Comprehensive Immunogenetics.* Elsevier, 1981.

Hood L, Prahl J: The immune system: A model for differentiation in higher organisms. *Adv Immunol* 1971;**14**:291.

Ontogeny

Hunkapiller T, Hood L: Diversity of the immunoglobulin gene superfamily. *Adv Immunol* 1989;**44**:1.

Kincade, PW: Experimental models for understanding B lymphocyte formation. *Adv Immunol* 1987;**41**:181.

Lawton AR, Cooper MD: Ontogeny of immunity.

Chapter 1 in: *Immunologic Disorders in Infants and Children,* 3rd ed. Stiehm ER (editor). Saunders, 1988.

Stutman O: Ontogeny of T cells. *Clin Immunol Allergy* 1985;**5**:191.

Vogler LB, Lawton AR: Ontogeny of B cells and humoral immune functions. *Clin Immunol Allergy* 1985;**5**:235.

Williams AF: A year in the life of the immunoglobulin superfamily. *Immunol Today* 1987;**8**:298.

3

The Immune Response

Joel W. Goodman, PhD

The **immune response** is made up of a complex sequence of events; it is triggered by the introduction of a stimulus (immunogen or antigen) and usually culminates in the elimination of the provoking agent. Indeed, the primary function of the immune response is to discriminate between self and nonself and thereby to eliminate the latter, be it a pathogenic microorganism, a tissue allograft, or an innocuous environmental substance such as proteins in pollens, grasses, or food.

The immune response depends primarily on 3 major cell types: macrophages, thymus-derived lymphocytes (T cells), and bone marrow–derived lymphocytes (B cells). These interact with one another, either directly or via interleukins. In addition, the immune system is integrally connected with the complement, kinin, clotting, and fibrinolytic systems, all of which are involved in inflammation.

The interplay of these elements, which are still imperfectly understood despite the rapid pace of progress in immunology during recent years, can be bewildering to the uninitiated. The purpose of this chapter is to clarify a very complex subject by considering the essential elements of the immune response in a stepwise, simplified fashion, from the initial encounter with an immunogen to the final products of the response, which function to eliminate the antigenic stimulus.

INNATE & ADAPTIVE IMMUNITY

All living things are continually under environmental assault. There are 2 levels of defense against invasion by external agents: **innate immunity** and **adaptive immunity** (also known as acquired immunity) (Table 3–1). The principal differences betwen the two relate to specificity and immunologic memory, which are properties of acquired immunity only.

Innate Immunity

Innate immunity, sometimes called natural immunity, is present from birth and includes numerous nonspecific elements.

Body surfaces, especially skin, form the first line of defense against penetration by microorganisms. When penetration does occur, the invading organisms initially encounter other elements of the innate immune system. The enzyme lysozyme is widely distributed in secretions and can damage the cell walls of many bacteria. Similarly, the alternative complement pathway (see Chapter 14) is directly activated by a variety of bacteria; this may result in clearance of the bacteria via lysis or via facilitation of phagocytosis by macrophages (see Chapter 11), which possess receptors for certain components of the complement system, and by **polymorphonuclear neutrophils (PMN),** for which activated complement components are chemotactic. The serum concentration of certain proteins, called **acute-phase proteins,** increases during infection. One of these is **C-reactive protein (CRP),** so called because it binds to the C protein of pneumococci. This interaction activates the alternative complement pathway, which can then aid in eliminating the bacteria as described above.

Innate immunity against viruses, as opposed to bacteria, is implemented by natural killer NK cells and by **interferons.** NK cells are lymphocytes that are capable of binding to and killing virus-infected and tumor cells by a mechanism not yet understood (see Chapter 5). They are distinguishable from cytotoxic T lymphocytes (see below) on the basis of surface antigens and their failure to exhibit immunologic memory. NK cells are activated by interferons, which are also components of the innate immune system. Alpha and beta interferons (see Chapter 7) are produced by certain leukocytes and by virus-infected cells. Aside from their action on NK cells, interferons elevate the resistance of normal cells to viral infection and thus constitute a vital early defense mechanism against many viruses.

Adaptive Immunity

If the defenses provided by the innate immune system fail to fully prevent infection (or completely halt dissemination of nonliving immunogens), the adaptive immune response comes into

34

Table 3–1. Comparison of innate and adaptive immunity.

Property	Innate Immunity	Adaptive Immunity
Physical barriers	Skin and mucous membranes	None
Soluble factors	Enzymes (eg lysozyme and complement) Acute-phase proteins (eg CRP) Alpha and beta interferons	Antibodies Lymphokines
Cells	Macrophages, PMN, eosinophils, NK cells	T and B lymphocytes
Self-nonself discrimination	Yes	Yes
Specificity	No	Yes
Memory	No	Yes

play. Adaptive immunity is a more recent evolutionary development (see Chapter 2) than innate immunity and is distinguished by a remarkable specificity for the offending immunogen (see Chapter 8) and by its memory (ie, intensified responses upon subsequent encounters with the same or closely related immunogens). In this adaptive immune response, the foreign agent or immunogen triggers a chain of events that lead to the activation of lymphocytes and the production of antibodies and effector lymphocytes which are highly specific for the immunogen.

The principal players in adaptive immunity are **antigen-presenting cells (APC),** thymus-derived lymphocytes (T cells), and bone marrow–derived lymphocytes (B cells). T cells produce soluble molecules with many effects, and B cells eventually result in antibody formation. The roles of these important lymphocytes are described here, but a more detailed account of their properties is given in Chapters 2 and 5.

The Adaptive Immune Response

The adaptive immune response is triggered by the presence of a foreign agent that escapes early elimination by the innate immune system. A "grand scheme," necessarily somewhat oversimplified, of the major events in the adaptive immune response is shown in Figure 3–1. These events are considered in turn.

IMMUNOGENS & ANTIGENS

This subject is covered thoroughly in Chapter 8. Briefly, an **immunogen** is a molecule that can induce an immune response in a particular host. The term "antigen," which is frequently used interchangeably with immunogen, actually refers to the ability of a molecule to react with the products of adaptive immunity, particularly antibodies, not necessarily to its ability to induce their formation. Thus, although all immunogens are also antigens, the converse is not true.

In general, the more complex the foreign agent, the more distinct are the immunogens it contains. Thus, a single foreign molecule is a single immunogen, but foreign cells such as bacteria are composed of many immunogens, each of which may elicit a unique immune response. The foreign agent in Figure 3–1 is a virus, which usually contains several immunogenic proteins. Most immunogens are composed largely or exclusively of protein (lipoproteins, glycoproteins, nucleoproteins). Pure carbohydrates may be immunogenic, but they fall into a special class of immunogens called **T cell-independent antigens** (see Chapter 8).

The fate of an immunogen that penetrates the physical barriers of the innate immune system depends partially on its route of entry. In general, an immunogen may take 3 routes. If the immunogen enters the bloodstream, it is carried to the spleen, which becomes the principal site of the immune response. If the immunogen remains localized in the skin, a local inflammatory response ensues and it travels through afferent lymphatic channels to regional lymph nodes draining the affected area, which then serve as the major site of the immune response. Finally, the immunogen may enter the mucosal immune system in the respiratory or gastrointestinal tract (see Chapter 15), both of which have lymphoid tissue (tonsils and Peyer's patches) for mounting an immune response. Antibodies produced there are deposited locally, but immune lymphocytes from those organs may be transported via the thoracic duct to other lymphoid organs, thereby spreading the response systemically. There is always some trafficking of lymphocytes via the blood and lymphatics, so although a response may be initiated locally, it eventually spreads throughout the body (see Chapter 2).

Antigen Processing & Presentation

Responses to most immunogens, with the possible exception of T cell-independent antigens (see Chapter 8), require processing of the immunogen by APC. The reason for this is that T cells, which are the principal orchestrators and regulators of the immune response, ordinarily recognize immunogens only together with major histocompatibility complex (MHC) antigens (see Chapter 4) on the surfaces of other cells. Thus, the first steps in the immune response following entry of the im-

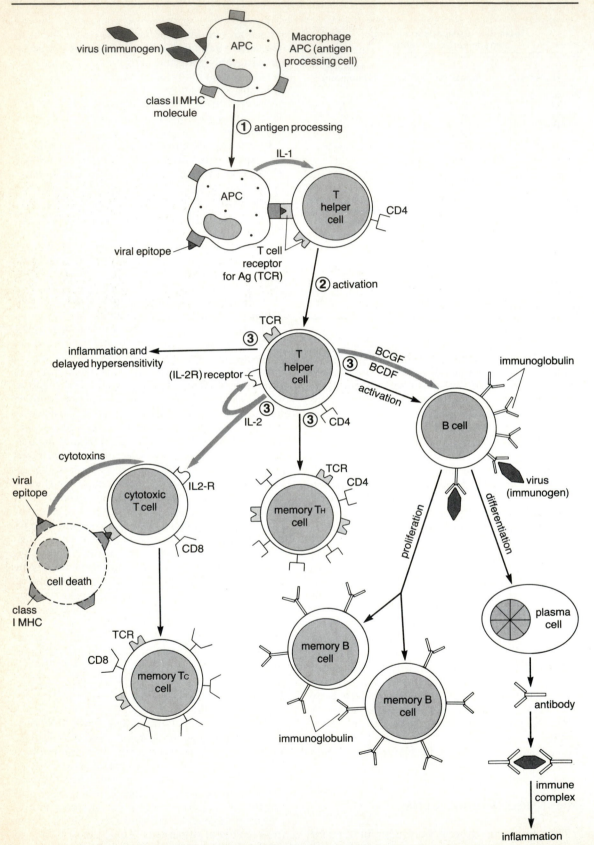

Figure 3-1. Grand scheme of adaptive immune system (see text for explanation).

munogen involve capture and processing of the immunogen by APC and presentation of a processed form of the immunogen in association with class II MHC molecules to a subset of T cells called **helper T (T**H**) cells** (Table 3–2).

Although all somatic cells express class I MHC proteins, relatively few cell types express class II proteins. Those that do include macrophages, dendritic cells in lymphoid tissue, Langerhans cells in the skin, Kupffer's cells in the liver, and microglial cells in central nervous system tissue, all of which are very similar and may have a common precursor. B cells, the precursors of antibody-secreting cells (plasma cells), also express class II MHC molecules. The common denominator among these diverse cells is the expression of class II antigens and hence their role as APC (Table 3–2).

These cells phagocytose or pinocytose the immunogen, which is then modified in endocytic vacuoles in the cytoplasm. The precise steps of antigen processing have not been definitively established and may range from denaturation and unfolding to proteolysis. If an agent undergoes proteolysis, fragments of the original immunogen (epitopes; see Chapter 8) become noncovalently associated with class II molecules and the complex is transported to the cell surface, where it is then accessible to the T cell (Fig 3–2). Only a limited number of the peptide fragments from a protein antigen are capable of associating with class II molecules to form an immunogenic complex. Such peptides are termed **immunogenic epitopes** (see Chapter 8). It is believed that all immunogenic epitopes become bound to a single binding site on the class II molecule.

Although it is unexpected, B cells, the precursors of antibody-secreting cells, can also present antigen to T cells. B cells not only express class II proteins but also have a very efficient capture mechanism for specific antigens through their immunoglobulin antigen receptors (see Chapter 5).

B cells alone are relatively poor activators of resting or virgin T cells when presenting antigens, possibly because such T cells require auxiliary activating factors, such as interleukins, that B cells fail to provide. However, B cells require only about one-thousandth as much immunogen as do macrophages for activating memory T cells. Because B cells specific for a particular immunogen are rare in an unimmunized individual and virgin T cells do not respond well to antigen presented by B cells, it is believed that macrophages probably play the predominant role as APCs in the initial, or primary, immune response, whereas B cells may dominate in the memory, or secondary, response (see below).

ACTIVATION OF HELPER T CELLS

TH cells are the principal orchestrators of the immune response because they are needed for the activation of the major effector cells in the response, ie, cytotoxic T (TC) cells and antibody-producing B cells. The activation of TH cells occurs early in the immune pathway (Fig 3–1) and requires at least 2 signals. One signal is provided by the binding of the T cell antigen receptor to the class II MHC-antigen complex on the APC. The second signal derives from interleukin-1 (IL-1), a soluble protein produced by the APC. Macro-

Table 3–2. Cells of the acquired immune system.

Cell Type	Antigen-Specific	Immunologic Functions	Distribution	Selected Markers
Antigen-presenting cells				
Macrophages	No		Wide	Class II MHC molecules
Dendritic cells	No		Lymphoid tissues	Class II MHC molecules
Langerhans cells	No		Skin	Class II MHC molecules
Kupffer's cells	No	Process and present antigen to T cells	Liver	Class II MHC molecules
Microglial cells	No		Central nervous system	Class II MHC molecules
B lymphocytes	Yes		Wide	Class II MHC molecules and surface immunoglobulin
T lymphocytes				
TH cells	Yes	Perform positive regulation	Wide	CD4
TC cells	Yes	Kill cells bearing foreign antigens	Wide	CD8
TS cells	Yes	Perform negative regulation	Wide	CD8
B lymphocytes	Yes	Produce antibody	Wide	Surface immunoglobulin

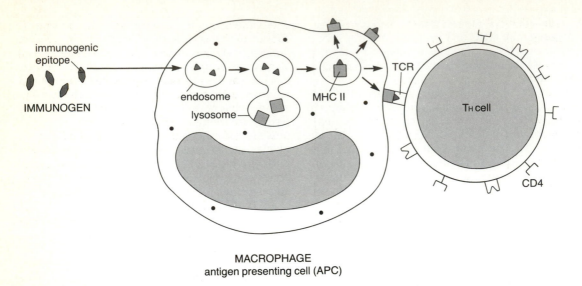

MACROPHAGE
antigen presenting cell (APC)

Figure 3-2. Uptake and processing of immunogen by APC. Fragmentation of the immunogen takes place in an acidic compartment (produced by fusion of endosome with lysosome), and the immunogenic epitope becomes associated with class II MHC molecules. This complex is transported to the cell surface, where it is accessible to TH cells specific for that particular epitope-class II combination. An immunogen usually has more than one epitope, each of which may be processed and presented in this manner. The initial contact between processed antigen and class II MHC is depicted as occurring in the endosome, but that is uncertain.

phages produce much more IL-1 than B cells do, which may account for their ability to activate virgin T cells.

Together, the 2 signals induce the expression of receptors for another lymphokine, IL-2, as well as the production of a battery of cell growth and differentiation factors (cytokines) that are important for triggering B cells and activating macrophages (Fig 3–3). IL-2 induces the growth of cells expressing IL-2 receptors, including the very same TH cells that produce it (autocatalytic effect) and TC cells that do not ordinarily produce it. Thus, the main function of IL-2 is to amplify the response initiated by contact of TH cells with APCs.

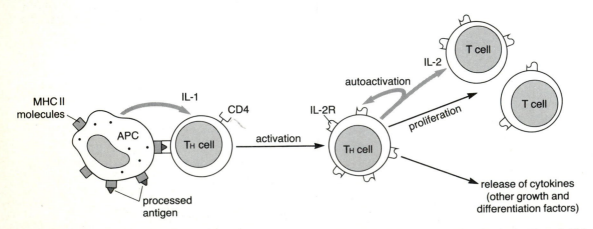

Figure 3-3. TH cell activation. The APC presents an epitope in the context of class II molecules in the TH cell. This interaction constitutes one of the 2 essential activating signals for the TH cell. The other is provided by IL-1 produced by the APC. The activated TH cell expresses IL-2 receptors and produces IL-2, which triggers growth of the TH cell and production of other lymphokines important in the activation of other cell types.

ACTIVATION OF CYTOTOXIC T CELLS

The activated TH cell is the key to further steps along the immune pathway, notably the triggering of TC cells, whose major function is the killing of cells that express foreign or nonself antigens, and B cells, which differentiate into antibody-producing plasma cells. The TC cell can be distinguished from the TH cell by the presence of CD8 rather than CD4 (Table 3–2) and by its recognition of foreign antigen in the context of class I rather than class II MHC molecules. CD4 and CD8 proteins on T cells have been shown to bind to class II and class I molecules, respectively, on APC, and thereby these CD molecules participate in T cell recognition of antigen-MHC complexes.

TC cells, like TH cells, also require 2 activating signals. One is provided by interaction of the T cell antigen receptors with a complex of a foreign epitope and class I MHC on the target cell; these cells may be virus-infected or tumor cells or foreign tissue grafts. The second signal is furnished by IL-2 produced by the activated TH cell. The activated TC cell then releases cytotoxins that kill the target cell (Fig 3–4).

ACTIVATION OF B CELLS

Antibody production requires both the activation of B lymphocytes and their differentiation into antibody-producing plasma cells. The sequence of events in this process can be visualized as follows. While the TH cell is being activated as described above, relevant B cells have also been engaging immunogen through their antigen receptors, which are membrane-bound forms of the antibodies they will later secrete (see Chapters 5 and 9). Antigen binding is followed by endocytosis of the antigen-receptor complex, which appears to furnish an activating signal; however, this is insufficient for full activation of B cells, which require additional signals from TH cells. These additional signals are lymphokines (BCGF and BCDF; see below) that are released by activated TH cells and have a short radius of activity. Thus, the relevant T and B cells must be in close proximity to participate in an immune response.

Because B cells can also function as APC, they process endocytosed antigen and transport immunogenic epitopes complexed with class II molecules to their surface. These complexes then activate T cells or induce the formation of memory T cells. Effector T cells can then deliver the appropriate lymphokines at close range, which affects other T and B cells and probably nonlymphoid cells as well (Fig 3–5).

B Cell–Stimulating Lymphokines

At least 2 lymphokines produced by TH cells are needed for growth and differentiation of B cells. The first lymphokine is descriptively called **B cell growth factor** (BCGF), which, in concert with antigen, stimulates proliferation of B cells. The second lymphokine, termed **B cell differentiation factor** (BCDF), induces activated B cells to differentiate into antibody-secreting plasma cells. Thus, the complete process of B cell activation and differentiation requires at least 3 signals, one provided by the immunogen and at least 2 furnished by TH cells. Other TH products may also be involved; the process has not yet been fully delineated.

A fraction of activated B cells proliferate but do not differentiate into plasma cells, possibly because they receive insufficient BCDF. Such B cells form a pool of **memory cells,** which can respond to subsequent encounters with the relevant immunogen. TH cells are also long-lived, providing memory in the T cell compartment of the immune system.

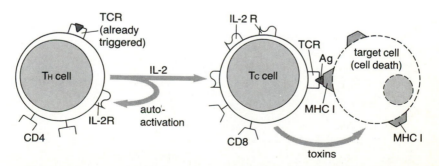

Figure 3-4. Activation of TC cell by antigen. A complex of MHC class I and processed antigenic epitope together with IL-2 produced by TH cells triggers activation in TC. The TC activated by the 2 signals secretes toxins that kill the target cell.

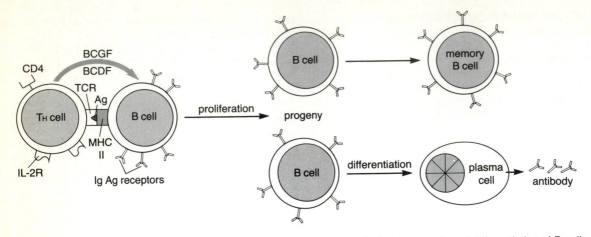

Figure 3-5. B cell–activation pathway. Signals from antigen and Tн cells induce growth and differentiation of B cells. Some B cells progress to the plasma cell stage and secrete antibody, while others form a pool of memory B cells.

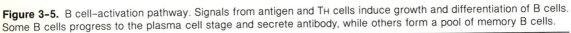

KINETICS OF THE IMMUNE RESPONSE

An individual's first encounter with a particular immunogen is called a **priming event** and leads to a relatively weak, short-lived antibody response designated the **primary immune response** (Fig 3-6). The response is divisible into several phases.

The **lag** or **latent phase** is the time between the contact with the immunogen and the detection of antibodies in the circulation, which averages about 1 week in humans. During this period, activation of T and B lymphocytes is taking place. The **exponential phase** marks a rapid increase in the quantity of antibodies in the circulation. Antibodies are secreted by plasma cells, the terminal phase of the pathway depicted in Figure 3-1. After an interval during which the antibody level remains relatively constant because synthesis and degradation are occurring at approximately equal rates (**steady-state phase**), the antibody level gradually declines (**declining phase**) as synthesis of new antibody wanes. The regulatory mechanisms involved in turning off the antibody response are considered below.

Subsequent encounters with the same immunogen lead to responses that are qualitatively similar to the primary response but manifest marked

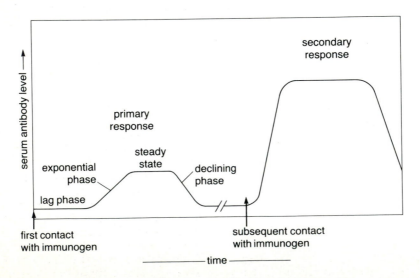

Figure 3-6. Primary and secondary immune responses.

quantitative differences (Fig 3–6). In the **secondary** or **anamnestic response,** the lag period is shortened, and antibody levels rise more rapidly to a much higher steady-state level (steeper slope), remaining detectable in serum for much longer periods. Memory T and B cells generated during the primary response are responsible for the more rapid kinetics and greater intensity and duration of secondary responses; this explains why booster injections of vaccines are so efficacious.

CLONAL SELECTION

The properties of the immune response are fully consistent with the theory of clonal selection proposed by Sir Macfarlane Burnet and for which he was awarded the Nobel Prize in medicine in 1960. The clonal selection theory postulates that virgin lymphocytes express antigen receptors before ever encountering antigen. Thus, the immune cell population is composed of a very large number of individual clones of lymphocytes, each with its own antigen receptor, permitting it to recognize and respond to only a very small part of the total universe of antigenic epitopes. The whole library of lymphocyte clones, however, is sufficiently diverse to deal with any potential immunogen. Antigen, then, serves as a selective agent in the immune response, recruiting only clones that recognize its epitopes, which are then selectively expanded without affecting the rest of the lymphoid population. Thus, primary and secondary responses are strictly specific for the provoking immunogen, and the kinetic differences between them are explicable in terms of the antigen-specific clones expanded during the primary response.

The clonal selection theory further proposes that immature lymphocytes which contact antigen are somehow eliminated predominantly in the embryonic thymus, whereas mature lymphocytes are responsive to their antigens. This aspect of the theory can account for self-nonself discrimination, because clones reactive with self antigens (autoreactive lymphocytes) would contact antigen early in development and be aborted. The basic tenets of clonal selection have been extensively confirmed experimentally and are now firmly established.

MECHANISMS OF ANTIGEN ELIMINATION

The ultimate function of the immune system is to seek and destroy alien substances in the body. This is accomplished in several different ways.

One, described above, is the direct killing of target cells expressing foreign antigens by activated Tc cells via elaboration of cytotoxins. Antibodies perform the task in a variety of ways, the most important of which are discussed below.

Toxin Neutralization

Antibodies specific for bacterial toxins or the venom of insects or snakes bind these antigenic toxins, thus causing inactivation and promoting elimination of the antigen-antibody complexes via the reticuloendothelial system. Because of their effectiveness, antibodies against toxins and venom are used to passively protect nonimmune individuals who have been exposed and are consequently at risk.

Virus Neutralization

Antibodies specific for epitopes on the surface of a virus may block the attachment of the virus to target cells, particularly if the antibodies bind at or close to the site of attachment on the virus. This mechanism is probably less important in defense against viral infection than the killing of virus-infected target cells by Tc cells.

Opsonization of Bacteria

Antibodies can coat bacteria, thereby promoting their clearance by macrophages, which have receptors for certain classes of antibodies (see Chapter 9). Binding to macrophages via these receptors facilitates phagocytosis of the coated antigen. The antibody in this situation is called an **opsonin.**

Activation of Complement

Certain classes of antibodies can activate the complement cascade when they are complexed with antigen (see Chapter 9). If the epitope is on the surface of a cell, such as a bacterium, activated complement can lyse the cell through its enzymatic activity (see Chapter 14). Some of the components of complement also have opsonic activity. They bind to the antigen-antibody complex and subsequently to receptors on macrophages, further facilitating phagocytosis of the coated antigen. Other components of activated complement are chemotactic for phagocytic neutrophils. Still other components cause the release of histamine by mast cells or basophils. The responses mediated by the complement system are complex and are involved in the induction of inflammation, which is itself a very important defense mechanism (see Chapters 11 and 12). Other enzyme systems that interact with the immune system in inflammation include the kinin system, the clotting system, and the fibrinolytic system (see Chapter 11).

Antibody-Dependent Cellular Cytotoxicity (ADCC)

The major class of antibodies, IgG (see Chapter 9) binds to a subclass of NK cells that expresses receptors for it. NK cells armed with antibody bind to the target cell, be it a bacterium or a tumor cell, and kill it with cytotoxins. This NK cell can be distinguished from the Tc cell by the fact that it does not express the CD8 marker and requires antibody for its activity.

INFLAMMATION & DELAYED HYPERSENSITIVITY

Another inflammatory response, **delayed-type hypersensitivity (DTH),** is mediated by a subset of TH cells. These T cells, following activation by APC, release lymphokines that attract and activate macrophages, setting up an inflammatory reaction. The response is called "delayed" because inflammatory responses mediated by antibody become apparent within minutes or hours, whereas DTH takes 24–48 hours to appear. The two are also distinguished by the nature of the cellular infiltrate: antibody complement-mediated inflammation features predominantly PMN, whereas DTH features mononuclear cells.

It is noteworthy that inflammatory responses have a "Jekyll-and-Hyde" characteristic. In addition to their value for the elimination of infectious agents, inflammatory responses may be mounted against normally innocuous environmental substances and thereby cause disease. Allergic reactions to poison oak and poison ivy are typical DTH reactions, whereas inflammatory responses to grasses, pollens, drugs, and antibiotics are more commonly triggered by antibodies (see Chapter 29).

REGULATION OF THE IMMUNE RESPONSE

We have now traced the adaptive immune response from its initiation by entry of the immunogen to the induction of effector functions of cellular and antibody immunity. After the elimination of the offending immunogen, the response is damped, thereby preventing uncontrolled activation of lymphocytes and unregulated production of antibody.

One regulatory mechanism is reflected by the declining phase of the antibody response (Fig 3–6). Negative regulatory mechanisms constrain the response, but positive regulation that heightens the response exists as well. The TH cell is the cardinal positive regulatory element in the immune response. Imbalances in the exquisitely tuned immune regulatory system may occur by virtue of genetic defects, infectious or neoplastic disease, or hormonal imbalance and may lead to immune deficiencies (see Chapter 23) or to a loss of self-nonself discrimination and autoimmunity (see Chapter 35). For example, acquired immunodeficiency syndrome (AIDS) results from depletion of the TH cell population by infection with human immunodeficiency virus (HIV), which cripples an individual's ability to mount immune responses, leading to susceptibility to normally innocuous microorganisms (opportunistic infection) and possibly to certain cancers, the most common of which is Kaposi's sarcoma. On the other hand, myasthenia gravis is an autoimmune disease caused by inappropriate production of antibodies reactive with the acetylcholine receptor, which blocks transmission of nerve impulses.

Major Regulatory Influences on the Immune Response

Many factors influence the intensity of the immune response. The dose and immunogenic potency of the antigen, its route of entry, and the presence or absence of adjuvants when vaccines are administered (see Chapter 8) all play a role in the magnitude and duration of the response. However, once the response is under way, there are 3 tightly interwoven major mechanisms that limit its growth and longevity (Fig 3–7).

A. Antibody: The production of antibody results in **feedback inhibition** of further production of the same antibody. This feedback inhibition may operate in several ways. The antibody could simply remove residual antigen, thus limiting the immunogenic stimulus. Levels of circulating antigen decline sharply following the appearance of antibodies in the circulation, as would be expected. However, antibodies may also limit the response through their role in **idiotypic regulatory circuits,** as described below.

B. Idiotype-Specific Regulation: Idiotypes are antigenic epitopes located in the antigen-binding regions of antibody molecules (see Chapter 9). An individual is believed to have on the order of 10^7 B cell clones, each genetically programmed to make its antibody possessing a unique profile of idiotypic epitopes (**idiotopes**). Upon immunogenic stimulation, the number of clones capable of recognizing epitopes on the antigen is expanded, as described above, and so the level of their particular idiotopes is elevated. This perturbation in the steady-state level of these idiotopes serves as an immunogenic stimulus, inducing anti-idiotype antibody responses. Therefore, despite being self antigens, idiotypes are apparently immunogenic when their level is increased, although the basis for this apparent contradiction of self tolerance is not clearly understood. It may be due to the min-

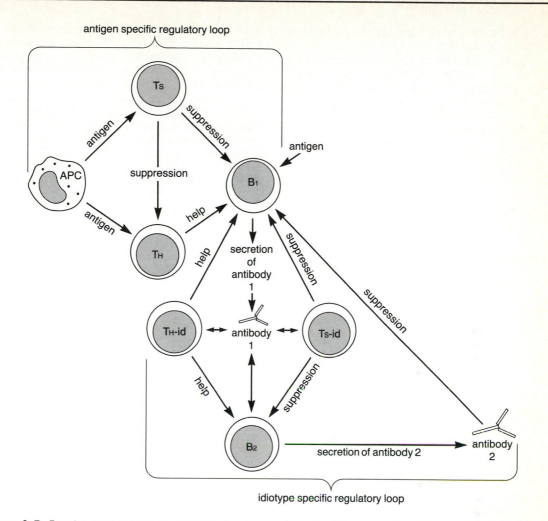

Figure 3-7. Regulatory circuits in the adaptive immune response involving suppressor Ts cells and idiotypes. The original antigen activates TH and Ts cells, which exert opposing influences on specific B cells (B₁). B₁ cells secrete antibody-1, which stimulates anti-idiotypic responses by TH (TH-id), Ts (Ts-id), and B₂ cells. Antibody-2 expresses idiotypes that may stimulate anti-id responses, and so on along the network.

ute quantity of any particular idiotype in the virgin lymphocyte population, which could escape notice as a "self-marker" during lymphocyte development.

Anti-idiotype antibodies have been shown to appear in the circulation of animals during the declining phase of a number of carefully studied immune responses; this suggests that they may be instrumental in turning off the response (Fig 3–7). It is also conceivable that reaction of anti-idiotype antibody with B cell (or T cell) antigen receptors serves as an immunogenic signal for the lymphocyte in much the same way that ordinary immunogens do. However, the appearance of anti-idiotype antibody in the course of a normal immune response has not been found to trigger a resurgence of antibody to the original immunogen.

If antibodies against exogenous immunogens have sets of idiotopes, anti-idiotype antibodies should have their own idiotypes and consequently induce anti-anti-idiotype responses, sometimes referred to as antibody-3 (anti-idiotype being antibody-2; Fig 3–7). These theoretic considerations led Nobel laureate Niels Jerne to propose that the lymphoid system is a closed interacting network of cells that communicate via idiotype–anti-idiotype recognition. In other words, every lymphocyte expresses idiotypes that will be recognized by the antigen receptors of other lymphocytes. Jerne further proposed that every possible epitope is represented in the total population of more than 10^7 idiotopes. He called idiotopes "internal images" of epitopes because they are structural parts of the antibody molecules themselves but resemble the epitopes of molecules outside the immune system (ie, on bacteria and viruses).

Some features of Jerne's idiotype network theory have been confirmed experimentally. As already mentioned, anti-idiotype antibodies arise normally during the course of immune responses, and in some instances it has been demonstrated that at least a fraction of the anti-idiotype antibody resembles the epitope that induced the original antibody response. It has been difficult to detect the successive waves of anti-idiotypes beyond antibody-3, possibly because the immunogenic signals diminish with increasing time from the original stimulus. Even though it has not been possible to verify the network in all details, it is believed to play an important role in immune regulation.

C. Suppressor T Cells: Another type of T cell we have not previously considered is able to suppress the activity of TH cells and may also act directly on B cells. These suppressor T cells (TS cells) express CD8, which distinguishes them from CD4 TH cells. Cytotoxic T cells also express CD8, but Ts cells do not appear to exert cytotoxic activity; they seem to be a distinct subset of T cells. Ts cells may be specific for the epitopes of exogenous antigens or for idiotype markers on the antigen receptors of B cells (antibodies) or T cells (Fig 3–7).

The mechanism of action of Ts cells is less clear than their existence, but they have been reported to secrete factors that can suppress the activities of TH and B cells. Thus, Ts cells and idiotypic regulation interface with each other in the complex control of the immune response, as depicted simplistically in Figure 3–7.

It can readily be visualized that such complex, delicately balanced, interacting regulatory networks may malfunction at any of a number of points. As mentioned above, a number of diseases have been associated, with varying degrees of certainty, with defects in these regulatory networks. Such diseases are treated in depth later in this volume and collectively represent one of the most intensive areas of biomedical research.

SUMMARY

There are 2 levels of protection against infection. Innate or natural immunity is present from birth, lacks specificity and memory, and consists of physical barriers such as skin and mucous membranes, certain enzymes, and phagocytic cells. Acquired or adaptive immunity is specific for the invading antigen, exhibits memory, and is based on the responses of T and B lymphocytes.

In the adaptive immune response, antigen is initially taken up and processed by APC, which express fragments of it called immunogenic epitopes complexed with class II MHC molecules to TH cells; these recognize features of both the epitope and the class II molecule.

Activated TH cells regulate the activities of other lymphocytes in a positive fashion through the secretion of soluble factors called lymphokines. One of these, IL-2, is an activating signal for Tc cells, which recognize antigens in the context of class I MHC molecules on target cells.

TH cells also furnish growth and differentiation signals to B cells, which then differentiate into antibody-secreting plasma cells.

The basis for memory in the immune response is the generation of antigen-specific TH and B cells following initial exposure to an antigen in the primary response. These memory cells are prepared to make amplified responses upon subsequent encounters with the same antigen in secondary, or anamnestic, responses.

Tc cells and antibodies use a variety of mechanisms to eliminate foreign antigens, some of which are integrally linked to inflammation.

The regulation of immune responses is accomplished through complex interacting networks involving antibody feedback, Ts cells, and idiotype–anti-idiotype interactions.

REFERENCES

Asherson GL, Colizzi V, Zembala M: An overview of T-suppressor cell circuits. *Annu Rev Immunol* 1986;**4**:37.

Goodman JW, Sercarz EE: The complexity of structures involved in T cell activation. *Annu Rev Immunol* 1983;**1**:465.

Kishimoto T, Hirano T: Molecular regulation of B lymphocyte response. *Annu Rev Immunol* 1988;**6**:485.

Singer A, Hodes RJ: Mechanisms of T-cell B-cell interaction. *Annu Rev Immunol* 1983;**1**:211.

von Boehmer H: The developmental biology of T lymphocytes. *Annu Rev Immunol* 1988;**6**:309.

The Human Major Histocompatibility Human Leukocyte Antigen (HLA) Complex

4

Benjamin D. Schwartz, MD, PhD

IMMUNE SYSTEM MECHANISMS

The immune system has evolved to protect the individual from a hostile environment containing innumerable viruses, bacteria, fungi, worms, and other parasites. To do so effectively, the immune system must distinguish between antigens against which an immune response would be beneficial and those against which it would be harmful. In other words, the immune system must discriminate "nonself" from "self." This crucial discrimination is achieved via the molecules of the major histocompatibility complex (MHC).

It now appears that every antigen, both nonself and self, is recognized by T cells only in conjunction with MHC molecules. Thus, CD4 (generally helper) T cells recognize antigens in conjunction with class II MHC molecules, whereas CD8 (generally cytotoxic) T cells recognize antigens in the context of class I MHC molecules (see below).

During embryogenesis, a process of T cell "education" occurs in the thymus, whereby T cells recognizing self antigens in the context of MHC molecules are eliminated and T cells potentially recognizing foreign antigens in the context of the individual's own MHC molecules are selected for survival. Breakdown in the elimination of self-recognition can result in autoimmune disease, whereas failure to recognize foreign antigens can lead to immunodeficiency with overwhelming infections and possibly uncontrolled spread of tumors.

The MHC Molecules

The MHC molecules are part of the immunoglobulin "supergene" family and appear to have evolved from the same primordial gene as immunoglobulin and T cell receptor molecules. Most probably as a result of repeated duplication and mutations of this primordial MHC gene during evolution, the genes encoding the MHC molecules are found clustered into a relatively small chromosomal region. It is this cluster of genes that constitutes the MHC.

The Human MHC

The human MHC was discovered in the mid-1950s, when leukoagglutinating antibodies were first found in the sera of both multiply transfused patients and 20–30% of multiparous women. Each antiserum gave a positive reaction with the cells of some but not all individuals, and different antisera reacted with the cells of different but overlapping populations of individuals. This pattern suggested that these antisera were detecting alloantigens (ie, antigens present on the cells of some individuals of a given species) that were the products of at least one polymorphic genetic locus.

Human Leukocyte Antigens (HLA Antigens)

The importance of matching these antigens for success in organ transplantation was soon realized and provided an important impetus for studying the genes that determine **human leukocyte antigens (HLA antigens).** Over the past 2 decades, the role played by the HLA complex in the regulation of human immune responses has become widely appreciated. By 1973, certain HLA antigens were found to be associated with specific diseases in a high proportion of cases. Together, these findings provided a second impetus for the study of the HLA complex.

The initial delineation of the HLA system resulted from cytotoxicity testing for identification of specific HLA antigens in this system, combined with the use of computers to codify reaction patterns of literally thousands of anti-HLA alloantisera. Recently, recombinant DNA methods have helped to delineate HLA genes and the amino acid sequence of many HLA molecules. Very recently, the elucidation of the crystal structure of an HLA molecule has provided insight into how HLA molecules function in an immune response. An international workshop now meets every 2–3 years to update the description of the organization and nomenclature of the HLA complex.

EVOLUTIONARY ORIGINS OF THE HLA COMPLEX

The origins of the MHC can be traced to the advanced invertebrates. It has been proposed that in these lower organisms, a recognition system arose that allowed individuals to distinguish self from nonself, especially in regard to other individuals of the species. Presumably, this recognition system prevented fusion of members of the species, which, in turn, promoted genetic diversity and dissemination of the species over a wider habitat.

Evidence for such a recognition system can be observed, for example, in tunicates. If a colony of sea squirts, which is an example of advanced invertebrates, is divided in half, each half will grow independently. If brought back into contact, the 2 colonies fuse and grow again as a single colony. In contrast, if 2 unrelated colonies of sea squirts are brought into contact, they almost never fuse. Rather, the cells at the contact point die, and a barrier of necrotic material results that keeps the 2 colonies separate. Furthermore, if this experiment is repeated with many different unrelated colonies, the vast majority of such fusions fail, suggesting that this recognition system is highly polymorphic.

This ability to distinguish self from nonself—and subsequent graft rejection of nonself—becomes increasingly evident as the phylogenetic ladder is ascended (see Chapter 2). These processes are reminiscent of syngeneic (self) and allogeneic (foreign) recognition phenomena seen in mammals and suggest the premium that nature has placed on self-recognition. It is likely that this primitive recognition system has evolved into the modern immune system, with the MHC functioning as a central element.

STRUCTURE, TISSUE DISTRIBUTION, & FUNCTION OF HLA MOLECULES

HLA molecules and the genes that encode them fall into 3 categories: classes I, II, and III. Class I and class II HLA molecules are cell surface glycoproteins and are members of the immunoglobulin supergene family, as shown by amino acid homologies. (This family includes a wide variety of cell surface molecules including immunoglobulins, T cell receptors, CD4, and CD8.)

The class I and class II molecules are distinguishable on the basis of their structure, tissue distribution, and function (Table 4–1). The class I molecules, also termed the classic histocompatibility molecules, include the HLA-A, -B, and -C molecules. Class II molecules include HLA-DR, -DQ, and -DP molecules.

The class III molecules include the second and fourth (C2 and C4) components of the classic complement pathway and properdin factor B of the alternative pathway. The class III HLA molecules are soluble and do not act as transplantation antigens, nor do they present antigen to T cells. The location of complement genes within the HLA complex remains unexplained (see Chapter 14).

1. CLASS I HLA MOLECULES

Structure of Class I HLA Molecules

The HLA-A, -B, and -C molecules each consist of a 2-chain structure. The heavy or α chain (MW 44,000) is a polymorphic glycoprotein determined by genes in the HLA complex on chromosome 6 and is noncovalently linked to a nonpolymorphic MW 12,000 protein, β_2-microglobulin, determined by a gene on chromosome 15. A schematic picture of a class I molecule is shown in Figure 4–1.

The entire molecule is anchored in the cell membrane by the MW 44,000 α chain. The α chain contains 338 amino acid residues and can be divided into 3 regions. Starting at the N-terminal end of the molecule, these regions are an extracellular hydrophilic region (residues 1–281), a transmembrane hydrophobic region (residues 282–

Table 4–1. Comparison of class I and II HLA.

Properties	Class I	Class II
Antigens included	HLA-A, -B, -C	HLA-D, -DR, -DQ, -DP
Tissue distribution	Ubiquitous on virtually every cell	Restricted to immunocompetent cells, particularly B cells, and macrophages
Functions	Present processed antigenic fragment to CD8 T cells. Restrict cell mediated cytolysis of virus-infected cells.	Present processed antigenic fragment to CD4 T cells. Necessary for effective interaction among immunocompetent cells.

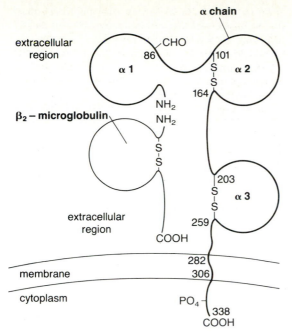

Figure 4-1. Schematic representation of a class I HLA molecule. The molecule consists of an MW 44,000 polymorphic transmembrane glycoprotein termed the α chain, which bears the antigenic determinant, in noncovalent association with an MW 12,000 nonpolymorphic protein termed β_2 microglobulin. The α chain has three extracellular domains termed α_1, α_2, and α_3. Abbreviations: NH$_2$, amino terminus; COOH, carboxy terminus; CHO, carbohydrate side chain; -SS-, disulfide bond; PO$_4$, phosphate. Numbers indicate amino acid residues where certain features are found (see text).

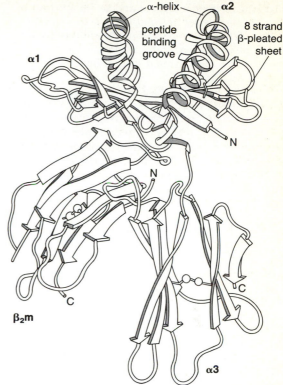

Figure 4-2. The diagrammatic crystalline structure of a class I HLA molecule (side view). The extracellular part of the molecule is depicted in side view with the portion distal to the cell membrane on top and the portion proximal to the membrane at the bottom. The transmembrane and intracytoplasmic domains are not shown. The β_2 microglobulin (β_2m) and α_3 domain support an interactive structure formed by the α_1 and α_2 domains. This interactive structure consists of a β-pleated sheet platform supporting two α helixes, which form a cleft that binds antigenic peptide fragments. β strands are shown as broad arrows; α helices are shown as ribbonlike structures. N indicates the amino terminus; C indicates the carboxy end.

306), and an intracellular hydrophilic region (residues 307–338). The extracellular region is divided into 3 domains termed $\alpha 1$, $\alpha 2$, and $\alpha 3$, which are composed of amino acid residues 1–90, 91–180, and 181–271, respectively. Comparison of the amino acid sequences of several HLA antigens has shown that the vast majority of the HLA antigenic determinants reside in the $\alpha 1$ or $\alpha 2$ domain.

Structure-Function Relationships of Class I HLA Molecules

The structure-function relationships of the class I molecule were advanced with the elucidation of the crystalline structure of the HLA-A2 molecule. A side view of the molecule is shown in Figure 4–2. β_2-Microglobulin and the $\alpha 3$ domain have a β-pleated sheet* structure similar to that of an immunoglobulin domain and form the lower part of the molecule. The $\alpha 1$ and $\alpha 2$ domains each consist of 4 β strands and an α helix, and they form the upper portion of the molecule. The 8 β strands of

these 2 domains form a β-pleated sheet that acts as a platform supporting the 2 α helices. These α helices create a groove or cleft that serves as the antigen-binding site to accept a peptide fragment appropriately processed from a larger antigen. Most of the polymorphism of class I molecules is

---

*A β-pleated sheet is a structure in which sections of a polypeptide chain or different polypeptide chains are aligned side by side and held together by hydrogen bonds to form a relatively flat surface or "sheet." The pleating maximizes the number of hydrogen bonds possible between the polypeptide chains.

localized to these α helices and to the portion of the β-pleated sheet platform that forms the floor of this cleft. Thus, the antigen-binding site varies from one class I molecule to another, and a given class I molecule can bind only a limited number of peptide fragments.

It should be emphasized that although the antigen-binding site of a class I molecule displays some selectivity in the peptide fragments it binds, this site is quite different from an immunoglobulin antigen-binding site that displays exquisite specificity. The 2 α helices, together with the bound antigenic fragment, make up a ligand recognized by the T cell receptor on a class I restricted CD8 T cell. A top view of the class I molecule, as it would appear to the T cell receptor of a CD8 T lymphocyte, is shown in Figure 4–3.

Function of Class I HLA Molecules

Class I HLA molecules are present on all nucleated cells, which is appropriate for their physiologic role. For an antigen to be recognized by a CD8 (generally cytotoxic) T lymphocyte, the antigen must be recognized in combination with a class I molecule. This phenomenon is termed **HLA restriction.** When, for example, a virus infects a cell, certain of the viral antigens are metabolized to peptide fragments that are then bound by the class I molecule and presented to CD8 cytotoxic (killer) T cells. The antigen receptor of a given T lymphocyte will recognize a particular viral peptide only in the context of a particular class I HLA molecule. These receptors do not recognize the *particular* viral peptide bound by a *different* class I molecule, a *different* viral peptide bound by the *particular* class I molecule, or the class I molecule *by itself*. Once recognition occurs, the cytotoxic T lymphocyte kills the target cell bearing the viral antigen. In the nonphysiologic condition of transplantation, it is the foreign class I molecules (with as yet unidentified bound peptides) that are recognized by the host CD8 T lymphocytes during graft rejection.

2. CLASS II HLA MOLECULES

The class II HLA-DR, -DP, and -DQ molecules are also 2-chain structures. Unlike the class I molecules, however, both chains are encoded by genes within the HLA complex.

Structure of Class II HLA Molecules

Each class II molecule is a heterodimer consisting of 2 glycoprotein chains, an α chain (MW 34,000) and a β chain (MW 29,000), in noncovalent association. Because the structures of all class II molecules are similar, the detailed structure of a class II HLA-DR molecule is described as the prototype.

The α chain and β chain are composed of 229 and 237 amino acids, respectively (Fig 4–4). Like the class I heavy chain, the α and β chains each consist of 3 regions: an extracellular hydrophilic region, a transmembrane hydrophobic region, and an intracellular hydrophilic region. The last 2 of these anchor the chains in the cell membrane.

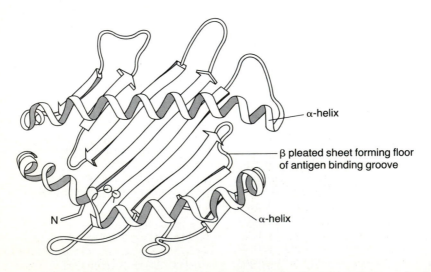

Figure 4–3. The diagrammatic crystalline structure of a class I HLA molecule (top view). The molecule is shown as the T cell receptor would see it. The antigen-binding site formed by the α helices (ribbonlike structures) and β-pleated strands (broad arrows) is shown. N indicates the amino terminus.

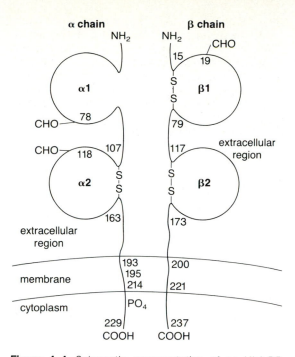

Figure 4–4. Schematic representation of an HLA-DR molecule. The molecule consists of an MW 34,000 glyco-protein (the α chain) in a noncovalent association with an MW 29,000 glycoprotein (the β chain). (Abbreviations and numbers are as in Fig 4–1.)

The extracellular hydrophilic region of the α chain contains 2 domains (residues 1–84 and 85–178), termed α1 and α2, respectively. The extracellular hydrophilic region of the β chain also contains 2 domains (residues 1–91 and 92–192), termed β1 and β2, respectively. The α2 and β2 domains both show significant homology to domains of immunoglobulin constant regions.

The structural features of the DQ and DP molecules are similar to those of DR. The DQ α and β chains have 234 and 229 amino acids, respectively, whereas the DP α and β chains each have 229 amino acids.

Although the crystalline structure of the class II molecules is not yet known, similarities between the structures of class I and class II molecules have allowed hypothetic models of class II structure to be generated by computer. It is thought that the class II α2 and β2 domains constitute the portion of the molecule proximal to the cell membrane that supports the portion distal to the cell membrane formed by the α1 and β1 domains. This latter portion is an interactive structure composed of 8 β strands and 2 α helices and is very similar to that created by the α1 and α2 domains of the class I molecule. The 2 α helices and a portion of the β-pleated sheet of the class II molecule also form a cleft or groove.

The polymorphism of the class II molecules is located in this cleft, resulting in different antigen-binding sites for each class II molecule. Thus, a given class II molecule can bind only a limited number of antigenic peptide fragments. This binding site of the class II molecule therefore shows some selectivity for antigens, but it lacks the fine specificity of an immunoglobulin antigen-binding site.

A top view of the class II α1 and β1 domains, as it would appear to a T cell receptor on a CD4 T lymphocyte, is shown in Figure 4–5. A processed antigenic peptide fragment can be accepted by the antigen-binding groove created by the 2 α helices and the platform. The α helices and antigenic peptide fragment then make up the ligand recognized by the receptor on CD4 T lymphocytes. Constraints on the recognition of the class II antigenic peptide complex by CD4 T lymphocytes are similar to those on the recognition of the class I antigenic peptide complex by CD8 T lymphocytes.

Function of Class II HLA Molecules

Class II HLA molecules have a limited cellular distribution. They are found chiefly on immunocompetent cells, B lymphocytes, antigen-presenting cells (macrophages and dendritic cells), and, in humans, activated T cells. In addition, cells that do not normally express class II molecules (such as resting T cells, endothelial cells, and thyroid cells) can be induced to express them. This abnormal expression has been postulated as an important element of one theory to account for HLA-disease associations (see below).

The function of class II molecules is to present processed antigenic peptide fragments to CD4 T lymphocytes during the initiation of immune responses. Just as CD8 T lymphocytes recognize peptide fragments only in the context of a class I molecule (see above), CD4 (generally helper) T lymphocytes recognize peptide fragments only in the context of class II molecules (Fig 4–6). In the nonphysiologic condition of bone marrow transplantation, class II molecules that have bound unidentified antigenic peptides on the host cells elicit a response from the engrafted donor T cells, resulting in a graft-versus-host reaction.

NOMENCLATURE & GENETIC ORGANIZATION OF THE HLA SYSTEM

Nomenclature & Genetic Loci

The nomenclature of the HLA system is devised by the HLA Nomenclature Committee of the World Health Organization. The entire histocompatibility complex is termed the HLA complex. It occupies a segment of approximately 3500 kilo-

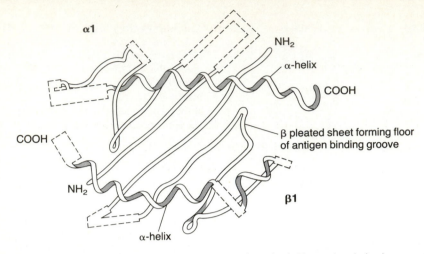

Figure 4–5. The crystalline structure of a class II HLA molecule (top view). The molecule is shown as it might appear to a T cell receptor. The antigen-binding site formed by the α chain α_1 domain and β chain β_1 domain consists of the β-pleated sheet platform (thin strands) supporting two α helices (ribbonlike structures) and is very similar to that of the class I molecule. NH_2 indicates the amino terminus; COOH indicates the carboxy end.

bases (kb) on the short arm of chromosome 6. Figure 4–7 schematically depicts the current map of the HLA complex, showing the genetic regions containing the various HLA loci. A **locus** is the position of a given gene on the chromosomes. The positions of the regions with respect to one another and to the centromere, as well as the approximate distances between regions, are shown in kilobases.

The HLA-A, -B, and -C gentic loci determine the class I molecules, which bear the class I antigens, and the HLA-DR, -DQ, and -DP genetic subregions, each of which contains several additional loci, determine the class II molecules, which bear the class II antigens (see above for an explanation of classes I and II).

Several other genetic regions are part of the HLA complex. The complement or HLA class III

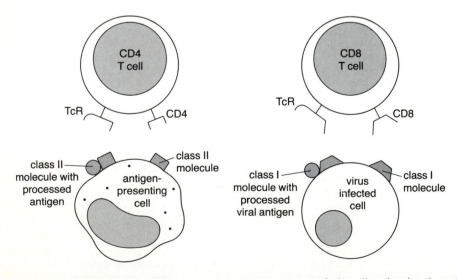

Figure 4–6. CD4 T cells (left) recognize processed antigen in the context of class II molecules through the T cell receptor and recognize an epitope on the nonpolymorphic region of the class II molecule through CD4. In contrast, CD8 T cells (right) recognize processed antigen in the context of class I molecules through their T cell receptor and an epitope on the nonpolymorphic region of the class I molecule through CD8.

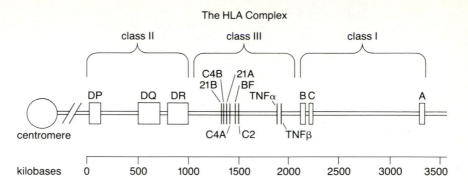

Figure 4-7. The HLA complex. The HLA complex is found on the short arm of chromosome 6. Locations of various MHC classes are indicated by brackets. The locations of these genes have been determined by molecular biologic techniques. Distances are given in kilobases. 21A and 21B are 21-hydroxylase A and B, respectively. BF is properidin factor, and BG is the alternative complement pathway. C2, C4A, and C4B are complement components. TNFα and TNFβ are tumor necrosis factor α and β, respectively. The DP, DQ, and DR subregions each contain multiple loci.

region has been mapped between the HLA-B and -DR regions and contains genes for the second and fourth components (C2 and C4) of the classic complement pathway and properdin factor B (BF) of the alternative pathway. The genes determining 21-hydroxylase A and B of the steroid biosynthetic pathway are also found here. The genes for

tumor necrosis factors α and β (lymphocytotoxin) have recently been mapped between the complement and HLA-B regions.

The HLA system is extremely polymorphic, having multiple alternative forms or alleles of the gene at each known locus (Table 4-2). For example, there are at least 24 distinct alleles at the

Table 4-2. Complete listing of recognized HLA specificities.

A	B		C	D	DR	DQ	DP
A1	B5	B51(5)	Cw1	Dw1	DR1	DQw1	DPw1
A2	B7	Bw52(5)	Cw2	Dw2	DR2	DQw2	DPw2
A3	B8	Bw53	Cw3	Dw3	DR3	DQw3	DPw3
A9	B12	Bw54(w22)	Cw4	Dw4	DR4	DQw4	DPw4
A10	B13	Bw55(w22)	Cw5	Dw5	DR5	DQw5(w1)	DPw5
A11	B14	Bw56(w22)	Cw6	Dw6	DRw6	DQw6(w1)	DPw6
Aw19	B15	Bw57(17)	Cw7	Dw7	DR7	DQw7(w3)	
A23(9)	B16	Bw58(17)	Cw8	Dw8	DRw8	DQw8(w3)	
A24(9)	B17	Bw59	Cw9(w3)	Dw9	DR9	DQw9(w3)	
A25(10)	B18	Bw60(40)	Cw10(w3)	Dw10	DRw10		
A26(10)	B21	Bw61(40)	Cw11	Dw11(w7)	DRw11(5)		
A28	Bw22	Bw62(15)		Dw12	DRw12(5)		
A29(w19)	B27	Bw63(15)		Dw13	DRw13(w6)		
A30(w19)	B35	Bw64(14)		Dw14	DRw14(w6)		
A31(w19)	B37	Bw65(14)		Dw15	DRw15(2)		
A32(w19)	B38(16)	Bw67		Dw16	DRw16(2)		
Aw33(w19)	B39(16)	Bw71(w70)		Dw17(w7)	DRw17(3)		
Aw34(10)	B40	Bw70		Dw18(w6)	DRw18(3)		
Aw36	Bw41	Bw72(w70)		Dw19(w6)			
Aw43	Bw42	Bw73		Dw20	DRw52		
Aw66(10)	B44(12)	Bw75(15)		Dw21	DRw53		
Aw68(28)	B45(12)	Bw76(15)		Dw22			
Aw69(28)	Bw46	Bw77(15)		Dw23			
Aw74(w19)	Bw47			Dw24			
	Bw48	Bw4		Dw25			
	B49(21)	Bw6		Dw26			
	Bw50-(21)						

[1]See text for explanation. Numbers in parentheses indicate parent HLA antigen from which these antigens split (see text and Table 4-4).

HLA-A locus and at least 50 distinct alleles at the HLA-B locus. Each allele determines the structure of a glycoprotein chain. The products of the HLA-A, -B, -C, -DR, -DQ, and -DP alleles are all cell surface molecules that carry their own antigenic determinants, which are detectable by various in vitro histocompatibility tests (see Chapter 21).

The 7 groups of antigens officially recognized by the HLA Nomenclature Committee are HLA-A, -B, -C, -D, -DR, -DQ, and -DP. These are designated by the locus (for class I) or subregion (for class II) determining the antigenic specificity and a number; thus, HLA-A1 is the number 1 specificity determined by a gene at the HLA-A locus, and HLA-DR3 is the number 3 specificity determined by the HLA-DR subregion. Antigens that have not yet been officially recognized are designated by a "w" (for "workshop") placed before the number, eg, HLA-DRw1. Official recognition results in the elimination of the "w," eg, HLA-DR1. The entire listing of officially and tentatively recognized HLA-A, -B, -C, -D, -DR, -DQ, and -DP antigens is presented in Table 4–2.

HLA Public & Private Antigens

HLA antigens found on a single molecule (and no other) are termed **HLA private antigens.** In contrast, **HLA public antigens** are determinants common to several HLA molecules each of which additionally bears a distinct HLA private antigen. HLA-Bw4 and -Bw6 are the best-known examples of HLA public antigens, and one or the other is found on every molecule determined by HLA-B alleles. The distribution of the HLA-Bw4 and -BW6 public antigens on HLA-B molecules bearing HLA-B private antigens is shown in Table 4–3.

Several HLA antigens initially thought to be single private antigens were later found to be a group of 2 or 3 closely related antigens, each of narrower specificity. These latter antigens are termed "splits" of the original broad-specificity

Table 4-4. Splits of HLA antigens.

Original Broad Specificities	Splits
A9	A23, A24
A10	A25, A26, Aw34, Aw66
Aw19	A29, A30, A31, A32, Aw33, Aw74
A28	Aw68, Aw69
B5	B51, Bw52
B12	B44, B45
B14	Bw64, Bw65
B15	Bw62, Bw63, Bw75, Bw76, Bw77
B16	B38, B39
B17	Bw57, Bw58
B21	B49, Bw50
B21	B49, Bw50
Bw22	Bw54, Bw55, Bw56
B40	Bw60, Bw61
Bw70	Bw71, Bw72
Cw3	Cw9, Cw10
DR2	DRw15, DRw16
DR3	DRw17, DRw18
DR5	DRw11, DRw12
DRw6	DRw13, DRw14
DQw1	DQw5, DQw6
DQw3	DQw7, DQw8, DQw9
Dw6	Dw18, Dw19
Dw7	Dw11, Dw17

antigens. Biochemical analysis has indicated that splits are, in fact, closely related structural variants. In Table 4–2, HLA antigens that are splits are followed in parentheses by their original broad antigen. Thus, for example, the terms HLA-A25(10) and -A26(10) indicate that HLA-A25 and -A26 are splits of HLA-A10. Conversely, HLA-A10 can be considered a public antigen on the HLA molecules bearing the private HLA-A25 and -A26 antigens. Table 4–4 lists the currently recognized splits of the broad-specificity antigens.

Conversely, HLA private antigens can be organized into groups based on apparent serologic cross-reactivity between members of the group. These groups are termed **cross-reactive groups (CREGs).** Thus, for example, the B7-CREG includes HLA-B7, -Bw22 (subsequently split into -Bw54, -Bw55, and -Bw56), -B27, -B40 (subsequently split into -Bw60 and -Bw61), and -Bw42. For at least 3 of the CREGs (B5-, B7-, and B15/B17-CREG), the basis for the cross-reactivity is a public HLA antigen common to all members of the CREG. It is assumed that the cross-reactivity between members of other CREGs will also be explained by the presence of public antigens.

Organization of the Class II Region

The organization of the class II region (also called the HLA-D region) has recently been clarified (Fig 4–8). It contains 3 distinct subregions, DR, DQ, and DP, each of which contains multiple

Table 4-3. Private B-locus antigens associated with the public HLA-Bw4 and HLA-Bw6 antigens.[1]

Bw4
B5, B13, B17, B27, B37 B38(16), B44(12), Bw47, B49(21), B51(5), Bw52(5), Bw53, Bw57(17), Bw58(17), Bw59, Bw63(15), Bw77(15)
Bw6
B7, B8, B14, B18, Bw22, B35, B39(16), B40, Bw41, Bw42, B45(12), Bw46, Bw48, Bw50(21), Bw54(w22), Bw55(w22), Bw56(w22), Bw60(40), Bw61(40), Bw62(15), Bw64(14), Bw65(14), Bw67, Bw70, Bw71(w70), Bw72(w70), Bw73, Bw75(15), Bw76(15)

[1]Numbers in parentheses indicate parent HLA molecules from which these antigens split (see text and Table 4–4).

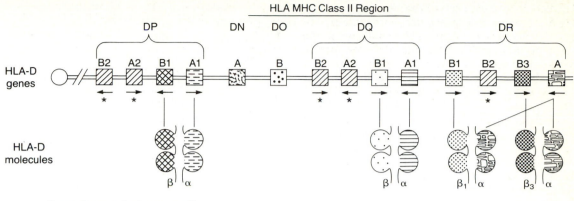

* pseudogenes (not expressed)

Figure 4–8. The HLA-D region and the molecules it encodes. The organization of the genes within each of the 3 defined subregions, DP, DQ, and DR is shown. Genes encoding α chains or genes with homologous nucleotide sequences are designated A, whereas genes encoding β chains or genes with homologous nucleotide sequences are designated B. The number of DRB genes depends on the DR type. DRB2, DQA2, DQB2, DPA2, and DPB2 genes are pseudogenes. The A gene of DN and the B gene of DO are not currently known to be transcribed in vivo. Pairs of class II genes that determine class II molecules are shown. The direction of transcription (5′ to 3′) is given under the genes (arrows). Most haplotypes determine four distinct class II molecules.

genetic loci. There are also 2 newly discovered subregions, termed DN (formerly DZ) and DO, each of which contains a single genetic locus. It should be recalled that each class II HLA molecule consists of 2 distinct chains, termed α and β, that form a heterodimer. Both the α and β chains of a given class II molecule are determined by genes within the corresponding subregion. For example, the HLA-DQα and -DQβ chains are both determined by genes within the DQ subregion (Fig 4–8).

Class II genes that determine α chains, as well as genes with related sequences, are designated by the letter "A," while class II genes that determine β chains, and genes with related sequences, are designated by the letter "B." If 2 or more A or B genes are present within a given subregion, they are designated by a number following the letter, eg, HLA-DRB1 and -DRB3, and HLA-DQA1 and -DQA2.

A. HLA-DR Subregion: The DR subregion contains a single HLA-DRA gene. The number of DRB genes varies with the DR type, but the most common configuration has 3 DRB genes, designated DRB1, DRB2, and DRB3 (or DRB4). (A given DR subregion will contain DRB3 or DRB4, but not both.) DRB2 is a pseudogene; ie, it is not expressed. The product of the DRA gene, the DRα chain, can combine individually with the products of both the DRB1 and the DRB3 (or DRB4) genes, the DRβ1 and the DRβ3 (or DRβ4) chains, to produce 2 distinct DR molecules,

DRαβ1 and DRαβ3 (or DRαβ4). The DRα chain is virtually nonpolymorphic, whereas the DRβ chains are highly polymorphic; thus, the DRβ chain is responsible for determining the DR antigen or DR type. The DRαβ1 molecules bear the DR specificities DR1–DRw18 (see Table 4–2), whereas the DRαβ3 molecules bear the DRw52 specificity and the DRαβ4 molecule bears DRw53. DRw52 and DRw53 are generally associated with particular subsets of DR specificities DR1–DRw18 (Table 4–5).

B. HLA-DQ Subregion: The DQ subregion contains 2 sets of genes: DQA1 and DQB1, and DQA2 and DQB2. DQA2 and DQB2 are pseudogenes. As products of the DQA1 and DQB1 genes, the DQα and DQβ chains combine to form the DQαβ molecule. In contrast to the DR molecules, both the DQα and β chains are polymorphic. However, it appears that the DQβ chain is the major determinant of the DQ type or antigen. The DQαβ molecules bear DQ specificities DQw1–DQw9. Because each individual has 2 DQ

Table 4–5. HLA-DRw52- and HLADRw53-associated DR antigens.

DRw52
   DR3, DR5, DRw6, DRw8, DRw11(5), DRw12(5), DRw13(w6), DRw14(w6), DRw17(3), DRw18(3)
DRw53
   DR4, DR7, DR9

subregions, one on each of the two chromosomes 6, and because DQ genes are codominantly expressed (see below), the fact that both the α and β chains of the DQ molecule are polymorphic allows individuals who are DQ heterozygotes (ie, who have 2 different DQA1 genes and 2 different DQB1 genes) to actually express 4 distinct DQ molecules by *cis*- and *trans*-pairing (Fig 4–9). *cis*-Pairing refers to the association of the α and β chains determined by genes on the same chromosome, and *trans*-pairing refers to the pairing of α and β chains encoded, respectively, by genes on opposite chromosomes. The molecules formed by *trans*-pairing are also called **hybrid molecules** and may be important in HLA-disease associations (see below).

C. HLA-DP Subregion: The HLA-DP subregion also contains 2 sets of genes: HLA-DPA1 and -DPB1, and HLA-DPA2 and -DPB2. HLA-DPA2 and -DPB2 are pseudogenes. The HLA-DPA1 and -DPB1 genes determine the DPα and β chains, respectively, which combine to form the DPαβ molecule. The DPα chain displays limited polymorphism (2 forms have been described to date), whereas the DPβ chain is highly polymorphic and appears to determine the DP antigen or type. Because both DPα and β chains display polymorphism, *cis*- and *trans*-pairing can occur, resulting in the expression of 4 distinct DP molecules in DP heterozygotes. The DP molecules bear DP antigens DPw1–DPw6.

D. Other Class II Subregions: The DN subregion contains a single HLA-DNA gene, and the DO subregion contains a single HLA-DOB gene. Neither of these genes has been found to be expressed in vivo, although expression has been induced in vitro. No function for these genes is presently known. It should be noted that there are no specific class II genes encoding the HLA-D antigens. The HLA-D antigens are defined by a cellular reaction termed the **mixed leukocyte reaction (MLR;** see Chapter 21). It is now thought that the antigenic determinants recognized during this reaction are actually antigenic epitopes present on the HLA-DR, -DQ, and possibly the -DP molecules. The highest correlation appears to be between the HLA-D and -DR antigens (Table 4–6).

Class III MHC Antigens

The complement components (see also Chapter 14) determined by the complement loci in the class III region also display polymorphism. There are 4 alleles determining the 4 alternative forms of properdin factor B (BF) that can be distinguished by their electrophoretic mobility: a common fast form (BF*F), a common slow form (BF*S), a rare fast form (BF*F1), and a rare slow form (BF*S1). There are C2 alleles determining the 2 common forms of C2 (C2*C and C2*A) and a rare deficiency allele (C2*QO). The C4 locus has actually been duplicated, so that there are 2 distinct C4 genetic loci, designated C4A (formerly Rogers), which determines the electrophoretically more acidic group of C4 components; and C4B (formerly Chido), which determines the electrophoretically more basic group of C4 components. There are 7 common structural alleles and one deficiency allele at the C4A locus and 3 common

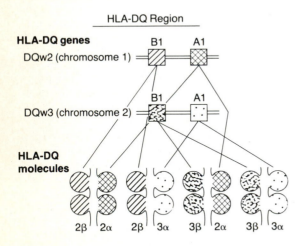

HLA-DQ Region

HLA-DQ genes

DQw2 (chromosome 1)   B1   A1

DQw3 (chromosome 2)   B1   A1

HLA-DQ molecules

2β 2α | 2β 3α | 3β 2α | 3β 3α

Figure 4–9. *cis*- and *trans*-pairing of HLA-DQα and β chains. Both DQα and Dβ chains are polymorphic. An individual who is heterozygous at both the DQA1 locus and DQB1 locus will have 2 different DQα chains and 2 different DQβ chains. Either of the α chains can pair with either of the β chains to give 4 different DQ αβ molecules. The middle 2 molecules, which contain an α chain and a β chain encoded by DQ subregions on different chromosomes, are termed hybrid molecules and result from *trans*-pairing (see text). The specific class II HLA antigens, DQw2 and DQw3, are used for illustrative purposes. The outer molecules 2βα and 3βα are formed by *cis*-pairing (see text).The B2 and A2 pseudogenes are omitted from the chromosome.

Table 4-6. HLA-DR and -D associations.

DR Antigen	Associated D Antigen(s)
DR1	Dw1, Dw20
DRw15(2)	Dw2, Dw12
DR216(2)	Dw21, Dw22
DR3	Dw3
DR4	Dw4, Dw10, Dw13, Dw14, Dw15
DRw11(5)	Dw5
DRw13(w6)	Dw6, Dw18, Dw19
DRw14(w6)	Dw9, Dw16
DR7	Dw7, Dw11, Dw17
DRw8	Dw8
DR9	Dw23
DRw52	Dw24, Dw25, Dw26

Table 4-7. Common alleles at the HLA-linked complement loci.

BF	C2	C4A	C4B
BF*F	C2*C	C4A*1	C4B*1
BF*S	C2*A	C4A*2	C4B*2
BF*F1	C2*QO	C4A*3	C4B*3
BF*S1		C4A*4	C4B*QO
		C4A*5	
		C4A*5	
		C4A*6	
		C4A*7	
		C4A*QO	

structural alleles and one deficiency allele at the C4B locus. Table 4-7 presents a listing of the known common alleles at each of the HLA-linked complement loci.

Haplotype, Codominance, & Inheritance

Because of their close linkage, the combination of alleles at each locus on a single chromosome is usually inherited as a unit. This unit is referred to as the **haplotype.** Because individuals inherit one chromosome from each parent, each individual has 2 HLA haplotypes. All HLA genes are codominant, so both alleles at a given HLA locus are expressed, and 2 complete sets of HLA antigens, one from each parent, can be detected on cells. Based upon mendelian inheritance, there is a 25% chance that 2 siblings will share both haplotypes, a 50% chance that they will share one haplotype, and a 25% chance that they will share no haplotype and thereby be completely HLA-incompatible (Fig 4-10).

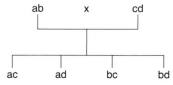

Figure 4-10. Inheritance of HLA haplotypes. A haplotype is the combination of alleles at each locus on a single chromosome that is inherited as a unit. Haplotype designations in the figure are given as a, b, c, and d. The maternal haplotypes are a and b, and the paternal haplotypes are c and d. Offspring of this mating (ab × cd) inherit one of the 2 possible haplotypes from each parent and so will have haplotypes ad, ab, bc, and bd. There is a 25% chance that 2 offspring will be HLA-identical (eg, ac and ac), a 25% chance that they will be totally HLA-nonidentical (eg, ac and bd), and a 50% chance that they will be HLA-semi-identical (eg, ac and ad).

Linkage Disequilibrium

Because human matings are random, the frequency of finding a given allele at one HLA locus with a given allele at a second HLA locus should simply be the product of the frequencies of each allele in the population. However, certain combinations of alleles are found with a frequency far exceeding that expected. This phenomenon is known as **linkage disequilibrium** and is quantitated as the difference (Δ) between the observed and expected frequencies.

As an example, the HLA-B8 allele and the HLA-DR3 allele are found in the North American white population with frequencies of 0.09 and 0.12, respectively. Thus, the expected frequency with which the HLA-B8-DR3 haplotype should be found is 0.09×0.12, or 0.0108. However, this haplotype is found with a frequency of approximately 0.0740, almost 7 times the expected frequency, for a Δ of $0.0740 - 0.0108 = 0.0632$. Table 4-8 lists some common examples of linkage disequilibrium. Several hypotheses have been offered in an attempt to explain the phenomenon of linkage disequilibrium, including (1) a selective advantage of a given haplotype, (2) migration and admixture of 2 populations, (3) inbreeding, and (4) random drift of the gene pool.

IMMUNE RESPONSE GENES

Immune response (Ir) genes were originally described in animal models as genes that determine whether an individual can respond immunologically to a particular foreign antigen. Classic genetic techniques mapped the Ir genes to the vicinity of the class II MHC genes, and it was postulated that the respective class II molecules were in fact the protein products of Ir genes.

An extrapolation of the crystal structure of the class I molecules to the class II molecules and an understanding of the antigen-binding site of class

Table 4-8. Examples of linkage disequilibrium in Caucasians.

Haplotypes	Δ ($\times 10^3$)[1]
HLA-A1, B8	53.2
HLA-A2, B44	14.8
HLA-B27, Cw1	9.0
HLA-B27, Cw2	19.9
HLA-B7, DR2	36.8
HLA-B8, DR3	61.3
HLA-DR2, DQw1	93.6
HLA-DR3, DQw2	37.4
HLA-DR4, DQw3	87.5

[1]Δ is the difference between observed and expected frequencies of the haplotype that results from linkage disequilibrum.

II molecules have in essence confirmed this postulate and established the mechanism by which class II molecules can mediate the effect of Ir genes.

The variation of the antigen-binding site among different class II molecules and hence the variation in the ability of a given class II molecule to bind a given antigenic peptide fragment predict that only certain class II molecules can present particular antigens. These variations also account for the observation that only certain individuals, ie, those who inherit the appropriate class II genes, can respond to a given foreign substance.

Multiple examples of Ir gene effects in humans are known. Two of the most striking are the IgE antibody response to short ragweed antigen Amb a V (Ra5), which is highly associated with HLA-DR2; and the IgE antibody response to short ragweed antigen Amb a VI (Ra6), which is highly associated with HLA-DR5. Although currently unproved, it is thought that peptides derived from the ragweed antigens bind to these class II molecules.

HLA & DISEASE

Diseases associated with HLA antigens have several common characteristics. In general, these diseases (1) have unknown cause and unknown pathophysiologic mechanism, (2) have a hereditary pattern of distribution but weak penetrance and thus do not have an absolute association with a given HLA antigen, (3) are associated with immunologic abnormalities, and (4) have little or no effect on reproduction.

Methods Demonstrating HLA-Disease Associations

Both population and family studies have been used to demonstrate the relationship between marker genes within the HLA complex and various disease states. These 2 types of studies yield different types of information. Population studies determine the statistical associations to be made between a particular HLA marker gene and a particular disease. Such associations cannot be interpreted as proof of genetic linkage between a disease susceptibility gene and the HLA marker gene, because association does not necessarily indicate genetic linkage, nor does linkage necessarily indicate association. For example, if a disease susceptibility gene is on a chromosome other than chromosome 6 and therefore not linked to HLA, but the presence of a particular HLA antigen is necessary for the phenotypic expression of that disease susceptibility gene, then an HLA-disease association would be established.

Conversely, a gene such as phosphoglucomutase 3 (PGM_3) is on chromosome 6 and therefore linked to HLA, but no HLA-specific association of disease with PGM_3 is found. In contrast to population studies, family studies can demonstrate linkage between a disease susceptibility gene and the HLA marker. Because population studies are easier to perform, most of the data on HLA and disease derive from this type of study.

Expressions of Risk in HLA-Disease Associations

The association of a particular disease with a particular HLA antigen is quantitated by calculating the relative risk (RR). This can be defined as the chance an individual with the disease-associated HLA antigen has of developing the disease compared with an individual who lacks that antigen. It is calculated by using the following formula:

$$RR = \frac{p^+ \times c^-}{p^- \times c^+}$$

where p^+ = the number of patients possessing the particular HLA, antigen
c^- = the number of controls lacking the particular HLA, antigen
p^- = the number of patients lacking the particular HLA, antigen and
c^+ = the number of controls possessing the particular HLA antigen

The higher (above 1) the relative risk, the more frequent is the antigen within the patient population.

In contrast, the absolute risk (AR) is the chance an individual who possesses the disease-associated HLA antigen has of actually developing the disease. It is calculated by the following formula:

$$AR = \frac{p^+}{c^+} \times P$$

where p^+ and c^+ are as above for the relative risk, and
P = prevalence of the disease in the general population.

Ankylosing Spondylitis as Prototype Disease Associated With HLA-B27

The prototype of HLA-disease associations, ankylosing spondylitis with HLA-B27, can be used to illustrate these concepts. Ninety percent of Caucasian patients with ankylosing spondylitis in the United States possess HLA-B27, compared with approximately 9% of Caucasian controls. The relative risk is therefore $p^+c^-/p^-c^+ = (90 \times 91)/(10 \times 9) = 91$. Thus, an HLA-B27-positive individual has 91 times the risk that an HLA-B27-negative individual has of developing the disease. The prevalence of clinically apparent severe ankylosing spondylitis is approximately 0.4%. The absolute risk is calculated as $90/9 \times 0.004 = 0.04$. Therefore, of 100 HLA-B27-positive individuals, only 4 will actually develop clinically severe ankylosing spondylitis.

Because there is usually a significant difference in the frequency of a given antigen among different racial groups, it is always necessary to compare a patient group with a control population of the same race. Thus, for example, HLA-B27 is found in 48% of black patients with ankylosing spondylitis in the USA, compared with 2% of black controls in the USA, yielding a relative risk of 37 for this population.

Multiple Genetic & Disease Associations

In some cases, a disease may be associated with antigens determined by 2 different HLA loci. The actual association is frequently only with one antigen, but an apparent association with the second antigen is seen because of the phenomenon of linkage disequilibrium between the genes determining the 2 antigens (see above). The actual or primary association can usually be ascertained by statistically testing each antigen for disease association in the absence of the influence of the second antigen.

Antigens determined by almost all HLA loci have human disease associations. Thus, for example, idiopathic hemochromatosis has been associated with HLA-A3, ankylosing spondylitis with HLA-B27, rheumatoid arthritis with HLA-DR4, Sjögren's syndrome with DRw52, insulin-dependent diabetes mellitus with DQw8, celiac disease with a DP restriction fragment length polymorphism, and systemic lupus erythematosus with complement-deficient haplotypes. Selected HLA-disease associations are presented in Table 4–9.

The majority of diseases have been associated with class II antigens, and this association almost certainly reflects the role of the class II molecules in presenting processed antigenic fragments to CD4 T lymphocytes. Of interest is that several documented or presumed autoimmune diseases have been found to be associated with HLA-DR3 (Table 4–10). Most recently, specific class II region restriction endonuclease fragments have been associated with particular diseases.

Hypotheses To Explain HLA-Disease Associations

Several hypotheses, including the 5 discussed below, have been advanced to explain HLA-disease associations. Four of these apply equally to HLA class I and class II antigens, and one applies only to class II molecules.

The first 4 hypotheses will be illustrated by using the example of ankylosing spondylitis and

Table 4–9. Selected HLA-disease associations in Caucasian patients.

Disease	Antigen	Approximate RR
Ankylosing spondylitis	B27	81.8
Reiter's syndrome	B27	40.4
Acute anterior uveitis	B27	7.98
Rheumatoid arthritis	DR4	6.4
Juvenile rheumatoid arthritis Seropositive	DR4	7.2
	Dw4	25.8
	Dw14	47
	Dw4/Dw14	116
Pauciarticular	DR5	2.9
Systemic lupus erythematosus (Caucasian patients)	DR2	3.0
	DR3	2.7
	C4A Null	5.4
	C4A deletion	5.5
Behçet's disease	B5	3.3
Sjögren's syndrome	DR3	5.6
Graves' disease	DR3	3.8
Insulin-dependent diabetes mellitus	DR4	6.3
	DR3	3.3
	DR3/4	33
	DR2	.25
	DQw8	31.8

HLA-B27. It should be immediately emphasized that these examples are purely speculative and that, except where noted, there is no evidence to support this speculation.

A. HLA Molecules Are Receptors of Etiologic Agents: Particular HLA molecules may act as receptors for etiologic agents such as viruses, toxins, or other foreign substances. Support for this hypothesis comes from the observation that other cell surface molecules act as receptors for viruses; eg, CD4 acts as a receptor for human immunodeficiency virus (HIV). If, for example, HLA-B27 is the receptor for a virus that causes ankylosing spondylitis, B27-positive indi-

Table 4–10. Diseases of known or presumed autoimmunity associated with HLA-DR3.

Systemic lupus erythematosus
Sicca syndrome
Myasthenia gravis
Dermatitis herpetiformis
Insulin-dependent diabetes mellitus
Graves' disease
Idiopathic Addison's disease
Celiac disease
Autoimmune chronic active hepatitis

viduals will be at increased risk for ankylosing spondylitis but can develop the disease only if they are exposed to the virus.

B. HLA Is Selective for Antigenic Peptides: The antigen-binding groove of only particular HLA molecules can accept the processed antigenic peptide fragment that is ultimately responsible for causing disease. If HLA-B27 is the only class I molecule that can accept a particular etiologic peptide for presentation to a CD8 T cell, only individuals with B27 will be predisposed to disease.

C. T Cell Receptor Determines Disease Predisposition: The T cell antigen receptor is actually responsible for disease predisposition, but because T cell recognition is restricted by an HLA molecule, and apparent association is seen between the disease and HLA. Suppose that all B27-positive individuals can form a particular B27-processed antigen complex but that only certain of these individuals possess B27-restricted T lymphocytes with the appropriate T cell receptor to recognize this complex. If the recognition of this complex by these T cells leads to ankylosing spondylitis, then only the individuals with these particular T cells can develop the disease. Although the antigen receptors on the T cells are ultimately responsible for the development of disease, an apparent association with HLA-B27 is observed because of the HLA-B27 restriction of these T cells.

D. Causative Agents Mimic HLA Molecules: The disease-associated HLA antigen is immunologically similar to the causative agent for the disease. This molecular mimicry hypothesis involves 2 alternatives. The first holds that because of the similarity between the causative agent and the HLA antigen, the etiologic agent is regarded as self, no immune response is mounted, and the causative agent produces disease without any interference from the host immune system. The second alternative suggests that the causative agent is regarded as foreign, and a vigorous immune response is mounted against the etiologic agent. Because of the similarity of the agent and the HLA antigen, the immune response is turned against the HLA antigen and this "autoimmune" response then produces disease. This theory has gained support from the following observations. HLA-B27 has been associated with Reiter's disease as well as ankylosing spondylitis. Reiter's disease in a B27-positive individual follows bouts of dysentery caused by certain strains of *Shigella flexneri*. These disease-producing *Shigella* strains contain a plasmid that encodes a protein with a stretch of 5 amino acids identical to a stretch of 5 amino acids in HLA-B27. Because only B27-positive individuals share this structural and immunologic similarity with the etiologic organism, only

these individuals are predisposed to disease according to the molecular mimicry hypothesis.

E. Expression of Class II MHC Molecules Is Aberrant: The last hypothesis relates only to diseases associated with class II HLA molecules. It postulates that the induction of class II expression on the surface of cells that do not normally express class II molecules is responsible for disease. Tissue-specific molecules on the surface of cells are constantly undergoing turnover and degradation. If the cells do not express class II molecules, degradation of the molecules to potentially antigenic peptides has no consequences. However, if these cells are induced to express class II molecules, the degradation of the tissue-specific molecules could lead to "antigen processing." A peptide fragment from the tissue-specific molecule would be bound by the antigen-binding site of the class II molecule, thereby forming an immunogenic complex and initiating an immunologic response against the tissue-specific molecule. If only certain class II molecules (eg, HLA-DR3) can bind these tissue-specific molecular fragments, then disease associations with HLA will be seen. Such a scenario has been postulated for the form of hyperthyroidism known as Graves' disease, in which antibodies directed against the receptor for thyroid-stimulating hormone are present and which is associated with HLA-DR3.

Other Diseases With Strong HLA Associations

The associations of insulin-dependent diabetes mellitus and rheumatoid arthritis with HLA are particularly instructive regarding several points.

A. Insulin-Dependent Diabetes Mellitus: This disease is negatively associated with HLA-DR2 (RR = 0.25), so that the presence of HLA-DR2 is protective against the development of disease. In contrast, the disease is positively associated with HLA-DR3 (RR = 3.3) and HLA-DR4 (RR = 6.3) but is even more highly associated with HLA-DR3/DR4 heterozygosity (RR = 33). Thus, there is something about this heterozygous state that particularly predisposes to insulin-dependent diabetes mellitus.

HLA-DR4 is in linkage disequilibrium with DQw3, and HLA-DR3 is in linkage disequilibrium with DQw2. Thus, the majority of HLA-DR3/DR4 heterozygotes will also be HLA-DQw2/DQw3 heterozygotes. Because both the DQα and β chains are polymorphic, DQw2/DQw3 heterozygotes will possess 2 hybrid molecules—DQw2αDQw3β and DQw3αDQw2β—not detected in other individuals (Fig 4–8). It is possible that one of these hybrid molecules is actually responsible for predisposition to disease.

HLA-DQw3 has recently been "split" into DQw7 (formerly DQw3.1) and DQw8 (formerly

DQw3.2). Further analysis has indicated that insulin-dependent diabetes mellitus is highly positively associated with HLA-DQw8 but negatively associated with HLA-DQw7. Sequence analysis has revealed that the HLA-DQw8 β chain has an alanine residue at position 57, whereas the HLA-DQw7 β chain has an aspartic acid at this position. Additional sequence data indicate that DQβ chains found in other haplotypes positively associated with insulin-dependent diabetes mellitus lack an aspartic acid at position 57, whereas DQβ chains present in haplotypes negatively associated with the disease possess this aspartic acid. Thus, a single amino acid appears to be crucial in the predisposition to this disease. Similar findings can be anticipated with respect to other diseases.

B. Rheumatoid Arthritis: Rheumatoid arthritis is highly associated with HLA-DR4 and particularly with 2 of the 5 subtypes of HLA-DR4, termed Dw4 and Dw14 (Table 4–5). In addition, it is associated with DR1. Sequence analysis indicates that the β chains of the Dw14 subtype of DR4 and DR1 share identical amino acid sequences from residues 67–78 in a highly polymorphic region of the molecule that is found in the α helix of the antigen-binding site.

This finding suggests that particular regions (eg, residues 67–78) or "antigenic epitopes" of molecules rather than entire molecules are responsible for predisposition to disease. It has been further proposed that such regions may be transferred between distinct HLA molecules by a mechanism termed **gene conversion.** Gene conversion, although not well defined mechanistically, is thought to be similar to recombination, but genetic information is transferred only in one direction. This observation of shared epitopes may also be one explanation for the lack of absolute associations between HLA and disease.

It should be emphasized that HLA-associated diseases are a heterogeneous group, that different mechanisms may be operating in different HLA-associated diseases, and that more than one mechanism may be operating concurrently to produce disease. Further studies are necessary to clarify these issues.

SUMMARY

The HLA complex contains a number of genes that are crucial in the initiation, regulation, and implementation of an immune response. It is the most highly polymorphic complex known in mammalian species. It contains the HLA-A, -B, and -C genes, which encode the class I HLA molecules, and the HLA-DR, -DQ, and -DP subregions, which encode the class II HLA molecules.

The class I and II HLA molecules are each 2-chain structures. The HLA-encoded class I α chain has 3 extracellular domains and is associated with a non-HLA-encoded chain, β_2-microglobulin. The class II α and β chains are both encoded by the HLA complex, and each contains 2 extracellular domains.

The demonstrated structure of the class I molecule and the presumed structure of the class II molecule indicate that the interactive portion of the molecules consists of a β-pleated sheet platform upon which rest 2 α helices. These 2 α helices form the sides and the β-pleated sheet forms the floor of a cleft or groove that is the antigen-binding site. Processed antigenic peptide fragments can fit into this groove. Because most of the polymorphism of the class I and II molecules is localized to the α helices and the portion of the β-pleated sheet that is the floor of the groove, the antigen-binding site varies from one HLA molecule to another. This observation explains why different HLA molecules bind different antigenic fragments; it also explains Ir gene effects and HLA-disease associations.

The class I molecules have a ubiquitous tissue distribution and present processed antigenic peptide fragments to CD8 (predominantly cytotoxic) T lymphocytes, whereas class II molecules have a distribution limited to immunocompetent cells and present processed antigenic peptide fragments to CD4 (predominantly helper) T lymphocytes.

Because of their role in the immune response, many HLA antigens have been associated with predisposition to particular diseases; the majority of such associations involve class II HLA antigens. The magnitude of the association is quantitated by the relative risk. Although very little is known about the etiology or pathogenesis of the HLA-associated diseases, several models have been proposed to explain the mechanism by which the HLA molecules may be involved. Recent evidence suggests that single amino acid changes in crucial regions of an HLA molecule can alter disease predisposition and that regions of identical amino acid sequence (epitopes) found on different HLA molecules may be responsible for disease predisposition.

REFERENCES

General

Dupont B (Editor): *Histocompatibility Testing 1987.* Vol 1 of: *Immunobiology of HLA.* Springer-Verlag, 1989.

Dupont B (editor): *Immunogenetics and Histocom-*

patibility. Vol. 2 of: *Immunobiology of HLA.* Springer-Verlag, 1989.

McDevitt HO: The HLA system and its relation to disease. *Hosp Pract* (July 15) 1985;**20**:57.

Schwartz, BD et al (editors): Workshop on the immunogenetics of the rheumatic diseases. *Am J Med* 1988;**85(Suppl 6A)**:1. [Entire issue.]

Nomenclature & Genetic Organization
of the HLA System

Bohme J et al: HLA-DR beta genes vary in number between different DR specificities, whereas the number of DQ beta genes is constant. *J Immunol* 1985;**135**:2149.

Carroll MC et al: A molecular map of the human major histocompatibility complex class III region linking complement genes C4, C2, and factor B. *Nature* 1984;**307**:237.

HLA Nomenclature Committee: Nomenclature for factors of the HLA system, 1987 *Immunogenetics* 1988;**28**:391.

Möller G (editor): Molecular genetics of class I and II MHC antigens. (2 parts.) *Immunol Rev* 1985;**84**:1 and **85**:1. [Entire issues.]

Spies T et al: Structural organization of the DR subregion of the human major histocompatibility complex. *Proc Natl Acad Sci USA* 1985;**82**:5165.

Trowsdale J, Campbell RD: Physical map of the human HLA region. *Immunol Today* 1988;**9**:34.

Structure, Tissue Distribution, & Function

Babbitt BP et al: Binding of immunogenic peptides to Ia histocompatibility molecules. *Nature* 1985;**317**:359.

Bjorkman PJ et al: Structure of the human class I histocompatibility antigen, HLA-A2. *Nature* 1987;**329**:506.

Brown JH et al: A hypothetical model of the foreign antigen-binding site of class II histocompatibility molecules. *Nature* 1988;**332**:845.

Buss S, Sette A, Grey HM: The interaction between protein-derived immunogenic peptides and Ia. *Immunol Rev* 1987;**98**:116.

Marrack P, Kappler J: T cells can distinguish between allogeneic major histocompatibility complex products on different cell types. *Nature* 1988;**332**:840.

McMichael AJ et al: HLA restriction of cell-mediated lysis of influenza virus-infected human cells. *Nature* 1977;**270**:524.

Möller G (editor): Structure and function of HLA-DR. *Immunol Rev* 1982;**66**:1. [Entire issue.]

Ir Genes

Marsh DG, Meyers DA, Bias WB: The epidemiology and genetics of atopic allergy. *N Engl J Med* 1981;**305**:1551.

HLA & Disease

Möller G (editor): HLA and disease susceptibility. *Immunol Rev* 198;**70**:1. [Entire issue.]

Tiwari JL, Terasaki PI (editors): *HLA and Disease Associations.* Springer-Verlag, 1985.

Todd JA, Bell JI, McDevitt HO: HLA-DQ beta gene contributes to susceptibility and resistance to insulin-dependent diabetes mellitus. *Nature* 1987;**329**:599.

Cells of the Immune Response: Lymphocytes & Mononuclear Phagocytes

5

Lewis Lanier, PhD

Lymphocytes and **mononuclear phagocytes** play a central role in the immune response. These cell types are responsible for both innate and acquired immunity against bacterial and viral pathogens. In addition to cell-mediated immune functions, they are the source of a vast array of secreted proteins that influence the growth and development of many body tissues. Moreover, in addition to their beneficial role in protection against microbial pathogens, these cells may adversely affect normal body tissues during the course of certain autoimmune diseases. In this chapter, an overview of the functions of various types of lymphocytes and mononuclear phagocytes is presented.

Leukocytes (white blood cells) are a heterogeneous group of cells that mediate immune responses. Leukocytes are found predominantly in the blood, bone marrow, and lymphoid organs (eg, spleen, thymus, tonsils, and lymph nodes), as well as in epithelium and elsewhere. Classification of leukocytes was first based on morphologic criteria, principally nuclear size and shape and histochemical staining characteristics of the cytoplasm. Three major cell types were distinguished: **granulocytes, lymphocytes,** and **monocytes** (Fig 5–1).

Granulocytes (10–15 μm in diameter), also referred to as polymorphonuclear leukocytes, have a multilobular nucleus and abundant granules in the cytoplasm. Three subtypes of granulocytes exist: **neutrophils, basophils,** and **eosinophils.** When stained with Giemsa dye, the granules of neutrophils appear blue-gray, those of basophils blue, and those of eosinophils red. Lymphocytes are small (7–12 μm in diameter) mononuclear spherical cells typically containing very little cytoplasm that stains pale blue with Giemsa dye. Monocytes (10–30 μm in diameter) are also mononuclear; they have a characteristic kidney-shaped nucleus and more cytoplasm than lymphocytes do.

Blood monocytes differentiate when stimulated by various substances into **macrophages.** Like monocytes, macrophages are mononuclear cells, but they also possess more abundant cytoplasm with predominant intracellular vacuoles and granules and are pleomorphic. Certain types of macrophages, called **histiocytes,** are resident in spleen, lung (alveolar macrophages), liver (Kupffer's cells), skin (Langerhans cells), and other tissues.

I. LYMPHOCYTES

Although morphologic and biophysical properties have provided a useful classification for the major groups of leukocytes, these groups do not consist of homogeneous populations. Monoclonal antibodies directed against cell surface antigens have demonstrated identifying heterogeneity, particularly within lymphocytes. On the basis of expression of cell surface markers, 3 distinct lineages of lymphocytes have been identified: T cells, B cells, and natural killer (NK) cells. Moreover, the presence or absence of certain cell surface markers has been used to delineate stages of differentiation, states of cellular activation, and functionally distinct subsets of lymphocytes.

A series of International Human Leukocyte Differentiation Antigen Workshops has established a unified nomenclature for the most commonly studied cell surface antigens (Table 5–1).

T cells, B cells, and NK cells are distinguished primarily by their antigen receptors and by certain characteristic cell surface markers called clusters of differentiation (CD; Fig 5–2). T cells recognize antigens by a membrane structure called the CD3/T cell antigen receptor complex (the CD3/TCR complex), whereas B cells recognize antigens by using surface immunoglobulin molecules. (The structure and function of the CD3/TCR complex are discussed in Chapter 6.) Although the recogni-

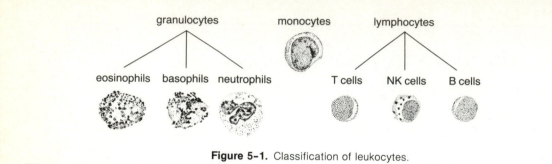

Figure 5–1. Classification of leukocytes.

Table 5–1. Leukocyte differentiation antigen nomenclature.

CD[1]	MW	Predominant Leukocyte (Function)	Frequently Used Antibodies
1a	49,000	Thymocytes, Langerhans cells	αLeu 6, T6
1b	45,000	Thymocytes, Langerhans cells	
1c	43,000	Thymocytes, Langerhans cells	
2	50,000	T and NK cells	αLeu 5, T11
2R	50,000	Activation-related epitope of CD2	T11-3, 9.1
3	20,000–30,000	T cells (T cell-antigen receptor complex)	αLeu 4, T3
4	60,000	T cell subset (class II MHC interaction, HIV receptor)	αLeu 3, T4
5	67,000	T cells and B subset	αLeu 1, T1
6	120,000	T cells	T12
7	40,000	T and NK cells, platelets	αLeu 9, 3A1
8α	32,000	T and NK subsets (class I MHC interaction)	αLeu 2, T8
8β		T subset	
9	24,000	Pre-B, monocytes, platelets	
10	100,000	Pre-B cells, cALL[3] (enkephalinase)	αCALLA,J5
11a	180,000	Leukocytes (cellular adhesion)	αLFA-1α
11b	160,000	Myeloid cells, NK cells, T subset (complement receptor type 3)	αCR3, OKM1
11c	150,000	Myeloid cells, NK cells, T subset (complement receptor type 4)	αLeuM5
12		Monocytes, granulocytes, platelets	
13	150,000	Granulocytes, monocytes (aminopeptidase N)	
14	53,000	Monocytes	αLeuM3, Mo2
15	CHO[4]	Granulocytes	αLeuM1
16	50,000–70,000	NK cells, granulocytes, T subset (IgG-Fc receptor type III)	αLeu 11,3G8
17	Lipid	Granulocytes, monocytes, platelets (lactoceramide)	
18	95,000	Leukocytes (β subunit of CD11a, b, c)	αLFA-1β
19	95,000	B cells	αLeu 12, B4
20	35,000	B cells	αLeu 16,B1
21	140,000	B cells (complement receptor type 2)	αCR2, B2
22	135,000	B cells	αLeu 14
23α	45,000	B cells (IgE-Fc receptor type II)	αLeu 20
23β	45,000	B cells, monocytes, eosinophils, T subset	
24	65,000, 55,000, 65,000	B cells, granulocytes	
25	55,000	Activated lymphocytes, monocytes (low-affinity IL-2 receptor)	αIL2-R, TAC-1
26	130,000	T cells (dipeptidyl peptidase IV)	5.9, Ta1
27	55,000	T cells, plasma cells	
28	44,000	T cell subset	9.3
29	135,000	Leukocytes, platelets	4B4, VLA-β
30	120,000	Activated B, T cells	
31	130,000–140,000	Monocytes, granulocytes, platelets gpLLa[5]	
32	40,000	Monocytes, granulocytes, platelets, B cells (IgC-Fc receptor type II)	
33	67,000	Myeloid leukemia	
34	115,000	Hematopoietic stem cells	αHPCA-1
35	220,000	Granulocytes, monocytes (complement receptor type 1)	
36	85,000	Monocytes, platelets	
37	40,000–45,000	B cells	
38	45,000	Subsets of leukocytes	αLeu 17, OKT10
39	80,000	B cells, macrophages	
40	50,000	B cells	

Table 5–1 (cont'd). Leukocyte differentiation antigen nomenclature.

CD[1]	MW	Predominant Leukocyte (Function)	Frequently Used Antibodies
41a	125,000	Platelets gpIIb/IIIa	
41b		Platelets gpIIb	
42a	145,000	Platelets gpIX	
42b		Platelets gpIb	
43	95,000	T cells, granulocytes	
44	65,000–85,000	Leukocytes (homing receptor)	Hermes
45	180,000–220,000	Leukocytes	HLE-1
45R	220,000	T subset, NK cells, B cells	αLeu 18, 2H4
45R0	180,000	T subset, activated T	UCHL-1
46	55,000–66,000	Leukocytes, platelets	
47	47,000–52,000	Leukocytes, platelets	
48	41,000	Leukocytes	
w[6]49a	210,000	Leukocytes, platelets (cell adhesion)	VLA-1α
w49b	165,000	Leukocytes, platelets (cell adhesion)	VLA-2
w49c	135,000	Leukocytes, platelets (cell adhesion)	VLA-3
w49d	150,000	Leukocytes, platelets (cell adhesion)	VLA-4
w49e	135,000	Leukocytes, platelets (cell adhesion)	VLA-5
w49f	120,000	Leukocytes, platelets (cell adhesion)	VLA-6
w50	140,000/108,000	Leukocytes	
w51	120,000	Leukocytes, platelets (vitronectin receptor α chain)	
w52	25,000–30,000	Leukocytes	CAMPATH-1
53	32,000–40,000	Leukocytes	
54	85,000	Activated B and T, macrophages (CD11/CD18 ligand, rhinovirus receptor)	ICAM-1
55	73,000	Leukocytes (delayed accelerating factor)	
56	140,000–200,000	NK cells, T subset	αLeu 19, NKH1
57	CHO	T and NK subsets	αLeu 7
58	45,000–60,000	Leukocytes (CD2 ligand)	LFA-3
59	18,000–20,000	Leukocytes, platelets	MEM-43
w60	120,000	T subset, platelets (GD3 ganglioside)	
61	114,000	Platelets gpIIIa	
62	150,000	Platelets	
63	53,000	Platelets	
64	75,000	Monocytes, macrophages (IgG Fc receptor type I)	
w65		Granulocytes, monocytes (fucoganglioside)	
66	180,000–200,000	Granulocytes	
67	100,000	Granulocytes	
68	110,000	Macrophages	
69	28,000–32,000	Activated lymphocytes	αLeu 23
w70		Activated lymphocytes	Ki-24
		Reed-Sternberg cells	
71	90,000	Proliferating cells (transferrin receptor)	
72	43,000/39,000	B cells	
73	69,000	B, T subset (ecto-5′ nucleotidase)	
74	41,000, 35,000/33,000	B cells, monocytes (invariant chain)	
w75		B cells, T cell subset	
76	85,000/67,000	B cells, T cell subset, granulocytes	
77		Activated B cells	
w78		B cells	αLeu 21

[1]CD, cluster of differentiation.
[2]α, antibody to. . . .
[3]cALL, common acute lymphocytic leukemia.
[4]CHO carbohydrate antigen.
[5]gp, glycoprotein.
[6]w is the provisional (Workshop) designation.

tion structure(s) of NK cells has not been identified, these cells use neither T cell antigen receptors nor immunoglobulins. T, B, and NK cells mediate a vast array of cellular functions in immune responses. Their distribution in the body is given in Table 5–2.

T LYMPHOCYTES

Development of T Lymphocytes in the Thymus

T cells are the special lineage of lymphocytes that arise from maturation of stem cells in the thy-

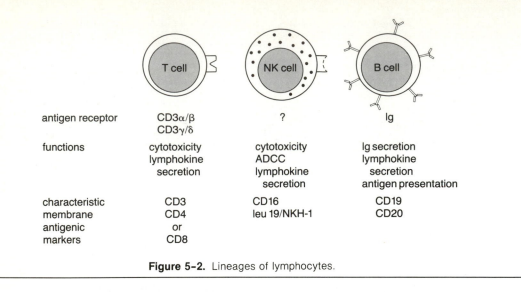

	T cell	NK cell	B cell
antigen receptor	CD3α/β CD3γ/δ	?	Ig
functions	cytotoxicity lymphokine secretion	cytotoxicity ADCC lymphokine secretion	Ig secretion lymphokine secretion antigen presentation
characteristic membrane antigenic markers	CD3 CD4 or CD8	CD16 leu 19/NKH-1	CD19 CD20

Figure 5–2. Lineages of lymphocytes.

mus; hence the name "T" cells. The central role of the thymus is the rearrangement and productive expression of the T cell receptor (TCR) genes and the subsequent selection of the antigen receptor repertoire that enables mature T cells to recognize foreign but not usually self antigens. Progenitor cells from either bone marrow or fetal liver enter the thymus and undergo stages of differentiation, resulting in the migration of mature T lymphocytes into the blood and peripheral lymphoid tissues (eg, spleen, lymph nodes, lymphatic system, and tonsils).

A complex series of changes in genotype and phenotype accompany the maturation of T cells in the thymus (Fig 5–3). The earliest recognizable thymocyte, the **pro-T cell,** can be identified by expression of certain antigens on the cell surface (eg, CD2 and CD7) and by the presence of CD3ε protein in the cytoplasm (but not on the cell surface). Pro-T cells differentiate into **pre-T cells** by rearrangement of δ-, γ-, and β-TCR genes. First, γ/δ-TCR-bearing cells arise from pre-T cells that productively rearrange and express γ- and δ-TCR genes. Pre-T cells destined to generate α/β-TCR-bearing T cells then rearrange α-TCR genes,

thereby deleting the δ-TCR genes between the Vα and Cα genes on the chromosome.

Thymocytes that express CD3/α/β-TCR on the cell surface and react with self antigens are usually deleted from the population by an unknown process. Other CD3/α/β-TCR-bearing thymocytes are "educated" to recognize antigenic peptides only when associated with self MHC proteins by a process that also has not yet been delineated. Most thymocytes fail in this selection process and die within the thymus; only a minority successfully differentiate into mature T lymphocytes and migrate to the peripheral lymphoid organs and blood. In peripheral blood, about 70% of lymphocytes are T cells.

Markers of Thymic Lymphocytes

Molecules other than the CD3/TCR complex are involved in thymic differentiation of T lymphocytes and can also be used as markers to identify stages of maturation (Fig 6–3). Pro-T cells express CD2 and CD7 on the cell surface; these immature thymocytes lack CD3, CD4, and CD8. As they mature, the majority of pro-T and pre-T lymphocytes begin to express CD1, CD4, and CD8 markers, usually within the thymic cortex.

Subsequently, these CD4+8+ immature thymocytes express low levels of the CD3 α/β-TCR complex and then undergo selection and "education." A proportion of the relatively immature CD4+8+ cells lose expression of either CD4 or CD8 to become CD4+8− or CD4−8+; the amount of CD3/TCR on the cell surface is increased, and the CD1 molecule is lost. These more mature thymocytes are found predominantly in the cortex and have a phenotype similar to that of T cells in the periph-

Table 5–2. Distribution of lymphocytes.

Tissue	Percentage of Lymphocytes (normal range)		
	T cells	B cells	NK cells
Blood	65–75	5–10	5–15
Thymus	>95	<1	<1
Lymph node	70–80	10–20	<1
Spleen	20–30	40–50	1–5

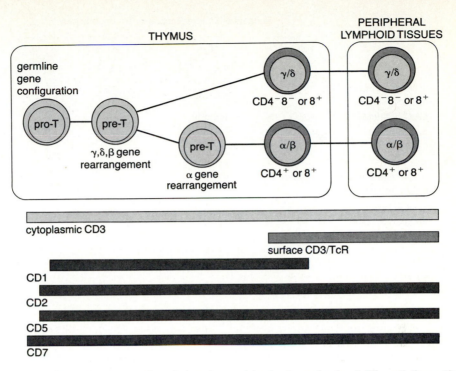

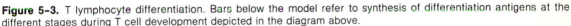

Figure 5–3. T lymphocyte differentiation. Bars below the model refer to synthesis of differentiation antigens at the different stages during T cell development depicted in the diagram above.

eral lymphoid tissues. They presumably represent the population from which truly mature α/β-TCR T cells arise. γ/δ-TCR-bearing thymocytes apparently do not follow this maturation pathway and do not coexpress CD4 and CD8 during differentiation. α/β-TCR- and γ/δ-TCR-bearing T cells probably then represent distinct lineages of T lymphocytes that arise from a common progenitor. Their precise relationship, however, has not been fully delineated. α/β-TCR-bearing T cells are the predominant T cell type in the thymus and peripheral lymphoid tissues after birth, constituting nearly all of both CD3 thymocytes and mature, peripheral T cells.

Function of T Cells in Immune Responses

T cells initiate the immune response, mediate antigen-specific effector responses, and regulate the activity of other leukocytes by secreting soluble factors. Effector functions of T cells include **cell-mediated cytotoxicity** and **cell-mediated immunity,** also known as delayed-type hypersensitivity (DTH). Augmentation of B and T cell activation and differentiation (ie, helper or amplifier function), suppression of an immune response (suppressor function), and secretion of potent cytokines, including gamma interferon and interleu-

kins (see Chapter 7), constitute the regulatory effects of T cells on many leukocytes as well as on other nonimmune cells in the body (Fig 5–4).

A correlation exists between the expression of membrane antigens and the functional activities of T cells. Mature T lymphocytes can be subdivided on the basis of expression of CD4 or CD8 antigens on the cell surface. $CD4^+8^-$ and $CD4^-8^+$ T cells represent some 70% and 25%, respectively, of the total T cell population in blood and peripheral lymphoid tissues. Minor subsets of T cells can express $CD4^-8^-$ or $CD4^+8^+$ phenotypes and account for the remaining 4% and 1%, respectively, of total mature T cells. CD4 and CD8 are membrane glycoproteins that bind to class II and class I major histocompatibility complex (MHC) antigens, respectively.

Recognition of Antigen by T Lymphocytes

T cells usually do not react with intact protein antigens, but rather bind to antigens that are processed into small peptides and bound to major histocompatibility complex (MHC) antigens on the cell surface of an antigen-presenting cell or target cell. Antigen-presenting cell (APC) is a general term to describe any cell (including monocytes, macrophages, B cells, dendritic cells, and some T

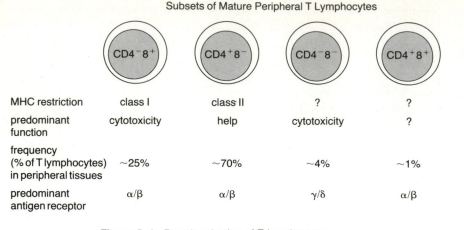

Figure 5–4. Functional roles of T lymphocytes.

cells) that can internalize and degrade a protein antigen into peptide fragments and then present these peptides on the cell surface membrane bound to self MHC antigens. Both class I (HLA-A, -B, -C) and class II (HLA-DR, -DP, -DQ) structures bind peptides for interaction with α/β-TCR. Natural ligands for the γ/δ-TCR have not been defined, but it is likely that these receptors will also bind peptide antigens. The CD3/TCR complex on the cell surface of T cells binds to the peptide/MHC on the APC. This interaction generates an activation signal for the T cells. The initial phase of signal transduction results in activation of phosphodiesterases that hydrolyze phospholipid phosphatidylinositol bisphosphate to generate diacylglycerol and inositol triphosphate, which is subsequently metabolized to inositol bisphosphate, inositol phosphate, and inositol. Inositol triphosphate rapidly increases intracellular free Ca^{2+} levels, and diacylglycerol stimulates protein kinase C activity. These early activation events are necessary, but not sufficient, for the subsequent induction of lymphokine secretion and proliferation. Usually, a cosignal is required. In some cases, cytokines produced by the APC (eg, interleukin-1 from monocytes) may provide cofactors that result in production of lymphokines and growth factors by T cells and, ultimately, cellular proliferation. The mechanism of these cosignals in T cell activation is not well understood.

Antigen-driven proliferation is an important feature of the immune system. Given the extent of the antigen receptor repertoire, only a few T cells in the total population will specifically react with any given antigen prior to immunization; however, exposure to antigen, usually in conjunction with other cofactors or cytokines that facilitate

the process (eg, IL-1), results in preferential clonal proliferation and expansion of these specific effectors. A consequence of exposure to antigen is the generation of memory T cells. Memory T cells are capable of self-renewal, resulting in the generation of cells that rapidly respond to reexposure to the antigen, following years or even decades after the primary stimulation (eg, tetanus immunization). Although the mechanism of this process is unknown, it is an essential and unique aspect of the immune response.

Cytotoxic-Suppressor T Cells

CD4$^-$8$^+$ T cells mediate most antigen-specific cytotoxicity—the ability to kill other cells that are perceived as foreign, eg, virus-infected or allogeneic cells introduced into the host by transplantation. CD4$^-$8$^+$ T cells recognize peptide antigens bound to class I MHC molecules on the cell surface of the target. During viral infection, viral peptides bind to self MHC molecules within the cytoplasm of the virus-infected target cell and are transported to the cell surface for recognition by cytotoxic T lymphocytes (CTL). In transplantation, allogeneic MHC molecules are themselves recognized as antigens by the CTL. Activated CTL destroy the target cell by a process that is not well-defined.

As a consequence of activation, CD4$^-$8$^+$ T cells also release **lymphokines** (eg, IL-2, gamma interferon), which can augment immune responses by other B and T lymphocytes. In addition to their cytotoxic function, CD4$^-$8$^+$ T cells can suppress immune responses, possibly by the release of soluble factors that interfere with the function of other immune cells. Because of these functions, the CD4$^-$8$^+$ T cell population is often referred to as the **T cytotoxic-suppressor subset (Tc/s).** This is an oversimplification, however, because cytotoxic and suppressive functions can also be mediated by other T cells, including the $CD4^+8^-$ and $CD4^-8^-$ T subsets. Moreover, whether suppression and cytotoxicity are mediated by independent cells within the $CD4^-8^+$ T population or, alternatively, represent functions mediated by the same cell has not been determined.

Helper T Cells

$CD4^+8^-$ T lymphocytes make up the subset referred to as the helper or helper/inducer T (TH or TH/I) cells because of their ability to augment B cell responses and to amplify the cell-mediated responses effected by $CD4^-8^+$ T cells. Under certain circumstances, $CD4^+8^-$ T cells can also mediate cytotoxicity and immune suppression. $CD4^+8^-$ T lymphocytes usually recognize peptide antigens that are bound to class II MHC glycoproteins present on the surface of an antigen-presenting cell. After exposure to peptide-MHC, $CD4^+8^-$ T cells are activated and proliferate.

Activated $CD4^+8^-$ T cells secrete soluble factors that influence effector functions mediated by other leukocytes. For example, antigen-stimulated $CD4^+8^-$ cells secrete IL-2, which, in turn serves as a growth factor for antigen-independent polyclonal proliferation of other T cells and augments cytotoxic activity mediated by CTL and NK cells.

IL-4, also secreted by T cells activated by antigens, augments the growth of B cells and other T cells, enhances CTL function, and induces the expression of Fc receptors for IgE on B cells and monocytes. However, IL-4 can also inhibit the activation of B and NK cells by IL-2. Many other cytokines (eg, IL-2, -3, -4, -5, and -6, granulocyte macrophage colony-stimulating factor (GM-CSF), tumor necrosis factor (TNF), and gamma interferon) are produced by antigen-specific stimulation of $CD4^+8^-$ T lymphocytes (see Chapter 7). Thus, the $CD4^+8^-$ T cells provide regulatory factors that either augment or suppress functions mediated by the entire immune system.

Minor T Cell Subsets

The role of the minor $CD4^-8^-$ and $CD4^+8^+$ T subsets is less clear. Culture of mature $CD4^+8^-$ T cells in IL-4 induces the expression of CD8 on the cell surface, suggesting a possible explanation for in vivo $CD4^+8^+$ cells. The physiologic consequence of this process is unknown, but it may permit cells to interact with both class I and II MHC antigens, thus facilitating immune responses. Unlike the majority of $CD4^+8^-$, $CD4^-8^+$, and $CD4^+8^+$ T lymphocytes that express an α/β-TCR, most $CD4^-8^-$ T cells possess a γ/δ-TCR. Although the natural antigens recognized by $CD4^-8^-$ γ/δ-TCR T cells have not been identi-

fied, these cells can mediate cell-mediated cytotoxicity and secrete cytokines such as IL-2, IL-4, and gamma interferon after activation.

Relationship of Cell Surface Markers With Stages of Differentiation or Activation

Lymphoid tissues contain a diverse collection of T cells that differ in terms of stage of differentiation, prior exposure to antigen, and state of activation as reflected by the heterogeneity of their cell surface marker expression within the T cell population in these tissues. It was previously thought that expression of different antigenic phenotypes reflected the existence of distinct lineages of T cells with unique functions; however, recent studies indicate that these phenotypes relate to the state of differentiation or state of activation of the cells (Fig 5–5).

Activation of T lymphocytes via either antigen-specific or antigen-independent (eg, cytokine, mitogen) stimulation alters the phenotype of the cells. Expression of new cell surface markers is induced, some markers are lost, and the amounts of other markers may be increased or decreased. For example, deliberate activation of T cells by stimulation of the CD3/TCR complex induces de novo synthesis of class II MHC antigens; the early activation antigen, CD69; and receptors for IL-2 (CD25) and transferrin. Activation increases the amount of CD2, CD18, CD26, CD29, CD38, CD44, CD45RO, CD54, and CD58 on the cell surface and results in down-regulation of CD45R antigens. Thus, the antigenic phenotype of T cells appears to reflect the stage of differentiation or activation rather than identifying a unique lineage within the T cell population.

B LYMPHOCYTES

Immunoglobulin as Antigen Receptor

B cells express **immunoglobulin** on the cell surface membrane. Immunoglobulin is responsible for binding of antigen, subsequent cellular activation, and the secretion of soluble immunoglobulin into serum and tissues. Unlike the TCR, which usually recognizes only peptide antigens bound to MHC molecules, immunoglobulins on B cells are able to bind directly and with high affinity to intact antigens, including glycoproteins, glycolipids, polysaccharides, peptides, and virtually any immunogenic molecule.

Immunoglobulins are glycoproteins composed of 2 disulfide-bonded **heavy (H) chain** subunits, each of which is linked by interchain disulfide bonds to a **light (L) chain,** forming a tetramolecular complex. In humans, 2 L chain genes, desig-

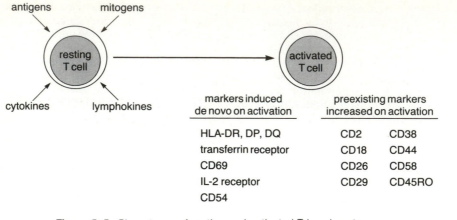

markers induced de novo on activation	preexisting markers increased on activation	
HLA-DR, DP, DQ	CD2	CD38
transferrin receptor	CD18	CD44
CD69	CD26	CD58
IL-2 receptor	CD29	CD45RO
CD54		

Figure 5–5. Phenotypes of resting and activated T lymphocytes.

nated κ and λ, are on chromosomes 2 and 22, respectively; the H chain locus is present on chromosome 14. Like the T cell antigen receptor, immunoglobulin H and L chains are composed of variable (V), joining (J), and constant (C) genes that rearrange during B cell development. H genes also possess diversity (D) elements. The human H chain locus contains several C region elements: μ, δ, $\gamma 1$–$\delta 4$, ϵ, $\alpha 1$, and $\alpha 2$. Numerous (>100) V_H and V_L genes and a high rate of V-region somatic mutation allow for an extensive repertoire of antigen recognition that is expanded further by junctional diversity.

Isotype Switching of Immunoglobulin in B Cells

B cells initially express a single RNA transcript containing both μ and δ segments that are processed into separate μ and δ H chain mRNA by alternative splicing, allowing a single B cell to express both IgM and IgD with an identical V region and hence the same antigenic specificity. Although a single B cell expresses a unique immunoglobulin V_H and V_L throughout its life, as a consequence of maturation the V/J segment may be "switched" to other 3′ C region elements by somatic recombination, with resulting deletion of the intervening genetic material including the μ and δ C segments. This allows for the generation of immunoglobulin with identical specificity (V regions) but diverse effector functions contributed by the different H chain isotypes. These C region elements differ with respect to binding of complement components, interaction with Fc receptors, and transfer of immunoglobulin across membranes (eg, placenta).

Differentiation of B Cells

B lymphocytes arise from progenitor cells in the bone marrow. B cells rearrange immunoglobulin genes during the early stages of maturation (Fig 5–6). During this process, the pre-B cells first rearrange immunoglobulin heavy chain genes and then rearrange light chain genes. When functional H and L chains are both synthesized, immunoglobulin is expressed on the cell surface. These immunoglobulin-expressing cells are referred to as **virgin B cells** because they possess competent immunoglobulin on the membrane but have not yet interacted with antigen. At this stage, B cells migrate from the bone marrow into the blood and peripheral lymphoid tissues.

The stages of B cell maturation are reflected by changes in the expression of several cell surface differentiation antigens (Fig 5–6). After interaction of antigen with surface immunoglobulin, B cells are activated and ultimately mature into **plasma cells,** which are responsible for production of large quantities of immunoglobulin, which is secreted. After the same exposure to antigen, some B cells live for years and are thus referred to as **memory B cells.** These cells are responsible for the rapid **recall responses** observed after reexposure to antigens previously recognized by the immune system.

Activation & Function of B Cells

Antigen-specific activation of B cells occurs after binding of antigen to membrane immunoglobulin independent of the action of APC. A second signal is provided by soluble factors released from monocytes or T cells. This results in activation via the phosphatidylinositol pathway and

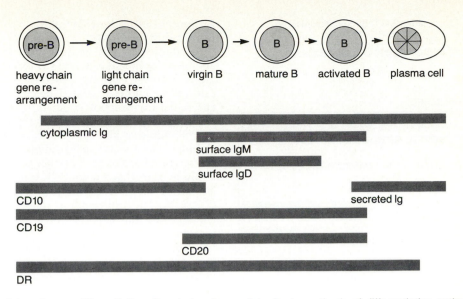

Figure 5–6. B lymphocyte differentiation. Bars below the model refer to synthesis of differentiation antigens at the different stages during B cell development depicted in the diagram above.

subsequent clonal expansion similar to activation of T cells. Two general types of antigen have been described: **T cell-independent antigens** and **T cell-dependent antigens.** B cells encountering T cell–independent antigens are capable of proliferation and immunoglobulin secretion in the absence of Tн cells. These antigens are often carbohydrates or antigens expressing multiple repeating determinants that permit extensive cross-linking of the surface immunoglobulin on the B cells.

In contrast, response to T cell-dependent antigens requires interaction between B and T cells for subsequent immunoglobulin production. Tн cells recognize the antigen and produce several soluble mediators, including IL-4 and -5 and other cytokines that augment or help B cells to respond. Depending upon the nature of the antigen and the availability of T cell-generated cytokines, immunoglobulin **isotype switching** occurs.

Plasma Cells & Memory B Cells

When provided with the appropriate factors, B cells ultimately differentiate into plasma cells, which secrete large amounts of soluble immunoglobulin into the serum or tissue. In the plasma cell, the immunoglobulin RNA transcripts are truncated by mRNA splicing to delete the transmembrane segment of the molecule, permitting immunoglobulin secretion rather than attachment to the cell membrane. After primary exposure to antigen, memory B cells are generated. In addition to producing immunoglobulin, B cells also may secrete certain cytokines (eg, IL-6) that affect the growth and differentiation of B cells and other lymphocytes.

NATURAL KILLER (NK) CELLS

Phenotypic Characteristics of NK Cells

NK cells are a subset of lymphocytes that arise from a precursor cell in the bone marrow. Mature NK cells are present in blood, bone marrow, and spleen but are infrequent in the lymph nodes or thymus. The exact developmental relationship of NK cells to T and B lymphocytes is unknown. However, NK cells are clearly a distinct lineage; children with **severe combined immunodeficiency disease (SCID),** a disorder that prevents the development of mature B and T lymphocytes, possess normal mature NK cells. Moreover, NK cells rearrange neither immunoglobulin nor T cell antigen receptor genes. NK cells can be identified by the presence of certain characteristic differentiation antigens (Fig 5–7). All NK cells express CD56 and CD16 but lack expression of the CD3/TCR. Most mature NK cells are large granular lymphocytes (LGL), as are some T cells. In normal individuals, NK cells make up 10–15% of lymphocytes in peripheral blood and 1–2% of lymphocytes in spleen.

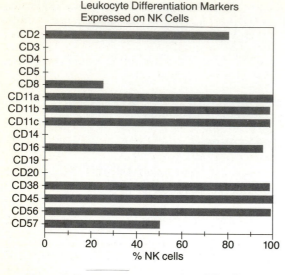

Figure 5–7. Antigens expressed on NK cells.

Function of NK Cells

NK cells were originally defined by their ability to kill certain tumor cells (referred to as **NK activity**) without deliberate tumor cell immunization of the host. Unlike most CTL, NK cells recognize and kill both autologous (self) and allogeneic tumors without requiring recognition of MHC antigens on the target cell. This **MHC-unrestricted cytotoxicity** is not confined to NK cells, however; a small subset of T lymphocytes can also mediate this function. It has been suggested that this NK activity may be important in immune surveillance by preventing metastasis of tumors through the blood, although this remains controversial.

The most important role of NK cells is probably in defense against viral infection. NK cells kill virus-infected host cells but not normal uninfected cells. In very rare cases, NK cells are absent; these patients have been reported to be particularly susceptible to certain viral infections, such as cytomegalovirus infection and varicella. Because NK cells do not require prior exposure to the antigen to respond, they may provide the initial antiviral defense during the latent period before development of antibodies and antigen-specific CTL.

Unlike T and B lymphocytes, NK cells do not possess antigen specificity and do not acquire immune memory after an initial exposure to a virus-infected or tumor cell. The membrane receptors on NK cells responsible for recognition of tumor and virus-infected cells have not yet been identified.

Antibody-Dependent Cellular Cytotoxicity (ADCC)

In addition to NK activity, NK cells mediate **antibody-dependent cellular cytotoxicity (ADCC)**, the mechanism whereby a cytotoxic effector cell can kill an antibody-coated target cell. Binding and signal transduction occur through a cell surface receptor that is located on the cytotoxic effector cells and that binds the Fc region of immunoglobulin. The effector cells mediating ADCC were formerly referred to as "K (killer cells"; however, it now appears that a unique "K cell" does not exist. Rather, most ADCC in peripheral blood is mediated by NK cells and a small subset of T lymphocytes that express CD16, an Fc receptor that preferentially binds complexes of human IgG1 and IgG3. Thus, ADCC provides a mechanism for NK cells to use the antigen-binding specificity of antibodies to direct their killing activity.

NK Cell Activation by Cytokines

Resting NK cells isolated from normal individuals kill only a limited range of tumors (the K562 erythroleukemia is the prototype "NK-sensitive" tumor); however, NK cells can be activated by certain cytokines to increase their cytotoxic activity and proliferate. For example, after a few hours of exposure to IL-2 in tissue culture, NK cells acquire the capacity to kill essentially all tumor cell types without damaging most normal tissues. This phenomenon is called **lymphokine-activated killer (LAK)** activity. Although some T lymphocytes can also mediate this activity, NK cells are responsible for most of it.

In addition to increasing cytotoxic activity, IL-2 acts as a growth factor and directly induces the proliferation of NK cells. Patients treated with IL-2 demonstrate an elevated level of NK cells in peripheral blood, and these circulating IL-2-activated NK cells are capable of killing a broad spectrum of tumor cell types. The cytotoxic activity of NK cells can also be increased by alpha interferon and, to a lesser extent, by gamma interferon. Interferons are frequently induced during viral infection, so they may play a role in the antiviral immunity mediated by NK cells.

Other Functioning NK Cells

NK cells mediate a variety of immune factors other than cytotoxicity. After appropriate stimulation (eg, interaction with certain tumors, virus-infected cells, bacterial products, lymphokines, or immunoglobulin complexes), NK cells secrete several cytokines, including gamma interferon, TNF, serine esterases, GM-CSF. These cytokines can influence the function of other mature lymphocytes and monocytes in peripheral lymphoid tissues and affect the development of immature hematopoietic cells in bone marrow. They can either augment or suppress the function and development of these cell types, depending on the circumstances.

II. MONOCYTES & MACROPHAGES

DIFFERENTIATION & PHENOTYPE

Monocytes and macrophages develop from immature hematopoietic progenitor cells in the bone marrow. These progenitor cells can give rise to erythrocytes, granulocytes, megakaryocytes, or monocytes, depending upon the signals provided by CSF or certain interleukins.

The monocyte progenitor is the monoblast, which develops into a promonocyte and then a monocyte in the bone marrow. Mature monocytes enter the circulation, and a proportion exit from the blood and develop into resident macrophages in the spleen, lymph nodes, liver, lung, thymus, peritoneum, nervous system, skin, and other tissues.

MONOCYTE IDENTIFICATION

Monocytes and macrophages can be identified by morphology, expression of certain cell surface differentiation antigens, and the presence of characteristic enzymes in the cytoplasm. Human monocytes and macrophages express class II MHC antigens (HLA-DR, -DP, and -DQ), gamma interferon receptor, aminopeptidase N (CD13), receptors for complement components (complement receptor types 1 [CD35], 3 [CD11b], and 4 [CD11c]), and receptors for the Fc region of IgG (IgG-Fc receptor types I (CD64) and II (CD32)). Mature monocytes express high levels of a relatively monocyte-specific antigen, CD14; however, expression of this antigen is lost when the monocytes differentiate into macrophages. Histocytochemical studies have shown that monocytes and macrophages possess nonspecific esterases, lysozyme, alkaline phosphodiesterase, and peroxidase and that the amount and intracellular localization of these substances change during monocyte-macrophage differentiation and activation.

FUNCTION OF MONOCYTES & MACROPHAGES

The term "macrophage" originated from the observation that these cells engulf and ingest for-

eign matter, a process designated **phagocytosis** (ingestion of small soluble substances is called **pinocytosis**). A major role of monocytes and macrophages in an inflammatory response is to eliminate bacteria and other pathogens by this process (see Chapters 11 and 12).

IMMUNE RESPONSES & MONOCYTES

Monocytes and macrophages can serve as APC for T lymphocytes by ingesting and degrading foreign antigen in phagolysosomes into peptides that bind to MHC glycoproteins for presentation on the cell surface. Because human monocytes and macrophages express both class I (HLA-A, -B, and -C) and class II (HLA-DR, -DP, and -DQ) MHC glycoproteins, they are able to present antigen to CD8 and CD4 T lymphocytes, respectively. Activated lymphocytes, in turn, secrete factors that affect monocyte and macrophage function and differentiation.

Monocyte and macrophage development is affected by the secretion of cytokines (CSF), lymphokines (IL-2, IL-3, and IL-4), and interferons by activated T lymphocytes. For example, gamma interferon produced by activated T cells stimulates and increases the amount of MHC glycoproteins on monocytes and macrophages, allowing for more efficient antigen presentation.

Cytokines produced by monocytes and macrophages similarly affect the response of lymphocytes. Prostaglandin E, for example, inhibits lymphocyte function and proliferation, whereas IL-1 acts as a potent cosignal with antigen for activation and proliferation of T lymphocytes. Thus, monocytes and macrophages are of central importance in initiation and regulation of immune responses, as well as being major sources of secretory proteins for many tissues and organs.

SUMMARY

The immune system contains several cell types, including lymphocytes, mononuclear phagocytes (monocytes, macrophages), and granulocytes. These cells mediate distinct immune functions and secrete a great variety of soluble substances that regulate the immune system as well as inflammation and functions in other tissues and organs.

Three distinct types of lymphocytes exist: T cells, B cells, and NK cells. T and B cells can recognize more than 10^{11} different antigens by using their membrane glycoprotein receptors, the T cell antigen receptor and immunoglobulin, respectively. These receptors are generated by somatic recombination of genetic elements during T and B cell development in the thymus and bone marrow, respectively.

Immunoglobulin on B cells directly binds many types of antigens, including proteins, carbohydrates, lipids, and small quantities of chemicals. In contrast, T cell antigen receptors bind only peptide antigens that are bound to class I or II MHC molecules or APC. Binding of antigen receptors of either B or T cells results in activation and proliferation and in the release of soluble factors that inhibit or augment other aspects of the immune response.

Subsets of T cells interact with antigen bound to either class I (HLA-A, -B, and -C) or class II (HLA-DR, -DP, and -DQ) MHC structures. CD8 T cells usually react with peptide class I MHC complexes and are principally mediators of cellular cytotoxicity or killing. CD4 T cells react with peptide-class II MHC complexes and are the predominant mediators of lymphokine secretion, which augments or suppresses the response of other lymphocytes.

An important and probably unique feature of B and T lymphocytes is immunologic memory, whereby they remember prior exposure to antigen and respond rapidly after reexposure to the same antigen.

The third type of lymphocyte, the NK cell, does not have immunologic memory and does not express an antigen receptor resulting from gene rearrangement. NK cells recognize and kill virus-infected cells and certain tumors by an unknown process. Unlike T lymphocytes, NK cells do not require the presence of MHC glycoproteins on the target to recognize and kill a virus-infected cell or tumor.

Lymphocytes and mononuclear phagocytes act in concert to respond rapidly to eliminate the foreign antigen and then to regulate the response after the antigen has been eliminated.

REFERENCES

Lymphocytes

Allison JP, Lanier LL: Structure, function, and serology of the T-cell antigen receptor complex. *Annu Rev Immunol* 1987;**5**:503.

Clevers H et al: The T cell receptor/CD3 complex: a dynamic protein ensemble. *Annu Rev Immunol* 1988;**6**:629.

Kishimoto T, Hirano T: Molecular regulation of B lymphocyte response. *Annu Rev Immunol* 1988;**6**:485.

McMichael AJ et al (editors): *Leucocyte Typing IV.* Oxford Univ Press, 1989.

Miyajima A et al: Coordinate regulation of immune and inflammatory responses by T cell-derived lymphokines. *FASEB J* 1988;**2**:2462.

Sanders ME, Makgoba MW, Shaw S: Human naive and memory T cells: reinterpretation of helper-inducer and suppressor-inducer subsets. *Immunol Today* 1988;**9**:195.

Trinchieri G: Biology of natural killer cells. *Adv Immunol* 1989;**47**:187.

Monocytes & Macrophages

Clark SC, Kamen R: The human hematopoietic colony-stimulating factors. *Science* 1987;**236**:1229.

Hamilton TA, Adams DO: Molecular mechanisms of signal transduction in macrophages. *Immunol Today* 1987;**8**:151.

Werb Z et al: Secreted proteins of resting and activated macrophages. In: *Handbook of Experimental Immunology,* 4th ed. Vol 2. Weir DM et al (editors). Blackwell, 1986.

The T Cell Receptor 6

Joan Goverman, PhD and Jane R. Parnes, MD

T and B lymphocytes are responsible for the ability to recognize an invasion of foreign materials or antigens in the body. These cells are capable of recognizing an almost limitless variety of foreign cells and substances and, at the same time, exhibiting exquisite specificity. For example, a person immunized against smallpox can resist infection by smallpox but not by other viruses. T cells are specially suited for dealing with infections within the cells of the host; in contrast, B cells recognize free or soluble antigen through cell surface–bound immunoglobulin with no requirement except antigen-receptor complementarity. To carry out this function, T cells have unique properties for antigen recognition.

T cells recognize antigen only when it is presented on the cell surface of an antigen-presenting cell (APC), where it must be associated with polymorphic cell surface polypeptides encoded within the major histocompatibility complex (MHC). The requirement for simultaneous recognition of MHC molecules with antigen provides a mechanism for ensuring that T cells come into action only when they touch another cell. This is important because T cells regulate or kill other cells through cell-to-cell contacts, unlike B cells, whose secreted antibodies act at a distance. T cells are said to be self-MHC-restricted because they recognize antigen only when it is associated with self as opposed to nonself MHC proteins. The actual ligand of the T cell receptor (TCR) is composed of a small fragment of a foreign antigen complexed to some of the polymorphic residues within an MHC molecule (Fig 6–1). The receptor appears to contact portions of both the antigen peptide fragment and the MHC. The TCR is assisted in binding its ligand by accessory molecules, CD4 or CD8, which are expressed on the T cell surface and also bind MHC molecules. However, these accessory molecules appear to bind to a nonpolymorphic region of the MHC molecule, whereas the TCR interacts with both polymorphic residues of MHC proteins and antigenic determinants. Thus, TCRs exhibit a tremendous amount of di-

versity to correspond to the wide array of antigens encountered in the life span of the host. The molecular structure of the TCR and the mechanisms used in generating diversity are the subject of this chapter. Correlations of TCR genes with particular diseases and approaches toward treating these diseases through immunotherapy are briefly discussed.

STRUCTURE & DIVERSITY OF THE T CELL RECEPTOR

The TCR is a disulfide-linked heterodimer composed of α and β glycoprotein chains (MW 40,000–50,000). Both chains are composed of 2 domains: the amino-terminal portion consists of a region of variable amino acid sequence (V region) and the carboxy-terminal portion consists of a region of constant amino acid sequence (C region) (Fig 6–2). The region domains associate with each other to form an antigen-binding "pocket," whereas the C region domains anchor the receptor to the T cell membrane and presumably participate in initiating the effector function of the cell. The TCR is noncovalently associated on the cell surface with CD3, a complex of at least 5 polypeptides that may participate in mediating activation signals. CD3 is functionally important because it is required for the expression of the TCR on the cell surface. T cells, in fact, can be activated directly by antibodies specific for the CD3 complex.

Like immunoglobulin genes, the genes that encode the TCR α and β chains are formed from the joining together of separate genetic elements. The sequence encoding the V region of the α chain is formed from a V and a J (joining) gene segment, whereas that encoding the V region of the β chain is formed from a V, a D (diversity), and a J gene segment (Fig 6–3). These gene segments rearrange during T cell ontogeny within the thymus by deletion of intervening DNA to form a contiguous V gene. As with immunoglobulin gene rearrangement, this process is dependent upon the presence

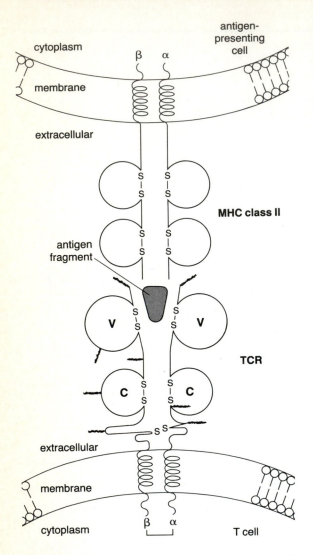

Figure 6–1. Complex of antigen fragment and class II MHC molecule forming the ligand of the TCR. See the legend to Fig 6–2 for an explanation of structural details of the TCR.

but closely linked clusters, in each of which the C region gene is preceded by a series of J segments and one D segment (Fig 6–3). The number of possible $V_\alpha J_\alpha$ and $V_\beta D_\beta J_\beta$ combinations therefore provides for the enormous diversity generated by the rearrangement process. In addition, there are 2 mechanisms directly linked to rearrangement that generate even more diversity. First, the endpoints of the rearranging gene segments are flexible, causing variation in the amino acid sequence between the joining gene segments. Second, nucleotides can be either deleted or added randomly (N region diversity) at the junctions of rearranging gene segments. These mechanisms, together with the random pairing of α and β chains, account for much of the diversity potential of the TCR repertoire. In contrast to immunoglobulin genes, TCR genes do not appear to diversify by means of somatic mutation of the rearranged genes.

Determination of the molecular structure of the TCR has yielded several insights into the nature of the dual specificity for antigen and MHC. Extensive analysis of T cells with defined specificity has shown that there is no absolute correlation between V gene usage and recognition of either antigen or MHC determinants. Thus, the TCR is not composed of separate binding sites for antigen and MHC but, rather, appears to recognize its ligand as a single antigenic complex, much like an antibody. The phenomenon of self MHC restriction is most probably a result of developmental influences of the thymus during T cell ontogeny rather than of germline-encoded, unique structural properties of the receptor.

A second receptor present on the surface of early thymocytes and a small subset of peripheral T cells has been characterized. It is also a disulfide-linked heterodimer composed of a γ and δ chain. These chains also consist of V and C regions and are encoded by rearranging gene segments. The diversity potential of the γ/δ receptor appears to be limited relative to that of the α/β receptor. The function of cells expressing the γ/δ receptor and the ligand for the receptor are unknown, although many demonstrate non-MHC-restricted killing of target cells.

When an α/β-TCR on a CD4 lymphocyte binds to its specific peptide antigen-class II MHC molecule combination on an APC, a trimolecular complex is formed that transmits a signal to the CD4 lymphocyte. The signal initiates a series of biochemical reactions within the cell, resulting in subsequent biologic responses (Fig 6–4). The critical biochemical events are (1) hydrolysis of phosphatidylinositol biphosphate to form inositol triphosphate and diacylglycerol, (2) influx of Ca^{2+} into the cell cytoplasm, and (3) activation of protein kinase C. Ca^{2+} and protein kinase C act as second messengers, probably in conjunction with other

of specific DNA sequences adjacent to the rearranging gene segments. Sequences encoding the V region are joined to those encoding the C region after transcription by means of mRNA splicing. The rearrangement of gene segments to form the TCR gene allows for the generation of the enormous diversity of receptors. There are at least 50 V_α gene segments and an estimated 100 or more J_α gene segments for encoding of the α chain. Similarly, for the β chain there are at least 60 V gene segments, two D gene segments, and 13 J gene segments. There are also 2 closely related C region genes for β, and these are located in 2 separate

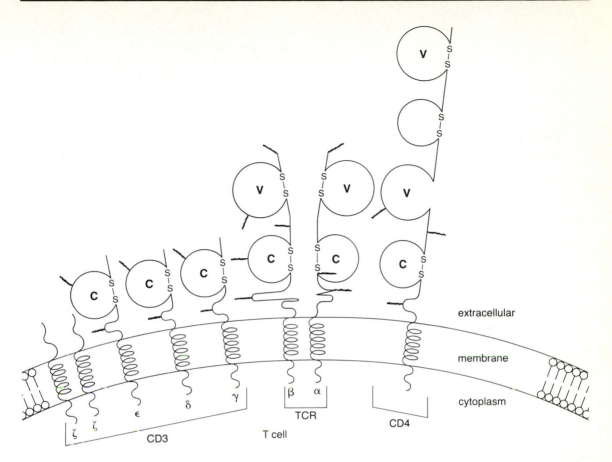

Figure 6-2. Structure of TCR α and β polypeptides. The variable (V) and constant (C) domains and positions of disulfide bonds (SS) are shown. The sites of N-linked glycosylation are marked (〰〰). The transmembrane region is shown (ⵣⵣⵣⵣ) traversing the plasma membrane. The polypeptide chains of the adjacent CD3 and CD4 molecules are also shown.

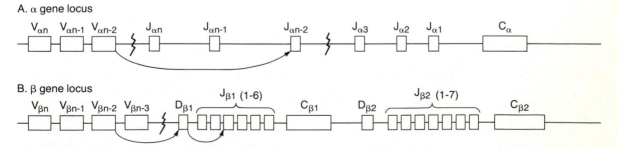

Figure 6-3. Organization of the TCR genes. **A:** α chain gene organization. Only a few of the multiple V and J gene segments are shown. The arrow indicates one potential rearrangement between a V and a J segment. **B:** β chain gene organization. A few of the multiple V gene segments are shown. All D and J gene segments are indicated. One potential rearrangement is illustrated. The $D_{\beta1}$ gene segment could also rearrange to a J in the $J_{\beta2}$ gene cluster. In both panels the jagged lines indicate separation of the DNA on either side by very large distances.

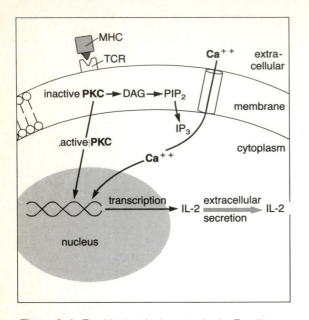

Figure 6-4. The biochemical events in the T cell membrane and cytoplasm initiated by activation of the TCR by the antigen fragment-class II MHC complex. See the text for further explanation. PKC, Protein kinase C; DAG, diacylglycerol; PIP_2, phosphatidylinositol biphosphate; IP_3, inositol triphosphate.

receptor-generated signals not yet identified, to induce the transcription of the interleukin-2 (IL-2) gene. Production of IL-2 by the lymphocyte and its secretion results in clonal proliferation of the CD4 lymphocyte.

THE T CELL RECEPTOR & DISEASE

The specific somatic recombinational events that T cells undergo during ontogeny lead to corresponding specific rearrangement patterns on Southern blots of T cell genomic DNA. These patterns have been used to determine the cell type of origin of certain cancers, to determine whether a variety of T cell neoplastic disorders are clonal or polyclonal in origin, and, combined with analysis of cell surface markers, to determine the developmental stage of neoplastic T cells. The specificity of these rearrangements within T cell leukemias, coupled with new technologies for amplifying specific DNA sequences, potentially could provide a means of determining the presence or absence of small numbers of residual leukemic cells after therapy and of monitoring the duration of remissions. However, the fidelity of this approach to diagnosis needs further study (See Chapter 48).

In addition to the presence of clonal TCR gene rearrangements in T cell leukemias, specific chromosomal translocations and inversions have been observed with high frequency in such disorders. In particular, inversions and translocations involving chromosome 14 band q11 are particularly common in the malignant cells in T cell leukemias and have also been seen in T cell clones from patients with ataxia-telangiectasia (who often develop T cell chronic lymphocytic leukemia associated with such chromosomal abnormalities). The region involved in these chromosomal rearrangements contains the TCR α chain gene, and the breakpoints have been found to occur within the α chain J region, presumably because of mistakes in the normal process of TCR gene rearrangement. The other breakpoint in many of these translocations or inversions involves the sequence downstream of the immunoglobulin heavy chain locus on chromosome 14 band q32. It is possible that the latter sequence is responsible for tumorigenesis. Reciprocal translocations involving the human TCR β chain locus on chromosome 7 band q34 have also been found, although with lower frequency, in a variety of T cell leukemias or lymphomas and appear to be specific for this type of neoplasia. The mechanisms by which these gross chromosomal rearrangements involving TCR genes leads to neoplastic growth are not known.

The possible role of the TCR in autoimmune disorders has recently been the subject of intense investigation because of the potential for monoclonal antibody therapy. If specific TCR V region (or perhaps D or J segment) expression can be shown to correlate with specific autoimmune diseases, either in a population with such a disorder or within a given individual, treatment of the disease with monoclonal antibodies specific for the particular TCR (or TCR element) might be possible. The most promising evidence for the role of specific TCRs in a human autoimmune disease occurs in rheumatoid arthritis, in which particular TCR β chain rearrangements predominate in T cells cultured from the synovia of individuals with advanced disease. The specific rearrangements seen in these cultured cells differ from one individual to another. If these β chain genes play an important role in the pathogenesis of the destructive joint changes of rheumatoid arthritis, therapy directed against the specific β chain proteins would have to be individualized for each patient depending upon the particular V gene segment(s) involved. This type of therapy has already been used successfully to prevent and cure experimental allergic encephalomyelitis, a T cell autoimmune disease in mice that is the experimental model of multiple sclerosis in humans. Application of such therapy to human autoimmune disorders is an exciting possibility for the future.

SUMMARY

The TCR is a 2-chain molecule that recognizes foreign antigens bound to self MHC proteins. This dual specificity focuses the attention of T cells on cell-bound antigens. The specificity and diversity of the TCR arises from the large number of germline V gene segments that undergo somatic recombination during T cell development to form a complete TCR gene. Not only has the recent explosion of knowledge about the TCR contributed to our knowledge of T cell function, but it has also provided diagnostic tools for T cell neoplastic diseases and the potential for specific immunotherapy of autoimmune disorders.

REFERENCES

General

Allison JP, Lanier LL: Structure, function, and serology of the T-cell antigen receptor complex. *Annu Rev Immunol* 1987;**5**:503.

Wilson RK et al: Structure, organization and polymorphism of murine and human T-cell receptor α and β chain gene families. *Immunol Rev* 1988; **101**:149.

Structure & Diversity of the TCR

Concannon P et al: Diversity and structure of human T-cell receptor β-chain variable region genes. *Proc Natl Acad Sci USA* 1986;**83**:6598.

Tillinghast J, Behlke M, Loh D: Structure and diversity of the human T-cell receptor β-chain variable region genes. *Science* 1986;**233**:879.

Toyonaga B et al: Organization and sequences of the diversity, joining, and constant region genes of the human T-cell receptor β chain. *Proc Natl Acad Sci USA* 1985;**82**:8624.

Yoshikai Y et al: Organization and sequences of the variable, joining, and constant region genes of the human T-cell receptor α chain. *Nature* 1985; **316**:837.

The TCR & Disease

Acha-Orbea H et al: Limited heterogeneity of T cell receptors from lymphocytes mediating autoimmune encephalomyelitis allows specific immune intervention. *Cell* 1988;**54**:263.

Baer R et al: The breakpoint of an inversion of chromosome 14 in a T-cell leukemia: sequences downstream of the immunoglobulin heavy chain locus are implicated in tumorigenesis. *Proc Natl Acad Sci USA* 1987;**84**:9069.

Smith SD et al: Clinical and biologic characterization of T-cell neoplasias with rearrangements of chromosome 7 band q34. *Blood* 1988;**71**:395.

Stamenkovic I et al: Clonal dominance among T-lymphocyte infiltrates in arthritis. *Proc Natl Acad Sci USA* 1988;**85**:1179.

Waldmann TA: The arrangement of immunoglobulin and T cell receptor genes in human lymphoproliferative disorders. *Adv Immunol* 1987;**40**:247.

7

Cytokines

Joost J. Oppenheim, MD, Francis W. Ruscetti, PhD, & Connie Faltynek, PhD

Over the past 25 years, an important group of peptide mediators has been detected, characterized, and purified. These mediators, termed **cytokines,** function as up- and down-regulators of immunologic, inflammatory, and reparative host responses to injury. Many of these hormone-like polypeptides are secreted in the course of immunologic and inflammatory responses. Cytokines produced by lymphocytes are called **lymphokines,** whereas the peptides produced by monocytes or macrophages are called **monokines.** Cytokines function as intercellular signals that regulate local and, at times, systemic inflammatory responses. Cytokines are distinct from endocrine hormones since they are produced by a number of cells rather than by specialized glands. Cytokines are not usually present in serum and generally act in a paracrine (ie, locally near the producing cells) or autocrine (ie, directly on the producing cells) rather than in an endocrine manner on distant target cells. Cytokines modulate reactions of the host to foreign antigens or injurious agents by regulating the growth, mobility, and differentiation of leukocytes and other cells.

Although some transformed lymphocyte, macrophage, keratinocyte, and fibroblast cell lines spontaneously secrete cytokines into the culture medium, normal resting cells and most cell lines must be stimulated to produce cytokines. T or B lymphocytes obtained from immunized donors can be specifically activated by antigens to produce lymphokines. Many cytokines are simultaneously produced by activated cells and are difficult to isolate from one another. Now that many of the genes encoding the cytokines have been cloned, it is clear that there are multiple dissimilar and genetically unrelated cytokines.

Cytokines generally are synthesized and secreted peptides or glycoproteins with molecular weights (MW) ranging from 6000 to 60,000. They are extremely potent compounds that act at concentrations of 10^{-10}–10^{-15}mol/L to stimulate target cell functions following specific ligand-receptor interactions. This high specific activity has facilitated cytokine detection by bioassays, but the small quantities produced have impeded their purification. Nevertheless, characterization of cytokines has progressed at a phenomenal rate because of recent technologic developments: (1) the use of cell clones that produce large amounts of limited numbers of cytokines; (2) the development of high-performance liquid chromatography (HPLC) techniques; (3) the availability of monoclonal antibodies for neutralization and detection; (4) immunoaffinity purification; and, especially, (5) the use of gene cloning techniques.

A single purified cytokine can have multiple effects on the growth and differentiation of many cell types. Consequently, cytokines may exhibit considerable overlap in their biologic effects on lymphoid, myeloid, and connective tissue target cells. In addition, biologically distinct cytokines may have similar effects by initiating the production of a cascade of identical cytokines or of one another.

This chapter will focus on a discussion of the more pivotal cytokines that amplify the afferent and efferent limbs of the immune and inflammatory responses: IL-1 to IL-8, tumor necrosis factor (TNF), interferons (IFN), colony-stimulating factors (CSF), and other growth and chemotactic factors (Table 7–1).

INTERLEUKIN-1 (IL-1)

IL-1 consists of 2 distinct peptides that have a multiplicity of immunologic, inflammatory, and reparative activities. These include effects on lymphoid and nonlymphoid cells (Fig 7–1). In 1972, a **lymphocyte-activating factor (LAF),** which was mitogenic for murine thymocytes, was discovered in the supernatant of cultures of adherent human peripheral blood cells and murine splenocytes. Human LAF was also *comitogenic* in that it synergistically enhanced the proliferative

Table 7–1. Characteristic properties of cytokines.

Cytokine	MW	Principal Cell Sources	Primary Type of Activity	Preeminent Effects
IL-1	17,500	Macrophages and others (see Table 7–2)	Immunoaugmentation.	Inflammatory and hemato-poietic
IL-2	15,500	T lymphocytes and LGL	T and B cell growth factor.	Activates T and NK cells
IL-3	14,000–28,000	T lymphocytes	Hematopoietic growth factor.	Promotes growth of early mye-loid progenitor cells
IL-4	20,000	TH cells	T and B cell growth factor; promotes IgE reactions.	Promotes IgE switch and mast cell growth
IL-5	18,000	TH cells	Stimulates B cells and eosinophils	Promotes IgA switch and eo-sinophilia
IL-6	22,000–30,000	Fibroblasts and others	Hybridoma growth fac-tor; augments inflam-mation.	Growth factor for B cells and polyclonal immunoglobulin production
IL-7	25,000	Stromal cells	Lymphopoietin.	Generates pre-B and pre-T cells and is lymphocyte growth factor
IL-8	8,800	Macrophages and others	Chemoattracts neutro-phils and T lympho-cytes.	Regulates lymphocyte homing and neutrophil infiltration
G-CSF	18,000–22,000	Monocytes and others	Myeloid growth factor.	Generates neutrophils
M-CSF	18,000–26,000	Monocytes and others	Macrophage growth factor.	Generates macrophages
GM-CSF	14,000–38,000	T cells and others	Monomyelocytic growth factor.	Myelopoiesis
IFN α IFN β IFN γ	18,000–20,000 25,000 20,000–25,000	Leukocytes Fibroblasts T lymphocytes and NK cells	Antiviral, antiprolifera-tive, and immunomo-dulating.	Stimulates macrophages and NK cells Induce cell membrane anti-gens (eg, MHC)
TNFα LT = TNFβ	17,000 18,000	Macrophages and others T lymphocytes	Inflammatory, immu-noenhancing, and tu-moricidal.	Vascular thromboses and tu-mor necrosis
TGFβ	25,000	Platelets, bone, and others	Fibroplasia and immu-nosuppression.	Wound healing and bone re-modeling

response of murine thymocytes to lectins such as concanavalin A (Con A) or phytohemagglutinin (PHA).

In 1974, it was reported that cultured human monocytes also secreted a **B cell–activating factor (BAF)** that stimulated antibody production by T cell-depleted murine splenocytes. Subsequent analyses revealed that the biochemical properties of LAF and BAF were similar and that they also resembled the structure of pyrogenic macrophage-derived factors called **endogenous pyrogens.** In 1979, these factors were all renamed interleukin-1 (IL-1). IL-1 is detected by bioassays of its comito-genic effect on thymocytes, IL-1-reactive cell lines, or, more recently, by enzyme-linked immu-nosorbent assay (ELISA).

IL-1 Producers & Inducers

IL-1 is produced by 11 types of macrophages, irrespective of their tissue of origin, as well as by keratinocytes, dendritic cells, astrocytes, micro-glial cells, normal B lymphocytes, cultured T cell clones, fibroblasts, neutrophils, endothelial cells, and smooth muscle cells. However, IL-1-like fac-tors are produced by virtually all nucleated cell types. Although a number of cell lines produce low levels of IL-1 constitutively, most normal cells must be stimulated by a variety of agents to pro-

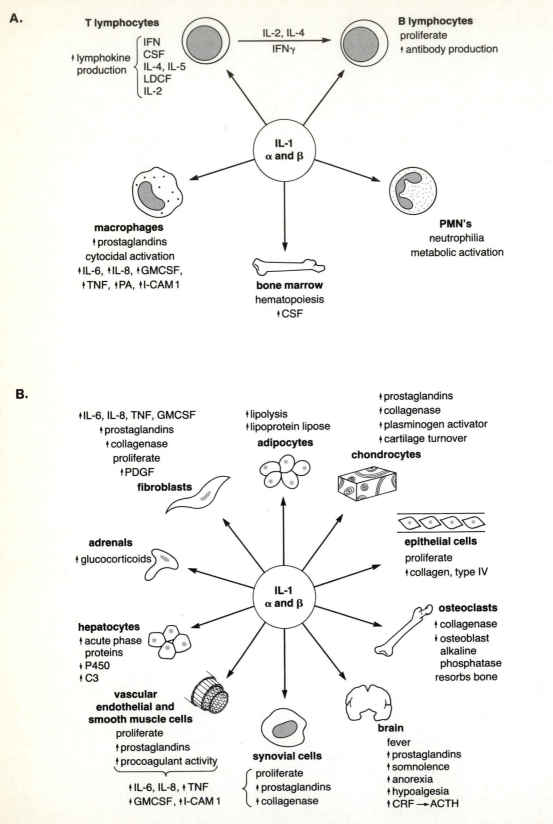

Figure 7–1. A: Actions of IL-1 on hematopoietic and lymphoid tissues. **B:** Actions of IL-1 on nonlymphoid tissues.

duce IL-1. IL-1 production by these cells is stimulated by diverse agents, including adjuvants such as lipopolysaccharide (LPS) and muramyl dipeptide (MDP), injurious ultraviolet irradiation, urate or silicate particles, aluminum hydroxide, and microorganisms. Agents that activate lymphocytes can stimulate macrophages to produce IL-1 either by direct contact between the cells, which is genetically controlled by class II major histocompatibility complex (MHC) molecules (see Chapter 4), or by producing lymphokines such as TNF, CSF, or IFN γ which stimulate macrophages.

The nature of the stimulant determines whether IL-1 accumulates predominantly at intracellular sites or is released into the extracellular environment. Latex particles, LPS, and zymosan, for example, stimulate increases in both the intracellular and extracellular levels of IL-1, whereas silica particles and phorbol myristate acetate (PMA) predominantly stimulate the extracellular release of IL-1. The intrinsic cellular factors that regulate the release of IL-1 are unidentified, but cell injury appears to be one cause.

IL-1 is found in some tissues in the absence of noxious stimuli. For example, amniotic fluid and urine contain significant levels of IL-1, and IL-1β. mRNA expression and production occur in the skin and adult brain. At the time of the luteal phase of the menstrual cycle and during strenuous exercise, IL-1 levels are elevated in human plasma.

Specific antagonists of IL-1 production are of considerable therapeutic interest because IL-1 is implicated in chronic inflammatory diseases. Corticosteroids, already in wide use as anti-inflammatory agents, inhibit IL-1 production by macrophages. Prostaglandins, which are themselves mediators of inflammation, appear to inhibit the release of IL-1 from macrophages. Thus, prostaglandin E_2 (PGE$_2$), for example, a product of the cyclooxygenase pathway, exerts a negative effect on IL-1 production. Conversely, inhibitors of the lipoxygenase pathway reduce the amount of IL-1 released, and leukotrienes appear to stimulate IL-1 production (see Chapter 13).

Structure-Function Studies of IL-1

IL-1 exists in 2 molecular forms called IL-1α and IL-1β. Two distinct IL-1 genes coding for IL-1α and IL-1β have been identified in all species to date (Table 7-2). Human IL-1α and IL-1β, which exhibit 45% homology at the nucleotide level and only 26% homology at the amino acid level, are antigenically distinct. Despite this, the potency and activities of IL-1α and IL-1β are virtually identical, and they bind with equal affinity to the same cell surface receptors. Many cell types express both IL-1 genes, but ratios of IL-1α to IL-1β can vary widely; eg, human monocytes produce predominantly IL-1β, whereas keratinocytes produce largely IL-1α.

IL-1α and IL-1β are initially translated as propeptides (MW 31,000) that are enzymatically processed to yield a soluble form (MW 17,000) at

Table 7-2. Properties of human inflammatory cytokines.

Property	IL-1	TNF
Chromosome	2	6
Proform	271 amino acids (IL-1α), 269 amino acids (IL-1β)	236 amino acids (TNFα), 204 amino acids (TNFβ)
Mature form	159 amino acids (IL-1α), 153 amino acids (IL-1β)	157 amino acids (TNFα), 171 amino acids (TFNβ)
Cell sources	Macrophages, keratinocytes, endothelial cells, fibroblasts, astrocytes, B and T cells	Macrophages, T and B lymphocytes, Keratinocytes, Fibroblasts, endothelial cells, astrocytes (TNFα); T lymphocytes (T$_H$1 subset), EBV B cell lines (TNFβ)
Receptor	60–80-kDa glycoprotein $K_d = 10^{-10}$ mol/L 50–5000 sites/cell	80-kDa glycoprotein $K_d = 10^{-10}$ mol/L 1000–10,000 sites/cell
In vivo effects	Local neutrophilic infiltration Delayed-type hypersensitivity Fibroplasia and angiogenesis Endogenous pyrogen Acute-phase reactants Neutrophilia Radioprotection Adjuvant and antimicrobial agent	Local neutrophilic infiltration Schwartzman reaction and necrosis of tumors Endogenous pyrogen Acute-phase reactants Cachexia, neutrophilia Radioprotection Adjuvant Angiogenesis

or beyond the outer cell membrane, which then acts extracellularly. Biologically active IL-1α, but not IL-1β, has been detected on the surface of cells and can thus participate in interactions during cell-to-cell contact.

Receptors for IL-1

IL-1 acts on target cells via high-affinity receptors on the plasma membrane. The numbers of such receptors vary from about 100 on T cells to a few thousand on fibroblasts, but the affinity is relatively constant ($K_d = 10^{-10}$ mol/L), suggesting that most cell types have a common IL-1 receptor. The extracellular piece of the IL-1 receptor belongs to the immunoglobulin gene superfamily. There are a 21-amino-acid transmembrane region and a 217-amino-acid cytoplasmic tail. Expression of IL-1 receptors on the cell surface is down-regulated by internalization following binding of IL-1. In contrast, both glucocorticoids and prostaglandins increase the expression of functional IL-1 receptors on some human cell types, eg, fibroblasts and B cells, but not on T cells, monocytes, or neutrophils. The critical intracellular events following binding of IL-1 to its receptor are still unidentified, although elevated levels of diacylglycerol, cyclic AMP (cAMP), G proteins, and ornithine decarboxylase have been detected in some cell types.

Inhibitors of Activities of IL-1

IL-1 activity can be regulated by endogenous factors that affect cytokine production by modulating either receptor expression or signal transduction after receptors are triggered. Potent nonspecific antagonism to the actions of IL-1 is attributed to transforming growth factor β (TGFβ), corticosteroids, and α melanocyte-stimulating hormone (αMSH). An inhibitory factor in urine of myelogenous leukemia patients specifically competes with IL-1 binding to receptors for IL-1. Pharmacologic inhibition of IL-1 activity (eg, by corticosteroids) may be useful in controlling some inflammatory reactions.

Immunologic & Inflammatory Effects of IL-1 & TNF

TNF also consists of 2 distinct peptides with multiple immunologic and local as well as systemic inflammatory activities. These also include effects on lymphoid and nonlymphoid cells (Fig 7–2). TNFα was first described as an activity in serum that induces hemorrhagic necrosis in certain tumors in vivo and was later independently discovered as **cachectin,** a circulating mediator of wasting during parasitic disease. TNFα is produced by activated macrophages and other cells and has a broad spectrum of biologic actions on many immune and nonimmune target cells. **Lym-**

photoxin, which is primarily a product of T lymphocytes, has also been called TNFβ. TNFα and TNFβ bind to the same receptor on target cells and consequently have the same biologic activities.

TNFα & TNFβ Genes & Their Products

The gene for human TNFα is located within or near the MHC genes on the short arm of chromosome 6, closely linked to the gene for TNFβ (Table 7–2). The degree of homology between TNFα and TNFβ is 46% at the nucleotide level and 28% at the amino acid level. The precursor form of TNFα consists of 236 amino acids. Prior to or during secretion, 79 N-terminal amino acids are enzymatically removed from the pro form to yield the MW-17,400 soluble mature TNFα. Although TNFα and the MW-20,000 TNFβ do not cross-react immunologically, they bind equally well to the same receptors. Since tumor cell killing by formaldehyde-fixed and activated macrophages can be blocked by monoclonal antibodies to TNFα, an active membrane-associated form of TNFα has been proposed.

TNF Inducers & Producers

Many cell types can produce TNFα. Monocyte-macrophages produce TNFα in response to PMA, LPS, Sendai virus, MDP, tumor cells, mycoplasmas, or BCG (bacilla Calmette-Guérin) (Table 7–2). Lymphocytes can be stimulated by antigens or mitogens to produce TNFβ, but lymphocytes and natural killer (NK) cells can also produce some TNFα. A number of endogenous mediators are also active inducers of TNF; these include IL-3 (for mast cells), IL-1, TNF itself, GM-CSF, CSF-1, leukotriene B$_4$ (LTB$_4$), platelet-activating factor (PAF), and IFN γ in conjunction with LPS (for macrophages) (see Table 7–1 for abbreviations).

Receptors for TNF

Between 1000 and 10,000 high-affinity receptors for TNF per cell have been observed on various cells (K_d is approximately 2×10^{-10}–6×10^{-10} mol/L). Cross-linking studies revealed TNF-binding structures of MW 60,000–80,000 on human cells. The action of TNF is considerably augmented by IFN γ on several target cell types, at least in part by increasing TNF receptor expression. The intracellular effects of TNF are still largely unknown.

Immunologic Activities of IL-1 & TNF

The multifaceted effects of the major "broad-spectrum" inflammatory mediators, namely IL-1 and TNF, can be reviewed together. Although the high-affinity receptors for IL-1 and TNF, which

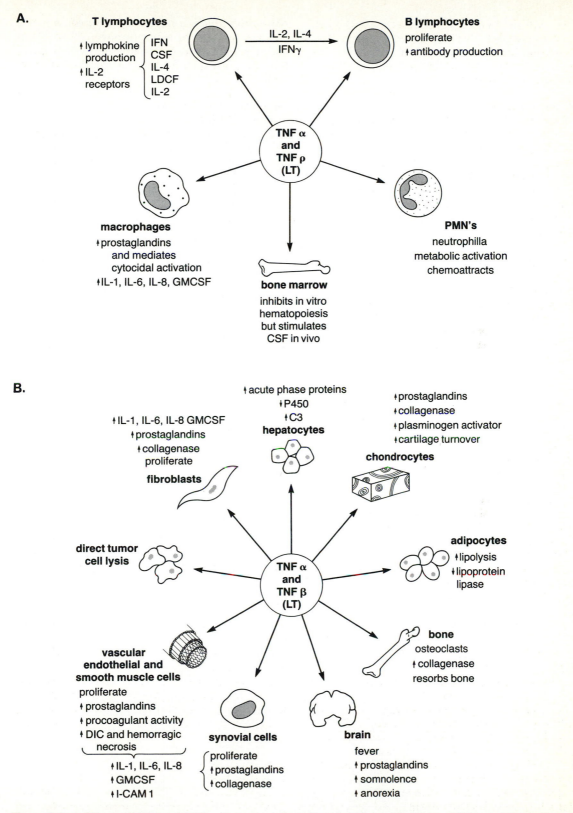

Figure 7-2. *A:* Effects of TNFα and β (LT) on hematopoietic and lymphoid tissues. *B:* Effects of TNFα and β on nonlymphoid tissues.

have been detected on virtually all nucleated cell types, are structurally completely unrelated, these 2 cytokines show a remarkably high degree of overlap in their in vitro immunologic and nonimmunologic activities (Table 7–3). Although the in vivo effects of IL-1 and TNF also exhibit some similarities, TNF has more in vivo toxic, vascular occlusive, and antitumor effects, whereas IL-1 is more protective against lethal mediation and is a greater mobilizer of bone turnover (Table 7–3). Differences in the rate and site of in vivo production, as well as half-life and distribution, may account for the differences in these in vivo effects.

IL-1 augments immunologically mediated inflammatory reactions. It promotes the proliferation of T lymphocytes by enhancing the produc-

Table 7–3. Comparison of target cells and actions of IL-1 and TNF/LT.

Target Cells or Tissues	Effects	IL-1α, β	TNF/LT
T lymphocytes	Enhance IL-2 receptor expression	+	+
	Induce lymphokine production	+ +	+
	Act as thymocyte comitogen	+ +	+
B lymphocytes	Enhance antibody production	+	+
	Promote B cell proliferation	+	+
Neuroendocrine cells	Release CRF to Pituitary ACTH adrenal cortico-steroids	+	−
	Induce prostaglandin-mediated fever	+	+
	Induce somnolence and anorexia	+	+
Neutrophils	Act as chemoattractants	−	+
	Increase adhesiveness, phagocytosis, ADCC, oxygen intermediates	−	±
	Cause degranulation and enzyme release		
Monocytes and macrophages	Act as chemoattractant	−	±
	Induce prostaglandins, IL-1, IL-6, GM-CSF, and IL-8	+	+
	Coactivate to cytocidal state	+	+ +
Endothelial cells and vascular smooth muscle	Increase adhesiveness (I-CAM1)	+	+ +
	Induce procoagulant activity, IL-1, IL-6, GMC-SF, plasminogen activator inhibitor, prostaglandins, and MHC	+	+ +
	Act as mitogenic and angiogenic agents	+	+ +
Osteoblasts	Decrease alkaline phosphate levels	+ +	+
Osteoclasts	Cause bone resorption (increase collagenase)	+	+
Chondrocytes	Increase cartilage turnover	+	+
Fibroblasts/synovial cells	Act as mitogen agents and express oncogenes	+	+
	Induce prostaglandins, IL-1, IL-6 collagenase, GM-CSF, and IL-8	+	+
Hepatocytes	Induce some acute-phase reactants	+	+
	Decreased cytochrome P450 and Increase C3	+	+
	Increase Plasma Cu, decrease Plasma Fe + Zn	+	+
Hematopoietic cells	Inhibit some precursor cell proliferation and differentiation	−	+
	Stimulate precursor cells	+	−
Tumor cells and virus-infected cells	Selectively act as cytostatic/cytocidal agents	+	+ +
Adipocytes	Decrease lipoprotein lipase levels	+	+ +
	Increase lipolysis	+	+ +
Epithelial cells	Act as mitogenic agents	+	N.D.[1]
	Secrete collagen type IV	+	N.D.
Pancreatic β Cells	Modulate insulin levels	+	−
Dendritic Cells	Increase T cell activation	+	N.D.

[1]N.D., No reported data.

tion of T lymphocyte-derived lymphokines such as IL-2 and IL-2 receptors on T cells. In addition, IL-1 augments the capacity of accessory antigen-presenting cells (APC) to activate T cell-dependent immune responses. Although the immunologic effects of TNF are not as well established as those of IL-1, TNF also is comitogenic for thymocytes and induces IL-2 receptors. Both IL-1 and TNF have been shown to augment B cell proliferation, surface immunoglobulin receptor expression, and antibody production. Injection of either IL-1 or TNF together with an antigen has an adjuvant effect on T cell-dependent antibody responses.

Inflammatory Activities
of IL-1 & TNF

TNF has more potent in vitro effects than IL-1 on neutrophils, monocytes, and endothelial cells. Higher concentrations (approximately 1000 U/ml) of TNF, but not of IL-1, are chemotactic for neutrophils, and TNF activates the neutrophil respiratory burst and degranulation. Similarly, TNF (but not IL-1) is said to be chemotactic in vitro for monocytes. However, both IL-1 and TNF can augment the capacity of monocytes to produce other inflammatory mediators such as prostaglandins, IL- 6, and the neutrophil-attracting peptide, which has been renamed IL-8. In addition, IL-1 and, to an even greater degree, TNF increase the adhesiveness of endothelial cells by inducing the expression of cell membrane adhesion molecules such as intrinsic cell adhesion molecule type 1 (I CAM-1). These differences may account for the greater vascular and in vivo antitumor effects of TNF.

Injection of IL-1 induces local acute inflammatory responses that begin within 1 hour and peak within 3–4 hours. Initially, neutrophils adhere to endothelial cells and marginate along blood vessel walls. This is followed by neutrophil infiltration and edema from extravasation of fluids into the tissues. In contrast, slow release of IL-1 from ethylene vinyl acetate copolymer disks implanted into a subcutaneous site results in delayed-type hypersensitivity (DTH) granuloma formation with considerable mononuclear cell infiltration, fibrosis, and new blood vessel formation. Intradermal injections of TNF also produce acute inflammation with neutrophil infiltration.

Both IL-1 and TNF are mitogenic for endothelial cells and have in vivo angiogenic activity. TNF and, to a lesser degree, IL-1 stimulate endothelial cells and to produce prostaglandins, IL-6, and procoagulant factor (tissue factor III), which has the capacity to initiate the clotting cascade. These local coagulation and inflammatory effects block the blood supply and may account for the unique capacity of TNF to cause infarcts and hemorrhagic necrosis of tumors, the property that led to the initial discovery of TNF.

The hemorrhagic Shwartzman reaction has been attributed to TNF because endotoxin shock can be blocked by the administration of antiserum to TNF. The Shwartzman reaction is a usually fatal disseminated intravascular coagulopathy (DIC) that occurs after systemic exposure to endotoxin followed within 24 hours by a second dose of intravenous endotoxin. Repeated injections of IL-1 are reported to yield local Shwartzman reactions. Low doses of IL-1 act synergistically with TNF to induce the hemorrhagic shock of a Shwartzman reaction.

Neuroendocrine Effects
of IL-1 & TNF

IL-1 and TNF act alone and together to induce a number of other systemic inflammatory reactions such as hypothalamus-mediated fever and hepatocyte-mediated acute-phase responses. IL-1, but not TNF, has been reported to stimulate the hypothalamus to produce corticotropin-releasing factor (CRF), which stimulates the release of adrenocorticotropic hormone (ACTH) from the pituitary; this, in turn, induces the production of glucocorticoids by the adrenals. IL-1 thereby initiates a negative regulatory feedback loop, since glucocorticoids suppress the production of both IL-1 and TNF. In addition, TNF as well as IL-1 can induce IL-6, which, in turn, stimulates the production of ACTH, potentially elevating the plasma levels of glucocorticoids.

Glucocorticoids have the capacity to increase IL-1 receptor (IL- 1R) expression, but not TNF receptor expression, on human B lymphocytes. The capacity of glucocorticoids to increase IL-1R expression on B cells suggests that IL-1 may participate in the reported capacity of these steroids to act as polyclonal B lymphocyte activators in vitro and in vivo. This paradoxical up-regulation of IL-1R on B lymphocytes by otherwise immunosuppressive steroids may serve to further suppress inflammation by diverting the immune response from cellular immunity. Thus, steroids seem to favor humoral immunity at the expense of cell-mediated immunity, thereby diminishing inflammation.

Connective Tissue Effects
of IL-1 & TNF

Both IL-1 and TNF stimulate alkaline phosphatase activity in osteoblasts, induce osteoclasts to resorb bone and chondrocytes to increase cartilage turnover, and activate proliferation by fibroblasts and synovial cells. Increased levels of IL-1 and TNF are found in inflammatory joint fluids. Fibrosis and thickening of tissues in joints can be mediated by these cytokines.

Effects of IL-1 & TNF on Hematopoiesis

IL-1 is identical to hematopoietin-1, a factor that synergizes with CSF to stimulate early bone marrow hematopoietic progenitor cells to form giant colonies with high proliferative potential (HPP colonies). In addition, IL-1 induces the production by bone marrow stromal cells of a number of the hematopoietic CSF as well as receptors for CSF-1. TNF also actively induces CSF production by bone marrow stromal cells and macrophages but does not promote HPP colonies. Both TNF and IL-1 administration induce a considerable bone marrow-derived neutrophilia. TNFα, if given 1 day prior to lethal radiation, is radioprotective. However, IL-1 is more effective as a radioprotective agent at lower concentrations than TNFα. Furthermore, IL-1 and TNF show additive or synergistic radioprotective effects, suggesting that their mechanisms of action differ.

Other Activities of IL-1 & TNF

IL-1 stimulates epithelial-cell proliferation and function, eg, production of collagen type IV, whereas the effect of TNF on epithelial cells is unknown. IL-1, but not TNF, selectively affects pancreatic β cells and causes changes in plasma insulin levels. Both TNF and IL-1 exhibit indirect antiviral effects that are mediated in part by the induction of IFN β. TNF and LT are cytostatic and cytocidal for a number of tumor cells in vitro. TNF is cytocidal for a wider variety of tumor cells and kills them more rapidly than does IL-1. The hallmark of the cachectin (or wasting) activity of TNF is probably related to the ability of TNF to increase lipoprotein lipase activity and hence lysis of fat cells. However, IL-1 is also reported to have this capability.

Overall, the considerable overlap in the broad spectrum of activities of these cytokines results in a rather perplexing redundancy in intercellular communications. The redundancy provides alternative pathways for mobilizing host reactions in emergencies, and it enhances efficiency, since IL-1 and TNF exhibit many synergistic interactions. This results in an enormous amplification of the effects of relatively small amounts of these cytokines when both are produced.

INTERLEUKIN-2

IL-2 is an MW-15,400 peptide consisting of 133 amino acids and an essential internal disulfide bond. It exerts numerous immunologic effects by stimulating proliferation and lymphokine production by T cells, B cells, and NK cells. In 1976, a polypeptide hormone, initially called **T cell growth factor (TCGF)**, was found to stimulate human T cell proliferation and to enable T cells to grow continuously in culture. The discovery of TCGF not only made it possible to study the factors involved in T lymphocyte growth but also provided a valuable tool for studying cellular and humoral immunity in vitro. The ability to propagate and develop clones from single normal T cells that maintained their specific immunologic functions has greatly facilitated biochemical and molecular studies of the development, properties, and regulation of immunocompetent T cells.

Molecular Properties of IL-2

Human, primate, and mouse IL-2 have been purified to homogeneity. IL-2 is a single protein (MW 15,000), but the presence of variable amounts of carbohydrate results in higher-MW forms of IL-2. Because recombinant IL-2, which lacks carbohydrate groups, is as active as natural IL-2, carbohydrates are not necessary for IL-2 activity.

Molecular studies with cloned complementary DNA (cDNA) from various human sources and other species indicate that there is only a single gene for IL-2 and that it is located on human chromosome 4. There is little or no homology between the sequence of IL-2 and other sequenced growth factors.

Receptors for IL-2

An initial signal, the antigen, is presented on accessory cells to T cells. This step is required to activate lymphocytes to maximally respond to IL-2. Resting T lymphocytes do not proliferate in response to the same low concentrations (10–20 pmol) of IL-2 that result in maximal proliferation of such antigen-activated T cells. Consequently, antigens and lectins such as PHA are mitogenic for T cells because they cause some T cells both to produce IL-2 and to become maximally responsive to IL-2. This IL-2-responsive state is based on the development of lymphocyte membrane IL-2 receptors that satisfy all the criteria of hormone receptors: (1) a high-affinity binding constant of about 10^{-12} mol/L; (2) binding that is saturable at 20 minutes at 37 °C; and (3) specificity of ligands for target cells. There is a close correlation between the concentration of IL-2 causing lymphocyte proliferation and the concentration that lead to significant IL-2 binding.

A monoclonal antibody, designated **anti-Tac** (for a *T C*ell *A*ctivation antigen that specifically recognizes the the alpha chain of the human IL-2 receptor) suppresses IL-2 mediated proliferation of previously activated T cell lines and blocks activation of peripheral blood lymphocytes by antigens or lectins. The IL-2 receptor was characterized by radioisotopically labeling IL-2 receptor-bearing cell lines followed by immunoprecipitation of IL-2 receptor with anti-Tac. The molecule is a glycoprotein of MW 55,000–60,000.

Characterization of Another IL-2-Binding Protein Distinct From Tac

Several different leukemia cell lines or clones of these cell lines bind IL-2 in the absence of any detectable cell surface Tac antigen via another IL-2-binding protein (MW 75,000). In fact, 3 IL-2-binding affinities have now been identified: The Tac antigen (p55) binds IL-2 with a K_d of 10^{-8} mol/L; the MW-75,000 protein (p75) binds with an intermediate-affinity K_d of 10^{-9} mol/L, and a third receptor binds with a high-affinity K_d of 10^{-11} mol/L and is a complex of the other 2 proteins. A number of studies suggest that p75 can function alone and transmit a biologic signal in response to binding IL-2. The sole function of the Tac moiety seems to be the formation of high-affinity IL-2 receptors by complexing with p75, called the beta chain of the IL-2 receptor thereby increasing the sensitivity and rapidity of the lymphocytic response (Table 7–4). The precise nature of the complex between these 2 IL-2-binding proteins is unknown. In a hypothetic model of this complex, p75 has an intracytoplasmic domain responsible for signaling, and one molecule of IL-2 binds to one molecule of both binding proteins.

IL-2 Production & Detection

Freshly isolated resting T cells do not express IL-2 mRNA, nor do they contain IL-2 protein. The production of IL-2 by normal T lymphocytes requires that cells be activated by antigens or poly-

clonal T cell activators. Other pathways of T cell and thymocyte activation, such as ligand binding to CD2 surface receptors, also stimulate IL-2 production.

Studies of isolated subpopulations of lymphocytes and thymocytes show that antigens induce IL-2 from CD4 helper T (TH) cells. However, potent polyclonal mitogens and class I MHC alloantigens can stimulate the CD8 T lymphocytes to produce IL-2. Medullary thymocytes stimulated with T cell mitogens secrete low levels of IL-2. In addition, a subset of large granular lymphocytes (LGL) that bear the CD2 and CD6 markers and are related to NK cells can be induced by lectins such as PHA or by CSF and IFN γ to produce IL-2.

The assay of IL-2 uses tritiated thymidine incorporation to measure the growth-supporting effects on IL-2-dependent human or murine cytotoxic T cell lines. Human IL-2 is active on mouse cells; therefore, the murine cell line CTLL has been most widely used. The precise IL-2 concentration in an experimental sample is determined by comparison with a standard containing a known amount of IL-2. There is a radioimmunoassay for IL-2, but it is less sensitive than the bioassay and the antibodies used can react to inert IL-2, giving potentially false values. A radioreceptor assay in which purified IL-2 receptors are used is being developed.

Intracellular Regulation of IL-2 Production

After activation of T cells, de novo transcription and translation precede the appearance of secreted IL-2. In normal human lymphocytes stimulated with PHA, IL-2 mRNA accumulates at 4 hours, reaches a peak at 12 hours, and sharply declines thereafter. The rapid shutoff of IL-2 mRNA production, together with its short half-life (1–2 hours) in vivo, ensures that IL-2 production is very transient. Removal of the activating signal leads to a decay in IL-2 mRNA levels owing to a cessation of transcription. It has recently been demonstrated that the A + T- rich region of the 3′ untranslated mRNA for inducible cytokines such as IL-2 imparts instability to mRNA and shortens its half- life. The rapid decline in IL-2 mRNA that is always seen in activated normal cells, despite persistent stimulation and transcription of the gene, suggests that repressive protein(s) is also induced. This intricate control mechanism, which ensures the transience of IL-2 mRNA, is important in the regulation of immune reactivity by ensuring the decay of IL-2 after antigen is removed from the reaction.

Role of IL-2 in T Cell Activation

The induction of lymphocyte proliferation involves 2 steps (Fig 7–3). The first step, called **com-**

Table 7–4. Properties of the human IL-2 receptor.

High-Affinity Complex
1. Composed of 2 heterologous subunits
2. Transiently expressed
3. Internalized by IL-2, induced by antigen, IL-2, TNF, and IL-4
4. Conveys protein-kinase C activitation, [$Ca2^+$], and pH changes
5. Enhances cell-mediated functions (eg, lymphokine production)
6. Signals S-phase progression

P75
1. Participates in high-affinity complex
2. Responsible for internalization of complex
3. Present alone on a few resting T cells and LGL
4. At high IL-2 doses, yields signal transduction and gene activation

p55
1. Participates in high-affinity complex
2. Transient expression increased by IL-2
3. Induced by IL-2, TNF, IL-4, and IL-6
4. No signal transduction
5. No defined function by itself

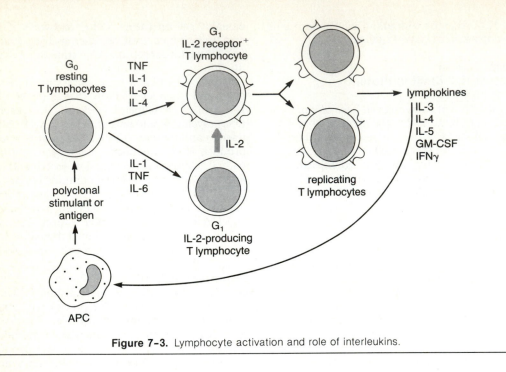

Figure 7-3. Lymphocyte activation and role of interleukins.

---

petence, is initiated by an exogenous signal delivered to the quiescent T cell by mitogen or antigen. This leads to partial activation of the T cell, resulting in an increase in size, induction of transcription of certain genes, and passage from the G_0 phase to the early G_1 phase in the cell cycle. However, the first signal by itself is not sufficient to stimulate growth. A second, endogenous, signal is needed to induce cell cycle progression, with transition to the S phase and ultimately to cell division. In the second step, the binding of IL-2 to its high-affinity receptor is required for progression of the T cell through the cell cycle. Both anti-IL-2 and anti-Tac antibodies can inhibit this T cell growth. T cells are unique in that both IL-2 and its receptor are synthesized de novo following initial activation.

Lymphocytes express maximal levels of high-affinity IL-2 receptors for only a brief period following exposure to specific antigen. The subsequent decline in receptor expression is unusual because it occurs independently of the presence of IL-2, indicating that there is another mechanism of receptor regulation besides IL-2-mediated receptor down-regulation. It also means that there is only a finite period for immune T cell clones to expand. Consequently, T lymphocyte proliferation ceases and the cells arrest in the G_1 phase, even in the presence of saturating concentrations of IL-2. Readdition of antigen causes the reappearance of optimal numbers of IL-2 receptors on the lymphocytes, enabling cells to again grow in response to IL-2. These events can be repeated; they describe the cyclical nature of normal T cell growth in vivo and underscore the constant need for stimuli (ie, antigens) to induce IL-2 receptors necessary for continuous proliferation of T cell clones in vitro.

IL-2-Induced Cytokine Production

The addition of IL-2 to purified activated T cells promotes several cellular functions besides proliferation (Table 7–5). T lymphocytes activated by IL-2 produce other lymphokines including IFN γ; lymphotoxin; B cell growth and differentiation factors such as IL-4, IL-6, BCGF, and BCDF; hematopoietic growth factors such as IL-3, IL-5, and GM-CSF; and TGF β. IL-2-activated T cells can also exhibit enhanced cytotoxicity. These various functions are amplified even further by the capacity of IL-2 to clonally expand the pool of antigen-reactive cells. A model for the development of immune reactivity of T cells incorporates the concept that an initial signal is required for IL-2 production and IL-2 receptor expression (Fig 7–3).

T Cell Clones & Lines
Dependent on IL-2

IL-2 preferentially supports the growth of CD8 Tc cells, but CD4 TH cells and a few CD8 Ts cell lines also have been grown. In addition to the ca-

Table 7–5. Properties of human IL-2.

Origin
1. Activated peripheral T cells
2. Activated medullary thymocytes
3. Activated subset of LGL

Target Cell Specificity for Proliferative Stimulus
1. Activated mature T cell subsets
2. Activated LGL
3. Activated B cells

Biologic Effects
1. Binds to specific receptors on T cells, B cells, and monocytes
2. Promotes entry into the S phase, except monocytes
3. Stimulates lymphokine secretion
4. Enhances macrophage cytocidal state
5. Augments immunoglobulin production
6. Activates natural killer activity of LGL

Biochemical properties
1. MW 15,400
2. 133 amino acids
3. Isoelectric point 8.0

pacity of these cloned cells to release IL-2, they appear to cooperate with histocompatible adherent cells in the presence of specific antigen to release a variety of other lymphokines.

The continuous IL-2-dependent lymphocyte lines developed from normal cells that have been used for IL-2 bioassays (such as the widely used CTLL-2 line) are actually cell variants that spontaneously express high levels of receptors for IL-2. Successive generations of cells constitutively express IL-2 binding sites and therefore need only IL-2 to grow. CTLL is used for bioassays because it responds only to IL-2, unlike cell lines that respond to other growth factors such as IL-4. In the absence of IL-2, these cells cease to proliferate, and they die within 12–24 hours.

Interactions of IL-2 With Non-T Cells

Freshly isolated large granular lymphocytes (LGL), which exhibit antigen- nonspecific NK cell activity, do not express the MW-55,000 Tac antigen (a part of the IL-2 receptor). Nevertheless, they can be stimulated by IL-2 to proliferate, to produce other lymphokines, and to exhibit enhanced NK activity. This response to IL-2 requires the expression of the p75 IL-2-binding protein on the unstimulated LGL. After in vitro incubation, LGL also begin to express both p55 Tac antigen and the high-affinity IL-2 receptor complex.

High-affinity receptors for IL-2 have also been found on B lymphoblasts. Activated normal as well as some transformed B lymphoblasts, but not resting B cells, express about 30% as many Tac antigen receptors for IL-2 as do activated T cells. IL-2 can induce both increased antibody production and proliferation by purified normal B lymphocytes but at higher (2- to 3-fold) doses of IL-2.

Monocytes and macrophages also normally express a low density of the p55 Tac antigen. In mice, myeloid precursors, mast cells, and monocytes possess only low-affinity receptors for IL-2. Activation of macrophages by IFN γ or LPS, however, results in the development of high-affinity IL-2 receptors consisting of p75 and the p55 Tac antigen. Addition of IL-2 to these activated macrophages results in the activation of the Tac, GM-CSF, and G-CSF genes and also augments the tumoricidal activities of these macrophages.

In Vivo Effects of IL-2

Intravenously injected recombinant IL-2 is rapidly cleared from the circulation of humans, with a half-life of 3–22 minutes. Part of the clearance may be due to absorption by activated T cells, but the kidneys constitute the main clearance site. However, ligation of renal arteries prolongs the serum half-life only transiently, and only breakdown products of IL-2 are recovered in the urine, suggesting the existence of alternative clearance sites for IL-2. Based on the molarity of IL-2 required to half-maximally bind receptors, 15,000–25,000 units must be given intravenously to human subjects to obtain effects on the immune system. Continuous intravenous infusion results in sustained high levels of IL-2. These high doses of recombinant IL-2 have elicited multiple toxic side effects. One of the most important of these is the "vascular leak syndrome," wherein infusion of recombinant IL-2 leads to a rapid accumulation of extracellular fluid and hence to ascites and pulmonary edema. IL-2 stimulates the production of cytokines capable of activating endothelial cells, leading to vascular permeability. High levels of IL-2 elevate the serum levels of ACTH and cortisol; this elevation leads to immunosuppressive effects. Intraperitoneal and subcutaneous injections of IL-2 lead to more prolonged serum concentrations of >2 U/mL at about 2 and 6 hours, respectively, so that these routes of administration permit the use of lower doses with less toxic side effects.

Toxins (eg, diphtheria toxin) fused to growth factors (eg, IL-2) have exciting therapeutic potential for deletion of antigen-reactive T cells. IL-2 toxin has been shown to be very selective and to have potent toxic effects (50% maximum effective dose (ED_{50}) of 10–50 pmol) against a number of cell lines, particularly human T-cell lymphotrophic virus type I (HTLV-I)- associated cells in vitro. Such a toxin could be used in treatment of acute T cell leukemia and other IL-2-bearing neoplasias.

Immunotherapy with IL-2 and lymphokine-activated killer (LAK) cells is discussed in Chapter 57.

INTERLEUKIN-4 & -5

This section addresses IL-4 and IL-5, 2 other lymphokines with TCGF and BCGF activities; however, IL-3, which acts as a multi-CSF, will be discussed subsequently with the other hematopoietic CSF.

Cloned murine CD4 TH lymphocyte lines can be separated into 2 distinct subsets based on their capacity to produce lymphokines. Only the murine TH1 subset secretes IL-2, IFN γ, and lymphotoxin (TNFβ), whereas the TH2 subset and mast cells secrete IL-4 and IL-5. The properties of these lymphokines are shown in Table 7–6. The human analogues of these TH subsets have not yet been identified.

IL-4

IL-4 (Fig 7–4) was initially detected and its gene was cloned by using its B cell growth activity for assay. IL-4, formerly designated BCGF-I, is mitogenic for B cells that have previously been activated by T cell–dependent antigens, T cell–independent antigens, or anti-immunoglobulin antisera. IL-4 synergizes with IL-2 to stimulate B cell growth. Although it is not a growth factor for resting B cells, IL-4 induces rapid increases in B cell surface expression of class II MHC antigens and Fc receptors for IgE. It is also a major regulator of immunoglobulin isotype expression. IL-4 induces IgE and IgG1 production and decreases IgG2b and IgG3 production by LPS- stimulated B cells. Thus, IL-4 promotes immunoglobulin isotype switching to the C-ε and C-γ 1 genes and therefore may be important in the etiology of atopic allergies.

Like other cytokines, IL-4 also acts on nonlymphoid cells. It is mitogenic for T lymphocytes and supports the growth of mast cell lines. Furthermore, IL-4 costimulates, with CSF, the growth of hematopoietic precursors and induces the differentiation of more mature myeloid cells. It is a potent activator of macrophage cytocidal functions and induces the expression of cell surface class II MHC antigens on macrophages as well as B lymphocytes.

IL-5

IL-5 (Fig 7–4) was first detected and its gene was later cloned on the basis of its T cell-replacing activity (TRF) and B cell growth activity (BCGF-II) for the BCl-1 lymphoma line. Recombinant murine IL-5 has been shown to promote the growth of activated B cells and to combine with IL-2 to promote B cell proliferation. IL-5 promotes antibody production by B cells, particularly of the IgA isotype. Thus, IL-5 favors isotype switching to the C-α gene. IL-5 has modest mitogenic effects on T cells. In addition, it induces the differentiation of bone marrow precursors into eosinophils and supports the growth of eosinophilic cell lines and induction of Tc.

Therefore, by producing IL-4 and IL-5, murine TH2 cells promote IgE and IgA production as well as mast cell and eosinophil growth and differentiation. This suggests that TH2 cells participate preferentially in the development of antibodies for atopic reactions and for host defense against parasitic diseases. In contrast, the lymphokines produced by TH1 cells selectively engage in host defense against viral, microbial, and neoplastic diseases, since IL-2, interferons, and TNFβ promote macrophage activities such as cytotoxicity and phagocytosis, mediate DTH reactions, and

Table 7–6. Properties of IL-4 and IL-5

Property	IL-4	IL-5
Size of mature form	20 kDa	18 kDa
Cell sources	TH cells, mast cells	TH cells
Cell targets and activities	Acts as comitogen for B cells Enhances Ia and FcRε expression on B cells Promotes switch to IgG1 and IgE (decreases IgG2b and IgG3) Acts as mast cell stimulant Comitogen for thymocytes Activates macrophages Stimulates hematopoiesis	Acts as costimulant of B cell proliferation and differentiation Enhances IL-2 receptor expression Promotes switch to IgA Stimulates BCl-1 growth Stimulates eosinophils Acts as comitogen for thymocytes
Size of receptors	60 kDa	46.5 kDa

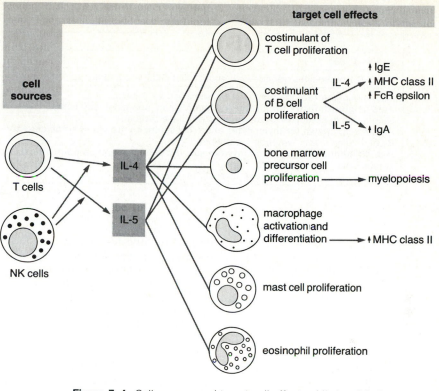

Figure 7–4. Cell sources and target cell effects of IL-4 and IL-5.

favor IgG1a production. In fact, IFN γ and IL-4 generally have opposing effects on immunoglobulin production; IFN γ will favor the production of IgG3 at the expense of IL-4 induction of IgG or IgE. The homologous subpopulations of TH1 and TH2 cells and their products remain to be identified in humans.

INTERLEUKIN-6

Properties of IL-6

IL-6 was initially called IFN β_2 on the basis of its presumed antiviral activity and its cross-reactivity with some antisera to IFN β. However, more recent studies show that IL-6 has little or no antiviral activity and therefore should not be considered an interferon. IL-6 is a cytokine with multiple biologic activities on a variety of cells (Table 7–7). Cloning of the genes coding for molecules expressing these various biologic activities revealed that the protein product of a single gene possesses all these activities. This substance is now most commonly called IL-6.

The gene for IL-6 is located on human chromosome 7. The reported MW of IL-6 ranges between 22,000 and 30,000, owing in part to differential glycosylation and phosphorylation of a single protein. IL-6 can be produced by many cells, including T and B lymphocytes, monocytes, endothelial cells, epithelial cells, and fibroblasts. A variety of stimuli including TNF, IL-1, platelet-derived growth factor, antigens, mitogens, and bacterial endotoxin (LPS) induce the production of IL-6.

IL-6 Receptor

There is a wide range of IL-6-responsive target cells that bear specific high-affinity IL-6 receptors. These include Epstein-Barr virus (EBV)-transformed B cell lines, plasma cell lines, myelomonocytic cell lines, and normal resting T lymphocytes. IL-6 receptors are present on activated but not resting B cells, which accounts for the ability of IL-6 to induce differentiation of preactivated but not resting B cells. Reported dissociation constants (K_d) are in the range of 10^{-10}–10^{-12} mol/L, and there are 10^2–10^4 receptors per cell.

The gene encoding the IL-6 receptor has been cloned and has a domain similar to one in the immunoglobulin gene superfamily. Unlike the receptors for many growth factors, the IL-6 receptor does not have a tyrosine kinase domain.

Table 7-7. Properties of IL-6.

Property	IL-6
Chromosome	7
MW of mature form	22,000–30,000
Cell sources	T and B lymphocytes, monocytes, endothelial cells, epithelial cells, fibroblasts
Cell targets and activities	Acts as cofactor for immunoglobulin secretion by B cells Acts as growth factor for myelomas, hybridomas, and plasmacytomas Stimulates hepatocytes to produce acute-phase proteins Acts as comitogen for thymocytes and T cells inhibits growth of some carcinoma and non-B-cell leukemia and lymphoma cell lines Has differentiation effects on myelomonocytic cell lines and on normal hematopoietic precursor cells Stimulates pituitary ACTH and adrenal glucocorticoids

Activities of IL-6

IL-6, as a B cell stimulatory factor, is a differentiation or maturation agent that promotes the ability of activated cells of the B cell lineage to secrete immunoglobulins. IL-6 is also a growth factor for hybridomas, plasmacytomas, and EBV-transformed peripheral blood B cells. Recently, it has been demonstrated that freshly isolated human myeloma cells both produce IL-6 and express IL-6 receptors. Moreover, anti-IL-6 antibodies inhibit the growth of the myeloma cells in vitro, suggesting that IL-6 may function as an autocrine signal in the process of uncontrolled proliferation during myeloma.

In contrast to these stimulating properties, IL-6 performs antiproliferative activities for carcinoma and non-B-cell leukemia and lymphoma cell lines. In vivo administration of IL-6 increases neutrophil counts. It also has differentiation effects on myelomonocytic cell lines and on normal hematopoietic precursor cells, and it augments colony formation by hematopoietic cells.

In the acute inflammatory response to infection or trauma, the liver responds by altering the synthesis of several plasma proteins known as acute-phase proteins. IL-6, as a **hepatocyte-stimulating factor (HSF),** induces the synthesis of acute-phase proteins, including C-reactive protein, α_1-antichymotrypsin, α_1-acid glycoprotein, fibrinogen, and C3 while inhibiting the synthesis of proteins such as prealbumin and albumin. The expression of some of these acute-phase proteins is also modulated by IL-1 or TNF, which combine synergistically with the HSF activity of IL-6. In addition, administration of high doses of IL-6 also produces fever by stimulating the hypothalamic fever center; IL-6 is therefore an endogenous pyrogen.

IL-6, as a T cell-activating factor or T cell costimulant, can provide, at least in part, the second (antigen-nonspecific) signal that is required in addition to antigen or mitogen for T cell activation. IL-6 has been shown to augment proliferation of thymocytes and monocyte-depleted preparations of peripheral blood T lymphocytes stimulated with suboptimal doses of PHA via both IL-2-dependent and IL-2-independent pathways. It enhances both IL-2 production and expression of receptors for IL-2.

As is apparent, IL-1, TNF, and IL-6 have some overlapping biologic activities (Tables 7–1 and 7–2). Since IL-1 and TNF are potent inducers of IL-6, it will be of interest to determine which biologic activities ascribed to IL-1 or TNF are actually mediated by IL-6.

INTERLEUKIN-7

IL-7, an MW-25,000 cytokine that acts predominantly on T and B lymphocyte progenitors, has recently been identified. Murine and human IL-7 have both been purified, and the genes have been cloned and expressed. IL-7 is produced by stromal cells of the bone marrow. It stimulates pre-B cells and is a costimulant of early thymocytes. Therefore, it can be considered a lymphopoietin. In addition, it is a costimulant together with polyclonal lectins of mature T cells but not of mature B cells. In vivo administration of IL-7 to mice stimulates predominantly B cell hyperplasia of the spleen and lymph nodes. However, IL-7 also promotes in vivo recovery from cyclophosphamide toxicity by stimulating myeloid precursors and megakaryocytes to produce colony-forming units and platelets. Consequently, IL-7 also appears to have hematopoietic activities.

INTERFERONS

In 1957, it was discovered that a soluble factor produced by cells exposed to inactive virus was able to transfer "interference" of viral replication to fresh cells. It was therefore named "interferon" the interferons have since been shown to be a large family of secreted proteins having antiviral activity. Moreover, they also have potent antiproliferative and immunomodulatory activities. The interferons are produced by most cells of vertebrate species in response to viral infection or other selected stimuli.

Assays for Interferon

The commonly used assays for interferon are antiviral bioassays that measure inhibition either of virus production or of the cytopathic effect of virus on cultured cell lines. The more recent development of radioimmunoassays or other ligand-binding tests has facilitated the quantification and identification of interferons.

Interferon Types & Induction

Many proteins with various degrees of structural homology have the property of inducing an antiviral state in target cells and therefore are, by definition, interferons. The interferons can be divided into antigenically distinct types and classified according to their primary cell of origin or according to the stimulus for induction, as shown in Table 7–8.

A. Type I Interferons (IFN α and IFN β): These are induced by viral infections or artificially by a double-stranded RNA such as poly(I·C). Most type I interferons are characterized by being stable at pH 2.0. IFN α, which is produced primarily by leukocytes, consists of multiple subspecies that are antigenically related. One human IFN α gene family has at least 14 functional nonallelic members. The amino acid sequences of these human IFN α subspecies are about 80% homologous. A second family of IFN α genes has also been identified in the human genome. The antigenically distinct IFN β is the major interferon synthesized by nonleukocytic cells, including fibroblasts, although it can also be produced by leukocytes. The amino acid sequence of IFN β is approximately 30% homologous with that of the IFN α family.

B. Type II Interferon (IFN γ or Immune Interferon): This is produced during immune reactions by antigen-, mitogen-, or lectin-stimulated T lymphocytes or by LGL with NK activity. Type II interferon is labile at pH 2.0, a property often used as a simple method of identification.

Although the reasons for the genetic diversity of the interferons in humans are unknown, different interferons are not equally potent in each of their diverse activities, and the various types of interferon may be differentially active on different cell types and at different times in various organs or tissues.

Activities of Interferons

The interferons induce an antiviral state that protects the target cells against most types of viruses (Fig 7–5). In addition, the interferons have potent cellular effects (Table 7–9), primarily inhibition of cell proliferation. Interferons can either inhibit or enhance cell differentiation, depending on the cell type and the dose of interferon. The interferons are also potent immunomodulatory agents and play important roles in normal host defense.

Immunomodulatory Effects of Interferon

The immunomodulatory activities of interferon are mediated by its effects on the cells responsible for host defense, ie, macrophages, T and B lymphocytes, and LGL with NK activity.

A. Activation of Macrophages: The interferons increase bactericidal and tumoricidal capabilities of macrophages and augment their accessory cell functions. The interferons possess the activities described as **macrophage-activating factor (MAF)** and **monocyte migration inhibitory factor (MIF),** although other proteins may also have these activities.

Table 7–8. Classification of human interferons.

Interferon	Principal Cellular Source	Inducing Stimulus	MW of Natural Monomeric Form	Chromosome Number	
				IFN	Receptor
Type I					
IFN α	Leukocytes	Virus or double-stranded RNA	18,000–20,000	9	21
IFN β	Fibroblasts	Virus or double-stranded RNA	23,000	9	21
Type II (Immune)					
IFN γ	T lymphocytes, LGL	Antigen or mitogen	20,000–25,000	12	6

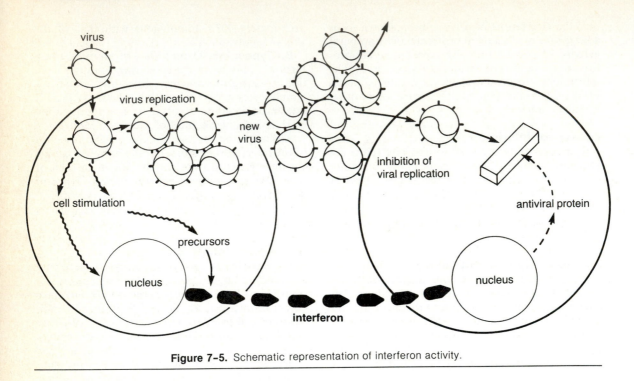

Figure 7–5. Schematic representation of interferon activity.

Macrophages that have been activated in vitro by IFN α show morphologic evidence of maturation such as enlargement, increased spreading, pseudopod formation, and vacuolization beginning in vitro at 1 hour and peaking in 48–72 hours. The activation of macrophages by IFN α, β, or γ is accompanied by increased expression of receptors for the Fc portion of immunoglobulins

Table 7–9. Effects of interferons on cellular functions.

Inhibit
Cell proliferation
Tumor growth
Fibroblast-adipocyte differentiation

Enhance
Promyelocytic and monoblastic leukemic cell differentiation
Phagocytosis by macrophages
Accessory cell functions of macrophages (IFN γ > IFN α, β)
Endotoxin-induced IL-1 secretion by macrophages (IFN γ > α, β)
Generation of CTL
Activity of NK cells
Expression of class I and II MHC antigens and Fc receptors

Mixed Effects
Erythroleukemic cell differentiation
Production of antibodies
Cell-mediated immune phenomena

(FcR). This increase in FcR expression promotes both increased phagocytosis of immune complexes and increased capacity of the macrophages to lyse antibody-coated bacteria, parasites, and tumor cells by ADCC, in which antibody molecules couple macrophages to target cells by binding to their FcR and antigenic sites, respectively.

The induction of antigen-specific, T lymphocyte-mediated immune responses requires "presentation" of antigen in conjunction with a class II MHC antigen by an accessory cell to a Th cell. IFN γ and, to a much lesser degree, IFN α and β maintain the expression of class II MHC antigen on the surface of macrophages as well as on other cell types. In addition, IFN γ can boost the level of class II antigen expression above resting levels. Owing at least in part to increased expression of class II MHC antigen, macrophages pretreated with IFN γ thus exhibit significantly enhanced accessory cell functions, which enable them to activate T lymphocytes more effectively.

B. Effects of Interferon on Lymphocytes: Interferon can either augment or suppress cellular and humoral immunity, depending on the dose, time of administration, and genetic makeup of the recipient. In general, in vivo administration of interferon or interferon inducers before or concomitant with antigenic sensitization has considerable inhibitory effects, whereas administration of interferon after antigenic sensitization augments both cellular and humoral immune responses. The latter observation is probably of greater physiologic relevance, since IFN γ is produced in vivo relatively late in the normal course of an immune response. The inhibitory and stimulatory effects of all the interferons can also be demonstrated in vitro. For example, higher preexposure doses of interferon or simultaneous addition of interferon suppresses lymphocyte proliferation and in vitro antibody production, whereas low doses of interferon or late addition can enhance lymphocyte proliferation and antibody production. IFN α, β, and γ also have both positive and negative effects on such cell-mediated immunologic phenomena as delayed hypersensitivity, graft-versus-host response, and mixed leukocyte reactions.

The mechanisms by which interferons augment cellular and humoral immunity are complex and are partly based on increased class II MHC antigen expression, increased class I antigens on CTL targets, increased production of other cytokines such as IL-1, and direct effects on T and B cell differentiation. The immunosuppressive effects of interferons may be due in part to their antigrowth activity.

C. Effects of Interferon on NK Cell Activity: NK cell activity is mediated by the cytotoxic effects of LGL in the absence of prior sensitization against virus-infected cells, certain tumor cell lines, and normal hematopoietic cells. Both in vitro and in vivo administration of IFN α or β or interferon inducers enhance the NK cell activities of LGL. Paradoxically, pretreatment of some target cells with interferon makes them less susceptible to NK cytolysis, again emphasizing the complexities of the actions of the interferons in the immune system.

Molecular Mechanisms of Action of Interferon

In contrast to antibodies that react with and neutralize viruses directly, the interferons establish an antiviral state and act as antiproliferative and immunodulatory agents by inducing the synthesis of cellular proteins and altering the metabolism of target cells. In this regard, the interferons are similar in their mechanism of action to polypeptide hormones and growth factors.

A. Interferon Receptors: The initial event in the action of the interferons is their binding to specific receptors on the cell surface. All type I interferons can bind to a single type of interferon receptor, whereas type II interferon binds to a different receptor. Most cell types respond to interferon, and interferon receptors are therefore present on most cells. The binding of the interferons to their receptors is primarily of high affinity, with K_d in the range of 10^{-10}–10^{-11} mol/L. The binding is saturable, with up to 7000 type I and 13,000 type II interferon receptors per cell on some cultured cell lines. However, some cells express far fewer interferon receptors; eg, small resting T lymphocytes have only 250 IFN α and 500 IFN γ high-affinity receptors per cell.

The type II interferon receptor was recently purified, monoclonal antibodies were prepared, and the cDNA for the receptor was cloned. Current evidence suggests that a single type of IFN γ-binding protein exists; however, other species-specific proteins besides the IFN γ-binding protein are required for the response to IFN γ. To date, the type I interferon receptor has not been purified to homogeneity, nor has its gene been cloned.

After the binding of the interferons to cell surface receptors, the interferon-receptor complexes cluster in coated pits and are internalized by receptor-mediated endocytosis. At least part of the internalized interferon is degraded in lysosomes. The biochemical events that transduce the signal from the cell surface interferon receptor to the rest of the cell to produce the various biologic responses to interferon are not defined. There is evidence for a role for protein kinase C in some of the actions of the interferons; however, nuclear receptors for the interferons have been described, and the results of several studies have suggested that signals for some of the responses to the interferons may be generated following ligand internalization.

B. Interferon-Induced mRNAs and Proteins: The interferons exert their biologic effects by modulating the synthesis of several specific mRNAs and proteins. Interferon-induced proteins include, among others, the MHC antigens and 2 enzymes: a protein kinase and 2'-5' oligo(A) (2-5A) synthetase. The protein kinase phosphorylates the small subunit of protein synthesis initiation factor type 2. After activation by double-stranded RNA, the 2–5A synthetase synthesizes small 2'-5' oligoadenylates that bind to and activate a latent endoribonuclease. Therefore, 2 enzymes participate in the antiviral and perhaps antimitogenic effects of the interferons. Several lines of evidence indicate that there are different but intersecting biochemical pathways for the establishment of the different biologic responses to type I and II interferons.

In Vivo Role of Interferon in Disease States

Interferon activity cannot normally be detected in tissues or serum but appears rapidly during viral infections. Interferon also transiently appears in the sera of animals with a systemic hypersensitivity reaction following intravenous administration of a large dose of a relevant antigen. It has been detected in the sera of some patients with clinically active autoimmune diseases including systemic lupus erythematosus, rheumatoid arthritis, scleroderma, and Sjögren's syndrome. The serum interferon activity from systemic lupus erythematosus patients has been identified as a mixture of IFN γ and IFN α.

Interferon plays a protective role in viral diseases, since addition of interferon or interferon inducers can halt the development of viral diseases. Moreover, anti-interferon antibodies exacerbate viral infections. Interferons are protective as antiviral agents even in immunodeficient subjects; however, the effects of interferon are not all beneficial. Overexpression or inappropriate expression of IFN α or β has been shown to have deleterious effects in mice. The interferon component of the host antiviral response, in excess, may cause aberrant autoimmune states or self-destructive host inflammatory responses.

Clinical experience with interferons as therapeutic agents is discussed in Chapter 62.

HEMATOPOIETIC COLONY-STIMULATING FACTORS

Colony-stimulating factors (CSF) are the cytokines that stimulate a limited number of pluripotent stem cells, present predominantly in the bone marrow, to produce large numbers of platelets, erythrocytes, neutrophils, monocytes, eosinophils, and basophils, most of which are short-lived in the blood. The CSF were named according to the type of target cells that form colonies in soft agar. Consequently, IL-3, otherwise known as **multi-CSF,** acts on pluripotent stem cells to produce all types of hematopoietic cells. GM-CSF acts on a bipotential stem cell (the colony forming unit in culture (CFU-C)) to produce mononuclear phagocytes and granulocytes; G-CSF principally causes granulocyte precursor proliferation; M-CSF is a mononuclear phagocyte progenitor

growth factor; and erythropoietin is a stimulator of erythroid development. However, in vivo administration of purified recombinant CSF frequently leads to effects that extend beyond the known in vitro activities of these cytokines; presumably this is based on their capacity to produce a cascade of other cytokines and to stimulate the functional activities of leukocytes (Table 7–10). In addition to maintaining homeostasis, these cytokines marshall bone marrow responses to environmental stress such as infection or trauma. For example, in defense against microorganisms, the number of granulocytes increases from 10^9 per day to as many as 2×10^{11}.

Both progenitors and mature progeny of lymphoid and myeloid cells require stimulation by several hemopoietins for proliferation and differentiation. The various CSF have totally unrelated protein sequences and apparently use distinct receptors, although these distinct receptors may be functionally linked on the target cell populations. Despite these differences, these growth factors have many overlapping functions and induce quite similar biologic responses in some cells, particularly in the production of mature granulocytes and macrophages (Table 7–10). The significance of this overlapping system is not entirely clear. It may be a fail-safe system, or the differences in cellular sources of these proteins may reflect different roles in steady-state maintenance or immune amplification of hematopoiesis.

A number of other cytokines have recently been found to influence hematopoiesis. They include IL-1, TNF, IL-4, IL-5, IL-6, and IL-7 and are discussed above. Whether these cytokines act directly or indirectly (by stimulating the production of CSF or receptors for CSF) must be defined. Overall, the hematopoietic growth factors alone or in combination are not just mitogenic stimuli but have 4 distinct actions on target cells: (1) enhanced survival, (2) growth stimulation, (3) dif-

Table 7–10. Human hematopoietic growth factors.

Name	Protein Size (kDa)	Cellular Sources	Cells Stimulated
G-CSF	18–22	Monocytes, fibroblasts	Neutrophils
GM-CSF	14–38	T cells, endothelial cells, fibroblasts, monocytes	Neutrophils, monocytes, eosinophils, erythroid cells, megakaryocytes
IL-3 (Multi-CSF)	14–28	T cells	Neutrophils, monocytes, eosinophils, basophils, erythroid cells, megakaryocytes
M-CSF	18–26[1] 35–45[1]	Monocytes, T and B cells Fibroblasts, endothelial cells, epithelial cells	Megakaryocytes
Erythropoietin	30–34	Kidney cells	Erythroid cells

[1]Protein is dimeric.

ferentiation commitment, and (4) functional activation of end-stage cells.

Immune amplification of leukocyte development may be controlled primarily at the level of cytokine production. Some of the genes encoding these hematopoietins are not normally expressed. IL-2, IL-3, IL-4, and IL-5 are produced only when T lymphocytes are stimulated by specific antigens such as microbial proteins. G-CSF and GM-CSF are produced by both fibroblasts and endothelial cells after stimulation by products of activated macrophages such as IL-1 and TNF. Activated macrophages can also produce their own hematopoietins.

Biologic Activities of the CSF

It is not clear how the wide array of hematopoietic cells develop from a single cell type. The majority of pluripotent stem cells are not actively going through the cell cycle. IL-6 and IL-1 have been implicated in stimulating the entry of these cells into the cell cycle, whereas other factors, such as TGFβ take the stem cells out of cycle. Furthermore, it is not clear what regulates the commitment of the stem cell to differentiate to a specific cell lineage. The evidence supports a random selection by hematopoietic factors, but other regulatory factors may be required.

Both IL-3 and GM-CSF support the development of multipotent colonies (colony forming units giving rise to granulocytes, erythrocytes,

monocytes, and megakaryocytes (CFU-GEMM)). although IL-3 seems to stimulate the more primitive progenitor cells. After treatment with 5-fluorouracil, IL-3-responsive cells are detectable earlier than GM-CSF-responsive cells. G-CSF, M-CSF, IL-5, and erythropoietin represent a class of molecules whose function is restricted to one specific lineage. For example, G-CSF stimulates the growth and differentiation of pure neutrophil colonies in semisolid media. In addition, it stimulates the functional activities of mature neutrophils by enhancing superoxide anion production, phagocytosis, and ADCC. Thus, G-CSF stimulation makes neutrophils much more efficient in killing bacteria.

Therapeutic Applications of CSF

New techniques in molecular biology have made possible the cloning and expression of the hematopoietin genes. This has provided large numbers of these molecules for study in the clinic. The preclinical studies of hematopoietins have revealed fewer toxic side effects than for agents such as TNF, IL-1, and IL-2. Thus, these molecules appear to have therapeutic potential in 2 areas: (1) stimulating production of blood cells in patients in whom one or more of the formed blood elements are abnormally low, and (2) boosting host defenses against microbial invasion. Hematopoietic dysfunction, such as granulocytopenia, is the major cause of death in cancer patients undergo-

Table 7–11. Properties of human TGFβ.

Property	TGFβ
Chromosome	Long arm of chromosome 19
Proform	391 amino acids
Mature Form	112 amino acids TGFβ1 or CIF-A, 25-kDa homodimer TGFβ2 or CIF-B, 25-kDa homodimer TGFβ1,2, 25-kDa heterodimer TGFβ3, 25-kDa homodimer
Cell sources	Platelets, placenta, kidney, bone, and T and B lymphocytes
Cell target and activities	Is chemotactic and mitogenic, for fibroblasts Enhances collagen, fibronectin and collagenase synthesis Stimulates osteoclastic bone resorption Is mitogenic for osteoblasts Inhibits proliferation of endothelial cells, epithelial cells, smooth muscle cells, T and B lymphocytes, early hematopoietic stem cells, fetal hepatocytes, and keratinocytes Inhibits mixed leukocyte reaction, generation of CTL Suppresses NK and lymphocytic-activated killer cell development
Receptor	280 kDa with 65 K_d and 85 K_d chains Murine 3T3 fibroblasts express 80,000 receptors/cell; lymphocytes have only 250 receptors/cell.
In vivo effects	Enhances wound repair Causes angiogenesis and fibroplasia

ing chemotherapy or radiotherapy. Since there is no present method to elevate granulocyte counts, the ability of GM-CSF and G-CSF to stimulate the production and function of neutrophils could aid in the management of iatrogenic suppression of neutrophilic granulocytes. In addition, preclinical studies have shown that GM-CSF and G-CSF can protect against lethal bacterial septicemia, suggesting that these molecules would be therapeutic in bacterial infections. Eventually, combinations of the regulators will be used for maximal effectiveness (see also Chapter 62).

TGFβ

TGFβ was initially discovered as a cofactor with TGFα that promoted anchorage-independent growth of rat kidney fibroblasts and enabled them to grow in a non-contact-inhibited manner. Thus, TGFβ is a growth factor for fibroblasts and promotes wound healing. However, it has consider-

able antiproliferative activity and acts as a negative regulator of immunity and hematopoiesis (Table 7–11). It is produced by many cell types, including activated macrophages and T lymphocytes. There are at least 3 forms of TGFβ (TGFβ1, 2, and 3). These 3 gene products react with the same high-affinity cell surface receptors that are expressed in widely varying numbers by many cell types.

TGFβ has antiproliferative effects on a wide variety of cell types, including epithelial cells, endothelial cells, smooth muscle cells, fetal hepatocytes, early myeloid progenitor cells, and T and B lymphocytes (Fig 7–6). TGFβ at 10^{-10}–10^{-12} mol/L blocks the proliferative effects of IL-2 on T and B cells, of BCGFs on B cells, and of IL-1 on thymocytes. In addition, TGFβ inhibits T cell-dependent polyclonal antibody production, mixed leukocyte reactions, and the in vitro generation of CTL. It also inhibits the induction of NK cell ac-

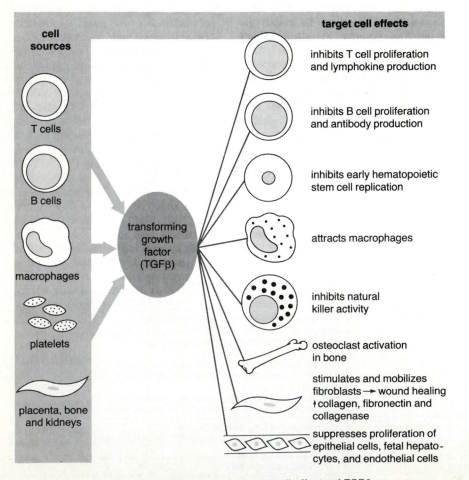

Figure 7–6. Cell sources and target cell effects of TGFβ.

tivities and the induction of lymphokine-activated killer cells by IL-2. Consequently, as a late product of activated T cells, TGFβ is unique in that it can act as a negative-feedback regulator that can dampen immunologically mediated inflammatory reactions.

SUMMARY

Exogenous as well as endogenous agents that induce or inhibit cytokine production or action can modulate immunologic reactions. Exogenous stimuli are of primary importance as inducers of endogenous cytokines. Most cytokines are produced by many cell types in response to noxious or physiologic stimuli, whereas lymphokines are produced only by lymphocytes and have largely immunoregulatory functions.

Lymphokines that are produced largely by T cells and by LGL, including IL-2, IL-4, IL-5, and IFN γ, act predominantly on lymphoid cells and are immunologically induced regulators of the immune response. However, IL-2, IL-4, and IL-5 can also modulate the function of a variety of other leukocytes such as macrophages, mast cells, and eosinophils, respectively; IFN γ also acts on a broad spectrum of cells in addition to lymphoid cells. In contrast, IL-3 is a lymphokine that acts as a hematopoietic growth factor. The other cytokines that modulate the activities of lymphoid and nonlymphoid cells are produced by many cell types and consist of IL-1, IL-6, IL-7, IL-8, TNF, IFN α, IFN β, and TGFβ. They presumably represent intercellular signals that enable connective tissues, skin, nervous system, and other tissues to communicate with the immune system.

Cytokines, in turn, regulate each other by competition, interaction, and mutual induction in a series of lymphokine cascades and circuits with positive or negative feedback effects. For example, cytokines such as IL-1 and IL-2 induce the production of other cytokines such as TNF and interferon. Furthermore, IL-1 and IL-2 induce each other reciprocally. Less well known, but perhaps equally important, are observations that even mesenchymal growth factors such as TGFβ can induce IL-1 production by macrophages.

In addition to cytokine regulation of cytokines, neuroendocrine hormonal peptides such as endorphins and corticosteroids, as well as products of the lipoxygenase and cyclooxygenase pathway, can have agonistic or antagonistic effects on some cytokine activities. The effects of cytokines can also be regulated at the level of cell membrane receptors. Agents that influence cytokine receptor expression modulate the activities of these mediators. Thus, a complex network of endogenous ligand-receptor interactions is involved in regulating host defense mechanisms. The therapeutic use of cytokines is still in its infancy. However, some disease states have already been shown to respond to interferon and IL-2. Agonists and antagonists of the cytokines and their receptors will probably play an important role in the eventual therapy of inflammatory, infectious, autoimmune, and neoplastic diseases.

REFERENCES

General
Aarden LA et al: Revised nomenclature for antigen-nonspecific T cell proliferation and helper factors. *J Immunol* 1979;**123**:2978.
Gillis S (editor): *Recombinant Lymphokines and Their Receptors.* Marcel Dekker, 1987.
Pick E (editor): *Lymphokines.* Vols 9–14. Academic Press, 1984–1987.

Interleukin-1
Dinarello CA: Biology of interleukin-1. *FASEB J* 1988;**2**:108.
Durum SK, Oppenheim JJ, Neta R: Role of interleukin-1. In: Oppenheim JJ, Shevach EM (editors): *Textbook of Immunophysiology.* Oxford University Press (in press).
Mizel SB: Interleukin-1 and T cell activation. *Immunol Today* 1987;**8**:330.
Neta R, Oppenheim JJ: Why should internists be interested in IL-1? *Ann Intern Med* 1988.
Oppenheim JJ et al: There is more than one IL-1. *Immunol Today* 1986;**7**:45.

Tumor Necrosis Factor
Beutler B, Cerami A: Cachectin and tumor necrosis factor as two sides of the same biological coin. *Nature* 1986;**320**:584.
Beutler B et al: Control of cachectin (tumor necrosis factor) synthesis: mechanism of endotoxin resistance. *Science* 1986;**232**:977.
Carswell EA et al: An endotoxin-induced serum factor that causes necrosis of tumors. *Proc Natl Acad Sci USA* 1975;**72**:3666.
Le J, Vilcek J: TNF and IL-1: Cytokines with multiple overlapping biological activities. *Lab Invest* 1987;**56**:234.
Old LJ: Tumor necrosis factor (TNF). *Science* 1985;**230**:630.
Paul NL, Ruddle NH: Lymphotoxin. *Annu Rev Immunol* 1988;**6**:407.

Interleukin-2, -4, and -5
Greene WC, Leonard WJ: The human IL-2 receptor. *Annu Rev Immunol* 1986;**4**:69.
Kishimoto T, Hirano T: Molecular regulation of B lymphocyte response. *Annu Rev Immunol* 1988;**6**:485.

Paul WE, Ohara J: B cell stimulatory factor-1/interleukin-4. *Annu Rev Immunol* 1987;**5:**429.

Rosenberg S, Lotze M: Cancer immunotherapy using IL-2 and IL-2- activated lymphocytes. *Annu Rev Immunol* 1985;**4:**681.

Smith K: The two-chain structure of high-affinity IL-2 receptors. *Immunol Today* 1987;**8:**11.

Smith KA: Interleukin-2: inception, impact and implications. *Science* 1988;**240:**1169.

Interferons

DeMaeyer E, DeMaeyer-Guignard J: *Interferons and Other Regulatory Cytokines.* Wiley, 1988.

Faltynek CR, Kung H-F: The biochemical mechanisms of action of the interferons. *Biofactors* 1988;**1:**277.

Friedman RM, Vogel SN: Interferons with special emphasis on the immune system. *Adv Immunol* 1983;**34:**97.

Pestka S et al: Interferons and their actions. *Annu Rev Biochem* 1987;**56:**727.

Taylor-Papadimitriou J: The effects of interferon in the growth and function of normal and malignant cells. In: *Interferons from Molecular Biology to Clinical Application.* Burke DC, Morris AG (editors). Cambridge University Press, 1983.

Vilcek J, DeMaeyer E (editors): *Interferon 2: Interferons and the Immune System.* Elsevier/North-Holland, 1984.

Interleukin-6

Billiau A: Interferon B2 as a promoter of growth and differentiation of B cells. *Immunol Today* 1987;**8:**84.

Kawano M et al: Autocrine generation and requirement of BSF-2/IL-6 for human multiple myelomas. *Nature* 1988;**332:**83.

Revel M: Interleukin-6. In: *Monokines and Other Non-Lymphocytic Cytokines.* Powanda M et al (editors). Liss, 1988.

Wong GC, Clark SC: Multiple actions of IL-6 within a cytokine network. *Immunol Today* 1988;**9:**137.

Hematopoietic Cytokines

Clark S, Kamen R: Human hematopoietic colony-stimulating factors. *Science* 1987;**236:**1229.

Golde D, Glasson J: Myeloid growth factors in inflammation. In: *Inflammation: Basic Principles & Clinical Correlates.* Gallin J, Goldstein I, Snyderman R (editors). Raven Press, 1988.

Ihle JN: Lymphokine regulation of hematopoietic development. In: *Textbook of Immunophysiology.* Oppenheim JJ, Shevach EM (editors). Oxford University Press (in press).

Metcalf D: Molecular biology and functions of granulocyte-macrophage colony-stimulating factors. *Blood* 1986;**67:**257.

Metcalf D: Role of colony-stimulating factors in resistance to acute infections. *Immunol Cell Biol* 1987;**65:**35.

Transforming Growth Factor β

Ellingsworth LR: Effect of growth factors on immunity and inflammation. In: *Textbook of Immunophysiology.* Oppenheim JJ, Shevach EM (editors). Oxford University Press (in press).

Sporn MB et al: TGFβ biological function and chemical structure. *Science* 1986;**233:**532.

Other Cytokines

Goodwin RG et al: Human interleukin-7: molecular cloning and growth factor activity on human and murine B-lineage cells. *Proc Natl Acad Sci USA* 1989;**86:**302.

Matsushima K et al: Molecular cloning of a human monocyte-derived neutrophil chemotactic factor (MDNCF) and the induction of MDNCF mRNA by IL-2 and TNF. *J Exp Med* 1988;**167:**1883.

Peveri P et al: A novel neutrophil-activating factor produced by human mononuclear phagocytes. *J Exp Med* 1988;**167:**1547.

Immunogenicity & Antigenic Specificity

Joel W. Goodman, PhD

8

Immunogenicity is a property that allows a substance to induce a detectable immune response (humoral or cellular or, most commonly, both) when introduced into an animal. Such substances are called "immunogens." The older term "antigen" now refers to agents that can react with antibodies evoked by immunogens, whether or not they are themselves immunogenic. It follows that all immunogens are also antigens, although the converse is not true. Low-molecular-weight compounds, including many drugs and antibiotics, are nonimmunogenic but, when coupled to immunogenic proteins, give conjugates that can raise antibodies against the low-molecular-weight component. This component can react with such an antibody by itself (see the section below on haptens) and thus is antigenic but not immunogenic.

The term **epitope** refers to the part of an antigen that combines with specific antibody or T cell receptor. The term "antigenic determinant" was previously used to connote what we now call an epitope. These terms are in contrast with the term "immunogenic determinant," which connotes immunogenicity, not merely antigenicity.

IMMUNOGENS

Chemical Nature of Immunogens

The most potent immunogens are macromolecular proteins, but polysaccharides, synthetic polypeptides, and other synthetic polymers such as polyvinylpyrrolidone are immunogenic under appropriate conditions (see below). Although pure nucleic acids or lipids have not been shown to be immunogenic, antibodies that react with them may be induced by immunization with nucleoproteins or lipoproteins. Antibodies reactive with DNA appear spontaneously in the serum of patients with systemic lupus erythematosus (see Chapter 36).

Requirements for Immunogenicity

Immunogenicity is not an inherent property of a molecule, as are its physicochemical characteristics, but is operationally dependent on the experimental conditions of the system. These include the immunogen, the mode of immunization, the organism being immunized, and the sensitivity of the methods used to detect a response. The factors that confer immunogenicity on molecules are complex and incompletely understood, but it is known that certain conditions must be satisfied in order for a molecule to be immunogenic.

A. Foreignness: The immune system somehow discriminates between "self" and "nonself," so that only molecules that are foreign to the animal are normally immunogenic. Thus, albumin isolated from the serum of a rabbit and injected back into the same or another rabbit will not generate the formation of antibody. Yet the same protein injected into other vertebrate animals is likely to evoke substantial amounts of antibody depending on the dose of antigen and the route and frequency of injection.

B. Molecular Size: Extremely small molecules such as amino acids or monosaccharides are not immunogenic, and it is generally accepted that a certain minimum size is necessary for immunogenicity. However, there is no specific threshold below which all substances are inert and above which all are active, but rather a gradient of immunogenicity with molecular size. In a few instances, substances with molecular weights of less than 1000 have proved to be immunogenic, but as a general rule molecules smaller than molecular weight 10,000 are only weakly immunogenic or not immunogenic at all. The most potent immunogens are macromolecular proteins with molecular weights greater than 100,000.

C. Chemical Complexity: A molecule must possess a certain degree of chemical complexity to be immunogenic. The principle has been illustrated very clearly with synthetic polypeptides. Homopolymers consisting of repeating units of a single amino acid are poor immunogens regardless of size, whereas copolymers of 2 or—even better—3 amino acids may be quite active. Once again, it is difficult to establish a definite threshold, and the general rule is that immunogenicity increases with structural complexity. Aromatic amino acids contribute more to immunogenicity than nonaromatic residues, since relatively simple random polypeptides containing tyrosine are better antigens than the same polymers without tyrosine, and immunogenicity is proportionate to the tyrosine content of the molecule. Also, the attachment of tyrosine chains to the weak immunogen gelatin, which is poor in aromatic amino acids, markedly enhances its immunogenicity.

D. Genetic Constitution of the Animal: The ability to respond to a particular antigen is a function of the way the immune response is controlled genetically. It has been known for some time that pure polysaccharides are immunogenic when injected into mice and humans but not when injected into guinea pigs. Much additional information has accrued from the use of inbred strains of animals. As one of many examples, strain 2 guinea pigs respond readily in an easily detectable manner to poly-L-lysine, whereas strain 13 guinea pigs do not. The ability to respond is inherited as an autosomal dominant trait. Many analogous examples have been described in humans, and the genetic control of the human immune response is discussed in Chapter 4.

E. Method of Antigen Administration: Whether an antigen will induce an immune response depends on the dose and the mode of administration. A quantity of antigen that is ineffective when injected intravenously may evoke a copious antibody response if injected subcutaneously in adjuvant (see below). In general, once the threshold is exceeded, increasing doses lead to increasing—but less than proportionate—responses. However, excessive doses may not only fail to stimulate antibody formation; they can also establish a state of specific unresponsiveness or tolerance.

ADJUVANTS

The response to an immunogen can be enhanced if it is administered as a mixture with substances called **adjuvants.** Adjuvants function in one or more of the following ways: (1) by prolonging retention of the immunogen, (2) by increasing its effective size, or (3) by stimulating the influx of populations of macrophages and/or lymphocytes. A number of adjuvants have been

used in experimental animals, the most potent being Freund's complete adjuvant (CFA), a water-in-oil emulsion containing killed mycobacteria. CFA presumably works by providing a depot for the immunogen and by stimulating macrophages and certain lymphocytes, but its very strong inflammatory effect precludes its use in humans. A muramyl dipeptide constituent of mycrobacterial cell walls has also been found to possess adjuvant activity. The most widely used adjuvant in humans is a suspension of aluminum hydroxide on which the immunogen is adsorbed (alum precipitate). This adjuvant increases the effective particle size of the immunogen, promoting its presentation to lymphocytes (see Chapter 5).

EPITOPES

Although strong immunogens are large molecules, only restricted portions of them are involved in actual binding with antibody combining sites. Such areas, which determine the specificity of antigen-antibody reactions, are designated epitopes (previously called antigenic determinants). The number of distinct determinants on an antigen molecule usually varies with its size and chemical complexity. Estimates of the number of epitopes on an antigen have been made on the basis of the number of antibody molecules bound per molecule of antigen. Such measurements provide minimum values, since steric hindrance may prevent simultaneous occupation of all sites. Furthermore, antibody populations from different animals are likely to vary in specificity, and variations also occur in specificities of a single individual at different times. This means that antibodies specific for all epitopes of an antigen molecule may not be present in a particular antiserum. Typical results for this approach are about 5 epitopes for hen egg albumin (MW 42,000) and as many as 40 for thyroglobulin (MW 700,000). However, it has been found that virtually any region on the exposed surface of a protein may serve as an epitope.

Size & Location of Epitopes

Antibody complementarity is directed against limited parts of the antigen molecule. Numerous studies with homopolymers of sugars or amino acids or multichain polymer-protein conjugates indicate that an epitope is of the order of 4–6 amino acid or sugar residues (Fig 8–1). The weight of evidence also indicates that the entire exposed surface of a protein may be antigenic. Therefore, large proteins express many potential epitopes. However, a given individual will make antibodies against only a small subset of the total. For exam-

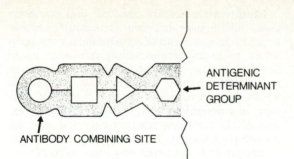

Figure 8–1. A view of the "lock-and-key" complementariness between an antigenic determinant group and an antibody combining site. The determinant can be considered to be composed of discrete subunits, which may be amino acids in a peptide chain or sugars in a saccharide chain. The antibody combining site is then composed of subsites, each of which can accommodate a discrete subunit of the antigenic determinant. (Reproduced, with permission, from Goodman JW: Antigenic determinants and antibody combining sites. In: *The Antigens*. Vol 3. Sela M [editor]. Academic Press, 1975.)

A cardinal factor in the selection of epitopes is exposure of the structure to the aqueous environment and therefore to the immune apparatus. The terminal side chains of polysaccharides represent the most potent epitope regions of that class of compounds. The principle has been demonstrated most vividly with multichain synthetic polypeptides having sequences of alanine on the outside and tyrosine-glutamic acid closer to the backbone, or the reverse (Fig 8–2). Antibodies to the former were largely alanine-specific, whereas the latter evoked antibodies with a predominant specificity for tyrosine-glutamic acid sequences. The most exposed region was preferred as the determinant in each instance. The same is generally true for globular proteins. A feature of proteins that correlates well with accessibility and has had predictive value for identifying epitopes is the **hydrophilicity** of local regions within the protein. The greater the average hydrophilicity, the higher the likelihood that the region will be antigenic.

In addition to accessibility, which is an intrinsic feature of the antigen, host factors play important roles in epitope selection and probably account for the different specificity patterns in antisera from different individuals. A large body of evidence attests to the genetic control of antibody specificity to a given antigen. Some of the earliest evidence accrued from a comparison of the specificity of anti-insulin antibodies from strain 2 and strain 13 guinea pigs, which are uniformly di-

ple, as noted above, a given antiserum to hen egg albumin has specificity for no more than about 5 epitopes. Since the total number when comparing different antisera is much greater, there is obviously a selection of potential epitopes in any given immunization.

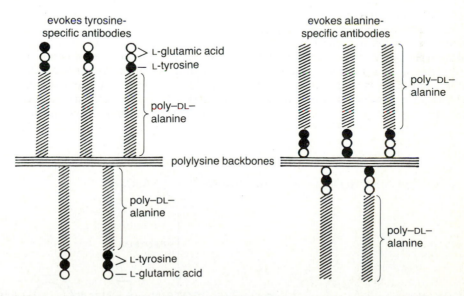

Figure 8–2. *Left:* A multichain copolymer in which L-tyrosine and L-glutamic acid residues are attached to multi-poly-DL-alanyl-poly-L-lysine(poly-[Tyr,Glu]-poly-DL-Ala-poly-Lys). *Right:* Copolymer in which tyrosine and glutamic acid are attached directly to the polylysine backbone with alanine peptides on the ends of the side chains. Horizontal lines: poly-L-lysine; diagonal hatching: poly-DL-alanine; closed circles; L-tyrosine; open circles: I-glutamic acid. (From Sela M: Antigenicity: Some molecular aspects. *Science* 1969;**166**:1365. Copyright© 1969 by the American Association for the Advancement of Science.)

rected against opposite ends of the insulin molecule. Outbred populations are more difficult to study, but the principle that genetic makeup strongly influences epitope selection has been clearly established (see Chapter 4).

Haptens

Much of our understanding of the specificity of antigen-antibody reactions derives from the pioneering studies of Karl Landsteiner in the early years of the 20th century with small, chemically defined substances which are not immunogenic but can react with antibodies of appropriate specificity. They are called haptens, from the Greek word *haptein,* "to fasten." Landsteiner covalently coupled the diazonium derivatives of a wide variety of aromatic amines to the lysine, tyrosine, and histidine residues of immunogenic proteins (Fig 8-3). The conjugated proteins raised antibody specific for the azo substituents, as demonstrated by the capacity of the free hapten to bind antibody. The conjugated hapten therefore becomes a partial or complete epitope. The total epitope may include amino acids in the protein to which the hapten is linked. The protein, called the **carrier,** has its set of native or integral epitopes as well as the new ones introduced by the conjugated hapten (Fig 8-4).

Although most haptens are small molecules, macromolecules may also function as haptens. The definition is based not on size but on immunogenicity.

The use of hapten-protein conjugates has spotlighted the remarkable diversity of immune mechanisms as well as the exquisite structural specificity of antigen-antibody reactions. Virtually any chemical entity may serve as an epitope if coupled to a suitably immunogenic carrier. Even antibodies with specificity for metal ions have been produced in this way.

Landsteiner's studies showed that antibody could distinguish between structurally similar haptens. In one series of experiments, antibodies raised to *m*-aminobenzenesulfonate were tested for their ability to bind with other isomers of the homologous hapten and related molecules in which the sulfonate group was replaced by arsonate or carboxylate groups (Table 8-1). As expected, the strongest reaction occurred with the homologous hapten. The compound with the sulfonate group in the *ortho* position was somewhat poorer than the *meta* isomer but distinctly better than the *para* isomer. The substitution of arsonate for sulfonate resulted in very weak binding with antibody. Although both substituents are negatively charged and have a tetrahedral structure, the arsonate group is bulkier because of the larger size of the arsenic atom and the additional hydrogen atom. The benzoate derivatives are also negatively charged, but the carboxylate ion has a planar rather than tetrahedral 3-dimensional configuration and shows even less affinity for the antisulfonate antibody.

The reaction of antibody with an antigen or hapten other than the one that induced its formation is called a **cross-reaction.** Thus, the reaction of anti-*m*-aminobenzenesulfonate with any of the other compounds in Table 8-1 is a cross-reaction. Cross-reactions almost invariably have a lower binding affinity than homologous reactions between antibody and its inducing antigen.

Studies of this kind have shown that antibody recognizes the overall 3-dimensional shape of the epitope group rather than any specific chemical property such as ionic charge. It is believed that epitopes and antibody combining sites possess a structural complementariness which may be figuratively visualized as a "lock-and-key" arrangement (Fig 8-1). The electron cloud box of the antibody site is contoured to match that of the

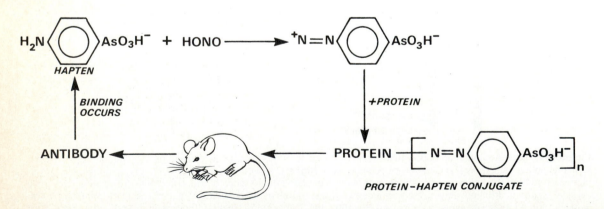

Figure 8-3. The preparation of hapten-protein conjugates and their capacity to induce the formation of antihapten antibody to the azophenylarsonate group in this example.

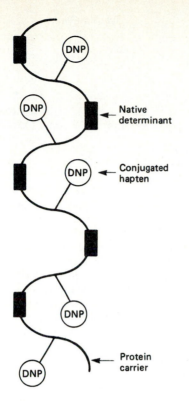

Figure 8-4. Diagrammatic illustration of a hapten-protein conjugate. The protein has several native or integral antigenic determinants denoted by thickened areas. The conjugated dinotrophenyl (DNP) hapten introduces new antigenic determinants.

Table 8-1. Effect of variation in hapten structure on strength of binding to *m*-aminobenzenesulfonate antibodies.

	ortho	meta	para
R = sulfonate	+ +	+ + +	±
R = arsonate	−	+	−
R = carboxylate	−	±	−

Strength of binding is graded from negative (−) to very strong (+ + +). (From Landsteiner K, van der Scheer J: On cross reactions of immune sera to azoproteins. *J Exp Med* 1936; **63**:325.)

epitope, with the affinity of binding directly proportionate to the closeness of fit. The startling diversity of the antibody response is perhaps more comprehensible if antibody specificity is viewed as directed against a molecular shape rather than a particular chemical structure.

Immunodominance

Given a particular epitope, which may be the size of a tetrapeptide, the amino acid subunits of that epitope will contribute unequally to binding with antibody. The degree of the influence on reactivity is a measure of the immunodominance of the component.

Antibody specificity may be directed against conformational or sequential features of antigens. The former usually holds for globular proteins and helical structures. For example, polymers of the tripeptide L tyrosyl-L alanyl-L glutamic acid form an α-helix under physiologic conditions. The same tripeptide can be attached to a branched synthetic polypeptide (Fig 8–5). The tripeptide itself does not possess an ordered configuration. Antibodies to the 2 polymers do not cross-react, and the tripeptide binds antibodies produced against the branched polymer but not those made against the helical polymer. The immunodominant element of the helical polymer is its conformation. Antiserum against human hemoglobin A_1 combines better with the oxygenated form than with the reduced form, and this has been attributed to the difference in quaternary structure between the 2 forms. There are many examples of conformation-dependent antibody specificity.

Epitopes whose specificity is dictated by the sequence of subunits (amino acids or sugars) within the epitopes rather than by the macromolecular superstructure of the antigen molecule are designated **sequential epitopes.** In such cases, components of the epitope can act as haptens and bind with antibody, the reaction being demonstrable either directly, by such techniques as equilibrium dialysis or fluorescence quenching, or indirectly, by inhibition of the reaction between antigen and antibody. Sequential epitopes may be composed of terminal or internal sequences of macromolecules, or they may be artificially added to carriers, as in the case of the tripeptide Tyr-Ala-Glu. Characterization of the antigenic structure of several proteins has shown that sequential epitopes are always localized in hydrophilic regions of the molecule, where exposure to the aqueous environment is maximal.

When the epitope is a terminal sequence, the terminal residue of the sequence is almost invariably the immunodominant subunit. Again, many examples exist to illustrate this point, which was recognized by Landsteiner when he showed that the terminal amino acid of peptides coupled to a

Tyr–Ala–Glu

Tyr
Ala
Glu

Glu
Ala
Tyr

← DL–Ala
← Lys

(Tyr–Ala–Glu)ₙ
(MW 100,000; *a*-helix)

(75,000 MW; multichain)

Figure 8-5. A synthetic branched polymer in which peptides of sequence Tyr-Ala-Glu are attached to the amino groups of side chains in multi-poly-DL-alanyl-poly-L-lysine *(left)* and a periodic polymer of the tripeptide Tyr-Ala-Glu *(right)*. (From Sela M: Antigenicity: Some molecular aspects. *Science* 1969;**166**:1365. Copyright© 1969 by the American Association for the Advancement of Science.)

protein carrier exerted a dominant effect on specificity. Goebel made the same observation with glycosides conjugated to protein carriers. In general, then, it may be concluded that all epitopes exhibit a gradient of immunodominance. When the epitope is composed of a terminal sequence, the gradient decreases from the most exposed portion inward.

In addition, epitopes may be continuous or discontinuous. If antibodies bind to a contiguous sequence of amino acids, the epitope is continuous. A discontinuous epitope, on the other hand, is composed of residues that are separated from one another in the sequence of the protein but are brought into proximity by tertiary folding. There are numerous examples of discontinuous epitopes in proteins. Conformational epitopes may be continuous or discontinuous, but sequential epitopes are always continuous.

IMMUNOGENIC DETERMINANTS

Immunogens are normally large molecules, and immunogenicity is, within limits, a function of molecular size and complexity. A characteristic of immunogens is their capacity to induce cellular immunity mediated by T lymphocytes (see Chapter 5), which haptens are unable to do. It is believed that an immunogen must possess at least 2 determinants to stimulate antibody formation, which is the function of another line of lymphocytes, B cells. At least one determinant must be capable of triggering a T cell response. Our concern here is with structural determinants of immunogens that interact with T and B lymphocytes. Early studies with small, well-defined immunogens supported the interpretation that specificities of the 2 cell types may be directed against different determinants of the antigen molecule. In recent years, more than 50 epitopes that activate T cells have been found on large proteins.

The pancreatic hormone glucagon consists of only 29 amino acids but is immunogenic. It has been functionally dissected into component determinants that interact with T cells (immunogenic determinants) and with antibody (haptenic determinants). Using isolated tryptic peptides of the hormone, it was found that antibodies recognized a determinant or determinants in the amino terminal part of the molecule, whereas T lymphocytes responded only to the carboxy-terminal fragment (Fig 8-6). The latter was therefore identified as the immunogenic or "carrier" portion of the molecule and the former as the haptenic region.

Several synthetic molecules about the size of a single antigenic determinant induce an almost purely cellular immune response, with little or no antibody production, but are capable of acting as carriers for conjugated haptens in much the same fashion as macromolecular immunogens are. One such unideterminant immunogen is the compound L-tyrosine-*p*-azobenzenearsonate (ABA-Tyr). Despite its molecular weight of only 409, ABA-Tyr

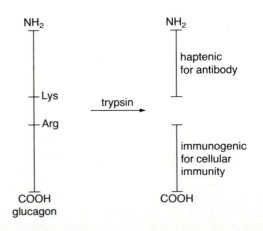

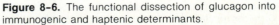

Figure 8-6. The functional dissection of glucagon into immunogenic and haptenic determinants.

induces cellular immunity with little or no antibody production in a variety of animal species. A hapten such as the dinitrophenyl group can be coupled to ABA-Tyr through a spacer group (6-aminocaproic acid) to produce a bideterminant or bifunctional immunogen (Fig 8–7). This antigen induces antibody specific for the dinitrophenyl haptenic determinant and cellular immunity directed against the ABA-Tyr immunogenic determinant. The concept of archetypal bifunctional immunogens has recently been applied to construction of synthetic peptide vaccines against infectious agents (see below).

Experiments with analogs of immunogenic determinants, designed along the lines of Landsteiner's classic studies on the specificity of antihapten antibodies, have shown that cellular (T cell) responses to antigens are as exquisitely specific as antigen-antibody reactions.

Recent findings indicate that in some instances different determinants on a protein antigen may activate different functional subpopulations of T cells (see Chapter 5). For example, different fragments of myelin basic protein induce suppression and immunity in rodents. Immunity is manifested as an autoimmune allergic encephalomyelitis. Animals presensitized with the suppressor-inducing fragment and subsequently challenged with the intact molecule did not develop encephalomyelitis. A determining factor in the selective activation of suppressor or helper T cells by particular determinants appears to be the genetic constitution of the animal. Thus, the same region (though perhaps not the identical determinant) of hen egg lysozyme induces suppression in strain B10 mice but helps in strain B10.A mice. Another example is the induction of suppression or help by a random synthetic copolymer of glutamic acid, alanine, and tyrosine in different inbred strains of mice.

The selective activation of help or suppression is being actively investigated, because it may eventually offer a rationale for manipulating the immune response in humans to such clinically important antigens as histocompatibility antigens, tumor antigens, and allergens.

THYMUS-INDEPENDENT ANTIGENS

A certain type of molecule may be immunogenic without the apparent participation of T lymphocytes. Such molecules appear to be able to directly trigger B lymphocytes (antibody-producing cells). Their characteristic feature is a structure that consists of repeating units. Bacterial polysaccharides and some polymerized proteins are thymus-independent antigens. However, not all repeating unit polymers behave this way. Poly-L-lysine, for example, is a thymus-dependent antigen in responder guinea pigs despite its simple, repetitive structure.

The mechanism by which thymus-independent antigens act is still unclear, but the immune response to such antigens differs from the response to more typical thymus-dependent antigens in that the antibody produced is largely or exclusively of the IgM class and little or no immunologic memory is engendered. Recent careful analysis of the responses to these antigens indicates that many, if not all, do require some degree of T cell help, although significantly less than that required by conventional thymus-dependent antigens. Therefore, it may be more accurate to consider them as thymus-efficient rather than as thymus-independent antigens.

SYNTHETIC VACCINES

Two promising new approaches to vaccine development have emerged in the modern era of biomedical technology. One is the cloning of genes coding for important surface proteins of infectious agents, with production of large quantities of the desired protein by microorganisms transfected with the gene. A recombinant vaccine containing the major surface protein of the hepatitis B virus has recently been approved and marketed.

The other approach is the chemical synthesis of short peptides from the known sequences of proteins from infectious organisms. The peptides

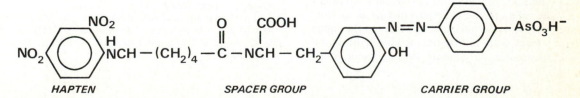

Figure 8–7. The bifunctional antigen dinitrophenyl-6-aminocaproyl-L-tyrosine-p-azobenzenearsonate.

may be linked to carriers, thereby becoming "synthetic antigens." This approach is predicated on the assumption that antibodies induced to short peptides of the order of 6–15 amino acids will react with the homologous sequences in the native proteins. Indeed, it has been shown that antibodies to many peptides representing sequences from the exposed surfaces of folded proteins, where they are accessible to antibody, do react with the native molecules, although the affinities of binding may be lower than with the peptides themselves. These findings offer promise for the manufacture of synthetic vaccines that are based on the hapten-carrier principle for use in human and animal prophylaxis. However, an important consideration is that immunologic memory in the response to hapten-carrier conjugates is directed primarily at the carrier, which bears the immunogenic determinants. Since the carriers are different in the synthetic vaccine and the native protein from which the peptide came, an encounter with the infectious agent following immunization with the synthetic vaccine should elicit little or no memory. Although sufficiently high antibody titers raised by the vaccine could provide substantial protection even without memory, this does represent a serious limitation for this type of vaccine.

An innovative way around the dilemma was taken in the design of a malaria vaccine based on the bifunctional immunogen concept discussed above. A helper T cell determinant on the circumsporozoite protein of *Plasmodium falciparum* was identified, synthesized, and covalently coupled to a second peptide representing the major haptenic determinant of the protein. The bifunctional conjugate elicited high-titer antibody responses in mice and induced anamnesis to the native protein. Although this vaccine technology is still in its infancy, it may signal the wave of the future.

SUMMARY

The immunologic properties of molecules include immunogenicity and antigenicity. Immunogenicity refers to the ability to induce an immune response, whereas antigenicity refers to the capacity to react with antibodies produced in an immune response. In general, immunogenicity is a function of foreignness of the immunogen to the individual being immunized, and increases with increasing molecular size and chemical complexity. However, peptides composed of only 8 or so amino acids can be immunogenic. The response to immunogens can be enhanced by adjuvants.

The subunit of an immunogen that actually binds with antibody is an antigenic determinant, or epitope. Large proteins possess many epitopes. The binding between antibody and antigen is exquisitely specific, but cross-reactions can occur between antibodies and other compounds bearing structurally related epitopes.

It is possible to raise antibodies to virtually any small compound (hapten) by coupling it to an immunogenic carrier and using the conjugate for immunization. The hapten is one of many epitopes of the complex conjugate and will react by itself with antibodies directed against it.

A number of immunogenic determinants or epitopes have been identified on immunogens. These structures are similar in size to antigenic determinants, but they trigger T cell responses and are responsible for immunogenicity. They may prove useful in the fabrication of relatively simple synthetic vaccines.

REFERENCES

Benjamin DC et al: The antigenic structure of proteins: A reappraisal. *Annu Rev Immunol* 1984;**2**:67.

Good MF et al: The T cell response to the malaria circumsporozoite protein: An immunological approach to vaccine development. *Annu Rev Immunol* 1988;**6**:663.

Goodman JW: Antigenic determinants and antibody combining sites. Page 127 in: *The Antigens*. Vol 3. Sela M (editor). Academic Press, 1975.

Goodman JW: Modelling determinants for recognition by B cells and T cells. *Prog Allergy* 1989;**56** (in press).

Goodman JW, Sercarz EE: The complexity of structures involved in T cell activation. *Annu Rev Immunol* 1983;**1**:465.

Goodman JW et al: Antigen structure and lymphocyte activation. *Immunol Rev* 1978;**39**:36.

Landsteiner K: *The Specificity of Serological Reactions*. Harvard Univ Press, 1945.

Lerner RA: Synthetic vaccines. *Sci Am* (Feb) 1983;**248**:66.

Livingston AM, Fathman CG: The structure of T cell epitopes. *Annu Rev Immunol* 1987;**5**:477.

Reichlin M: Amino acid substitution and the antigenicity of globular proteins. *Adv Immunol* 1975;**20**:71.

Sela M: Antigenicity: Some molecular aspects. *Science* 1969;**166**:1365.

Immunoglobulin Structure & Function

9

Joel W. Goodman, PhD

The immunoglobulins are proteins with antibody activity; ie, they combine specifically with the substance that elicited their formation (immunogen or antigen; see Chapter 8), and they make up the humoral arm of the immune response. With the possible exception of "natural" antibody, antibodies arise in response to foreign substances introduced into the body. They are therefore products of induced responses. The immunoglobulins, which circulate in body fluids, comprise a heterogeneous family of proteins, they account for approximately 20% of the total plasma proteins. In serum electrophoresis, the majority of immunoglobulins migrate as "gamma globulins," a historic but now archaic term.

The 2 hallmarks of immunoglobulins are the *specificity* of each for one particular antigenic structure and their *diversity* as a group, which meets the challenge of a vast array of antigenic structures in the environment. In addition to specifically binding antigens, the immunoglobulins express secondary biologic activities, which are important in defense against disease, eg, complement fixation, transplacental passage, and facilitation of phagocytosis. They are heterogeneous with respect to these activities, which are independent of the antigen-binding function of immunoglobulin molecules. This chapter explains how the structure of immunoglobulins accounts for their specificity, diversity, and secondary biologic activities.

BASIC STRUCTURE & TERMINOLOGY

Immunoglobulins are glycoproteins composed of 82–96% polypeptide and 4–18% carbohydrate. The polypeptide component possesses almost all of the biologic properties associated with antibody molecules. Antibodies are bifunctional molecules in that they bind specifically with antigen and also initiate a variety of secondary phenomena, such as complement fixation and histamine release by mast cells, which are independent of their specificity for antigen. Antibody molecules are extremely heterogeneous, as might be expected in view of their enormous diversity with respect to antigen binding and their different biologic activities. This heterogeneity is easily demonstrated by serologic, electrophoretic, and amino acid sequence methods and severely hampered early structural studies.

Two major discoveries ushered in the period of detailed structural study of antibodies. The first was the finding that enzymes and reducing agents could be used to digest or dissociate immunoglobulin molecules into smaller components. The second was the realization that the electrophoretically homogeneous proteins found in serum and urine of patients with multiple myeloma were related to normal immunoglobulins. These myeloma proteins were found to be structurally homogeneous. They are also called monoclonal proteins, since they are synthesized by single clones of malignant plasma cells. A clone here refers collectively to the progeny of a single lymphoid cell.

Our present understanding of immunoglobulin structure is based collectively on studies of monoclonal and normal proteins. The discussion of the details of immunoglobulin structure is introduced with a list of definitions of the relevant terms used here and in Figs 9–1 and 9–2.

List of Definitions

Basic unit (monomer): Each immunoglobulin contains at least one basic unit or monomer comprising 4 polypeptide chains (Fig 9–1).

H and L chains: One pair of identical polypeptide chains contains approximately twice the number of amino acids, or is approximately twice the molecular weight, of the other pair of identical polypeptide chains. The chains of higher molecular weight are designated **heavy (H) chains** (Fig 9–1) and those of lower molecular weight **light (L) chains.**

V and C regions: Each polypeptide chain con-

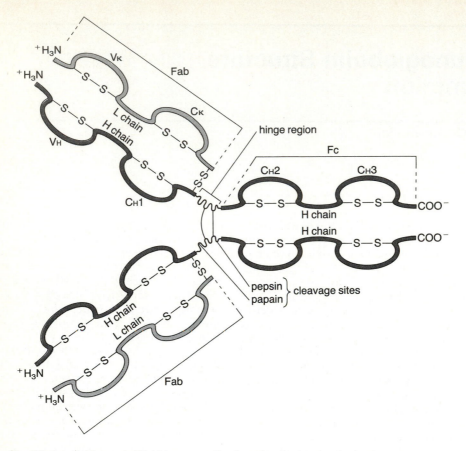

Figure 9–1. Simplified model for an IgG1 (κ) human antibody molecule showing the basic 4-chain structures and domains (V_H, C_H1, etc). V indicates the variable region; C indicates the constant region. Sites of enzyme cleavage by pepsin and papain are shown. Note portions of inter- and intrachain desulfide bonds.

tains an amino-terminal portion, the **variable (V) region;** and a carboxy-terminal portion, the **constant (C) region.** These terms denote the considerable heterogeneity or variability in the amino acid residues in the V region compared with the C region.

Domains: The polypeptide chains do not exist 3-dimensionally as linear sequences of amino acids but are folded by disulfide bonds into globular regions called domains. The domains in H chains are designated V_H and C_H1, C_H2, C_H3, and C_H4; and those in L chains are designated V_L and C_L.

Antigen-binding site: The part of the antibody molecule that binds antigen is formed by only small numbers of amino acids in the V regions of H and L chains. These amino acids are brought into close proximity by the folding of the V regions.

Fab and Fc fragments: Digestion of an immunoglobulin G (IgG) molecule by the enzyme pa-

pain produces 2 Fab (antigen-binding) fragments and one Fc (crystallizable) fragment.

Hinge region: The area of the H chains in the C region between the first and second C region domains (C_H1 and C_H2) is the hinge region. It is more flexible and is more exposed to enzymes and chemicals. Thus, papain acts here to produce Fab and Fc fragments.

F(ab)′₂ fragment: Digestion of an IgG molecule by the enzyme pepsin produces one F(ab)′₂ molecule and small peptides. The F(ab)′₂ molecule is composed of 2 Fab units and the hinge region, with intact inter-H chain disulfide bonds, since pepsin cleaves the IgG molecule on the carboxy-terminal side of the these bonds.

Disulfide bonds: Chemical disulfide (–S–S–) bonds between cysteine residues are essential for the normal 3-dimensional structure of immunoglobulins. These bonds can be interchain (H chain to H chain, H chain to L chain, L chain to L chain) or intrachain.

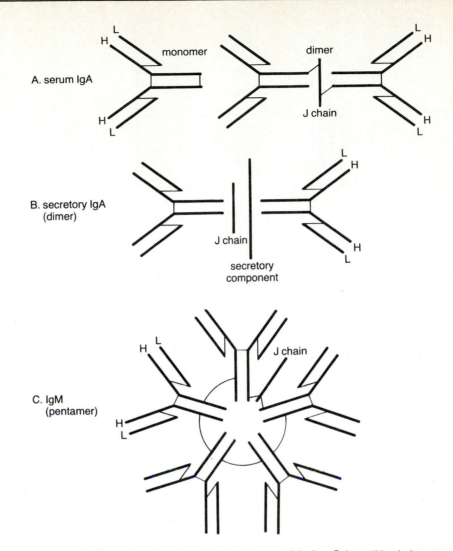

Figure 9-2. Highly schematic illustration of polymeric human immunoglobulins. Polypeptide chains are represented by thick lines; disulfide bonds linking different polypeptide chains are represented by thin lines.

Classes: There are 5 classes of immunoglobulins, designated IgG, IgA, IgM, IgD, and IgE (Table 9–1). They are defined by antigenic differences in the C regions of H chains. IgG, IgA, and IgM have been further subdivided into subclasses on the basis of relatively minor antigenic differences in C_H regions.

L chain types: L chains are divided into κ and λ types on the basis of antigenic determinants. Akin to the subclasses of H chains 4 subtypes of λ chains have been found.

Isotypes: These are the antigenic differences that characterize the class and subclass of H chains and the type and subtype of L chains. Each normal individual expresses all the isotypes characteristic of the species inasmuch as each isotype occupies a distinctive genetic locus in the genome.

Allotypes: These are polymorphic (allelic) forms of H and L chains that exhibit a mendelian pattern of inheritance. The antigenic determinants that characterize allotypes are usually localized to C regions. Thus, a particular isotype may have several alternative (allelic) structures.

Idiotypes: These are antigenic determinants that distinguish one V domain from all other V domains.

S value: The S value refers to the sedimentation coefficient of a protein, measured by the technique of Svedberg. S values of normal immunoglobulins range from 6S to 19S (Table 9–1). In general, the larger the S value of a protein, the higher its molecular weight.

Polymers: Immunoglobulins composed of more than a single basic monomeric unit are

Table 9-1. Properties of human immunoglobulin chains.

Designation	H Chains					L Chains		Secretory Component	J Chain
	γ	α	μ	δ	ϵ	κ	λ	SC	J
Classes in which chains occur	IgG	IgA	IgM	IgD	IgE	All classes	All classes	IgA	IgA, IgM
Subclasses or subtypes	1,2,3,4	1,2	1,2	…	…	…	1,2,3,4	…	…
Allotypic variants	Gm(1)–(25)	A2m(1), (2)	…	…	…	Km(1)–(3)[2]	…	…	…
Molecular weight (approximate)	50,000[1]	55,000	70,000	62,000	70,000	23,000	23,000	70,000	15,000
V region subgroups	$V_HI–V_HIV$					$V_\kappa I–V_\kappa IV$	$V_\lambda I–V_\lambda VI$		
Carbohydrate (average percentage)	4	10	15	18	18	0	0	16	8
Number of oligosaccharides	1	2 or 3	5	?	5	0	0	?	1

[1]60,000 for γ3.
[2]Formerly Inv(1)–(3).

termed polymers. The main examples are IgA dimers (2 units) and trimers (3 units) and IgM pentamers (5 units).

J chain: This is a polypeptide chain that is normally found in polymeric immunoglobulins.

Secretory component: IgA molecules in secretions are most commonly composed of 2 IgA units, one J chain, and an additional polypeptide, the secretory component.

FOUR-CHAIN BASIC UNIT

Immunoglobulin molecules are composed of equal numbers of heavy and light polypeptide chains, which can be represented by the general formula $(H_2L_2)_n$. The chains are held together by noncovalent forces and usually by covalent interchain disulfide bridges to form a bilaterally symmetric structure (Fig 9–1). It has been shown that all normal immunoglobulins have this basic structure, although some, as we shall see, are composed of more than one 4-chain unit.

Each polypeptide chain is made up of a number of loops or domains of rather constant size (100–110 amino acid residues) formed by the intrachain disulfide bonds (Fig 9–1). The N-terminal domain of each chain shows much more variation in amino acid sequence than the others and is designated the variable region to distinguish it from the other relatively constant domains (collectively called the constant region in each chain). The zone where the variable and constant regions join is termed the "switch" region.

Immunoglobulins are rather insensitive to proteolytic digestion but are most easily cleaved about midway in the heavy chain in an area between the first and second constant region domains (C_H1 and C_H2) (Fg 9–1). The enzyme papain splits the molecule on the N-terminal side of the inter-heavy chain disulfide bonds into 3 fragments of similar size: 2 Fab fragments, which include an entire light chain and the V_H and C_H1 domains of a heavy chain; and one Fc fragment, composed of the C-terminal halves of the heavy chains. If pepsin is used, cleavage occurs on the C-terminal side of the inter-H chain disulfide bonds, yielding a large $F(ab)'_2$ fragment composed of about 2 Fab fragments. The Fc fragment is extensively degraded by pepsin. The region in the H chain susceptible to proteolytic attack is more flexible and exposed to the environment than the more compact, globular domains and is known as the "hinge" region. Antigen-binding activity is associated with the Fab fragments or, more specifically, with the V_H and V_L domains, while most of the secondary biologic activities of immunoglobulins (eg, complement fixation) are associated with the Fc fragment.

HETEROGENEITY OF IMMUNOGLOBULINS

As already noted, immunoglobulin molecules comprise a family of proteins with the same basic molecular architecture but with a vast array of antigen-binding specificities and different biologic activities. These different activities are, of course, reflections of structural differences dictated by the amino acid sequence of the polypeptide chains. This structural heterogeneity has been an obstacle for protein chemists, but plasmacytomas of human and murine origin provide homogeneous (monoclonal) immunoglobulins that have greatly facilitated the study of the amino acid sequence of antibody molecules. Furthermore, it is now possible to produce at will virtually unlimited quantities of monoclonal antibodies of prescribed antigen specificity by somatic cell fusion of plasmacytoma cells with normal antibody-producing cells from immunized animals (see Chapter 18). The monoclonal antibodies produced by such somatic cell hybrids, or "hybridomas," are being used on a vast scale as diagnostic reagents.

Light Chain Types

All L chains have a molecular weight of approximately 23,000 but can be classified into 2 types, kappa (κ) and lambda (λ), on the basis of multiple structural differences in the constant regions, which are reflected in antigenic differences (Table 9–1). The 2 types of L chains have been demonstrated in many mammalian species. Indeed, the amino acid sequence homologies between human and mouse κ chains are much greater than those between the κ and λ chains within each species, indicating that the 2 types separated during evolution prior to the divergence of mammalian species.

The proportion of κ to λ chains in immunoglobulin molecules varies from species to species, being about 2:1 in humans. A given immunoglobulin molecule always contains identical κ or λ chains, never a mixture of the two.

Heavy Chain Classes

Five classes of H chains have been found in humans, based again on structural differences in the constant regions detected by serologic and chemical methods. The different forms of H chain, designated γ, α, μ, δ and ϵ (Table 9–1), vary in molecular weight from 50,000 to 70,000, the μ and ϵ chains possessing 5 domains (one V and four C) rather than the 4 of γ and α chains. The δ chain has an intermediate molecular weight which is believed to be due to an extended hinge region. Likewise, the $\gamma3$ chain has an extended hinge region consisting of about 60 amino acid residues, including 14 cysteines, which account for the large number of inter-heavy chain disulfide bonds in IgG3 (Fig 9–3).

The class of the H chain determines the class of the immunoglobulin. Thus, there are 5 classes of immunoglobulins: IgG, IgA, IgM, IgD, and IgE. Two γ chains combined with either two κ or two λ L chains constitute an IgG molecule, the major class of immunoglobulins in serum. Similarly, two μ chains and two L chains form an IgM subunit; IgM molecules are macroglobulins which consist of 5 of these basic 4-chain subunits (Fig 9–2). IgA is polydisperse, comprising 1–5 such units. The other classes (IgD and IgE), like IgG, consist of a single 4-chain unit. The classification and properties of immunoglobulins and their component polypeptide chains are summarized in Tables 9–1 and 9–2.

Subclasses of Polypeptide Chains

Most of the H chain classes have been further subdivided into **subclasses** on the basis of serologic or physicochemical differences in the constant regions. However, H chains representing the various subclasses within a class are much more closely related to each other than to the other classes. For example, there are 4 subclasses of γ chain in humans, $\gamma 1$, $\gamma 2$, $\gamma 3$, and $\gamma 4$ (Table 9–2), which yield IgG1, IgG2, IgG3, and IgG4 subclasses of immunoglobulin G molecules, respectively. The C regions of these γ chains are much more homologous to each other than to those of α, μ, δ, or ϵ chains. In some species, the charge spectra of the IgG subclasses differ sufficiently to permit their isolation by electrophoretic techniques. This is not true for human IgG subclasses, which have been recognized by serologic and chemical methods, facilitated by the existence of myeloma proteins and monoclonal antibodies.

A noteworthy aspect of the structural differences between the immunoglobulins subclasses is the number and arrangement of interchain disulfide bridges (Fig 9–3). In IgA2, the L chains are covalently linked to each other instead of to the H chains so that L–H binding is entirely by noncovalent forces. In other immunoglobulins, the

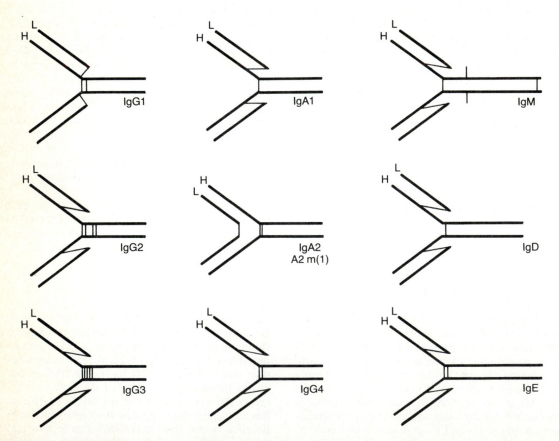

Figure 9-3. Distribution of interchain disulfide bonds in various human immunoglobulin classes and subclasses. H chains are represented by long thick lines and L chains by short thick lines. Disulfide bonds are represented by thin lines. The number of inter-heavy chain disulfide bonds in IgG3 may be as large as 14.

Table 9-2. Properties of human immunoglobulins.

	IgG	IgA	IgM	IgD	IgE
H chain class	γ	α	μ	δ	ϵ
H chain subclass	$\gamma1, \gamma2, \gamma3, \gamma4$	$\alpha1, \alpha2$	$\mu1, \mu2$		
L chain type	κ and λ	κ and λ	κ and λ	κ and λ	κ and λ
Molecular formula	γ_2L_2	$\alpha_2L_2{}^1$ or $(\alpha_2\text{-}L_2)_2SC^2J^3$	$(\alpha_2L_2)_5J^3$	δ_2L_2	ϵ_2L_2
Sedimentation coefficient (S)	6–7	7	19	7–8	8
Molecular weight (approximate)	150,000	160,000[1] 400,000[4]	900,000	180,000	190,000
Electrophoretic mobility (average)	γ	Fast γ to β	Fast γ to β	Fast γ	Fast γ
Complement fixation (classic)	+	0	+ + + +	0	0
Serum concentration (approximate; mg/dL)	1000	200	120	3	0.05
Serum half-life (days)	23	6	5	3	2
Placental transfer	+	0	0	0	0
Reaginic activity	?	0	0	0	+ + + +
Antibacterial lysis	+	+	+ + +	?	?
Antiviral activity	+	+ + +	+	?	?

[1] For monomeric serum IgA. [3] J chain.
[2] Secretory component. [4] For secretory IgA.

L–H bond may be formed close to the junction of the V_H and C_H1 domains or, alternatively, near the junction between C_H1 and C_H2 in IgG1.

As for L chains, κ chains do not exhibit C region subclasses, but 4 distinct λ chain forms have been discerned in humans which have apparently arisen by tandem gene duplication. These are called subtypes to distinguish them from H chain subclasses, which determine the subclass of the intact molecule. Since all H chains may be combined with any of the L chains, the latter play no role in determining the class or subclass of immunoglobulin. Put another way, the complete repertoire of κ and λ chains is found in each immunoglobulin subclass.

Allotypic (Allelic) Forms of Heavy & Light Chains

Some H and L chain isotypes bear genetic markers that are inherited in typical mendelian fashion. These alternative forms at a given genetic locus are called **allotypes.** In humans, allelic forms have been found for γ and α H chains and κ L chains. The allotypes associated with γ chains are designated "Gm" (for gamma), those associated with α chains are termed "Am," and those associated with κ L chains are called "Inv" (abbreviation of a patient's name). Thus far, allotypic forms of λ L chains or the H chains of IgM, IgD, and IgE have not been found.

Allotypy has been detected by using homologous (same species) antisera that react with antigenic determinants foreign to the immunoglobulins of the host. For example, mothers may become immunized to paternal allotypic determinants on fetal immunoglobulins during the course

of pregnancy. Alternatively, immunization may result from blood transfusions. Another source of detecting reagents has been the sera of some patients with rheumatoid arthritis, which contain "rheumatoid factors" reactive with IgG from some (not all) normal individuals (see Chapter 36). Such rheumatoid factors detect allotypic determinants. The structural differences that account for allotypic determinants usually involve only one or, at most, several amino acid substitutions in the constant regions of H and L chains.

SECRETORY COMPONENT & J CHAIN

Immunoglobulins are present not only in serum but also in various body secretions such as saliva, nasal secretions, sweat, breast milk, and colostrum. IgA is the predominant immunoglobulin class in the external secretions of most species. IgA usually exists in human serum as a 4-chain unit with a molecular weight of approximately 160,000 (7S). This unit may polymerize to give disulfide-bonded polymers with 8-chain, 12-chain, or larger structures. The IgA in secretions consists of two 4-chain units associated with one of each of 2 additional chain types, the secretory component and the J chain (Tables 9–1 and 9–2). The secretory component is associated only with IgA and is found almost exclusively in body secretions. The J chain is associated with all polymeric forms of immunoglobulins that contain 2 or more basic units. Fig 9–2 shows simplified models of secretory IgA and various polymeric serum immunoglobulins. Evidence suggests that binding of an

IgA to secretory component or J chain (or both) may promote the polymerization of additional monomeric 4-chain basic units. The secretory component may exist in free form or bound to IgA molecules by strong noncovalent interactions. The binding does not usually involve covalent bonding, although disulfide bonds have been implicated in a small fraction of human secretory IgA molecules. The secretory component is synthesized by nonmotile epithelial cells near the mucous membrane where secretion occurs. Its function may be to enable IgA antibodies to be transported across mucosal tissues into secretions.

The secretory component is a single polypeptide chain with a molecular weight of approximately 70,000. The carbohydrate content is high but not precisely known (Table 9–1). Its amino acid composition differs appreciably from that of every other immunoglobulin polypeptide chain, including J chain. No close structural relationship exists between the secretory component and any immunoglobulin polypeptide chain. Indeed, secretory component can be found free in secretions of individuals who lack mesaurable IgA in their serum or secretions.

J chain is a small acidic polypeptide that is synthesized by cells which secrete polymeric immunoglobulins.

Quantitative mesurements indicate that there is a single J chain in each IgM pentamer or polymeric IgA molecule. J chain is covalently bonded to the penultimate cysteine residue of α and μ chains. Whether or not J chain is required for the proper polymerization of the IgA and IgM basic unit is controversial. Polymeric immunoglobulins of certain lower vertebrates such as nurse shark and paddlefish are apparently devoid of J chain. These observations indicate that J chain is not an absolute requirement for polymerization of the immunoglobulin basic units. Nevertheless, the presence of J chain does facilitate the polymerization of basic units of IgA and IgM molecules into their appropriate polymeric forms.

CARBOHYDRATE MOIETIES OF IMMUNOGLOBULINS

Significant amounts of carbohydrate are present in all immunoglobulins in the form of simple or complex side chains covalently bonded to amino acids in the polypeptide chains (Table 9–1).

The function of the carbohydrate moieties is poorly understood. They may play important roles in the secretion of immunoglobulins by plasma cells and in the biologic functions associated with the C regions of H chains.

The attachment in most cases is by means of an N-glycosidic linkage between an N-acetylglu-cosamine residue of the carbohydrate side chain and an asparagine residue of the polypeptide chain. However, other linkages have also been observed, including an O-glycosidic linkage between an amino sugar of an oligosaccharide side chain and a serine residue of the polypeptide chain. In general, carbohydrate is found in only the secretory component, the J chain, and the C regions of H chains; it is not found in L chains or the V regions of H chains. Exceptions to this rule have been found in a small number of myeloma proteins. The secretory component has more carbohydrate than either the α chain or the L chain; this accounts for the higher carbohydrate content in secretory IgA than in serum IgA. Studies on monoclonal immunoglobulins indicated that IgM and IgE generally have an average of 5 oligosaccharides each; IgG, one oligosaccharide; and IgA, 2 or 3 oligosaccharides. This agrees with the overall carbohydrate content of immunoglobulins, since IgM, IgD, and IgE have the largest amounts of carbohydrate, followed by IgA and then by IgG (Table 9–1). However, these studies were performed on a limited number of monotypic immunoglobulins. In view of the findings that (1) different myeloma proteins of the same class or subclass may differ from one another in carbohydrate content, (2) an individual myeloma protein occasionally exhibits microheterogeneity with respect to its carbohydrate content, and (3) V regions of a small number of immunoglobulin polypeptide chains contain carbohydrate, it is incorrect to assume that all immunoglobulins belonging to a given class or subclass have the same number of oligosaccharide side chains.

BIOLOGIC ACTIVITIES OF IMMUNOGLOBULIN MOLECULES

As already noted, immunoglobulins are bifunctional molecules that bind antigens and, in addition, initiate other biologic phenomena which are independent of antibody specificity. These 2 kinds of activity can each be localized to a particular part of the molecule; antigen binding to the combined action of the V regions of H and L chains, and the other activities to the C regions of H chains. These latter activities, some of which are listed in Table 9–2, will be considered in this section.

Immunoglobulin G (IgG)

In normal human adults, IgG constitutes approximately 75% of the total serum immunoglobulins. Within the IgG class, the relative concentrations of the 4 subclasses are approximately as follows: IgG1, 60–70%; IgG2, 14–20%; IgG3, 4–8%; and IgG4, 2–6%. These figures vary somewhat from individual to individual and correlate weakly with the presence of certain H chain C region allotypic markers. Thus, the capacity of a given individual to produce antibodies of one or another IgG subclass may be under genetic control.

IgG is the only class of immunoglobulin that can cross the placenta in humans, and it is responsible for protection of the newborn during the first months of life (see Chapter 17). The subclasses are not equally endowed with this property, IgG2 being transferred more slowly than the others. The adaptive or biologic value of this inequality, if any, is obscure.

IgG is also capable of fixing serum complement (see Chapter 14), and once again the subclasses function with unequal facility in the following order: IgG3 > IgG1 > IgG2 > IgG4. IgG4 is completely unable to fix complement by the classic pathway (binding of C1q) but may be active in the alternative pathway. The specific location of the C1q binding site on the IgG molecule appears to reside in the C_H2 domain.

Macrophages bear surface receptors that bind IgG1 and IgG3 and their Fc fragments. The passive binding of antibodies by such Fc receptors is responsible for "arming" macrophages, which can then function in a cytotoxic fashion (see Chapter 12). Fc receptors on macrophages also facilitate phagocytosis of particulate antigens, such as bacteria, which are coated with antibody, a phenomenon known as **opsonization** (Fig 9–4). The specific location of the Fc receptor binding site on IgG1 and IgG3 molecules seems to be in the C_H3 domain.

The major differences between the subclasses of human IgG are summarized in Table 9–3.

Immunoglobulin A (IgA)

IgA is the predominant immunoglobulin class in the mucosal immune system (see Chapter 15).

Each secretory IgA molecule consists of two 4-chain basic units and one molecule each of secretory component and J chain (Fig 9–2). The molecular weight of secretory IgA is approximately 400,000. Secretory IgA provides the primary defense mechanism against some local infections owing to its abundance in saliva, tears, bronchial secretions, the nasal mucosa, prostatic fluid, vaginal secretions, and mucous secretions of the small intestine. The predominance of secretory IgA in membrane secretions led to speculation that its principal function may not be to destroy antigen (eg, foreign microbial organisms or cells) but rather to prevent access of these foreign substances to the general immunologic system. However, secretory IgA has been shown to prevent viruses from entering and infecting host cells. Hence, it may be important in antiviral defense mechanisms.

IgA normally exists in serum in both monomeric and polymeric forms, constituting approximately 15% of the total serum immunoglobulins.

Immunoglobulin M (IgM)

IgM constitutes approximately 10% of normal immunoglobulins and normally exists as a pentamer with a molecular weight of approximately 900,000 (19S). IgM antibody is prominent in early immune responses to most antigens and predominates in certain antibody responses such as "natural" blood group antibodies. IgM (with IgD) is the major immunoglobulin expressed on the surface of B cells. IgM is also the most efficient complement-fixing immunoglobulin, a single molecule bound to antigen sufficing to initiate the complement cascade (see Chapter 14).

Immunoglobulin D (IgD)

The IgD molecule is a monomer, and its molecular weight of approximately 180,000 (7–8S) is slightly higher than that of IgG. This immuno-

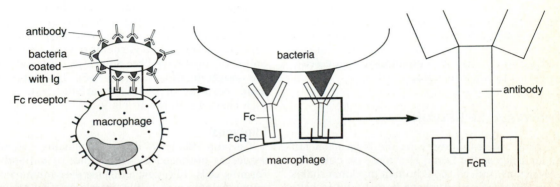

Figure 9–4. Schematic representation of phagocytosis of an antibody-coated bacterium. Note the Fc receptor (FcR) on the macrophage and its binding to the Fc portion of antibody and bound antigen (the bacterium).

Table 9-3. Properties of human IgG subclasses.

	IgG$_1$	IgG$_2$	IgG$_3$	IgG$_4$
Abundance (% of total IgG)	70	20	6	4
Half-life in serum (days)	23	23	7	23
Placental passage	+++	+	+++	+++
Complement fixation	++	+	+++	−
Binding to Fc receptors	+++	+	+++	−

globulin is normally present in serum in trace amounts (0.2% of total serum immunoglobulins). It is relatively labile to degradation by heat and proteolytic enzymes. There are isolated reports of IgD with antibody activity toward certain antigens, including insulin, penicillin, milk proteins, diphtheria toxoid, nuclear antigens, and thyroid antigens. However, the main function of IgD has not yet been determined. IgD (with IgM) is the predominant immunoglobulin on the surface of human B lymphocytes at certain stages of their development, and it has been suggested that IgD may be involved in the differentiation of these cells.

Immunoglobulin E (IgE)

The identification of IgE antibodies are reagins and the characterization of this immunoglobulin class marked a major breakthrough in the study of the mechanisms involved in allergic diseases (see Chapters 11 and 29). IgE has a molecular weight of approximately 190,000 (8S). It constitutes only 0.004% of the total serum immunoglobulins but binds with very high affinity to mast cells via a site in the Fc region. Upon combination with certain specific antigens called allergens, IgE antibodies trigger the release from mast cells of pharmacologic mediators responsible for the characteristic wheal-and-flare skin reactions evoked by the exposure of the skin of allergic individuals to allergens. IgE antibodies provide a striking example of the bifunctional nature of antibody molecules. "Allergen" is an alternative term used by allergists for any antigen that stimulates IgE production. IgE antibodies bind allergens through the Fab portion, but the binding of IgE antibodies to tissue cells is a function of the Fc portion. Like IgG and IgD, IgE normally exists only in monomeric form. It may also be important in defense against parasitic infections.

THE VARIABLE REGION

The V regions, comprising the N-terminal 110 amino acids of the L and H chains, are quite heterogeneous. Indeed, no 2 human myeloma chains from different patients have been found to have identical sequences in the V region. However, distinct patterns are discernible, and V regions have been divided into 3 main groups based on degree of amino acid sequence homology. These are the V_H group for H chains, V_κ group for κ L chains, and V_λ group for λ L chains. These V region groups are associated with the appropriate C region subclasses or subtypes for that particular polypeptide only. For example, a V_H sequence will be found only on an H chain, never on a κ or λ L chain, and so forth. However, a particular V_H sequence may associate with any C_H class (γ, α, μ, δ, or ε). The genes coding for associated V and C regions are probably linked (see Chapter 10).

V Region Subgroups

When the sequences of the V regions of κ chains are compared, they can be further divided into 4 subgroups which have substantial homologies. The subgroups differ from one another principally in the length and position of amino acid insertions and deletions and bear much closer structural homology to each other than to λ or H chain V regions. Similar subdivisions have been made in H chain V regions and λ chain V regions.

Hypervariable Regions

The V regions are not uniformly variable across their spans but consist of relatively invariant positions, which define the type and subgroup to which the V region belongs, as well as highly variable zones or "hot spots." A plot of the known variations versus position in the sequence reveals 3 or 4 peaks, depending on the chain type. These peaks of extreme variability are known as **hypervariable regions** and have been shown to be intimately involved in the formation of the antigen-binding site. L chains appear to have 3 hypervariable regions, while H chains have 4, although only 3 of the 4 have been shown to contribute to the antigen-binding site (Fig 9–5). The approximate locations of the hypervariable regions in each chain are shown in Fig 9–6.

Idiotypes

The term "idiotype" denotes the unique V region sequences produced by each clone of antibody-forming cells. Idiotypic antigenic determinants of immunoglobulin molecules were identified by immunizing animals with specific antibodies raised

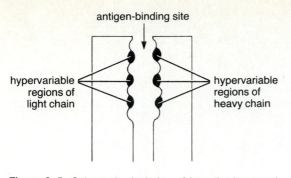

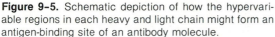

Figure 9-5. Schematic depiction of how the hypervariable regions in each heavy and light chain might form an antigen-binding site of an antibody molecule.

against a particular antigen in genetically similar animals. The only antigenic differences between the immunoglobulins of the donor and recipient were the unique V region sequences related to the specificity of the antibody. Thus, responses were restricted to such determinants. It is also possible to immunize across species lines to obtain anti-idiotype antisera, but in this case the antisera must be carefully absorbed with immunoglobulins from the donor species to render them specific for idiotypic markers.

In some cases, the reaction between anti-hapten antibody and anti-idiotypic antisera raised against that anti-hapten antibody can be inhibited by the hapten, indicating that the idiotypic antigenic determinants are close to or within the antigen-binding site of the antibody molecule. An antibody to idiotypic determinants is therefore regarded as an immunologic marker for the antibody combining

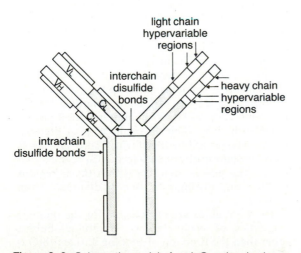

Figure 9-6. Schematic model of an IgG molecule showing approximate positions of the hypervariable regions in heavy and light chains.

site. Although it is not yet formally proved, idiotypic determinants are believed to be associated with hypervariable regions, which determine antibody specificity.

It seems legitimate to extend the term "idiotype" to any combination of a particular L chain V region with a particular H chain V region. That is, any such combination will express a unique idiotypic specificity. Since any L chain may combine with any H chain and a common pool of V_H regions is shared by the 5 different classes of H chains, it follows that idiotypic determinants may be shared by different immunoglobulin classes. Idiotypic determinants are heritable, at least in some cases, as observed in certain inbred strains of mice.

THE THREE-DIMENSIONAL STRUCTURE OF IMMUNOGLOBULINS

Although the inference that the polypeptide chains of immunoglobulin molecules are folded into compact globular domains separated by short linear stretches was derived initially from amino acid sequence studies, confirmation of this structural model required examination of crystallized immunoglobulins or their component parts by x-ray diffraction analysis (Fig 9-7). This work has shown that all domains have a characteristic pattern of folding, regardless of their origin. Thus, V region and C region domains from L chains and H chains all have a very similar appearance. In addition, there is close physical approximation between corresponding domains, ie, V_H and V_L, C_H1 and C_L, and the identical H chain domains in the Fc portion. X-ray diffraction analysis of a crystallized myeloma protein complexed with hapten (see Chapter 8) revealed that the contact points between antigen and the antibody-combining site are located in the hypervariable regions of the H and L chains.

Other evidence in favor of the domain model has come from limited proteolysis of immunoglobulins, in which the major products appear to consist of one or more domains (as expected, based on the model, since the areas between the domains are more exposed and consequently more susceptible to enzymatic attack). It has also been found that some of the proteins present in patients with H chain disease (see Chapter 48) have large deletions involving the entire C_H1 domain.

All domains, including those from the same polypeptide chain, different polypeptide chains, the same molecules, and different molecules, show a significant degree of amino acid homology. This led to the hypothesis that all immuno-

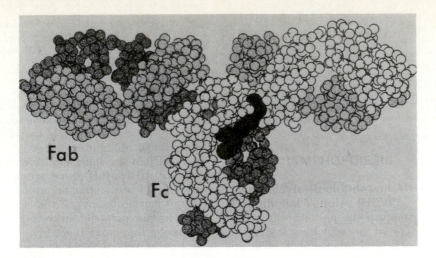

Figure 9–7. Three-dimensional structure of the immunoglobulin molecule. (Reproduced, with permission, from Silverton EW, Navia MA, Davies DR: Three-dimensional structure of an intact human immunoglobulin *Proc Natl Acad Sci USA* 1977;**74:**5140.)

globulin polypeptide chains evolved by a process of tandem gene duplication from a common ancestor that was equivalent to one domain.

CELL SURFACE IMMUNOGLOBULINS

Although, as noted earlier, IgM and IgD constitute the predominant membrane immunoglobulins, all classes of immunoglobulins have been found on the surfaces of B lymphocytes, where they function as antigen receptors. The membrane and secreted forms of μ, δ, and γ chains (and presumably α and ϵ chains as well) differ in structure. The membrane forms have an additional carboxy-terminal sequence of approximately 40 amino acid residues, which begins with a highly acidic sequence of 12–14 residues and terminates with a strikingly hydrophobic sequence of about 26 residues. The hydrophobic portion of the segment is believed to represent the transmembrane component anchoring the heavy chain in the cell membrane. It is similar in hydrophobicity and length to known transmembrane segments of other proteins, and it satisfies the requirements for the formation of a membrane-spanning alpha helix.

Whereas the acidic part of the membrane segment shows little amino acid sequence homology between heavy chain classes, the hydrophobic sequences of μ and γ chains show substantially greater homology than do the constant-region domains of those classes. This sequence conservation is puzzling, because transmembrane segments of other proteins seem to have little in common besides length and hydrophobicity.

SUMMARY

Immunoglobulins are glycoproteins and have a basic symmetric 4-chain structure composed of 2 identical heavy (H) and 2 identical light (L) chains, which are covalently joined by disulfide bonds. The chains are folded into domains consisting of about 100 amino acids, each of which is stabilized by an internal disulfide bond. The first domains of the H and L chains vary in structure (V domains) and make up the antigen-binding site. Thus, each immunoglobulin molecule has at least 2 identical binding sites (ie, it is bivalent). The structural variation between the V domains of different antibodies accounts for their specificity and diversity. The unique structure of each antibody V region is referred to as its idiotypic profile. The other domains make up the constant (C) regions of the 2 types of L chain (κ and λ) and the H chains. The 5 classes of immunoglobulins are distinguished by their H chain C (C_H) regions. Several classes are further divided into subclasses based on minor differences in the C_H regions. Allotypes are genetic markers within the C regions which can distinguish one individual from another.

The C_H regions are responsible for the biologic properties of each class of immunoglobulins, other than the function of binding antigen. IgG is the predominant class in serum and the only one that crosses the placenta and confers immunity on the fetus. It is also capable of fixing complement and promoting phagocytosis (opsonization). IgM exists in the pentameric form and fixes complement most efficiently. It is the earliest immunoglobulin to appear on the surface of developing B lymphocytes. IgA is the only class found in external secretions, where it is called secretory IgA and appears to be an efficient antiviral antibody. IgD is found on B lymphocytes at certain stages of their development and appears to be involved in their differentiation. IgE is responsible for many common allergies. It binds to receptors on mast cells and triggers degranulation of the cells upon contact with antigen. IgE may protect against parasitic infections.

REFERENCES

Alzari PM et al: Three-dimensional structure of antibodies. *Annu Rev Immunol* 1988;**6**:555.

Amos B (editor): *Progress in Immunology. I.* Academic Press, 1971.

Brent L, Holborow J (editors): *Progress in Immunology, II.* North-Holland, 1975.

Capra JD, Kehoe JM: Hypervariable regions, idiotypy, and the antibody-combining site. *Adv. Immunol* 1975:**20**:1.

Cunningham AJ (editor): *The Generation of Antibody Diversity: A New Look,* Academic Press, 1976.

Davie JM et al: Structural correlates of idiotypes. *Annu Rev Immunol* 1986;**4**:147.

Davies DR, Metzger H: Structural basis of antibody function. *Annu Rev Immunol* 1983;**1**:87.

Eisen HN: *Immunology.* Harper & Row, 1974.

Gergely J, Medgyesi GA (editors): *Antibody Structure and Molecular Immunology.* North-Holland, 1975.

Hilschmann N, Craig LC: Amino acid sequence studies with Bence Jones protein. *Proc Natl and Acad Sci USA* 1965;**53**:1403.

Hood L, Prahl JW: The immune system: A model for differentiation in higher organisms. *Adv Immunol* 1971;**14**:291.

Kehry M et al: The immunoglobulin μ chains of membrane-bound and secreted IgM molecules differ in their C-terminal segments. *Cell* 1980;**21**:393.

Koshland ME: The coming of age of the immunoglobulin J chain. *Annu Rev Immunol* 1985;**3**:425.

Mestecky J, Lawton AR (editors): *The Immunoglobulin A System.* Plenum Press, 1974.

Möller G (editor): Immunoglobulin D: Structure, synthesis, membrane representation and the function. *Immunol Rev* 1977; No. 37. [Entire issue.]

Natvig JB, Kunkel HG: Immunoglobulins: Classes, subclasses, genetic variants, and idiotypes. *Adv. Immunol* 1973;**16**:1.

Nisonoff A, Hopper JE, Spring SB: *The Antibody Molecule.* Academic Press, 1975.

Padian EA et al: Model-building studies of antigen-binding sites: The hapten-binding site of MOPC-315. *Cold Spring Harbor Symp Quant Biol* 1976;**41**:627.

Poljak RJ et al: Three-dimensional structure and diversity of immunoglobulins. *Cold Spring Harbor Symp Quant Biol* 1976;**41**:639.

Porter RR: Structural studies of immunoglobulins. *Science* 1973;**180**:713.

Spiegelberg HL: Biological activities of immunoglobulins of different classes and subclasses. *Adv Immunol* 1974;**19**:259.

Williams SF, Barclay AN: The immunoglobulin superfamily—domains for cell surface recognition. *Annu Rev Immunol* 1988;**6**:381.

Wu TT, Kabat EA: An analysis of the variable regions of Bence Jones proteins and myeloma light chains and their implications for antibody complementarity. *J Exp Med* 1970;**132**:211.

10   Immunoglobulin Genetics

Tristram G. Parslow, MD, PhD

To contend with the almost unlimited variety of antigens that it may encounter, the human immune system is able to produce an estimated 10^8 different antibody molecules, each with a unique specificity for antigen. How can so many different antibody proteins be encoded in the genes of every human being? The source of this diversity of antibodies lies in the structure of the immunoglobulin genes and in the remarkable ability of B cells to create and modify these genes by rearranging their own chromosomal DNA.

IMMUNOGLOBULIN GENES ARE FORMED THROUGH DNA REARRANGEMENT

The antigen specificity of an antibody is determined by amino acid sequences within its paired heavy (H) and light (L) chain variable (V) domains, which together form the antigen-binding site (see Chapter 9). To produce antibodies with many different specificities, the immune system must have the genetic capability to produce a very large number of different V domain sequences. The sequence of the constant (C) region, on the other hand, is generally the same for all H or L chains of a given immunoglobulin isotype and has no effect on antigen specificity. In fact, the entire family of immunoglobulin proteins consists of a relatively small number of different C region domains linked in various combinations with an almost unlimited assortment of V region sequences.

In 1965, Dreyer and Bennett first recognized that these interchangeable combinations of protein domains must be the result of an active reshuffling of gene fragments that takes place within the B cell chromosomes. This was a revolutionary insight, because it implied that a cell could efficiently manipulate its chromosomes to change the structure of genes that it had inherited. However, this proved to be only a part of the story: nearly a decade later, Tonegawa made the remarkable discovery that the inherited chromosomes contain no immunoglobulin genes at all, but only the building blocks from which these genes can

be assembled. Since that time, elegant molecular studies by Tonegawa and others have revealed in detail the extraordinary events that give rise to an immunoglobulin gene.

As with most human genes, the information that codes for an immunoglobulin protein is dispersed along the DNA strand in multiple coding segments (**exons**) that are separated by regions of noncoding DNA (**introns**); after the gene is transcribed into RNA, the introns are removed from the transcript and the exons are joined by RNA splicing. Unlike nearly all other genes, however, the immunoglobulin DNA sequences that are found in germ cells or other nonlymphocyte cell types do not exist as intact, functional genes. This is because the exons that code for V domains are normally broken up along the chromosome into still smaller gene segments; these segments each lack some of the features needed for proper RNA splicing and so cannot function individually as exons. Before a developing B cell can begin to synthesize immunoglobulin, it must fuse 2 or 3 of these gene segments to assemble a complete V region exon. This fusion of gene segments is achieved through a highly specialized process that requires cutting, rearrangement, and rejoining of the chromosomal DNA strands. The enzymatic machinery that is needed to carry out this process of immunoglobulin gene rearrangement is found only in developing lymphocytes.

LIGHT CHAIN GENES

The kappa (κ) L chain genes are the simplest and will be considered first. All of the genetic information needed to produce κ chains lies within a single locus on chromosome 2 (Fig 10–1). The C domain of the protein (amino acid residues 109–214) is encoded by an exon called C_κ, and only one copy of this exon is found on the chromosome. The sequence encoding any given V domain, however, is contained in 2 separate gene segments called the variable (V_κ) and joining (J_κ) segments. The V_κ segment encodes approximately the first 95 amino acids of the V domain; the shorter J_κ

unrearranged kappa locus

$V_{\kappa 1}$ $V_{\kappa 2}$ $V_{\kappa 3}$ $V_{\kappa n}$ J_1 J_2 J_3 J_4 J_5 C_κ

V/J joining

rearranged kappa gene

V/J_3 C_κ

transcription

primary transcript

RNA splicing

kappa mRNA

V J_3 C_κ

Figure 10–1. The assembly and expression of the κ L chain locus. A DNA rearrangement event fuses one V segment (in this example, $V_{\kappa 2}$) to one J segment ($J_{\kappa 3}$) to form a single exon. The V/J exon is then transcribed together with the unique C_κ exon, and the transcript is spliced to form mature κ mRNA. Note that any unrearranged J segments on the primary transcript are removed as part of the intron during RNA splicing.

achieved by specific enzymatic deletion of the chromosomal DNA that normally separates the 2 segments. Transcription can then begin at one end of the V segment and pass through both the fused V_κ/J_κ exon and the nearby C_κ exon. When transcribed together, these 2 exons contain all of the information needed to synthesize a particular κ protein.

The organization of the κ genes thus accounts for the unusual properties of this L chain protein family. Because there is only one C_κ exon, for example, all κ proteins must have identical C region sequences. On the other hand, because the cell can choose from among many alternatives V_κ and J_κ segments and can join these together in various combinations, a large number of different V domain sequences can result. For example, 100 V_κ and 5 J_κ segments could give rise to 500 (100 × 5) different V domains. This reshuffling process, known as "combinatorial joining," is the most important source of light chain protein diversity.

Lambda L chains arise from a similar gene complex on chromosome 22. Joining of V_λ and J_λ segments occurs in a manner identical to that of the κ segments. A given chromosome 22, however, may contain 6–9 slightly different copies of the C_λ exon (corresponding to various subclasses of λ protein), each with a nearby J_λ segment. A V segment may fuse to any of these alternative J_λ segments, and the resulting V_λ/J_λ exon can then be transcribed together with the adjacent C_λ exon. The B cell selects only one of the available J_λ segments for V/J joining, and in so doing, it determines which C_λ subclass will be expressed (Fig 10–2).

segment codes for the remaining 13 (amino acids 96–108). In contrast to the single C_κ exon, multiple V_κ and J_κ segments are present, each with a somewhat different DNA sequence. The 5 J_κ segments are clustered near the C_κ exon, whereas at least 100 different V_κ segments lie scattered over a region that spans more than 2 million base pairs of DNA (roughly 1% of the length of chromosome 2). This wide separation between the V_κ and J_κ segments is found in the DNA of all nonlymphoid cells. When an immature hematopoietic cell becomes committed to the B lymphocyte lineage, however, it selects one V_κ and one J_κ segment and fuses these to form a single continuous exon. In most cases, this process of "V/J joining" is

HEAVY CHAIN GENES

All immunoglobulin H chains are derived from a single region on chromosome 14 (Fig 10–3). Each H chain C region is encoded by a cluster of several short exons. The μ C region, for example,

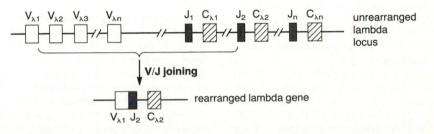

Figure 10–2. Assembly of a λ L chain gene. An individual λ locus contains 6–9 alternative C_λ exons, each with a nearby J_λ segment. In this example, DNA rearrangement fuses $V_{\lambda 1}$ with $J_{\lambda 2}$; the resulting gene will produce L chains that contain the $\lambda 2$ C region.

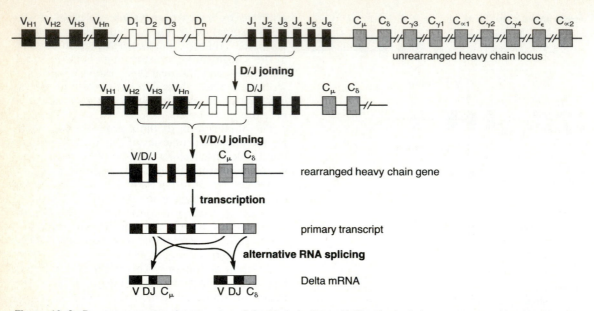

Figure 10–3. Rearrangement and expression of the H chain locus. Unlike the L chain genes, assembly of an H chain V region exon requires 2 sequential DNA rearrangement events involving 3 different types of gene segments. The D_H and J_H segments are joined first and are then fused to a V_H segment. Nine alternative C region sequences are present; of these, however, only the C_μ and C_δ sequences are initially transcribed. The primary transcript can be spliced in either of 2 ways to generate mRNAs that encode μ or δ H chains with identical V domains. This diagram is highly schematic: each C_H sequence is actually composed of multiple exons whose aggregate length is more than 3 times longer than that of the V/D/J exon.

is divided among 5 exons known collectively as the C_μ sequence. C region (C_H) sequences for each of the 9 heavy chain isotypes are arrayed in tandem along the chromosome in the following order: C_μ, C_δ, $C_{\gamma3}$, $C_{\gamma1}$, $C_{\alpha1}$, $C_{\gamma2}$, $C_{\gamma4}$, C_ϵ, $C_{\alpha2}$; only a single copy of each is present. The 6 J_H segments and a few hundred V_H segments (the exact number is unknown) are arranged in a manner analogous to those of the κ gene. In contrast to the L chain genes, however, a third type of gene segment, called the diversity (D_H) segment, must also be used in forming an H chain V region. At least 20 of these D_H segments, each coding for 2 or 3 amino acids, lie between the J_H and V_H segments on the unrearranged chromosome. In assembling the H chain gene, lymphocytes must complete 2 DNA rearrangement events, first bringing together one D_H and one J_H segment and subsequently linking these to a V_H segment (a sequence termed **V/D/J joining**).

Use of the D_H segment greatly increases the amount of H chain diversity that can be produced. For example, 200 V_H, 10 D_H, and 6 J_H segments could give rise to 12,000 (200 × 10 × 6) different H chain V domains, and these, when combined with 500 κ chain V domains, could form 6 million (500 × 12,000) different antigen-binding sites! Even using a relatively small number of gene

segments, then, the immune system can generate enormous antibody diversity through combinatorial joining.

THE MOLECULAR BASIS OF IMMUNOGLOBULIN GENE REARRANGEMENT

Active gene rearrangements of the type that produce V/J and V/D/J joining were first thought to be a unique property of the immunoglobulin genes. More recently, however, identical rearrangements have been found to give rise to genes that encode the antigen receptors of T lymphocytes, a diverse family of proteins which are functionally and genetically similar to immunoglobulins in many respects (see Chapter 6). There is evidence that rearrangement of both these gene families is carried out by the same molecular machinery: a presumably complex system of enzymes and other proteins known collectively as the **V/(D)/J recombinase.** This term must be used operationally because none of the enzymes involved in recognizing, cleaving, or religating the various gene segments has yet been purified and characterized.

V/(D)/J recombinase activity is found almost

exclusively in cells that are undergoing the early stages of B and T cell development. Potential sites for DNA rearrangement by the recombinase appear to be marked by the presence of a pair of short DNA sequences (7 and 9 base pairs, respectively) that are found adjacent to each unrearranged V, D, or J segment and are deleted in the course of rearrangement. The relative positions and orientations of these short sequences help to ensure that segments are joined in the proper order and alignment to produce a functional exon.

OTHER SOURCES OF ANTIBODY DIVERSITY

Additional diversity of V region sequences arises because the V/(D)/J rearrangement process is somewhat imprecise, so that the site at which one segment fuses with another can vary by a few nucleotides. As a result, the DNA coding sequence that remains at the junction between any 2 segments can also vary. Moreover, during assembly of a H chain gene, a few nucleotides of random sequence (called N regions) are often inserted at the points of joining between the V, D, and J segments; these insertions are thought to be produced by terminal deoxynucleotidyl transferase (TdT), an enzyme that is present in immature lymphocytes. The variations in gene sequence that result from imprecise joining or from the insertion of N regions contribute substantially to overall antibody diversity. At the same time, however, these processes greatly increase the risk that 2 segments may be joined in an improper translational reading frame, resulting in a nonfunctional gene. In practice, such unsuccessful rearrangements occur frequently and generally cannot be reversed or repaired; they represent a cost paid by the immune system in exchange for greater potential gene diversity.

Fully assembled V/J and V/D/J exons in lymphocytes have also been found to undergo point mutation at an unusually high rate, a phenomenon termed **somatic hypermutation.** Occasionally, such mutations alter the specificity or the affinity of the antibody molecule.

THE HEAVY CHAIN ISOTYPE SWITCH

When first assembled, a V/D/J exon is transcribed together with the nearby C_μ exon to form μ H chain RNA. Exons corresponding to the other H chain isotypes lie farther downstream and are not transcribed. To express these other isotypes, the H chain gene must undergo a different type of DNA rearrangement known as isotype switching,

in which a new C_H sequence is placed adjacent to the original V/D/J exon. This is accomplished through a specific DNA deletion process that removes all of the intervening C_H sequences (Fig 10–4). Although isotype switching bears some resemblance to V/(D)/J joining, these 2 processes are thought to occur through different enzymatic pathways. In particular, switching takes place in cells that are no longer able to carry out V/(D)/J rearrangements (see below) and occurs at sites located several hundred bases away from the V/D/J and C_H exons themselves. Switching does not change the structure of the V/D/J exon and so does not affect antigen specificity.

Thus, V regions for all of the H chain classes are assembled from a single common pool of V_H, D_H, and J_H segments; once assembled, the V/D/J exon can then be linked to any one of the C region sequences through the process of isotype switching. By this means, the effector function of an antibody can be changed without altering its specificity for antigen. Because isotype switching occurs by deletion of one or more C_H regions, it is irreversible. The selection of a new C_H isotype may be influenced by lymphokines or other factors acting upon the B cell; for example, the microenvironment found in Peyer's patches of the gut appears to favor switching to $C_{\alpha 1}$, resulting in the production of IgA.

In general, only the C_H region nearest the V/D/J exon can be expressed. One major exception to this rule is the C_δ sequence, which lies very near

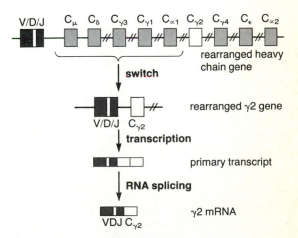

Figure 10–4. The H chain isotype switch. To express an isotype other than μ or δ, the fully assembled H chain locus undergoes an additional DNA rearrangement event that places a new C_H sequence adjacent to the V/D/J exon. This occurs by deletion of the intervening C_H exons and is carried out by an enzymatic pathway distinct from that of V/D/J rearrangement. In the example shown, the gene switches to the $C_{\gamma 2}$ isotype.

the C_μ region and is often transcribed along with the V/D/J and C_μ exons. The resulting RNA can be spliced to yield either μ or δ mRNA, enabling the cell simultaneously to express IgM and IgD antibodies that have identical V domain sequences. Such coexpression of IgM and IgD on the surface membrane is a common phenotype among B lymphocytes.

IMMUNOGLOBULIN GENE REARRANGEMENTS & B CELL ONTOGENY

The DNA rearrangements that assemble immunoglobulin genes occur only at a very early stage in B cell development and follow a strict develop-mental sequence (Fig 10–5). Joining of the D_H and J_H segments is one of the earliest events in the ontogeny of a B cell and occurs simultaneously on both copies of chromosome 14. The cell then attempts to join a V_H segment to the fused D_H/J_H segment on one chromosome. If this first attempt succeeds in producing a functional gene, the cell begins to synthesize μ (and perhaps also δ) H chains encoded by the rearranged gene. At this early stage of development (known as the pre-B stage), the H chains remain within the cytoplasm of the cell and are not displayed on the surface membrane. Through a mechanism that is not well understood, the expression of H chain protein is thought to inhibit any further rearrangement of H chain genes in the cell. If, however, the first rearrangement is not successful, a second attempt

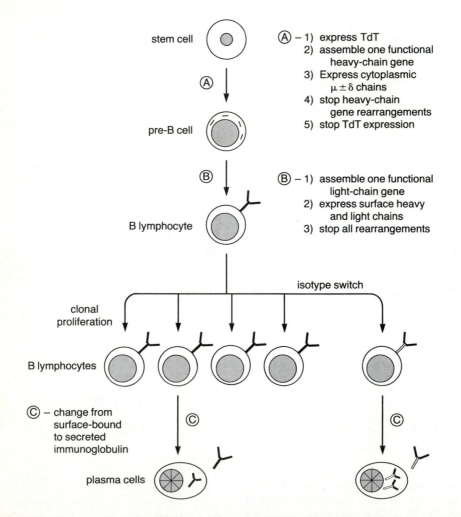

Figure 10–5. Major genetic events in B cell ontogeny. The sequence of events that marks the progression from each stage of development to the next is listed (A–C). Note that the ability to perform V/(D)/J rearrangements is lost by the time the cell becomes a mature B lymphocyte. Isotype switching does not change the antigen specificity of an immunoglobulin.

at V/D/J assembly can be made by using the other chromosome 14.

L chain gene rearrangements do not begin until the cell is actively producing cytoplasmic H chain protein (ie, after H chain V/D/J rearrangements have ceased). V/J joining is then attempted on each chromosome 2 or 22 in succession, until a functional κ or λ gene is produced. As soon as either type of L chain protein appears, the cell loses the ability to perform additional V/J rearrangements. The cell then enters the B lymphocyte stage of development, in which the H and L chain proteins are expressed together as disulfide-linked heterodimers on the cell surface membrane but are not secreted in appreciable quantities.

As mentioned above, successful assembly of a single H or L chain gene prevents all other genes of that type from undergoing rearrangement in the same cell. Consequently, only one H chain and one L chain gene can give rise to protein in any individual B lymphocyte, a phenomenon termed **allelic exclusion.** Moreover, when the lymphocyte divides, chromosomes bearing the active rearranged genes are passed on to its progeny, and the daughter cells continue to express these genes without performing further V/J or V/D/J rearrangements. For this reason, all of the immunoglobulin molecules produced by a given B lymphocyte and its progeny have identical antigen specificity and L chain isotype (κ or λ), a phenomenon known as **clonal restriction.** The diversity of antibody molecules produced by the immune system as a whole reflects cellular diversity, ie, the fact that innumerable B cell precursors each rearrange their genes independently and in different combinations, resulting in a large assortment of clones, each of which possesses a unique antigenic specificity.

The immunoglobulins on the surface membrane of a B lymphocyte serve as receptors for specific antigens. Mature lymphocytes tend to be quiescent cells and do not proliferate under ordinary circumstances. If, however, a B lymphocyte comes into contact with an antigen that can bind to its surface immunoglobulins, this binding stimulates the cell to undergo rapid clonal proliferation, producing daughter cells which bear identical surface-bound immunoglobulin. Many of these cells then undergo a final step in differentiation to become plasma cells, which secrete large amounts of this same immunoglobulin to form circulating antibodies. Such antigen-dependent proliferation and secretion form the essential basis of a humoral immune response. It is important to bear in mind that the specificity of this response depends upon the allelic exclusion and clonal restriction of immunoglobulin expression: each clone of lymphocytes can respond only to antigens that can bind to its unique pair of H and L chains,

and all of the antibodies secreted by the activated clone are directed against that particular antigen.

Although the H chain class also tends to be maintained during clonal B cell proliferation, isotype-switching rearrangements can still occur, occasionally giving rise to a daughter cell that expresses a different class of H chains and passes this new trait along to its progeny. More subtle changes in the H chain protein also determine whether an immunoglobulin will be membrane-bound or secreted. The final 2 exons of each C_H sequence encode a short hydrophobic tail, which serves to anchor the carboxyl terminus of the H chain onto the cell surface membrane. When a lymphocyte matures into a plasma cell, however, the H chain mRNA that it produces lacks these final exons; as a result, the immunoglobulins are secreted from the cell as soluble antibodies.

CLINICAL ASPECTS

Apart from their role in generating antibody diversity, immunoglobulin gene rearrangements are gaining increasing importance in clinical diagnosis and research. Rearrangement of these genes can be detected by using a technique known as **Southern blotting,** after its inventor, E. M. Southern (Fig 10–6). For this purpose, DNA is extracted from a population of cells contained, for example, in a tissue biopsy or sample of peripheral blood. The DNA is then digested with one or more restriction enzymes, a type of bacterial endonuclease that cleaves the long chromosomal DNA at defined sites to produce an array of shorter DNA fragments of various lengths. Next, these fragments are separated according to length by electrophoresis through an agarose gel and are treated with alkali to melt apart the complementary strands of the double helix in each fragment. A sheet of nylon or other suitable material is then pressed against the gel; the denatured DNA fragments bind tightly to the nylon and are drawn out of the gel. When the nylon is peeled away, it retains on its surface the immobilized DNA fragments, still arranged according to length, as they had been in the gel, but now exposed and accessible to further analysis. DNA fragments that contain a particular gene sequence can then be identified by their ability to bind specific DNA probes. Such probes simply consist of radioisotopically labeled single-stranded DNA molecules whose sequence is complementary to a portion of the gene in question and which are therefore capable of binding to the gene under appropriate conditions by base-pairing. Because the probe is radioactive, the fragments to which it binds can be identified by autoradiography, and the lengths of these frag-

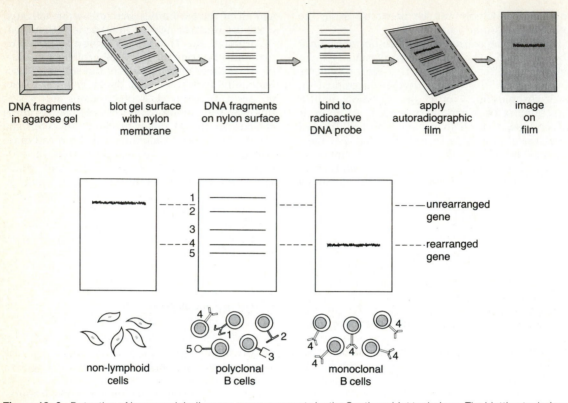

Figure 10-6. Detection of immunoglobulin gene rearrangements by the Southern blot technique. The blotting technique (*A*) is described in the text; it can be used to determine the size of DNA restriction fragments that encompass a specific gene. DNA rearrangement in lymphocytes alters the sizes of fragments bearing the immunoglobulin genes; the sizes of the immunoglobulin-specific fragments are characteristic of each B cell clone. This provides a means of detecting B cells and of assessing the clonal composition of B cell populations (*B*). DNA isolated from nonlymphoid cells contains only unrearranged immunoglobulin genes, whereas DNA from normal lymphocyte populations reveals many different rearranged genes—one from each of the many independent B cell clones. Detection of a only a single rearranged gene suggests that a lymphocyte population is monoclonal and therefore possibly malignant.

ments can be estimated by their positions along the agarose gel.

If all of the cells in a population contain DNA of identical sequence, the restriction enzyme should cleave at identical sites in the DNA of each cell. The fragment on which any particular gene resides will then have the same length for every cell and will appear as a single band on the autoradiogram. This is true of most cellular genes and of the unrearranged immunoglobulin loci found in nonlymphoid cells. Gene rearrangement in lymphocytes, however, dramatically changes the DNA sequences in and around an immunoglobulin locus and thus alters the size of the fragment that encompasses the locus (Fig 10–6). Because the size of the altered fragment varies according to the structure of the rearranged gene, its position on the Southern blot can serve as a distinctive "molecular fingerprint" that is unique to each B cell clone. By using the Southern blot to estimate the proportion of identically rearranged immuno-

globulin genes in DNA extracted from a population of lymphocytes, it is possible to determine whether any single B cell clone predominates—a possible indication of cancer (see Chapter 48). This technique also provides a sensitive means for detecting the recurrence of a malignant clone after treatment. Moreover, because immunoglobulin gene rearrangements occur almost exclusively among lymphoid cells, their presence can provide compelling evidence that an undifferentiated cancer is of lymphoid origin.

Just as importantly, errors in immunoglobulin gene rearrangement are now thought to contribute to the genesis of several major types of leukemia and lymphoma. For example, the cells of Burkitt's lymphoma, a B-lymphocytic cancer, usually contain a specific chromosomal abnormality called t(8,14), in which a portion of chromosome 8 has been translocated onto chromosome 14 (Fig 10–7). In this translocation, chromosome 14 breaks within the immunoglobulin H chain locus, while

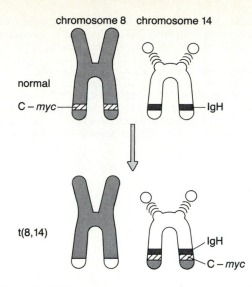

Figure 10-7. The t(8,14) chromosomal anomaly of Burkitt's lymphoma. A reciprocal exchange of genetic material occurs that involves the distal ends of the long arms of chromosomes 8 and 14. This transposes the c-*myc* proto-oncogene from chromosome 8 into the active immunoglobulin H chain locus on chromosome 14 and is thought to contribute to the development of a cancer.

the breakpoint on chromosome 8 coincides with a cellular proto-oncogene known as c-*myc*. As a result, the c-*myc* gene is moved to a position directly adjacent to the H chain gene. It is thought that this proximity to the active H chain locus alters the expression of the proto-oncogene and so contributes to malignant transformation. Less commonly, Burkitt's lymphoma may lack t(8,14) and instead exhibit a closely related anomaly in which the c-*myc* locus is translocated into the κ or λ L chain gene on chromosome 2 or 22. A different type of anomaly, called t(14,18), is observed in more than 85% of patients with follicular lymphoma, the most common human B cell cancer; here, the putative proto-oncogene *bcl-2* on chromosome 18 is translocated into the H chain locus on chromosome 14. In some of these translocations, chromosome breakage in the affected immunoglobulin locus occurs directly beside a J segment; this strongly implies that the translocation results in part from an error in immunoglobulin gene rearrangement.

SUMMARY

The remarkable properties of immunoglobulin genes provide a basis for understanding many as-

pects of B cell differentiation and of the humoral immune response. Through the active DNA rearrangements that assemble V/(D)/J exons or mediate isotype switching, the immune system is able to generate almost unlimited antibody diversity from a relatively small amount of chromosomal DNA. All of the immunoglobulin produced by an individual B lymphocyte, however, has identical antigen specificity. This specificity is determined by the structures of its V region exons and is established during the early stages of B cell ontogeny. Thereafter, V/(D)/J rearrangements cease, and the proliferative and secretory activity of each B cell clone depends upon the nature of antigens that it may subsequently encounter.

REFERENCES

Immunoglobulin Gene Organization & Rearrangements

Dreyer WJ, Bennett JC: The molecular basis of antibody formations: A paradox. *Proc Natl Acad Sci USA* 1965;**54**:864.

Honjo T, Alt FW, Rabbitts TH (editors): *Immunoglobulin Genes.* Academic Press, 1989.

Leder P: The genetics of antibody diversity. *Sci Am* (May) 1982:102.

Tonegawa S: Somatic generation of antibody diversity. *Nature* 1983;**302**:575.

Mechanism & Ontogeny of Gene Rearrangements

Akira SJ, Okazaki K, Sakano H: Two pairs of recombination signals are sufficient to cause immunoglobulin V-(D)-J joining. *Science* 1987;**238**:1134.

Lieber MR et al: Developmental stage specificity of the lymphoid V(D)J recombination activity. *Genes Dev* 1987;**1**:751.

Yancopoulos GD, Alt FW: Regulation of the assembly and expression of variable-region genes. *Annu Rev Immunol* 1986;**4**:339.

Other Sources of Antibody Diversity

French DL, Laskov R, Scharff MD: The role of somatic hypermutations in the generation of antibody diversity. *Science* 1989;**244**:1152.

Landau N et al: Increased frequency of N-region insertion in a murine pre-B-cell line infected with a terminal deoxynucleotidyl transferase retroviral expression vector. *Mol Cell Biol* 1987;**7**:3237.

Max EE et al: Variation in the crossover point of kappa immunoglobulin gene V-J recombination: Evidence from a cryptic gene. *Cell* 1980;**21**:793.

Heavy Chain Isotype Switch & Immunoglobulin Secretion

Blattner FR, Tucker PW: The molecular biology of immunoglobulin D. *Nature* 1984;**307**:417.

Cebra JJ, Komisar JL, Schweitzer PA: CH isotype "switching" during normal B-lymphocyte development. *Annu Rev Immunol* 1984;**2**:493.

Early P et al: Two mRNAs can be produced from a

single immunoglobulin μ gene by alternative RNA processing pathways. *Cell* 1979;**20**:313.

Gene Rearrangements in Clinical Immunology

Arnold A et al: Immunoglobulin-gene rearrangements as unique clonal markers in human lymphoid neoplasms. *N Engl J Med* 1983;**309**:1593.

Bakhshi A et al: Lymphoid blast crises of chronic myelogenous leukemia represent stages in the development of B-cell precursors. *N Engl J Med* 1983;**309**:826.

Cleary ML, Warnke R, Sklar J: Monoclonality of lymphoproliferative lesions in cardiac-transplant recipients. *N Engl J Med* 1984;**310**:477.

Chromosomal Translocations & Oncogenesis

Croce CM, Nowell PC: Molecular basis of human B cell neoplasia. *Blood* 1985;**65**:1.

Tsujimoto Y et al: The t(14;18) chromosome translocations involved in B-cell neoplasms result from mistakes in VDJ joining. *Science* 1985;**229**:1390.

Mechanisms of Inflammation

11

Abba I. Terr, MD

The immune response generates a population of T lymphocytes and antibodies with specificity for recognizing an antigen on subsequent encounters. When the same antigen or a cross-reacting antigen containing the same antigenic epitope is subsequently encountered, several events may occur, known collectively as **effector mechanisms.** These are as follows.

Neutralization. The antibody blocks a toxic site on a microorganism or a chemical toxin, either by direct reaction with the toxic site or by steric hindrance, thereby preventing toxic damage to the host.

Cytotoxicity. The antibody lyses the cell containing the antigenic epitope through various mechanisms, such as complement-induced lysis or antibody-dependent cellular cytotoxicity (ADCC).

Cytostimulation. An autoantibody reacting with a host cell receptor stimulates metabolic processes within a cell by activating the receptor, thereby simulating a normal ligand, such as a hormone.

Inflammation. The reaction of specific T lymphocyte or antibody with antigen causes the recruitment of inflammatory cells and endogenous mediator chemicals. In some cases, the normal function of the organ or tissue is altered by an increase in vascular permeability and by contraction of visceral smooth muscle.

CLASSIFICATION

This chapter will describe the 3 principal classes of immunologically induced inflammation. The classification used here is based on the nature of the initiating immune response: (1) T cell-mediated generation of cytokines, (2) antigen-antibody complex-mediated generation of factors derived from the complement system, and (3) IgE antibody-mediated release of active chemicals from mast cells. A fourth type of inflammation, called cutaneous basophil hypersensitivity, will be mentioned only briefly, because its importance in human inflammation is not known. Although these mechanisms will be described separately, they can and often do operate simultaneously and synergistically in the in vivo immune response. Each class of inflammation is characterized by a particular histologic pattern with a cellular infiltration in the target tissue.

However, inflammation is a response that is not limited to just immunologic stimuli. The cells and chemical mediators of inflammation can be activated by nonimmunologic physical means, such as injury, trauma, heat, or environmental or endogenous tissue-damaging chemicals. Furthermore, inflammatory reactions that are induced immunologically may be accompanied by other immunologic effector responses, such as antigen neutralization and cytotoxicity.

PROTECTIVE & DELETERIOUS EFFECTS

Immunologically induced inflammation begins with the specific recognition of the antigen, but the events that ensue have no immunologic specificity. Although inflammation is an efficient means of protection against invading pathogenic microorganisms and recovery from infection, ie, protective immunity, the cells and chemical mediators participating in inflammation are also capable of damaging tissues and interfering with the functioning of organs within the host. The deleterious effects of inflammation are expressed as hypersensitivity (allergy) when immunologically induced inflammation is directed to a causative antigen that is not intrinsically harmful. Examples of antigens that can produce hypersensitivity include drugs, inhaled pollen grains or dust particles, ingested foods, and plant oils or chemicals in contact with the skin. In these cases, the tissues that are damaged and the organ functions that are disrupted are generally innocent bystanders with regard to the immune response directed at the foreign antigen. The harmful consequences of immunologically induced inflammation are also expressed in autoimmune diseases, wherein the effector mechanisms are misdirected to a host cell, possibly because of a defect in immune regulation.

METHODS OF STUDY

The accumulated knowledge about the mechanisms of human inflammation has been derived from many sources, including the analysis of tissue pathology, cytology, and biochemistry of mediators in tissues and body fluids during both naturally acquired and experimentally induced exposures to antigens. Historically, the first experimental model system of inflammation was the localized cutaneous reaction to an intradermal injection of antigen, ie, the skin test. This simple procedure, first used almost 100 years ago, continues to provide much essential information about the mechanisms of the various classes of inflammation (Table 11–1). Immunologic mechanisms have been determined by the technique of passive transfer skin testing, in which mixed populations of cells, purified lymphocyte preparations, serum, purified immunoglobulins, or immunoglobulin subclasses have been transferred from the sensitized (immunized) donor to a previously unimmunized recipient. The relevant mediators are analyzed by studying the effects of specific inhibitors of mediators on antigen-induced skin test reactions or by testing fluid obtained from suction-induced blisters of the skin test site.

This chapter will give a broad outline of the immunologic events that lead to inflammation. The inflammatory cells are discussed in more detail in Chapter 12, mediators of hypersensitivity in Chapter 13, cytokines that operate as mediators

in cell-mediated immunity in Chapter 7, and the complement system in Chapter 14.

CELL-MEDIATED IMMUNITY

Cell-mediated immunity (CMI) is also known as delayed hypersensitivity or delayed-type hypersensitivity (DTH). These terms describe the same immunologic phenomenon, so the one used depends upon whether the effect on the host is protective or harmful. CMI and DTH refer to inflammation generated by the reaction of antigen with its corresponding antigen-specific T lymphocyte. In the previously immunized (sensitized) individual, the effector T cells that produce CMI and that can passively transfer that same antigen-specific immunity are known as T_{DH} cells, a term which described the cell's activity and not a cell surface marker.

Mechanisms

The T lymphocyte responds on exposure to antigen only when the antigen is processed by an antigen-presenting cell (APC) (such as a macrophage) yielding peptide fragments and only in the context of the class II MHC molecule expressed on the surface of the APC along with the antigen peptide fragments (see Chapter 6). Exposure of the T_{DH} cell to antigen for induction of CMI requires the same processing of antigen and genetically restricted presentation. Only in this way is the T_{DH} cell activated. Activation of a small number of T_{DH} cells results in the production and secretion of lymphokines. The action of these lymphokines on other cells both amplifies the size of the specific T_{DH} cell population and recruits

Table 11–1. Classes of immunologically induced inflammation sharing the time course, cellular composition, relevant mediators, and immunologic mechanisms as reflected in the cutaneous response to skin testing.

Type of Inflammation	Skin Test Terminology	Time of Maximal Reaction (Hours)	Principal Inflammatory Cells	Primary Mediator	Immunologic Mechanisms of Inflammation
1. CMI, DTH	Delayed	36	Lymphocytes, macrophages (granuloma)	Lymphokines	T_{DH} cell, cytokine, activated macrophage
2. Immune complex	Late	8	Polymorphonuclear neutrophils	Complement	Antigen-antibody complex, complement activation, neutrophil chemotaxis
3. IgE Immediate phase	Immediate	0.25	Eosinophils	Histamine, leukotrienes	Mast cell, fixed IgE, mediators
Late phase	Late	6	Eosinophils, neutrophils	PAF, other mediators	Chemotaxis from mast cell
4. Cutaneous basophil hypersensitivity	Delayed	36	Basophils	Unknown	Unknown

other immunologically nonspecific lymphocytes and other inflammatory cells. Although identification of the relevant lymphokines in this response is currently incomplete, certain functional activities can be described.

The cells attracted by lymphokine-induced chemotaxis include monocytes, granulocytes, B and T lymphocytes, and basophils. Activation of macrophages by lymphokines with macrophage-activating factor (MAF) not only causes these cells to express class II MHC molecules, but also enhances their phagocytic and bactericidal activities. Vasodilation occurs, effectively enhancing the availability of cells from the circulation. The coagulation-kinin system is activated, so that fibrin is formed and deposited. This material is probably important in a localization of the inflammatory reaction, and it gives the characteristic induration of the cutaneous DTH. These events are depicted in Figure 11–1.

Histopathology

The microscopic appearance of CMI is characteristic, and its occurrence in a number of clinical diseases suggests that this particular immunologic mechanism is involved in the pathogenesis. There is a mononuclear cellular infiltration with monocytes and lymphocytes (often in a perivascular distribution) and granulocytes. In addition, fibrin deposition, edema, and tissue destruction occur. In advanced lesions there may be liquefaction of tissue, called caseation necrosis. A hallmark of CMI is the granuloma, a focal accumulation of monocytes, lymphocytes, neutrophils, plasma cells, and epithelioid giant cells that probably arises from coalescence of cells of the monocyte-macrophage series. The granuloma is considered to be the end result of CMI in which an antigen has persisted at the site because of low solubility and degradability, thereby causing persistent local antigenic stimulation. Granulomas occur in CMI from infections, in DTH to metals and organic particles, and in the disease sarcoidosis, in which the antigen is unknown.

Clinical Manifestations

A state of CMI/DTH is acquired naturally during the course of many infections, artificially by immunization, and through contact by many different sensitizing chemicals on the skin and mucous membranes.

Immunity to infection by obligate intracellular pathogenic organisms is mediated by CMI. The variety of organisms provoking this type of immunity is extensive and includes viruses, *Chlamydia,* fungi, bacteria, protozoa, and helminthic parasites. A major consequence of CMI in the primary infection is localization of the infection. However, as mentioned above, persistent antigenic stimulation in a granulomatous lesion may lead to tissue necrosis and systemic spread of organisms.

Hypersensitivity diseases mediated by DTH are discussed in Chapter 33. The primary disease in this category is allergic contact dermatitis. In this disease, the sensitizing antigens are usually haptens, which complex with skin protein carrier molecules before being processed by Langerhans cells in the skin. Examples of common contact sensitizers are pentadecyl catechol in the oil from poison ivy and nickel in jewelry.

Allograft rejection and the graft-versus-host reaction are complex immunologic phenomena that involve the class II MHC antigen as the target for rejection, but other antigenic cellular molecules and other immunologic effector mechanisms, especially cytotoxicity, are also involved. In a similar fashion, CMI participates along with other effector responses in tumor immunity and in autoimmune diseases.

Regulation

An active feedback inhibition regulating the extent of CMI is suggested by experimental evidence obtained with guinea pigs. The inhibitory effect appears to be antigenically nonspecific. A state of

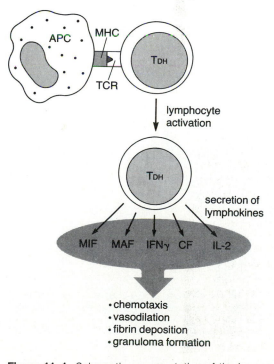

Figure 11–1. Schematic representation of the immunologic events in cell-mediated inflammation. Abbreviations: APC, antigen-presenting cell; MHC, major histocompatibility complex; TCR, T cell receptor; MIF, monocyte migration inhibitory factor; MAF, macrophage-activating factor; IFNα, alpha interferon; CF, complement fixation; IL-2, interleukin-2.

nonspecific depression of cellular immunity occurs in humans under certain circumstances and has been referred to as **anergy.** Anergy may accompany diseases with extensive granulomata, such as miliary tuberculosis, severe coccidioidomycosis, lepromatous leprosy, and sarcoidosis. It also occurs in Hodgkin's disease. A temporary loss of CMI occurs during the acute phase of certain viral infections such as measles. Anergy is usually defined as the absence of DTH skin tests to a panel of commonly encountered antigens or loss of a previously positive DTH skin test. Until the mechanism of anergy becomes known, the term should be considered an operational one without necessarily implying a mechanism.

IMMUNE COMPLEX-MEDIATED INFLAMMATION

Immune complex-mediated inflammation refers to the inflammatory cell response that occurs following a reaction of antigen and antibody and the subsequent activation of the complement system. Complement-generated inflammation functions both in immunity and in hypersensitivity. The 2 cardinal expressions of hypersensitivity in this case are the cutaneous Arthus reaction and systemic serum sickness. Both of these immunologic reactions were first recognized in the early 1900s, and since then the pathogenesis of immune-complex phenomena has been extensively studied by using rabbits. Rabbit models that apply to human diseases include the Arthus reaction on the skin, "one-shot" serum sickness, and chronic serum sickness produced by daily intravenous injections of antigen.

Mechanisms

The antigen may be either a high-molecular-weight protein, ie, a "complete antigen," or a hapten. However, the conditions necessary for complement activation require binding of the hapten to a host carrier protein. The chemical nature of the antigen is probably not as critical as its mode of exposure to the antibody. The reaction is antigen dose-related, especially in the serum sickness on first exposure to antigen, when the likelihood of this reaction increases with increasing dose of antigen. A prolonged period of antigen exposure also enhances the likelihood of serum sickness. An antigen with a net ionic charge could enhance the localization of the antigen-antibody complex to certain tissue sites bearing the opposite charge.

A. Complement-Activating Antibodies: The antibody must be capable of activating complement. IgM antibodies and IgG antibodies of all subclasses except for IgG4 activate the comple-

ment system through the classical pathway. IgM antibodies are more efficient than are IgG antibodies by virtue of their higher valence, permitting the development of large complexes with antigen. IgA antibodies activate complement through the alternative pathway. IgE antibodies have no effect on the complement system and therefore are not involved in this type of immune complex reaction, although it is possible that antigen-IgE antibody complexes have other pathogenic properties. IgD antibodies are not known to produce any form of inflammation.

B. Immune-Complex Formation: In the usual model of immune complex-mediated inflammation, antigen-antibody complexes cross-linked in a lattice fashion are formed in the circulation and secondarily deposited in tissues. In experimentally induced serum sickness with complexes formed at various points in the in vitro precipitin reaction (Fig 11–2), the complexes formed in moderate antigen excess are of the most effective size for activating complement and, furthermore, have the most prolonged residence in the circulation. Complexes formed in far antigen or antibody excess are small, because saturation of all antibody- or antigen-binding sites, respec-

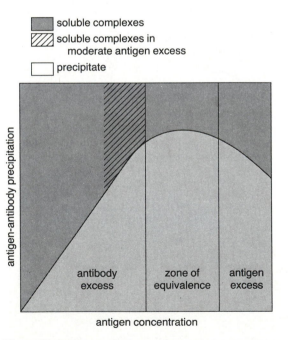

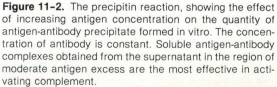

Figure 11–2. The precipitin reaction, showing the effect of increasing antigen concentration on the quantity of antigen-antibody precipitate formed in vitro. The concentration of antibody is constant. Soluble antigen-antibody complexes obtained from the supernatant in the region of moderate antigen excess are the most effective in activating complement.

tively, prevents multiple cross-linking required for lattice formation.

C. Immune-Complex Deposition: Soluble complexes of antigen and antibody formed in the circulation are deposited in various tissues. If the immune complexes are large enough, they become trapped, particularly on the basement membrane of the glomerulus and in blood vessels, where they deposit on the internal elastic lamina. The localization to these tissues may also depend on other secondary factors such as blood flow turbulence and the ionic charge of the immune complex. The size of the complex, however, appears to be the predominant factor in tissue localization. In the cutaneous Arthus reaction, a high concentration of immune complexes is generated locally because the antigen is injected directly into the skin, thereby creating focal deposits in blood vessels. In diseases in which antibody is formed to a cellular autoantigen, the immune complex is formed by deposition of antibody on the cell-fixed antigen at that tissue site, rather than being deposited as an immune complex from the circulation.

D. Complement Activation: Complement activation can be initiated through either the classical or alternative pathway, depending on the immunoglobulin class of antibody within the immune complex (see Chapter 14). The principal inflammatory factor derived from the complement cascade appears to be C5a, which is chemotactic for neutrophils from the circulation and from surrounding tissues. The resulting vasculitis is made up of several elements (Fig 11–3). Neutrophils release lysosomal enzymes and generate toxic oxidants in the process of phagocytizing the immune complex, thereby causing destruction of the internal elastic lamina of the blood vessel wall. Blood vessel endothelial cells swell and prolifer-

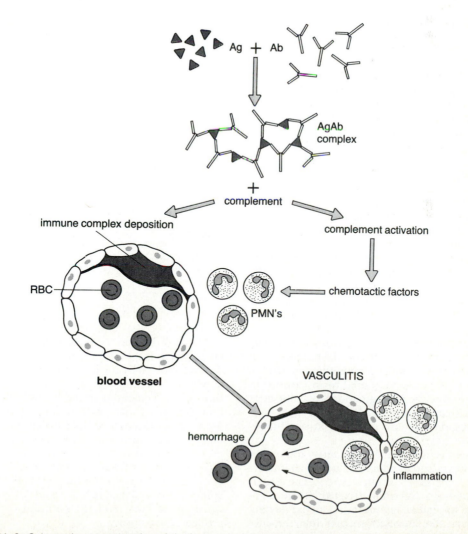

Figure 11–3. Schematic representation of the immunologic events in immune complex-mediated inflammation.

ate, and there is aggregation of platelets. Later, mononuclear cells infiltrate the area, but the mechanism of their attraction is unknown.

E. Control Mechanism: Recently a possible control mechanism has been described which could limit the extent of immune-complex inflammation. It has been shown that immune complexes are solubilized by C3 convertase. This enzyme is formed by activation of C3 by factor B of the alternative complement pathway. When C3 convertase is bound to immune complexes at equivalence, C3 fragments dissociate antigen-antibody binding, thereby breaking up the immune complex.

F. Normal Immune-Complex Formation: Small quantities of immune complexes are formed normally in the absence of disease. The antigens responsible for these normal antigen-antibody complexes are not all known, although at least some are antigens from ingested foods. Other environmental antigens and possibly autoantigens could be responsible for these normal circulating complexes. Nevertheless, they are promptly eliminated through phagocytosis by cells of the mononuclear phagocyte system (formerly called the reticuloendothelial system), which contain receptors for the Fc portion of IgG and for C3. Immune-complex disease therefore requires (1) large amounts of antigen; (2) generation of immune complexes large enough to activate complement; and (3) in some cases, impaired function of the mononuclear phagocyte system, possibly because of an abnormality of the Fc receptor.

Clinical Manifestations

In immunity, immune-complex inflammation is accompanied by other complement-mediated phenomena such as opsonization, immune adherence, and ADCC of bacteria and other microorganisms by antibodies to surface antigens on these pathogens. In certain hypersensitivity states, on the other hand, immune complex inflammation is recognized as an important isolated pathogenic mechanism.

A. Arthus Reaction: The Arthus reaction as described for rabbit skin occurs in humans as a frequent consequence of immunotherapy for allergy; it is present in a very mild form, consisting of edema and tissue inflammation but with little or no significant vasculitis. It appears occasionally as a response to insect bites or injected medications.

A single injection of a large quantity of foreign protein antigen into a rabbit produces a characteristic acute "one-shot" serum sickness. The associated immunologic events are depicted in Figure 11–4. During an initial equilibration phase lasting 12–24 hours, the injected antigen load reaches equilibrium between the circulation and extravas-

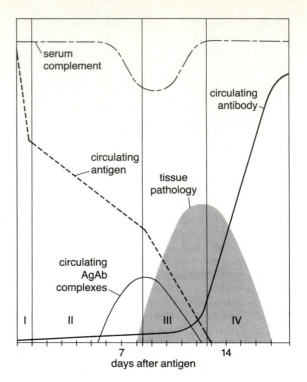

Figure 11-4. Immunologic events in experimental "one-shot" serum sickness in rabbits. The pathogenesis of human serum sickness is similar. A single high dose of antigen is given intravenously on day 0. Phase I: Equilibration of antigen between blood and tissues. Phase II: Primary antibody response. Near the end of this phase, antibody combines with antigen, forming circulating immune complexes. Phase III: Tissue pathology and progression of clinical disease. Circulating complexes activate complement and deposit in tissues. The serum complement level falls transiently, and residual antigen is rapidly cleared from the blood. Phase IV: Remission. Antigen is no longer available, and the level of circulating antibody rises. No further immune complexes form, complement levels return to normal, pathologic lesions repair, and symptoms subside.

cular space as the immune response begins. Over the next 5–7 days, as the primary antibody response takes place, residual antigen is slowly degraded. This is followed by the immune elimination phase, in which circulating antigen is rapidly cleared because newly generated antibody enters the circulation, combines with antigen, and forms circulating antigen-antibody complexes. During this brief phase of several days, circulating immune complexes can be detected in the serum, and this is reflected by a transient drop in the level of serum complement. It is during this phase that immune complexes are deposited in tissues, complement activation occurs, and the pathologic events described above ensue.

B. Serum Sickness: The clinical symptoms

of serum sickness, described in more detail in Chapter 32, include fever, lymphadenopathy, arthralgias, and dermatitis. The final phase begins when free antigen is no longer available, immune complexes no longer form, the serum complement level returns to normal, and free antibody appears in the circulation. No new pathologic lesions develop, and healing with gradual subsidence of symptoms takes place. Serum sickness was once a common reaction to the administration of large quantities of foreign hyperimmune serum used to treat a variety of infectious and toxic diseases prior to the era of antibiotic therapy. Today, heterologous serum is no longer used to treat infections, but it is used in transplantation as a source of anti-lymphocyte or anti-thymocyte antibodies and experimentally as a source of antibodies to specific lymphocyte antigens, such as CD3 for therapeutic immunomodulation. Serum sickness also occurs as an allergic reaction to penicillin and during the prodromal phase of some viral infections, most notably viral hepatitis.

C. Autoimmune Diseases: In 2 autoimmune diseases, thyroiditis and Goodpasture's syndrome, a localized form of immune-complex inflammation results from the action of anti-thyroglobulin antibodies and anti-glomerular basement membrane antibodies, respectively.

An experimental chronic serum sickness can be induced in rabbits by daily intravenous infusions of a quantity of antigen calculated to maintain a prolonged state of moderate antigen excess, based on quantitative antibody determinations. In animals requiring small doses of antigen because of a relatively weak antibody response, this disease model produces membranous glomerulonephritis; in animals requiring large daily doses of antigen because of a brisk antibody response, the predominant lesion is an immune alveolitis in the lungs. These experiments have been used as a model for the pathogenesis of systemic lupus erythematosus, rheumatoid arthritis, polyarteritis nodosa, and other diseases of unknown etiology that are characterized by the presence of circulating immune complexes and vasculitis. The serum sickness model cannot be used to explain all of the pathology and clinical manifestations of these diseases, and the antigen responsible for vasculitis in these conditions is unknown. Solubilization of immune complexes by C3 convertase, discussed above, could explain the frequent occurrence of systemic lupus erythematosus in patients with inherited complement deficiencies.

IgE-MEDIATED INFLAMMATION

IgE-mediated inflammation refers to the inflammatory response mediated by the reaction of antigen with IgE antibodies that occupy receptor sites on mast cells. The interaction of antigen with these cell-fixed antibodies causes the mast cell to degranulate, release certain preformed mediators, and generate other mediators de novo. The result is a 2-phase response, with an initial immediate effect on blood vessels, smooth muscle, and secretory glands, followed by a later cellular inflammatory response. This type of inflammatory response is commonly known as immediate hypersensitivity.

Mechanisms

IgE-mediated inflammation is common. Antigens include a variety of environmental inhaled and ingested allergens; drugs given by injection, inhalation, or orally; and certain microorganisms, especially helminths. The antigen may be complete or haptenic, and its physicochemical nature is probably not important, because known antigens include proteins, carbohydrates, low-molecular-weight organic compounds, and metals. The dose of antigen, however, is important. In contrast to immune complex-mediated inflammation, IgE antibodies are typically formed to very small doses of antigen, and once these antibodies are formed, extremely small quantities of antigen are sufficient to evoke a response.

A. IgE Antibody: The unique feature of IgE antibodies is a structural component of the ϵ heavy chains that binds specifically to a high-affinity receptor (FcϵRI) on the mast cell surface membrane. There is no similar structure on other immunoglobulin heavy chains that can either stimulate the mast cell receptor or block the occupation of the receptor by IgE antibodies. The chemistry of this reactive portion of the IgE antibody is currently unknown, but it involves the normal conformation of the intact molecule and is destroyed by heating at 56°C for 4 hours.

B. Mast Cells and Basophils: The mast cells and basophils both bear the surface FcϵRI at high density. The average number of receptors has been calculated at 270,000 per basophil, but the number on mast cells has not been determined. The high affinity of this receptor for IgE is reflected by an equilibrium constant (K_a) of 2.8×10^{-9} mol/L. Binding is reversible, but the dissociation constant is low. This explains the very small quantities of IgE antibody required for response and the persistence of that response. Despite the high affinity, the binding of IgE antibody to its receptor is noncovalent. IgE antibodies in circulation are in equilibrium with antibodies on mast cells and basophils. Recently it has been shown that both human and rodent IgE antibodies can react with the human mast cell receptor, but it is not known whether human IgE antibody can occupy the rodent mast cell receptor.

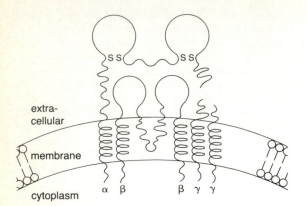

Figure 11–5. The high-affinity mast cell receptor for IgE (FcεRII).

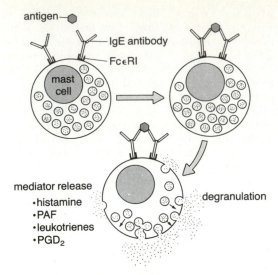

Figure 11–6. Schematic representation of the immunologic events in IgE-mediated inflammation.

The high-affinity mast cell receptor for IgE is composed of 4 polypeptide chains (Fig 11–5). The α chain (MW 50,000) contains the binding site for IgE and is exposed on the cell surface. It contains 2 domains and has 30% carbohydrate. The β chain (MW 30,000) is located entirely within the cell membrane. There are 2 identical disulfide-linked γ chains on the cytoplasmic aspect of the cell surface membrane. A different low-affinity (K_a 10^{-5} mol/L) receptor (FcεRII) is present on eosinophils, monocyte-macrophages, lymphocytes, and platelets. This receptor is expressed when those cells are activated, and it plays no known role in the release of mediators of inflammation.

Cellular events of IgE-mediated inflammation are depicted in Figure 11–6. A multivalent antigen (or hapten-carrier complex) reacts with 2 or more IgE antibodies occupying FcεRI receptors; this results in physical bridging of the receptors owing to receptor motion in the plane of the cell membrane, which is in a relatively fluid state. Receptors bound to antigen in this way migrate and form a cap on one pole of the cell. Receptor motion is believed to be the initial signal for mast cell activation.

C. Mediators: Once the cell is activated, generation and release of mediators are accompanied by a rapid series of intracellular biochemical events. The first of these is activation of membrane-associated enzymes serine oxidase, phospholipase C, and adenylate cyclase. This is followed by the same methyltransferase reaction that accompanies ligand-receptor activation in many other cell systems. The critical action of phospholipase C on inositol phospholipids and methylation of membrane phospholipids precedes the influx of extracellular calcium ion into the cell. The initial enzyme reactions are maximal within 15 seconds after the antigen-IgE antibody union has taken place, and calcium uptake is maximal within 2–3 minutes.

Other intracellular reactions include mobilization of protein kinase C from the cytosol to the cell membrane, where it is activated, and an increase in intracellular cyclic AMP (cAMP). The effect of these intracellular enzyme reactions is the fusion of membranes of the cytoplasmic granules with each other and with the mast cell membrane; this is reflected microscopically as degranulation. Preformed mediators, such as histamine, are present within these granules prior to exposure of the cell to antigen and are therefore released from the cell. Active membrane-associated mediators, such as the products of arachidonic acid (prostaglandins and leukotrienes), are then generated.

The variety of mediators that are described in more detail below have different effects on different end organs (blood vessels, smooth muscles, afferent nerve endings, and secretory glands). However, the release of mediators from mast cells follows a clear biphasic course of an immediate response that is maximal at 15–30 minutes and a later response that is maximal at 6 hours.

D. Immediate and Late Phases: The immediate response is mediated principally by the effects of histamine and leukotrienes from the mast cell. The late response requires a number of mediators, of which platelet-activating factor (PAF) is probably the most important, although the arachidonic acid metabolites (leukotrienes and prostaglandins) are probably also important. The late response is characterized by recruitment of inflammatory cells, especially neutrophils and eosinophils. Eosinophils release major basic protein, whereas neutrophils, eosinophils, and mast cells release lysosomal enzymes.

Pathology

The immediate response consists grossly of erythema, localized edema in the form of a wheal, and pruritus, all of which can be explained by the actions of histamine. The microscopic pathology consists of vasodilation and edema with a mild cellular infiltrate initially of granulocytes followed by eosinophils. The late response appears grossly as erythema, induration, heat, burning, and itching. Microscopically, neutrophils predominate, along with edema, degranulated mast cells, and a perivascular distribution of eosinophils. There are some mononuclear cells and free eosinophilic granules in the later stages. Fibrin deposition probably occurs transiently. There are no signs of immunoglobulin or complement deposition.

Clinical Manifestations

IgE-mediated inflammation is responsible for atopic allergy (hay fever, asthma, and atopic dermatitis), systemic anaphylaxis, and allergic urticaria. It is at least in part responsible for immunity to infestation by helminths. It may play a facilitative role as a "gatekeeper" in immune complex–mediated immunity and CMI because of its ability to provide rapid vasodilation, resulting in the formation of a portal of entry into tissues for circulating soluble factors and cells.

CUTANEOUS BASOPHIL HYPERSENSITIVITY

Cutaneous basophil hypersensitivity, formerly known as Jones-Mote hypersensitivity, is a form of inflammation that at present has uncertain significance. It is elicited by protein antigens, which, when injected into the skin, cause a localized area of swelling which is softer than that of DTH, and it is pruritic. It generally follows the same time course as DTH, but it differs histologically from DTH, since there is prominent infiltration with basophils, but no granulomas or other characteristics of DTH. It can be transferred passively with serum or B cells, indicating that it is an antibody-mediated phenomenon and not CMI, although T cells might be required for its expression. Its clinical significance is unknown. The presence of basophils in renal allografts suggests that it may be

involved as one component of the transplant rejection phenomenon.

SUMMARY

The inflammatory response is the primary means by which the immune system functions in immunity. Inflammation is also responsible for hypersensitivity reactions and for many of the clinical effects of autoimmunity.

There are 3 principal pathways of immunologically induced inflammation. CMI/DTH involves the interaction of antigen with the effector T lymphocyte, causing the generation of lymphokines that give rise to a mononuclear cellular inflammation and the formation of granulomas. Immune complex–mediated inflammation involves the interaction of antigen with antibody of certain immunoglobulin isotypes that activate the complement cascade. This generates a variety of chemotactic factors that induce neutrophilic inflammation and vasculitis. IgE-mediated inflammation involves the interaction of antigen with IgE antibodies occupying mast cell receptors. Activation of the mast cell releases mediators with effects on blood vessels, smooth muscles, and secretory glands, causing changes in vascular permeability and the functioning of visceral organs.

The inflammation in infectious, allergic, and autoimmune diseases may involve one or more of these immunologically induced inflammatory pathways.

REFERENCES

Barnett EV: Circulating immune complexes: Their biologic and clinical significance. *J Allergy Clin Immunol* 1986;**78**:1089.

Bielory L et al: Human serum sickness: A prospective analysis of 35 patients treated with equine anti-thymocyte globulin for bone marrow failure. *Medicine* 1988;**67**:40.

Boros DL, Yoshida T (editors): *Basic and Clinical Aspects of Granulomatous Diseases.* North Holland Publishing Co, 1980.

Buhner D, Grant JA: Serum sickness. *Dermatol Clin* 1985;**3**:107.

Dvorak HF, Galli SJ, Dvorak AM: Expression of cell-mediated hypersensitivity in vivo: Recent advances. *Int Rev Exp Pathol* 1980;**21**:119.

Erffmeyer JE: Serum sickness. *Ann Allergy* 1986; **56**:105.

Galli SJ, Askenase PW: Cutaneous basophil hypersensitivity. Pages 321–369 in: *The Reticuloendothelial*

System. Philips SM, Escobar MR (editors). Plenum, 1986.

Ishizaka T, Ishizaka K: Activation of mast cells for mediator release through IgE receptors. *Prog Allergy* 1984;**34:**188.

Metzger H et al: The receptor with high affinity for immunoglobulin E. *Annu Rev Immunol* 1986;**4:**419.

Naguwa SM, Nebon BL: Human serum sickness. *Clin Rev Allergy* 1985;**3:**117.

Serafin WE, Austen KF: Current concepts: Mediation of immediate hypersensitivity reactions. *N Engl J Med* 1987;**317:**30.

Van Es LA: Factors affecting the deposition of immune complexes. *Clin Immunol Allergy* 1981;**1:**281.

Inflammatory Cells: Structure & Function

12

David H. Broide, MB, ChB

The inflammatory response, like the immune response, can be generated both from cells (neutrophils, eosinophils, basophils, macrophages, mast cells, platelets, and endothelium) and from circulating proteins (components of the complement, coagulation, fibrinolysis, and kinin pathways) (see Chapter 13). The cellular inflammatory response is the mechanism by which the body defends against infection and repairs tissue damage. However, persistent inflammation can result in disease states and thus be detrimental to the host. The clinical expression depends on the site (lung, joint, or blood vessel) and cellular nature (neutrophil or eosinophil) of the inflammatory response. To rapidly activate the cellular inflammatory response and to protect the body from the potent cellular inflammatory mediators, these mediators are stored either preformed in cytoplasmic granules or as phospholipids available to be newly generated in the cell surface membrane. Furthermore, there is both a mobile (circulating) and a stationary (noncirculating) cellular inflammatory capacity. Thus, in the inflammatory response, a distinction can be made between short-lived circulating inflammatory cells (neutrophils, eosinophils, and basophils) and cells that preexist in the tissue as long-lived resident noncirculating inflammatory cells (mast cells and macrophages) (Table 12–1). For some inflammatory cells (neutrophils and macrophages) the primary function is phagocytosis, and for others (mast cells and basophils) it is the secretion of inflammatory mediators. The phagocytic cells, by eliminating particles or organisms that have gained access to the host, act as a protective barrier between the environment and the host. In contrast, the secretory cells contain both inflammatory mediators, which increase vascular permeability, and chemotactic factors, which recruit other inflammatory cells, thus contributing to host defense either by amplifying the effects of the phagocytic cells or by having a direct effect on target cells.

This chapter will describe the ultrastructure and identification of each of the inflammatory cells, as well as their subtypes, receptors, and cellular changes during inflammation (activation, degranulation, and metabolism).

NEUTROPHILS

Polymorphonuclear neutrophils are the predominant leukocytes in the circulation, where they have a brief existence between their formation in the bone marrow and their subsequent phagocytic and microbicidal activity in the tissue sites of inflammation. They are primarily responsible for maintaining normal host defenses against invading microorganisms, being the major cellular elements in most forms of acute inflammation, particularly during the earlier stage of the inflammatory response. Their cytoplasmic granules contain a potent array of digestive enzymes, which may either remove tissue debris or act intracellularly or extracellularly to kill and degrade microorganisms. To perform their function in tissues, neutrophils are equipped to adhere to vascular endothelium, diapedese through the walls of small blood vessels, and migrate toward particles to be ingested (**chemotaxis**). In a coordinated, sequential series of steps, they can recognize, attach to, and engulf particles (**phagocytosis**); discharge cytoplasmic granule contents into phagocytic

Table 12–1. Inflammatory Cells.[1]

Circulating	Tissue Resident
Neutrophils	Mast cells
Eosinophils	Macrophages
Basophils	Endothelium
Platelets	

[1]The cells participating in the inflammatory response can be categorized into (1) circulating and (2) noncirculating, tissue-resident inflammatory cells. Another useful way to classify inflammatory cells, as either primary phagocytic cells (macrophages, neutrophils) or primary secretory cells (mast cells, basophils), has the potential disadvantage of ignoring the secretory capacity of primary phagocytic cells such as macrophages.

vacuoles (**degranulation**); and generate a burst of oxidative metabolism. Phagocytosed micro-organisms, coated with complement and specific antibody (**opsonization**), are killed by a combination of neutrophil-generated toxic oxygen radicals and cytotoxic cytoplasmic granule-derived proteins.

Origin & Tissue Distribution

Neutrophils are bone marrow-derived members of the granulocyte series, which arise from pluripotential stem cells in the bone marrow. Stromal cells in the bone marrow produce specific glycoprotein colony-stimulating factors termed granulocyte colony-stimulating factor (G-CSF), granulocyte-macrophage colony-stimulating factor (GM-CSF), and interleukin 3 (IL-3) (see Chapter 7). These factors stimulate neutrophil progenitor cells in the bone marrow to proliferate and differentiate into mature neutrophils. The mature cells remain in the marrow storage compartment for approximately 5 days and then circulate for about 10 hours before entering the tissues at sites of inflammation. It has been estimated that more than 100 billion neutrophils enter and leave the circulation of a 70 kg person daily under normal conditions. This enormous turnover can be increased up to 10-fold during an acute infection.

Ultrastructure & Identification

The neutrophil has a characteristic segmented, multilobe (2–5 lobes) nucleus, which contains densely clumped chromatin and no nucleoli. The neutrophil cytoplasm contains fine granules that stain pink with Wright's stain. In contrast, Wright-stained eosinophil and basophil cytoplasmic granules are larger and stain bright orange (eosinophils) or purplish-black (basophils). The mature neutrophil is conspicuously deficient in rough endoplasmic reticulum, which indicates that the synthesis of new protein is not an important function.

Enzymes associated with neutrophil cytoplasmic granules are capable of hydrolyzing a wide variety of both natural and synthetic substrates, including simple and complex polysaccharides, proteins, and lipids. These enzymes are important in maintaining normal host defenses and in mediating inflammation. Two major types of neutrophil cytoplasmic granules are distinguishable by their morphology, staining characteristics, enzyme content, and order of synthesis during myeloid development. Primary granules are also known as **azurophil granules** because of their blue appearance on Wright's stain. They contain myeloperoxidase and other lysosomal hydrolases, and they appear in the cytoplasm of neutrophils during the promyelocyte stage of development, arising from the concave surface of the Golgi com-

plex. Secondary granules, also known as **specific granules,** are formed from the convex surface of the Golgi complex during the myelocyte stage of development and contain predominantly lysozyme and iron-binding lactoferrin. Azurophil granules, which are more dense and generally larger than the peroxidase-negative specific granules, contain all the neutrophil myeloperoxidase, β-glucuronidase, elastase, and cathepsin G, whereas specific granules contain all the neutrophil lactoferrin. Specific granules outnumber azurophil granules 3:1. The neutrophil ultrastructure is shown in Fig 12–1.

Receptors

A. Immunoglobulin Fc Receptors: Approximately 75–90% of peripheral blood neutrophils have cell surface receptors for the Fc portion of IgG (FcγR) (Table 12–2). There are 3 distinct FcγR's, 2 of which are present on neutrophils. They have apparent molecular weights of 42,000 and 50,000–70,000. The heavier one preferentially binds to antigen-IgG antibody complexes or IgG-coated particles. Binding of immune complexes to this neutrophil FcγR exceeds the binding by the corresponding monomeric IgG. It has been hypothesized that either IgG antibodies in immune complexes have more binding sites available to attach to neutrophil FcγR's or the complexes produce allosteric changes in the conformation of immunoglobulin molecules, thereby

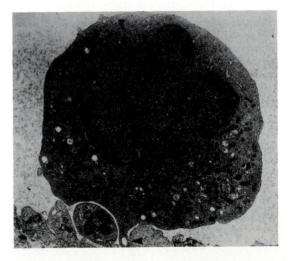

Figure 12–1. Electron micrograph of a neutrophil depicting its characteristic morphology. The nucleus is hypersegmented with abundant heterochromatin and no nucleoli. The cytoplasm contains cytoplasmic granules of heterogeneous size and electron density. The neutrophil is in the process of diapedesing between endothelial cells (arrow). (Courtesy of Henry C Powell, University of California, San Diego.)

Table 12–2. Inflammatory-cell immunoglobulin Fc receptors.

Receptor	Present on:					
	Neutrophils	**Monocytes**	**Mast Cells**	**Basophils**	**Eosinophils**	**Platelets**
IgM	−	−	−	−	−	−
IgG						
IgG1	+	+	−	?	+	+
IgG2	+	+	−	−	?	+
IgG3	+	+	−	−	?	+
IgG4	+	+	−	−	?	+
IgA	+	+	−	−	?	−
IgD	−	−	−	−	+	−
IgE	−	+	+	+	+	+
FcϵRI	−	−	+	+	−	−
FcϵRII	−	+	?	?	+	+

[1]Symbols: +, receptor present; −, receptor absent; ?, presence unknown.

altering the tertiary structure of immunoglobulin and exposing sites capable of interacting with the neutrophil FcγR. Both types of neutrophil FcγR bind to multivalent forms of IgG, but exhibit weak or undetectable binding to monomeric IgG. In addition to IgG receptors, neutrophils have Fc receptors for IgA but appear to lack Fc receptors for IgE and IgD. Studies attempting to demonstrate binding of IgM to human neutrophils have generally not been successful.

B. Complement Receptors: Activation of either the classic complement pathway by antigen-antibody reactions or the alternative complement pathway by certain bacterial products generate complement fragments, which are able to amplify the inflammatory response by attracting and activating neutrophils. Complement fragment C3b mediates these effects through neutrophil cell surface complement receptors, which are described in Chapter 14.

In addition to receptors for IgG and C3b, neutrophils contain receptors for f-Met-Leu-Phe (FMLP), leukotriene B$_4$ (LTB$_4$), hematopoietic growth factors (GM-CSF and G-CSF), and complement fragments C5a and C3a.

Adherence & Chemotaxis

Peripheral blood contains 2 exchangeable pools of neutrophils, a central circulating axial pool and a marginal pool moving slowly along the vascular endothelium. One of the earliest events in acute inflammation is an increase in the adherence of circulating neutrophils to vascular endothelium. In response to IL-1 and other inflammatory mediators, endothelial cells become adhesive for neutrophils. Although the molecular nature of the endothelium-neutrophil adherence is at present incompletely understood, it is known that adherence of neutrophils to cells and surfaces is mediated partly by a related group of cell surface glycoproteins that include the CR3 receptor (C3bi), lymphocyte function antigen-1 (LFA-1), and p150,95. In addition, neutrophils possess receptors for the extracellular matrix components laminin and fibronectin, which could facilitate the attachment of neutrophils to host tissue or microbial surfaces.

There are a large number of chemotactic factors that can recruit neutrophils to sites of tissue inflammation. The best-characterized of these are FMLP, LTB$_4$, and C5a. They are derived from cellular as well as circulating plasma sources, including proteins (C5a and C567 derived from the complement pathway, fibrin fragments, and collagen fragments), enzymes (plasma kallikrein and C3bBb derived from the alternative complement pathway), lipids (LTB$_4$, platelet-activating factor [PAF]), synthetic N-formyl methionyl peptides (derived from bacterial protein and mitochondrial protein breakdown). Cellular sources of factors chemotactic for neutrophils include bacteria, macrophages, lymphocytes, platelets, and mast cells. At nanomolar concentrations of chemotactic factors, neutrophils respond by an increase in adhesiveness, an increase in chemotactic factor receptor number, and the release of specific cytoplasmic granule contents, and they are primed for the oxidative burst.

In contrast to tissue eosinophils, which are present in normal tissues at epithelial surfaces in contact with the environment, the neutrophil is not normally found in tissues unless recruited from the circulation to sites of tissue inflammation.

Phagocytosis

The internalization of extracellular substances by invagination of the plasma membrane (**endocytosis**) can be further defined as **phagocytosis** (the ingestion of particulate material) or **pinocytosis** (the internalization of fluids and solutes) (Fig 12–2). Attachment of a neutrophil to a suitable small particle results in the formation at the site of attachment of pseudopodia, which surround the particle and ultimately fuse at its distal pole. The neutrophil cell surface then completely

1. neutrophil maintains viability

(a) 'regurgitation during feeding'

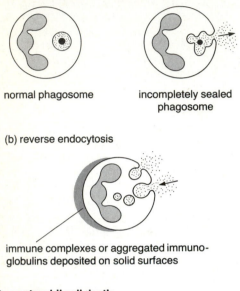

normal phagosome   incompletely sealed
                          phagosome

(b) reverse endocytosis

immune complexes or aggregated immunoglobulins deposited on solid surfaces

2. neutrophil cell death

(a) cell death

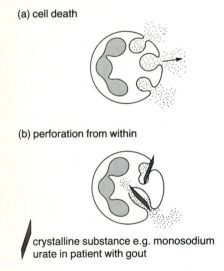

(b) perforation from within

crystalline substance e.g. monosodium
urate in patient with gout

Figure 12–2. Neutrophil events during phagocytosis and degranulation. See the text for a description.

surrounds the engulfed particle, forming a phago-cytic vesicle or **phagosome,** which moves into the cell and fuses with intracellular cytoplasmic gran-ules. This provides a local environment in which the opportunity for particle degradation by cy-toplasmic granule enzymes in the phagosome is enhanced. Phagocytosis requires metabolic energy and an active cytoplasmic contractile protein sys-tem. Although neutrophils are capable of phago-cytosing particles in the absence of IgG antibody

or complement, phagocytosis is stimulated by the presence of both C3b and IgG antibody, which have separate but synergistic roles in phagocyto-sis. Activation of the neutrophil C3b receptor pri-marily promotes recognition and attachment of bound or adherent particles, whereas occupation of the neutrophil IgG receptor by antibody ap-pears necessary for optimal phagocytosis.

Degranulation

Neutrophil cytoplasmic granules (modified ly-sosomes) contain a potent array of destructive en-zymes, which may act either inside or outside the neutrophil. Since mature neutrophils are deficient in their ability to synthesize new protein mole-cules, the cytoplasmic granules cannot be regener-ated once they have been lost. Intracellular degran-ulation, the "internal digestive system" of the neutrophil, is not a uniform process, as neutrophil azurophil and specific cytoplasmic granules dis-charge their contents at different rates during phagocytosis. During phagocytosis, neutrophil cy-toplasmic granule membranes fuse with the mem-branes of the phagocytic vacuole. The process of neutrophil degranulation involves discharge of the neutrophil cytoplasmic granule contents into the newly formed **phagolysosome.** The formation of phagolysosomes is crucial to host defense, as the ingested microorganisms are killed and digested within phagolysosomes. Although the contents of neutrophil cytoplasmic granules most often are discharged intracellularly into phagosomes, in certain circumstances they can be released extra-cellularly. The extracellular degranulation of neu-trophils could contribute significantly to inflam-mation, as neutrophils are richly endowed with a variety of neutral and acidic proteases that are collectively capable of activating complement, of generating kinins, of enhancing vascular perme-ability, and of degrading elastin, collagen, and a variety of other proteins. The mechanisms of neutrophil extracellular degranulation include neutrophil cell death as well as the extrusion of neutrophil cytoplasmic granule contents from incompletely sealed neutrophil phagosomes, open at their external borders to the extracellular space (Fig 12–2).

Neutrophils can also degranulate in the absence of phagocytosis when stimulated by immune com-plexes or aggregated immunoglobulins deposited on solid surfaces. This process is termed "reverse endocytosis," during which the merger of neutro-phil cytoplasmic granules with the plasma mem-brane results in the discharge of granule constitu-ents directly to the outside of the cell. This mechanism of cytoplasmic granule release from neutrophils could be pertinent to the pathogenesis of tissue injury in several diseases in which im-mune complexes are deposited upon cell surfaces or extracellular structures such as vascular basement membrane.

Oxidative Metabolism

Oxygen-derived free radicals generated by the neutrophil play an important role as microbicidal oxidants as well as mediators of inflammation and tissue injury (Table 12–3). The bulk of oxygen consumed by stimulated neutrophils is converted directly to superoxide anion radicals (O_2^-) by the enzyme NADPH oxidase. The superoxide is rapidly converted to hydrogen peroxide and hydroxyl radicals, which provide most of the microbicidal activity within the phagosome and extracellular environment. Additional oxidants such as hypochlorous acid and free chlorine are formed in the presence of hydrogen peroxide, halide, and neutrophil cytoplasmic granule–derived myeloperoxidase. The neutrophil is able to protect itself from the injurious effects of toxic oxygen radicals by the presence in the neutrophil cytosol of potent protective enzymes and scavengers such as superoxide dismutase, catalase, and the glutathione peroxidase-reductase cycle.

The generation of toxic oxidants in neutrophils is stimulated immunologically by a variety of microorganisms coated with the appropriate antibody (opsonin). Other stimuli include concanavalin A, FMPL, NaF, phorbol myristate acetate, C5a, the calcium ionophore A23187, serum-activated zymosan particles, latex beads, and various microorganisms coated with appropriate opsonins. As is the case with degranulation, enhanced oxidative metabolism by neutrophils can be stimulated in the absence of phagocytosis. The neutrophil respiratory oxidant burst is associated with increased oxygen consumption, superoxide generation, the emission of light (chemiluminescence), and increased glucose oxidation via the hexose monophosphate pathway.

Heterogeneity

Morphologically indistinguishable circulating neutrophils are heterogeneous in density, cell surface antigens, Fc receptor expression, and functional properties (eg, surface adherence, response to chemoattractants, aggregation, and phagocytosis). The origin and significance of this neutrophil heterogeneity are at present unknown. Whether the evidence for neutrophil heterogeneity reflects distinct stem cells or represents functional maturational differences within a common cell line awaits further study.

MAST CELLS

Mast cells are tissue cells with a prominent role in IgE-mediated inflammation. They are especially abundant in tissues at host-environment interfaces in organs such as the skin (10^4 mast cells/mm^3), lungs (10^6 mast cells/g, gastrointestinal tract, and nasal mucous membrane. They are thus strategically positioned to interact rapidly with inhaled or ingested antigens and to secrete a potent array of proinflammatory preformed and newly generated mediators, which produce increased vascular permeability, smooth muscle contraction, and mucus secretion. In addition, mast cell-derived factors are chemotactic for other inflammatory cells including eosinophils, neutrophils, and mononuclear cells (see Chapter 13).

Ultrastructure & Receptors

Mast cells are characterized by the presence of the high-affinity cell surface IgE receptor (FcϵRI) and histamine-containing cytoplasmic granules (50–200 per cell) (Table 12–2). Mast cells are relatively large (10–15 μm in diameter). They possess a single round or oval, eccentrically located nucleus and membrane-bound cytoplasmic granules (0.1–0.4 μm in diameter) that are smaller than the cytoplasmic granules of basophils (1.0–1.2 μm in diameter). Although mast cells and basophils both have histamine-containing cytoplasmic granules and high-affinity cell surface IgE receptors, mast cells differ from basophils in morphology, mediator content, and sensitivity to pharmacologic modulation. In tissues, human mast cells are vari-

---

Table 12–3. Generation of toxic oxygen products by the respiratory oxidant burst in leukocyte phagolysosomes.[1]

I. Electron transfer by oxygen burst

$$Glucose + NADP^+ \xrightarrow{\text{hexose monophosphate pathway}}$$

$$Pentose\ PO_4 + NADPH$$

$$NADPH + O_2 \xrightarrow{\text{NADPH oxidase}} NADP^+ + \boxed{O_2^-}$$

II. Spontaneous generation of toxic oxygen products

$$2O_2^- + 2H^+ \longrightarrow H_2O_2 + \boxed{^1O_2}$$

$$O_2^- + H_2O_2 \longrightarrow \boxed{\cdot OH} + OH^- + \boxed{^1O_2}$$

III. Peroxidase generation of halogenating compounds

$$H_2O_2 + Cl^- \xrightarrow{\text{peroxidase}} \boxed{OCl^-} + H_2O$$

$$OCl^- + H_2O \longrightarrow {}^1O_2 + Cl^- + H_2O$$

[1]The toxic products that kill bacteria during phagocytosis are shown in outline. O_2^-, superoxide anion; $^1O_2$, singlet oxygen; $\cdot OH$, hydroxyl free radical; OCl^-, hypochlorous anion. The leukocyte contains protective enzymes superoxide dismutase and catalase (equations not shown).

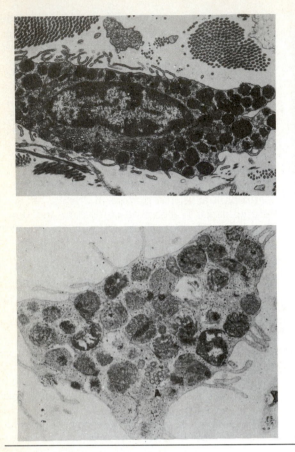

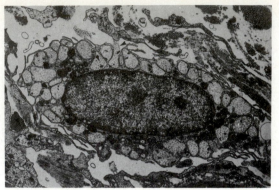

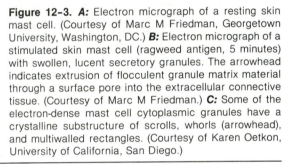

Figure 12–3. A: Electron micrograph of a resting skin mast cell. (Courtesy of Marc M Friedman, Georgetown University, Washington, DC.) **B:** Electron micrograph of a stimulated skin mast cell (ragweed antigen, 5 minutes) with swollen, lucent secretory granules. The arrowhead indicates extrusion of flocculent granule matrix material through a surface pore into the extracellular connective tissue. (Courtesy of Marc M Friedman.) **C:** Some of the electron-dense mast cell cytoplasmic granules have a crystalline substructure of scrolls, whorls (arrowhead), and multiwalled rectangles. (Courtesy of Karen Oetkon, University of California, San Diego.)

able in shape, appearing as round, oval, or spindle-shaped cells. Electron-microscopic analysis of human mast cells (Fig 12–3) reveals cytoplasmic granules that are heterogeneous in substructural pattern and exhibit scroll-like configurations, amorphous electron-dense granular zones, and highly ordered crystalline arrays. Individual cytoplasmic granules are frequently characterized by more than one of these patterns in sharp juxtaposition. During IgE-mediated mast cell activation, the crystalline structure of human skin and lung mast cell cytoplasmic granules is lost. The mast cell plasma membrane possesses numerous cell surface projections. The identification of mast cells by light microscopy is assisted by their characteristic staining properties. Mast cell cytoplasmic granules contain preformed mediators, including anionic proteoglycans. When stained with toluidine blue, the proteoglycans give the mast cell granule a metachromatic red or violet color.

IgE-mediated mast cell degranulation (described in Chapter 11) is characterized by a series of events, including enlargement of cytoplasmic granules, granule solubilization (disorganization and electron lucency of granules), and membrane fusion of adjacent cytoplasmic granules and the cell surface membrane. The conduits formed between the cytoplasmic granules and the outer cell membrane permit communication of the solubilized cytoplasmic granules with the extracellular space. Mast cell cytoplasmic granules contain much larger amounts of histamine ($5 \ \mu g/10^6$ cells) than do basophils ($1 \ \mu g/10^6$ cells).

Subtypes

The concept of mast cell heterogeneity was initially defined for the rat small intestine by the identification of a population of mucosal type mast cells differing in their staining and fixation properties from those of the rat connective tissue mast cell. Mucosal mast cells have subsequently been shown to differ from connective tissue mast cells in their T cell dependence, preformed cytoplasmic granule mediators (proteoglycan, protease), mediators generated from arachidonic acid, and functional responses to secretagogues (neuropeptides, compound 48/80) and antiallergic compounds.

Evidence for human mast cell heterogeneity is less conclusive. However, histochemical and biochemical analysis of mast cells derived from skin, lungs, nose, and intestines shows that there are 2 types of mast cells, which differ in content of the 2 cytoplasmic granule neutral proteases, tryptase and chymase. T mast cells contain tryptase and are the predominant type of mast cells in the lungs and gastrointestinal mucosa, whereas TC mast cells contain both tryptase and chymase and are the predominant mast cell type in the skin and gastrointestinal submucosa. The T lymphocyte dependence of T but not TC mast cells is suggested from studies of patients with congenital or acquired T lymphocyte defects (ie, patients with combined immunodeficiency or AIDS) in whom there is a deficiency of T mast cells in the gastrointestinal mucosa.

BASOPHILS

Basophils are circulating neutrophils with many of the functional properties of tissue mast cells. Mature basophils (5–7 μm in diameter) are the smallest cells in the granulocyte series. Basophils share with mast cells high-affinity IgE receptors and cytoplasmic granules containing histamine, but differ from mast cells in that they differentiate and mature in the bone marrow, circulate in the blood, and are not normally found in connective tissue (Table 12–4). The morphology of basophils also distinguishes them from mast cells. Basophils possess lobular bilobed or multilobed nuclei, peripherally condensed nuclear chromatin, and electron-dense aggregates of cytoplasmic glycogen (Fig 12–4). In contrast, mast cells have a single eccentric nucleus and uniformly distributed cell surface membrane processes, and they lack both the peripherally condensed nuclear chromatin and the electron-dense aggregates of cytoplasmic glycogen that are present in basophils. Another distinguishing feature between mast cells and basophils is the presence of 2 surface membrane proteins, Charcot-Leyden crystal protein and major basic protein, in the cell surface membrane of basophils but not mast cells. The basophil cell surface membrane is smooth, has occasional, irregularly distributed, short, blunt folds or uropods, and contains an average of 270,000 high-affinity receptors for IgE (Table 12–2). Basophils contain

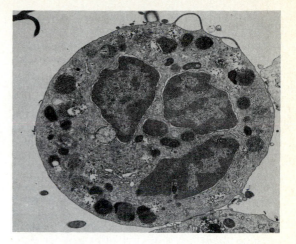

Figure 12–4. Electron micrograph of a peripheral blood basophil. The basophil has a multilobed nucleus and a smooth cell surface with occasional irregularly distributed short blunt folds or uropods. (Courtesy of Marc M Friedman.)

fewer cytoplasmic granules than mast cells and make up 0.2–1% of nucleated cells in bone marrow and peripheral blood.

Small to moderate numbers of basophils are found in a variety of inflammatory conditions involving the skin (late phase skin reaction to allergen, cutaneous basophil hypersensitivity reactions, lesions of bullous pemphigoid), small intestine (Crohn's disease), kidneys (allergic interstitial nephritis, renal allograft rejection), nose (allergic rhinitis), and eyes (allergic conjunctivitis). Although mast cells have an established role in IgE-mediated inflammation, the importance of basophils in immunity and hypersensitivity has yet to be determined.

EOSINOPHILS

Eosinophils are found in the tissues in many diseases, but predominantly in 2 forms of inflamma-

Table 12–4. Structural characteristics distinguishing basophils from mast cells[1]

Characteristic	Basophils	Mast Cells
Size	5–7 μm	10–15 μm
Nucleus	Lobular bilobed or multilobed nucleus with peripherally condensed nuclear chromatin	Single nucleus
Cytoplasm	Contains electron-dense aggregates of cytoplasmic glycogen not present in mast cells	Electron-dense, histamine-containing, membrane-bound secretory granules are smaller than cytoplasmic granules of basophils
Cell surface	Smooth with occasional irregularly distributed short blunt folds or uropods	Numerous cell surface projections
Distribution	Primarily circulating in blood	Tissue resident

[1]Mast cells and basophils are the only inflammatory cells with histamine-containing cytoplasmic granules and high-affinity cell surface IgE receptors

tion: allergy and parasitic infection. Eosinophils, like basophils and neutrophils, are bone-marrow-derived granulocytes, which can be distinguished from the other 2 members of the granulocyte series on the basis of morphology, staining properties, mediator content, and association with differing disease states. Although the eosinophil stem cell is not morphologically identifiable, the eosinophil promyelocyte is clearly distinguishable from the promyelocyte of neutrophils and the basophils by its characteristic cytoplasmic granules. The life span of an eosinophil is relatively short; it has a bone marrow maturation time of 2–6 days, a circulating half-life of 6–12 hours, and a connective tissue residence time of several days. The number of circulating blood eosinophils, which make up about 1–3% of circulating leukocytes, is a very small portion of the total body eosinophil count. It is estimated that for every circulating eosinophil, there are approximately 200 mature eosinophils in the bone marrow and 500 eosinophils in connective tissue. Although a precise model of human eosinophil proliferation and differentiation in vivo is not possible at present, in vitro studies suggest that hematopoietic growth factors such as GM-CSF, IL-3, and IL-5 (eosinophil-differentiating factor) are important factors in regulating eosinophilopoiesis.

Ultrastructure

The eosinophil nucleus is bilobed and lacks a nucleolus (Fig 12–5). The most distinctive feature of eosinophils is their specific or secondary cytoplasmic granules, which contain an electron-dense crystalloid core surrounded by a less dense matrix. Human eosinophils have approximately

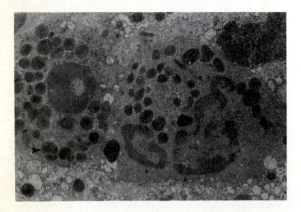

Figure 12–5. Electron micrograph of 2 tissue eosinophils depicting their distinct bilobed nuclei (small arrowheads) lacking nucleoli. The cytoplasm contains characteristic specific or secondary granules with a central electron-dense crystalline core running parallel to the long axis of the cytoplasmic granules (large arrowhead). The electron-dense core of the cytoplasmic granules is surrounded by a less electron-dense matrix.

200 secondary cytoplasmic granules per cell, one-tenth the number present in neutrophils. Eosinophils also have primary cytoplasmic granules, which are round, uniformly electron-dense, and characteristically seen in promyelocytes. Human eosinophils are slightly larger than neutrophils, being approximately 12–17 μm in diameter. The cytoplasmic granules are often spherical or ovoid and are 0.5 μm in diameter. The high content of a biochemically distinct peroxidase and the presence of at least 3 other basic proteins are the distinguishing features of the eosinophil cytoplasmic granules. One of these, the major basic protein, has a strong affinity for acidic dyes such as eosin, resulting in the characteristic intense red staining of the eosinophil cytoplasmic granules.

Receptors

A. Immunoglobulin Fc Receptors: A low-affinity IgE receptor (FcϵRII) identified on human eosinophils has a 100-fold-lower affinity to IgE than does the high-affinity IgE receptor (FcϵRI) present on mast cells and basophils, but its affinity for IgE is comparable to the affinity of FcγR for IgG (Table 12–2). Unlike other Fc receptors sequenced to date, FcϵRII is not a member of the immunoglobulin gene superfamily, but belongs to a primitive superfamily of vertebrate and invertebrate lectins (including CD23, the transferin receptor, the invariant chain of class II MHC antigens, influenza virus neuraminidase, and β-galactosidase 2,6-sialyltransferase). A common feature of this family of molecules is their unusual membrane orientation, with a cytoplasmic amino terminus and an extracellular carboxy terminus.

Approximately 10–30% of eosinophils from normal individuals have IgG receptors. Activation of the eosinophil IgG receptor with IgG-coated schistosomula or Sepharose-coated beads induces degranulation and the release of the newly generated mediator LTC$_4$. The generation of the eosinophil-derived LTC$_4$, in response to IgG activation, is increased up to 10-fold in "activated" hypodense eosinophils compared with normodense eosinophils (see below).

B. Complement Receptors: In normal individuals approximately 40–50% of eosinophils compared with 90% of neutrophils display complement receptors. The percentage of eosinophils bearing complement receptors is increased in the hypereosinophilic syndrome, helminth infections, and atopy. This suggests that activation of eosinophil complement receptors in these disorders may play a role in the inflammatory response of the eosinophil. The eosinophil CR3 receptor (which binds C3bi) appears to be more important than the CR1 receptor in mediating adherence and parasite cytotoxicity to antibody-schistosomula targets.

Activated Eosinophils

When peripheral blood eosinophils are separated on a density gradient, a subpopulation of low-density or "hypodense" eosinophils can be separated from normal or "normodense" eosinophils. Evidence that the hypodense eosinophils are cells that have been activated and degranulated in vivo includes (1) an altered expression of cell surface antigenic determinants, (2) an increased expression of IgG and IgE Fc receptors, (3) altered oxidative metabolism, (4) increased generation of LTC_4 after incubation with IgG-coated particles, and (5) an increased capacity to kill schistosomula of the parasite *Schistosoma mansoni* in vitro. Peripheral blood "activated" hypodense eosinophils have been found in patients with atopy, asthma, chronic helminthic infections, the idiopathic hypereosinophilic syndrome, and neoplasms. Eosinophils can be activated by vascular endothelium, T cell-derived cytokines (GM-CSF, IL-3, and IL-5), and monocyte-macrophage-derived cytokines (IL-1 and tumor necrosis factor [TNF]).

Effector Function

Helminthic (metazoan) parasites, especially those with tissue-dwelling phases, are associated with a prominent blood and/or tissue eosinophilia. This does not occur in protozoan infections. Eosinophil chemotactic and activating factors derived from mast cells, monocytes, and T lymphocytes appear to regulate eosinophil effector function in killing parasites. In vitro a number of parasites, including *Trichinella,* schistosomes, and *Fasciola,* can be killed or damaged by eosinophils. As the parasite represents a large, noningestible microorganism to the eosinophil, eosinophil cytotoxicity requires direct eosinophil-parasite cell contact. In vivo studies have shown that eosinophils accumulate around parasites in tissues and deposit toxic cytoplasmic granule contents on tissue parasites. The eosinophil, with its cationic secondary cytoplasmic granules and potent generated oxidants, is well equipped to destroy these multicellular organisms.

The role of eosinophilic inflammation in allergy has been studied most thoroughly in the pathogenesis of the airway inflammatory response in asthma. The hexagonal, bipyramidal Charcot-Leyden crystals, first found in 1872 in the sputum of patients with asthma, are "footprints" of the eosinophil inflammatory response in the airway. The Charcot-Leyden crystal is a protein with lysophospholipase activity derived from the eosinophil cell surface membrane. Major basic protein liberated from eosinophil cytoplasmic granules has been shown to be toxic to respiratory epithelium, and its levels are elevated in the sputum and bronchoalveolar lavage fluid of asthmatic patients.

Although eosinophils are able to function as phagocytes, they are less efficient than neutrophils both in the rate of phagocytosis and in the quantity of material ingested. Eosinophils are able to ingest bacteria, fungi, mycoplasmas, inert particles, and antigen-antibody complexes in vitro, but conclusive evidence for a functional role as phagocytic cells in vivo is still awaited.

MACROPHAGES

Macrophages share with neutrophils a central role in host defense against infection, which includes ingesting and killing invading organisms and releasing a number of factors involved in host defense and inflammation. They also function as antigen-presenting cells (APC) during the development of specific immunity (see Chapter 5). They are similar to neutrophils in their phagocytic capacity and in their potent array of cytoplasmic granule-derived hydrolytic enzymes and production of toxic oxygen metabolites. In contrast to neutrophils, macrophages have long life spans, can differentiate in situ, respond to external stimuli with a relatively slow and sustained time course, and usually become prominent in inflammatory lesions after the first 8–12 hours. Macrophages and neutrophils differ in their distribution of cytoplasmic granuloenzymes, reuse phagolysosomes to reconstruct their plasma membranes, and secrete nonlysosomal proteins.

Monocyte-Macrophage Formation

The cells in the mononuclear phagocyte system (previously termed the reticuloendothelial system) include promonocytes and their precursors in the bone marrow, monocytes in the circulation, and tissue macrophages. In the bone marrow, over a period of approximately 6 days, a committed progenitor cell termed "colony-forming unit granulocyte macrophage" (CFU-GM) differentiates under the influence of locally produced colony-stimulating factors (CSF) into a monoblast. The monoblast differentiates into a promonocyte and subsequently is released into the circulation as a monocyte. Monocytes are large cells with an oval, indented, or "folded" nucleus possessing lacy to strandlike chromatin and plentiful, gray-blue cytoplasm containing fine azurophilic granules. Human monocytes, circulating in the bloodstream, have a half-life of about 1–3 days. Migration of monocytes into the different tissues appears to be a random phenomenon in the absence of localized inflammation. Compared with neutrophils, monocytes have a much smaller bone marrow reserve, a longer intravascular half-life, and a larger extravascular tissue compartment. The tissue macrophage arises either by immigration of monocytes from the blood (probably the predominant mechanism) or by proliferation of precursors in local sites. Macrophages differ from monocytes in their relative enzymatic activities, their phagocytic capacities, and their cell surface membrane characteristics. The macrophage cell surface membrane has more immunoglobulin and complement receptors than the precursor monocyte does. During differentiation of monocytes to macrophages, azurophilic peroxidase-containing cytoplasmic granules are lost and lysosymes containing hydrolytic enzymes become prominent. Monocytes are richly endowed with myeloperoxidase, whereas tissue macrophages are not.

In the presence of helper T cells, macrophages may become actively endocytic cells organized into structures (granulomas) that are the hallmark of delayed hypersensitivity reactions. Macrophages that have accumulated at a site of chronic inflammation often differentiate further to form epithelioid cells, or they may fuse to form multinucleated giant cells.

Ultrastructure & Receptors

The ultrastructure of the macrophage is shown in Fig 12–6. The macrophages of the liver (Kupffer cells), lungs (alveolar macrophages), connective tissue (histiocytes), bone (osteoclasts), skin (Langerhans cells), central nervous system (microglial cells), and serous cavities (pleural and peritoneal macrophages) all belong to the mononuclear phagocyte series. Characteristic features of macrophages include the ability to adhere to glass, phagocytose, ruffle their membranes, display immunoglobulin Fc receptors, and stain positively

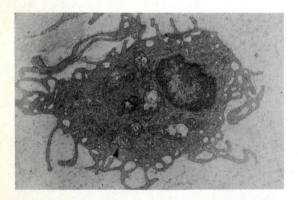

Figure 12–6. Electron micrograph of a macrophage revealing a cell with a single nucleus and cytoplasm containing modest numbers of mitrochondria (arrowhead). The numerous cell surface projections (filopodia) are consistent with the motile nature of this phagocytic cell. (Courtesy of Henry C Powell.)

for nonspecific esterase and peroxidase. The macrophage samples and senses its environment through specific cell surface membrane receptors, which include receptors for immunoglobulin and complement (IgG, IgE, C3b, C5a), hematopoietic growth factors (M-CSF, GM-CSF), lipoproteins, peptides, and polysaccharides (Table 12–2). Binding of agonists to these receptors is the initial step in the series of actions that eventuate in macrophage proliferation, chemotaxis, phagocytosis, secretion, or oxygen consumption. Occupancy of these receptors can activate the macrophage to secrete soluble products (including IL-1, hydrolytic enzymes, and products of oxidative metabolism) that endow the macrophage with the capacity to exert pro- or anti-inflammatory effects on the function of other cell types.

Activation

Activated macrophages exhibit morphologic, metabolic, and functional differences from resting macrophages. In its most commonly accepted sense, an "activated" macrophage is one that has an enhanced capacity to kill facultative intracellular microorganisms or tumor cells. During an infection, specific effector T lymphocytes, sensitized to antigens from the infecting organism, release soluble factors, such as gamma interferon and GM-CSF, that can activate macrophages. In this manner the induction of macrophage activation is immunologically specific (T cell-microbial antigen interaction), whereas its expression (macrophage activation) is nonspecific and consists, in essence, of an enhanced antimicrobial capacity. Macrophages are attracted to sites of inflammation by chemotactic factors derived from serum (C5a), lymphocytes, neutrophils, and fibroblasts. As with the neutrophil, phagocytosis is influenced by the presence of opsonins for the invading microorganism (IgG, complement, and perhaps fibronectin) as well as by the inherent surface properties of the microorganism. Macrophage activation is evident from morphologic changes (larger size, ruffling of the plasma membrane, increased formation of pseudopods, increased number of pinocytic vesicles), metabolic changes (increased glucose metabolism and respiratory oxidant burst), and functional changes (more vigorous migration in response to chemotactic factors, increased microbicidal activity) exhibited by the activated macrophage.

Phagocytosis & Secretion

Macrophages are able to internalize material external to the cell (endocytosis) by means of phagocytosis (the ingestion of particulate material) or pinocytosis (the ingestion of soluble materials). The generation of pinocytic vesicles is a constitutive event, which proceeds without known exogenous stimuli in an energy-dependent manner. In this way large amounts of the plasma membrane are continually recycled, allowing a constant reutilization of the plasma membrane and its receptors, as well as allowing a constant flow of solutes into the cell. Particle ingestion by macrophages is usually accompanied by a respiratory oxidant burst similar to that in neutrophils and eosinophils. Macrophage phagocytosis requires the expenditure of metabolic energy in the form of high-energy phosphate. The source of high-energy phosphate is creatine phosphate in the macrophage, compared with ATP in the neutrophil.

In addition to their role as phagocytic cells, macrophages are secretory and regulatory cells. The macrophage is an extraordinarily active secretory cell, having the capacity to produce approximately 100 different substances affecting the inflammatory response. Some of the macrophage products are secreted constitutively (lysosome, lipoprotein lipase), whereas others follow ligand-receptor interaction. Some ligands, such as immune complexes, trigger secretion in seconds to minutes after macrophage stimulation, whereas others, including lymphocyte mediators, require days after the stimulus for macrophage secretion.

In general, the antimicrobial spectrum of macrophages exceeds that of neutrophils, although neutrophils kill many organisms more rapidly than do macrophages. In addition to antimicrobial activity, macrophages subserve a number of important effector functions including antitumor function, immunoregulatory function, wound healing, and selective removal of autologous cells (senescent cells, cells targeted by autoimmune reactions, and metabolically defective cells). Macrophages can also play an important role in the resolution of acute inflammation. In addition to secreting extracellular proteases, which help liquefy the residual inflammatory exudate, macrophages phagocytose cellular debris, inflammatory exudate, and senescent neutrophils.

PLATELETS

Platelets, which arise in the bone marrow from megakaryocyte cytoplasm and thus lack a nucleus, are the smallest circulating cells (2 μm in diameter). Unstimulated platelets, which contain 3 types of cytoplasmic granules (dense bodies, α granules, and lysosomal granules), circulate as flattened disks remaining within the intravascular space during their 10-day life span. Platelet activation is characterized by a change in platelet morphology, platelet aggregation, generation of arachidonic acid metabolites (prostaglandins G_2 and H_2, thromboxane A_2), and secretion of platelet cytoplasmic granule contents. Although the content of preformed cytoplasmic granule mediators in platelets resembles that in other secretory inflammatory cells, the confinement of platelets to the intravascular compartment (intact platelets are rarely found extravascularly at inflammatory sites) suggests that platelets have a more limited role than the other cells in inflammation. This does not exclude the possibility that intravascularly activated platelets generate inflammatory mediators which might exert their effects at extravascular sites of tissue inflammation.

The role of platelets in inflammatory reactions is therefore not as well defined as that of the neutrophil, eosinophil, macrophage, or mast cell. However, activated platelets may contribute to inflammatory responses by releasing clotting and growth factors, amines, and lipids with vasoactivity, as well as neutral and acid hydrolases. Activated platelets may also aggregate and serve as foci that trap responding leukocytes and help produce vascular occlusion. Platelets are able to interact with the immune system through platelet cell surface FcγR and FcϵRII. The interaction of platelets with components of the immune system includes platelet binding of IgG and generation of platelet-derived proinflammatory mediators in response to IgG-immune complex platelet activation. Platelets also express 6×10^4 FcϵRII per cell (Table 12–2). Activation of FcϵRII on the platelet induces the formation of a factor cytotoxic to parasites (probably hydrogen peroxide or oxygen metabolites), but it does not lead to the release of the contents of the platelet cytoplasmic granules, nor to platelet aggregation. Activation of the platelet FcϵRII also induces production of PAF, a potent inflammatory mediator. The platelet therefore may play a role in cellular inflammation, in addition to its role in hemostasis and thrombosis.

ENDOTHELIUM

Recent evidence has led to the appreciation that endothelial cells are not merely conduit cells lining blood vessels and thus passive bystanders in the inflammatory response, but, rather, are actively involved in modulating the inflammatory response of the circulating inflammatory cells. Endothelial cells "activated" by various inflammatory cytokines (IL-1, TNF) exhibit increased adhesivity for many circulating inflammatory cells (monocytes, neutrophils). This increased endothelial adhesivity is probably important in recruiting circulating inflammatory cells to sites of tissue inflammation. Endothelial cells are also capable of secreting the cytokines IL-1 and GM-CSF, which are important modulators of the inflammatory response (see Chapter 7).

SUMMARY

Although the inflammatory cells differ in morphology, mediator content, stimuli for cell activation, and time course for mediator release, they do have many features in common. These common cellular features include common receptors (immunoglobulin and complement), cytoplasmic granules containing potent hydrolytic enzymes, the generation of arachidonic acid metabolites, and the ability to phagocytose or secrete. As tissue inflammation may be mediated by serum proteins or inflammatory cells, the control of the interrelated feedback systems is important to host defense. Cellular inflammation is a double-edged sword, being a crucial form of host defense but having serious deleterious effects if it is either inadequately or excessively activated.

In attempting to define the precise roles played by the different cell types in inflammation, important advances have been made in characterizing the structure and function of purified populations of the various inflammatory cells. However, the local environment in inflamed tissues represents a complex milieu in which many different inflammatory cells and serum proteins are present, raising the possibility of important modulating effects, which will not be recognized when only pure cell populations are studied. Despite the complexity of the inflammatory responses, it seems likely that there is considerable coordination and cooperation between the different cell types, which is mediated through inflammatory mediators and shared common receptors (ie, immunoglobulin and complement). Further characterization of the various inflammatory cells and their subtypes will assist in improving our understanding of the complex cellular interactions involved in cellular inflammation.

REFERENCES

Neutrophils

Cohen AM, et al: In vivo stimulation of granulopoieses by recombinant human granulocyte colony-stimulating factor. *Proc Natl Acad Sci USA* 1987;**84**:2484.

Goetzl EJ, Goldstein IM: Granulocytes. Chap 19, pp 322–345, in: *Textbook of Rheumatology,* 3rd ed. Kelley WN et al (editors). Saunders, 1989.

Lehrer RI et al: Neutrophils and host defense. *Ann Intern Med* 1988;**109**:127.

Malech HL, Gallin JI: Neutrophils in human diseases. *N Engl J Med* 1987;**317**:687.

Metcalf D: The molecular biology and functions of the granulocyte-macrophage colony-stimulating factors. *Blood* 1986;**67**:257.

Sklar LA: Ligand-receptor dynamics and signal amplification in the neutrophil. *Adv Immunol* 1986;**39**:95.

Macrophages

Adams DO: Molecular interactions in macrophage activation. *Immunol. Today* 1989;**10**:33.

Clark SC, Kamen R: The human hematopoietic colony-stimulating factors. *Science* 1987;**236**:1229.

Henson PM et al: Phagocytic cells: Degranulation and secretion. Chap 22, pp 363–390, in: *Inflammation: Basic Principles and Clinical Correlates.* Gallin JI et al (editors). Raven Press, 1988.

Johnston RB Jr: Current concepts in immunology: Monoctyes and macrophages. *N Engl J Med* 1988;**318**:747.

Roska AK, Lipsky PE: Monocytes and macrophages. Chap 20, pp 346–366, in: *Textbook of Rheumatology,* 3rd ed. Kelley WN et al (editors). Saunders, 1989.

Stossel TP: The molecular biology of phagocytes and the molecular basis of non-neoplastic phagocyte disorders. Chap 14, pp 499–533, in: *The Molecular Basis of Blood Diseases.* Stamatoyannopoulos G. et al (editors). Saunders, 1987.

Unanue ER, Allen PM: The basis for the immunoregulatory role of macrophages and other accessory cells. *Science* 1987;**236**:551.

Mast Cells & Basophils

Charlesworth EN et al: Cutaneous late phase response to allergen. Mediator release and inflammatory cell infiltration. *J Clin Invest* 1989;**83**:1519.

Helm B et al: The mast cell binding site on human immunoglobulin E. *Nature* 1988;**331**:180.

Irani AA et al: Two types of human mast cells that have distinct neutral protease compositions. *Proc Natl Acad Sci USA* 1986;**83**:4464.

Lemanske RF Jr, Kaliner M: Late-phase IgE-mediated reactions. *J Clin Immunol* 1988;**8**:1.

Schwartz LB et al: Tryptase levels as an indicator of mast cell activation in systemic anaphylaxis and mastocytosis. *N Engl J Med* 1987;**316**:1622.

Serafin WE, Austen KF: Mediators of immediate hypersensitivity reactions. *N Engl J Med* 1987;**317**:31.

Stevens RL, Austen KF: Recent advances in the cellular and molecular biology of mast cells. *Immunol Today* 1989;**10**:381.

Stevens RL et al: Biochemical characteristics distinguish subclasses of mammalian mast cells. Pages 183–203, in: *Mast Cell Differentiation and Heterogeneity.* Befus AD, Bienenstock J, Denburg JA (editors). Raven Press, 1986.

Eosinophils

Campbell HD et al: Molecular cloning, nucleotide sequence, and expression of the gene encoding human eosinophil differentiation factor (interleukin 5). *Proc Natl Acad Sci USA* 1987;**84**:6629.

Gleich GJ: Current understanding of eosinophil function. *Hosp Pract* 1988;**23**:137.

Gleich GJ, Adolphson CR: The eosinophil leukocyte: Structure and function. *Adv Immunol* 1986;**39**:177.

Rothenberg ME et al: Eosinophils co-cultured with endothelial cells have increased survival and functional properties. *Science* 1987;**237**:645.

Wardlaw AJ, Kay AB: The role of the eosinophil in the pathogenesis of asthma. *Allergy* 1987;**42**:321.

Platelets

Ginsberg MH: Role of platelets in inflammation and rheumatic disease. *Adv Inflamm Res* 1986;**2**:53.

Kunicki TJ, George JN (editors): *Platelet Immunobiology: Molecular and Clinical Aspects.* Lippincott, 1989.

Endothelium

Jaffe EA: Cell biology of endothelial cells. *Hum Pathol* 1987;**18**:234.

Mediators of Inflammation

Stephen I. Wasserman, MD

The various inflammatory cells discussed in Chapter 12 mediate their responses by releasing or generating chemical compounds or by recruiting other cells to release or activate additional chemical mediators. Our current knowledge of the chemistry, sources, actions, and mechanisms of generation of inflammatory mediators comes largely from studies of allergic diseases, especially IgE-mediated hypersensitivity.

Mediators of inflammation therefore are endogenous chemicals arising from the activation of inflammatory cells by an immune reaction. They are also released or generated from direct stimulation of the cells by cytokines or releasing factors or by exogenous drugs or chemicals. Mediators may be classified by function: (1) those with vasoactive and smooth-muscle-constricting properties, (2) those that attract other cells and are termed chemotactic factors, (3) enzymes, (4) proteoglycans, and (5) reactive molecules generated from the metabolism of oxygen (Table 13–1).

VASOACTIVE & SMOOTH-MUSCLE-CONSTRICTING MEDIATORS

Histamine

Histamine is a vasoactive and smooth-muscle-constricting mediator that is found preformed in the granules of mast cells and basophils (Fig 13–1). Other mediators with these properties are generated from inactive precursors following cell activation. Histamine is generated in this site by the action of histidine decarboxylase upon the amino acid histidine. Mast cells and basophils store approximately 5 and 1 μg of histamine/10^6 cells, respectively. Histamine may make up as much as 10% of the weight of the granule of these cells. It is bound through ionic linkages to proteoglycans and proteins within the mast cell and basophil granule and is particularly tightly bound to mast cell heparin. It is displaced from its binding sites in the granule by exposure to an increased ionic concentration. Levels of histamine in the

blood are highest in the morning and lowest in the late afternoon; they approximate 0.3 ng/mL. A small proportion of histamine, approximating 12–16 μg/24 h, is excreted unchanged in the urine, and the remainder is excreted as metabolic products of the action of histamine methyltransferase and diamine oxidase.

Histamine is found almost exclusively throughout the organism in mast cells and basophils, and therefore tissue levels are particularly high in the intestine, lungs, and skin. Histamine is released from its cellular stores when the cells are activated immunologically by the action of antigen on cell-bound IgE antibodies or when they are activated by nonimmunologic mechanisms, as described in Chapter 11. Increased amounts occur in the circulation of patients with mastocytosis, and the levels are further elevated during attacks of this disorder. Elevated blood levels may also be detected during anaphylaxis, asthma, and a variety of physical urticarias. Increases in local concentrations of histamine have been identified in bronchoalveolar lavage fluid of patients experiencing allergic reactions during allergen provocation or during experimental provocation of asthma and in blister fluids of patients with experimentally induced urticaria.

Histamine exerts its physiologic action by interacting with one of 3 separate target cell receptors, termed H1, H2, and H3 (Table 13–2). The primary H1 functions of histamine, identified by the inhibitory effects of the classic antihistamines, are (1) contraction of smooth muscle of bronchi, intestine, and uterus, and (2) augmentation of vascular permeability between post-capillary venular endothelial cells. Other H1 actions of histamine include pulmonary vasoconstriction, elevation of intracellular levels of cyclic GMP, augmentation of nasal mucus production, enhanced leukocyte chemokinesis, and production of prostaglandins from lung tissue. Stimulation of the H2 receptor augments gastric acid secretion, stimulates airway mucus production, augments intracellular levels of cyclic AMP, inhibits leukocyte chemokinesis,

Table 13–1. Mediators.

Vasoactive and smooth-muscle-constricting mediators
  Preformed
    Histamine
  Generated
    Arachidonic acid metabolites (PGD_2, LTC_4)
    PAF
    Adenosine
Chemotactic mediators
  Eosinophil-directed
    ECF-A
    ECF oligopeptides
    PAF
  Neutrophil-directed
    HMW-NCF
    LTB_4
    PAF
  Monocyte-directed
    Uncharacterized
  Basophil-directed
    Uncharacterized
  Lymphocyte-directed
    Uncharacterized
Enzymatic mediators
  Neutral proteases
    Tryptase—all mast cells
    Chymase—connective-tissue mast cells
  Lysosomal hydrolases
    Arylsulfatase
    β-Glucuronidase
    β-Hexosaminidase
  Other Enzymes
    Superoxide dismutase
    Peroxidase

Table 13–2. Histamine receptors.

Receptor	Histamine Actions
H1	Increased post-capillary venular permeability Smooth muscle contraction Pulmonary vasoconstriction Increased cGMP levels in cells Enhanced mucus secretion Leukocyte chemokinesis Prostaglandin production in lungs
H2	Enhanced gastric acid secretion Enhanced mucus secretion Increased cAMP levels in cells Leukocyte chemokinesis Activation of suppressor T cells
H3	Histamine release inhibition Histamine synthesis inhibition

and stimulates suppressor T lymphocytes. Stimulation of the H3 receptor has been best studied in central nervous tissue, where it inhibits the release and blunts the synthesis of histamine. Co-stimulation of H1 and H2 receptors causes maximal vasodilatation, cardiac irritability, and pruritus.

The clinical consequences of the release of histamine or its instillation into tissue include wheal-and-flare reactions in the skin associated with pruritus and flushing, bronchoconstriction and mucus secretion in the airways, intestinal cramping, gastric acid and enzyme release, intestinal mucus production, hypotension, and cardiac dysrhythmias. H1 actions of histamine can be blunted through the use of any of the large number of H1-directed antihistamines (see Chapter

63); H2 actions can be prevented by a number of compounds (eg, cimetidine and ranitidine); and H3 actions can be blocked by certain investigational compounds not available as drugs.

Metabolites of Arachidonic Acid

Prostaglandins and leukotrienes, products of the enzymatic cyclo-oxygenation and lipoxygenation, respectively, of arachidonic acid derived from cell membrane phospholipid, are two major families of inflammatory mediators (Fig 13–2). Their actions are broad, varying with the target tissue, and encompass vasoactive, smooth-muscle-active, and chemotactic properties.

Arachidonic acid, a 20-carbon, 4-double-bond fatty acid, is liberated from membrane phospholipids either through the sequential action of phospholipase C and diacylglycerol lipase or by the direct action of phospholipase A_2 upon membrane phospholipid. Once liberated, arachidonic acid is

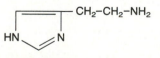

histamine

Figure 13–1. Chemical structure of histamine.

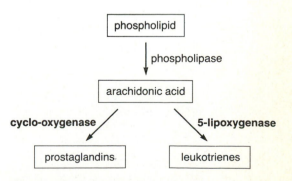

Figure 13–2. Derivation of prostaglandins and leukotrienes from arachidonic acid by the enzymes cyclo-oxygenase and 5-lipoxygenase, respectively.

reesterified or metabolized by either the cyclo-oxygenase or lipoxygenase pathways.

A. Cyclo-oxygenase Products: The product of cyclooxygenase action upon arachidonic acid in mast cells is prostaglandin D₂ (PGD₂) (Fig 13–3). Basophils, on the other hand, do not generate cyclo-oxygenase products of arachidonic acid. Connective tissue-type mast cells, when activated, appear to preferentially generate PGD₂ from liberated arachidonic acid. As is true of other prostaglandins, PGD₂ production is inhibited by nonsteroidal anti-inflammatory drugs, which, however, do not alter the release of other mast cell mediators. PGD₂ induces more prolonged erythema and wheal-and-flare vasopermeability responses in skin than histamine does.

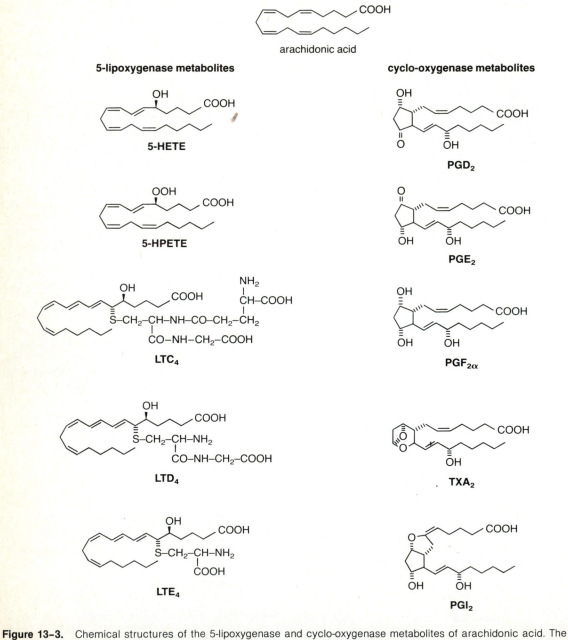

Figure 13–3. Chemical structures of the 5-lipoxygenase and cyclo-oxygenase metabolites of arachidonic acid. The compounds depicted in the figure are physiologically active mediators of inflammation.

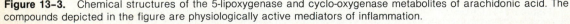

It also mediates a neutrophil infiltrate into skin and augments chemotaxis and chemokinesis of leukocytes in vitro. The systemic flushing and hypotensive episodes in patients with systemic mastocytosis have been attributed to this arachidonic acid product.

B. Lipoxygenase Products: When arachidonic acid is metabolized via the lipoxygenase pathway, a family of compounds is generated that contains 4 principal biologically active compounds, termed leukotrienes: leukotriene B_4 (LTB_4), LTC_4, LTD_4, and LTE_4 (Fig. 13–3). These are the predominant products of mucosal mast cells. LTB_4 is a dihydroxylated product with chemotactic potency (see below). LTC_4 is generated from lipoxygenase-modified arachidonic acid following the addition of the tripeptide glutathione; it forms one of the moieties of what was once termed "slow-reacting substance of anaphylaxis." The sequential modification of the terminal amino acids on the Cys-Gly-Glu tripeptide leads to the production of LTD_4 and LTE_4. This modification occurs through the action of γ-glutamyltranspeptidase and a variety of other peptidases found in biologic materials. These modified lipoxygenase products, known as the sulfidopeptide leukotrienes, are potent inducers of smooth muscle contractility, bronchoconstriction and mucus secretion in the airway, and the wheal-and-flare reaction in the skin. When injected intravenously, they may cause hypotension and cardiac dysrhythmias. The leukotrienes are several-hundredfold more potent on a molar basis than is histamine and are therefore believed to have an important role in the genesis of allergic disorders. At present, there are no inhibitors of leukotrienes that are sufficiently selective for clinical use.

Platelet-Activating Factor

Platelet-activating factor (PAF) is generated from a complex lipid that is stored in the precursor state in cell membranes. This lipid has a glycerol backbone modified in 3 ways: (1) on the first carbon of the glycerol backbone is located a long-chain alcohol molecule, usually of 16–18 carbons; (2) the second position in the storage form is generally arachidonic acid; and (3) on the third carbon is a phosphorocholine moiety (Fig 13–4). The activation of cells leads to the liberation of the arachidonic acid from the 2-position, and the addition at this site of an acetate group leads to the generation of fully active PAF. This molecule was originally named because it activates rabbit platelets. More recently, it has been determined that it has a number of other biologic effects, but the original descriptive name has been retained.

The biologic activity requires a long-chain alcohol of 16–18 carbons in the 1-position, the acetate group in the 2-position, and the phosphorocholine

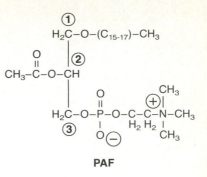

Figure 13–4. Chemical structure of platelet-activating factor (PAF). The biologically active moieties 1, 2, and 3 are discussed in the text.

moiety. PAF activates a variety of cell types, including platelets, whose mechanism of activation involves induction of aggregation and release of platelet granule constituents. It also activates neutrophils and eosinophils, causing the release of granular constituents, and is the most potent eosinophil chemoattractant yet described. When it is injected intravenously, its effects on those target cells are evidenced by transient neutropenia, thrombocytopenia, and basopenia. In addition, intravenous injection is associated with marked hypotension. When injected in the skin, PAF causes a wheal-and-flare reaction and leukocyte infiltration. When inhaled, it causes bronchoconstriction, an eosinophil infiltrate, and a state of nonspecific bronchial hyperreactivity that may persist for days to weeks following a single administration. Many of the actions of PAF are platelet-dependent, so that abrogation of platelets in animal models diminishes the ability of PAF to alter pulmonary resistance and compliance, although without affecting its ability to attract leukocytes or to induce hypotension or cardiac depression. In vivo, PAF is rapidly degraded by an acid-labile acetylhydrolase enzyme found in plasma, and it can also be degraded by a variety of phospholipases present in cells and tissues throughout the body.

Inhibitors of PAF action have been identified in biologic extracts from the Gingko tree, and a variety of other compounds are currently being studied for inhibition of this interesting molecule, but none are yet available for clinical use.

Adenosine

Adenosine is a nucleoside that is liberated from mast cells following the utilization of ATP during the degranulation process (Fig 13–5). It may be degraded by adenosine deaminase or may be taken up again by the cell and phosphorylated into

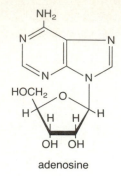

adenosine

Figure 13-5. Chemical structure of adenosine.

AMP. The blood levels of adenosine approximate 0.3 μmol/L, a concentration at which this molecule is minimally biologically active. These levels increase during hypoxia and antigen bronchoprovocation challenge of patients with asthma. Adenosine interacts with 2 receptors, termed A1 and A2, on cell surfaces. The A2 receptor is linked to elevations in intracellular levels of cyclic AMP and is blocked by methylxanthine drugs, further supporting a role for adenosine in asthma. When inhaled, adenosine causes bronchoconstriction, which can be inhibited by antihistamine. In vitro, adenosine does not cause mast cell mediator release, but it potentiates IgE-induced mast cell mediator release through an action on mast cell adenosine A2 receptors. This potentiation is believed to occur through a protein phosphorylation step, whose exact properties remain to be elucidated. Adenosine is also capable of inducing fluid and electrolyte secretion from intestinal epithelia.

CHEMOTACTIC MEDIATORS

Mast cells and basophils generate and release compounds that are capable of interacting with other leukocytes in augmenting their nonspecific or directed migration and are therefore termed **chemotactic mediators.** Some of these mediators are cell-specific, whereas others are directed at a variety of lymphocyte populations.

Eosinophil Chemotactic Mediators

It has long been known that immediate hypersensitivity reactions are associated with peripheral blood and tissue eosinophilia. For this reason, eosinophil chemotactic factors were the first to be investigated and identified. Two low-molecular-weight tetrapeptides of the sequence Val-Gly-Ser-Glu and Ala-Gly-Ser-Glu were isolated and termed collectively the eosinophil chemotactic factor of anaphylaxis (ECF-A). These molecules are very weak chemoattractant substances for eosinophils and are capable of augmenting eosinophil expression of complement receptors and of PAF synthesis. Molecules of similar molecular weight and charge have been identified in the blood of patients undergoing experimental bronchoprovocation challenge and patients with physical urticaria. Another family of chemotactic mediators of molecular weight between 1500 and 3000, which are presumed to be peptides, have also been identified in experimental model systems of asthma and urticaria. They are also capable of attracting eosinophils in vitro, but their other biologic potencies have yet to be investigated. The most potent eosinophil chemoattractant factor yet identified is PAF (see above). This molecule, although capable of attracting a variety of leukocytes, demonstrates at concentrations of 10^{-6}–10^{-11} mol/L a dose-dependent chemoattractant effect for eosinophils, far more potent than any other mediator yet identified.

Neutrophil-Directed Chemoattractant Factors

Three main molecular species capable of modulating neutrophil chemokinesis and chemotaxis are generated during mast cell mediated reactions. A protein of MW 660,000, termed high-molecular-weight neutrophil chemotactic factor (HMW-NCF), is the most unusual of these. It has been identified during experimental induction of physical urticaria and allergen-mediated bronchoconstriction. The molecule appears in the circulation very shortly after experimental challenge and during the late phase of IgE-mediated reactions. Its release is inhibited by pretreatment of allergic subjects with cromolyn, but its exact cell source and biologic role remain to be identified. It causes a transient neutrophilic leukocytosis and an increased expression of complement receptors upon neutrophils. Two low-molecular-weight mediators capable of modulating neutrophil chemotaxis are also generated by mast cells: (1) LTB$_4$, the dihydroxy product of the action of the lipoxygenase pathway upon arachidonic acid, and (2) PAF. These molecules are active at 10^{-6}–10^{-10} mol/L, similar in potency to C5a and much greater than any other neutrophil chemoattractant molecules. The exact role of these molecules in activating neutrophils during inflammation remains to be identified. However, as the chemotactic activation of neutrophils is associated with the production of toxic oxygen species (see below), their relevance to allergic inflammation may be more pertinent than previously assumed.

ENZYMATIC MEDIATORS

A variety of enzymes are present in mast cell and basophil granules and are released upon activation of these cells. Two major categories have been identified: (1) neutral proteases and (2) lysosomal hydrolases.

Neutral Proteases

Human and animal mast cells contain several neutral proteases, which not only are useful in characterizing the cells and identifying them in tissue, but also are believed to have important biologic properties. The first to be identified is a tryptic protease present in all mucosal and connective-tissue mast cells. This is a 4-chain heterodimer of MW 144,000, with trypsin-like potency. This enzyme makes up 25–50% of the granular protein in mast cell granules and is resistant to the action of circulating antiproteases. It is stabilized by its binding to granular heparin, and its biologic activity rapidly decays when this binding is broken. Although tryptase possesses some tryptic specificity, it differs from trypsin in the molecules that it cleaves, and therefore one cannot predict which substrates are susceptible to its action. It is known to cleave C3, to generate C3a, and to alter many of the blood-clotting proteins, but it is inactive on C5. A number of protease effects have been identified within supernatants of challenged human mast cells, including activation of kallikrein and cleavage of kininogen.

A second neutral protease with the specificity of chymotrypsin has also been identified and localized to human connective tissue but not mucosal mast cells. It is also abundant in the mast cell granule and may make up 10–20% of the granule protein in connective tissue mast cells. It may be distinguished from the tryptic protease by its lower molecular weight (26,000–30,000) and by its specificity for peptide substrates. One of its substrates appears to be angiotensinogen, but its natural substrate remains to be clearly elucidated, and its role in allergic pathophysiology is uncertain. Another mast-cell-neutral protease, carboxypeptidase A, has also been identified, and it, too, is richly present in mast cell granules.

Acid Hydrolases

A number of acid hydrolases, which are broadly distributed in primary lysosomes of a number of cells, are also found in mast cells. These hydrolases include β-hexosaminidase, which has been used as a marker of mast cell activation in vitro, β-glucuronidase, and arylsulfatase. Superoxide dismutase and peroxidase have been found in mast cell granules. It is speculated that these enzymes are capable of degrading ground substances such as chondroitin sulfates, but their specific functions are unknown.

PROTEOGLYCANS

The structural matrix of mast cell and basophil cytoplasmic granules contains chemical compounds known as **proteoglycans**, which are important in the storage and release of mediators from these cells. The major granular proteoglycan found in human mast cells is heparin. This proteoglycan (MW 60,000) is found at levels of approximately 5 μg/10^6 cells; it is an anticoagulant, and is also capable of modulating tryptase action. It is believed to act as a structural matrix for granular protein and amine binding. In addition to heparin, a highly sulfated granular proteoglycan, chondroitin sulfate E, is present in mast cells, whereas basophils contain chondroitin sulfates A and C. These compounds appear not only to act as structural molecules, but also to provide binding sites for the other mediators present within the mast cell granule.

TOXIC OXYGEN MOLECULES

Toxic oxygen molecules are liberated by activation of neutrophils, eosinophils, and probably also mast cells. Furthermore, mast cell chemoattractant molecules permit these cells to interact with neutrophils and eosinophils. As described in Chapter 12 (Table 12–3), NADPH oxidase donates an electron to oxygen to generate superoxide anion, which itself can interact with hydrogen ion to form hydrogen peroxide. Although the superoxide anion is short-lived, hydrogen peroxide is a rather stable molecule that can further mediate extracellular events, possibly leading to the generation of the hydroxyl radical, particularly in the presence of iron or other metal catalysts. In the presence of peroxidase, either myeloperoxidase from the neutrophil or the unique eosinophil peroxidase, hydrogen peroxide and a halide ion can generate a variety of hypohalous acids of the structure HOX. These molecules are capable of adding their halide ion, such as chloride, to a variety of biologic substrates, and they are believed to be important in biologic reactions in killing microorganisms. Other biologic reactions may be a consequence of the generation of hypohalous acids, for example, the generation of chloramines, which are relatively strong oxidants. Thus, the activation of the neutrophil, the eosinophil, or, presumably, the mast cell can lead to the sequential generation of superoxide anion, hydrogen peroxide, hydroxyl radical, hypohalous acid, and chloramines through the intercession of enzymes including NADPH oxidase and myeloperoxidase in the presence of a variety of metal ions as catalysts.

MEDIATOR INTERACTIONS

The panoply of mediators generated in allergic reactions and their overlapping biologic effects suggest that they may well interact in a synergistic or additive fashion. Known interactions include the interaction of histamine and leukotrienes, the interaction of heparin and tryptase, and, in cascade fashion, the induction of prostaglandins by histamine. Undoubtedly, other interactions remain to be discovered.

THE BIOLOGIC ROLE OF MEDIATORS

The best evidence for the role of mediators in allergic disease has come from studies of patients who are known to be sensitive to specific antigens and who are challenged by bronchoprovocation with aerosolized allergen. This causes acute bronchoconstriction within a few minutes of inhalation of antigen and spontaneous recovery within 30–60 minutes. In at least half of the subjects, a second, late-phase, IgE-mediated response occurs, which may begin within 2–4 hours and may persist for 4–18 hours (see Chapter 12).

In the early (immediate)-phase reaction, there is bronchial mucosal edema, erythema, mucous secretion, and bronchoconstriction. This reaction is accompanied by the release of histamine and a variety of neutrophil and eosinophil chemoattractants into the blood and the release of histamine, leukocyte chemoattractants, PGD_2, and sulfidopeptide leukotrienes in the bronchoalveolar lavage fluid. The late bronchial inflammatory reaction is accompanied in the blood by chemoattractant factors for neutrophils and eosinophils and by the evidence of neutrophil and particularly eosinophil infiltration into the airways. It appears, therefore, that the early reaction is dependent on vasoactive and bronchospastic mediators, particularly histamine, PGD_2, PAF, sulfidopeptide leukotrienes, and adenosine. Since potent H1 antihistamines and nonsteroidal anti-inflammatory drugs blunt this early-phase response, it is likely that PGD_2 and histamine play a role in its expression. Although there are no specific inhibitors of the late-phase reaction, leukocyte infiltration is an impor-

tant component, so PAF and other leukocyte chemoattractants probably play a major role in its expression.

More recent work has indicated that the mast cell growth and differentiation promoting cytokines, IL-3, IL-4, and GM-CSF, as well as other cytokines such as histamine-releasing factor generated from macrophages and lymphocytes, may activate mast cells to generate mediators. Therefore, the role of mast cells in inflammation may not be restricted to antigen-IgE antibody systems, but they may also interact with inflammatory systems dependent upon macrophages and lymphocytes. Although the participation of each of the mediators discussed above in the inflammatory responses in immunity and hypersensitivity has been well documented, the role, if any, of these mediators in normal physiologic functioning and homeostasis of the organism is unknown.

SUMMARY

The mediators of immediate hypersensitivity possess a sufficiently broad biologic spectrum of activity and potency to play a major role in human disease. Asthma, allergic rhinitis, and urticaria clearly owe their signs, symptoms, and chronicity to these mediators. Many other inflammatory disorders such as rheumatoid arthritis, vasculitis, and inflammatory bowel disease have, at least in the past, had manifestations due to these mediators. Important roles for these compounds in wound repair, angiogenesis, osteoporosis, and neural functioning have been suggested by well-controlled investigations. Clearly, the next decade holds extraordinary promise in expanding and elucidating the role for mediators of immediate hypersensitivity in health and disease.

REFERENCES

Wasserman SI: Mast cell mediators in the blood of patients with asthma. *Chest* 1985;**87**:13S.

Wasserman SI: Mediators of immediate hypersensitivity. *J Allergy Clin Immunol* 1983;**72**:101.

Wasserman SI: Platelet activating factor as a mediator of bronchial asthma. *Hosp Pract* 1988;**23**:49.

Weiss SJ: Toxic effects of neutrophils. *N Engl J Med* 1989;**320**:365.

Complement & Kinin

14

Michael M. Frank, MD

Complement activation, kinin generation, blood coagulation, and fibrinolysis are physiologic processes that occur through sequential cascadelike activation of enzymes normally present in their inactive forms in plasma. Although they are 4 distinct systems and perform different functions, they interact with each other and with various cell membrane proteins. The first two—complement and kinin—are the subjects of this chapter because of their involvement in immunologic effector responses.

THE COMPLEMENT SYSTEM

Complement is a collective term used to designate a group of plasma and cell membrane proteins that play a key role in the host defense process. Table 14–1 lists the major proteins, their molecular weights, and their serum concentrations.

FUNCTIONS OF COMPLEMENT

This complex system, which now numbers more than 25 proteins, acts in at least 3 major ways. The first and best-known function of the system is to cause lysis of cells, bacteria, and enveloped viruses. The second is to mediate the process of opsonization, in which foreign cells, bacteria, viruses, fungi, etc, are prepared for phagocytosis. This process involves the coating of the foreign particle with specific complement protein fragments that can be recognized by receptors for these fragments on phagocytic cells. Interaction with these receptors leads to binding of the particle to the cell membrane of the phagocyte, the first step in the phagocytic process.

The third function of the complement proteins is the generation of peptide fragments that regulate features of the inflammatory and immune response. These proteins play a role in vasodilatation at the site of inflammation, in adherence of the phagocytes to blood vessel endothelium and egress of the phagocyte from the vessel, in directed migration of phagocytic cells into areas of inflammation, and, ultimately, in clearing infectious agents from the body. Most of the early-acting proteins of this system are present in the circulation in an inactive form. The proteins undergo sequential activation to ultimately cause their biologic effects.

PATHWAYS OF COMPLEMENT ACTIVATION

Two major pathways of complement activation operate in plasma. A general scheme of the system is shown in Fig 14–1. The first complement activation pathway to be discovered is termed the **classic complement pathway.** Under normal physiologic conditions, activation of this pathway is initiated by antigen-antibody complexes. The second pathway, known as the **alternative complement pathway,** was discovered more recently, although phylogenetically it probably is the older activation pathway. It does not have an absolute requirement for antibody for activation. Both pathways function through the interaction of proteins termed components. Both proceed by means of sequential activation and assembly of a series of proteins, leading to the formation of a complex enzyme capable of binding and cleaving a key protein, C3, which is common to both pathways. Thereafter, the 2 pathways proceed together through binding of the terminal components to form a membrane attack complex, which ultimately causes cell lysis.

NOMENCLATURE

The proteins of the classic pathway and the terminal components are designated by numbers fol-

Table 14-1. Molecular weights and serum concentrations of complement components.

Classic Pathway Component	Molecular Weight	Serum Concentration ($\mu g/mL$)
C1q	410,000	70
C1r	85,000	34
C1s	85,000	31
C2	95,000	25
C3	195,000	1,200
C4	206,000	600
C5	180,000	85
C6	128,000	60
C7	120,000	55
C8	150,000	55
C9	79,000	60
Alternative pathway component		
Properdin	153,000	25
Factor B	100,000	225
Factor D	25,000	1
Inhibitors		
C1 Inhibitor	105,000	275
Factor I	105,000	34
Regulatory proteins		
C4-binding protein	560,000	8
Factor H	150,000	500

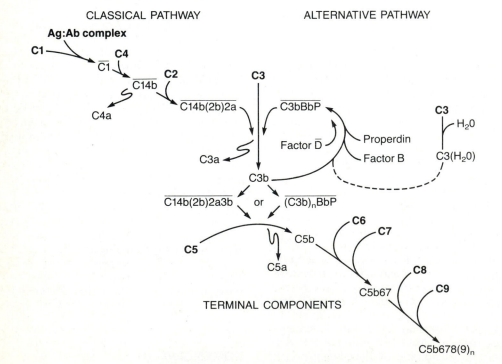

Figure 14-1. The complement cascade.

lowing the letter C. Proteins of the alternative pathway are generally given letter designations, as are other proteins that have major regulatory effects on the system. Under certain circumstances, which will be discussed briefly below, the pathways can be activated by nonimmunologic mechanisms, leading to the generation of biologically active products.

The proteins of each pathway interact in a precise sequence. When a protein is missing, as occurs in some of the genetic deficiencies, the sequence is interrupted at that point. The early steps in the activation process are associated with the assembly of complement cleavage fragments to form enzymes that bind the next proteins in the sequence to continue the reaction cascade. These enzymes are designated with a bar placed over the symbol of the component to indicate active enzymatic activity.

THE CLASSIC COMPLEMENT PATHWAY

The Function of Antibody & C1

In most cases, the classic pathway is initiated by the binding of antibody to an antigen. A single molecule of IgM antibody on an antigenic surface or 2 side-by-side molecules of IgG of the appropriate subclasses bind and activate C1, a macromolecular complex composed of 3 proteins—C1q, C1r, and C1s—held together in the presence of calcium ion. Binding to the antibody occurs via the C1q portion of the molecule. If the antibody-binding sites (epitopes) on a target antigen are too low in density for proper arrangement of antibody molecules, C1 binding may not occur. This is seen with erythrocytes coated with anti-Rh$_0$ (D) antibody. Although complement-activating subclasses of IgG are formed in response to this antigen, complement is not usually activated and has no role in the destruction of erythrocytes coated with anti-Rh$_0$ (D) antibody, because the proper complement-binding antibody doublets are not formed. The ability of antigen-antibody complex to interact with the C1q subcomponents of C1 serves as the basis for a group of assays used to detect immune complexes in serum samples: the C1q-binding assays. C1q is bound by IgM, IgG1, IgG2, and IgG3. It is not bound by IgG4, IgE, IgA, or IgD, so these antibody isotypes do not activate the classic pathway.

Nonimmunologic Classic Pathway Activators

It is of interest that a number of nonimmunologic activators of the classic pathway exist. Certain bacteria (eg, certain *Escherichia coli* and *Sal-*

monella strains of low virulence) and viruses (eg, parainfluenza virus) interact with C1q directly, causing C1 activation and, in turn, classic pathway activation in the absence of antibody. Such an interaction obviously would aid the host natural defense process. Other structures, eg, the surface of urate crystals, myelin basic protein, denatured DNA, bacterial endotoxin, and polyanions such as heparin, also may activate the classic pathway directly. Such activation by urate crystals is thought to contribute to the inflammation and pain associated with gout.

For simplicity, a series of block diagrams showing the interaction of the components is depicted in Figure 14–2. C1q is shown as a molecule with a central core and 6 radiating arms, each of which ends in a podlike structure. Each C1q molecule is composed of 18 separate polypeptide chains, divided into 3 chain types with 6 chains of each type. The amino-terminal segments of these chains closely resemble collagen and have a triple-helix, collagenlike structure. Thus, the arms of C1q are highly flexible. The globular heads contain the carboxy-terminal ends of the polypeptide chains and bind to the C$_H$2 domain of the appropriate immunoglobulin. The enzymatic potential of C1 resides in the C1r and C1s chains, which are associated with the collagenlike portion of the molecule. Each chain has a molecular weight of about 85,000 and is a proenzymatic form of a serine protease. There are one C1q, 2 C1r, and 2 C1s chains making up each C1 macromolecular complex.

Mechanism of C1 Activation

Binding of C1 to antibody is followed by activation of C1r and, in turn, C1s. This activation is associated with cleavage of the 2 identical C1r chains and of the 2 C1s chains. Each chain is cleaved into long and short fragments, with the appearance of an enzymatic site on the short fragment. It is believed that the function of the activated C1r enzyme, $\overline{\text{C1r}}$, is to cleave C1s, which then develops enzymatic activity. $\overline{\text{C1s}}$ cleaves the next portion in the sequence, C4 (Figs 14–1 and 14–2).

C4 & C2

C4 is a 3-chain molecule. The largest of the 3 chains, the α chain, is cleaved at a single site by $\overline{\text{C1s}}$, with the release of a small peptide, C4a. The larger peptide, consisting of most of the α chain together with the β and γ chains of C4, binds to the target cell to continue the complement cascade. Binding involves the formation of a covalent amide or ester bond between the target cell and the α chain of C4 (see the discussion of chemistry under C3 below). In the presence of magne-

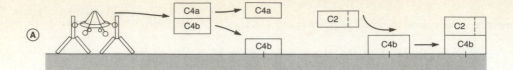

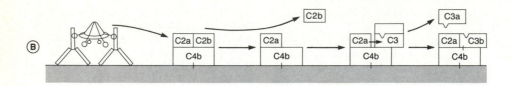

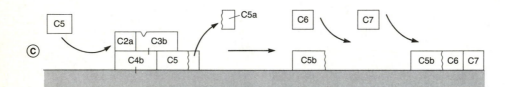

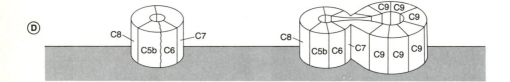

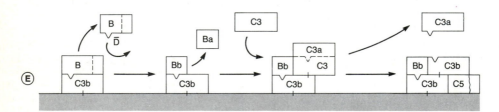

Figure 14-2. Diagram of the complement cascade. **A:** The classic complement pathway. A doublet of IgG antibody molecules on a surface can bind and activate C1, a 3-part molecule composed of C1q, C1r, and C1s. C1q has a core and 6 radiating arms, each of which ends in a pod. The pod recognizes and binds to the Fc fragment of the IgG. Upon activation the C1 binds and cleaves C4. The small fragment, C4a, is released. The large fragment binds to the target to continue the cascade. In the presence of magnesium ion, C2 recognizes and binds to C4b. **B:** Once C2 is bound to C4b, it can be cleaved by C1. A small fragment, C2b, is released, and the large fragment, C2a, remains bound to the C4b. This newly formed complex of 2 protein fragments can now bind and cleave C3. This molecule is, in turn, cleaved into 2 fragments, C3a and C3b. The small fragment, C3a, is released, and the large fragment, C3b, can bind covalently to a suitable acceptor. C3b molecules that bind directly to the C4b continue the cascade. **C:** The complex formed of C2a, C4b, and C3b can bind and cleave C5. A small fragment of C5, C5a, is released. The large fragment, C5b, does not bind covalently. It is stabilized by binding to C6. When C7 binds the complex of C5b, C6 and C7 becomes hydrophobic. It is partially lipid-soluble and can insert into the lipid of the cell membrane bilayer. **D:** When the C5b67 binds C8, a small channel is formed in the cell membrane. Multiple molecules of C9 can bind and markedly enlarge the channel. The channel has a hydrophobic outer surface and a hydrophilic central channel that allows passage of water and ions. **E:** The alternative complement pathway. In the presence of magnesium ion, C3b on a surface can bind factor B, just as C4b can bind C2. Factor D, a fluid-phase factor, can cleave bound factor B into 2 fragments, Ba and Bb. Ba is released. The C3bBb complex can now bind an additional molecule of C3 and cleave it, just as C4b2a can bind and cleave C3. C3a is released, and the new complex of C3bBbC3b, usually written (C3b)2Bb, can bind C5 to continue the cascade.

sium ion, C4b on a target cell is capable of interacting with and binding the next component in the series, a single-chain molecule of MW 95,000, termed C2. C2 binds to C4b and, in the presence of $\overline{C1s}$, is cleaved. The larger cleavage fragment of C2 (C2a), which contains the enzymatic site, remains in complex with C4b to continue the complement cascade. The complex of C4b and C2a develops a new capacity: the ability to bind and cleave the next component in the series, C3. For this reason it is termed the classic pathway C3 convertase. The peptide complex $\overline{C4b2a}$ is unstable and decays with loss of the C2 peptide from C4b as an enzymatically inactive fragment from its binding site on the C4b. Target-bound C4b can accept another C2 and, in the presence of active C1, will regenerate a convertase capable of continuing the complement cascade. These early steps in the classic pathway are under tight regulation, as discussed below.

C3

The C3 convertase of the classic pathway as described above binds and activates C3, a glycoprotein (MW 195,000) present at a concentration of 1.2 mg/ mL of plasma. The molecule has 2 disulfide-linked chains, termed α and β (MW 120,000 and 75,000, respectively). Like C4, C3 contains an internal thiolester bond buried in a hydrophobic pocket that links 2 amino acids in the α chain, twisting the α chain into a strained configuration. On cleavage of the thiolester, the molecule undergoes a major conformational change, which alters its biochemical properties. When C3 is activated by the $\overline{C4b2a}$ convertase, a peptide, C3a (MW 9,000), is cleaved from the α chain. The internal thiolester is exposed to the surrounding medium and is immediately cleaved. The half-life of the intact but reactive thiolester is in the range of 30–60 microseconds. It will interact with any suitable acceptor in the environment. Suitable acceptors include molecules that have reactive hydroxyl or amino groups on their surface. If the thiolester does not form a covalent bond with an acceptor, the reactive group interacts with water, is hydrolyzed, and can no longer form a covalent bond with the target. A particle coated with C3b is opsonized and may interact with cells with C3b receptors (see the section on receptors below). To continue the complement cascade sequence, it appears that C3b must interact directly with target C4b, forming a covalently bound complex. C3b also has a strong tendency to interact with IgG present in the area of activation. The dimer formed from C3b and the IgG molecule is a more potent opsonin than is C3b alone (see the section on opsonization below).

THE CLASSIC PATHWAY C5 CONVERTASE

The complex on a target surface consisting of C4b, C2a, and C3b ($\overline{C4b2a3b}$) has a newly expressed enzymatic activity: it can coordinate with and cleave C5. Again, 2 fragments, C5a and C5b, are formed, with C5a being the smaller. In this case the larger fragment does not have an internal thiolester linkage and cannot form a covalent bond with the target. It remains associated with the $\overline{C4b2a3b}$ complex and is available to interact with later components. It is C5b that initiates that segment of the complement cascade that leads to membrane attack.

In summary, the early steps of the complement cascade lead to the generation of a series of enzymatically active peptides and peptide complexes. As each complex is formed, it has a different specificity from the preceding complex, interacting with the next protein in the complement cascade. Each enzyme will interact with multiple molecules of the next substrate protein in the cascade of reactions either until it decays, as occurs with $\overline{C4b2a}$ and $\overline{C4b2a3b}$, which interact with C3 and C5, respectively, or until it is inhibited by regulatory proteins present on cells or in plasma. Thus, there is a potential for considerable biologic amplification; a limited number of antigen-antibody complexes will lead to the activation of large numbers of complement molecules.

THE ALTERNATIVE COMPLEMENT PATHWAY

C3 not only acts as a centrally important component of the classic pathway but also is the key component in the functioning of the alternative pathway. As described above, C3 can have 2 molecular forms: a native form that circulates in plasma with an intact thiolester, and a conformationally altered form, $C3(H_2O)$, in which the thiolester bond has been hydrolyzed. Once the conformational change has occurred, $C3(H_2O)$ in the presence of magnesium ion can interact with another circulating protein, factor B of the alternative pathway—a protein analogous to C2. Factor B has similar thermostability properties to C2 and requires magnesium ion to interact with its ligand, conformationally altered C3. The genes for factor B and C2 are located side by side on chromosome 6. It is reasonable to believe that C2 arises from a gene duplication of factor B. In the presence of factor D, a C1-like serine protease, the factor B bound to $C3(H_2O)$, is cleaved. Thus, in many respects the alternative pathway is like the classic pathway. Conformationally altered $C3(H_2O)$ resembles C4b; factor D resembles C1 in its function, although it has no binding site for the target and therefore is much less efficient in function. Factor B, acting much like C2, binds to altered C3 and is cleaved. Together, these proteins form an alternative pathway C3 convertase that can bind and activate C3, much as the classic pathway convertase binds and activates C3. As in the classic pathway, the activated C3 is cleaved into C3a and C3b. C3b with a cleaved thiolester has the same general conformation as $C3(H_2O)$. C3b binds factor B, and in the presence of factor D, it continues alternative pathway activation.

Thus, whereas the classic pathway proceeds in a fashion that is strictly sequential (C1 being required before C4, before C2, etc.), the alternative pathway activation is in many ways circular. C3 in the circulation is slowly hydrolyzed to $C3(H_2O)$. In the altered conformation it interacts with factors B and D of the alternative pathway to form a C3-cleaving enzyme that will bind fresh C3 and form C3a and C3b. The newly formed C3b can, of course, bind to suitable acceptors on targets and can itself continue alternative pathway activation. Thus, the slow cleavage of C3 in the circulation acts as a nidus to initiate alternative pathway activation. Once again, control proteins under normal circumstances prevent this nidus, which appears to form physiologically at all times, from inducing massive alternative pathway activation.

Alternative Pathway Amplification

The ability of hydrolyzed C3 to interact with alternative pathway components to form C3a and C3b and continue alternative pathway activation is termed the "feedback amplification system." The alternative pathway convertase (C3bBb) is extremely unstable and decays rapidly under normal physiologic conditions. Such rapid decay would markedly reduce its effectiveness. Properdin, a protein in plasma, binds to the alternative pathway convertase and stabilizes it, thus slowing its decay and allowing it to continue the complement cascade.

Cobra Venom Factor

It is interesting that for years investigators have used a protein derived from cobra venom (cobra venom factor) to activate complement. Recent investigation has shown that this protein is a fragment of cobra C3 and is a physiologic analogue of C3b in this reptile. This protein, when added to human plasma, activates complement just as C3b, derived physiologically, activates the alternative pathway. C3b generated by complement activation in normal serum is under tight regulatory control by plasma proteins, as mentioned below. However, cobra venom factor is not inhibited by these regulators and therefore can induce massive complement activation.

THE LATE COMPONENTS C5–9 & THE MEMBRANE ATTACK COMPLEX

As described above, C5 is bound and then cleaved by either the alternative or classic pathway convertase into C5a and C5b. C5a is released. Its biologic activity is described in a later section. C5b continues the lytic sequence; however, it does not form a covalent bond with the surface of its target. C5b is rapidly inactivated unless it is stabilized by binding to the next component in the cascade, C6. The C5b6 complex now can bind C7, the third protein involved in membrane attack. The C5b67 complex becomes increasingly hydrophobic and will interact with nearby membrane lipids. It is capable of inserting into the lipid bilayer of cell membranes. In that location, one C5b67 complex can accept one molecule of C8 and multiple molecules of C9, ultimately forming a cylinderlike structure, C5b678(9)n, which has been termed the **membrane attack complex (MAC)** (Fig 14–3). This structure has a hydrophobic outer surface, which associates with the membrane lipid of the bilayer, and a hydrophilic core through which small ions and water can pass. The ionic environment of the extracellular fluid then communicates with that inside the cell, so that once this complex is inserted into the membrane, the cell cannot maintain its osmotic and chemical equilibrium. Water enters the cell because of the high internal oncotic pressure, and the cell swells and bursts. The assembly of C5b–C8 appears to form a small membrane channel that is increasingly enlarged and stabilized by the binding of multiple molecules of C9. One lesion penetrating the erythrocyte membrane is sufficient to destroy the cell. Cells with more complex metabolic machinery can internalize and destroy complement lesions that form on the cell surface, thereby providing some protection against complement attack.

CONTROL MECHANISMS

The complement system has evolved to aid in the host defense process by directly damaging invading organisms and by producing tissue inflammation. Maintaining tight regulatory control of this system is of critical importance to prevent complement-mediated destruction of the individual's own tissues. When complement is involved in causing disease, it usually is functioning normally but is misdirected, ie, damaging to the host tis-

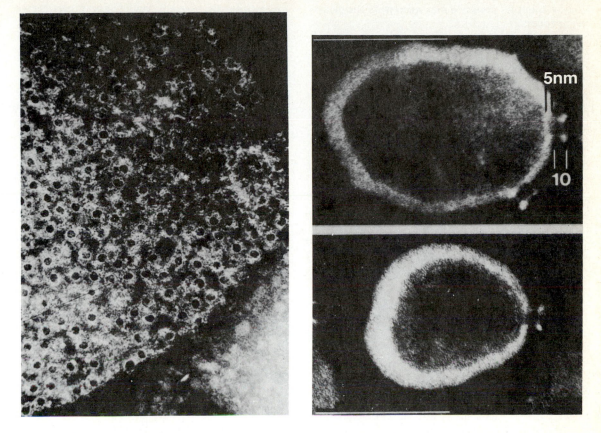

Figure 14-3. Lysis of cells by C5b-9, the MAC. **Left:** Surface of cells lysed by antibody and complement. Note the surface lesions. (Micrograph courtesy of R Dourmashkin.) **Right:** Two views of the purified lesions allowed to attach to lipid micelles. The hollow cylinder formed by the C5b-9 has allowed the electron-dense dye to enter the lipid droplet. (Photograph courtesy of S Bhakdi.)

sues. Many control proteins have evolved to defend against this attack.

The C1 Inhibitor

The first of these, C1 inhibitor (C1INH), recognizes activated $\overline{\text{C1r}}$ and $\overline{\text{C1s}}$ and destroys their activity. This glycoprotein (MW 105,000) not only inhibits $\overline{\text{C1r}}$ and $\overline{\text{C1s}}$, but also acts as an inhibitor of activated Hageman factor (see below) and all of the enzyme systems activated by Hageman factor fragments. Thus, C1INH regulates enzymes formed during activation of the kinin-generating system, the clotting system, and the fibrinolytic system. In each of these systems C1INH binds physically to the active site of the enzyme to destroy its activity and thereby is consumed. Interestingly, during this process the C1 is dissociated, with the C1INH binding to each of the C1r and C1s enzymatic sites and freeing C1q of its subunits. Since C1INH is consumed when acting as an inhibitor, 2 genes are necessary to provide the

relatively high plasma concentration of the protein gene product required for effective inhibitor activity. A relative deficiency occurs in patients with hereditary angioedema, who have a defect in one of the 2 genes responsible for formation of C1INH. These patients have one-half to one-third the normal level of C1INH and have frequent attacks of angioedema—painless swelling of deep cutaneous tissues—whose cause is still uncertain. It may arise from activation of the kinin-generating system or from activation of the complement system, with generation of peptides that cause vascular leakage.

C4-binding Protein, Factor I, & Factor H

C4-binding protein (C4BP) and a second protein, factor I, are responsible for regulation of C4b. C4BP binds to C4b and facilitates cleavage by the proteolytic enzyme factor I. On target surfaces, C4BP is not required for C4b cleavage by factor I, but its presence may accelerate the cleavage process.

Factor I also is responsible for the cleavage of C3b (Fig 14–4). In this case the required cofactor is termed factor H. Factor H acts as an obligate cofactor in the fluid phase and as an accelerator of C3 cleavage on cell surfaces (see Fig 14–4). In the presence of factors H and I, the C3b or C3(H₂O) α-chain is cleaved at 2 sites to form a partially degraded molecule, iC3b. This molecule, although inactive in continuing the complement cascade, is active in phagocytosis and will be discussed further below. Under the appropriate conditions, as discussed below, factor I can cleave iC3b further to form a molecule termed C3dg, which also interacts with specific receptors that recognize this C3 degradation peptide.

Vitronectin (S Protein)

Yet another control protein, S protein (also called vitronectin), interacts with the C5b67 complex as it forms in the fluid phase and interacts with its membrane-binding site to prevent the binding of C5b67 to biologic membranes. Following binding of S protein to fluid-phase C5b67, binding of C8 and C9 to the fluid-phase complex

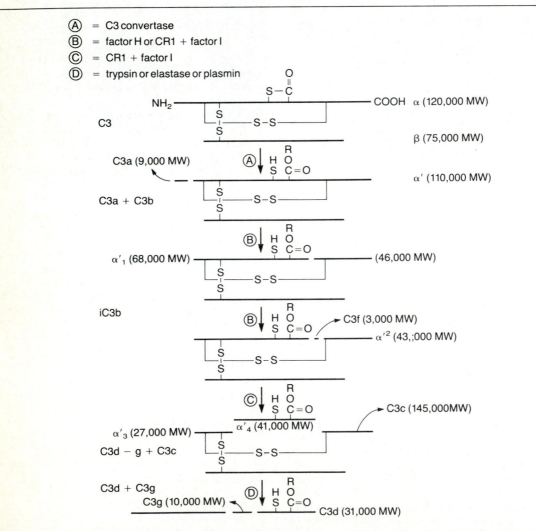

Figure 14–4. The C3 degradation pathway. The α and β chains of C3 are shown. Activation of C3 with the formation of C3a and C3b by the C3 convertases is shown (step A). C3b is degraded to iC3b by the action of factor H or CR1 plus factor I (step B). Two forms of iC3b have been described differing in loss of a 3-kDa fragment. In the presence of CR1 and factor I, C3c is released and C3dg remains target bound (step C). C3dg can be further degraded to C3d by proteolytic enzymes (step D). Specific cellular receptors exist for each of these fragments.

can proceed, but the complex does not insert into lipid membranes and does not lyse cells.

In the control of complement attack against host tissue, it would be beneficial if complement proteins such as C3b were rapidly degraded when bound to host cells but not degraded when bound to the surface of a microorganism. A process for accomplishing this goal has evolved. When deposited on a microorganism, C3b is often in a "protected site," which is protected from the action of the control proteins factors H and I. The C3b persists to activate the alternative pathway and destroy the organism. In contrast, on host cells C3b interacts with factors H and I and is degraded. The biochemical basis for this protection of C3b on an organism surface is not yet completely understood, but appears to relate to the presence of charged carbohydrates such as sialic acid on mammalian cells, facilitating the binding of factor H.

GENETIC CONSIDERATIONS

Most of the genes encoding proteins of the classic and alternative pathways have been cloned, and their amino acid sequences have been determined. Moreover, the activation peptides have been studied in some detail. Allotypic variants of many of the proteins have been found that show genetic polymorphisms, as demonstrated by differences in surface charge. Almost all of the variants of complement proteins show autosomal codominant inheritance at a single locus. The genes for C4, C2, and factor B are located within the major histocompatiblity locus on the short arm of chromosome 6 in humans and are termed class III histocompatibility genes. The significance of the intimate localization of histocompatibility genes and complement genes is unknown at present.

Interestingly, there are 2 C4 loci on each chromosome; thus, there are 4 C4 genes. The 2 loci code for proteins termed C4A and C4B, which differ in functional activity. Individuals with at least one null allele at one of the C4 loci are fairly common and are thought to be prone to the development of autoimmune disease. Genes for many of the regulatory proteins that interact with C4 and C3 are grouped as a supergene family on chromosome 1. This family is now known to encode factor H, C4-binding protein, decay-accelerating factor, CR1, and CR2. The gene products of this family have a 60-amino-acid domain made up of shorter repeating segments that repeat multiple times in the molecule. They presumably originate from a common gene precursor. See Chapter 28 for a discussion of inherited complement component deficiencies with associated syndromes.

BIOLOGIC CONSEQUENCES OF COMPLEMENT ACTIVATION IN INFLAMMATION

In general, the larger fragments formed during complement component cleavage tend to continue the complement cascade, and the smaller fragments mediate features of inflammation. For example, the cleavage of C3 and C5 generates C3a and C5a fragments, which consist of the first 77 and 74 amino acids of the C3 and C5 α chains, respectively. Cleavage of C4 generates C4a, a MW 77,000 amino acid fragment from the α-chain of C4. All of these small activation peptides have anaphylatoxic activity; they cause smooth muscle contraction and degranulation of mast cells and basophils, with consequent release of histamine and other vasoactive substances that induce capillary leakage. C5a is the most potent of these anaphylatoxins.

C5a and C3a also have important immunoregulatory effects on T cell function, either stimulating (C5a) or inhibiting (C3a) aspects of cell-mediated immunity.

C5a has profound effects on phagocytic cells. It is strongly chemotactic for neutrophils and mononuclear phagocytes, inducing their migration along a concentration gradient toward the site of generation. It increases neutrophil adhesiveness and causes neutrophil aggregation. In addition, it dramatically stimulates neutrophil oxidative metabolism and the production of toxic oxygen species, and it triggers lysosomal enzyme release from a variety of phagocytic cells. Cellophane membranes used in renal dialysis machines and membrane oxygenators may activate the alternative pathway with C5a generation. This, in turn, may lead to neutrophil aggregation, embolization of the aggregates to the lungs, and pulmonary distress. It is suspected that C5a generation plays an important deleterious role in the development of adult respiratory distress syndrome.

The life span of these biologically potent peptides, C3a and C5a, is limited by a serum carboxypeptidase that cleaves off the terminal arginine from the peptides, in most cases markedly reducing their activity.

COMPLEMENT PROTEINS ASSOCIATED WITH CELL MEMBRANES

Receptors & Regulatory Molecules

On the surface of most cells are complement receptors, ie, interactive membrane proteins with important regulatory properties. Receptors for the C1q component of C1 have been identified on neutrophils and monocytes, the majority of B lymphocytes, and a small population of lymphocytes lacking both B and T cell markers. Binding via this receptor has been shown to activate cells for a variety of cellular functions, including phagocytosis and oxidative metabolism. C1q can also augment the cytotoxicity of human peripheral blood lymphocytes to antibody-sensitized chicken erythrocytes and supports antibody-independent cytolytic activity by certain lymphoblastoid cell lines. The C1q receptor does not interact with C1q in intact C1, but interacts once the C1 has been dissociated by the C1 inhibitor.

A. THE C3 RECEPTORS: The best-studied receptors are those that recognize C3 fragments (Table 14–2). Importantly, these receptors do not recognize native circulating C3 and are not blocked by the normal plasma protein. Receptors exist for C3b, iC3b, and C3dg. These receptors have a characteristic cellular distribution, with the C3b receptor (termed CR1) being prominent on erythrocytes, granulocytes, mononuclear phagocytes, and B lymphocytes in humans. In contrast, the C3bi receptor (CR3) is present only on phagocytic cells. The C3d receptor (CR2) is present on lymphoblastoid cells and B lymphocytes. These receptors bind the various C3 fragments as indicated. If the C3 is bound to an antigen or target particle, the antigen or target will bind via the C3

ligand to the surface of cells with the receptor. For phagocytic cells, binding of the target to the phagocyte surface can augment the ingestion process.

Thus, CR1 and CR3 are both important in the process of phagocytosis. However, they also serve several other functions. They both act as cofactors for the further degradation of C3 fragments by the serum enzyme factor I. In each case, C3 fragment bound to the receptor can be cleaved by factor I to the decay fragment C3dg. This fragment is not formed in the absence of complement receptors. CR3 plays a major role in cell adherence; phagocytes from CR3-deficient patients have marked abnormalities in adherence and ingestion. CR3 is one member of a family of proteins termed "integrens." Other members of the CR3 group of proteins are LFA1 and p150/95, the latter being a protein that binds C3b and C3dg and that has recently been identified as CR4. All members of the CR3 family are 2-chain proteins with the same β chain. Presumably, the β chain is important in membrane localization of the protein. Recently, a number of children with deficiency of all of the CR3 proteins have been identified. They present with a history of delayed separation of the umbilical cord at birth and frequent soft-tissue and cutaneous infections by a variety of organisms, especially staphylococci and *Pseudomonas aeruginosa*.

CR2 is a receptor for the C3d and C3dg frag-

Table 14–2. Cellular receptors for C3 fragments.

Designation	Complement Component Recognized	Protein Structure	Cells	Function
CR1	C4b/C3b, iC3b	1 chain (MW 165,000–240,000)	Erythrocytes, phagocytes, B lymphocytes, some glomerular podocytes, eosinophils, Langerhans cells	Aids target cell ingestion by phagocytes; acts as cofactor in the metabolism of C3b, allowing factor I to cleave C3b to C3dg.
CR3	iC3b	2 chains, α (MW 170,000) and β (MW 95,000)	Phagocytes	Aids in ingestion; important in adherence of cells to surface; acts as cofactor for further degradation of C3bi.
CR2	C3d, C3dg	1 chain (MW 140,000)	B lymphocytes, some T cells, epithelial cells, follicular dendritic cells, NK and ADCC effector lymphocytes	On B cells, has immunoregulatory properties; site of attachment of Epstein-Barr virus to lymphocytes and epithelial cells.
CR4	iC3b, C3dg	2 chains, α (MW 150,000) and β (MW 95,000)	Kupffer cells, other phagocytes	Not well studied; presumably aids in attachment and metabolism of C3 coated targets.
C3aR	C3a, C4a	?	Neutrophils, T cells, goblet cells, smooth muscle, mast cells, monocytes, eosinophils	Immunoregulation, anaphylatoxin (see text).
C3eR	C3e	?	Neutrophils	Causes release of PMN from marrow stores.

ments of C3. It is present on B lymphocytes and nasal epithelial cells. It appears to function on B lymphocytes to facilitate differentiation. Interestingly, it serves as the site for attachment and cellular penetration of the Epstein-Barr virus.

B. Regulatory Molecules: Several other cellular membrane proteins act not as receptors but rather to control untoward complement activation. **Decay-accelerating factor (DAF)** is a single-chain membrane protein (MW 70,000) that is a potent accelerator of C3 convertase decay, but, unlike CR1 and CR3, it has no factor I cofactor activity. Functionally, the protein acts to limit membrane damage if, by chance, complement is activated at the cell surface. C8-binding protein, also known as **homologous restriction factor (HRF),** acts to prevent successful completion and membrane insertion of the MAC. This membrane protein therefore acts to prevent cell lysis at yet another step in the complement cascade. It is called homologous restriction protein because it recognizes C8 and C9 of the same species far better than it recognizes late components of other species. Human homologous restriction protein on cells will prevent the action of human C8 and C9 on those cells far better than it will prevent the action of C8 and C9 from other species. Any potential advantage of this function is completely obscure.

Interestingly, DAF and HRF are bound to the cell surface by a **phosphoinositide glycosidic linkage** rather than by a transmembrane domain within the amino acid backbone of the protein. This phosphoinositide linkage is reported to give the protein far greater lateral mobility within the cell membrane, increasing its ability to intercept damage-causing complement complexes. In patients with paroxysmal nocturnal hemoglobinuria, phosphoinositide-linked proteins are incorrectly assembled or inserted into cellular membranes of hematologic cells, rendering these cells exquisitely sensitive to complement-mediated lysis.

Another protein, **membrane cofactor protein (MCP;** formerly glycoprotein 45–70), is present on most blood cells but not on erythrocytes. This protein, a product of the supergene C4b/C3b-binding family, acts as a cofactor to facilitate the cleavage of C3b and iC3b by factor I. It does not accelerate convertase decay or bind with sufficient affinity to act as a receptor.

THE KININ CASCADE

The kinin-generating system is a second important mediator-forming system in blood. Here there is one major final product, **bradykinin,** a nonapeptide with potent activity causing increased vascular permeability, vasodilatation, hypotension, pain, contraction of many types of smooth muscle, and activation of phospholipase A_2 with attendant activation of cellular arachidonic acid metabolism.

PROTEINS OF THE KININ CASCADE

There are 4 elements of the bradykinin-generating system: **Hageman factor, clotting factor XI, prekallikrein,** and **high-molecular-weight kininogen.** Factor XI circulates as a complex with high-molecular-weight kininogen in a molar ratio of 2:1. Prekallikrein also circulates in a complex with high-molecular weight kininogen in a molar ratio of 1:1. In contrast, Hageman factor circulates as an uncomplexed single-chain plasma protein.

STEPS IN KININ ACTIVATION

On interaction with a negatively charged surface such as is supplied experimentally by glass or naturally by many biologically active materials like the lipid A of gram-negative bacterial endotoxin, Hageman factor is cleaved and activated. The cleaved Hageman factor (HFa) has proteolytic activity and can cleave additional molecules of Hageman factor to generate more HFa. Cleavage of the single chain of Hageman factor (MW 80,000) yields heavy and light chains (MW 50,000 and 28,000, respectively) that remain linked by disulfide bonds. The active enzymatic site of Hageman factor resides in its light chain. Cleavage is also catalyzed by other proteolytic enzymes, particularly kallikrein. HFa can interact with the complex of factor XI and high-molecular weight kininogen to activate factor XI to factor XIa. This, in turn, can activate the intrinsic coagulation cascade. HFa can also interact with the high-molecular-weight kininogen–prekallikrein complex to cleave the single-chain prekallikrein into a 2-chain molecule (kallikrein), with the chains associated via a disulfide linkage. The cleaved molecule now has proteolytic enzymatic activity associated with the lower-molecular-weight chain. To facilitate these cleavages of both factor XI and prekallikrein, high-molecular-weight kininogen complexes are bound to the surface, presumably near the Hageman factor.

AMPLIFICATION & REGULATION OF KININ GENERATION

Active kallikrein is capable of further cleaving HFa, with further degradation of the heavy chain

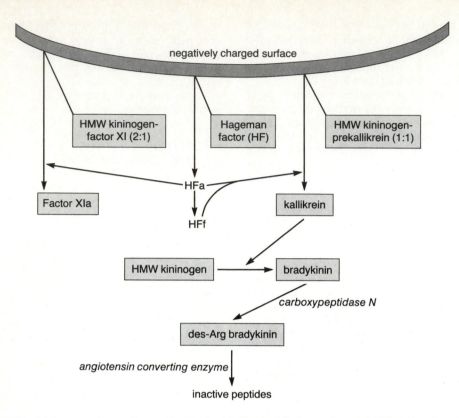

Figure 14–5. The kinin-generating pathway. Emphasized is the fact that complexes of high-molecular-weight (HMW) kininogen with both factor XI and prekallikrein associate on a surface with Hageman factor. The Hageman factor activates and in turn is responsible for the activation of factor XI and prekallikrein. Active kallikrein cleaves high-molecular-weight kininogen to release bradykinin.

but not the light chain. The resulting molecule, HFf, remains capable of activating the high-molecular-weight kininogen–prekallikrein complex, but it does not remain surface-bound and does not interact efficiently with the high molecular weight kininogen–factor XI complex. Prekallikrein is also a single-chain glycoprotein that is converted to an active form by cleavage within a disulfide bridge, resulting in a 2-chain molecule with the chains linked by disulfide bonds. The enzymatic site resides in the light chain, and the surface-binding site is on the heavy chain. Active kallikrein can cleave high molecular weight kininogen at several sites to release bradykinin from the kininogen. Bradykinin has a short half-life, interacting with carboxypeptidase N, which removes the C-terminal arginine to form the molecule termed des-Arg bradykinin. Des-Arg bradykinin no longer has the smooth muscle-contracting activity of bradykinin and cannot induce capillary plasma leakage when injected into skin, but it retains some of its vascular effects. Des-Arg bradykinin is, in turn, cleaved by angiotensin-converting en-

zyme to form low molecular weight peptides with consequent loss of biologic activity.

PLASMA INHIBITORS OF KININ GENERATION

The inhibitors of this mediator-generating system include C1 inhibitor, α_2-macroglobulin, and α_1-antitrypsin. C1 inhibitor and α_2-macroglobulin are the principal inhibitors of active kallikrein, with C1 inhibitor contributing most to inhibitory activity. C1 inhibitor and α_1-antitrypsin are the 2 major inhibitors of factor XIa, and C1 inhibitor is the principal inhibitor of active Hageman factor.

LOW-MOLECULAR-WEIGHT KININOGEN & TISSUE KALLIKREINS

A low molecular weight kininogen also exists in plasma. This protein has an identical heavy chain to that of high molecular weight kininogen. Low molecular weight kininogen can act as a source of bradykinin, but it is not easily cleaved by kallikrein. However, there are tissue kallikreins—low molecular weight kallikreins found in multiple tissues—that can cleave low molecular weight kininogen to lysylbradykinin (bradykinin with an additional linked lysine). Presumably, lysylbradykinin undergoes the same degradation pathway as does bradykinin.

FUNCTIONS OF KININS IN DISEASE

The physiologic role of the kinin-generating system is uncertain, and in only a few cases do we understand its role in disease. Free bradykinin and lysylbradykinin have been found in nasal secretions during rhinitis and viral nasal inflammation, and it is reasonable to believe that both blood and tissue kallikreins contribute to its presence. It is believed that kinins, via their ability to cause smooth muscle contraction and capillary leakage, contribute to asthma, but this is by no means proven at this time. Kinin generation has been found following antigen challenge of human lung fragments passively sensitized with specific IgE antibody, but the exact pathways involved in its generation are still uncertain. It has also been suggested that release of tissue kallikreins and activation of the kinin system is responsible for the severe pain of pancreatitis. The kinin-generating system has been reported to be involved in edema formation in hereditary angioedema, because kinins are present in fluid from suction-induced blisters over angioedema areas and because levels of circulating prekallikrein fall during attacks of this disease. Nevertheless, the kinin-forming system has not yet been conclusively proved to be responsible for the attacks of edema in hereditary angioedema.

REFERENCES

General
Borsos T: *The Molecular Basis of Complement Action.* Appleton-Century-Crofts, 1970.
Frank MM, Fries LF: Complement. Pages 679–702 in: *Fundamental Immunology,* 2nd ed. Paul WE (editor). Raven Press, 1989.
Harrison RA, Lachmann PJ: Complement technology. Chapter 39 in: *Handbook of Experimental Immunology,* 4th ed. Vol. 1. Weir DM (editor). Blackwell, 1986.

Classic Pathway
Cooper NR: The classical complement pathway: activation and regulation of the first complement component. Page 151 in: *Advances in Immunology.* Academic Press, 1985.
Kerr MA: The second component of human complement. *Methods Enzymol* 1981;**80**:54.
Tack BF: The β-Cys-γ-Glu thioester bond in human C3, C4, and α_2-macroglobulin. *Springer Semin Immunopathol* 1983;**6**:259.
Ziccardi RJ: The first component of human complement (C1): Activation and control. *Springer Semin Immunopathol* 1983;**6**:213.

Alternative Pathway
Pangburn MK, Muller-Eberhard HJ: The alternative pathway of complement. *Springer Semin Immunopathol* 1984;**7**:163.

Membrane Attack Complex
Mayer MM et al: Membrane damage by complement. *Crit Rev Immunol* 1981;**2**:133.
Muller-Eberhard HJ: The membrane attack complex of complement. *Annu Rev Immunol* 1986;**4**:503.

Control Mechanisms
Bock SC et al: Human C1 inhibitor: primary structure, with DNA cloning, and chromosomal localization. *Biochemistry* 1986;**25**:4292.
Frank MM, Gelfand JA, Atkinson JP: Hereditary angioedema: The clinical syndrome and its management. *Ann Intern Med* 1976;**84**:580.

Genetic Considerations
Alper CA, Rosen FS: Genetics of the complement system. Page 141 in: *Advances in Human Genetics.* Vol. 7. Harris H, Hirschhorn K (editors). Plenum, 1976.
Campbell RD et al: Structure, organization and regulation of the complement genes. *Annu Rev Immunol* 1988;**6**:161.

Biologic Effects
Goldstein IM: Complement: Biologically active products. Page 55 in: *Inflammation: Basic Principles and Clinical Correlates.* Gallin JE, Goldstein IM, Snyderman R (editors). Raven Press, 1988.
Hugli TE: Biochemistry and biology of anaphylatoxins. *Complement* 1986;**3**:111.
Hugli TE: Structure and function of the anaphylatoxins. *Springer Semin Immunopathol* 1984;**7**:193.
Reid KBM et al: Complement system proteins which interact with C3b or C4b. *Immunol Today* 1986;**7**:230.
Schapira M et al: Biochemistry and pathophysiology of human C1-inhibitor: Current issues. *Complement* 1986;**2**:111.

Cell Membrane Receptors & Regulatory Molecules
Berger M, Gaither TA, Frank MM: Complement receptors. *Clin Immunol Rev* 1983;**1**:471.
Pangburn MK, Schreiber RD, Muller-Eberhard HJ: Deficiency of an erythrocyte membrane protein with complement regulatory activity in paroxys-

mal nocturnal hemoglobinuria. *Proc Natl Acad Sci USA* 1983;**80:**5430.

Ross GD, Medof ME: Membrane complement receptors specific for bound fragments of C3. *Adv Immunol* 1985;**37:**217.

Schifferli JA, Ng YC, Peters DK: The role of complement and its receptor in the elimination of immune complexes. *N Engl J Med* 1986;**315:**488.

Zalman LS et al: Deficiency of the homologous restriction factor in paroxysmal nocturnal hemoglobinuria. *J Exp Med* 1987;**165:**572.

Kinins

Colman RW: Contact systems in infectious disease. *Rev Infect Dis* 1989;**4(suppl):**689.

Proud D, Kaplan AP: Kinin formation: Mechanisms and role in inflammatory disorders. *Annu Rev Immunol* 1988;**6:**49.

The Mucosal Immune System

15

Warren Strober, MD, and Stephen P. James, MD

The mucosal immune system is composed of the lymphoid tissues that are associated with the mucosal surfaces of the gastrointestinal, respiratory, and urogenital tracts. It has evolved under the influence of the complex and distinctive antigenic array present in mucosal areas and may be distinguished from the systemic (internal) immune system by a number of features. These include (1) a mucosa-related immunoglobulin, IgA; (2) a complement of T cells with mucosa-specific regulatory properties or effector capabilities; and (3) a mucosa-oriented cell traffic system for cells initially induced in the mucosal follicles to migrate to the diffuse mucosal lymphoid tissues underlying the epithelium. This last feature leads to the partial segregation of mucosal cells from systemic cells; thus, the mucosal immune system is a somewhat separate immunologic entity.

FUNCTIONS

The primary function of the mucosal immune system is to provide for host defense at mucosal surfaces. In this role it operates in concert with several nonimmunologic protective factors, including (1) a resident bacterial flora that inhibits the growth of potential pathogens; (2) mucosal motor activity (peristalsis and ciliary function) that maintains the flow of mucosal constituents, reducing the interaction of potential pathogens with epithelial cells; (3) substances such as gastric acid and intestinal bile salts that create a mucosal microenvironment unfavorable to the growth of pathogens; (4) mucus secretions (glycocalyx) that form a barrier between potential pathogens and the epithelial surfaces; and, finally, (5) substances such as lactoferrin, lactoperoxidase, and lysozyme that have inhibitory effects on one or another specific microorganism. Optimal host defense at the mucosal surface depends on both intact mucosal immune responses and nonimmunologic protective functions. Thus, antibiotic therapy that eliminates normal flora may result in infection, despite the existence of an intact immune system; mucosal infections are common in congenital and acquired immunodeficiency states even in the presence of normal nonimmunologic protective factors.

A second but equally important function of the mucosal immune system is to prevent the entry of mucosal antigens and thus protect the systemic immune system from inappropriate antigenic exposure. This occurs both at the mucosal surface, by preventing the entry of potentially antigenic materials, and in the circulation, by providing for the clearance of mucosal antigens via a hepatic clearance system. In addition, the mucosal immune system contains regulatory T cells that down regulate systemic immune responses to antigens which breach the mucosal barrier. Abnormalities of this aspect of mucosal immune function may be important in the development of autoimmunity.

ANATOMY

The mucosal immune system is a quantitatively important part of the immune system. The human gastrointestinal tract contains as much lymphoid tissue as the spleen does. The system can be morphologically and functionally subdivided into 2 major parts: (1) organized tissues consisting of the mucosal follicles (also called gut-associated lymphoid tissues [GALT] and bronchus-associated lymphoid tissues [BALT]) and (2) a diffuse lymphoid tissue consisting of the widely distributed cells located in the mucosal lamina propria (see Fig 15–1 and Chapter 2). The former (or organized) tissues are "afferent" lymphoid areas, where antigens enter the system and induce immune responses, and the latter or diffuse tissues are "efferent" lymphoid areas, where antigens interact with differentiated cells and cause the secretion of antibodies by B cells or induce cytotoxic reactions by T cells. As mentioned above, the 2 parts of the mucosal immune system are linked by a mucosal "homing" mechanism, so that sensi-

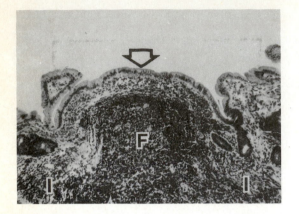

Figure 15-1. Histologic section of a human Peyer's patch lymphoid nodule from the terminal ileum. Antigens are taken up from the lumen through the follicle epithelium (arrow) for processing in the dome. The follicle (F) and its germinal center are composed largely of B cells. The interfollicular areas (I), composed of T cells, contain both high endothelial venules from which T lymphocytes enter follicles and lymphatics through which lymphocytes leave Peyer's patches. Magnification × 72. (Courtesy of Robert L Owen.)

tized cells from the lymphoid follicles travel to the diffuse lymphoid areas, where they can best interact with their inciting antigens. Finally, both the organized and the diffuse mucosal lymphoid areas are highly antigen-dependent; their numbers are remarkably reduced in germ-free states and expanded under conditions of increased antigenic stimulation.

Mucosal Lymphoid Aggregates

Mucosal lymphoid aggregates are morphologically different from those of the systemic lymphoid system. They receive antigen via the epithelium rather than through the lymphatic or blood circulation. More particularly, antigen enters through specialized epithelial cells called M cells (membranous cells) in the epithelium overlying the lymphoid aggregates (Fig 15-2).

A. M cells: M cells are flattened epithelial cells characterized by poorly developed brush borders, a thin glycocalyx, and a cytoplasm rich in pinocytotic vesicles, but they are virtually devoid of the proteolytic machinery found in absorptive epithelial cells. Antigen transport by M cells involves (1) initial binding to the M cell surface via as yet undefined binding sites, (2) uptake into pinocytotic vesicles, (3) vesicular transport across the cell body, and, finally, (4) release of material in an undegraded form into the subepithelial area.

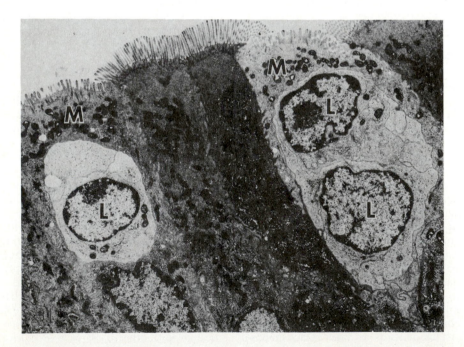

Figure 15-2. Transmission electron micrograph of the epithelium of a rat Peyer's patch lymphoid follicle. M cells (M) have short, irregularly shaped microvilli and surround intraepithelial lymphoid cells (L). Magnification × 6300. (Courtesy of Robert L Owen, MD).

Such transport is applicable to widely disparate substances including particulates (viruses, bacteria, and protozoa) and soluble proteins. However, neither binding nor uptake is totally indiscriminate. For instance, there is some evidence that the transport of bacteria by M cells is inhibited by specific antibodies, which may interact with bacterial determinants necessary for binding to M cells. This fact may explain the lack of uptake of resident microorganisms into M cells. Furthermore, some organisms that bind to M cells are taken up, whereas others are not. The ability to be taken up by M cells may have an impact on the virulence of an organism. For example, viral binding to and uptake by M cells may be an obligate means of entry of the organism and therefore a positive virulence factor, whereas uptake leading to antibody formation and immune elimination of the organism has a negative impact on virulence.

B. Dome Cells: The area just below the epithelium of the lymphoid aggregate (the so-called dome area) is rich in cells bearing class II major histocompatibility complex (MHC) antigens (macrophages, dendritic cells, and B cells) and therefore is rich in cells capable of antigen presentation following exposure to antigens in vitro or via oral antigen feeding in vivo. For this reason, any lack of response following oral antigen administration is not due to a lack of antigen-presenting cells in mucosal lymphoid aggregates (see the discussion of oral unresponsiveness below). M cells do not bear class II MHC antigens and are therefore probably not involved in antigen presentation; on the other hand, absorptive epithelial cells, particularly in the presence of inflammation, do express class II MHC antigens and have been shown to have antigen-presenting function in vitro.

The dome areas also contain many T cells. Although most of these cells bear CD4, a number bear neither CD4 nor CD8. This latter population may correspond to the cells recently identified as contrasuppressor cells (see the discussion of IgA regulation below).

C. Follicles: Below the dome area is the follicular zone, which contains the germinal centers. B cells predominate in this region, although scattered T cells are also present. As in other germinal centers, the B cells are highly differentiated and bear surface IgD; however, unlike other germinal-center B cells, a large fraction (up to 40%) bear surface IgA. Thus, the lymphoid aggregates of the mucosal immune system form the site of IgA B cell development, but the mucosal follicle is conspicuous for the absence of the terminally differentiated IgA B cells (IgA plasma cells), presumably because such cells leave the follicle before differentiating into plasma cells. The interfollicular areas between and around the follicles are also rich in T cells; most of the small population of CD8 T cells in mucosal lymphoid aggregates are found in these areas.

Diffuse Mucosal Lymphoid Tissue

The diffuse lymphoid tissues of the mucosal immune system consist of cell populations present in 2 separate compartments: the **intraepithelial lymphocyte (IEL) compartment** and the **lamina propria lymphocyte (LPL) compartment.**

A. Intraepithelial Lymphocytes: The IEL are, as the name implies, a population of cells lying above the basement membrane, among the epithelial cells. Although this population is numerically smaller than the lamina propria cell population, it is nonetheless considerable, there being 6–40 IEL/100 epithelial cells under normal conditions and a larger number in various inflammatory states. The IEL population is phenotypically heterogeneous, consisting for the most part of CD3 and CD2 T cells that are also predominantly of the CD8 phenotype. Recently it has been shown that proliferation of human IEL can be induced by stimulation of these cells via the CD2 receptor but not the T cell receptor. The reason for such activation requirements is as yet unknown.

Studies with mice suggest that IEL have specialized immune effector functions, including natural killer (NK) cell activity, specific cell cytotoxicity, secretion of gamma interferon (IFN-γ) with an increase in epithelial cell expression of class II MHC antigens, and expression of γ/δ T cell receptors.

B. Lamina Propria Lymphocytes: The lymphocyte population beneath the epithelial layer in the lamina propria, the LPL, is distinguished from the IEL population in being about equally divided between B cells and T cells. The B cell population is dominated by IgA B cells (and plasma cells), but IgM, IgG, and IgE B cells (and plasma cells) are also present (in descending order of frequency). In IgA deficiency, IgM rather than IgA cells are the predominant cells in the gastrointestinal mucosa and the number of IgG B cells is not increased; on the other hand, in various inflammatory diseases of the mucosa (eg, ulcerative colitis), the population of B cells producing each of the isotypes, particularly those producing IgG, is increased. In both normal and diseased mucosal tissue, the B cell population is composed of cells that display spontaneous immunoglobulin secretion in vitro.

The mucosal T cell population is composed of both CD4 and CD8 cells, with the former being twice as numerous as the latter, just as in peripheral blood. Recent evidence suggests that these cells have undergone prior activation. This is supported by the findings that lamina propria T cells contain IL-2 receptor (IL-2R) mRNA, have increased class II MHC and IL-2R expression, and have high expression of mRNA for IL-2 and IFN-γ. Activated CD4 T cells act as helper cells in vitro; it is not surprising that the CD4 lamina propria T cells provide more help and less suppression than do the corresponding CD4 cells in other tissues. These findings and recent data that CD4 lamina propria T cells respond to specific antigens by secreting "helper" lymphokines rather than by proliferating have led to the concept that lamina propria T cells are a class of memory T cells.

Lamina Propria Macrophages

Cells with typical macrophage morphology are found in the diffuse mucosal areas throughout the mucosal immune system. In these areas they tend to be concentrated in the more superficial parts of the mucosa just below the epithelium. They may derive from the mucosal lymphoid aggregates (as do mucosal lymphocytes), because cells with monocyte morphology are found in the intestinal lymphatics that drain the intestinal tissue. A high proportion of lamina propria macrophages bear class II MHC and other surface markers associated with phagocytic cell activity, which suggests that they are in a more highly activated state than are the corresponding cells in other lymphoid areas. These cells probably are important in nonspecific host defense. In addition, they may produce cytokines (IL-1, IL-6) necessary for local B cell differentiation and other immune processes.

Lamina Propria NK & Lymphokine-Activated Killer (LAK) Cells

Cells bearing NK cell markers (CD16, CD56) are sparse in the lamina propria, and NK activity is difficult to demonstrate in LPL populations unless procedures to enrich for NK cells are used. On the other hand, definite, albeit low (as compared with the level in spleen or peripheral blood cells) NK activity is seen in primate and rodent LPL populations, which suggests that the lack of NK activity in human lamina propria is due in part to the fact that human habitats and habits are not conducive to stimulation of mucosal NK cells, even though the potential for such stimulation does exist. In contrast to cells having NK function, cells with lymphokine-activated killer (LAK) function are easily demonstrated among the LPL. LAK cells are either CD8 T cells or NK cells that manifest antigen-nonspecific cytotoxicity when exposed to IL-2. Because the lamina propria lacks cells with NK markers, the LAK activity in this population is likely to be mediated by T cells or other undefined cells. Finally, the LPL population contains CD8 T cells that can be activated by allogeneic cells, anti-CD3 antibody, and mitogens to manifest cytolytic or suppressor function; these cells probably originate from precursor cells induced in the mucosal aggregates, although some might arise locally. Cytotoxicity is mediated by CD57-negative cells in the lamina propria but by CD57-positive cells in blood, showing that mucosal cytolytic effector cell populations may sometimes be phenotypically different from corresponding populations in the systemic immune system.

Lamina Propria Mast Cells

The mucosal areas are rich in mast cell precursors, which rapidly differentiate into mature mast cells when they are appropriately stimulated. Through their release of mediators, mast cells constitute an important mechanism by which inflammatory cells rapidly enter mucosal tissues and participate in local host defense.

In humans, mast cells in mucosal tissue have relatively small amounts of histamine and tryptic protease, whereas those in connective tissue contain relatively large amounts of histamine and possess both tryptic and chymotryptic proteases. Differential mast cell development in these 2 tissues may depend on the types of cells and cytokines present in their local environments. In this regard, mast cell precursors differentiate into mucosal mast cells under the influence of lymphokines secreted by T cells such as IL-3, whereas connective-tissue mast cells appear to require these factors as well as a factor(s) produced by fibroblasts. This may account for the rapid appearance of mast cells in mucosal tissues infected with nematode parasites, since presumably the parasites can stimulate mucosal T cells to secrete lymphokines that cause differentiation of mast cell precursors into mucosal mast cells. Thus, the significance of the mucosal mast cell type to the mucosal immune system (and to the body as a whole) may lie in its unique capacity to rapidly expand in number under the influence of a T cell-derived signal.

IMMUNOGLOBULIN A

Structure & Function

The central role of IgA in the mucosal immune response is one of the distinguishing features of the mucosal immune system. This is based on the fact that IgA has a number of properties that allow it to function more efficiently than other immunoglobulins in the mucosal environment.

The biochemical structure, genetics, and synthesis of IgA are discussed in Chapter 9. The features of this immunoglobulin that relate to its function in mucosal immunity are discussed here.

IgA is quantitatively the most important of the immunoglobulins, having a synthetic rate exceeding that of all other immunoglobulins combined when secretory as well as circulating IgA is taken into account. In humans it is encoded by 2 genes that lie in the immunoglobulin region of the genome downstream of each of two blocks of γ and ε heavy-chain genes. The first IgA gene encodes IgA1, the predominant circulating IgA (ca 80% of the total), as well as a major component of the IgA in mucosal secretions. The second IgA gene encodes IgA2, the IgA that is particularly abundant in the secretions, especially those of the distal gastrointestinal tract (ca 60% of the total). IgA1 differs from IgA2 in being susceptible to cleavage in its hinge region by proteases secreted by a number of different bacteria. Such cleavage can lead to markedly reduced functional activity; however, given the fact that IgA2 is also present in the part of the mucosa where IgA protease-producing bacteria reside, such proteases probably have little effect on the host defense function of the IgA system as a whole. Another difference between IgA1 and IgA2 is that the latter occurs in 2 allotypic forms, IgA2(m1) and IgA2(m2), which, in turn, are distinguished from one another by the fact that IgA2(m1) lacks interchain (H-L) disulfide bonds.

IgA manifests 3 structural features that relate specifically to its role as the mucosal immunoglobulin (Fig 15–3).

A. IgG Polymerization: The IgA heavy chain, in common with the IgM heavy chain, has an extra cysteine residue–containing C-terminal domain. This domain permits IgA to interact with a bivalent (or multivalent) molecule, also produced by B cells, known as J (joining) chain to form IgA dimers and trimers. IgA polymerization is important to IgA function because polymerized IgA (pIgA) has an increased capacity to bind to and agglutinate antigens.

B. Secretory Component: Only dimerized IgA can react with secretory component (SC), a protein (MW 95,000) produced by epithelial cells. SC acts as a transport receptor for IgA and becomes part of the secreted IgA molecule (see discussion below). It renders the IgA molecule less susceptible to proteolytic digestion and more mucophilic, thus enhancing the ability of the IgA molecule to interact with potential pathogens and to prevent their attachment to the epithelial surface. In addition, the IgA hinge region contains a glycosylated, proline-rich region that is generally more resistant to proteolysis by mammalian proteases than is IgG. On this basis, IgA has greater survivability in the gastrointestinal lumen than IgG or other immunoglobulins have. Such survivability, as already mentioned, is enhanced by the presence of secretory component.

C. Fc Region Properties: The Fc domain of IgA is characterized by certain unique properties, both positive and negative. Unlike the IgM or IgG Fc region, the IgA Fc region does not react with components of either the classic or alternative complement pathway, except possibly when the IgA is highly polymerized or is in the form of an immune complex; even in the latter instance, it does not bind C3b and therefore does not recruit inflammatory cells and mediators. In addition, although IgA facilitates phagocytosis and other phagocytic cell functions in the presence of specific antigen, it actually down-regulates phagocytosis in the absence of the antigen.

These facts suggest that free IgA (ie, IgA not associated with antigen) has anti-inflammatory effects. This, of course, is a highly useful property in an area of the body that is replete with materials that can induce excessive inflammatory responses.

IgA has certain pro-inflammatory features as well. Its Fc region binds to lactoferrin and lactoperoxidase and thereby enhances the function of these nonspecific host defense elements. There is also evidence that IgA can interact via its Fc region with Fc receptors to mediate antibody-dependent cellular cytotoxicity reactions (ADCC).

Transport

As noted above, the capacity of dimeric IgA to bind to SC enhances it effectiveness as a mucosal immunoglobulin. More importantly, however, SC is the key factor in an IgA transport system in allowing the mucosal immune system to focus IgA at mucosal sites (Fig 15–4). The sequence of events occurring during IgA transport involves first the binding of polymeric IgA to SC (via a covalent interaction) on the basolateral surface of the epithelial cell (or hepatocyte, as noted below), followed by endocytosis of IgA into vesicles, movement of IgA-containing vesicles to the apical surface of the cell, and, finally, release of IgA-SC complexes into the mucosal lumen. This final step requires cleavage of the SC receptor molecule so that the receptor for IgA becomes part of the secreted IgA molecule. Cellular synthesis and translocation of SC is independent of the presence of IgA and usually exceeds the amount necessary for transport, leading to the secretion of free (unbound) SC.

IgA transport mediated by SC occurs in the epithelium of the digestive tract, the salivary glands, the bronchial mucosa, and the lactating mammary glands. It also occurs in the uterine epithelium, where it is regulated by the effects of estrogen on SC synthesis by uterine epithelial cells. IgA transport mediated by SC also takes place in the liver, in which case it results in secretion of IgA into the bile. This involves the biliary epithelial cells but not hepatocytes, as in rodents, implying that SC-mediated transport is less important in humans

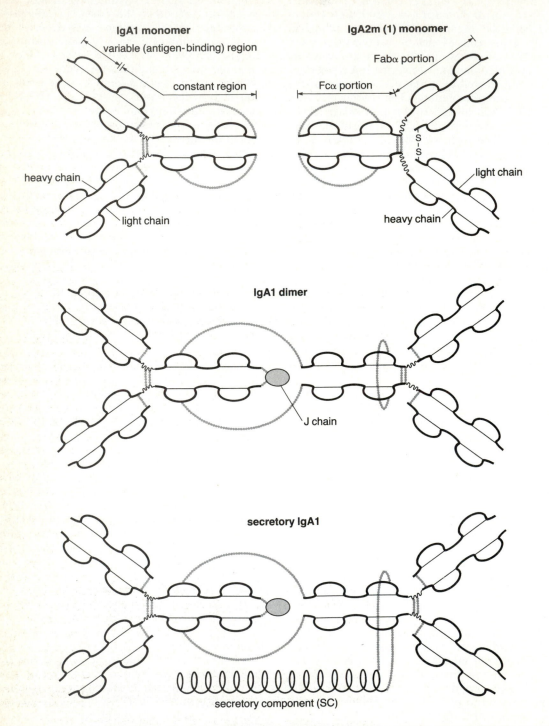

Figure 15-3. Diagrammatic representation of IgA structural forms. Hatched areas indicated immunoglobulin domains. Beads indicate disulfide bonds. In the actual IgA dimer and secretory IgA molecule, the J chain and secretory component molecules are intertwined with Cα heavy chains.

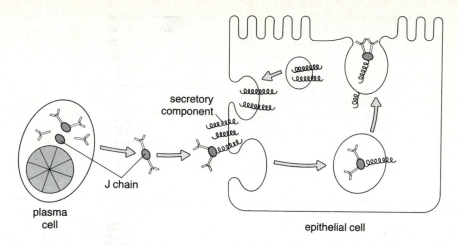

Figure 15–4. SC-mediated transport of IgA across the epithelial cell. Synthesis of SC (indicated as spirals) is independent of the transport process, and SC is released onto the luminal surface whether or not it is bound to IgA. Transport of IgA by this process does not result in its degradation.

than in certain other species. However, lessened SC-mediated transport in humans is compensated for by other hepatic uptake mechanisms. In this regard, IgA1 can be internalized by hepatic cells via asialoglycoprotein receptors as well as by Fc receptors.

Hepatic uptake of IgA may be one mechanism by which IgA secreted into the circulation is redirected back to the mucosa in species with well-developed SC-mediated hepatic transport capabilities, possibly to clear the circulation of potentially damaging antigenic material that has penetrated the mucosal barrier and become bound to circulating IgA. This mechanism has, in fact, obtained limited support from experiments in animals, but further study is necessary to establish its validity in humans.

Immune Exclusion

The ability of IgA to undergo SC-mediated transport or other clearance mechanisms facilitates the process of immune exclusion, whereby the mucosal immune system prevents the entry of antigenic molecules that could potentially evoke harmful immune responses. First, IgA molecules delivered into the secretions by SC-mediated transport can bind to antigens at the mucosal surface and thus lead to their entrapment in the mucus layer and their degradation by proteases before they become bound to and taken up by epithelial cells. That IgA antibody is best suited to this function is shown by the fact that individuals with selective IgA deficiency (ie, those who have low IgA levels and normal IgM and IgG levels) show increased absorption of macromolecules and high levels of circulating immune complexes

following ingestion of antigens. This may be the cause of the increase in autoimmunity associated with IgA deficiency. Second, there is good evidence in animals and some evidence in humans that injected antigens become bound to circulating IgA and are then cleared in the liver via SC-mediated transport. Thus, the mucosal immune system either prevents the entry of potentially harmful antigens to the circulation via the mucosa or facilitates their removal from the circulation. This has the effect of limiting the immune response to the antigens present in the mucosal area to the regulated response occurring in the mucosal immune system itself, as discussed below.

Secretory versus Circulating IgA

In recent years in vivo and in vitro studies of IgA synthesis and catabolism have allowed insights into the source of IgA present in various body compartments. The results of these studies show that in humans most circulating IgA is produced in the bone marrow and is in the form of IgA1 monomers, whereas secretory IgA is produced mainly at mucosal sites (either as IgA1 or IgA2 dimers or polymers). Polymeric IgA (whether IgA1 or IgA2) is more rapidly catabolized than monomeric IgA because polymeric IgA is subject to additional clearance mechanisms such as SC-mediated transport and asialoglycoprotein receptor-mediated uptake. In rats and rabbits, polymeric IgA accounts for about half of the circulating IgA, although most IgA delivered into the circulation is polymeric IgA. This is explained by the fact that in these species SC-mediated transport in the liver is a quantitatively important process and thus polymeric IgA is more rapidly cleared than monomeric IgA. The importance of hepatic clearance of polymeric IgA in rats and rabbits is underscored by the observation that in these species (but not in humans) biliary obstruction leads to increased IgA levels.

The separate origin of mucosal and circulating IgA in humans has led Conley and Delacroix to suggest that the IgA system in humans is bipartite, ie, is composed of 2 relatively independent synthetic centers that are separately regulated. An alternative view more in keeping with the concept that the bone marrow is not an inductive site for IgA B cells is that the IgA1 B cells that produce IgA in the marrow originate in the mucosa and secondarily colonize the marrow to form a separate (but subordinate) locus of IgA-producing B cells. In any case, the monomeric IgA1 arising from the bone marrow in humans may provide a selective advantage in that such IgA may be better suited than other forms of IgA to mediate the clearance of mucosal antigens from the circulation (as discussed above). This is because a monomeric IgA1 molecule may form smaller, more nonpathogenic complexes with circulating antigens than polymeric IgA, yet retain the capacity to undergo removal via interaction with appropriate receptors in the liver.

PRODUCTION OF OTHER IMMUNOGLOBULINS IN THE MUCOSA

Immunoglobulins other than IgA also play a role in the mucosal immune system. Mucosal synthesis of IgM, which can be transported across the epithelial cell via the SC-mediated mechanism, is measurable and physiologically significant. Its capacity to act as a mucosal immunoglobulin is underscored by the fact that it usually replaces IgA adequately to produce mucosal immunity in individuals with selective IgA deficiency. Mucosal synthesis of IgG, on the other hand, is quite low in most mucosal areas, and IgG cannot be transported across the epithelium. Nevertheless, it does have a mucosal role. It is synthesized in substantial amounts in the distal pulmonary tract and is an important antibody class in pulmonary secretions, which it probably enters by passive diffusion. IgE is also synthesized in mucosal tissues, particularly during parasitic infection or during certain pathologic (allergic) states. However, there is no preferential localization of IgE B cells in the mucosa and the number of B cells synthesizing IgE is small, as it is in other tissues. Recent studies with rats suggest that the mucosa may be an important site for IgE B cells during neonatal development.

REGULATION OF IgA SYNTHESIS AT MUCOSAL SITES

Several factors are involved in the preferential synthesis of IgA in mucosal follicles rather than in other lymphoid areas. Cells derived from mucosal lymphoid aggregates (Peyer's patches), but not those from the spleen, have the capacity to induce secretory IgM (sIgM)-positive B cells to undergo isotype switching to sIgA-positive B cells in vitro. Cells bringing about the isotype switching were identified as T cells, but it remains possible that other cells, including mucosal macrophages and stromal cells, also play a role (Fig 15–5). Although it is presumed that the switch cells produce an

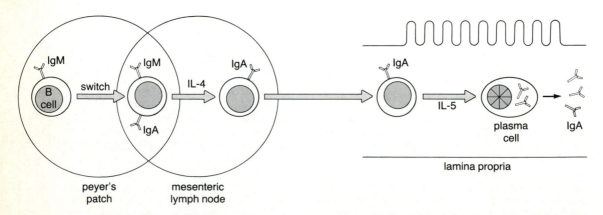

Figure 15–5. Regulation of the IgA response. This involves switching events on the mucosal follicle (Peyer's patch) and then a series of post-switch regulatory events in the mesenteric lymph node and lamina propria. The latter events are known to involve IL-4 and IL-5.

IgA-specific switch cytokine or lymphokine, such a material has yet to be identified. It is known, however, that neither IL-4 nor IL-5 can perform this function in the IgA system, unless perhaps they act in conjunction with other factors.

A second mechanism that accounts for the predominance of IgA B cells in the mucosal lymphoid aggregates involves the fact that B cells in mucosal areas come under the influence of post-isotype switch IgA-specific signals, ie, signals that favor terminal differentiation of IgA B Cells (Fig 15–5). A class of T cells that bear Fc receptors specific for IgA (FcαR) and that enhance post-switch differentiation of sIgA-bearing B cells have been identified. It is thought that such cells act through the release of IgA-binding factors which act on sIgA-positive B cells. There is evidence that certain T cells secrete IL-5, which, along with other lymphokines such as IL-6, may have preferential effects on IgA B cell differentiation. Either of these types of T cells having effects on IgA B cell differentiation may be more abundant in mucosal areas than elsewhere and may therefore act in concert with switch cells to lead to preferential IgA B cell maturation in the mucosal follicles.

Other types of IgA class-specific regulatory cells have been reported. One such cell is the "contrasuppressor" T cell obtained from Peyer's patches. These cells appear to counteract the effects of suppressor T cells on IgA responses to a greater extent than they counteract the effects of suppressor T cells on IgG or IgM responses. There is also a suppressor T cell that bears IgA-specific Fc receptors and that down-regulates IgA responses in a class-specific fashion. Cells of this type are induced in mice and humans bearing IgA plasmacytomas or myelomas, and in mice they mediate suppression of responses elicited by oral antigen administration. Thus, T cells bearing IgA-Fc receptors can act as both IgA-specific helper and suppressor cells and are, in this sense, analogous to cells having both positive and negative regulatory effects on IgE responses.

ORAL UNRESPONSIVENESS

The mucosal immune system responds negatively to the vast number of antigens from foods and normal bacterial flora in the mucosal environment. This unresponsiveness prevents the system from being overwhelmed by the antigens.

Oral unresponsiveness is more complete for antigens on the surface of erythrocytes, those associated with bacteria and viruses, and most protein antigens than it is for thymus-independent antigens and complex particulate antigens (including live viruses). This may explain why the mucosal system mounts immune responses to potential pathogens while remaining generally unresponsive to food antigens. Oral unresponsiveness is both B cell (antibody) and T cell mediated, but not necessarily to the same degree in all cases.

Adoptive transfer experiments with animals show that one cellular mechanism underlying oral unresponsiveness is the strong tendency for antigenic stimulation via mucosal follicles to induce **antigen-specific** suppressor T cells in Peyer's patches. However, it is not clear why suppressor circuits are initiated more readily in the mucosal system than elsewhere. The presence of **antigen-nonspecific** suppressor cells may be a second mechanism of oral unresponsiveness. Evidence for this comes from the observation that in animals that are genetically unresponsive to lipopolysaccharide (LPS; a B cell mitogen), oral responses to certain antigens are increased, suppressor T cell responses following oral challenge are reduced, and the phenomenon of oral unresponsiveness does not occur. Although the mechanism is unknown, it is significant that in the "normal" LPS-rich (B cell mitogen-rich) environment of the mucosa, antigen-nonspecific regulatory cells play an important role in down-regulating responses to specific antigens. A third possible mechanism is clonal inhibition (or clonal anergy) resulting from direct effects of antigens on B or T cells in mucosal follicles. Peyer's patches in sheep are sites of massive cell turnover and death; these cells may be undergoing negative clonal selection, just as they do in the thymus.

Abnormalities of oral unresponsiveness may relate to certain immunologic diseases. First, oral unresponsiveness appears to be decreased in several autoimmune mouse strains, which suggests that inappropriate reactivity to one or another antigen in the mucosal system may be a factor in the development of autoimmunity. This possibility gains credence from recent evidence that autoantibodies are structurally related to antibodies against simple antigenic determinants commonly present in the mucosal environment. Second, oral unresponsiveness is reduced in young children, resulting in hypersensitivity to certain oral antigens such as milk proteins. Third, genetically determined defects associated with oral unresponsiveness may form the basis of gluten-sensitive enteropathy or the inflammatory bowel diseases (see Chapter 40).

MUCOSAL HOMING

A characteristic feature of the mucosal immune system is the homing capability of cells developing in the mucosal follicles (Fig 15–6). As mentioned

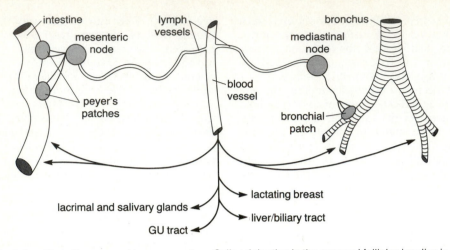

Figure 15–6. Cell traffic in the mucosal immune system. Cells originating in the mucosal follicles localize in subepithelial areas of many mucosal tissues. The ability to do so is governed by specific receptor-ligand interactions involving receptors on lymphoid cells and ligands on endothelial cells.

above, this mechanism acts to limit and focus the mucosal immune response to mucosal tissues. Studies of mucosal cell traffic show that B lymphoblasts arising in mesenteric or bronchial lymph nodes selectively localize to mucosal areas and that the majority (70–90%) of the localizing B cells are IgA B cells. T lymphoblasts from mesenteric node and thoracic duct lymph also localize to mucosal sites, both to the lamina propria and to the IEL compartment; however, compared with B cells, a smaller proportion of T cells arising in the mucosal follicles have this property. Small resting (or memory) B cells and T cells arising in the mucosal follicles also recirculate in the mucosal immune system.

Mucosal homing is not an antigen-trapping mechanism. Mucosal lymphoblasts migrate to antigen-free intestinal grafts in extraintestinal sites. Antigen challenge to an isolated area of mucosa results in the appearance of antigen-reactive cells in equal numbers at both exposed and nonexposed areas of mucosa, indicating that cell migration is not directed by antigen. After cells have migrated into the lamina propria, however, antigen does cause them to become sessile (fixed in tissue) and to proliferate. In fact, antigen-specific responses are enhanced at intestinal sites that have been previously exposed to antigen and reduced elsewhere in the intestine.

There is a growing body of data supporting the idea that mucosal homing is initiated by interactions between specific homing receptors on Peyer's patch-derived lymphocytes and ligands for such receptors on endothelial cells (addressins). These interactions are followed by cellular penetration of the endothelium and the entry of cells into mucosal tissue proper. Thus, the capacity of a Peyer's patch lymphocyte to home to the lamina propria can be explained by the selective induction of homing receptors on lymphocytes developing at this site.

BREAST MILK IMMUNOLOGY

The lactating breast is an important component of the mucosal traffic "loop" and ensures that mucosal immunoglobulins and cells are available to protect the neonate during a critical period of relative immunologic incompetence. The concentration of IgA in initial breast secretions (colostrum) is extremely high, averaging 50 mg/mL (versus 2.5 mg/mL in adult serum). However, it falls rapidly to serum levels after the first 4 days, in part owing to the dilutional effect of increased secretion volume. The IgA of breast milk originates from IgA B cells in breast tissue, which migrated there from gastrointestinal and respiratory mucosal follicles. Such migration is dependent on as yet unidentified changes in breast tissue brought about by the action of hormones. The locally synthesized IgA is then transported across the epithelium by an SC-mediated transport mechanism.

Human colostrum and milk are rich in antibodies to a variety of organisms. The beneficial effect of such antibodies may not be obvious in developed countries, but it is readily apparent in underdeveloped countries, where exposure to environmental pathogens is much greater. In addition to protecting the newborn from infection, breast milk antibodies may play a role in establishing the normal flora and in preventing the uptake of certain macromolecules. The latter effect may be relevant to the development of allergies, but this is not yet certain.

Breast milk secretion also contains a significant number of cells, and its ingestion results in the transfer of as many as 10^8 cells/d to the newborn. Most of the cells in breast milk are macrophages and granulocytes, but small numbers of B and T lymphocytes are also present. The macrophages are functionally active and contain ingested IgA; thus, they may be a vehicle for the delivery of IgA to critical areas. Although the T cells are present in small numbers, they are able to transfer specific immune reactivity; suggesting that these cells gain entry to the newborn circulation.

SUMMARY

The antigenic environment of the mucosa is a chaotic mix of virtually the entire antigenic universe, to which may be added potential mitogens that could further stimulate the mucosal system. In this situation it is essential that the relevant immune system be capable of discriminating between stimuli that have possible pathogenic import and those that are harmless and would merely engage the system in a fruitless and wasteful response. The mucosal immune system is shaped to fulfill this need. On the one hand, it has a highly focused response to stimuli, which produces antibodies that interact with and eliminate potential pathogens, without at the same time evoking undue inflammation. Such responses also help to prevent entry and to facilitate clearance of unwanted antigens. On the other hand, it also elaborates suppressor elements that interact with ubiquitous antigens and thus down regulate responses both in the mucosal areas and in systemic lymphoid tissues. In pursuing these somewhat opposing goals, the mucosal immune system fulfills an important and critical "gatekeeper" function of the immune system, which ensures the integrity of the internal milieu.

REFERENCES

General

Mestecky J, McGhee J: Immunoglobulin A (IgA): Molecular and cellular interactions involved in IgA biosynthesis and immune response. *Adv Immunol* 1987;**40**:153.

Strober W, Brown WR: The mucosal immune system, In: *Immunological Diseases,* 4th ed. Samter M (editor). Little, Brown, 1988.

Antigen-Presenting Cells

Ermak TH, Owen RL: Differential distribution of lymphocytes and accessory cells in mouse Peyer's patches. *Anat Rec* 1986;**215**:144.

Richman LK, Graeff AS, Strober W: Antigen presentation by macrophage-enriched cells from the mouse Peyer's patch. *Cell Immunol* 1981;**62**:110.

M Cells

Sneller MC, Strober W: M cells and host defense. *J Infect Dis* 1986;**154**:737.

Intraepithelial Lymphocytes

Ernst PB, Befus AD, Bienenstock J: Leukocytes in the intestinal epithelium: An unusual immunological compartment. *Immunol Today* 1985;**6**:50.

Mucosal Mast Cells

Befus AD et al: Mast cells from the human intestinal lamina propria. *J Immunol* 1987;**138**:2604.

Irani AA et al: Two types of human mast cells that have distinct neutral protease compositions. *Proc Natl Acad Sci USA* 1986;**83**:4464.

Lamina Propria Lymphocytes

Fiocchi C et al: Modulation of intestinal immune reactivity by interleukin 2: Phenotypic and functional analysis of lymphokine-activated killer cells from human intestinal mucosa. *Dig Dis Sci* 1988;**33**:1305.

James SP et al: Intestinal lymphocyte populations and mechanisms of cell mediated immunity. *Immunol Allergy Clin N Am* 1988;**8**:369.

IgA Structure & Transport

Conley ME, Delacroix DL: Intravascular and mucosal immunoglobulin A: Two separate but related systems of immune defense? *Ann Intern Med* 1987;**106**:892.

Kilian J, Mestecky J, Russel MW: Defense mechanisms involving Fc-dependent functions of immunoglobulin A and their subversion by bacterial immunoglobulin A proteases. *Microbiol Rev* 1988;**52**:296.

Underdown BJ, Schiff JM: Immunoglobulin A: Strategic defense initiative at the mucosal surface. *Annu Rev Immunol* 1986;**4**:389.

Walker WA: Antigen handling by the small intestine. *Clin Gastroenterol* 1986;**15**:1.

Regulation of IgA Synthesis

Harriman GR et al: The role of IL-5 in IgA B cell differentiation. *J Immunol* 1988;**140**:3033.

Kawanishi H, Saltzman LE, Strober W: Mechanisms regulating IgA class-specific immunoglobulin production in murine gut-associated lymphoid tissues. *J Exp Med* 1983;**157**:433.

Kiyono H et al: Isotype-specific immunoregulation. IgA-binding factors produced by Fcα receptor-positive T cell hybridomas regulate IgA responses. *J Exp Med* 1985;**161**:731.

Oral Unresponsiveness

Mowat AM: The regulation of immune responses to dietary protein antigens. *Immunol Today* 1987; **8**:93.

Mucosal Cell Homing

Bienenstock J et al: Regulation of lymphoblast traffic and localization in mucosal tissues, with emphasis on IgA. *Fed Proc* 1983;**42**:3213.

Jalkanen S et al: Human lymphocyte and lymphoma homing receptors. *Annu Rev Med* 1987;**38**:467.

Breast Milk

Ogra PL, Losonsky GA, Fishaut M. Colostrum-derived immunity and maternal-neonatal interaction. *Ann NY Acad Sci* 1983;**409**:82.

Physiologic & Environmental Influences on the Immune System

16

Abba I. Terr, MD, Devendra P. Dubey, PhD, Edmond J. Yunis, MD,
Raymond G. Slavin, MD, & Robert H. Waldman, MD

The immune system has developed a high intrinsic capacity for recognizing and dealing with foreign substances. This capacity is controlled by a series of internal processes of self-regulation. In the intact host, however, the immune system has anatomic and physiologic relationships with other systems of the body, and there is a potential for it to be adversely or beneficially affected by environmental influences.

In contrast to the current wealth of information about the immune system itself, there is relatively little information about the relationship between the immune system, other physiologic systems, and the environment. Available data are very incomplete, but research interest in many of these areas is gaining momentum. This chapter will cover a selected group of topics dealing with external and internal influences on the immune system. These include psychoneuroimmunology, aging, nutrition, environmental chemicals, and uremia.

PSYCHONEUROIMMUNOLOGY

Abba I. Terr, MD

For many years a few investigators have been studying the interrelationships among the immune system, the nervous system, the endocrine glands, and psychologic behavior. There is evidence from clinical observations and experimentation and from animal studies that the immune response and its various effector mechanisms are regulated and modulated in part by neuroendocrine influences, in addition to internal regulation by its own feedback inhibition, regulatory lymphocytes, and the anti-idiotype network. The nervous system/immune system interaction appears to be bidirectional, and it is influenced by and expressed in behavioral and emotional terms. There are some important similarities between central nervous system and immune system function. Both respond to environmental stimuli, the nervous system sensing physical signals and the immune system sensing chemical structures.

Much of the research in this area deals with the effect of stress on the immune response. In this context, stress is usually defined as the host response to an adverse environmental event or stimulus, called a stressor, and the effects are related to inability to cope with the stressor. Coping mechanisms are defined subjectively and include both internal psychologic mechanisms and external social support systems.

ANATOMIC CONNECTIONS BETWEEN THE NERVOUS AND IMMUNE SYSTEMS

Although a direct nervous system/endocrine anatomic connection between the hypothalamus and the pituitary has been well established for some time, a similar study of innervation of the immune system has been undertaken only recently. There are, in fact, nerve endings in the thymus, spleen, and lymph nodes, primarily sympathetic efferents. In both humans and animals, autonomic nervous system fibers to the thymus appear embryologically before immature T cells do. In the bone marrow, spleen, and lymph nodes, the nerve endings appear in locations rich in T cells but not B cells.

PHYSIOLOGIC INTERRELATIONSHIPS

The nervous and immune systems are comparable in a number of ways. Both are characterized by a diversity of cell types and by cell-to-cell transmission of information by soluble factors such as lymphokines (in the immune system) and neurotransmitters (in the nervous system). Both systems have the capacity for short-lived and long-lived memory. Opportunities for cross-communication are becoming increasingly evident. Lymphocytes and macrophages have receptors capable of responding to the neurotransmitters acetylcholine and norepinephrine, endorphins, enkephalins, and a number of endocrine hormones including adrenocorticotropic hormone (ACTH), corticosteroids, insulin, prolactin, growth hormone, estradiol, and testosterone. Lymphocytes, in turn, are capable of producing and secreting ACTH and endorphinlike compounds, which could act as an autocrine feedback regulator of lymphocyte functions.

Neurons in the brain, particularly in the hypothalamus, can recognize immunocyte products (including prostaglandins, interferons, and interleukins) and chemical mediators from inflammatory cell products (including histamine and serotonin).

ANIMAL EXPERIMENTS

Short-term animal experiments have been performed primarily with rodents and primates. The relevance of these results to humans is obviously tenuous because of small but significant differences in the immune responses and obviously enormous differences in psychologic makeup. Many animal experiments have involved the effect of acute stressors on antibody responses, antibody-induced effects such as anaphylaxis, mitogen responses, and quantitative changes in circulating immunoglobulins and lymphocytes. Stressors have included physical stimuli, such as electric shock, loud noise, and acceleration, and purely psychologic stressors, such as infant-mother separation, peer separation, restraints, and overcrowding. Results have been mixed. Although early experiments showed that antibody production was increased after low-voltage electric shock, more recent studies have generally shown an early inhibition of antibody production, mitogenic responses of lymphocytes, and reduced lymphocyte counts. Longer-term experiments generally show that these effects are transient; this suggests that adaptation occurs. Immunologic effects are most pronounced when the animal is stressed in an inescapable condition, possibly stimulating the phenomenon of poor coping in humans. Some reports suggest that stressed animals have an increased incidence of infections and enhanced growth of injected syngeneic tumor cells. Since the immunologic measurements of lymphocyte counts and lymphocyte responses are usually performed with circulating cells, the effect of stress is caused at least in part by stress-induced glucocorticoid lymphopenia. However, a slight but reproducible suppressive effect on the immune response occurs in adrenalectomized animals. The results on tumor growth may reflect changes in vascularity or hormone effects independent of any effect on the immune system itself.

There are several compelling reports of Pavlovian conditioning of the immune response. Rats given saccharin as a conditioned stimulus along with the immunosuppressant drug cyclophosphamide as an unconditioned stimulus (but used in this case to produce nausea) were later fortuitously discovered to be conditioned for immune suppression with saccharin alone. This observation led to a series of experiments in which both antibody-mediated immunity and cell-mediated immunity (CMI) were depressed by conditioning. In a reverse type of experiment, conditioning was also used successfully to significantly reduce the dose of cyclophosphamide required to control systemic lupus in mice. Mediators from immunologically sensitized mast cells have also been released in vivo by a conditioned stimulus of an odor in guinea pigs and an audiovisual stimulus in rats.

The presence of an immune response on the brain has been shown by the fact that norepinephrine synthesis in the hypothalamus (as well as in the spleen) is inhibited at the peak of an induced immune response to a foreign antigen. Follow-up experiments showed that the inhibition was related to soluble factors secreted by lymphocytes, but the nature of these factors has not yet been determined.

Hemispheric lateralization of the central nervous system control of immunity is shown by the effect of experimental lesions in the cerebral neocortex. Left-sided neocortical lesions in mice caused a reduction in the number of spleen cells, T cell-dependent responses, natural killer (NK) cells, lymphokines, and regulatory T cells, whereas right-sided lesions produced the opposite effect. B cells and macrophages were not affected.

Finally, an interesting series of experiments reveals that immune responses were altered when surgical lesions were induced in the brain. Lesions in the anterior hypothalamus of mice inhibited immune responses, whereas lesions in the amygdala or hippocampus enhanced them, possibly via neural influences on spleen suppressor cell activity. In other studies, an induced immune response in mice produced changes in the electrical activity of brain neurons, an effect that was probably mediated by lymphokines.

A variety of endocrine hormones administered to different animals cause differing effect on immune responses. In general, glucocorticoids, androgens, estrogen, and progesterone inhibit antibody production, whereas growth hormone, thyroxine, and insulin enhance it. The effect of autonomic neurotransmitters is likewise a dual one, with parasympathetic agonists increasing and sympathetic agonists decreasing antibody production and cytotoxicity.

STUDIES IN HUMANS

Anecdotal reports based on clinical observations have long suggested that psychologic factors, particularly stressful life events, influence diseases related to the immune system. Clinicians and patients alike have long suspected that symptoms of infections and allergies are worsened by stressful events. Graves' disease is reported to appear after separation or loss of a close family member. A number of retrospective studies on bereavement suggest that it is associated with a susceptibility to diabetes, ulcerative colitis, rheumatoid arthritis, systemic lupus erythematosus (SLE), and cancer. However, spousal bereavement has also been associated with occurrence of schizophrenia, coronary artery disease, sudden accidents, and death.

The designs of clinical studies have usually taken one of 2 forms: cross-sectional analysis of immune responses in a susceptible population and prospective case-control studies.

Several investigators have used spousal bereavement to study immunologic changes secondary to a stressful life event in otherwise normal individuals. A prospective study of husbands of women with advanced breast cancer found that lymphocyte responses to mitogens diminished during the first 2 months following the wife's death, although total lymphocyte and lymphocyte subset counts, delayed-type hypersensitivity (DTH), and circulating levels of cortisol, prolactin, growth hormone, and thyroid hormone remained normal. In some studies, there are reports of an increase in the severity of respiratory infections accompanying these functional lymphocyte changes, but this information is based on patient reports rather than objective evidence. In general, possible confounding factors of weight loss, changes in diet, sleep alteration, lack of exercise, and use of drugs were not monitored.

The stress produced in first-year dental students as a result of their academic examinations produced a significant drop in salivary IgA secretion. In these studies it was noted that the basal secretory levels and response to stress correlated with the personality traits of each student. Those with an inherent need for personal relationships tended to have higher levels of secretory IgA. In another report, the stress of examinations caused a decrease in circulating CD4 cells and NK cell activity in medical students; this effect was most marked in students who expressed loneliness. Other studies have shown that although anxiety and depression may inhibit some manifestations of the immune response, subjects who coped well with stress showed an increase in NK cell activity. The significance of such observations for host defense is unclear. Although experiments using Pavlovian conditioning have not been done with human subjects, there are a number of anecdotal reports of suppression of immediate and delayed skin tests to allergens induced by hypnosis or meditation.

THE IMMUNOLOGY OF PSYCHIATRIC ILLNESS

In recent years an emphasis in psychiatry research has shifted to a search for a biologic, rather than a psychologic, cause for many psychiatric diseases, especially for the major depressive disorders. Depressive disease, also called affective disorder, has a 1–2% prevalence in the general population, is characterized by dysphoria, and may be accompanied by somatic symptoms. It may manifest as simple unipolar depression or as alternating manic-depressive bipolar disease. Immunologic studies are confounded by the fact that increased release of corticosteroids from the pituitary is a feature of major depressive disorder as well as a response to a wide range of stresses that may produce temporary depression in normal individuals. Case-control studies on depression have shown variable effects on circulating lymphocytes. On balance, counts of circulating lymphocytes and their subsets are not consistently changed, although mitogenic responses are often reported to be diminished. Controlling for the effects of diet and activity makes studies on this group of patients difficult. The investigators usually discontinue administration of antidepressant medications prior to obtaining blood samples for study, but a possible effect of drug withdrawal has not been carefully investigated.

Patients with schizophrenia also show variable and inconsistent changes in circulating lymphocyte concentrations. Mitogen responses were normal in patients with agarophobia and panic attacks. One interesting report showed evidence of a possible human leukocyte anitgen (HLA) linkage in a family study of depression, regardless of whether the disease was unipolar or bipolar. The association suggested that an HLA-associated gene may be involved in the susceptibility to the disease, which probably requires other factors for clinical expression.

NEUROPSYCHIATRIC STUDIES IN IMMUNOLOGIC DISEASES

This area has received much less research attention. An organic psychosis can occur in some forms of autoimmune disease, such as SLE, but the relevance of this to psychiatric illness in general is obscure. Recent clinical trials of recombinant lymphokines have revealed, in some cases, side effects including psychiatric symptoms. For example, interferon therapy characteristically produces a picture of depression with fatigue, drowsiness, disorientation, lethargy, withdrawal, and electroencephalogram (EEG) abnormalities.

A recent provocative report that certain immune diseases—autoimmune thyroiditis, celiac disease, regional ileitis, ulcerative colitis, childhood atopic allergy, and myasthenia gravis—are significantly more common among those who are naturally left-handed is reminiscent of the animal studies showing hemispheric dominance in immune responses, but these results should be considered preliminary.

SUMMARY

Clinical and experimental psychoneuroimmunology studies to date confirm the long-standing belief that the immune system does not function completely autonomously. The findings suggest many exciting research opportunities, but few if any conclusions can yet be drawn about the interrelationships of psychiatric and immunologic factors that can be applied to the diagnosis and treatment of specific diseases.

AGING & NUTRITIONAL EFFECTS ON IMMUNE FUNCTIONS IN HUMANS

Devendra P. Dubey PhD,
& Edmond J. Yunis, MD

The elderly are more susceptible than younger adults to develop certain infectious diseases with increased severity, and they are at greater risk of developing cancer and autoimmune diseases. This suggests that immune deficiencies may be a feature of the aged population. Studies generally agree that there is a decline in immune functions in older individuals but disagree about which specific immune functions are impaired. The conflicting results may be due to methodologic differences, differences in the selection of subjects for study, and lack of an accepted definition of "old"

and "young." The changes in immune function due to disease may further confound the determination of intrinsic age-related decline in the immune function.

This section describes the age-related changes in the thymus, T cell responses to mitogens and antigens, lymphokine production, antibody production, and NK cell function. The T cell response to PHA, CMI, and T cell–dependent antibody production significantly decline, whereas T cell–independent antibody production is not significantly affected in healthy aged individuals.

AGING

The Thymus & Aging

The thymus plays a central role in T cell maturation and proliferation. One of the better-known phenomena associated with aging is the involution of the thymus. Morphologic studies reveal that although the weight and volume of the thymus may show large variations among individuals, they increase until 6 months of age and thereafter remain constant, although the morphology of the thymus changes significantly.

Structurally, the thymus can be divided into 4 major regions: epithelial cortex, cortex, corticomedullary region, and medulla. The outer region of the cortex contains many macrophages and large blastlike lymphocytes. The inner cortex and medulla contain medium-sized and smaller lymphocytes as well as Hassall's corpuscles. In addition to lymphoid cells, the thymus contains nonlymphoid cells: cortical and medullary epithelial cells, interdigitating reticulum cells, macrophages, and mast cells. Blood vessels are found in the cortex and medullary region and characteristically possess epithelial cells in the adventitia, which serves as a blood-thymus barrier. Hematopoietic stem cells from bone marrow travel through the bloodstream and enter the thymus through the epithelial cell lining of the cortex (Fig 16-1). Prothymocytes (or pre-T cells) differentiate within the microenvironment of the thymus. In the thymus 4 peptide hormones, thymulin, thymosin a, thymosin β, and thymopoietin, are synthesized. These hormones are involved in the proliferation and differentiation of T cells. In addition, direct contact with the thymic epithelium, which expresses HLA antigens, is required for the generation of functional T cells and their education to recognize antigens of the major histocompatibility complex (MHC) region. The thymus is believed to be linked with the central nervous system, the endocrine system, and the immune system and thus to participate in the regulation of immune function by a complex network of interactions. The most significant change in the

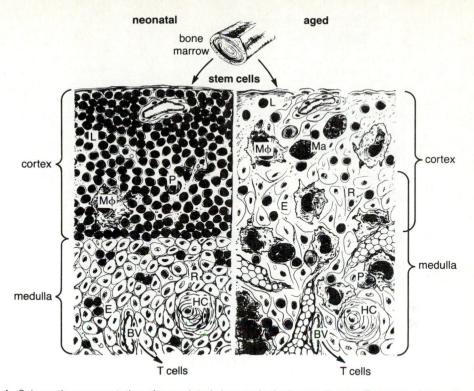

Figure 16–1. Schematic representation of age-related changes in the human thymus. The cortex is heavily populated with lymphocytes (L) in neonatal thymus, and the medulla contains Hassall's corpuscles (HC) and fewer lymphocytes. The aged thymus is involuted and atrophied and contains fat cells. The cortex has fewer lymphocytes, infiltrated with macrophages (Mφ) and mast cells (mα). The medulla is relatively unaffected. The stem cells that migrate to the thymus encounter the epithelial cells (E), which express class I and II antigens on their surface. Class I antigen is weakly expressed on the thymocytes in the cortical region and strongly expressed on thymocytes in the medullary region. It differentiates into mature T-cells with CD4 and CD8 antigen expression

thymus during aging is a decrease in the mass of the organ, in the number of lymphocytes, and in thymic hormone production (Fig 16-2).

T & B Lymphocyte Changes & Aging

The total number of lymphocytes and the number of T and B cells in the peripheral blood do not change with age. The relative proportions of CD4 and CD8 T cells are both slightly reduced with age. The reduction in CD4 cells is somewhat greater than in CD8 cells, resulting in lowered CD4/CD8 cell ratios. It is possible that although the changes are numerically small, they may be important to immune regulation. T lymphocyte proliferation is low in response to mitogens in the aged, without a corresponding reduction in the number of T cells.

The autologous mixed-lymphocyte reaction is considered an in vitro model with which to study T-T interaction in which both helper T (CD4) and suppressor/cytotoxic (CD8) cell functions are generated. The autologous mixed-lymphocyte response of lymphocytes from the aged is significantly lower than that of lymphocytes from the young, and could not be corrected by the addition of interleukin-2 (IL-2).

Other T cell functions defective in the elderly population are the ability to respond to or to stimulate allogeneic and autologous lymphocytes in mixed-lymphocyte reactions, reduced generation of cytotoxic T cells, and reduced capability to reject primary allografts and tumor cells. The level of interferon produced by lymphocytes from elderly donors exposed to herpes simplex virus is decreased.

The B cell responsiveness to pokeweed mitogen is dependent on T cell subsets. Lymphocytes from aged donors exhibit a lower frequency of pokeweed mitogen-induced plaque-forming cells in comparison with those from young subjects. This apparent decrease in B cell function could be due to an age-related decline in helper T cell function. This is supported by the observation that in the elderly population the proportion of CD45R, a

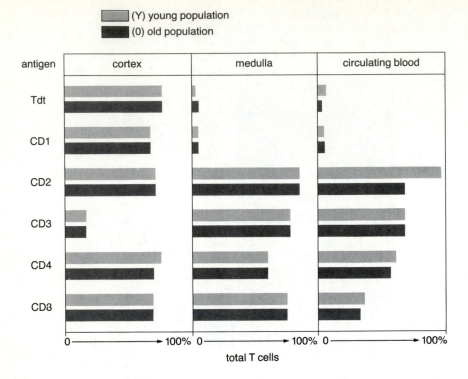

Figure 16–2. Age-dependent changes in the human thymocytes and peripheral blood lymphocytes. Immature thymocytes are found in the cortex. These cells express terminal deoxyribonucleotidyl transferase (Tdt). The expression of this enzyme is lost when thymocytes become mature. CD1 antigen is lost in the medullary region. The percentage of CD2- and Cd3-positive cells increases when the cells move from the cortex to the medulla. In the cortex CD4 is coexpressed with CD8. In the medulla, CD4 and CD8 antigens are expressed on different cells. A small percentage of cells in the medulla coexpress CD4 and CD8 antigens. With age there may be a slight decrease in the number of mature CD3 cells and an increase in the number of immature CD1 cells.

subset of CD4 T cells, is significantly lower than in younger age groups.

Activation of T cells plays a crucial role in the responsiveness of the host to a foreign antigen. Some of the early activation events are stimulation of phospholipase C and protein kinase C, mobilization of intracellular calcium, IL-2 production and its receptor expression, and activation of proto-oncogenes such as c-*myc* and c-*myb*. A defect in T cell responses to mitogen or antigens may reflect a defect in one or more steps of signal transduction. T cells of older people respond poorly to mitogen or antigen stimulation. Studies have not revealed any defect in the antigen-presenting capacity or other stimulatory characteristics of macrophages of older people. However, a defect in IL-2 production as well as expression of both high-affinity and low-affinity IL-2 receptors has been observed, and T cell proliferation cannot be restored by addition of exogenous IL-2. The binding of IL-2 receptor with the ligand (IL-2) and internalization of this complex are also impaired. A similar reduction in c-*myc*

gene expression in activated T cells has been reported. Definitive information on the other early steps in signal transduction, such as calcium mobilization and protein kinase C activation, is still lacking.

Humoral Immunity & Aging

An increased frequency of infections and autoimmune diseases is observed among the elderly. One of the most common causes of morbidity and mortality in this population is infections caused by certain bacteria such as *Streptococcus pneumoniae* and *Escherichia coli*. Polyclonal hyperimmunoglobulinemia and increased levels of autoantibodies are also common. The lack of a response to bacterial infection may be due to an age-related defect in antibody function. Although the total concentration of immunoglobulins remains unchanged with age, there is an increase in the level of IgA and IgG antibodies. Antibody responses to specific antigens such as flagellin, purified protein derivative (PPD), hepatitis B virus, and multivalent influenza virus vaccines are decreased. The subpopulation of CD8 T cells in the elderly population has been shown to decrease with age, suggesting that loss of regulatory suppressor T cell activity may explain the occurrence of autoantibodies in the elderly.

Recent studies show a decrease in the NK lytic activity but an increase or no change in the number of NK cells as defined by CD16 and CD57 (Leu 7) markers in healthy elderly individuals. However, others have observed a decrease in activity as well as in the number of NK cells in this age group.

SUMMARY

The functions of the immune system show some evidence of decline with age. Involution of the thymus is accompanied by reduced production of thymic hormones and an increase in the number of immature lymphocytes. The DTH response is reduced. Although the number of circulating T lymphocytes in peripheral blood does not show any significant decrease with age, a small decrease in the proportion of subsets of T cells responsible for immune regulation may lead to a reduced responsiveness to foreign antigens and increased autoimmunity. There is an age-dependent decline in in vitro T cell responses to mitogens such as PHA and concanavalin A. IL-2 and gamma interferon (IFN-γ) production by T cells is reduced. No change in the antigen-presenting capacity of macrophages has been observed. Data on NK cell activity of old individuals are controversial, and further study is needed. B cells do not show any significant decrease in number but have a reduced capacity to form hemolytic plaques by antibody secretion and are diminished in T cell–dependent antibody production. This reflects a possible defect in T cell subsets that regulate antibody production.

The importance of these changes is not yet clear. Many other factors, such as nutritional deficiency and stress, that may suppress immune function could induce immune deficiency and render older people vulnerable to life-threatening infections, autoimmunity, and cancers.

NUTRITION

Proteins, carbohydrates, lipids, vitamins, and minerals are essential for human maintenance and growth. Qualitative and quantitative changes in these nutrients may significantly affect the functions of the immune system. Cells of the immune system, when activated, are metabolically very active and synthesize and secrete molecules that are involved in cell-cell interaction. Thus, either a deficiency or an excess of specific nutrients can influence the synthesis of these molecules, thereby altering the regulation of immunity.

Malnutrition is a common cause of immune deficiency, with a particularly significant effect on CMI, phagocytosis, and the complement system. It may have long-term reversible or irreversible effects, depending on its severity and duration. Malnourishment of the mother can lead to nutritional deficiencies in utero that may affect the newborn's ability to respond to infections at birth. This in utero deficiency may involve both CMI and humoral immunity. In severe protein-calorie malnutrition, the humoral response and antibody production may return to a normal level after the subject is maintained on an adequate diet, but the deficiency in CMI may persist.

Protein-Calorie Malnutrition

Chronic nutritional deficiency may lead to different kinds of diseases such as kwashiorkor and marasmus. Kwashiorkor is an extreme case of protein-calorie malnutrition. Marasmus, a milder form of the disease, is a clinical manifestation of protein, fat, vitamin, or mineral deprivation during the early part of life. Patients with these diseases have a higher than normal incidence of bacterial and parasitic infections. Severe thymic atrophy is seen in malnourished children, especially in patients with kwashiorkor and to a lesser extent in those with marasmus. A severe case of kwashiorkor leads to acute thymic involution accompanied by loss of corticomedullary differentiation, a reduced number of thymocytes, and various degrees of depletion of lymph node germinal centers and paracortical cells in peripheral lymphoid tissues. The degree of thymic atrophy depends on the duration and severity of the nutritional deficiency. Lymphoid organs such as the thymus and lymph nodes become smaller, and there is lymphopenia, impaired response to PHA, low NK activity, and decreased cutaneous DTH reactions. These findings suggest that protein-calorie malnutrition affects CMI (Table 16–1). The effects of protein-calorie malnutrition on humoral immunity are less severe. B cell numbers and immunoglobulin levels are not affected significantly, but the antibody response may vary with the antigen and the form in which it is given. Although serum IgA levels are normal in protein-calorie-malnourished individuals, secretory IgA levels are low, suggesting that synthesis of secretory component by epithelial cells is impaired. In many cases, hypergammaglobulinemia of the IgM type is present. Patients with kwashiorkor characteristically have hypoproteinemia and hypoalbuminemia and yet

Table 16–1. Effects of protein deficiency
on immune functions.

Cell-Mediated Immunity
Decreased cutaneous DTH, delayed skin homograft rejection, decreased thymic hormone activity.

Reduced circulating CD3 cells and CD4 subsets; increased relative proportion of TdT immature T cells.

Suppressed T cell responses to mitogens such as PHA and concanavalin A; reduced autologous mixed-lymphocyte reaction response.

Humoral Immunity
Normal level of serum antibody, reduced antibody response to T cell–dependent antigen (eg, sheep erythrocytes), secretion but normal T cell–independent antibody production.

Nonspecific Immune Functions
Normal antigen processing by macrophages; reduced phagocytosis.

Impaired PMN activity.

Table 16–2. Effects of vitamin deficiencies
on immune functions.

Nutritional Status	Immune Effects
Vitamin A deficiency	Atrophy of thymus and spleen, decreased DTH decrease in circulating leukocytes and lymphocytes, reduced T and B cell responses to certain mitogens and antigens, reduced secretory IgA production; high infection rate; effect reversible after treatment with vitamin A.
Vitamin B$_6$ (pyridoxine) deficiency	Decreased DTH, prolonged survival of skin homografts; reduced T and B cell numbers, decreased antibody-forming cells, reduced phagocytic activity of neutrophils; impaired thymic epithelial cell functions. Mothers with B$_6$ deficiency have fetuses with much smaller thymus and spleen, and the newborns have reduced CMI.
Vitamin B$_{12}$ deficiency	Decreased DTH, reduced T and B cell responses to mitogens and antigens, impaired phagocytic and bactericidal capacity of PMN; in humans, pernicious anemia with autoimmune phenomena.
Vitamin D deficiency	No consistent effects.
Vitamin E deficiency	Decreased DTH, decreased T and B cell responses to mitogens, decreased immunoglobulin production.
Folic acid deficiency	Decreased DTH, suppressed T cell responses to mitogens, reduced antibody production, no effect on PMN activity.
Vitamin C deficiency	No significant effect on T or B cell functions, temporary decrease in vitamin C in macrophages and PMN, reduced phagocytic capacity; the effect is reversible.

have relatively high levels of serum immunoglobulins.

Protein-calorie malnutrition also impairs macrophage functions and polymorphonuclear-neurophil (PMN) activity. Although cell numbers and phagocytosis may remain normal, the oxidative and glycolytic activity of these cells is significantly reduced. Since protein-calorie malnutrition may be accompanied by mineral, vitamin, fat, and carbohydrate deficiencies, it is important that the effects of deficiency or excess of these individual nutritional components on immune functions also be understood.

Vitamin Deficiency

Deficiencies in immune function due to protein-calorie deficiency may result from a lack of adequate vitamins. In vitro studies show that vitamins are involved in the synthesis of DNA and proteins as well as in the regulation of cell proliferation and maturation of immune cells. Table 16-2 describes the reported effects of vitamin deficiencies on immune function.

Trace Element Deficiency

Trace elements are essential for adequate nutrition. The deficiency or excess of copper, iron, zinc, manganese, or selenium in the diet generally suppresses immune function (Table 16–3), rendering the host vulnerable to infections and other disorders.

A. Iron: Lymphoid cells need iron for metabolic activities such as cell division, electron transport, and oxidation and reduction reactions. Iron is transported from extracellular fluids to the cell by the iron-binding protein transferrin. The iron-transferrin complex enters immune cells by binding with transferrin receptors and is transported inside the cells via endocytosis. The observation that patients with protein-calorie malnutrition invariably suffer from iron deficiency and a high frequency of infection suggests that an iron deficiency may impair the functioning of lymphoid cells.

B. Copper: A deficiency of copper is also associated with protein-calorie malnutrition and appears to occur more frequently with kwashiorkor than with marasmus. Menkes' kinky-hair syndrome is a fatal genetic disease, which is due to defective copper metabolism and reduced synthesis of ceruloplasmin. It results in an increase in

Table 16-3. Effects of trace element deficiency on immune functions.

Condition	Immune Status
Mn deficiency	Decreased CMI, reduced levels of serum immunoglobulin, reduced antibody-forming cells.
Fe deficiency	Decreased DTH reaction, reduced T cell mitogenic response, reduced lymphokine production by activated T cells; reduced antibody production, reduced phagocytosis by PMN.
Zn deficiency	Depressed DTH reactions, thymic atrophy, decrease in thymic hormone activity, decreased number of T cells and CD4 cells, reduced proliferation responses to PHA, increased number of CD8 cells; reduced NK cell activity, increased monocyte activity; decreased chemotaxis of monocytes and PMN.
Cu deficiency	Reduced function of monocytes.
Se deficiency	Decreased CMI, suppressed T cell response to mitogens and antigens, decreased phagocytosis by monocytes and macrophages.

the frequency of infection mainly as a result of defective functioning of the immune system.

C. Zinc: The discovery of nutritional zinc deficiency in the pathogenesis of several diseases such as sickle cell anemia, renal disorders, and the genetic disorder acrodermatitis enteropathica provided the impetus for a study of the mechanism of zinc-induced changes in cell metabolism and immunity. Zinc is an important cofactor for a large number of enzymes involved in DNA synthesis, such as DNA polymerase and thymidine kinases, which, in turn, regulate cellular functions. Zinc deficiency causes a profound immune deficiency state in both humans and mice. Mice maintained on low-zinc diets during in utero development have an immune deficiency state, which was reversed when they were maintained on a diet supplemented with zinc.

D. Selenium: Selenium has profound effects on tumor development. Dietary supplementation of selenium, along with vitamin E, inhibits tumorigenesis and retards tumor growth in animals. A lack of selenium has been found to be associated with decreased CMI.

Fatty Acids

Fatty acids are the building blocks of several classes of lipids (neutral fatty acids, cholesterol esters, glycolipids), all of which make up to various degrees the structural components of the cell membranes. Various effects of deficiency have been associated with immunity (Table 16-4). The fluidity of these membranes is regulated to some extent by their cholesterol content, as is the maintenance of the structural and functional integrity of the cell.

Fatty acids are either unsaturated or saturated. The unsaturated fatty acid relevant to immune function is arachidonic acid. Prostaglandins, the product of arachidonic acid, play an important role in immunoregulation such as T cell proliferation and NK cell function. Lipids are precursors of vitamins A, E, K, and D as well as cholesterol. Biosynthesis of these vitamins and cholesterol is affected by the presence of exogenous lipids and cholesterol. In in vitro studies, high levels of cholesterol have been found to suppress immune function by inhibiting the cholesterol synthesis needed for the normal functioning of the immune cells. An excess in polyunsaturated fatty acids in the diet is highly immunosuppressive. One of the possible mechanisms of immunosuppression by fatty acids is that the polyunsaturated fatty acids influence membrane fluidity and hence the cell surface receptor distribution and function. Also, it has been suggested that since the polyunsat-

Table 16-4. Effects of fatty acid status on immune functions.

Fatty Acid Type	Effect when Deficient	Effect when in Excess
Polyunsaturated	Reduced humoral response for both T cell-dependent and T cell-independent antigens; decreased membrane fluidity.	Immunosuppression, delayed rejection of skin grafts, suppressed DTH, reduced lymphocyte response to mitogens and antigens, reduced chemotactic and phagocytic activity of neutrophils.
Saturated	Rarely encountered.	In vitro inhibition of lymphocyte response to some antigens and mitogens.
Cholesterol	Rarely encountered.	Inhibition of humoral and cutaneous hypersensitivity to antigens; reduced lymphocyte and macrophage function.

urated fatty acids linoleic acid and arachidonic acid are precursors of prostaglandins, the excess production of these immunoregulatory molecules may suppress T cell and NK cell function.

SUMMARY

Nutrition plays an important role in the maintenance of health. Both malnutrition and excess food intake enhance the incidence of infections and possibly cancers. Changes in CMI and humoral immunity are significantly modulated by nutrition. Nutritional deficiencies, such as protein-calorie deficiency, vitamin deficiency, trace-metal deficiency, and excess fatty acids, have profound effects on immune functions such as DTH, T cell responses to mitogens, antibody production, and NK activity. Some of these immune deficiencies are reversible with nutritional supplements.

THE EFFECT OF ENVIRONMENTAL CHEMICALS ON THE IMMUNE SYSTEM

Robert H. Waldman, MD

In recent years there has been concern about possible genetic, oncologic, and immunologic effects of industrial and agricultural chemicals. The chemicals suspected of having possible immunologic toxicity belong primarily to 2 major categories: halogenated hydrocarbons and heavy metals.

Human exposure can be occupational (eg, farmers exposed to pesticides, or workers who treat wood with pentachlorophenol), environmental (eg, contamination of well water with trichloroethylene), or accidental (eg, the explosion at Seveso, Italy, which contaminated the countryside with dioxins). Publicity regarding these exposures has led to considerable discussion by the general public and by the medical community about the magnitude of the effect of environmental chemicals on immunity.

This section reviews the state of knowledge about the effects of these chemicals on the human immune system, examines the magnitude of the problem as it relates to the immune system, and presents general principles for evaluating the medical and lay literature on this topic.

EVALUATION OF EXPOSED PERSONS

Because intentional exposure is not possible, evaluating the effects of potentially toxic chemicals on the human immune system is based on clinical observations and laboratory testing of persons accidentally exposed. Clinical observation is directed to finding evidence of increased susceptibility to infection in general and opportunistic infections in particular and of the specific cancers that occur in known varieties of immunodeficiency.

Opportunistic infections are discussed in detail in Chapter 56, but they can be conveniently classified in 2 ways. One is by the type of organism: (1) disease caused by organisms that do not cause disease in normal hosts, eg, *Pneumocystis carinii;* (2) severe and generalized disease caused by organisms that normally cause mild, local disease, eg, *Candida albicans;* and (3) reactivation of disease that is normally quiescent eg, varicella-zoster infection. The second classification is by the type of immune abnormality. As examples, pyogenic bacteria are common pathogens in antibody deficiencies, whereas reactivation of tuberculosis occurs in depressed CMI. Cancers associated with immune deficiencies are discussed in more detail in Chapter 47. There is no evidence for a generalized increase in common cancers (lung, breast, prostate) in immunosuppressed patients, but there is an increase in a few rare cancers, eg, Kaposi's sarcoma and extranodal B cell non-Hodgkin's lymphoma (see Chapter 47).

The second way to evaluate effects of potentially toxic chemicals on the immune system is by laboratory testing. Measurement of immunologic factors in the laboratory is undoubtedly helpful in evaluating patients who have opportunistic infections. A more dubious use of the laboratory is in the evaluation of healthy people, or patients with vague and subjective complaints. There are many limitations in laboratory testing, and this topic is covered in detail in Chapter 22. One must ensure that newer tests have been well standardized, especially for the ages of the people being tested; that the necessary conditions for handling the specimens are used; and that the laboratory carrying out the tests has had enough experience to be reliable. It should be remembered that the reference range is generally established to include 95% of normal individuals. Therefore, if 10 tests are performed (a white count and differential is a total of 7 tests) on a patient, there is a 50% chance of one or more "abnormalities." Also, it should be remembered that many drugs commonly taken by patients, eg, aspirin and oral contraceptives, as well as the common cold and other viral infections, may have clinically insignificant but measurable effects on immunologic laboratory testing. Pregnancy, stress, and aging also have measurable effects.

The high incidence of laboratory "abnormalities" means that to be significant with respect to an effect of chemicals on the human immune system, the changes should have some degree of consistency from patient to patient or from epidemiologic study to epidemiologic study. For example, if one patient has all normal tests except for an increased serum IgM level, another patient has high NK cell activity, another has a slightly low mitogen stimulation with pokeweed mitogen, etc, one must conclude that there is no pattern and therefore probably no effect of the chemical(s).

ANIMAL TESTING OF TOXIC CHEMICALS

The use of animal toxicity studies for evaluating the effects of chemicals on the human immune system has the same inherent limitations of all animal toxicity studies: (1) there are interspecies differences in sensitivities to agents; (2) the dosages used are usually much greater than those to which humans are exposed; (3) observed changes in short-term toxicity experiments may be transient and not clinically significant; and (4) the effects may be secondary; eg, the chemical may cause gastrointestinal effects, leading to undernutrition with secondary immunologic abnormalities.

Selection of animal species and strains for immunotoxicity experiments is usually based on traditional toxicology studies in which changes in the gross and microscopic pathology of visceral organs, weight, mortality, etc, are observed. The test chemical is given in a short-term, high-dose exposure, usually by ingestion or injection. Extrapolation of the results to long-term, low-dose exposure is entirely speculative.

Animal studies have shown effects on antibody production and T cell function of halogenated hydrocarbons, such as dioxins and dibenzofurans, and of polychlorinated biphenyls and pentachlorephenol. However, the effect of the last 2 is most probably due to contamination by small amounts of the first 2 classes of chemicals.

EPIDEMIOLOGIC STUDIES

There have been several epidemiologic studies of human exposure to potentially toxic chemicals, and these can conveniently be divided into those involving occupational exposure and those following accidents. Examples of occupational exposures include workers in the wood-treating industry (exposed to pentachlorophenol), those in the dry-cleaning industry (trichloroethylene and perchloroethylene), and those manufacturing transformers (polychlorinated biphenyls). Much attention has been given to the exposure of military personnel to dioxin (Agent Orange) during the Vietnam War. The level of exposure was chronic and generally low to moderate, ie, higher than the background exposure of the general public, but not as high as the exposure of those involved in accidents described below. This is evidenced by the rarity of chloracne, a hallmark of high levels of exposure to halogenated hydrocarbons.

There is no evidence in any group described above, or of any similar group, of clinically significant immunosuppression. No increase has been seen in opportunistic infections or immunologically related cancers, nor has any other abnormality been found that could be related to the immune system. Similarly, laboratory testing has revealed no significant or consistent abnormalities. One large, well-controlled study of Air Force personnel exposed to Agent Orange showed no laboratory abnormalities in immune factors in the exposed group compared with the control group, and yet the tests were sensitive enough to pick up significant differences between smokers and nonsmokers.

There have been epidemiologic studies of populations exposed to accidental chemical spills. Examples of these are several industrial accidents leading to exposure of workers and, in the Seveso accident, inhabitants of the surrounding area to dioxins; the people of Times Beach, Missouri, who were exposed to dioxins; and rice oil ("Yusho") accidents in Japan and Taiwan, where polychlorinated biphenyls accidentally contaminated cooking oil. These accidents are usually, but not always, higher-dose exposures (the exposed persons in several instances developed chloracne) and are more acute. There were transient changes in some laboratory tests of immune functions in children who had suffered intense exposure after the Seveso accident, those exposed to the contaminated rice oil in Japan and Taiwan, and the inhabitants of Times Beach. In some, there were minor abnormalities in immunoglobulin levels, which later returned to normal. There have also been effects on some tests of CMI, such as depression of DTH skin test responses, which also returned toward normal. In addition, methodologic questions have been raised regarding some of these studies, particularly the data on skin test responses of the inhabitants of Times Beach.

SUMMARY

There is concern about potential toxicity to the immune system from environmental or occupational exposure to a variety of chemicals. The current methodology used to evaluate human immunotoxicity has many shortcomings, but clinical observations do not support a widespread fear that "toxic" chemicals in our work or general environments are harmful to our immune systems.

IMMUNOLOGIC EFFECTS OF UREMIA

Raymond G. Slavin, MD

A number of clinical features of uremia point to abnormalities in immune function; these include a high rate of infection and an increased incidence of cancers. Up to 60% of patients with chronic renal failure suffer from severe infection, and 40% of deaths are thought to be due to infection. Studies of animals with experimentally induced uremia and of uremic patients have shown that immune functions may be markedly altered. It should be emphasized that many of the studies showing these changes are not conclusive, and, indeed, results are often contradictory. One reason for these discrepancies, especially in human studies, is that many factors may contribute to the apparent immune competency of patients with end-stage renal disease. These include hemodialysis, drugs, blood transfusions, duration of failure, and physiologic and metabolic disturbances associated with uremia. All of these may alter immune function. In addition, the immune response in patients with uremia is dependent to some extent on the particular antigen tested.

Table 16–5 summarizes the immune function factors that are probably affected by uremia. The most striking immune abnormalities of uremia occur in cell-mediated reactions. The uniform lymphocytopenia that occurs in acute and chronic uremia and involves mainly T cells appears to be due to an alteration of lymphocyte trafficking, with circulating lymphocytes being redistributed to the bone marrow.

In general, intrinsic cell defects appear to be less important than serum-mediated ones in inhibiting CMI. Washed uremic lymphocytes or uremic lymphocytes incubated in normal serum respond normally to mitogens such as PHA. Addition of uremic serum to normal or uremic lymphocytes significantly suppresses cellular responses. Several factors in uremic serum have been shown to be responsible for this type of immunosuppression. An in vivo correlate can be seen in adoptive transfer experiments in guinea pigs. Animals that were sensitive to tuberculin and that were then made uremic lost their tuberculin skin reactivity, but lymph node cells from these sensitized, nonresponding uremic animals could transfer DTH to normal animals. In contrast, lymph node cells from normal sensitized guinea pigs could not transfer sensitivity to uremic animals. This suggests that immunologically competent lymphocytes are present in uremic guinea pigs but are rendered nonresponsive in the presence of the uremic state.

The response of spleen cells from chronically uremic rats to mitogens is significantly suppressed compared with that of spleen cells from control animals. The suppression appears to be mediated by a suppressor cell, probably a monocyte, that is also present in the peritoneum and lungs of uremic rats and in the peripheral blood of uremic humans. Sera from uremic rats induces increased suppressor activity of normal spleen cells.

The reduced response of uremic lymphoid cells to mitogens and antigens may be due, in part, to the inability of uremic cells to act as antigen-presenting cells. In uremic rats, the antigen-presenting ability of macrophages is significantly diminished.

In the area of humoral antibody, a decrease in immunoglobulin levels is seen in uremic humans, with the most profound changes being found in IgM levels. Antibody production varies with the antigen presented. In the experimental animal model of uremia in the rat, antibody production to bovine serum albumin is suppressed, whereas anti-sheep erythrocyte antibody is not affected.

A decrease in neutrophil chemotaxis has been reported to occur in humans with uremia. Sera of uremic patients contain a chemotactic-factor inhibitor that is specific for several chemoattractants. The inhibitor reacts directly and irreversibly with the chemoattractants and is heat-labile. It thus resembles the chemotactic factor inhibitor present in low titers in normal human sera.

Table 16–5. Immune function abnormalities in uremia.

Immune Function	Abnormalities
CMI	Lymphocytopenia Impaired delayed skin reactivity Decreased in vitro lymphocyte proliferation Prolonged homograft survival Impaired graft-versus-host reaction
Humoral antibody	Decrease in immunoglobulin levels Decrease in antibody production
Chemotaxis	Decrease in neutrophil chemotaxis

SUMMARY

The increased rate of infection and the high incidence of cancer associated with chronic renal failure point to possible abnormalities of immune function in this condition. Studies of experimentally induced uremia in animals and of humans with chronic renal failure indicate that a variety of defects occur in CMI, antibody production, and neutrophil chemotaxis, with the most significant changes being in cell-mediated reactions.

REFERENCES

Psychoneuroimmunology

Ader R (editor): *Psychoneuroimmunology*. Academic Press, Orlando, 1981.

Besedovsky HO, DelRey AE, Sorkin E: What do the immune system and the brain know about each other? *Immunol Today* 1983; **4**:342.

MacQueen G et al: Pavlovian conditioning of rat mucosal MAST cells to secrete rat mast cell protease II. *Science* 1989; **243**:83.

Riley V: Psychoneuroendocrine influences on immunocompetence and neoplasia. *Science* 1981; **212**:1109.

Schleifer SJ et al: Depression and immunity. *Arch Gen Psychiatry* 1985; **42**:129.

Aging

Crawford J, Cohen HJ: Relationship of cancer and aging. *Clin Geriatr Med* 1987; **3**:419.

Deguchi Y et al: Age-related changes of proliferative response, kinetics of expression of protooncogenes after the mitogenic stimulation and methylation level of the protooncogene in purified human lymphocyte subsets. *Mech Ageing Dev* 1988; **44**:153.

Ford PM: The immunology of aging. *Clin Rheum Dis* 1986; **12**:1.

Krishnaraj R, Blandford G: Age-associated alterations in human natural killer cells. I. Increased activity per conventional and kinetic analysis. *Clin Immunol Immunopathol* 1987; **45**:268.

Lighart GJ et al: Admission criteria for immunogerontological studies in man: The Senieur protocol. *Mech Ageing Dev* 1986; **28**:47.

Mackinodan T et al: Cellular, biochemical and molecular basis of T-cell senescence. *Arch Pathol Lab Med* 1987; **111**:910.

Miller RG: Age-associated decline in precursor frequency for different cell-mediated reactions with preservation of helper and cytotoxic effect per precursor cell. *J Immunol* 1984; **132**:63.

Nordin AA, Proust JJ: Signal transduction mechanisms in the immune system. Potential implications in immunosenescence. *Endocrinol Metab Clin* 1987; **16(4)**:919.

Saltzman RL, Peterson PK: Immunodeficiency of the elderly. *Rev Infect Dis* 1987; **9**:127.

Weksler ME: The senescence of the immune system. *Semin Immunol* 1986; **16**:53.

Nutrition

Beisel WR: Simple nutrients and immunity. *Am J Clin Nutr* 1982; **35**:417.

Chandra RK: Malnutrition. Pages 187–203 in: *Immunodeficiency Disorders*. Chandra RK (editor). Churchill Livingstone, 1982.

Chandra RK: Nutrition and immunity. *Trop Geogr Med* 1988;**40**:546.

Chandra RK: *Trace Elements, Immune Response and Infections*. Wiley, 1983.

Good RA, Lorenz E: Nutrition, immunity, aging and cancer. *Nutr Rev* 1988;**46**:62.

Gross RL, Newberne PM: Role of nutrition in immunologic function. *Physiol Rev* 1980; **60**:188.

Laouri D, Kleinknecht C: The role of nutritional factors in the course of experimental renal failure. *Am J Kidney Dis* 1985;**5**:147.

Lipschitz DA: Nutrition, aging and the immunohematopoietic system. *Clin Geriatr Med* 1987;**3**:319.

Walford RL et al: Dietary restriction and aging: historical phases, mechanisms and current directions. *J Nutr* 1987; **117**:1650.

Environmental Chemicals

Dean JH, Murray MJ, Ward EC: Toxic modification of the immune system. In: *Cassarett and Doull's Toxicology: The Basic Sciences of Poisons*, 3rd ed. Doull J, Klaassen CD, Amdur MO (editors). Macmillan, in press.

Hoffman RE et al: Health effects of long-term exposure to 2,3,7,8-tetrachlorodibenzo-p-dioxin. *JAMA* 1986;**255**:2031.

Klemmer HW et al: Clinical findings in workers exposed to pentachlorophenol. *Arch Environ Contam Toxicol* 1980; **9**:715.

Masuda Y, Yoshimura H: Polychlorinated biphenyls and dibenzofurans in patients with Yusho and their toxicologic significance: A review. *Am J Ind Med* 1984;**5**:31.

Reggiani G: Localized contamination with TCDD—Seveso, Missouri and other areas. Page 303 in: *Halogenated Biphenyls, Terphenyls, Naphtholenes, Dibenzodioxins, and Related Products*. Kimbrough R (editor). Elsevier/North Holland, 1980.

Reggiani G: Medical problems raised by the TCDD contamination in Seveso, Italy. *Arch Toxicol* 1978;**40**:161.

Uremia

Mezzano S et al: Analysis of humoral and cellular factors that contribute to impaired immune responsiveness in experimental uremia. *Nephron* 1984; **36**:15.

Johnston MFM, Slavin RG: Mechanisms of inhibition of adoptive transfer of tuberculin sensitivity in acute uremia. *J Lab Clin Med* 1976;**87**:457.

Hayry P et al. Is uremia immunosuppressive in renal transplantation? *Transplantation* 1982;**34**:168.

Alevy YG, Slavin RG, Hutcheson PA: Immune response in experimentally induced uremia. I. Suppression of mitogen responses by adherent cells in chronic uremia. *Clin Immunol Immunopathol* 1981;**19**:8.

17 Reproductive Immunology

Daniel V. Landers, MD, Richard A. Bronson, MD, Charles S. Pavia, PhD, & Daniel P. Stites, MD

The last few decades have seen a rapid expansion in our knowledge of the immunology of the reproductive process. Advancing research in molecular biology and monoclonal antibody technology has helped to outline the complex nature of the immunologic events that surround fertilization, implantation, and intrauterine tolerance, growth, and development of the embryo. Immune responses to self antigins on sperm or alloantegins in females are associated with alterations in fertility. Over the years, investigators from around the world have begun to unravel the mystery of the fetal-maternal allograft. Although our understanding is far from complete, we have accumulated a tremendous amount of information about the immunologic events surrounding reproduction. Numerous alterations in the maternal immune response have been identified that evolve from the very beginning of gestation. A great deal has been uncovered regarding the success of the fetus as an allograft at both the maternal-fetal-placental interface and the more distant sites of fetal-maternal cell contact. Research efforts continue to further our understanding of the immune mechanisms of sperm penetration, sperm antibodies, and immune mechanisms involved in the maintenance of early pregnancy. These investigative efforts have led to new insights into contraceptive therapy, primary infertility, recurrent spontaneous pregnancy loss, and management of patients with allotransplants or tumors.

REPRODUCTIVE IMMUNOLOGY IN THE FEMALE

The exact mechanisms involved in the apparent success of the fetus as an allograft are only partially understood. Several hypotheses have been proposed, each of which is supported by substantial scientific investigation. The mechanisms that link the various hypotheses and the many signals and unknown factors that initiate and regulate the system as a whole remain unclear. The basic hypothesis remains that there exist both physical and humoral barriers to immune rejection of the fetus. This rather simplistic view has remained substantially unchallenged; however, our understanding at the molecular level has progressed. It is clear that for the fetus to avoid immune recognition and attack by the maternal immune system, the maternal immune response must be blunted, the fetal antigen stimulus must be suppressed, or, as is most likely, both must occur. In normal human allograft rejection, T lymphocytes play a major role in recognition and cytolysis of foreign antigen-bearing cells. This role is primarily undertaken by cytotoxic T lymphocytes (CTL). The fetal allograft must be protected against these effector cells. This may occur by a variety of mechanisms, which are discussed below.

REGULATION OF MATERNAL RECOGNITION OF THE FETAL ALLOGRAFT

The unique structure of the placenta provides an interface of maternal blood for exchange of gases and nutrients by the fetus. The hemochorial nature of the placenta provides direct exposure of the syncytiotrophoblast layer of the chorionic villi to maternal circulating lymphocytes. While the syncytiotrophoblasts come into direct contact with maternal T cells, including CTL, no apparent recognition or cytolytic events are evident. Numerous studies have shown that syncytiotrophoblast membranes do not express class I human leukocyte antigens (HLA antigens). This lack of antigenic expression may account for the lack of cytolytic response; however, many unexplained phenomena still exist. There are additional interfaces between maternal and trophoblastic tissue. Syncytiotrophoblasts are shed into the intervillous spaces and transported intravascularly to distant maternal sites, including the lungs, without causing an inflammatory or immune response at these sites. Furthermore, cytotrophoblasts are known to migrate to the uterine spiral arteries following implantation, and they eventually replace maternal endothelium at that site. Thus, maternal lymphocytes interface with histocompatibility antigens on endovascular trophoblast without stimulating a significant immune response. Other theoretic mechanisms of fetal protection exist; eg, that fetal antigens may be only weakly expressed, but the normal production of maternal antibodies to fetal erythrocytes, immunoglobulins, trophoblasts, and HLA contradict this hypothesis.

Two classes of trophoblast antigens have been identified. These unique antigens include trophoblastic antigen 1 (TA1) and the trophoblast-lymphocyte cross-reactive (TLX) antigens. TA1 may be involved in the immune protection afforded the fetus during pregnancy. Their levels in the blood of pregnant women increase as pregnancy progresses. These antigens have inhibitory effects on mixed-lymphocyte reactions without affecting nonspecific lymphocyte responses to mitogens. TLX antisera cross-react with unstimulated peripheral blood lymphocytes, placenta endothelium, and villous fibroblasts. These antigens are allogeneic and species-specific. Together, TA1 and the TLX antigens may function in normal pregnancy by inducing maternal production of antibodies that block the immune response to TA1. Thus, absence of TLX antigen recognition due to sharing of maternal-paternal TLX antigen profiles may not allow anti-TA1 activity and may lead to subsequent fetal rejection.

THE UTERUS AS A SITE FOR IMMUNE REACTIVITY

Although the uterus was once considered an immunologically privileged site, much experimental evidence indicates that both afferent and efferent limbs of the immune response are operative in this reproductive organ. When placed into the nonpregnant uterus, allografts are promptly rejected and cause hypertrophy of the draining para-aortic lymph nodes. A secondary response occurs when there is a local challenge with tissue of the same antigenic specificity. In addition, local alloimmunization in the uterine environment has a dramatic effect on subsequent reproductive capabilities. Increased numbers of embryos develop in pregnant animals whose uterine horns have been presensitized against paternal histocompatibility antigens and have already expressed the local "recall flare," a delayed hypersensitivity reaction. The immunologic basis for this unexpected result is unknown, although it suggests that maternal immune reactivity has a beneficial effect and may play a vital role in maternal-fetal coexistence.

Following sexual intercourse, allogeneic spermatozoa are not ordinarily recognized as foreign and are therefore not rejected in the immunocompetent maternal host. This may be related to the presence of nonspecific immunosuppressive factors in semen. A high-molecular-weight component present in human seminal plasma has a strong suppressive effect on mitogen, antigen, and allogeneic cell activation of human lymphocytes, whereas other substances in semen interfere with the microbicidal activity of antibody, complement, and granulocytes.

The events of implantation of the fertilized egg and ensuing invasion of uterine tissue by the trophoblast evoke an inflammatory reaction resulting in the formation of a highly specialized gestational tissue called the decidua. Besides possessing endocrinologic activity, decidual tissue may act as a selective barrier by preventing released fetal or trophoblastic antigens from reaching the neighboring afferent lymphatic vessels and by preventing access of sensitized maternal lymphocytes to the conceptus. The decidua may also release immunosuppressive factors and express natural killer (NK) activity very early during its development. The well-known fact that ectopic pregnancy can elicit decidual reactions in extrauterine sites suggests that this locally evoked reaction at the site of implantation and the later development of the placenta play key roles in maintaining the integrity of the fetus.

ALLOANTIGENICITY OF THE FETOPLACENTAL UNIT & AN IMMUNOLOGIC ROLE FOR THE PLACENTA

The placenta is a unique and complex organ. Its biologic existence is brief. Its structural elements are heterogeneous, and its functionally active cell types include the trophoblastic, lymphocytic, and erythroid series. Like the fetus, the placenta consists of tissue derived from 2 different parental genotypes. It produces protein and steroid hormones that regulate the physiologic activities of pregnancy. Concurrently, it acts as the fetal lung, kidneys, intestine, and liver. It is becoming evident that an immunologic role for this organ may be of paramount importance for the successful maintenance of mammalian pregnancy.

Both the maternal and paternal components of fetal transplantation antigens are expressed on cellular elements within the placenta. However, from an immunologic standpoint, the key question is whether transplantation antigens can be demonstrated on trophoblast membranes. These membranes are the interface in direct apposition to the maternal circulation in the human hemochorial placenta. As such, they present a direct challenge for both the afferent and efferent limbs of the immune response and could serve as the site of immune attack by immunologically competent maternal lymphocytes.

Whether or not transplantation antigens are expressed on trophoblasts has become a matter of intense controversy. The answer seems to be dependent upon the ontogenetic and phylogenetic expression of these antigens at various stages of gestation. It has been reported that placental antigens may be masked by histocompatibility or specific trophoblast antibodies, fibrinoid, fibrinomucoid, or immune complexes. Class I (HLA-A, -B, -C) antigens can be detected on early human placental cytotrophoblast, although it has been difficult to demonstrate any HLA antigens on other human trophoblast tissue, including the syncytiotrophoblast of the mature chorionic villus. Although class I MHC antigens are expressed on murine trophoblasts, it is not yet known whether transplantation antigens are present in an immunogenic form on mammalian trophoblast cells, an important key to our understanding of the many aspects of the immunologic interaction between mother and fetus. The demonstration that maternal lymphocytes are capable of killing cultured human trophoblast cells from their own placenta is evidence that trophoblast cells do display transplantation antigens. Extrauterine placental allografts are usually rejected by allogeneic recipients and provoke a state of alloimmunity—while transplants of trophoblast from early gestational tissue proceed to grow and develop unimpeded without eliciting a detectable rejection.

A variety of hormonal and immunologic events occurring during pregnancy could modulate maternal transplantation immunity against paternal antigens expressed on the placenta and trophoblast. Circulating alpha-fetoprotein, placental-ovarian steroids, protein hormones, and antibody have widely different concentrations in pregnancy serum than at their sites of production. These factors have been proposed as naturally occurring immunosuppressive factors. Although there is no firm evidence that these circulating factors adequately explain the cell regulatory events that occur in the maternal immune system, and the concentrations of gestational steroid and protein hormones in maternal serum never achieve a level that will suppress immunity in vivo, these substances, taken together, could exert a potent immunosuppressive effect at the fetal-maternal interface, where they are made and maintained at high levels throughout most stages of pregnancy. Interestingly, the trophoblast produces most of the major pregnancy-associated hormones that have been implicated as immunomodulators, which is consistent with evidence that trophoblastic cells themselves or soluble extracts or eluates of placental tissue inhibit various expressions of cell-mediated immunity.

Other immunologic properties have been ascribed to cells derived from the placenta. Trophoblastic tissue serves as an anatomic barrier between fetal and maternal tissues and thereby serves as the first line of defense against maternal antifetal alloimmunity. Maternal lymphocytes sensitized to fetal antigens could be excluded specifically, as are certain antibodies, or nonspecifically, by a generalized barrier to cellular traffic. During early gestation, the trophoblast actively invades and proliferates within the maternal decidua. Studies with mice show that different stages of the trophoblast are highly phagocytic and lymphoid cells from murine placentas mediate graft-versus-host (GVH) reactions, respond to mitogenic lectins, and synthesize antibodies. There is also some evidence that the placenta produces the antiviral agent interferon and the macrophage-derived immune factor interleukin-1. The expression of immunelike function by both trophoblastic elements and lymphoid stem cells may be one of several processes enabling the fetoplacental unit to protect itself from injury. This is accomplished by preventing harmful infectious agents and certain maternal antigens and antibodies from reaching the embryo and by limiting the passage of cells from mother to fetus. These defense mechanisms could be especially important during the early stages of in utero development, when the fetus is quite vulnerable since it has not yet acquired complete immune competence.

FETAL-MATERNAL EXCHANGE OF HUMORAL & CELLULAR COMPONENTS

The human placenta is hemochorial, which means that there is direct apposition between the maternal circulation and the syncytiotrophoblast that lines the chorionic villi of the placenta. Although fetus and mother are grossly separated, cells as well as soluble substances can pass through the placenta during gestation, particularly at the time of placental separation (Fig 17–1).

That such transplacental traffic results in allosensitization to transplantation antigens has been extrapolated from observations rather than proved by rigorously documented experiments. Syncytial trophoblast (more than 200,000 cells per day) is continuously released from the placenta and has been shown to circulate in human mater-

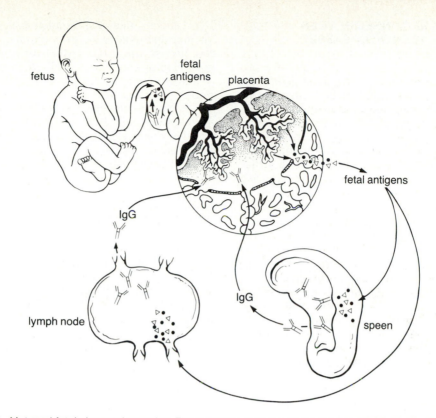

Figure 17–1. Maternal-fetal-placental complex. The anatomic features of the fetal-maternal relationship during pregnancy are depicted, with the placenta acting as a selective filter of leaking fetal or trophoblastic antigens that may sensitize maternal immune effector mechanisms. The passage of maternal immunity to the fetus is likewise regulated by the intervening layer of trophoblastic cells (where fetal and maternal tissues are in intimate proximity).

nal blood from the 18th week of gestation. Various blood elements that undoubtedly contain transplantation antigens can pass bidirectionally. This establishes adequate conditions for sensitization of the mother by fetal (paternal) transplantation antigens. Under experimental circumstances—or clinically after intrauterine blood transfusion—immunocompetent cells that gain entrance to the fetus can rarely cause GVH disease and runting. The placenta, then, provides only a partial barrier to transport of soluble or cellular elements and certainly should not be viewed as an absolute impediment to their traffic.

In addition, whereas under normal physiologic conditions the trophoblast seems to be invulnerable to immune attack, it is quite probable that some maternal reactivity to this tissue does arise, primarily to protect the pregnant host from extensive and otherwise unchecked growth and invasion of the trophoblast, as occurs in choriocarcinoma.

In the early stages of fetal development in primates, immune protection of the fetus is provided by maternally derived antibodies acquired exclusively by placental transmission. In other species,

immunoglobulins are transferred via the yolk sac or via intestinal absorption of colostrum during suckling. During gestation, only antibodies belonging to the IgG class are readily transferred from mother to fetus, and this process is most probably facilitated by the interaction of immunoglobulin molecules with Fc receptors present on the surface of trophoblastic membranes and other extraembryonic membrane components. With intrauterine infection, the fetus is capable of synthesizing IgM and IgA. The presence of high levels of these immuoglobulins in cord serum at birth is presumptive evidence of such infection.

The neonate is exposed to an environment that presents much greater risk of infection than was the case in the uterine shelter. Unless in utero infection has occurred, the newborn is usually not capable of mounting a quick and effective reaction against pathogenic organisms. Maternally acquired antibody provides initial protection against infection. The presence of maternal immunoglobulins in sufficiently high titer should protect against the initial invasion of certain pathogens that would otherwise multiply and disseminate without hindrance.

IMMUNOLOGIC CONSEQUENCES OF TRANSPLACENTALLY PASSED SUBSTANCES

Under certain circumstances, transferred maternal antibody is not beneficial to the fetus. This is most evident in hemolytic disease of the newborn mediated by either ABO or Rh blood group fetal-maternal incompatibilities. Situations involving ABO incompatibilities arise more frequently than does Rh hemolytic disease, but they usually take a milder course, with cases requiring transfusion being extremely rare. The disorder occurs primarily in blood group O mothers bearing fetuses of type A or B and is believed to be the result of the transfer of IgG anti-A or anti-B antibodies from mother to fetus. Although blood group A and group B women have antibody to type B and type A erythrocytes, respectively, these naturally occurring isoagglutinins are usually of the IgM class and therefore do not readily cross the placenta and cannot harm the fetus.

The more serious condition that can adversely affect fetal development results from Rh isoimmunization, which resembles the pathophysiology of ABO incompatibility yet manifests important immunologic differences. Rh antigens are expressed on blood cells only, whereas antigenic specificities related to A and B blood group determinants are widely distributed in nature and in the human body. During a pregnancy in which an Rh-negative mother is bearing an Rh-positive fetus, sensitization may occur if fetal erythrocytes cross into the maternal circulation via the placenta or when there is transplacental hemorrhage following the birth of the child or after an abortion. Alternatively, the mother could already be primed as a result of receiving an earlier transfusion of Rh-positive blood. Less than 1 mL of fetal blood can elicit a response. Maternal antibodies pass through the placenta, gain access to the fetal bloodstream, and cause the destruction of erythrocytes. Rh disease occurs rarely during the first pregnancy, with the vast majority of Rh-negative mothers becoming sensitized with increasing parity. The deleterious effects of isoimmunization can be prevented conveniently by administering Rh_0 (D) immune globulin to the mother immediately after delivery of her first Rh-positive child or following an abortion. The major suggested explanation for the action of anti-Rh immunoglobulins is that fetal erythrocytes present in the maternal circulation as a result of fetal detachment are destroyed and rapidly cleared, so that they are not available long enough to sensitize the mother effectively. Treatment must be administered after subsequent Rh-incompatible pregnancies, since there is no apparent development of tolerance following prophylactic therapy.

In certain situations, simultaneous ABO and Rh incompatibilities between mother and fetus may prevent the more destructive effects of Rh isoimmunization. The naturally occurring anti-A or anti-B antibodies in a group O, Rh-negative mother will effectively destroy Rh-positive erythrocytes crossing the placenta if the fetus is also of either group A or B blood type. The rapid removal of these cells by the already primed maternal immune system would make sensitization against Rh factor highly unlikely.

MATERNAL IMMUNE RESPONSE DURING PREGNANCY

Pregnancy has long been associated with a depression in cellular immunity, but the reason for this is far from clear. The human T lymphocyte is one of the major cellular components of the host defense response to foreign antigens, whether that antigen is an allograft, a virally infected cell, or any other foreign HLA antigen-bearing cell. The number and function of T cells change during pregnancy. Total lymphocyte counts fall during gestation; the maximal decrease occurs at 25–28 weeks of pregnancy. Most studies also show that T cell numbers are decreased. CD4 cells decrease and CD8 cells increase toward the end of pregnancy, resulting in a decrease in the CD4/CD8 cell ratio. Studies of NK cells during gestation show that although the number of these cells decreases, their level of activity is probably unchanged. In vitro tests of T cell function, using mitogens and mixed-lymphocyte reactions, show a decrease in proliferative response during pregnancy. T cell function in pregnancy has barely begun to be characterized.

Changes in humoral immunity also occur during gestation. The serum immunoglobulin concentrations increase, but alterations of specific immunoglobulin subclasses have not been well characterized.

MATERNAL-FETAL ANTIMICROBIAL IMMUNITY

Pregnant women seem to be at an increased risk of acquiring certain infectious diseases, particularly those controlled primarily by cell-mediated immunity (CMI). The pregnancy-related alteration in the immune response to infection includes changes in T lymphocyte subpopulations, polymorphonuclear leukocyte function, peripheral blood lymphocyte responses, serum immunoglobulin concentrations, immunosuppressive serum factors, and maternal immunologic recognition mechanisms. Although it has been assumed that these alterations relate in some way to maternal tolerance of the fetal allograft, it is not clear how they relate to pregnancy-specific alterations in susceptibility to infection.

A number of infectious agents are thought to behave differently in pregnant women, owing primarily to altered host defenses. These include some viral agents such as poliomyelitis virus, hepatitis A virus, influenza A virus, Epstein-Barr virus, variola virus, and cytomegalovirus; bacterial agents such as *Neisseria gonorrhoeae* and *Streptococcus pneumoniae;* parasites such as *Plasmodium* species; and fungi such as *Coccidioides immitis.*

The humoral immune alteration associated with pregnancy may play a role in this increased susceptibility. These changes involve a decrease in serum IgG concentration with advancing gestation. Some decrease in the levels of IgM and IgM-bearing lymphocytes has also been reported in the first trimester, but these levels do not continue to decrease with advancing gestation. The significance of these changes, however, is unclear, and they do not necessarily represent impaired humoral immunity. In fact, antibody production in response to infection during pregnancy is probably unaltered.

A variety of cellular immune functions are depressed during pregnancy as described above, including T cell numbers and functions; NK cell numbers and activity; and neutrophil, monocyte, and macrophage numbers. Among the agents thought to participate in this depression of CMI are steroid hormones produced in pregnancy, such as progesterone, estrogens, cortisol, alpha-fetoprotein, and uromodulin. Despite these alterations, there is little direct evidence to suggest significant alteration in the cellular component of the immune system during pregnancy. Furthermore, except for some notable exceptions such as rubella, cytomegalovirus infection, syphilis, and toxoplasmosis, the human fetus usually remains relatively unaffected by maternal infectious diseases.

IMMUNITY IN RECURRENT SPONTANEOUS ABORTION

Maternal immune recognition of the fetus is thought to play an important role in fetal acceptance. It is well known that an increased incidence of HLA antigen sharing between mates is associated with repeated spontaneous abortion when compared with normal fertile controls. In fact, the development of "hybrid vigor" may be related in part to polymorphism of HLA disparity between parents. The proposed theory is that an allogeneic incompatibility is necessary at an HLA or a closely linked locus for maternal recognition and development of fetal acceptance. If such a recognition is lacking, cell-mediated allograft rejection or antibody response to foreign fetal antigen may lead to fetal loss. Numerous studies have found an association between repeated spontaneous abortion and HLA-sharing between mates. Furthermore maternal recognition of the allogeneic paternal TA1 or TLX antigen may lead to a blocking antibody that prevents a response to TA1. If mates share TLX antigen profiles prohibiting the maternal recognition of paternal TLX antigen, anti-TA1 activity may lead to rejection of the fetus. This hypothesis has yet to be confirmed.

Many centers now perform maternal immunization with paternal or donor lymphocytes in patients with 3 or more primary spontaneous abortions. The success rate in reducing abortion has been reported to be as high as 50–89%. The presumed mechanism of success is that the woman produces antipaternal alloantibodies, which play a role in protecting the fetus from immune-mediated rejection. There remains a great deal of difficulty in sorting out which patients indeed have immune-mediated recurrent losses and theoretically will benefit from this approach and which patients have another cause for their losses.

REPRODUCTIVE IMMUNOLOGY IN THE MALE

Since males are not exposed to histoincompatible gametes during reproduction, immune alterations involving the male reproductive system are necessarily autoimmune. Experimentally, auto- or alloimmunization to spermatozoa can in fact result in relative infertility in either the female or the male. Naturally occurring autoimmune reactions to sperm are uncommon but have become increasingly recognized as a consequence of vasectomy and in infertile couples. Recent findings suggest that potentially harmful immune responses associated with spermatozoa as antigens are inhibited by naturally occurring local and systemic immunoregulatory mechanisms.

NATURAL IMMUNITY TO SPERMATOZOA

Sera obtained from normal, fertile animals of many species, including rabbits, mice, and humans, have been found to contain antibodies that react with sperm of their own species and, to a lesser degree, with sperm of other species. In the rabbit, these naturally occurring antibodies enter the uterine secretions, probably as transudates from serum. Sperm recovered from the reproductive tract of female rabbits have immunoglobulins on the head region detectable by immunofluorescence. Interestingly, vigorously moving sperm recovered from the uterus did not fluoresce, whereas immotile sperm and those that showed evidence of senescence—as judged by alteration in the appearance of the acrosome—were bound by immunoglobulins. It has been proposed that binding of this naturally occurring antibody to spermatozoa may play a role in their clearance from the female reproductive tract, perhaps abrogating the immune response in the female to sperm-associated antigens, and in maintaining a state of tolerance.

The mechanism by which antibody binding to spermatozoa occurs appears to be through Fc receptors that have been demonstrated on alcohol-fixed sperm of both rabbits and pigs but were not present on the surface of living sperm of those species. While binding of intact immunoglobulins of the IgG class was noted, Fab fragments obtained from digests of purified rabbit IgG failed to bind to sperm.

It has recently been demonstrated that an IgG preparation from serum of unimmunized rabbits mediates complement-dependent sperm immobilization. This finding suggests that a naturally occurring antibody directed against a specific sperm-associated antigen is also present within the sera of some normal fertile bucks. Cytotoxic sperm-reactive antibodies have been found in the sera of nonimmunized inbred mice. Normal serum lysed spermatozoa of all strains tested, in the presence of complement. A 3-layer indirect immunofluorescence technique using normal mouse serum, rhodamine-conjugated goat antimouse serum, and rabbit antigoat antiserum also gave a distinct surface membrane fluorescence over the whole head, principal piece, and end piece of the sperm tail from any strain when tested using living spermatozoa in suspension. Absorption of normal serum with mouse spermatozoa removed both immunofluorescent and cytotoxic activity. The cytotoxic titer of sperm-reactive antibody in normal mouse serum was low—in the range of 1:8.

Naturally occurring antisperm antibodies have been detected by indirect immunofluorescence in 90% of sera of children of both sexes before puberty. The incidence declines thereafter to about 60% and persists throughout life. These naturally occurring antibodies were readily absorbed by sperm and testicular extracts but not by other human tissues. The constant staining pattern with several hundred serum samples also suggested they were unlikely to be alloantibodies. They were directed against neither blood group antigens nor sperm-coating antigens, since the antibodies were not absorbed by seminal plasma. Of special importance, these sperm-reactive naturally occurring antibodies did *not* stain the surface of viable sperm in suspension but rather were directed against intracellular antigens. Sera possessing antiacrosomal antibodies, when absorbed with lyophilized *Staphylococcus aureus, Escherichia coli, Pseudomonas aeruginosa, Klebsiella pneumoniae,* and *Candida albicans,* no longer reacted with sperm by indirect immunofluorescence. In contrast, reactivity against other regions of the sperm surface was not absorbed by microorganisms.

The sera of children, female blood donors, pregnant women, and women from infertile couples have also been screened for naturally occurring sperm-reactive antibodies. Analysis of the immunofluorescent staining patterns and titers of these antibodies revealed that while 68% of children's sera were positive, only one of 84 samples tested was titered to 1:16 dilution. Similarly, for female blood donors, while 79% were positive, only 3 of 80 sera were positive at 1:16 or greater. Conversely, in women with unexplained infertility, 15 of 29 sera tested showed at least one sperm-reactive antibody at a titer 1:16 or greater. Interestingly, while 9 sera from infertile women with an immunofluorescence titer of at least 1:64 were tested by means of a microscopic sperm agglutination test, none were positive. The antibody-antigen system detected by immunofluorescence is different from that detected by sperm agglutination, again suggesting that naturally occurring sperm-reactive antibodies are not directed against antigens on the sperm surface.

The sera of 2115 male partners of infertile couples have been studied by a sperm agglutination test in a gel. Three percent were found to have sperm agglutinins with titers of 1:32 or greater. This low incidence of agglutinating antibodies contrasts markedly with the high incidence of antibodies reactive with sperm subsurface antigens.

Against this background of naturally occurring sperm-reactive antibodies, there has been much confusion over the role of antisperm antibodies in impaired human reproduction. The subsurface nature of Fc receptors, the mediation of immunoglobulin binding to sperm of many species via the Fc portion of the immunoglobulin molecule, and the absence of immunoglobulin binding to living human spermatozoa have not been fully appreciated. It is now clear that sera of normal fertile men and women do not contain antibodies directed against antigenic determinants of the sperm surface and that their presence is a reflection of an aberrant immune response that may lead—depending upon isotype, antibody specificity, and titer—to altered sperm function.

ETIOLOGY OF AUTOIMMUNITY TO SPERMATOZOA

Sperm Antigens

The expression of antigens on sperm is central to the consideration of their immunogenicity in the reproductive tract, much the same as is the presence of antigens on placental trophoblast. Sperm antigens could theoretically elicit either auto- or alloimmunity, and either type could result in partial or complete infertility. Alternatively, these antigens could be nonimmunogenic in the normal environment of the reproductive tract.

Autoimmune diseases of the testis may be prevented by sequestration of autoantigens on germ cells by the presence of a blood-testis barrier. However, not all such antigens appear to be sequestered, since they can be detected in seminiferous tubules, where they are accessible to circulating antibodies and T cells. Active systemic or local immunoregulatory mechanisms must then be operative. Such mechanisms might include (1) activity of suppressor cells, (2) nonspecific suppression in the testis, (3) failure of antigen presentation in the testis, or (4) lymphocyte trafficking bypassing the testis.

The specific antigens to which antisperm antibodies are directed have yet to be defined. Newer techniques in immunoaffinity chromatography are making their identification in the near future likely. Evidence exists that antisperm antibodies in some women may be directed against antigens adsorbed to the sperm surface from seminal plasma at the time of ejaculation. Whether seminal plasma components may also be autoantigenic is unknown.

That these sperm antigens are tissue-specific antigens rather than alloantigens is indicated by an inability to detect HLA expression on mature human spermatozoa and the finding that antisperm antibodies detected in serum of men with autoimmunity to sperm also react similarly with spermatozoa from a panel of normal fertile men. Following exposure to serum possessing sperm-reactive antibodies, unfixed frozen sections of human stomach, thyroid, ovary, and adrenal have failed to show evidence of IgG binding by immunofluorescence. The vast majority of sera from men with autoimmunity to sperm also are free of antithyroid and antinuclear antibodies as well as rheumatoid factor.

To determine whether sperm-immobilizing antibodies in women are directed against peptide or carbohydrate portions of sperm antigens, ejaculated sperm have been treated with periodic acid which denatures carbohydrates. In some instances this reduces the subsequent ability of antibodies to immobilize these sperm, which suggests a role for carbohydrate antigens. Protein antigens are also involved as targets for these antibodies, emphasizing the complex nature of the target molecules for immobilizing antibodies to sperm.

The only sperm-specific antigen well characterized at present is LDH-X, an isoenzyme of LDH restricted mainly to sperm. ABO blood group antigens are expressed on sperm only in secretors, and this important fact suggests that they are absorbed from seminal plasma. Whether these antigens are expressed in the absence of such absorption is clinically moot, as no evidence for antibodies to ABO antigens in infertility has been found. However, anti-blood group antibodies in sera of women may react with adsorbed blood group substances on sperm surfaces from secretory males giving false-positive antigen-antibody tests. The presence of Rh antigens and the haploid expression of the genes determining these blood group antigens remains controversial.

Histocompatibility antigens may be intrinsically expressed on sperm and not absorbed from seminal plasma. Ia antigens in the mouse are clearly detectable on sperm from epididymis and ductus deferentes, the regions of the male reproductive tract where seminal plasma has not yet been formed. Whether both parental haplotypes are expressed in sperm remains unresolved. The presence of HLA antigens on sperm is controversial. Recently, studies with monoclonal antibodies directed at framework determinants of HLA-A, -B, -C, and -D antigens and employing very sensitive radioimmunoassays and immunofluorescence assays failed to find any HLA antigens in epididymal or ejaculated sperm.

There is fragmentary evidence for weak expression of both class I and II HLA antigens of sperm as well as the presence of mRNA for class II HLA antigens. Evidence for the presence of HLA-D antigens, the probable human analogs of murine Ia antigens, has been derived primarily from the ability of sperm to stimulate lymphocytes in allogeneic mixed sperm lymphocyte cultures. Conclusions from these experiments have been criticized by some because the sperm stimulator cell population was contaminated with small numbers of other cells from the reproductive tract, especially leukocytes known to express HLA-D antigens. Serologic methods for HLA antigens that do not employ monoclonal reagents may harbor non-HLA antibodies, thereby giving false-positive results. A definitive resolution to this very important issue of HLA expression on sperm awaits further studies with these specific reagents.

H-Y antigen, which is encoded as a male-specific antigen by a gene on the Y chromosome and is central to primary sex differentiation, appears to be expressed on sperm. If sperm expressed exclusively either Y- or X-determined antigens, sex determination by antibodies directed at either X- or Y-bearing sperm would theoretically be possible. However, most investigators have not been able to show haploid expression of genes determining H-Y or H-X antigens on sperm. Thus, the possibility of exploiting haploid gene expression for sex determination appears remote.

Unresolved questions in the important area of sperm antigens include (1) whether transplantation antigens are expressed in a haploid or diploid mode, (2) the identity of a sperm-specific antigen, and (3) the definition of antigens that give rise to antibodies which cause infertility in males or females.

Sperm Antibodies

A high incidence of sperm-reactive antibodies has been detected in the sera of homosexual men. Oral sex or deposition of sperm within the rectum during intercourse may result in immunization to sperm antigens. The distribution of immunoglobulin isotypes of sperm-reactive antibodies in the sera of these homosexual men is quite different from that seen in heterosexual men from infertile couples. While tail-directed antibody of the IgG class, and, to a lesser extent, IgA, predominate in the latter group, head-directed IgMs are found more frequently in the sera of homosexuals. The nature of the antigens to which these antibodies are directed is unknown.

It has been suggested that genital tract infections may lead to the development of autoimmunity to sperm. However, such individuals may constitute only a small proportion of the total population of men in whom sperm-reactive antibodies are detected. In a study of 324 consecutive ejaculates submitted for semen analysis and sperm antibody studies, 46 were found to possess autoantibodies to sperm. The incidence of pyospermia (greater than 1 million PMN per milliliter), as judged by acridine orange staining and fluorescence microscopy, was comparable in the 2 groups at 10.8% and 15.2% of those antibody-negative versus antibody-positive. Four of 46 ejaculates of autoimmune men were found to have more than 5 million PMN per milliliter, versus 9 of 278 ejaculates that were antibody-negative. Although this observation does not preclude a prior acute infection, it suggests that chronic genital tract infection is an unlikely cause of autoimmunity to sperm. Most men studied also denied knowledge or symptoms of acute prostatitis or epididymitis.

Role of Seminal Plasma Lymphocytes

A large number of lymphocytes, ranging from 42,000 to 29 million, have been identified in the semen of normal heterosexual men. Recently, by using monoclonal T cell probes and immunoperoxidase staining, a population of intraepithelial CD8-positive suppressor T lymphocytes has been identified within the human epididymis. It has been postulated that these cells might play a role in preventing the development of autoimmunity to spermatozoa by acting locally to limit B cell differentiation and production of specific antibody against sperm-associated antigens. Alternatively, these T cells might suppress antigen processing and presentation by macrophages.

METHODS OF DETECTING SPERM-REACTIVE ANTIBODIES

Many techniques have been described over the years for detection of sperm-reactive antibodies in serum and other body fluids. It has become increasingly apparent that there are 2 sources of immunoglobulins within the male genital tract. These include those present as transudates from serum and those locally secreted. Therefore, circulating sperm-reactive antibodies may not be representative of those antisperm antibodies present in semen. Infertile couples were tested for the presence of antisperm antibodies, either when impaired sperm cervical mucus-penetrating ability was noted on postcoital testing despite normal semen analysis or in the face of idiopathic infertility. During a 5-year period, 1825 semen specimens were submitted to the Laboratory of Human Reproduction at North Shore University Hospital, Manhasset, NY. Sperm were washed free of seminal fluid by low-speed centrifugation and tested directly by immunobead binding for the presence of surface-bound immunoglobulins. Humoral antisperm antibodies were detected by incubation of known antibody-free spermatozoa (husband or donor) in dilute patient serum (1:4), following which sperm were washed free of serum and tested by immunobead binding. Autoantibodies were detected on the sperm surfaces in 13% of ejaculates. In 846 men, matched serum and semen specimens were studied, and humoral antibodies could be compared with those present within the genital tract. Twenty percent of men were found to have sperm-reactive antibodies in their blood without any detected on spermatozoa.

Although humoral antibodies may enter the seminal plasma as transudates, total immunoglobulin levels in semen are about 90% of those seen in serum. Male infertility has previously been noted in association with high titers of circulating anti-sperm antibodies. Indeed, in cases where sperm-reactive antibodies were present in blood but not detected within the ejaculate, serum immunobead-binding levels were low. Bearing in mind that immune phenomena wax and wane and that these men with low-grade autoimmunity to sperm require further surveillance, it would seem that the absence of antisperm antibodies in the ejaculate means that they do not provide an immune basis for infertility.

Conversely, 15% of men were found to have antibodies present on the sperm surface, but no antibodies were detected in serum. These antibodies are primarily of the IgA class, although IgGs may also be detected. The predominance of IgA antibodies in semen—and their absence in serum—suggests local production within the genital tract. Whether these autoantibodies originate in the accessory gland secretions (and are encountered by sperm at the time of ejaculation) or within the epididymis is unknown.

In combination, one-third of serologic tests performed to detect antisperm antibodies provided misleading information that could lead to an error in clinical management. These results emphasize the need to study the ejaculate directly rather than solely using serologic tests in the diagnosis of immune-mediated male infertility.

DETECTION OF SPERM-ASSOCIATED IMMUNOGLOBULINS

Several methods are now clinically available to determine whether spermatozoa themselves are immunoglobulin-bound. These include the mixed agglutination reaction, a direct antiglobulin assay using ^{125}I-radiolabeled heterologous antibody, direct enzyme-linked immunosorbent assay (ELISA), and immunobead binding. Although each of these tests allows one to determine, in a semiquantitative way, the extent of autoimmunity to sperm, immunobead binding in particular provides a measure of the proportion of spermatozoa in the ejaculate antibody bound by each of the 3 major immunoglobulin isotypes (IgG, IgA, and IgM). The precise amount of immunoglobulin associated with the individual spermatozoal surface, however, still cannot be determined by current methods.

DETECTION OF HUMORAL ANTIBODIES

Sperm Immobilization Tests

Antibodies absolutely dependent on complement to produce immobilization of sperm were initially described by Fjällbrant in 1965 and Isojima in 1968. In these assays, donor sperm from the male to be tested—or from a normal control—are washed and incubated with serial dilutions of heat-inactivated test serum or other secretions. These can be derived from the male to be tested or from female partners. A source of complement (usually fresh guinea pig serum) is added. A time end point for immobilization (Fjällbrant) of 90% sperm—or a percentage of motile sperm at a standard time (Isojima)—is compared microscopically with sperm incubated in control sera and complement alone. Complement-dependent immobilization, while highly specific in that false-positive reactions are uncommon, will not detect the presence of non-complement-fixing immunoglobulins. The degree of antibody present on the sperm surface also appears to play a role in the extent of complement-dependent immobilization. Results obtained from immobilization tests have a definite relationship to immunologic infertility. However, correlation of sperm-immobilizing antibodies with agglutinating antibodies is not perfect.

Since seminal plasma contains complement inhibitors, complement-dependent cytotoxicity tests cannot be applied to detection of autoantibodies to sperm in semen. Although sperm agglutination, antiglobulin tests, radiolabeled protein A, and ELISA have all been applied to the study of antisperm antibodies within the seminal plasma, they suffer from the fact that the majority of sperm-reactive antibodies present within the ejaculate may be cell-associated (sperm-bound) rather than cell-free. If antibody concentrations are limiting relative to the number of antigenic sites on the sperm surface, there may be no residual antibody within the seminal plasma despite its presence bound to spermatozoa. Those antibodies detected within seminal plasma may then not be reflective of immunoglobulins associated with sperm.

Sperm Agglutination Tests

Agglutination tests are a sensitive and specific means of detecting sperm antibodies. The 2 main procedures for sperm agglutination are the gelatin agglutination test of Kibrick and the microagglutination test read macroscopically. In the Franklin-Dukes method, no gelatin is used, and agglutination is read on slides or in a microtiter tray in the microscope. Agglutination may be primarily head-to-head or tail-to-tail, rarely head-to-tail. Tail-to-tail agglutination usually occurs in female sera and head-to-head in male sera. The antigens detected by this test are not fully characterized.

Failure to give careful attention to controls in sperm antibody tests has often led to misleading results, especially with relatively undiluted sera. Obviously, obtaining a standard source of viable human sperm presents difficulties. Known positive and negative control sera must be included.

Other Antibody Tests

In response to the need for assays that correlate better with clinical evidence of infertility, a variety of new tests have appeared.

While a number of ELISAs have been developed to detect the presence of sperm-reactive antibodies in serum or semen, there has recently been increasing dissatisfaction with this approach. A high incidence of "naturally occurring" sperm-reactive antibodies in the sera of fertile men and women of all ages poses a major problem of "immunologic background noise" for the ELISA. These antibodies, which react with subsurface components of spermatozoa, are not expected to interfere with the membrane-associated interaction of gametes that lead to successful fertilization. The method of fixing spermatozoa is critical in determining which antigens are "presented" to a test serum sample. In particular, when spermatozoa are air-dried, disruption of the sperm plasma membrane can provide access to internal antigens. A marked variation in the ability of an ELISA to detect sperm-reactive antibodies has been documented when spermatozoa were fixed in different manners, eg, air-drying to wells, glutaraldehyde fixation, reacting with test serum when living, or following freeze-thaw.

Another approach has been to utilize extracts of spermatozoa as the target antigens for ELISA. It has been hypothesized that lithium diiodosalicylate extracts those sperm membrane-associated antigens that are relevant to infertility. However, they may be absent or altered beyond recognition by antibody. When several laboratories, each utilizing its own ELISA methodologies, studied a group of clinically defined serum provided by the WHO Reference Bank, there was no uniformity of results between groups. Different ELISAs thus appear to detect different groups of sperm-reactive antibodies, and which of these antibodies are relevant to impaired reproduction remains unknown.

Ideally, those sperm-reactive antibodies detected by a particular laboratory method must be shown either by clinical studies or by in vitro gamete interaction to alter sperm function. A correlation has been found between the proportion of spermatozoa that bind immunobeads in ejaculates of men with autoimmunity to sperm and the number of spermatozoa seen within cervical mucus on postcoital testing. Sperm penetration into cervical mucus was nearly absent, despite the presence of normal numbers of motile sperm in the ejaculate, when more than 80% of sperm were antibody-bound. Conversely, increasing numbers of spermatozoa were noted at postcoital testing, as immunobead binding levels dropped 50%. The extent of autoimmunity to sperm, as reflected in the

proportion of sperm-binding immunobeads, also correlated with the chance that pregnancy would occur in couples when female causes of infertility had been addressed but no specific treatment had been offered the husband.

Mathur has introduced a new sensitive and specific assay for cytotoxic antisperm antibodies. This double-immunofluorescence test depends on diacetyl fluorescein, which stains viable sperm, and on ethidium bromide, which counterstains dead sperm. In the presence of complement, this assay can detect both auto- and isoantibodies to sperm in infertile couples. Results of the sperm cytotoxicity and passive hemagglutination studies were compared with those obtained by immunobead-binding, tray agglutination, and gel agglutination, in a group of clinically defined sera provided by the WHO Reference Bank. There was no correlation among assays, which suggests that a different group of antibodies was being detected by the former procedures. Emphasis must be placed on whether the results of particular methodologies correlate with impaired sperm function, either clinically or in the laboratory.

ROLE OF ANTISPERM ANTIBODIES IN INFERTILITY

Antisperm Immunity in the Male

Antibodies directed toward various sperm antigens can result in reduced fertility in men. Results from several large series on the presence of sperm agglutinins in fertile and infertile men place the cutoff point for a significant titer of sperm-agglutinating antibodies at approximately 1:32. In most such studies, the correlation between sperm agglutinins and complement-dependent immobilizing antibodies is reasonably high. However, the tendency is toward lower titers and fewer fertile individuals with positive immobilizing antibodies. Thus, immobilizing antibodies are quite specific. Although agglutinating antibodies are a sensitive index for infertility, their specificity is poor.

Evidence exists that sperm-reactive autoantibodies may impair sperm entrance into cervical mucus from seminal plasma. This can be shown both clinically at postcoital testing and in vitro. Spermatozoa obtained from known fertile donors and previously shown to be able to penetrate human cervical mucus failed to do so following incubation with antibody in vitro. The Fc portion of the immunoglobulin has been implicated in restricting sperm motion within cervical mucus, since donor spermatozoa bound to Fab fragments of sperm-reactive antibodies show no impairment of sperm penetration within cervical mucus. IgA-labeled sperm treated with an IgA protease that cleaves Fc fragments regain their ability to penetrate cervical mucus as well.

Spermatozoa bound by immunoglobulins at the acrosomal and postacrosomal regions of the sperm head may be impaired in their ability to fertilize eggs, even if they reach the site of fertilization within the distal ampulla of the uterine tube. Species-specific receptors for the zona pellucida have been identified on the plasma membrane of sperm and antibodies to sperm membranes block attachment to the zona in animal experiments. Spontaneously occurring autoantibodies in men from infertile couples directed against surface antigens of the sperm head have also been shown to impair the ability of human sperm to attach to the zona pellucida of nonliving human ova. In addition, diminished in vitro fertilization rates of human eggs with intact zona have been observed if the woman's serum used in culture medium had antisperm antibody titers of greater than 1:10 or if more than 70% of sperm were bound to autoantibodies.

Several laboratories have now reported the ability of antisperm alloantibodies in women—as well as autoantibodies in men—to impair penetration of zona-free hamster ova by human sperm. The penetrating ability of spermatozoa was diminished markedly in the presence of sperm-reactive antibodies which fixed complement but not when IgA non-complement-fixing sperm-reactive antibodies were present.

Recently a variety of cytokines from activated macrophages and lymphocytes have been shown to be toxic for preimplantation embryos. Lymphocytes from women sensitized to sperm could secrete these factors if the cells were activated by antigens on sperm. Gamma interferon is produced by lymphocytes exposed to antibody-coated sperm. The clinical consequences of embryocytotoxic cytokines would probably be unexplained infertility rather than recurrent abortions, since the fertilized egg would be damaged by the cytokines prior to implantation.

Most agglutinating antibodies to sperm in seminal plasma are of the IgA class and may exist only in seminal plasma, whereas immobilizing antibodies are predominantly IgG. IgM antibodies gain access to seminal plasma only when there is a significant inflammatory lesion in the reproductive tract or after vasectomy.

Other Consequences of Autoimmunity to Sperm in the Male

Despite the presence of high levels of autoantibodies to sperm within the reproductive tract, sperm output is not impaired, and the distribution of sperm concentrations within semen is similar to that seen in infertile men in the absence of autoimmunity to sperm.

A blood-testis barrier exists as tight junctional complexes between Sertoli cells, dividing the seminiferous tubule into basal and adluminal compartments. In the dark mink, naturally occurring orchitis is associated with breakdown of tight junctions between Sertoli cells, suggesting that the blood-testis barrier might become defective during seasonal regression of the testis. Experimental immunization of guinea pigs with testis extracts containing specific autoantigens has also been associated with the development of immune orchitis. Specific plasma membrane antigens may be present on both mature epididymal spermatozoa and earlier stages of sperm development within the testis. In humans, however, there is no evidence that autoimmunity to sperm—either occurring spontaneously in infertile couples or following vasectomy—is associated with the development of clinical orchitis. In a single study, a man with prostatic cancer destined to undergo orchiectomy was immunized with spermatozoa and the testis subsequently examined for evidence of orchitis. Only focal lesions were noted, suggesting that those antigens present on mature spermatozoa may not be expressed during development of precursor sperm within the testis. However, the cancer itself may have altered this individual's immune responsiveness to sperm antigens. The failure of vasectomy to be associated with the development of clinical orchitis in humans also suggests a different pattern in the stage-specific expression of antigens on primate sperm.

One study showed that spontaneously occurring sperm-reactive IgG antibodies in the sera of men from infertile couples failed to bind to intratesticular spermatozoa or spermatocytes within the seminiferous tubules. This result suggests that antibodies directed against antigens present on the surface of ejaculate sperm did not make their appearance until after the completion of spermatogenesis. Alternatively, loss of relevant antigens might have occurred following orchiectomy or in preparation of the tissues for study.

Several studies using in vitro correlates of cellular immunity to sperm in infertile individuals have been performed. These have for the most part given conflicting results. Neither lymphocyte transformation nor leukocyte inhibitory factor production has given consistent evidence for cellular sensitization in individuals with sperm immunity. Clearly, this is an important area requiring additional study.

Various forms of therapy have been employed to reduce antibodies to sperm in the male. These include systemic administration of adrenal corticosteroids, attempts at artificial insemination with washed sperm, and, in the case of antibodies in the female, the use of condoms to reduce antibody titers by reducing exposure to sperm. The success of all of these forms of treatment is limited. Further studies are needed to fully confirm their efficacy, especially in controlled clinical trials.

IMMUNOLOGIC CONSEQUENCES OF VASECTOMY

About a million vasectomies are performed annually in the USA. Antibodies and probably cellular immunity to sperm develop in most vasectomized men as a result of interaction of extravasated sperm antigens with the immune system. Sperm are autoimmunogenic, mainly because of their normal sequestration behind a blood-testis barrier and their late development relative to the establishment of self tolerance. The potential adverse consequences of this immune response to sperm include (1) systemic effects on other organ systems and (2) interference with fertility after reanastomosis of the vasa deferentia (vasovasostomy).

There is no doubt that vasectomy in humans leads to production of sperm antibodies. Most studies indicate a 60–70% incidence of sperm agglutinins in serum and a 30–40% incidence of immobilizing antibodies by 1 year following the procedure that persist for as long as 10 years in about half of the initially positive patients.

Granuloma formation due to local extravasation of sperm is relatively common, but the presence of granulomas correlates poorly with antibody to sperm. The antibodies that develop after vasectomy are tissue-specific and do not react with HLA-antigens. A recent study showed a strong association of HLA-A28 with production of sperm antibodies following vasectomy, suggesting a genetic predisposition. Normal semen contains little or no IgM, but its presence following vasectomy and with antibodies for sperm relates to the degree of chronic inflammation from extravasal spermatozoa.

Little is known about cellular immunity to sperm following vasectomy. Several studies in animals immunized with sperm or undergoing vasectomy have shown inconstant development of T lymphocyte responsiveness to sperm. In vitro cellular immune studies in humans are still inconclusive. The well-recognized in vitro immunoinhibitory action of seminal plasma may in fact prevent such responses in vivo. Much more needs to be learned about other components of the immune response to sperm following vasectomy.

There are no established adverse systemic immune effects in long-term studies of vasectomy in humans. Sex hormone levels are not influenced by vasectomy. A slight increase in antinuclear and anti-smooth muscle antibodies has been demonstrated in a few individuals. There is evidence for circulating immune complexes composed of sperm antigens and antibody following vasectomy in men.

Vasectomy can accelerate atherosclerosis in monkeys fed atherogenic diets. The postulated mechanism involves deposition of sperm-antisperm immune complexes in vascular intima followed by plaque formation. Large epidemiologic studies in the USA using case-controls (1512 subjects) or cohort analysis (1764 men) revealed no evidence for increased cardiovascular disease in a 6- to 7-year follow-up period. This has been confirmed by Danish workers as well. Nevertheless, continued immunologic and clinical monitoring of vasectomized men seems warranted.

A successful surgical method for reanastomosis of ligated vasa deferentia, termed vasovasostomy, has been developed. The presence of sperm antibodies in 60–70% of vasectomized men represents a potential threat to restoration of full fertility. There are conflicting studies about whether the presence of sperm antibodies results in decreased fertility in such individuals. However, the well-documented antifertility effects of high titers of sperm antibody make it likely that fertility may not be fully restored.

IMMUNOLOGIC FEATURES OF SEMINAL PLASMA

Seminal plasma contains a variety of potentially antigenic substances, particularly enzymes, on enzymatic proteins and nonproteinaceous substances. Immunoglobulins are also present but at much lower concentrations than in serum (IgG, 7–13 mg/dL; IgA, 2–6 mg/dL). IgM is not normally detectable. Other substances with potential regulatory effects in the immune system include transferrin, zinc, prostaglandins, and polyamines.

Several potentially important immunoinhibitory substances have been detected in seminal plasma. One of these substances has broad-spectrum immunosuppressive effects on lymphocyte function in vitro, including blocking proliferation of T cells stimulated by mitogen, antigen, and allogeneic cells. It also blocks in vitro T cell-dependent or -independent antibody products of B cells. Although this factor is apparently a macromolecule present in several species, direct evidence of an in vivo immunosuppressive effect is lacking.

Seminal plasma interferes with a variety of microbicidal functions including bactericidal and opsonic activity of serum or granulocytes for a variety of microorganisms, such as *Neisseria gonorrhoeae* and *Escherichia coli* but not *Staphylo-*

coccus aureus. The precise mechanism by which this inhibitory activity is mediated has not yet been determined. Complement activation is reduced by incubation with seminal plasma, which contains a large variety of proteases and protease inhibitors. It is interesting to speculate that the various immunoinhibitors in seminal plasma have a role in protecting sperm from immunologic attack in the female reproductive tract. In pathologic states, infectious agents may escape destruction in the reproductive tract at a consequence of inhibition of microbicidal action.

Anaphylaxis due to components of semen (either sperm or seminal plasma) is rare. Symptoms occur immediately following sexual intercourse and include urticaria, angioedema, and occasionally hypotension. Immediate hypersensitivity to intrinsic seminal plasma antigens has been demonstrated. Therapy consists of abstinence, use of a condom to prevent contact with semen, and desensitization. A patient with severe allergy to seminal plasma underwent normal pregnancy and delivery after artificial insemination with seminal plasma-free spermatozoa.

REFERENCES

General

Beer AE, Billingham RE: *The Immunobiology of Mammalian Reproduction.* Prentice-Hall, 1976.

Lewis JE, Coulam CB, Moore SB: Immunologic mechanisms in the maternal-fetal relationship. *Mayo Clin Proc* 1986;**61**:655.

Möller G: Immunology of feto-maternal relationship. *Immunol Rev* 1983;**75**:1.

Wegmann TG, Gill TJ: *Immunology of Reproduction.* Oxford Univ Press, 1983.

The Uterus as a Site for Immune Reactivity

Beer AE, Billingham RE: Host response to intrauterine tissue of cellular and fetal allografts. *J Reprod Fertil [Suppl]* 1974;**21**:59.

Stites DP, Erickson RP: Suppressive effect of seminal plasma on lymphocyte activation. *Nature* 1975;**253**:727.

Maternal Immune Response During Pregnancy

Carr MC, Stites DP, Fudenberg HH: Cellular immune aspects of the human fetal-maternal relationship. 3. Mixed lymphocyte reactivity between maternal and cord blood lymphocytes. *Cell Immunol* 1974;**11**:332.

Tallon DF et al: Circulating lymphocyte subpopulations in pregnancy: A longitudinal study. *J Immunol* 1984;**132**:1784.

Terasaki PI et al: Maternal-fetal incompatibility. 1. Incidence of HL-A antibodies and possible association with congenital anomalies. *Transplantation* 1970;**9**:538.

Youtananukorn V, Matangkasombut P: Specific plasma factors blocking human maternal cell-mediated immune reaction to placental antigens. *Nature* 1973;**242**:110.

Immunoregulation of Maternal Recognition of the Fetal Allograft

Faulk WP, McIntyre JA: Immune regulation in human pregnancy. *Adv Nephrol* 1986;**15**:35.

Kasakura S: A factor in maternal plasma during pregnancy that suppresses the reactivity of mixed leukocyte cultures. *J Immunol* 1971;**197**:1296.

Pavia CS, Stites DP: Humoral and cellular regulation of alloimmunity in pregnancy. *J Immunol* 1979;**123**:2194.

Stites DP, Siiteri PK: Steroids as immunosuppressants in pregnancy. *Immunol Rev* 1983;**75**:117.

Stites DP et al: Immunologic regulation in pregnancy. *Arthritis Rheum* 1979;**22**:1300.

Alloantigenicity of the Fetoplacental Unit & an Immunologic Role for the Placenta

Chatterjee-Hasrouni S, Lala PK: Localization of H-2 antigens on mouse trophoblast cells. *J Exp Med* 1979;**149**:1238.

Faulk WP et al: Antigens of human trophoblasts: A working hypothesis for their role in normal and abnormal pregnancies. *Proc Natl Acad Sci USA* 1978;**75**:1947.

Montgomery B, Lala PK: Ontogeny of the MHC antigens on human trophoblast cells during the first trimester of pregnancy. *J Immunol* 1983;**131**:2348.

Pavia CS, Stites DP: Transplantation antigen expression on murine trophoblast: Detection by induction of specific alloimmunity. *Cell Immunol* 1981;**64**:162.

Pavia CS, Stites DP: Trophoblast regulation of maternal-paternal lymphocyte interactions. *Cell Immunol* 1981;**58**:202.

Siiteri PK, Stites DP: Immunologic and endocrine interrelationships in pregnancy. *Biol Reprod* 1982;**26**:1.

Fetal-Maternal Exchange of Humoral & Cellular Components

Brambell FWR: *The Transmission of Passive Immunity from Mother to Young.* Vol 18 of: *Frontiers of Biology.* North-Holland, 1970.

Jenkinson EJ, Billington WD, Elson J: Detection of receptors for immunoglobulin on human placenta by EA rosette formation. *Clin Exp Immunol* 1976;**23**:456.

Solomon JB: *Foetal and Neonatal Immunology.* Vol 20 of: *Frontiers of Biology.* North-Holland, 1971.

Immunologic Consequences of Transplacentally Passed Substances

Scott JR, Beer AE: Immunological factors in first-pregnancy Rh isoimmunization. *Lancet* 1973;**1**:717.

Scott JS: Immunological diseases in pregnancy. *Prog Allergy* 1977;**23**:321.

Woodrow JG: Rh-immunisation and its prevention. *Nord Med* 1971;**85**:704.

Maternal-Fetal Antimicrobial Immunity

Loke YW et al: Characterization of phagocytic cells

isolated from the human placenta. *J Reticuloendothel Soc* 1982;**31**:317.

Miller ME, Stiehm ER: Immunology and resistance to infection. Page 27 in: *Infectious Diseases of the Fetus and Newborn Infant*. Remington JS, Klein JO (editors). Saunders, 1983.

Immunity and Spontaneous Abortions

Clark DA: What do we know about spontaneous abortion mechanisms? *Am J Reprod Immunol* 1989;**19**:28.

Gatenby PA et al: Treatment of recurrent spontaneous abortion by immunization with paternal lymphocytes: correlates with outcome. *Am J Reprod Immunol* 1989;**19**:21.

Mowbray JF, Underwood JL: Immunology of Abortion. *Clin Exp Immunol* 1985;**60**:1.

Mowbray JF et al: Controlled trial of treatment of recurrent spontaneous abortion by immunization with paternal cells. *Lancet* 1985;**1**:941.

Rocklin RE et al: Maternal-fetal relation: Absence of an immunologic blocking factor from the serum of women with chronic abortions. *N Engl J Med* 1976;**295**:1209.

Sargent IL, Wilkins T, Redman CW: Maternal immune response to the fetus in early pregnancy and recurrent miscarriage. *Lancet* 1988;**2**:1099.

Antigens on Spermatozoa

Anderson DJ, Bach DL, Yunis EJ: Major histocompatibility antigens are not expressed on human epididymal sperm. *J Immunol* 1983;**129**:452.

Bishara A et al: Human leukocyte antigens (HLA) class I and class II on sperm cells studied at the serological, cellular and genetic levels. *Am J Reprod Immunol and Microbiol* 1987;**13**:97.

Erickson RP, Lewis SE, Butley M: Is haploid gene expression possible for sperm antigens? *J Reprod Immunol* 1981;**3**:195.

Hoppe PC, Koo GC: Reacting mouse sperm with monoclonal H-Y antibodies does not influence sex ratio of eggs fertilized in vitro. *J Reprod Immunol* 1984;**6**:1.

Isojima S et al: Purification of human seminal plasma antigens relevant to sperm immobilization, agglutination and blocking fertilization. *Am J Reprod Immunol* 1985;**7**:139.

Isojima S: Recent advances in defining human seminal plasma antigens using monoclonal antibodies. *Am J Reprod Immunol* 1988;**17**:150.

Methods of Detecting Sperm-Reactive Antibodies

Bronson RA, Cooper GW, Rosenfeld DL: Correlation between regional specificity of antisperm antibodies to the spermatozoan surface and complement-mediated sperm immobilization. *Am J Reprod Immunol* 1982;**2**:222.

Bronson R et al: Detection of spontaneously occurring sperm-directed antibodies in infertile couples by immunobead binding and enzyme-linked immunosorbent assay. *Ann NY Acad Sci* 1984;**438**:504.

Jager S, Kremer J, Van Slochteren-Draaisma T: A simple method of screening for antisperm antibodies in the human male: Detection of spermatozoal

surface IgG with the direct mixed agglutination reaction carried out on untreated fresh human semen. *Int J Fertil* 1978;**23**:12.

Rodman TC et al: Naturally occurring antibodies reactive with sperm proteins: Apparent deficiency in AIDS sera. *Science* 1985;**228**:1211.

Rose NR et al: Techniques for detection of iso- and auto-antibodies to human spermatozoa. *Clin Exp Immunol* 1976;**23**:175.

Tung KSK et al: Human sperm antigens and antisperm antibodies. 2. Age-related incidence of antisperm antibodies. *Clin Exp Immunol* 1974;**25**:73.

Role of Antisperm Antibodies in Infertility

Alexander NJ: Antibodies to human spermatozoa impede sperm penetration of cervical mucus or hamster eggs. *Fertil Steril* 1984;**41**:433.

Bliel JD, Wassermann PM: Sperm-egg interactions in the mouse: Sequence of events and induction of the acrosome reaction by a zona pellucida glycoprotein. *Dev Biol* 1983;**95**:315.

Bronson RA, Cooper GW, Rosenfeld DL: Auto-immunity to spermatozoa: Effect on sperm penetration of cervical mucus as reflected by postcoital testing. *Fertil Steril* 1984;**41**:609.

Bronson RA, Cooper GW, Rosenfeld DL: Complement-mediated effects of sperm head-directed human antibodies on the ability of human spermatozoa to penetrate zona-free hamster egs. *Fertil Steril* 1983;**40**:91.

Bronson R, Cooper G, Rosenfeld D: Reproductive effects of sperm surface antibodies. Pages 417–436 in: *Male Fertility and Its Regulation*. Lobl T, Hafez ESE (editors). MTP Press, 1985.

Bronson RA, Cooper GW, Rosenfeld DL: Sperm-specific iso-antibodies and auto-antibodies inhibit binding of human sperm to the human zona pellucida. *Fertil Steril* 1982;**38**:724.

Bronson RA et al: The effect of IgA protease on immunoglobulins bound to the sperm surface and sperm cervical mucus penetrating ability. *Fertil Steril* 1987;**47**:985.

Haas GG, Cines DB, Schreiber AD: Immunologic infertility: Identification of patients with antisperm antibody. *N Engl J Med* 1980;**303**:722.

Jager S et al: Induction of the shaking phenomenon by pretreatment of spermatozoa with sera containing antispermatozoal antibodies. *Fertil Steril* 1981;**36**:784.

London SF, Haney AF, Weinberg JB: Diverse humoral and cell-mediated effects of antisperm antibodies on reproduction. *Fertil Steril* 1984;**41**:907.

Menge AC, Medley NE, Mangione CM: The incidence and influence of antisperm antibodies in infertile human couples on sperm cervical mucus interaction and subsequent fertility. *Fertil Steril* 1982;**38**:439.

Rümke P: Autoantibodies against spermatozoa in infertile men. *J Reprod Fertil [Suppl]* 1974;**21**:169.

Witkin SS, Sonnaband J: Immune response to spermatozoa in homosexual men. *Fertil Steril* 1983;**39**:337.

Wolf DP, Sokolski JE, Quigley MM: Correlation of human in vitro fertilization with the hamster egg bioassay. *Fertil Steril* 1983;**40**:53.

Yanagimachi R: Specificity of sperm-egg interactions. In: *Immunobiology of Gametes*. Edidin M, Johnson MH (editors). Cambridge Univ Press, 1977.

Yanagimachi R, Okada A, Tung KSK: Effects of anti-guinea pig serum antibodies on sperm-ovum interactions. *Biol Reprod* 1981;**24**:512.

Immunologic Consequences of Vasectomy

Clarkson TB, Alexander NJ: Long-term vasectomy: Effects on occurrence and extent of atherosclerosis in rhesus monkeys. *J Clin Invest* 1980;**65**:15.

Goldacre MJ, Holford TR, Vessey MP: Cardiovascular disease and vasectomy. *N Engl J Med* 1983;**308**:805.

Lepow IH, Crozier R (editors): *Vasectomy: Immunologic and Pathophysiologic Effects in Animal and Man*. Academic Press, 1979.

Linnet L, Hjort T, Fogh-Anderson P: Association between failure to impregnate after vasovasostomy and sperm agglutinins in semen. *Lancet* 1981;**1**:117.

Linnet L, Moller NP-H, Bernth-Petersen P: No increase in arteriosclerotic retinopathy or activity in tests for circulating immune complexes 5 years after vasectomy. *Fertil Steril* 1982;**37**:798.

Massey FJ et al: Vasectomy and health: Results from a large cohort study. *JAMA* 1984;**252**:1023.

Perrin EB et al: Long-term effect of vasectomy on coronary heart disease. *Am J Public Health* 1984;**74**:128.

Teuscher C, Wild GC, Tung KSK: Experimental allergic orchitis: The isolation and partial characterization of an aspermatogenic polypeptide (AP3) with an apparent sequential disease-inducing determinant(s). *J Immunol* 1983;**130**:2683.

Tung KSK et al: Genetic control of antisperm autoantibody response in vasectomized guinea pigs. *J Immunol* 1981;**127**:835.

Witkin SS, Zelikovsky G, Bongiovanni AM: Sperm-related antigens, antibodies and circulating immune complexes in sera of recently vasectomized men. *J Clin Invest* 1982:**70**:33.

Witkin SS et al: IgA antibody response to vasectomy. *Ann NY Acad Sci* 1983;**409**:890.

Immunologic Features of Seminal Plasma

Brooks GF et al: Human seminal plasma inhibition of antibody complement-mediated killing and opsonization of *Neisseria gonorrhoeae* and other gram-negative organisms. *J Clin Invest* 1981;**67**:1523.

Frick OL: Seminal fluid allergy. (Editorial.) *West J Med* 1982;**137**:122.

James, K. Hargreave TB: Immunosuppression by seminal plasma and its possible clinical significance. *Immunol Today* 1984;**5**:357.

Lord EM, Sensabaugh GF, Stites DP: Immunosuppressive activity of human seminal plasma. 1. Inhibition of in vitro lymphocyte activation. *J Immunol* 1977;**118**:1704.

Mukherjee DC et al: Suppression of epididymal sperm antigenicity in the rabbit by uteroglobulin and transglutaminase in vitro. *Science* 1983;**219**:989.

Olsen GP, Shields JW: Seminal lymphocytes, plasma and AIDS. *Nature* 1984;**309**:116.

Peterson BH et al: Human seminal plasma inhibition of complement. *J Lab Clin Med* 1980;**96**:582.

Witkin SS et al: Demonstration of 11S IgA antibody to spermatozoa in human seminal fluid. *Clin Exp Immunol* 1981;**44**:368.

Etiology of Immunity to Sperm

Dym M, Caviacchia JC: Further observations on the blood-testis barrier in monkeys. *Biol Reprod* 1977;**17**:390.

Hill JA, Florina H, Anderson DJ: Products of activated lymphocytes and macrophages inhibit mouse embryo development. *J Immunol* 1987;**139**:2250.

Kramer JM, Erickson RD: Analysis of stage-specific protein synthesis during spermatogenesis of the mouse by two-dimensional gel electrophoresis. *J Reprod Fertil* 1982;**64**:139.

Mahi-Brown CA, Yule TD, Tung KSK: Evidence for active immunological regulation in prevention of testicular autoimmune disease independent of the blood-testis barrier. *Am J Reprod Immunol* 1988;**16**:165.

Millette CG, Bellve AR: Selective partitioning of plasma membrane antigens during mouse spermatogenesis. *Dev Biol* 1980;**79**:319.

Ritchie AWS et al: Intra-epithelial lymphocytes in the normal epididymis: A mechanism for tolerance to sperm auto-antigens? *Br J Urol* 1984;**56**:79.

Tunk KSK et al: The black mink *(Mustela vision)*: A natural model of immunologic male infertility. *J Exp Med* 1981;**154**:1016.

Witkin SS: Production of interferon gamma by lymphocytes exposed to antibody-coated spermatozoa: A mechanism for sperm antibody production in females. *Fertil Steril* 1988;**50**:498.

Section II.
Immunologic Laboratory Tests

Clinical Laboratory Methods for Detection of Antigens & Antibodies

18

Daniel P. Stites, MD, & R. P. Channing Rodgers, MD

One of the major challenges for modern medicine is the translation of basic advances in immunochemistry and immunobiology into diagnostic and therapeutic procedures that will be useful in the practice of clinical medicine. In the clinical immunology laboratory, tests that utilize a great many of the recently elucidated principles of basic immunology can be performed on a wide variety of samples taken from patients. The results of these laboratory procedures are then used by practicing physicians in the diagnosis, treatment and prognosis of clinical disorders. Furthermore, qualitative and quantitative analysis of immune responses has led to better understanding of the pathogenesis of many clinical disorders. This understanding in turn has stimulated further basic scientific research in immunology. In fact, observations made by clinical investigators in immunology have frequently dramatically changed the course of basic research in immunology and related fields. An example is the impetus given to research on T cells and B cells by careful clinical descriptions of patients with thymic aplasia and hypogammaglobulinemia.

Over the past 2 decades, immunologic laboratory methods have gradually become increasingly more refined and simplified. Because of their inherent specificity and sensitivity, these methods have now achieved a central role in the modern clinical laboratory. The goals of laboratory medicine are to improve the availability, accuracy, and precision of a body of medically important laboratory tests, to ensure correct interpretation, and to assess the significance of new tests introduced into clinical medicine. With the marked proliferation of new laboratory tests employing immunologic principles, these methods of laboratory diagnosis have often been uncritically applied to clinical situations. A better understanding of the methods used in the immunology laboratory should provide the student and practitioner of medicine with a useful guide for correct application and interpretation of this body of knowledge.

In the present chapter, tests for the detection of antigens and antibodies in clinical practice are discussed. One should distinguish 2 separate uses of methods described. They can be used to detect immune responses and their pathology, or, alternatively, they can use immunologic principles for quantitative and qualitative detection of antigens or antibodies by analytic chemical methods. Most of the techniques described involve application in the clinical laboratory of the principles of immunochemistry discussed earlier in this book. This chapter and the following one are not meant to be comprehensive laboratory manuals. Rather, the principles of the various immunologic methods and their application to selected clinical problems are reviewed. It is hoped that careful study of the chapters in this section in conjunction with the first section of this book will provide the reader with a solid background for an enhanced understanding of the detailed discussions of clinical immunology and descriptions of specific tests used in various disorders presented in clinical chapters that follow.

The topics covered in this chapter include the following:

(1) Immunodiffusion
(2) Electrophoresis and immunoelectrophoresis
(3) Immunochemical and physiochemical methods
(4) Binder-ligand assays
(5) Immunohistochemical techniques (immunofluorescence)
(6) Agglutination
(7) Complement assays

(8) Monoclonal antibodies
(9) Predictive Value Theory

IMMUNODIFFUSION

The purpose of all immunodiffusion techniques is to detect the reaction of antigen and antibody by the precipitation reaction. Although the formation of antigen-antibody complexes in a semisolid medium such as agar is dependent on buffer electrolytes, pH, and temperature, the most important determinants of the reaction are the relative concentrations of antigen and antibody. This relationship is depicted schematically in Fig 18–1. Maximal precipitation forms in the area of equivalence, with decreasing amounts in the zones of antigen excess or antibody excess. Thus, formation of precipitation lines in any immunodiffusion system is highly dependent on relative concentrations of antigen and antibody. The **prozone phenomenon** refers to suboptimal precipitation which occurs in the region of antibody excess. Thus, dilutions of antisera must be reacted with fixed amounts of antigen to obtain maximum precipitin lines. The prozone phenomenon is a cause of misinterpretation of immunoelectrophoresis patterns in the diagnosis of paraproteinemias when large amounts of antibodies are present.

Immunoprecipitation is the simplest and most direct means of demonstrating antigen-antibody reactions. The application of immunoprecipitation to the study of bacterial antigens launched the field of serology in the first part of the 20th century. In 1946, Oudin described a system of single diffusion of antigen and antibody in agar-filled tubes. This important advance was soon followed by Ouchterlony's classic description of double diffusion in agar layered on slides. This method is still in use today and has many applications in the detection and analysis of precipitating antigen-antibody systems.

Immunodiffusion reactions may be classified as single or double. In single immunodiffusion, either antigen or antibody remains fixed and the other reactant is allowed to move and complex with it. In double immunodiffusion, both reactants are free to move toward each other and precipitate. Movement in either form of immunodiffusion may be linear or radial. Specific examples are discussed in the remainder of this section.

Immunodiffusion has a clinical application in the quantitative and qualitative analysis of serum proteins. Quantitative analysis of serum proteins is often done by more sensitive and automated methods such as nephelometry, ELISA, or RIA. Single radial diffusion in agar has largely been supplanted by these

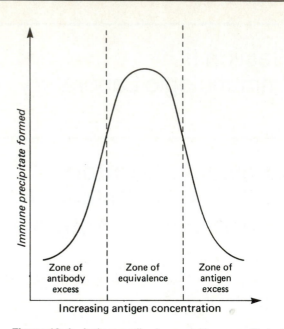

Figure 18–1. Antigen-antibody precipitin curve. Typical precipitin curve resulting from titration of increasing antigen concentration plotted against amount of immune precipitate formed. Amount of antibody is kept constant throughout.

methods, which do not rely on immunoprecipitation or diffusion.

METHODOLOGY & INTERPRETATION

Double Diffusion in Agar

This simple and extremely useful technique (also called **Ouchterlony analysis**) is based on the principle that when antigen and antibody diffuse through a semisolid medium (eg, agar) they form stable immune complexes, which can be analyzed visually.

The test is performed by pouring molten agar onto glass slides or into Petri dishes and allowing it to harden. Small wells are punched out of the agar a few millimeters apart. Samples containing antigen and antibody are placed in opposing wells and allowed to diffuse toward one another in a moist chamber for 18–24 hours. The resultant precipitation lines that represent antigen-antibody complexes are analyzed visually in indirect light with the aid of a magnifying lens. When antigen and antibody are allowed to diffuse in a radial fashion, an arc which approximates a straight line is formed at the leading edges of the diffusing antigen and antibody. Examples of patterns produced in simple double diffusion are shown in Fig 18–2.

Double diffusion is commonly performed by placing antigen and antibody wells at various angles for

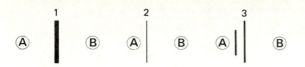

Figure 18–2. Reactions in simple double diffusion. In (1) antigen A and antibody B react equidistantly and intensely at equivalence. In (2) antigen A is present in reduced concentration or has not diffused as rapidly owing to size or charge, forming a precipitin line closer to the antigen well. In (3) a contaminant or impurity present in antigen A is reacting with antibody B.

comparative purposes. The 3 basic characteristic patterns of those reactions are shown in Fig 18–3. In addition to these 3 basic patterns, more complex interrelationships may be seen between antigen and antibody. The formation of a single precipitation line between an antigen and its corresponding antiserum can be utilized as a rough estimation of antigen or antibody purity. However, the relative insensitivity of the test and the limitation of immunodiffusion to *precipitating* antigen-antibody reactions partly restrict the applications of this technique. It is most useful in demonstrating the identity of serologic reactions to antigens from various infectious agents with antibodies of known positive reactivity.

Double immunodiffusion in agar can also be used for semiquantitative analysis in human serologic systems where the specificity of the precipitation lines has already been determined. Such an analysis is performed by placing antibody in a central well surrounded circumferentially by antigen wells (Fig 18–4). Serial dilutions of antigen are placed in the surrounding wells, and the development of precipitation lines can be taken as a rough measure of antigen concentration. Alternatively, this form of analysis is very useful in determining the approximate precipitating titer of an antiserum by simply reversing the location of antigen and antibody in the pattern (Fig 18–4).

Single Radial Diffusion

Double immunodiffusion is only semiquantitative. In 1965, Mancini introduced a novel technique employing single diffusion for accurate quantitative determination of antigens. This technique grew out of the simple linear diffusion technique of Oudin by means of the incorporation of specific antibody into the agar plate. Radial diffusion is based on the principle that a quantitative relationship exists between the amount of antigen placed in a well cut in the agar-antibody plate and the resulting ring of precipitation. The technique is performed as diagrammed in Fig 18–5.

In the method described originally by Mancini, the *area* circumscribed by the precipitation ring was proportionate to the antigen concentration. This end point method requires that the precipitation rings reach the maximal possible size, which often requires 48–72 hours of diffusion. Alternatively, the single radial diffusion method of Fahey allows measurement of the rings prior to full development. In this modification, the logarithm of the antigen concentration is proportionate to the *diameter* of the ring.

A standard curve is experimentally determined with known antigen standards, and the equation that describes this curve can then be used for the determination of antigen concentration corresponding to any diameter size (Fig 18–6). The sensitivity of these methods is in the range of 1–3 μg/mL of antigen.

An important clinical application of single radial diffusion is in the measurement of serum proteins—for example, immunoglobulin concentrations. A monospecific antiserum directed only at Fc or H chain determinants of the immunoglobulin molecule must be incorporated into the agar to determine immunoglobulin concentrations, since L (light) chain determinants are shared among immunoglobulin classes. Owing to the relatively low concentrations of IgD and IgE in human serum, this technique is used primarily to determine the other 3 immunoglo-

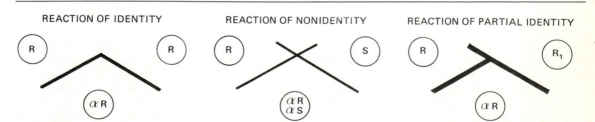

Figure 18–3. Reaction patterns in angular double immunodiffusion (Ouchterlony). R = antigen R, S = antigen S, R_1 = antigen R_1, αR = antibody to R, αS = antibody to S. Reaction of identity: Precisely similar precipitin lines have formed in the reaction of R with αR. Note that the lines intersect at a point. Reaction of nonidentity: Precipitin lines completely cross owing to separate interaction of αR with R and αS with S when R and S are non-cross-reacting antigens. Reaction of partial identity: αR reacts with both R and R_1 but forms lines that do not form a complete cross. Antigenic determinants are *partially* shared between R and R_1.

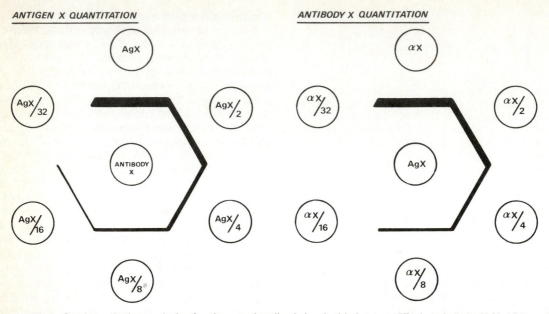

ANTIGEN X QUANTITATION

ANTIBODY X QUANTITATION

Figure 18–4. Semiquantitative analysis of antigen and antibody by double immunodiffusion. Antigen X (AgX) is serially diluted and placed circumferentially in wells surrounding the central well containing antibody against antigen X. Precipitin lines form with decreasing thickness until no longer visible at dilution of 1:32 of antigen X. On the right, a similar pattern is generated but with serial 2-fold dilutions of antibody X (αX). Formation of a single precipitin line indicates that a single antigen-antibody reaction has occurred.

bulin classes, IgG, IgA, and IgM. However, by decreasing the amount of specific anti-immunoglobulin antiserum placed in the agar, so-called "low-level" plates can be produced that have increased sensitivity for detection of reduced levels of serum immunoglobulins (IgG, IgA, IgM, and IgD).

There are a number of common pitfalls in the interpretation of single radial diffusion tests for immunoglobulin quantitation: (1) Polymeric forms of immunoglobulin such as occur in multiple myeloma or Waldenström's macroglobulinemia diffuse more slowly than native monomers, resulting in underestimation of immunoglobulin concentrations in these diseases. (2) High-molecular-weight immune complexes that may circulate in cryoglobulinemia or rheumatoid arthritis will result in falsely low values by a similar mechanism. (3) Low-molecular-weight forms such as 7S IgM in sera of patients with macroglobulinemia, systemic lupus erythematosus, rheumatoid arthritis, and ataxia-telangiectasia may give falsely high values. This phenomenon results from the fact that monomeric IgM diffuses more rapidly than the pentameric IgM parent molecule, which is used as the standard. (4) Reversed precipitation may occur in situations where the test human serum contains anti-immunoglobulin antibodies. In such a circumstance, diffusion and precipitation occur in 2 directions simultaneously and may result in falsely high values. This phenomenon has been well documented in the case of subjects with IgA deficiency

who have antibodies to ruminant proteins. These proteins cross the IgA-deficient intestinal mucosa, thereby gaining access to lymphatic tissues and stimulating anti-IgA responses. The problem of IgA quantitation in this circumstance can be avoided by using anti-immunoglobulin from rabbits (ie, a nonruminant species).

APPLICATIONS: SERUM IMMUNOGLOBULIN LEVELS IN HEALTH & DISEASE

Serum immunoglobulin levels are dependent on a variety of developmental, genetic, and environmental factors. These include ethnic background, age, sex, history of allergies or recurrent infections, and geographic factors (eg, endemic infestation with parasites results in elevated IgE levels). The patient's age is especially important in the interpretation of immunoglobulin levels. Normal human infants are born with very low levels of serum immunoglobulins that they have synthesized; the entire IgG portion of cord serum has been transferred transplacentally from the mother (Fig 18–7). If an infection occurs in utero, cord IgM and IgA are elevated. After birth, maternal IgG decays, resulting in a falling serum IgG level. This trend is reversed with the onset of significant autologous IgG synthesis. There is a gradual and progressive increase in IgG, IgA, and

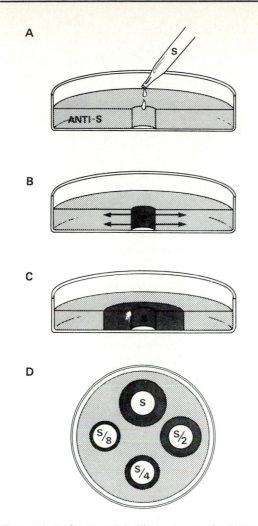

Figure 18–5. Single radial diffusion in agar (radial immunodiffusion). **A:** Petri dish is filled with semisolid agar solution containing antibody to antigen S. After agar hardens, the center well is filled with a precisely measured amount of material containing antigen S. **B:** Antigen S is allowed to diffuse radially from the center well for 24–48 hours. **C:** Where antigen S meets corresponding antibody to S in the agar, precipitation results. After reaction proceeds to completion or at a timed interval, a sharp border or a ring is formed. **D:** By serial dilution of a known standard quantity of antigen S—S/1, S/2, S/4, S/8—rings of progressively decreasing size are formed. The amount of antigen S in unknown specimens can be calculated and compared with standard in the timed interval (Fahey) method (Fig 18–6).

rum IgD concentrations have not clearly been associated with specific disease states. In fact, this immunoglobulin is the major B cell receptor for antigens and plays only a minor role as a circulating antibody. IgE levels, on the other hand, are useful in differential diagnosis of allergic, parasitic, and rare immunodeficiency states. Measurement of serum IgE levels requires sensitive methods such as RIA or enzyme-linked immunoassay. Measurement of serum IgG levels is particularly valuable in diagnosis and in monitoring immunoglobulin replacement in hypogamma-globulinemic patients.

Individual changes in serum immunoglobulins have been recorded in many diseases. A partial list of the instances of quantitative abnormalities in immunoglobulins is listed (Table 18–2). For a detailed discussion of immunoglobulin disorders, the reader is referred to Chapters 24 and 26, as well as other chapters in the Clinical section of this volume.

ELECTROPHORESIS & IMMUNOELECTROPHORESIS

Analysis of the heterogeneity in human serum proteins can be readily accomplished by electrophoresis. The separation of proteins in an electrical field was

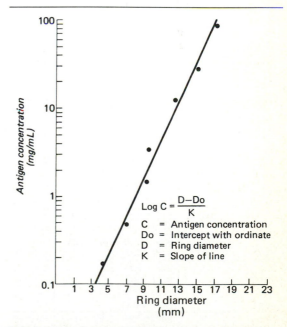

$$\text{Log } C = \frac{D - D_o}{K}$$

C = Antigen concentration
Do = Intercept with ordinate
D = Ring diameter
K = Slope of line

Figure 18–6. Standard curve for single radial diffusion. Relationship between ring diameter and antigen concentration is described by the line constructed from known amounts of antigen (Fig 18–5). Equation and curve for timed interval (Fahey) method.

IgM levels until late adolescence, when nearly normal adult levels are achieved (Fig 18–8). Furthermore, it is clear that there is a great deal of variability in immunoglobulin levels in the healthy population (Fig 18–8 and Table 18–1).

In routine practice, only IgG, IgA, IgM, and IgE levels are ordinarily measured. Abnormalities of se-

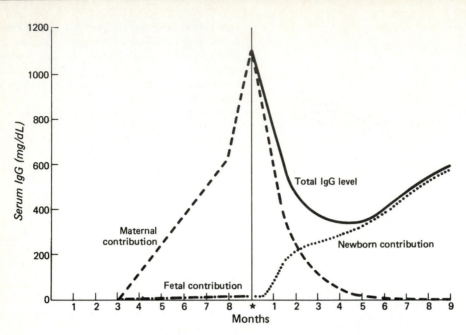

Figure 18–7. Development of IgG levels with age. Relationship of development of normal serum levels of IgG during fetal and newborn stages and maternal contribution. (Modified from Allansmith M et al: *J Pediatr* 1968;**72**:289.)

Table 18–1. Examples of levels of immune globulins in serum of normal subjects at different ages.[1]

Age	Number of Subjects	Level of IgG[2]		Level of IgM[2]		Level of IgA[2]		Level of Total γ-Globulin[2]	
		mg/dL (Range)	% of Adult Level	mg/dL (Range)	% of Adult Level	mg/dL (Range)	% of Adult Level	mg/dL (Range)	% of Adult Level
Newborn	22	1031 ± 200 (645–1244)	89 ± 17	11 ± 5 (5–30)	11 ± 5	2 ± 3 (0–11)	1 ± 2	1044 ± 201 (660–1439)	67 ± 13
1–3 months	29	430 ± 119 (272–762)	37 ± 10	30 ± 11 (16–67)	30 ± 11	21 ± 13 (6–56)	11 ± 7	481 ± 127 (324–699)	31 ± 9
4–6 months	33	427 ± 186 (206–1125)	37 ± 16	43 ± 17 (10–83)	43 ± 17	28 ± 18 (8–93)	14 ± 9	498 ± 204 (228–1232)	32 ± 13
7–12 months	56	661 ± 219 (279–1533)	58 ± 19	54 ± 23 (22–147)	55 ± 23	37 ± 18 (16–98)	19 ± 9	752 ± 242 (327–1687)	48 ± 15
13–24 months	59	762 ± 209 (258–1393)	66 ± 18	58 ± 23 (14–114)	59 ± 23	50 ± 24 (19–119)	25 ± 12	870 ± 258 (398–1586)	56 ± 16
25–36 months	33	892 ± 183 (419–1274)	77 ± 16	61 ± 19 (28–113)	62 ± 19	71 ± 37 (19–235)	36 ± 19	1024 ± 205 (499–1418)	65 ± 14
3–5 years	28	929 ± 228 (569–1597)	80 ± 20	56 ± 18 (22–100)	57 ± 18	93 ± 27 (55–152)	47 ± 14	1078 ± 245 (730–1771)	69 ± 17
6–8 years	18	923 ± 256 (559–1492)	80 ± 22	65 ± 25 (27–118)	66 ± 25	124 ± 45 (54–221)	62 ± 23	1112 ± 293 (640–1725)	71 ± 20
9–11 years	9	1124 ± 235 (779–1456)	97 ± 20	79 ± 33 (35–132)	80 ± 33	131 ± 60 (12–208)	66 ± 30	1334 ± 254 (966–1639)	85 ± 17
12–16 years	9	946 ± 124 (726–1085)	82 ± 11	59 ± 20 (35–72)	60 ± 20	148 ± 63 (70–229)	74 ± 32	1153 ± 169 (833–1284)	74 ± 12
Adults	30	1158 ± 305 (569–1919)	100 ± 26	99 ± 27 (47–147)	100 ± 27	200 ± 61 (61–330)	100 ± 31	1457 ± 353 (730–2365)	100 ± 24

[1]Reproduced, with permission, from Stiehm ER, Fudenberg HH: *Pediatrics* 1966;**37**:717.
[2]Mean ± 1 SD.

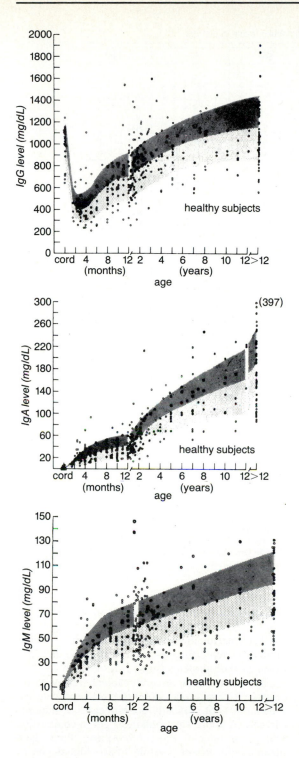

Figure 18–8. An example of variation of healthy subjects' serum levels of IgG, IgA, and IgM with age. Scattergrams of levels of IgG, IgA, and IgM in healthy subjects. Shaded areas are = 1 SD of the mean; each point represents one subject. (Reproduced, with permission, from Stiehm ER, Fudenberg HH: *Pediatrics* 1966; **37:**718.)

perfected in 1937 by Tiselius, who used free or moving boundary electrophoresis. However, owing to the relative complexity of this method, zone electrophoresis in a stabilizing medium such as paper or cellulose acetate has replaced free electrophoresis for clinical use.

In 1952, a 2-stage method was reported that combined electrophoresis with immunodiffusion for the detection of tetanus toxoid by antiserum. Shortly thereafter, the now classic method of immunoelectrophoresis was introduced by Williams and Grabar and by Poulik. In this technique, both electrophoresis and double immunodiffusion are performed on the same agar-coated slide. Immunoelectrophoresis has become an important tool for clinical paraprotein analysis as well as a standard method for immunochemical analysis of a wide variety of proteins. More recently, immunofixation electrophoresis and electroimmunodiffusion methods have been introduced. Various electrophoretic methods and examples of their uses in clinical immunodiagnosis are described in the following paragraphs.

ZONE ELECTROPHORESIS

Proteins are separated in zone electrophoresis almost exclusively on the basis of their surface charge (Fig 18–9). The supporting medium is theoretically inert and does not impede or enhance the flow of molecules in the electrical field. Generally, paper, agarose, or cellulose acetate strips are employed as supporting media. However, a major advantage of cellulose acetate is the speed of completion of electrophoretic migration (ie, 60–90 minutes compared with hours for paper). Additionally, cellulose acetate is optically clear; microquantities of proteins may be applied; and it is adaptable to histochemical staining procedures. For these reasons, cellulose acetate or agarose is preferred as the supporting medium for clinical zone electrophoresis.

In the technique itself, serum or other biologic fluid samples are placed at the origin and separated by electrophoresis for about 90 minutes, using alkaline buffer solutions. The strips are then stained for protein and scanned in a densitometer. In the densitometer, the stained strip is passed through a light beam. Variable absorption due to different serum protein concentrations is detected by a photoelectric cell and reproduced by an analog recorder as a tracing (Fig 18–9). Scanning converts the band pattern into peaks and allows for quantitation of the major peaks. Normal human serum is separated into 5 major electrophoretic bands, ie, albumin, α_1-globulin, α_2-globulin, β-globulin, and γ-globulin, by this method.

Applications

Zone electrophoresis is useful in the diagnosis of

Table 18–2. Serum immunoglobulin levels in disease.[1]

Diseases	IgG	IgA	IgM
Immunodeficiency disorders			
Combined immunodeficiency	↓↓↔↓↓↓	↓↓↔↓↓↓	↓↓↔↓↓↓
X-linked hypogammaglobulinemia	↓↓↔↓↓↓	↓↓↔↓↓↓	↓↓↔↓↓↓
Common variable immunodeficiency	↓↔↓↓↓	↓↔↓↓↓	↓↔↓↓↓
Selective IgA deficiency	N	↓↓↓	N
Protein-losing gastroenteropathies	N↔↓↓↓	N↔↓↓↓	N↔↓↓↓
Acute thermal burns	N↔↓↓↓	N↔↓↓↓	N↔↓↓↓
Nephrotic syndrome	N↔↓↓↓	N↔↓↓↓	N↔↓↓↓
Monoclonal gammopathies (MG)			
IgG (eg, G-myeloma)	N↔↑↑↑	N↔↓↓↓	N↔↓↓↓
IgA (eg, A-myeloma)	N↔↓↓↓	N↔↑↑↑	N↔↓↓↓
IgM (eg, M-macroglobulinemia)	N↔↓↓↓	N↔↓↓↓	N↔↑↑↑
L chain disease (ie, Bence Jones myeloma)	N↔↓↓↓	N↔↓↓↓	N↔↓↓↓
Chronic lymphocytic leukemia	N↔↓↓↓	N↔↓↓↓	N↔↓↓↓
Infections			
Infectious mononucleosis	↑↔↑↑	N↔↑	↑↔↑↑
AIDS	↑↑	↑↑	↑↑
Subacute bacterial endocarditis	↑↔↑↑	↓↔N	↑↔↑↑
Tuberculosis	↑↔↑↑	N↔↑↑↑	↓↔N
Actinomycosis	↑↑↑	↑↑	↑↑↑
Deep fungus diseases	N	N↔↑	N
Bartonellosis	↑	↓↔N	↑↑↔↑↑↑
Liver diseases			
Infectious hepatitis	↑↔↑↑	N↔↑	N↔↑↑
Laennec's cirrhosis	↑↔↑↑↑	↑↔↑↑↑	N↔↑↑
Biliary cirrhosis	N	N	↑↔↑↑
Chronic active hepatitis	↑↑↑	↑	N↔↑↑
Collagen disorders			
Lupus erythematosus	↑↔↑↑	N↔↑	N↔↑↑
Rheumatoid arthritis	N↔↑↑↑	↑↔↑↑↑	N↔↑↑
Sjögren's syndrome	N↔↑	N↔↑	N↔↑↑
Scleroderma	N↔↑	N	N↔↑
Miscellaneous			
Sarcoidosis	N↔↑↑	N↔↑↑	N↔↑
Hodgkin's disease	↓↔↑↑	↓↔↑	↓↔↑↑
Monocytic leukemia	N↔↑	N↔↑	N↔↑↑
Cystic fibrosis	↑↔↑↑	↑↔↑↑	N↔↑↑

N = normal, ↑ = slight increase, ↑↑ = moderate increase, ↑↑↑ = marked increase, ↓ = slight decrease, ↓↓ = moderate decrease, ↓↓↓ = marked decrease, ↔ = range.

[1]Modified and reproduced, with permission, from Ritzmann SE, Daniels JC (editors): *Serum Protein Abnormalities: Diagnostic and Clinical Aspects.* Little, Brown, 1975.

human paraprotein disorders such as multiple myeloma and Waldenström's macroglobulinemia (Fig 18–10). In these disorders, an electrophoretically restricted protein spike usually occurs in the γ-globulin region of the electrophoretogram. Since in zone electrophoresis the trailing edge of immunoglobulins extends into the β region and occasionally the α region, spikes in these regions are also consistent with paraproteinemic disorders involving immunoglobulins.

A marked decrease in serum γ-globulin concentration such as occurs in hypogammaglobulinemia can sometimes be detected with this technique (Fig 18–10). Reduction in IgA or IgM to very low levels cannot be detected by this method, since they represent such a relatively small fraction of total serum immunoglobulins. Free light chains are readily detectable in urine when present in increased amounts

such as in Bence Jones proteinuria of myeloma (Fig 18–11). Zone electrophoresis in agarose gels has also been useful in the diagnosis of certain central nervous system diseases with alterations in cerebrospinal fluid proteins (Fig 18–12 and Fig 43–3).

Oligoclonal bands in cerebrospinal fluid with restricted electrophoretic mobility have been detected in about 90% of clinically definite cases of multiple sclerosis. Agarose electrophoresis gel in conjunction with measurement of cerebrospinal fluid IgG/albumin ratios makes possible a fairly high degree of specificity for diagnosis of multiple sclerosis (see Chapter 43 and Fig 43–3).

Abnormalities in serum proteins other than immunoglobulins may also be detected by serum protein electrophoresis. Hypoproteinemia involving all serum fractions occurs during excessive protein loss, usually in the gastrointestinal tract. Reduction in al-

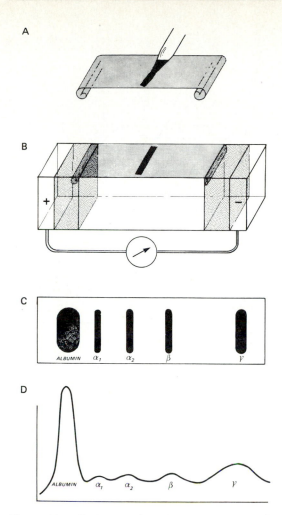

Figure 18–9. Technique of cellulose acetate zone electrophoresis. **A:** Small amount of serum or other fluid is applied to cellulose acetate strip. **B:** Electrophoresis of sample in electrolyte buffer is performed. **C:** Separated protein bands are visualized in characteristic position after being stained. **D:** Densitometer scanning from cellulose acetate strip converts bands to characteristic peaks of albumin, α_1-globulin, α_2-globulin, β-globulin, and γ-globulin.

bumin alone commonly occurs in many diseases of the liver, kidneys, or gastrointestinal tract or with severe burns. α_1-globulin decrease may indicate α_1-antitrypsin deficiency, and an increase reflects acute phase reactions occurring in many inflammatory and neoplastic disorders. Increase in α_2-globulins usually reflects the nephrotic syndrome or hemolysis with increased hemoglobin-haptoglobin in the serum. Because of its relative insensitivity, zone electrophoresis is almost always a presumptive screening test for serum protein abnormalities. Specific quantitative biochemical or immunologic tests must be performed to definitively identify the particular protein.

IMMUNOELECTROPHORESIS

Immunoelectrophoresis combines electrophoretic separation, diffusion, and immune precipitation of proteins. Both identification and approximate quantitation can thereby be accomplished for individual proteins present in serum, urine, or other biologic fluid.

In this technique (Fig 18–13), a glass slide is covered with molten agar or agarose in an alkaline buffer solution. An antigen well and antibody trough are cut with a template cutting device. The serum sample (antigen) is placed in the antigen well and is separated in an electrical field with a potential difference of approximately 3.3 V/cm for 30–60 minutes. Antiserum is then placed in the trough, and both serum and antibodies are allowed to diffuse for 18–24 hours. The resulting precipitation lines may then be photographed or the slide washed, dried, and stained for a permanent record.

A comparison of the relationship of precipitation lines developed in normal serum by immunoelectrophoresis and zone electrophoresis is shown in Fig 18–14.

Applications

In the laboratory diagnosis of paraproteinemias, the results of zone electrophoresis and immunoelectrophoresis should be combined. The presence of a sharp increase or spike in the γ-globulin region on zone electrophoresis strongly suggests the presence of a monoclonal paraprotein. However, it is necessary to perform immunoelectrophoresis to determine the exact H chain class and L chain type of the paraprotein. Several examples of the use of immunoelectrophoresis in demonstrating the identity of human serum paraproteins are shown in Fig 18–15.

Immunoelectrophoresis distinguishes polyclonal from monoclonal increases in γ-globulin (Fig 18–15). Additionally, decreased or absent immunoglobulins observed in various immune deficiency disorders can be analyzed with this technique. However, a further quantitative analysis such as single radial diffusion, nephelometry, or radioimmunoassay should be performed for measurement of immunoglobulin levels.

Immunoelectrophoresis can be used to identify L chains in the urine of patients with plasma cell dyscrasias or autoimmune disorders. Thus, with specific anti-κ and anti-λ antisera, the monoclonal nature of Bence Jones protein in myeloma can be confirmed.

Antisera to "free light chains" (κ or λ) obtained from urine of myeloma patients may occasionally reveal antigenic determinants not present on chains "bound" to chains. In H chain diseases, fragments of the immunoglobulin H chain are present in increased amounts in the serum (see Chapter 48). It was by careful analysis of immunoelectrophoretic patterns that Franklin initially discovered the existence of this rare but extremely interesting group of

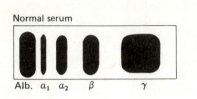

Normal serum

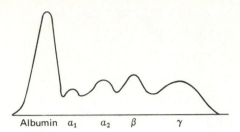

Alb. a_1 a_2 β γ

Albumin a_1 a_2 β γ

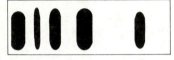

IgG myeloma with γ spike
and reduced albumin

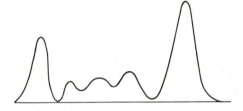

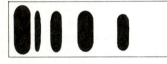

Waldenström's macroglob-
ulinemia with IgM spike

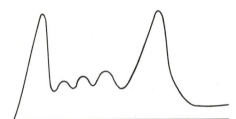

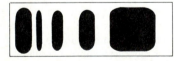

Polyclonal hypergammaglobulinemia

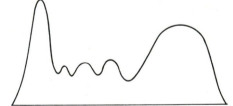

Hypogammaglobulinemia

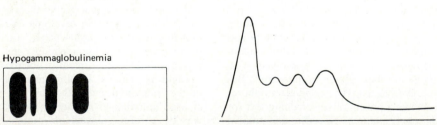

Figure 18–10. Zone electrophoresis patterns of serum immunoglobulin abnormalities in various diseases.

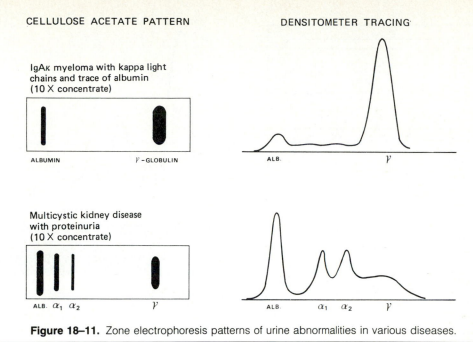

Figure 18–11. Zone electrophoresis patterns of urine abnormalities in various diseases.

disorders. Immunoelectrophoresis is also helpful in identifying increased amounts of proteins present in the cerebrospinal fluid in patients with various neurologic diseases.

Immunofixation Electrophoresis

This technique involves separation of proteins electrophoretically in a gel, followed by immunoprecipitation in situ with monospecific antisera

(Fig 18–16). Nonprecipitated proteins are removed by washing and the immunoprecipitation bands revealed with a protein stain. This method has been employed clinically to identify C3 conversion products and to identify paraproteins. The latter is especially helpful for low-level IgM or IgA components, which may be buried in an excess of normal IgG. There are several modifications of this basic method, such as overlay with radioactive or enzyme-linked

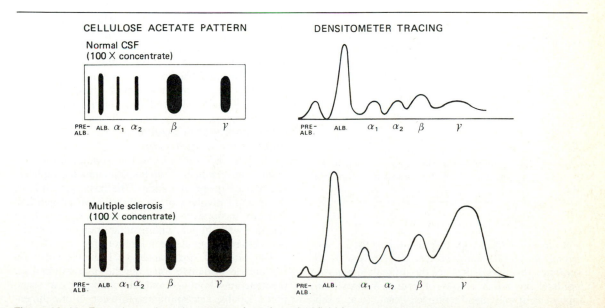

Figure 18–12. Zone electrophoresis patterns of cerebrospinal fluid from normal subject and multiple sclerosis patient.

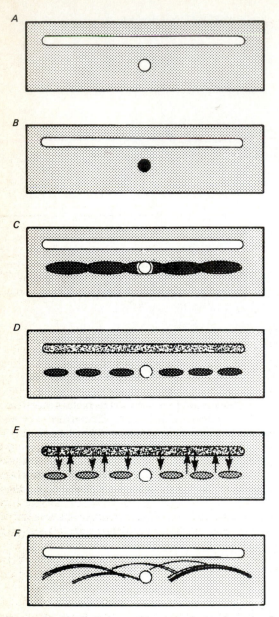

Figure 18–13. Technique of immunoelectrophoresis. **A:** Semisolid agar poured onto glass slide and antigen well and antiserum trough cut out of agar. **B:** Antigen well filled with human serum. **C:** Serum separated by electrophoresis. **D:** Antiserum trough filled with antiserum to whole human serum. **E:** Serum and antiserum diffuse into agar. **F:** Precipitin lines form for individual serum proteins.

antibodies that markedly increase the method's sensitivity. In clinical laboratories, its main use is for resolution of serum proteins in difficult diagnostic problems in which results of routine methods are equivocal. It may also be utilized generally as a substitute for immunoelectrophoresis.

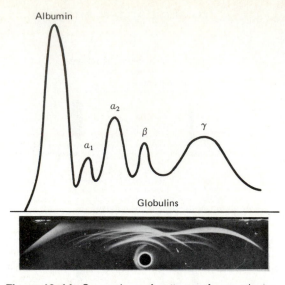

Figure 18–14. Comparison of patterns of zone electrophoresis and immunoelectrophoresis of normal human serum.

ELECTROIMMUNODIFFUSION

In immunodiffusion techniques described earlier in this chapter, antigen and antibody are allowed to come into contact and to precipitate in agar purely by diffusion. However, the chance of antigen and antibody meeting—and thus the speed of development of a precipitin line—can be greatly enhanced by electrically driving the 2 together. The technique of electroimmunodiffusion is useful in the serologic diagnosis of infectious diseases by serum **antigen** detection. Although numerous variations have been described coupling electrophoresis with diffusion, only 2 have as yet achieved any degree of clinical applicability. These are **one-dimensional double electroimmunodiffusion** (counterimmunoelectrophoresis) and **one-dimensional single electroimmunodiffusion** (Laurell's rocket electrophoresis).

One-Dimensional Double Electroimmunodiffusion

This method is also known as countercurrent immunoelectrophoresis, counterimmunoelectrophoresis, and electroprecipitation. The basic principle of the method involves electrophoresis of antigen and antibody in opposite directions simultaneously from separate wells in gel, with resultant precipitation at a point intermediate between their origins (Fig 18–17).

The principal disadvantages of double diffusion without electromotive force are the time required for precipitation (24 hours) and the relative lack of sensitivity. Double electroimmunodiffusion in one dimension can produce visible precipitin lines within 30 minutes and is approximately 10 times more sensitive than standard double diffusion techniques. However, this technique is only semiquantitative. Some of the antigens and antibodies detected by double electroimmunodiffusion are listed in Table 18–3.

One-Dimensional Single Electroimmunodiffusion

This method is also known as "rocket electrophoresis" or the Laurell technique. The principal application of this technique has been to quantitate antigens other than immunoglobulins. In this technique, antiserum to the particular antigen or antigens one wishes to quantitate is incorporated into an agarose supporting medium on a glass slide in a fixed position so antibody does not migrate. The specimen containing an unknown quantity of the antigen is placed in a small well. Electrophoresis of the antigen into the antibody-containing agarose is then performed. The resultant pattern of immunoprecipitation resembles a spike or rocket—thus the term rocket electrophoresis (Fig 18–18).

This pattern occurs because precipitation occurs along the lateral margins of the moving boundary of antigen as the antigen is driven into the agar containing the antibody. Gradually, as antigen is lost through precipitation, its concentration at the leading edge diminishes and the lateral margins converge to form a sharp point. The total distance of antigen migration for a given antiserum concentration is linearly proportionate to the antigen concentration. The sensitivity of this technique is approximately 0.5 μg/mL for proteins. Unfortunately, the weak negative charge of immunoglobulins prevents their electrophoretic mobility in this system unless special electrolytes and agar are employed. Several commercial systems are available for quantitating serum immunoglobulins and complement components with this technique.

IMMUNOCHEMICAL & PHYSICOCHEMICAL METHODS

Evaluation of serum protein disorders can usually be effectively accomplished by immunodiffusion and electrophoretic methods. Occasionally, more detailed study of immunologically relevant serum constituents is necessary. In this section, a number of the more complex immunochemical and physicochemical techniques are described that have proved to be important adjuncts in the characterization of serum protein and other disorders. These techniques may be available in the clinical laboratory and include column chromatography, measurement of se-

Table 18–3. Examples of clinical applications of double electroimmunodiffusion.

Cryptococcus-specific antigen in cerebrospinal fluid
Meningococcus-specific antigen in cerebrospinal fluid
Haemophilus-specific antigen in cerebrospinal fluid
Fibrinogen
Cord IgM in intrauterine infection
Carcinoembryonic antigen (CEA)
α_1-Fetoprotein
Fungal precipitins

rum viscosity, and methods to detect cryoglobulins, pyroglobulins, and immune complexes.

COLUMN CHROMATOGRAPHY

Chromatographic techniques are currently the most widely used methods for protein fractionation and isolation of immunoglobulins. In these techniques, a sample is layered on the top of a glass cylinder or column filled with a synthetic gel and is allowed to flow through the gel. The physical characteristics of protein molecules result in retention in the gel matrix to differing degrees, and subsequent elution under appropriate conditions permits protein separation.

Ion Exchange Chromatography

Ion exchange chromatography separates proteins by taking advantage of differences in their electrical charges. The functional unit of the gel is a charged group absorbed on an insoluble backbone such as cellulose, cross-linked dextran, agarose, or acrylic copolymers. Diethylaminoethyl (DEAE), a positively charged group, is the functional unit of anion exchangers used for fractionation of negatively charged molecules (Fig 18–19). Carboxymethyl (CM), negatively charged, is the functional unit of cation exchangers used for fractionation of positively charged molecules. Changing the pH of the buffer passing through the column affects the charge of the protein molecule. Increasing the molarity of the buffer provides more ions to compete with the protein for binding to the gel. By gradually increasing the molarity or decreasing the pH of the elution buffer, the proteins are eluted in order of increasing number of charged groups bound to the gel. DEAE-cellulose chromatography is an excellent technique for isolation of IgG, which can be obtained nearly free of all other serum proteins.

Gel Filtration

Gel filtration separates molecules according to their size. The gel is made of porous dextran beads. Protein molecules larger than the largest pores of the beads cannot penetrate the gel pores. Thus, they pass through the gel in the liquid phase outside the beads

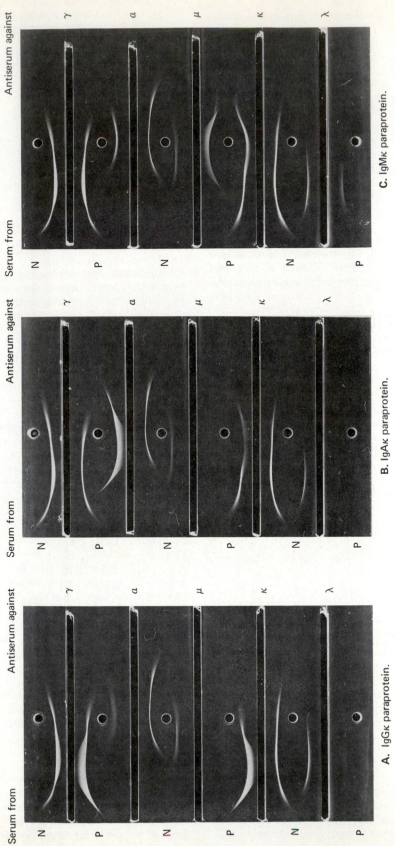

Serum from   Antiserum against

A. IgGκ paraprotein.

B. IgAκ paraprotein.

C. IgMκ paraprotein.

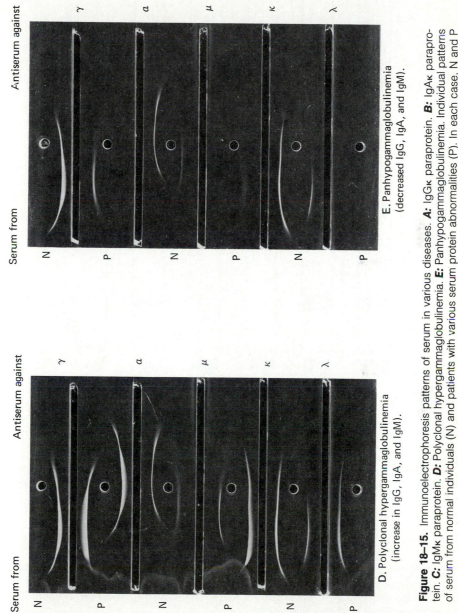

Figure 18–15. Immunoelectrophoresis patterns of serum in various diseases. *A:* IgGκ paraprotein. *B:* IgAκ paraprotein. *C:* IgMκ paraprotein. *D:* Polyclonal hypergammaglobulinemia. *E:* Panhypogammaglobulinemia. Individual patterns of serum from normal individuals (N) and patients with various serum protein abnormalities (P). In each case, N and P sera are reacted against antisera which are monospecific for γ, α, and μ heavy chains and κ and λ light chains.

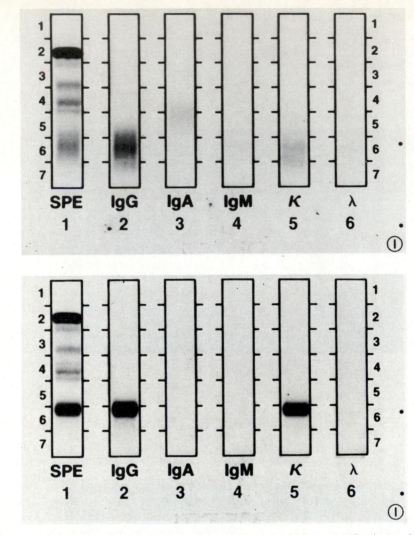

Figure 18–16. Immunofixation electrophoresis. **A:** Normal serum pattern. In lane 1 antibody to whole serum has detected normal serum proteins. In lanes 2–6 specific antibody to various light and heavy chains has detected the polyclonal immunoglobulins present in normal serum. The faint patterns for IgA, IgM, and κ reflect the relatively low concentrations of those molecules. **B:** IgG kappa paraprotein detected in serum from a patient with multiple myeloma. Note the very heavy IgG and kappa bands, which share the same position on the electropherogram. There is a reduction in other immunoglobulins, but other serum proteins are easily seen in lane 1.

and are eluted first. Smaller molecules penetrate the beads to varying extents depending on their size and shape. Solute molecules within the gel beads maintain a concentration equilibrium with solute in the liquid phase outside the beads; thus, a particular molecular species moves as a band through the column. Molecules therefore appear in the column effluent in order of decreasing size (Fig 18–20).

IgM can be easily separated from other serum immunoglobulins by gel filtration. Fig 18–21 shows the separation of the IgM and the IgG components of a mixed IgM-IgG cryoglobulin. Gel filtration is widely used also to separate H and L chains of immunoglobulins or to isolate pure Bence Jones proteins from the urine of patients with multiple myeloma.

Affinity Chromatography

Affinity chromatography uses specific and reversible biologic interaction between the gel material and the substance to be isolated. The specificity of the binding properties is obtained by covalent coupling of an appropriate ligand to an insoluble matrix, such as agarose or dextran beads. The gel so obtained is able to absorb from a mixed solution the substance

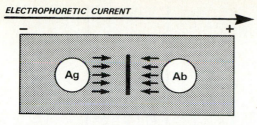

Figure 18–17. Double electroimmunodiffusion in one dimension. Antigen and antibody are placed in well and driven together with an electric current. A precipitin line forms within a few hours after beginning electrophoresis.

to be isolated. After unbound substances have been washed out of the column, the purified compound can be recovered by changing the experimental conditions, such as pH or ionic strength.

Antigen-antibody binding is one of the reactions that can be applied to affinity chromatography. When the gel material is coupled to an antigen, a specific antibody can be purified. Alternatively, when a highly purified antibody can be coupled to the gel, the corresponding antigen can be isolated.

Protein A is a protein isolated from the cell wall of some strains of *Staphylococcus aureus* that specifically reacts with IgG molecules of subclasses 1, 2, and 4. It is used as a specific ligand for isolation of IgG or for isolation of IgG3 from a mixture of IgG molecules of all subclasses.

Cell separation can also be achieved by affinity chromatography. Subpopulations of T and B lymphocytes have been defined by characteristic surface markers (see Chapters 5 and 19) that can react with specific ligands. For example, B cells that bear surface immunoglobulins can be separated on an anti-immunoglobulin column. Immunoglobulin-positive cells are retained on the gel, and desorption is achieved by running through the column a solution of immunoglobulins that compete with the cells.

SERUM VISCOSITY

The measurement of serum viscosity is a simple and valuable tool in evaluation of patients with paraproteinemia. Normally, the formed elements of the blood contribute more significantly to whole blood viscosity than do plasma proteins. However, in diseases with elevated concentrations of serum proteins, particularly the immunoglobulins, the serum viscosity may reach very high levels and result in a characteristic symptom complex—the hyperviscosity syndrome. Serum viscosity is determined by a variety of factors including protein concentration; the size, shape, and deformability of serum molecules; and the hydrostatic state (solvation), molecular charge, and temperature sensitivity of proteins.

In clinical practice, serum viscosity is measured in an Ostwald viscosimeter. A few milliliters of serum are warmed to 37 °C and allowed to descend through a narrow bore capillary tube immersed in a water bath at 37 °C. The rate of descent between calibrated marks on the capillary tube is recorded. The same procedure is repeated using distilled water. The relative serum viscosity is then calculated according to the following formula:

$$\text{Relative serum viscosity} = \frac{\text{Rate of descent of serum sample (in seconds)}}{\text{Rate of descent of distilled water (in seconds)}}$$

Normal values for serum viscosity range from approximately 1.4 to 1.9. Similar measurements can be performed with plasma instead of serum. However, fibrinogen present in plasma is a major determinant of plasma viscosity, and variations in this protein, especially in the presence of nonspecific inflammatory states, can markedly affect the results. For this reason, measurement of serum viscosity is preferred.

Serum viscosity measurements are primarily of use in evaluating patients with Waldenström's macroglobulinemia, multiple myeloma, and cryoglobulinemia. In myeloma, aggregation or polymerization of the paraprotein in vivo often results in hyperviscosity. In general, there is a correlation between increased serum viscosity and increased plasma volume. However, the correlation between levels of relative serum viscosity and clinical symptoms is not

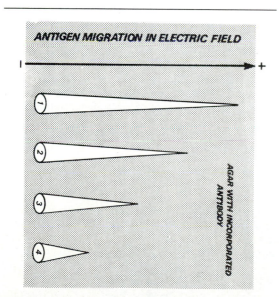

Figure 18–18. Single electroimmunodiffusion in one dimension (rocket electrophoresis. Laurell technique). Antigen is placed in wells numbered 1–4 in progressively decreasing amounts. Electrophoresis is performed and antigen is driven into antibody-containing agar. Precipitin pattern forms in the shape of a "rocket." Amount of antigen is directly proportionate to the length of the rocket.

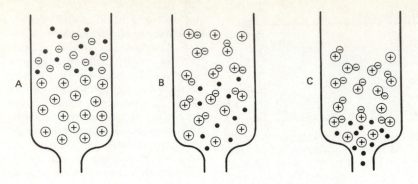

Figure 18–19. Principles of ion exchange chromatography. Three stages of protein separation by ion exchange chromatography are shown: **A:** The column bed is made up of a matrix of positively charged cellulose beads ⊕. **B:** The negatively charged molecules ⊖ in the protein mixture bind to the column and are retained. **C:** The neutral molecules ● pass between the charged particles and are eluted.

nearly as direct. Increased serum viscosity may interfere with various laboratory tests that employ flow-through devices such as Coulter counters and Technicon analyzers in clinical chemistry. Examples of disorders with increased serum viscosity are listed in Table 18–4.

CRYOGLOBULINS

Precipitation of serum immunoglobulins in the cold was first observed in a patient with multiple myeloma. The term "cryoglobulin" was introduced to designate a group of proteins which had the common property of forming a precipitate or a gel in the cold. This phenomenon was reversible by raising the temperature. Since those initial descriptions, cryoglobulins have been found in a wide variety of clinical situations. Purification and immunochemical analysis have led to classification of this group of proteins (Table 18–5). Type I cryoglobulins consist of a single monoclonal immunoglobulin. Type II cryoglobulins are mixed cryoglobulins; they consist of a monoclonal immunoglobulin with antibody activity against a polyclonal immunoglobulin. Type III cryoglobulins are mixed polyclonal cryoglobulins, ie, one or more immunoglobulins are found, none of which are monoclonal.

Technical Procedure for Isolation & Analysis

Blood must be collected in a warm syringe and kept at 37 °C until it clots. Serum is separated by centrifugation at 37 °C and then stored at 4 °C. When a cryoglobulin is present, a white precipitate or a gel appears in the serum after a variable period, usually 24–72 hours. However, the serum should be observed for 1 week to make certain that unusually late cryoprecipitation does not go undetected. The reversibility of the cryoprecipitation should be tested by rewarming an aliquot of precipitated serum.

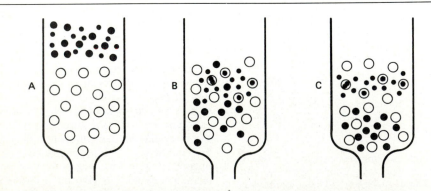

Figure 18–20. Principles of gel filtration chromatography. Three stages of protein separation by gel filtration are shown. A: Open circle ○ represents polymerized beads onto which a mixture of small ● and large ● protein molecules is layered. B: The molecules enter and pass through the column at different rates depending primarily on size and are separated by a simple sieving process. C: Larger molecules are eluted while smaller ones are retained.

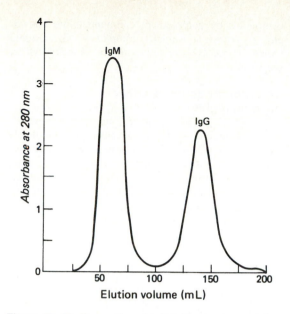

Figure 18–21. Separation of IgG-IgM mixed cryoglobulin by gel filtration. Two peaks are eluted from gel filtration column. The larger IgM molecules precede the smaller IgG molecules which were dissociated by dissolving the cryoprecipitate in an acidic buffer prior to application to the column. The absorbance at 280 nm measures relative amount of protein in various eluted fractions.

specific for γ, α, μ, κ, and λ chains. In this way, cryoglobulins can ordinarily be classified into the 3 types described above.

Clinical Significance

Type I and type II cryoglobulins are usually present in large amounts in serum (often more than 5 mg/mL). In general, they are present in patients with monoclonal paraproteinemias, eg, they are commonly found in patients with lymphoma or multiple myeloma. However, some are found in patients lacking any evidence of lymphoid malignancy, just as are "benign" paraproteins. Type III cryoglobulins indicate the presence of circulating immune complexes and are the result of immune responses to various antigens. They are present in relatively low concentrations (usually less than 1 mg/mL) in rheumatoid diseases and chronic infections (Table 18–5).

All types of cryoglobulins may be responsible for specific symptoms that occur as a result of changes in the cryoglobulin induced by exposure to cold. The symptoms include Raynaud's phenomenon, vascular purpura, bleeding tendencies, cold-induced urticaria, and even distal arterial thrombosis with gangrene.

Since type II and type III cryoglobulins are circulating soluble immune complexes, they may be associated with a serum sickness-like syndrome characterized by polyarthritis, vasculitis, glomerulonephritis, or neurologic symptoms. In patients with

The cryoprecipitate can be quantitated in several ways. Centrifugation of the whole serum in a hematocrit tube at 4 °C allows determination of the relative amount of cryoglobulin (cryocrit). Alternatively, the protein concentration of the serum may be compared before and after cryoprecipitation. The precipitate formed in an aliquot of serum may be isolated and dissolved in an acidic buffer and the cryoglobulin level estimated by the absorbance at 280 nm.

After isolation and washing of the precipitate, the components of the cryoglobulin are identified by immunoelectrophoresis or immunofixation electrophoresis. These analyses are performed at 37 °C, using antiserum to whole human serum and antisera

Table 18–4. Disorders with increased serum viscosity.

Waldenström's macroglobulinemia
Essential macroglobulinemia
Multiple myeloma
Cryoglobulinemia
Hypergammaglobulinemic purpura
Rheumatoid diseases associated with immune complexes or
    paraproteinemias
    Rheumatoid arthritis
    Sjögren's syndrome
    Systemic lupus erythematosus

Table 18–5. Classification of types of cryoglobulins and associated diseases.

Type of Cryoglobulin	Immuno-chemical Composition	Associated Diseases
Type 1 Monoclonal cryoglobulin	IgM IgG IgA Bence Jones protein	Myeloma, Waldenström's macroglobulinemia, chronic lymphocytic leukemia
Type II Mixed cryoglobulin	IgM-IgG IgG-IgG IgA-IgG	Myeloma, Waldenström's macroglobulinemia, chronic lymphocytic leukemia, rheumatoid arthritis, Sjögren's syndrome, mixed essential cryoglobulinemia
Type III Mixed polyclonal cryoglobulin	IgM-IgG IgM-IgG-IgA	Systemic lupus erythematosus, rheumatoid arthritis, Sjögren's syndrome, infectious mononucleosis, cytomegalovirus infections, acute viral hepatitis, chronic active hepatitis, primary biliary cirrhosis, poststreptococcal glomerulonephritis, infective endocarditis, leprosy, kala-azar, tropical splenomegaly syndrome

mixed essential IgM-IgG cryoglobulinemia, a rather distinctive syndrome may occur that is associated with arthralgias, purpura, weakness, and frequently lymphadenopathy or hepatosplenomegaly. This syndrome may be a sequela of hepatitis B infection. Glomerulonephritis is common. In some instances, it occurs in a rapidly progressive form and is of ominous prognostic significance.

Cryoglobulins may cause serious errors in a variety of laboratory tests by precipitating at ambient temperatures and thereby removing certain substances from serum. Complement fixation and inactivation and entrapment of immunoglobulins in the precipitate are common examples. Redissolving the cryoprecipitate usually does not fully restore activity to the serum, especially that of complement.

PYROGLOBULINS

Pyroglobulins are monoclonal immunoglobulins that precipitate irreversibly when heated to 56 °C. This phenomenon is different from the reversible thermoprecipitation of Bence Jones proteins and seems to be related to hydrophobic bonding between immunoglobulin molecules, possibly due to decreased polarity of the heavy chains. Pyroglobulins may be discovered incidentally when serum is heated to 56 °C to inactivate complement before routine serologic tests. Half of the cases involve patients with multiple myeloma. The remainder occur in macroglobulinemia and other lymphoproliferative disorders, systemic lupus erythematosus, and carcinoma and occasionally without known associated disease. They are not responsible for any particular symptom and have no known significance.

DETECTION OF IMMUNE COMPLEXES

The factors involved in deposition of immune complexes in tissues and production of tissue damage are discussed in Chapter 11. Subsequent chapters deal with the clinical manifestations of diseases associated with immune complexes, including rheumatic diseases (Chapter 36), hematologic diseases (Chapter 38), and renal diseases (Chapter 41). These clinical situations have in common the presence of detectable immune complexes in tissues or in the circulation.

Detection in Tissues

Immune complexes in tissues are detected by immunohistologic techniques using immunofluorescence or immunoperoxidase staining. The antisera used are specific for the immunoglobulin classes, complement components, or fibrin and, in selected cases, the suspected antigen.

Granular deposits of immunoglobulins usually ac-

companied by complement components are considered to represent immune complexes. The antigen moiety is rarely detected, since it is unknown in most cases.

Detection in Serum & Other Biologic Fluids

The presence of circulating immune complexes can be indirectly inferred when complement levels measured by C3 or CH_{50} are low or when serum is found to be anticomplementary during the performance of a serologic test using complement fixation. More selective means for detection of circulating immune complexes are available. Immune complex determination is used as a diagnostic criterion for various diseases, as an estimate of their severity, as an index to monitor the results of treatment in patients with immune complex diseases, and as a research tool in the investigation of the pathogenetic basis of immunologic diseases. A variety of methods exist to achieve maximum sensitivity, specificity, and reproducibility while keeping the technical procedure simple enough to be used as a routine test.

Methods in use are based on different biologic or chemical properties of immune complexes. As a result, they detect complexes of various sizes and properties, and none of the methods are satisfactory for all types. When possible, detection of circulating immune complexes should be done by several techniques (Table 18–6).

A. Physical Methods: Ultracentrifugation and gel filtration can be used, although they are not very sensitive methods and are usually used for separation rather than detection of immune complexes.

Cryoglobulins of types II and III, when detected in biologic fluids, represent immune complexes which can be easily isolated and characterized. However, cryoprecipitation is not a universal property of antigen-antibody complexes.

Table 18–6. Methods for detection of circulating immune complexes.

Physical methods
  Ultracentrifugation
  Gel filtration
  Cryoprecipitation
  Precipitation with polyethylene glycol
  Nephelometry
Interaction with rheumatoid factor or complement
  Precipitin reactions
  Inhibition of agglutination of IgG-coated latex particles
  Anticomplementary activity
  Solid-phase radioassay
  C1q binding test
  C1q deviation test
  Conglutinin binding test
Interaction with cell receptors
  Platelet aggregation test
  Inhibition of phagocytosis of labeled aggregates
  Inhibition of EAC rosette formation
  Raji cell test

Owing to their large size, immune complexes can be precipitated by high-molecular-weight polymers such as polyethylene glycol even at low concentrations of complexes which may leave soluble antigen or antibody as a residual in the reaction. Precipitated immune complexes are quantitated by measuring the protein content of the resolubilized precipitate (absorbance at 280 nm) or its concentration of immunoglobulins or complement components (radial diffusion).

B. Interaction With C1q, Rheumatoid Factor, or Conglutinin: Rheumatoid factor and C1q are able to agglutinate latex particles coated with aggregated IgG. When mixed with immune complexes, active sites on the Fc fragments of bound IgG are blocked, thereby preventing their subsequent agglutination by rheumatoid factor or C1q. Inhibition of the latex agglutination test can therefore be used for detection of immune complexes.

Binding of immune complexes to C1q leads to activation of the complement system, thereby depressing its hemolytic activity. This is the principle of the measure of anticomplementary activity of immune complexes in serum. The sample to be tested is freed from autologous complement activity by heat inactivation. It is then mixed in various dilutions with fresh normal serum which serves as a source of normal complement activity. Hemolytic activity (CH_{50}) of the fresh normal serum is measured with and without the addition of the sample. The anticomplementary activity is expressed as the percentage of reduction of CH_{50}.

Several techniques with radioisotopes or ELISA can be used to measure immune complex binding to C1q. For **solid-phase assay,** C1q is adsorbed on plastic polystyrene tubes. The sample is incubated in the coated tube, then washed out. The amount of immune complexes bound to C1q is estimated by binding of labeled anti-immunoglobulin antibody or by binding of labeled aggregated IgG onto free C1q. In the **liquid-phase assay,** the sample is incubated with soluble labeled C1q. In the C1q binding test, bound C1q is precipitated by polyethylene glycol and radioactivity measured in the precipitate. In the C1q deviation test, remaining free C1q is fixed on sensitized erythrocytes in such conditions that hemolysis does not occur. Radioactivity is measured in the erythrocyte pellet.

Conglutinin, a bovine serum protein, is known to react with fixed C3. This property is used in the **conglutinin binding test.** The sample is incubated with conglutinin, which is adsorbed onto plastic tubes. After washing, conglutinin-bound immune complexes are measured by the uptake of enzyme-conjugated or labeled anti-immunoglobulin antibody.

Clinical Usefulness

Initial enthusiasm regarding possible clinical ben-efits of measuring immune complexes has been tempered by their relative lack of diagnostic or prognostic specificity. Circulating complexes can occur in the absence of tissue deposition, and occasionally no serum complexes can be found despite tissue deposition. In addition, the considerable potential for uncovering causes of many idiopathic diseases by isolating and identifying the antigen in immune complexes has not yet been realized. Discrepancies among the results of various assays are common. Nevertheless, immune complexes have pathogenic roles depending on their size, immunoglobulin class, concentration, and affinity for cellular receptors. Most experts would probably agree that immune complex determinations are of little routine clinical utility.

NEPHELOMETRY

Nephelometry is measurement of light that is scattered from the main beam of a transmitted light source. This should not be confused with turbidimetry, which is the measurement of the decrease of light passing through a cloudy solution or suspension of material. In dilute solutions, the precipitation reaction between antigen and antibody produces increased reflection that can be measured by the scattering of an incident light. Devices to measure light scattering produced by reaction of diphtheria toxin and antitoxin were introduced by Libby in 1938, and this technique has received increasing application in the clinical laboratory.

Nephelometric determination of antigens is performed by addition of constant amounts of highly purified and optically clear specific antiserum to varying amounts of antigen. The resultant antigen-antibody reactants are placed in a cuvette in a light beam and the degree of light scatter measured in a photoelectric cell as the optical density (Fig 18–22). Accurate measurement of antigens can be made only in the ascending limb of the precipitin curve (Fig 18–1), where there is a direct linear relationship between antigen concentration and optical density. Thus, for accurate determination of solutions with high antigen concentrations, the samples are diluted to various concentrations.

There are several different approaches to applying nephelometry in the clinical laboratory. Automated immunoprecipitation employs a fluorometric nephelometer in line with a series of flow-through channels that allow for the measurement of multiple samples simultaneously. Laser nephelometers employ a helium-neon laser beam as a light source and sensitive detection devices to measure forward light scatter. Introduction of various electronic filters near the detection device ensures a high "signal-to-noise" ratio and a relatively high degree of sensitivity. A modified centrifugal fast analyzer equipped with a

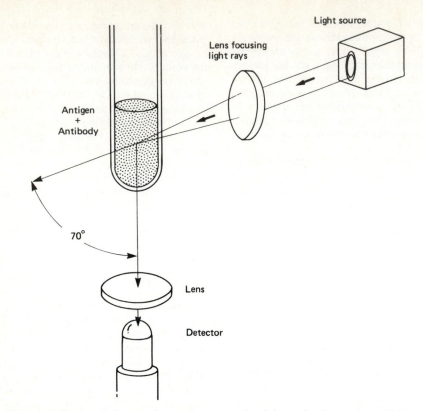

Figure 18–22. The principle of nephelometry for measurement of antigen-antibody reactions. Light rays from a laser or other high-intensity source are collected in the focusing lens and pass through the sample tube containing antigen and antibody. Light passing through the tube and emerging at a 70-degree angle is collected by another lens and focused into an electronic detector. This signal is converted to a digital recording of the amount of turbidity in the sample tube and can be mathematically related to either antigen or antibody concentration in the sample.

laser light source has also been employed for scatter measurements. This method has the potential advantages of speed, small amounts of reagents required, and versatility for other assays.

Nephelometry is theoretically a rapid and simple method for quantitation of many antigens in biologic fluids. Disadvantages of the technique include relatively high cost of optically clear, potent antisera of uniform specifications; high background resulting from sera containing lipids or hemoglobin; and the need for multiple dilutions, especially for high antigen concentrations. However, some of these potential sources of error are inherent in other immunoquantitative methods. Many of these inherent disadvantages can be overcome by the use of **rate nephelometry.** In this technique, a nephelometer electronically subtracts the background signal from that of an unreacted serum sample. More precise measurement of turbidity is achieved by taking several measurements rapidly during the ascending phase of the precipitation reaction. Nephelometers that combine many of these features are commercially available. The widespread use of such instruments—and nephelometric grade reagents—has made this method cheaper and applicable to many immunochemical determinations.

BINDER-LIGAND ASSAYS

One of the most important analytic methods developed in the past quarter century is binder-ligand assay (also known as **ligand assay, competitive protein-binding assay,** and **saturation analysis**). The first ligand assay method was **radioimmunoassay (RIA),** developed by Berson and Yalow in 1959 to detect and quantitate human insulin, utilizing human anti-insulin antibodies. Their discovery that the body manufactures antibodies against endogenous substances went against a fundamental dictum of the time, which held that the body could not make antibodies against itself. This discovery was in certain respects as important as the application of these antibodies to a new assay method. Simultaneously, Ekins developed an assay for human thyroid hormone by using thyroid-binding globulin isolated from a patient with elevated levels of this binding protein. The basic principle of his assay was the same, although it used a serum carrier protein rather than an antibody.

Since their inception, ligand assays have revolutionized disciplines within biology and medicine. One can quantitate hormones, drugs, tumor markers, and allergens and antibodies associated with allergy. The rapid detection of bacterial and viral antigens and antibodies in infectious diseases such as hepatitis and AIDS is possible.

Several features are common to nearly all types of binder-ligand assays. First, they all employ standards and compare these results with various unknown specimens for a concentration of a particular is sought. Second, reagents are separated into either a solid or liquid phase, either one of which may contain the binder or ligand. Third, some form of detection system is used to measure the interaction between ligand and binder. The details and variations of these common features are described below.

RADIOIMMUNOASSAY (RIA)

The chief goal of an assay is to determine the concentration of some molecule of interest, the **analyte.** Common to all of the ligand assays is the reaction of analyte with a binding protein, or **binder,** which most often is an **antibody.** In its role as a reactant with binder, the analyte is referred to as a **ligand.** Small analyte molecules are functionally **haptens,** which need to be conjugated to carriers to be rendered immunogeneic for the purpose of forming antibodies to be used for their detection. The free haptenic analyte can be detected by these antibodies in the absence of the carriers. In certain assay designs, binder can react with multiple distinct ligands, including the analyte.

There is a bewildering array of ligand assay methods; only one member of the ligand assay family, radioimmunoassay (RIA), will be described in full, followed by the broad chemical principles underlying some of the more important alternative ligand assay methods. Any ligand assay can be divided into 3 stages: calibration, interpolation, and quality control.

Calibration
A. The Binder-Ligand Reaction: A number of reaction vessels are established, each containing a small fixed concentration of binder and a small fixed concentration of radioisotopically labeled analyte known as the **label** or **tracer** (Fig 18–23). Calibration requires a set of dilutions of analyte of known concentration; these are referred to as the **standards**

or **calibrators.** Different known amounts of calibrator are then added to a series of antibody/label mixtures. The central event in RIA is the competition between the label and the unlabeled analyte for binding sites on an antibody. According to the degree of completion of the binder-ligand reaction, the assay is said to be either an **equilibrium assay** (the reaction is complete) or a **disequilibrium assay** (the reaction is incomplete). The label is divided into 2 categories by the reaction: label that is bound to antibody (the **bound fraction**) and label that is free in solution (the **free fraction**). As the amount of analyte increases relative to the small fixed amount of label present, an increasing fraction of the label will be free.

B. Partitioning and Separation: The bound and free fractions are subjected to a **partitioning step,** after which they are physically separated. Partitioning methods that sequester the binder and binder-ligand complexes include **salting out** of protein (using ammonium or sodium sulfate), **protein denaturation/precipitation** by solvent (such as methanol, ethanol, or acetone), and **precipitation** by polyethylene glycol or by a **second antibody** directed against the primary antibody. Immobilization of the binder to a **solid phase** such as the assay reaction tube or a macroscopic particle allows for rapid separation of bound and unbound label or analyte. A common method of removing the free fraction is **adsorption of free ligand** (using talc, charcoal, silica, ion exchange resin, cellulose, Sephadex, or fuller's earth).

Following partitioning, the bound and free fractions are subjected to **physical separation** by centrifugation or filtration during which a small degree of mixing of bound and unbound fractions can occur.

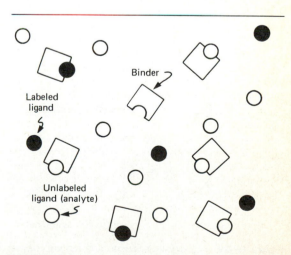

Figure 18–23. The binder-ligand reaction underlying RIA.

C. Measurement of Response: In radioassays, the measurement method is **radioactive counting,** the method for which depends upon the type of radiation emitted by the label. A **liquid scintillation counter** is used for alpha or beta emitters and a **solid crystal gamma counter** for gamma emitters. The final measurement, or some computed value derived from it, is known as the **response.** The choice of an appropriate response is dictated by the statistical requirements of data reduction. A commonly employed value in RIA is the ratio of bound to total label, or B:T.

D. Creation of a Calibration Curve: The physical and chemical steps taken thus far are referred to as the **analytic method** of the assay. A relationship between calibrator concentration and assay response must now be established. Most currently encountered assay calibration curves are roughly symmetric sigmoid curves when plotted using a logarithmic concentration axis (Fig 18–24).

This sort of curve can usually be characterized by the 4-parameter logistic equation

$$y = \left[\frac{a - d}{a + (x/c^b)}\right] + d \qquad \ldots (1)$$

where **a** is the upper asymptote, **d** is the lower asymptote, **c** is the concentration corresponding to the response **(a + d)/2,** and **b** is related to the slope at this point. Earlier workers used a simplified form of this equation, the **logit transformation,** which lends itself well to manual plotting. If one defines a new response value as **y' = (y − d)/(a − d),** the logit transformation proceeds as follows:

$$Y = \text{ligit }(y') = \ln\left[\frac{y'}{1 - y'}\right] \qquad \ldots (2)$$

Note the similarity of this approach to that of the von Krogh equation discussed later in this chapter. If the data really follow a symmetric sigmoid on the log-linear plot, then a plot of Y versus log concentration will be a straight line. The term **b** in the 4-parameter logistic equation is simply the slope of the line in the logitlog coordinate system.

Interpolation of Test Concentrations

Once a calibration relationship is in hand, we are ready to estimate the concentration of analyte in **test specimen "unknowns."** These specimens are processed just as the calibrators were, and a response is obtained. This response is used in conjunction with the calibration curve to find a **concentration estimate** corresponding to the observed response; this process is known as **interpolation.**

Quality Control & Error Computations

The goal in obtaining an analyte concentration estimate is generally to answer a question such as "Is the analyte concentration larger (or smaller) than a given dangerous or therapeutic level?" or "Is the concentration larger or smaller than some previously measured concentration?" Because random errors are involved in any measurement, an assay result should be accompanied by statistically determined **confidence limits** to aid in such judgments. Such confidence limits define a zone within which the results would be expected to fall at some stated level of probability. Furthermore, it is desirable to control the level of both random and systematic error in assay results, and so certain quality control procedures should be followed with each assay batch to allow the rejection of results likely to contain extraordinarily large error. There are many varieties of quality control tests: one of them relies upon use of quality control specimens of known concentration in each assay batch.

TYPES OF ANALYTIC METHODS

Radioisotopic Labels

There has been an explosion of methods based on various modifications of this initial assay scheme, arbitrarily divided according to their labeling methods.

A. Immunoradiometric Assay (IRMA): In this method, the binder (generally an antibody) is labeled rather than the ligand.

B. Sandwich Assay: There are numerous variations of this technique. In its most basic form, ligand reacts with an antibody that has been immobilized upon a solid surface. Then a radiolabeled second antibody is added, which reacts with ligand at a different site. This method has the potential advantage of added chemical specificity owing to the use of 2 distinct antigenic sites (Fig 18–25).

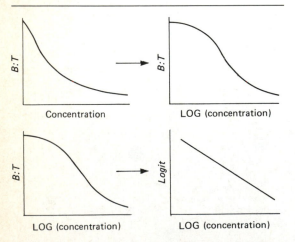

Figure 18–24. The logistic equation and the logit transformation. B:T = ratio of label bound to total label present.

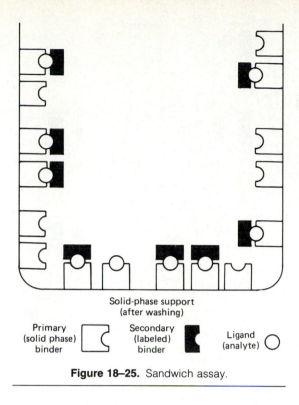

Figure 18–25. Sandwich assay.

approximately proportionate to analyte concentration. This method has been widely employed for therapeutic drug monitoring.

B. Enzyme-Linked Immunosorbent Assay (ELISA): This is an enzymatic variation on the sandwich assay method. One is attempting to detect an antibody, so the roles of binder and ligand are reversed (Fig 18–27). The solid-phase component is an antigen. The antibody to be detected binds to this component, and then a second, enzyme-labeled antibody directed against the antibody to be detected is added. The substrate of the enzyme is added, and a colored reaction product is produced which can be easily measured spectophotometrically.

Fluorometric Labels

A. Fluorescence Polarization Immunoassay (FPIA): The label is coupled by means of the analyte to a fluorescein derivative to form tracer molecules (Fig 18–28). When free in solution, tracer molecules tumble randomly and so rapidly that when excited by polarized light, emitted light is unpolarized. When the tracer is bound to an antibody, the tumbling is slowed and the emitted light is more polarized. The degree of polarization will reflect the amount of label that is bound. Thus far, only small analytes have been measurable by this means.

Other Methods

Other methods employ liposomes or erythrocytes as solid supports, nephelometry for particle detec-

Enzymatic Labels

A. Enzyme-Multiplied Immunoassay (EMIT): The label consists of ligand conjugated to an enzyme, which remains active (Fig 18–26). Binding of antibody to the enzyme-ligand complex inactivates the enzyme; the presence of free ligand (analyte) competes with the enzyme-ligand complex for antibody, increasing the resulting enzymatic activity. Over a limited range, the enzyme activity will be

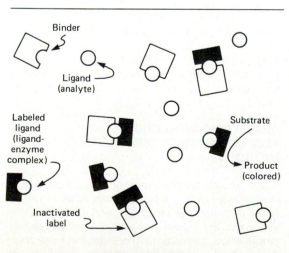

Figure 18–26. EMIT.

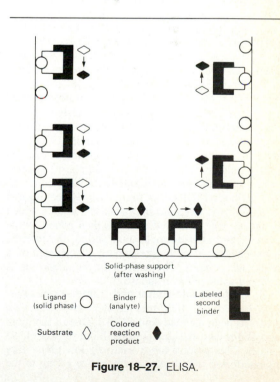

Figure 18–27. ELISA.

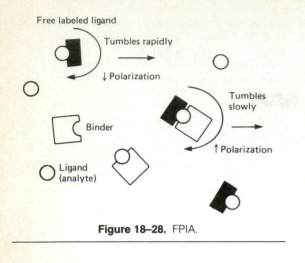

Figure 18–28. FPIA.

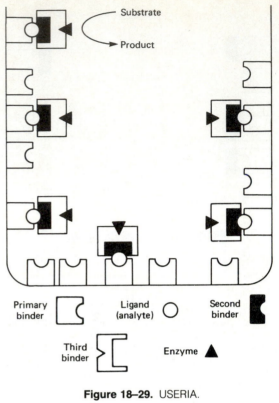

Figure 18–29. USERIA.

tion, metal atoms as labels (detected by atomic absorption), and electron-spin resonance ("spin labeling"). Enzymes from the blood-clotting cascade have been employed to produce a colored product from a chromogenic substrate as a response. Solid-phase systems have been sped up by the use of ultrasound to enhance the reaction rate of ligand with immobilized binder. Magnetic solid-phase support for antibody has been used to facilitate separation of bound and free fractions in an automated RIA method and in a manual sandwich assay. Bacteriophages have been employed as labels, as have chemiluminescent substances (luminol and its derivatives). The latex agglutination assay is now commonly employed for the rapid diagnosis of infectious agents. Microscopic latex spheres are coated with antibodies (or antigens), and agglutination (visible to the naked eye) is provoked by the presence of the corresponding antigen (or antibody).

A. Ultrasensitive Enzymatic Radioimmunoassay (USERIA): A method of detecting cholera toxin and rotavirus that was 1000-fold more sensitive than ELISA or RIA was described in 1979. The method combines aspects of radiometric and enzymatic methods (Fig 18–29). A solid-phase antibody is reacted with the analyte/standard, and then a second antibody is added. A third antibody, conjugated to an enzyme (alkaline phosphatase), is then added to the system. Tritiated AMP is then added to the system, and after an incubation period, the tritiated adenosine produced by the enzyme is separated on a Sephadex column. The activity of the adenosine is counted and used as response.

B. Biotin/Avidin-Enhanced Immunoassays: In this method, 1000-fold greater sensitivity than RIA has been claimed (Fig 18–30). One of the more straightforward designs requires biotinylation of the binder. This process has a relatively low probability of interfering with binder performance owing to the

chemically benign reaction (forming amide linkages) and to the low molecular weight (244) of biotin. There may be multiple biotin molecules per binder. The label, which may be enzymatic, radioisotopic, fluorometric, metallic, or of another type, is conjugated to avidin. Avidin is a small glycoprotein with an extremely high association constant for reaction with biotin. The label-avidin complex therefore associates with the binder. In another form, this assay employs avidin to bridge biotinylated binder-ligand complexes to a biotinylated label. Large complexes of avidin-biotin-label may also be attached to biotinylated binder. All of these methods are strategies for greatly increasing the amount of label per binder molecule.

COMPARING ANALYTIC PERFORMANCE OF DIFFERENT METHODS

The analytic performance of a given method is characterized by that assay's susceptibility to various forms of systematic error. For example, substances that mimic the presence of analyte or cross-react diminish assay specificity. Other substances can act as another binder or in some other way interfere with

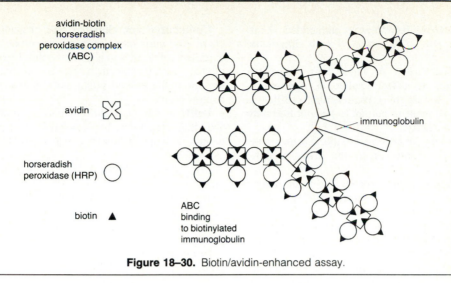

avidin-biotin
horseradish
peroxidase complex
(ABC)

avidin

horseradish
peroxidase (HRP)

biotin

immunoglobulin

ABC
binding
to biotinylated
immunoglobulin

Figure 18–30. Biotin/avidin-enhanced assay.

truthful measurement (**interference**). The amount of random error contained in the assay is expressed by the confidence limits around a particular assay determination. Random error determines the **sensitivity** of an assay, by which is meant the smallest amount of analyte that can be statistically distinguished from zero. It is best described in terms of the **lower detection limit,** which is the analyte concentration for which the confidence interval grazes zero. The precision of the assay, expressed as the width of the confidence interval, can be plotted against concentration to create an **imprecision profile,** which reveals assay error to be nonconstant; it is lowest at some point in mid-assay range and increases to either side.

It is difficult to compare the analytic performance of different ligand assay methods, since the workers involved often provide only scanty data, and many new methods are accompanied by exaggerated claims. A rigidly defined standard data reduction method would be of help, so that quantities such as analytic sensitivity and specificity would always be computed in the same manner.

Assay methods can be compared on the basis of the labeling method used. Two basic categories, **limited-reagent** (or **competitive**) **methods** and **excess-reagent** (or **noncompetitive**) **methods** are examples. RIA is an example of the former category; here, labeled ligand and unlabeled ligand compete for a limited amount of binder. The best achievable sensitivity of an RIA is of the order of 10^{-14} mol/L (this represents about 6×10^6 molecules in 1 mL of solution). A sandwich IRMA is an example of the latter category; a massive excess of labeled second antibody is added to the solid-phase binder-ligand complex. Reagent-excess methods are in principle capable of better sensitivity than limited reagent methods, but in practice IRMA has been less sensi-

tive than RIA. ELISA and USERIA have achieved sensitivities 1 and 2 orders of magnitude smaller than RIA. There are still analytes for which RIA is the only method available, as with vitamin B_{12}, and it seems likely that an array of different methods will remain in use for different applications.

There are alternative chemical methods, such as HPLC, for many analytes. An important principle of ligand assay must be borne in mind—it measures the chemical (generally immunochemical) reactivity rather than the physiologic or functional activity of an analyte. This has sometimes been an advantage, where much new knowledge has been gained about the various forms of drugs and hormones capable of cross-reacting with the intended analyte.

GLOSSARY OF ASSAY TERMINOLOGY

Accuracy: The degree to which an analyte concentration estimate corresponds to the true value. This is rarely knowable absolutely. Inaccuracy is caused by a combination of random and bias errors.

Analyte: The substance to be measured.

Analyte concentration estimate: The concentration of analyte in a test specimen which is estimated by the assay procedure. Also sometimes known as **dose,** a term from the earlier biologic assay field.

Analytic method: The physical and chemical manipulations to which calibrators and test specimens are subjected to produce their corresponding assay response values.

Analytic sensitivity: A vague term generally associated with the ability to detect small concentrations but in fact used with multiple meanings, which has provoked immense needless debate. The use of some mathematically defined term such as the **lower**

detection limit (see below) is recommended. Analogous to but not to be confused with **diagnostic sensitivity.**

Analytic specificity: A vague term associated with the ability to detect analyte as opposed to nonanalyte. The use of cross-reaction profiles is preferable. Analogous to but not to be confused with **diagnostic specificity.**

Batch: A single processing session in which a set of specimens is subjected to the assay analytic method.

Between-batch random error: The random error that accrues in an assay system, including within-assay random error and the additional sources of random error observed when comparing results obtained from repeated analysis of the same specimen in different batches of the same assay method.

Between-laboratory random error: The random error observed in measurements of the same specimen in different laboratories, including within-assay error, between-batch random error, and the additional sources of random error observed when comparing such results.

Bias: Systematic error. Causes include decay in the performance of the final detection device, specimen misidentification, decay of calibrators or test specimens, nonidentity of the chemical behavior of calibrators and test specimens (as with cross-reaction and interference), and others.

Calibration curve: The plotted or mathematically describable relationship between the response obtained from the analytic procedure and the analyte concentration.

Calibrators: Known concentrations of the analyte, used in creating the calibration curve. Also known as **standards.** There are multiple varieties.

Confidence interval: The analyte concentration range contained within a set of confidence limits.

Confidence limits: Statistically defined limits about an analyte concentration estimate, which reflect the random error inherent in the result. Example: 95% limits define a region within which, 95% of the time, the true estimate (in the absence of bias error) would be expected to fall (were the measurement with the accompanying computation of confidence limits to be repeated many times).

Continuous response assay: An assay in which the response varies over a continuous range of values, or a discrete range so large as to be well approximated by a continuous range, as in radioimmunoassay.

Cross-reaction: The reaction with the specific assay binding substance by some chemical entity other than the analyte, in such a way as to falsify the measured amount of analyte.

Cross-reaction profile: A plot of the bias error in the estimated concentration of analyte as a function of the concentration of a specified cross-reacting species, at a given fixed concentration of analyte.

Cumulative sum chart: A type of quality control chart. The cumulative sum of deviations (from the expected value) of some quality control parameter is plotted. Various statistical tests are available to determine if the plotted points may indicate a quality control problem.

Drift: A temporal shift in bias in assay results. This may sometimes be detected by placing quality control pool specimens at regular intervals in the assay batch.

Imprecision profile: A plot of imprecision (generally expressed as the width of a confidence limit of some specified level of certainty, and a given level of replication of calibrators and unknowns) versus analyte concentration. Also known as a **precision profile.**

Interference: Used in many different ways in clinical chemistry. For example, this term is used to refer to the bias error in a spectrophotometer reading produced by absorption of a given frequency of light by substances other than the one of primary interest. In ligand assays, the term usually refers to the presence of something that can mimic the chemical behavior of the binder, producing bias error. As an example, the presence of thyroid-binding globulin could interfere with a radioimmunoassay of thyroid hormone.

Interpolation: The process of reading the response for an unknown through the calibration curve to obtain an analyte concentration estimate.

Least squares (method of): A procedure for fitting a mathematical function to data in which the sum of the second powers of the vertical distances between the function and the data points is minimized.

Lower detection limit: The (statistically defined) lowest concentration distinguishable from the lowest calibrator concentration (the latter is generally zero). Should be reported along with its associated level of statistical confidence. Also referred to as the **minimum detection limit** or **minimum detectable dose.**

Outlier: Defined in 2 senses. First, a member of a replicate set that lies far from the other members of the set, presumably owing to some extraordinary error. Second, the mean of a replicate set for a calibrator that lies far from the calibration curve location suggested by the other calibrators, again presumably owing to some extraordinary error.

Parallelism testing: The process of determining whether the curve that can be drawn from the responses obtained from multiple dilutions of a test specimen can be superimposed upon the calibration curve by a simple multiplicative rescaling of the x axis of the test curve. Also referred to as **similarity testing,** which is perhaps more appropriate, since "parallelism testing" derives from the early days of biologic assay, when straight-line calibration relationships were employed.

Pooled response-error relationship: A response-error relationship obtained by pooling information from a number of consecutive assay batches (generally 10–30) so as to achieve better estimates of the expected error than would be possible with the limited information available in a single batch. Often used to estimate the imprecision profile.

Power function: Plot of the probability of rejection of an assay result as a function of the amount of error present (either bias or random) for a specified quality control test.

Precision: A qualitative term concerned with the reproducibility of a result and hence with its random error. Avoidance of this term is recommended; the use of some precisely defined mathematic expression of random error, such as a set of confidence limits with its associated level of statistical significance, is preferred.

Quality control chart: A plot of some assay performance parameter, most often the measurement obtained for a quality control pool, plotted chronologically on a flow chart. Statistical tests may be performed to ascertain if deviations from the average result would be so rare (if attributed to the usual amount of random error of the assay) as to represent a possible quality control problem. Also known as **Shewhart chart** and **Levey-Jennings chart.** See also **cumulative sum chart.**

Quality control pool: A large collection of material containing analyte stored so as to preserve it over a long period of time. Aliquots are taken and analyzed (with each assay batch in earlier assays, with decreasing frequency in some newer commercial assays) to assist in detecting exceptional error (particularly useful for bias).

Quantal response assay: An assay in which the response is some value which varies over a discrete range of values (example: 1, 2, 3, . . . n) rather than over a continuous range. An example is the type of biologic assay in which a small number of animals is employed and the response is the proportion of animals killed by a given dose of analyte. Requires statistical methods not discussed here.

Random error: Error arising from chance occurrences rather than systematic causes. Important sources in practice include pipetting, timing, and counting and detection errors. See also precision, imprecision, analytic sensitivity, lower detection limit, confidence limits.

Recovery: The amount of analyte detected when a known amount of calibrator is added to a previously assayed test preparation. Significant deviation from 100% suggests the presence of bias error.

Replicate: A repeated analysis of a calibrator, quality control specimen, or unknown, as when a specimen is said to be run in duplicate, triplicate, . . . n-tuplicate. The only source of information about random errors.

Residual: The vertical distance between a data point (in assay, this is often the mean of replicates obtained for a given calibrator concentration) and the mathematic equation fitted to it. If the residual is properly weighted for the amount of data it represents and for its variance, it is referred to as a **studentized residual.**

Response: Some mathematical function of the final measurement taken from the assay analytic method.

Response-error relationship: A plot of the error in the selected response versus the response.

Run: Assay jargon for the process of analyzing a single assay batch.

Standard deviation: A measure of the random error inherent in a set of measurements of the same quantity (equal to the square root of the variance). Although the standard deviation may be computed for any given set of numbers, it is interpretable in strict probabilistic terms only if the data are drawn randomly from a gaussian population.

Test specimen: A sample, generally a biologic fluid, an aliquot of which is presented to the assay process in order to determine the concentration of analyte present.

Unknown: Test specimen.

Upper detection limit: The (statistically defined) highest concentration distinguishable from the highest calibrator concentration. Should be reported along with its associated level of statistical confidence.

Valid analytic range: The range between the upper and lower detection limits.

Variance: A measure of the random error inherent in a set of measurements of the same quantity, equal to the second power of the standard deviation.

Weighting: The use of some estimate of random error in the process of regression so as to take into account the relative error of the data being fitted; the final fit will pay more attention to data of higher precision than to data of lower precision. In assay work, the inverse of the variance (estimated from a pooled response-error relationship) should be employed.

Within-assay random error: The random error observed in assay results analyzed in a single batch.

IMMUNOHISTOCHEMICAL TECHNIQUES

IMMUNOFLUORESCENCE

Immunofluorescence can be applied as a histochemical or cytochemical technique for detection and localization of antigens in cells or tissues. Specific antibody is conjugated with fluorescent compounds without altering its immunologic reactivity, resulting in a sensitive tracer of tissue antigens. The conjugated antibody is added to cells or tissues and becomes fixed to antigens, thereby forming a stable immune complex. Unbound antibody is removed by washing, and the resultant preparation is observed in a fluorescence microscope. This adaptation of a regular microscope contains a high-intensity light source, excitation filters to produce a wavelength capable of causing fluorescence activation, and barrier filters to remove interfering wavelengths of light. When observed in the fluorescence microscope against a dark background, antigens bound specifically to fluorescent antibody can be detected by their bright color.

Fluorescence is the emission of light of one color, ie, wavelength, while a substance is irradiated with light of a different color. The emitted wavelength is at a lower energy level than the incident or absorbed light (Fig 18–31). Fluorochromes such as rhodamine or fluorescein used in clinical laboratories have characteristic absorption and emission spectra. Fluorescein isothiocyanate (FITC) is a chemical form of fluorescein that readily binds covalently to proteins at high pH primarily through ϵ amino residues of lysine and terminal amino groups. Its absorption maximum is at 490–495 nm, and it emits its characteristic green color at 517 nm. Tetramethylrhodamine isothiocyanate, which emits red, has an absorption maximum at 550 nm and maximal emission at 580 nm (for rhodamine-protein conjugates). Consequently, different excitation and barrier filters must

be employed to visualize the characteristic green or red color of these fluorescent dyes. Generally, one wants to achieve an exciting wavelength nearly equal to that of the excitation maximum of the dye. Similarly, the barrier filter should remove all but the emitted wavelength spectrum. In practice, the actual brightness of fluorescence observed by the eye depends on 3 factors: (1) the efficiency with which the dye converts incident light into fluorescent light; (2) the concentration of the dye in the tissue specimen; and (3) the intensity of the exciting (absorbed) radiation.

Microscopes used for visualizing immunofluorescent specimens are modifications of standard transmitted light microscopes (Fig 18–32). In 1967, Ploem introduced an epi-illuminated system that employs a vertical illuminator and a dichroic mirror. In this system (Fig 18–33), the excitation beam is focused directly on the tissue specimen through the lens objective. Fluorescent light emitted from the epi-illuminated specimen is then transmitted to the eye through the dichroic mirror. A dichroic mirror allows passage of light of selected wavelengths in one direction through the mirror but not in the opposite direction.

There are several distinct advantages to the Ploem system. Fluorescence may be combined with transmitted light for phase contrast examination of the tissues, thereby allowing better definition of morphology and fluorescence. Also, interchangeable filter systems permit rapid examination of the specimen at different wavelengths for double fluorochrome staining, eg, red and green (rhodamine and

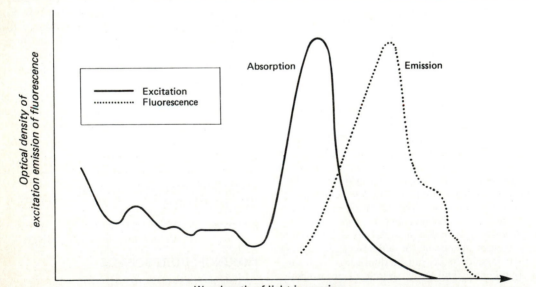

Figure 18–31. Absorption and emission spectra for a fluorescent compound.

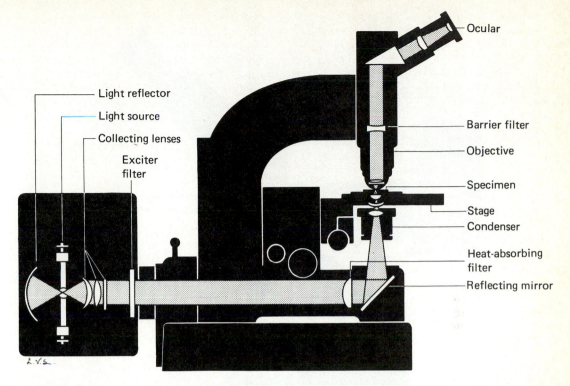

Ocular

Barrier filter

Objective

Specimen

Stage

Condenser

Heat-absorbing filter

Reflecting mirror

Light reflector

Light source

Collecting lenses

Exciter filter

Figure 18–32. Fluorescence microscope with transmitted light. Light beam is generated by a mercury vapor lamp, reflected by a concave mirror, and projected through collecting lenses to the exciter filter, which emits a fluorescent light beam. A reflecting mirror directs the beam from underneath the stage, through the condenser into the specimen. A barrier filter removes wavelengths other than those emitted from the fluorescent compound in the specimen, and the fluorescent pattern is viewed through magnification provided by the objective and ocular lenses.

fluorescein, respectively). This advantage in technique has resulted in superior sensitivity for examining cell membrane fluorescence in living lymphocytes.

Methodology & Interpretation

Virtually any antigen can be detected in fixed tissue sections or in live cell suspensions by immunofluorescence. It is the combination of high sensitivity and specificity, together with the use of histologic techniques, that makes immunofluorescence so useful. The steps involved in immunofluorescence include preparation of immune antiserum or purified antibodies, conjugation with fluorescent dye, and, finally, the staining procedure.

For immunofluorescence, an antiserum to the antigen one wishes to detect is raised in heterologous species. Pure monoclonal antibodies can be used and are prepared as described below. Antisera should contain milligram amounts of antibody per milliliter. Specificity must exceed a level detectable in ordinary double diffusion or immunoelectrophoretic techniques. More sensitive methods available include hemagglutination inhibition, RIA, and ELISA. Unwanted antibodies present in either conjugates or

antiglobulin reagents for the test can usually be removed with insoluble immunoabsorbents or avoided entirely by use of monoclonal antibodies.

After obtaining antiserum of high potency and appropriate specificity, the γ-globulin fraction can be prepared by ammonium sulfate precipitation and DEAE-cellulose ion exchange chromatography. It is necessary to partially purify serum γ-globulin, since subsequent conjugation should be limited to antibody as much as possible. This will increase the efficiency of staining and avoid unwanted nonspecific staining by fluorochrome-conjugated nonantibody serum proteins that can adhere to tissue components.

Conjugation of γ-globulin depends largely on the particular dye to be combined with the antibody molecule. From a clinical laboratory standpoint, only fluorescein, rhodamine, and some phycobiliproteins have been used widely. Fluorescein, in the form of FITC, or rhodamine, as tetramethylrhodamine isothiocyanate, is either reacted directly with γ-globulin in alkaline solution overnight at 4 °C or dialyzed against γ-globulin. Unreacted dye is then removed from the protein-fluorochrome conjugate by gel filtration or exhaustive dialysis. If necessary, the resultant conjugate can be concentrated by lyoph-

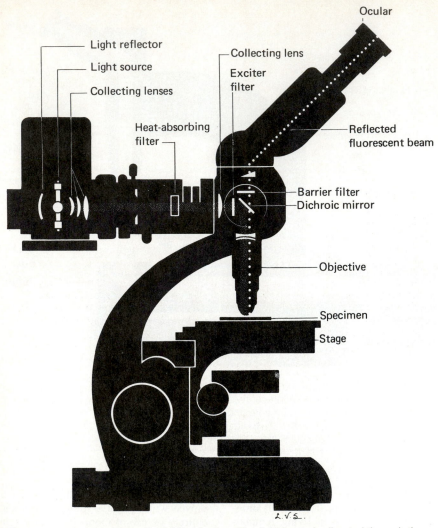

Figure 18–33. Fluorescence microscope with epi-illumination. The light beam is directed through the exciter filter and down onto the specimen. A dichroic mirror allows passage of selected wavelengths in one direction but not another. After reaching the specimen, the light is reflected through the dichroic mirror and emitted fluorescent light is visualized at the ocular.

ilization, pressure dialysis, or solvent extraction with water-soluble polymers. Thereafter, one must determine both the concentration of γ-globulin and the dye/protein or fluorescein/protein ratio of the compound. This is usually done spectrophotometrically with corrections for the alteration in absorbance of γ-globulin by the introduced fluorochrome.

Staining Techniques

A. Direct Immunofluorescence: (Figs 18–34 and 18–35.) In this technique, conjugated antiserum is added directly to the tissue section or viable cell suspension.

B. Indirect Immunofluorescence: This technique allows for the detection of antibody in the se-

rum. It eliminates the need to purify and individually conjugate each serum sample. The method is basically an adaptation of the antiglobulin reaction (Coombs test) or double antibody technique (Figs 18–34 and 18–35). Specificity should be checked as diagrammed and further established by blocking and neutralization methods (Fig 18–36).

Several additional variations in staining techniques have been used. These include a conjugated anticomplement antiserum for the detection of immune complexes containing complement or double staining with both rhodamine and fluorescein conjugates.

Immunofluorescence employing routine serologic procedures for the detection of antibody in human

DIRECT METHOD:

INDIRECT METHOD:

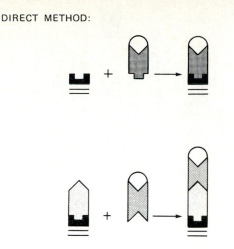

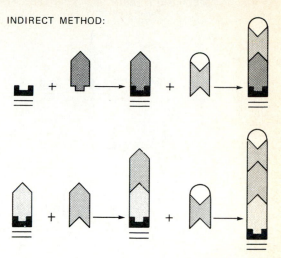

Figure 18–34. Mechanism of immunofluorescence techniques. *Direct Method.* ***(Top):*** Antigen in substrate detected by direct labeling with fluorescent antibody. ***(Bottom):*** Antigen-antibody (immune) complex in substrate labeled with fluorescent antiglobulin reagent. (Modified and reproduced, with permission, from Nordic Immunology, Tilburg, The Netherlands.)

Figure 18–35. Mechamism of immunofluorescence techniques. *Indirect Method.* ***(Top):*** Incubation of antigen in substrate with unlabeled antibody forms immune complex. Labeling performed with fluorescent antiglobulin reagent. ***(Bottom):*** Immune complex in substrate reacted with unlabeled antiglobulin reagent and then stained with fluorescent antiglobulin reagent directed at unlabeled antiglobulin. (Modified and reproduced, with permission, from Nordic Immunology, Tilburg, The Netherlands.)

LEGEND

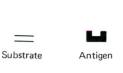

| Substrate | Antigen | Fluorescent antibody | Fluorescent antiglobulin | Immune complex | Unlabeled antibody | Unlabeled antiglobulin | Fluorescent heterologous antibody |

serum specimens has been widely applied (Table 18–7). Sensitivity is generally higher than with complement fixation and lower than with hemagglutination inhibition. Methods for detecting antibody by immunofluorescence include (1) the antiglobulin method, (2) inhibition of labeled antibody-antigen reaction by antibody in test serum, and (3) the anticomplement method.

C. Biotin-Avidin System: Avidin, a basic glycoprotein derived from egg albumin of MW 68,000, has a remarkably high affinity (10^{15} kcal/mol) for the vitamin biotin. Biotin can easily be covalently coupled to an antibody and then reacted with fluorochrome-coupled avidin. After reaction of antigen with unlabeled antibody, the biotin-labeled second antibody is added. Since many molecules of biotin can be coupled to an antibody, the subsequent addition of fluorochrome-labeled avidin results in a firm bond with exceedingly bright fluorescence.

Other advantages are lack of nonspecific binding of fluorochrome-coupled avidin to various substrates and general use of avidin conjugates in binding to biotin-labeled antibodies regardless of their species of origin or isotype.

Quantitative Immunofluorescence

Quantitative immunoassays using fluorochrome-labeled antigens and antibodies are available. The amount of light of a given wavelength emitted from a fluorescent specimen can be precisely measured by a microfluorometer. A number of assay methods have been introduced commercially in the field of quantitative immunofluorescence. Fluorescent immunoassay systems can be used to measure IgG, IgA, and IgM; C3 and C4; and antinuclear and anti-DNA antibodies. Immunoglobulins are measured by competitive binding of labeled specific antiserum for free and solid-phase antigen. The free antigen is

SPECIFICITY TESTS
Direct method:

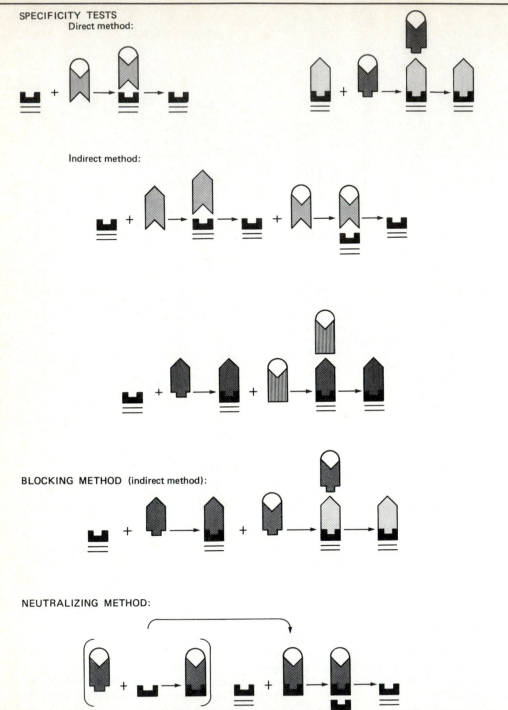

Indirect method:

BLOCKING METHOD (indirect method):

NEUTRALIZING METHOD:

Figure 18–36. Specificity tests. *Direct method.* **(Left):** Substrate antigen fails to react with fluorescent antiglobulin reagent. No fluorescence results. **(Right):** Immune complex-substrate fails to react with fluorescent antibody directed against unrelated antigen. No fluorescence results. *Indirect method.* **(Top):** Unlabeled specific antiglobulin is replaced by unrelated antibody. In second step, fluorescent antiglobulin cannot react directly with antigen in substrate that has not bound specific antiglobulin. No fluorescence results. **(Bottom):** First step performed by reacting specific antibody with substrate antigen. In second stage, the specific conjugate is replaced by unrelated fluorescent heterologous antibody. No fluorescence results. *Blocking method.* Substrate antigen is incubated with unlabeled specific antibody prior to addition of specific fluorescent antibody. Decreased fluorescence results. *Neutralizing method.* Substrate antigen is incubated with specific fluorescent antibody after it is absorbed with specific antigen in substrate. No fluorescence results.

Table 18–7. Clinical applications of immunofluorescence.

Identification of T and B cells in blood
Detection of autoantibodies in serum, eg, ANA
Detection of immunoglobulins in tissues
Detection of complement components in tissues
Detection of specific, tissue-fixed antibody
Rapid identification of microorganisms in tissue or culture
Identification of chromosomes of specific banding patterns
Identification of tumor-specific antigens on neoplastic tissues
Identification of transplantation antigens in various organs
Localization of hormones and enzymes
Quantitation of serum proteins and antibodies

present in patients' serum, whereas the bound immunoglobulin is fixed to a polymeric hydrophobic surface. The amount of fluorescent antibody bound to the solid-phase antigen is measured in a specially designed microfluorometer and converted to milligrams per deciliter by reference to a standard curve.

Serum antibodies to various cellular antigens such as DNA or nuclei can also be measured by an indirect fluorescence technique. Substrate (eg, DNA) is fixed to the polymer surface in solid phase and incubated with test sera. A second fluorescein antiimmunoglobulin reagent is then bound to the first antigen-antibody complex and the amount of bound fluorescence measured fluorometrically.

OTHER IMMUNOHISTOCHEMICAL TECHNIQUES

Enzyme-Linked Antibody

In this method an enzyme is conjugated to antibody directed at a cellular or tissue antigen. The resulting conjugate is then both immunologically and enzymatically active. Use of these conjugates is entirely analogous to that for direct or indirect immunofluorescence techniques.

Horseradish peroxidase is usually the enzyme chosen for coupling to antibody. Tissues are first reacted directly with antibody-enzyme conjugate or directly with enzyme-linked antiglobulin reagent following incubation with unlabeled immune serum. Thereafter, the tissue is incubated with the substrate for the enzyme. The enzyme in this case is detected visually by formation of a black color after incubation with hydrogen peroxide and diaminobenzidine. One advantage of this method is that ordinary light microscopes may be utilized for analysis of tissue sections. Furthermore, enzyme-coupled antibody can be used for ultrastructural studies in the electron microscope.

Additional immunohistochemical techniques have been developed for localization of tissue or cellular antigens. One in particular, the peroxidase-antiperoxidase (PAP) method, has been used in surgical pathology for detecting enzymes and tumor-related antigens. This is a 3-step method. First, fixed slides are stained with rabbit antiserum to a tissue antigen to be measured. Next, an anti-rabbit immunoglobulin that reacts with the first antibody is applied. Finally, an immune complex, consisting of rabbit antibodies to peroxidase combined with peroxidase, is added. This immune complex reacts with the anti-rabbit bridging antibody. A peroxidase substrate is added, which forms the colored reaction product.

Other techniques being developed include hapten-coupled antibodies, the use of staphylococcal protein A as an intermediate reagent, and systems with more than one immunoenzymatic reagent, ie, double staining. Fixation difficulties and standardization of readily available reagents still limit the wider application of these potentially powerful techniques.

Ferritin-Coupled Antibody

Ferritin, an iron-containing protein, is highly electron-dense. When coupled to antibody, it can be used for either direct or indirect tissue staining. Localization of ferritin-coupled antibody-antigen complexes in fixed tissue can then be achieved with the electron microscope. Other electron-dense particles such as gold or uranium can also be introduced chemically into specific antitissue antibodies. These reagents have also been applied in immunoelectron-microscopy.

Autoradiography

Radioactive isotopes such as ^{125}I that can be chemically linked to immunoglobulins provide highly sensitive probes for localization of tissue antigens. The antigens are detected visually after tissue staining by overlaying or coating slides with photographic emulsion. The appearance of silver grains as black dots has been used for subcellular localization of antigen both at light microscopic and ultrastructural levels. Autoradiography has also been applied to detection of proteins or immunoglobulins synthesized by cells in tissue culture.

Miscellaneous Methods

A variety of other methods have been described for localization of antigens in tissues. Many have not found widespread clinical application. In most cases, these techniques depend on secondary phenomena which occur as a result of the antigen-antibody interaction. These methods include the following:

(1) Complement fixation
(2) Conglutinating complement absorption test
(3) Antiglobulin consumption test
(4) Mixed hemadsorption
(5) Immune adherence
(6) Hemagglutination and coated particle reaction
(7) Immunoprecipitation

AGGLUTINATION

Agglutination and precipitation reactions are the basis of many techniques in laboratory immunology. Whereas precipitation reactions are quantifiable and simple to perform, agglutination techniques are only semiquantitative and somewhat more difficult. Important advantages of agglutination reactions are their high degree of sensitivity and the ability to assess endpoints visually. The agglutination of either insoluble native antigens or antigen-coated particles can be applied to measurement of a large variety of analytes.

According to Coombs, the 3 main requirements in agglutination tests are the availability of a stable cell or particle suspension, the presence of one or more antigens close to the surface, and the knowledge that "incomplete" or nonagglutinating antibodies are detectable with modifications, eg, antiglobulin reactions.

Agglutination reactions may be classified as either direct or indirect (passive). In the direct technique, a cell or insoluble particulate antigen is agglutinated directly by antibody. An example is the agglutination of group A erythrocytes by anti-A sera. Passive agglutination refers to agglutination of antigen-coated cells or inert particles which are passive carriers of otherwise soluble antigens. Examples are latex agglutination (fixation) for detection of rheumatoid factor and agglutination of DNA-coated erythrocytes for detection of anti-DNA antibody. Alternatively, **antigen** can be detected by coating latex particles or erythrocytes with purified **antibody** and performing so-called reversed agglutination. Another category of agglutination involves spontaneous agglutination of erythrocytes by certain viruses. This viral hemagglutination reaction can be specifically inhibited in the presence of antiviral antibody. Thus, viral hemagglutination can be used either to quantify virus itself or to determine by inhibition the titer of antisera directed against hemagglutinating viruses.

Inhibition of agglutination, if carefully standardized with highly purified antigens, can be used as a sensitive indicator of the amount of antigen in various tissue fluids. Hemagglutination inhibition using passive hemagglutination reactions can be semiautomated in microtiter plates and is sensitive for measuring antigens in concentrations of 0.1–10 µg/mL. With appropriate modification, passive hemagglutination with protein-sensitized cells can detect antibody at concentrations as low as 0.01 µg/mL.

AGGLUTINATION TECHNIQUES

Direct Agglutination Test

Erythrocytes, bacteria, fungi, and a variety of other microbial species can be directly agglutinated by antibody. Tests to detect specific antibody are carried out by serially titrating antisera in 2-fold dilutions in the presence of a constant amount of antigen. Direct agglutination is relatively temperature-independent except for cold-reacting antibody, eg, cold agglutinins. After a few hours of incubation, agglutination is complete and particles are examined either directly or microscopically for evidence of clumping. The results are usually expressed as a titer of antiserum, ie, the highest dilution at which agglutination occurs. Because of intrinsic variability in the test system, a titer usually must differ by at least 2 twofold dilutions ("2 tubes") to be considered significantly different from any given titer. Tests are carried out in small test tubes in volumes of 0.2–0.5 mL or in microtiter plates with smaller amounts of reagents.

Indirect (Passive) Agglutination Test

The range of soluble antigens that can be passively adsorbed or chemically coupled to erythrocytes or other inert particles has extended the application of agglutination reactions. Many antigens will spontaneously couple with erythrocytes and form stable reagents for antibody detection (Table 18–8). When erythrocytes are used as the inert particles, serum specimens often must be absorbed with washed, uncoated erythrocytes to remove heterophilic antibodies that would otherwise nonspecifically agglutinate them. The advantages of using erythrocytes for coating are their ready availability, sensitivity as indicators, and storage capabilities. Erythrocytes can be treated with formalin, glutaraldehyde, or pyruvic aldehyde and stored for prolonged periods at 4 °C.

A list of general methods available for coating antigens to erythrocytes is presented in Table 18–9. Treatment of erythrocytes with tannic acid increases the amount of most protein antigens subsequently adsorbed. This higher density of coated antigen greatly increases the sensitivity of the agglutination reaction. Although highly purified antigens are required for immunologic specificity, slightly dena-

Table 18–8. Substances that spontaneously adsorb to erythrocytes for hemagglutination.

Escherichia coli antigens
Yersinia antigens
Lipopolysaccharide from *Neisseria meningitidis*
Toxoplasma antigens
Purified protein derivative (PPD)
Endotoxin of *Mycoplasma* species
Viruses
Antibiotics, especially penicillin
Ovalbumin
Bovine serum albumin
DNA
Haptens, eg, DNCB

Table 18–9. Methods used to coat fresh and aldehyde-treated red blood cells with various antigens and antibodies for passive hemagglutination assay.[1]

Coupling Agent	Comments on Coupling	Antigens Commonly Coated
None	Simple adsorption	Penicillin, bacterial antigens including endo- and exotoxins, viruses, and ovalbumin.
Tannic acid	Adsorption possibly caused by changes analogous to enzymes. Most popular; usually satisfactory, but often difficult and unreliable.	A wide spectrum of antigens: serum proteins, microbial and tissue extracts, homogenates, thyroglobulin, and tuberculin proteins.
Bisdiazotized benzidine (BDB)	Chemically stable covalent azo bonds.	Proteins and pollen antigens.
1,3-Difluoro-4, 6-dinitrobenzene (DFDNB)	Adsorption after modification of cell membrane.	Purified proteins and chorionic gonadotropin.
Chromic chloride (CrCl₃)	Proteins bound to erythrocytes by the charge effect of trivalent cations.	Proteins.
Glutaraldehyde, cyanuric chloride, tetrazotized O-dianisidine	Cross-linking and covalent coupling.	Various proteins and certain enzymes.
Tolulene-2,4-diisocyanate	Covalently bound.	Proteins.
Water-soluble carbodiimide	Covalently bound.	Proteins.

[1]Modified and reproduced, with permission, from Fudenberg HH: Hemagglutination inhibition: Passive hemagglutination assay for antigen-antibody reactions. In: *A Seminar on Basic Immunology.* American Association of Blood Banks, 1971.

tured or aggregated antigens coat tanned erythrocytes best.

Agglutination tests may be performed in tubes or microtiter plates. In antisera with very high agglutination titers, a prozone phenomenon may obscure the results. The prozone phenomenon produces falsely negative agglutination reactions at high concentrations of antibody as a result of poor lattice formation and steric hindrance by antibody excess. However, the use of standard serial dilutions eliminates this difficulty. Since IgM antibody is about 750 times as efficient as IgG in agglutination, the presence of high amounts of IgM can influence test results.

HEMAGGLUTINATION INHIBITION

The inhibition of agglutination of antigen-coated red blood cells by homologous antigen is a highly sensitive and specific method for detecting small quantities of soluble antigen in blood or other tissue fluids. The principle of this assay is that antibody preincubated with soluble homologous or cross-reacting antigens will be "inactivated" when incubated with antigen-coated erythrocytes. Thus, the test proceeds in 2 stages (Fig 18–37). Antibody in relatively low concentration is incubated with a sample of antigen of unknown quantity. After combination with soluble antigen, antigen-coated cells are added and agglutinated by uncombined or free antibody. (The degree of inhibition of agglutination reflects the amount of antigen present in the original sample.) Controls, including samples of known antigen concentration and uncoated erythrocytes, must be employed. This hemagglutination inhibition method has been employed in the detection of HBsAg in hepatitis and in the detection of factor VIII antigen in hemophilia and related clotting disorders.

CLINICALLY APPLICABLE TESTS THAT EMPLOY AGGLUTINATION REACTIONS

Antiglobulin Test (Coombs Test)

The development of this simple and ingenious technique virtually revolutionized the field of immunohematology, and in various forms it has found widespread application in all fields of immunology. Antibodies frequently coat erythrocytes but fail to form the necessary lattice to produce agglutination. A typical example is antibody directed at the Rh determinants on human erythrocytes. However, the addition of an antiglobulin antiserum produced in a heterologous species (eg, rabbit anti-human γ-globulin) produces marked agglutination. Thus, the antiglobulin or Coombs test is used principally to detect subagglutinating or nonagglutinating amounts of antierythrocyte antibodies. However, more specific Coombs reagents directed at immunoglobulin classes, eg, anti-IgG, anti-IgA, or anti-L chains, may also be employed to detect cell-bound immunoglobulin. So-called non-gamma Coombs reagents which are directed against various complement components, eg, C3 or C4, may also produce erythrocyte agglutination in the case of autoimmune hemolytic anemia. In some instances of this disorder, only complement components are bound to the erythrocyte and the regular antiglobulin reaction is negative. The **direct Coombs test** detects γ-globulin or other serum proteins that are adherent to erythrocytes taken directly from a sensitized individual. The **indirect Coombs test** is a 2-stage reaction for detection of incomplete antibodies in a patient's serum. The serum in question is first incubated with test erythrocytes, and the putative antibody-coated cells are then agglutinated by a Coombs antiglobulin serum. The major applications of Coombs tests include

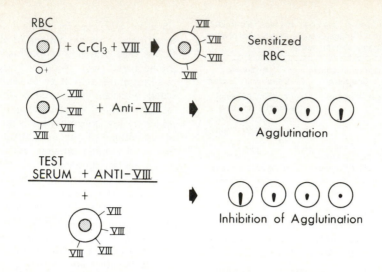

Figure 18–37. Hemagglutination inhibition. Human O + erythrocytes (RBC) are conjugated with coagulation factor VIII antigen by chromic chloride. The sensitized erythrocytes are reacted with specific antibody to factor VIII and are agglutinated. In the well of a V-shaped microtiter plate, agglutinated erythrocytes appear as discrete dots. Nonagglutinated cells form a streak when the plate is incubated at a 45-degree angle. Agglutination of sensitized red blood cells can be inhibited by the presence of homologous factor VIII antigen present in the test serum. With decreasing amounts of serum added to the test, the specific antibody agglutinates sensitized cells and forms a dot in the microtiter well. A semiquantitative estimation of the amount or titer of antigen in a test serum can be made in this way.

erythrocyte typing in blood banks, the evaluation of hemolytic disease of the newborn, and the diagnosis of autoimmune hemolytic anemia.

Bentonite Flocculation Test

Passive carriers of antigen other than erythrocytes have been widely used in serology for the demonstration of agglutinating antibody. Wyoming bentonite is a form of siliceous earth that can directly adsorb most types of protein, carbohydrate, and nucleic acid. After adsorption, many antigens are stable on bentonite for 3–6 months. Simple flocculation on slides with appropriate positive and negative control sera indicates the presence of serum antibody. Bentonite flocculation has been employed to detect antibodies to *Trichinella,* DNA, and rheumatoid factor.

Latex Fixation Test

Latex particles may also be used as passive carriers for adsorbed soluble protein and polysaccharide antigens. The most widespread application of latex agglutination (fixation) has been in the detection of rheumatoid factor. Rheumatoid factor is a pentameric IgM antibody directed against IgG (see Chapter 36). If IgG is passively adsorbed to latex particles, specific determinants on the IgG are revealed which then react with IgM rheumatoid factors. This method is more sensitive but less specific for rheumatoid factor than the Rose-Waaler test (see below).

Rose-Waaler Test

This passive hemagglutination test is also used for the detection of rheumatoid factor. Tanned erythrocytes (usually from sheep) are coated with subagglutinating amounts of rabbit IgG antibodies specific for sheep erythrocytes. Human rheumatoid factor will agglutinate these rabbit immunoglobulin-sensitized sheep erythrocytes by virtue of a cross-reaction between rabbit IgG and human IgG. The use of this test and latex fixation in the diagnosis of rheumatoid diseases (especially rheumatoid arthritis) is discussed in Chapter 36.

COMPLEMENT ASSAYS

Complement is one of the main humoral effector mechanisms of immune complex-induced tissue damage (see Chapter 14). Clinical disorders of complement function have been recognized for many decades, but their mechanism and eventual treatment have awaited elucidation of the complement sequence itself. The 9 major complement components of the classic pathway (C1–C9), several from the alternative pathway, and various inhibitors can now be measured in human serum. Clinically useful assays of complement consist primarily of CH_{50} or total hemolytic assays and specific functional or immunochemical assays for various components. Immunochemical means provide molecular concentrations in serum but do not provide data regarding the functional integrity of the various molecules.

It is worth emphasizing that the collection and storage of serum samples for functional or immunochemical complement assays present special problems as a result of the remarkable lability of some of the complement components. Rapid removal of serum from clotted specimens and storage at temperatures of $-70\ °C$ or lower are required for preservation of maximal activity.

Complement fixation or utilization, which occurs as a consequence of antigen-antibody reactions, provides a sensitive and useful means of detecting antigens or antibodies in serology.

HEMOLYTIC ASSAY

Specific antibody-mediated hemolysis of erythrocytes by complement is a relatively insensitive screening test for complement activity in human serum. However, it has limited usefulness, since a marked reduction in components is necessary to produce a reduction in the hemolytic assay. The hemolytic assay employs sheep erythrocytes (E), rabbit antibody (A) to sheep erythrocytes, and fresh guinea pig serum as a source of complement (C). Hemolysis is measured spectrophotometrically as the absorbance of released hemoglobin and can be directly related to the number of erythrocytes lysed. The amount of lysis in a standardized system employing E, A, and C describes an S-shaped curve when plotted against increasing amounts of added complement (Fig 18–38).

The curve is S-shaped, but in the mid-region, near 50% hemolysis, a nearly linear relationship exists between the degree of hemolysis and the amount of complement present. In this range, the degree of erythrocyte lysis is very sensitive to any alteration in complement concentration. For clinical purposes, measurement of total hemolytic activity of serum is taken at 50% hemolysis level. The CH_{50} is an arbitrary unit defined as the quantity of complement necessary for 50% lysis of erythrocytes under rigidly standardized conditions of sensitization with antibody (EA). CH_{50} test results are expressed as the reciprocal of the serum dilution giving 50% hemolysis. Variables that can influence the degree of hemolysis include erythrocyte concentration, fragility (age) of erythrocytes, amount of antibody used for sensitization, nature of the antibody (eg, IgG or IgM), ionic strength of the buffer system, pH, reaction time, temperature, and divalent cation (Ca^{2+} or Mg^{2+}) concentrations.

The value for CH_{50} units in human serum may be determined in several ways. Usually, one employs

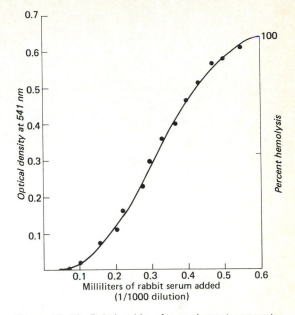

Figure 18–38. Relationship of complement concentration and erythrocytes lysed. Curve relating the percentage of hemolysis that results from increasing amounts of fresh rabbit serum (diluted 1:1000) as complement source is added to sensitized sheep erythrocytes (erythrocyte amboceptor [EA]). Hemolysis can be precisely determined by measuring the optical density of hemolysis supernates at 541 nm, the wavelength for maximal absorbance by hemoglobin.

the von Krogh equation, which converts the S-shaped complement titration curve into a nearly straight line.

The S-shaped curve in Fig 18–38 is described by the von Krogh equation:

$$X = K\left(\frac{Y}{1 - Y}\right)^{1/n}$$

where X = mL of diluted complement added,
Y = degree of percentage lysis,
K = constant,
n = 0.2 ± 10% under standard E and A conditions.

It is convenient to convert the von Krogh equation to a log form that renders the curve linear for plotting of clinical results (Fig 18–39):

$$\log X = \log K + \frac{1}{n}\ \log\ \frac{Y}{1 - Y}$$

The values of $Y/(1 - Y)$ are plotted on a log-log scale against serum dilutions. The reciprocal of the dilution of serum that intersects the curve at the value $Y/(1 - Y) = 1$ is the CH_{50} unit. Values for normal CH_{50} units vary greatly depending on partic-

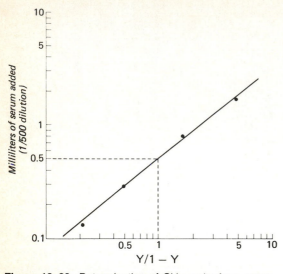

Figure 18–39. Determination of CH_{50} units from serum. Standard curve relating milliliters of serum 1:500 dilution to $Y/(1 - Y)$ from von Krogh equation. When $Y/(1 - Y)$ = 1.0, the percentage of lysis equals 50%. In the example shown, 0.5 mL of 1:500 serum dilution has produced $Y/(1 - Y)$ = 1.0 or 50% lysis. The CH_{50} value for this serum equals 1000, since 1 mL of serum would have 1000 lytic units.

ular conditions of the test employed. It should again be emphasized that the CH_{50} assay is relatively insensitive to reduction in specific complement components and may in fact be normal or only slightly depressed in the face of significant reduction in individual components.

MEASUREMENT OF INDIVIDUAL COMPLEMENT COMPONENTS

Functional Assays

Activation of the entire complement sequence of C1–C9 must occur to produce lysis of antibody-coated erythrocytes (EA). Thus, a general scheme can be proposed to determine the level of activity of individual complement components. Initially, one must obtain pure preparations of each of the individual components. These pure components are then added sequentially to EA until the step is reached just prior to the component to be measured. The test sample is added and the degree of subsequent erythrocyte lysis is then related to the presence of the later-acting components. Of course, all proximal components must be supplied in excess to measure more distally acting intermediates. Alternatively, the presence of genetically defined complement deficiencies has made available to the laboratory a further source of specifically deficient reagents for estimating individual component activity. A description

of the technique of functional assays for complement components and their inhibitors is found in the monograph of Rapp and Borsos.

Immunoassays for Complement Components

Antibodies can be prepared against most of the major complement components and compliment inhibitors, which allow immunochemical determination of complement components. Techniques that have been utilized for this purpose include electro-immunodiffusion (Laurell rocket electrophoresis), single radial diffusion, and rate nephelometry. Although immunologic assay of complement components is independent of their biologic function, alterations in the chemical composition of complement components during storage may alter their behavior in these immunoassays. For example, in storage, C3 spontaneously converts to C3c, which has a smaller molecular size than native C3. Thus, when single radial diffusion of the timed interval variety is used, stored serum will give falsely high estimates because more rapid diffusion produces a larger ring diameter. Crucial to accuracy in clinical laboratory tests for complement is reliability of standards. In general, commercial sera prepared from large normal donor pools are adequate. However, since complement components are thermolabile when stored above −70 °C, great care must be taken to ensure adequate refrigerated storage. In fact, the major source of error in complement determination is poor sample handling.

Measurement and significance of complement fragments or catabolic products are discussed in Chapter 14.

Significance of CH_{50} Units

A. Reduced Serum Complement Activity: Reduced amounts of serum complement activity have been reported in a variety of disease states (Table 18–10). The reduction in serum complement activity could be due to any one or a combination of (1) complement consumption by in vivo formation of antigen-antibody complexes, (2) decreased synthesis of complement, (3) increased catabolism of complement, or (4) formation of an inhibitor. Although complement has been demonstrated fixed to various tissues, eg, glomerular basement membrane, in association with antibody, tissue fixation of complement is apparently not an important mechanism in lowering serum complement activity. Isolated reduction in human serum levels of C1, C2, C3, C6, or C7 to 50% of normal only slightly reduces hemolytic activity. For this reason, many laboratories have switched from CH_{50} to a more simple immunochemical determination of C3. In general, the reduction of C3 correlates positively with CH_{50} activity reduction.

B. Elevated Complement Levels: Although complement levels are elevated in a variety of dis-

Table 18–10. Diseases associated with reduced hemolytic complement activity.

Systemic lupus erythematosus with glomerulonephritis
Acute glomerulonephritis
Membranoproliferative glomerulonephritis
Acute serum sickness
Immune complex diseases
Advanced cirrhosis of the liver
Disseminated intravascular coagulation
Severe combined immunodeficiency
Infective endocarditis with glomerulonephritis
Infected ventriculoarterial shunts
Hereditary angioneurotic edema
Hereditary C2 deficiency
Paroxysmal cold hemoglobinuria
Myasthenia gravis
Infective hepatitis with arthritis
Allograft rejection
Mixed cryoglobulinemia (IgM-IgG)
Lymphoma

Table 18–11. Diseases associated with elevated serum complement concentrations.

Obstructive jaundice
Thyroiditis
Acute rheumatic fever
Rheumatoid arthritis
Periarteritis nodosa
Dermatomyositis
Acute myocardial infarction
Ulcerative colitis
Typhoid fever
Diabetes
Gout
Reiter's syndrome

eases (Table 18–11), the significance of this observation is unclear. The most likely mechanism is overproduction.

The development of specific functional and immunologic methods for detecting complement components has led to the discovery of a variety of genetically determined disorders of the complement system. A discussion of the specific disease states which result from selective deficiency of the various complement components is found in Chapter 28.

COMPLEMENT FIXATION TESTS

The fixation of complement occurs during the interaction of antigen and antibodies. Thus, the consumption of complement in vitro can be used as a test to detect and measure antibodies, antigens, or both. The test depends on a 2-stage reaction system. In the initial stage, antigen and antibody react in the presence of a known amount of complement and complement is consumed (fixed). In the second stage, hemolytic complement activity is measured to determine the amount of complement fixed and thus the amount of antigen or antibody present in the initial mixture (Fig 18–40). The amount of activity remaining after the initial antigen-antibody reaction is

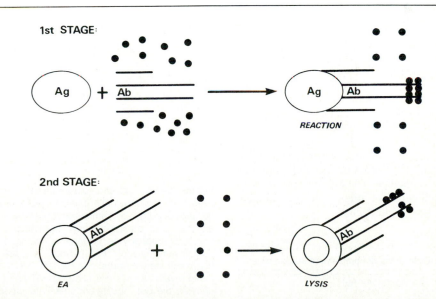

Figure 18–40. Principles of complement fixation. In the first stage, antigen (Ag) and antibody (Ab) are reacted in the presence of complement (●). The interaction of Ag and antibody fixes some but not all of the complement available. In the second stage, the residual or unfixed complement is measured by adding EA (erythrocyte amboceptor), which is lysed by residual complement. Thus, a reciprocal relationship exists between amounts of lysis in second stage and antigen present in the first stage.

back-titrated in the hemolytic assay (see above). Results are expressed as either the highest serum dilution showing fixation for antibody estimation or the concentration of antigen that is limiting for antigen determinations.

Extremely sensitive assays for antigen or antibody concentrations have been developed using microcomplement fixation. However, these assays are too cumbersome and complex for routine clinical laboratory use.

Complement fixation tests (Fig 18–40) have received widespread application in both research and clinical laboratory practice. Table 18–12 lists some of the applications of complement fixation for either antigen or antibody determination. It should be recalled that all complement assay systems involving functional tests can be inhibited by anticomplementary action of serum. This may result from antigen-antibody complexes, heparin, chelating agents, and aggregated immunoglobulins, eg, as in multiple myeloma.

MONOCLONAL ANTIBODIES

The production of monoclonal antibodies by somatic cell hybridization of antibody-forming cells and continuously replicating cell lines created a revolution in immunology. The technique of hybridoma formation described by Köhler and Milstein in 1975 has allowed preparation of virtually unlimited quantities of antibodies that are chemically, physically, and immunologically completely homogeneous since each antibody is synthesized from cells derived from a single clone. These molecules are then generally unencumbered by nonspecificity and cross-reactivity. In laboratory immunology, monoclonal antibodies are used to detect cellular and soluble antigens with RIA, ELISA, and IFA. Some well-established immunochemical methods such as immunodiffusion and immunoelectrophoresis probably do not require the degree of specificity afforded by monoclonal antibodies. The marrow specificity of monoclonal antibodies for single epitopes can theoretically limit their applicability.

Table 18–12. Applications of complement fixation tests.

Hepatitis-associated antigen (HBsAg)
Antiplatelet antibodies
Anti-DNA
Immunoglobulins
L chains
Wassermann test for syphilis
Coccidioides immitis antigen

TECHNIQUE OF MONOCLONAL ANTIBODY PRODUCTION

Hybridomas or somatic cell hybrids can readily be formed by fusing a single cell suspension of splenocytes or lymphocytes from immunized mice or rats to cells of continuously replicating tumor cells, eg, myelomas or lymphomas (Fig 18–41). The replicating cell line is selected for 2 distinct properties: (1) lack of immunoglobulin production or secretion, and (2) lack of hypoxanthine phosphoribosyl transferase (HPRT) activity. The cells are fused by rapid exposure to polyethylene glycol. Thereafter, 3 cell

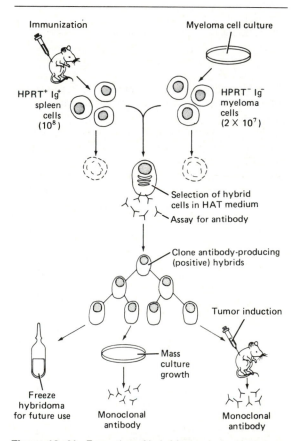

Figure 18–41. Formation of hybridomas between mouse cells and myeloma cells. Mouse myeloma cells that do not produce their own immunoglobulins and lack hypoxanthine and phosphoribosyl transferase (HPRT) are fused to splenocytes from an immunized mouse with polyethylene glycol. The hybrid cells are selected in hypoxanthine-aminopterin-thymidine (HAT) medium. Unfused myeloma cells are killed by HAT and unfused splenocytes die out. The hybridomas are cloned, and antibody is produced in tissue culture or by ascites formation. (Reproduced, with permission, from Diamond BA, Yelton DE, Scharff MD: Monoclonal antibodies: A new technique for producing serologic reagents. *N Engl J Med* 1981;**304**:1344.)

populations remain in culture: splenocytes, myeloma cells, and hybrids. The hybrids have the combined genome of the parent lines and eventually extrude chromosomes and acquire a diploid state. Selection for the hybrids is accomplished by awaiting natural death of the splenocytes. The myeloma cell line is killed, because in HAT medium, which contains hypoxanthine, aminopterin, and thymidine, HPRT cells cannot use exogenous hypoxanthine to produce purines. Aminopterin blocks endogenous synthesis of purines and pyrimidines, and the cells die. Hybrids begin to double every 24–48 hours, and colonies rapidly form.

The hybridoma cells are then cloned by limiting dilution methods and supernates assayed for antibody production, usually by ELISA or RIA. Recloning is performed to ensure monoclonality, and large numbers of cells are grown for antibody production. Extensive immunochemical and serologic studies are performed to ensure antibody specificity. Large quantities of antibody can be produced in serum-free tissue culture or in ascites fluid in syngeneic mice. Cells are stored in liquid nitrogen for further use.

Inter- as well as intraspecies hybridomas can be produced and propagated in long-term culture. For use in human therapeutic research, mouse hybridomas have usually been employed, but these regularly produce anti-murine antibody responses after infusions in humans. For this reason and for maximum specificity, human-to-human hybridomas have also been developed. Limitations in range of antibody specificities and technical difficulties in maintaining these hybridomas in culture need to be overcome.

Some examples of application of monoclonal antibodies in immunology are listed in Table 18–13.

COMPARATIVE SENSITIVITY OF QUANTITATIVE IMMUNOASSAYS

A major limitation of all quantitative immunoassays is their sensitivity. Exact lower limits of analyte detection vary with avidity, concentration, lots of antisera, temperature, length of reaction, and other factors. Nevertheless, it is useful to consider the approximate limits of sensitivity of various methods available in the clinical immunology laboratory. The most commonly employed techniques are listed in Table 18–14 in order of increasing sensitivity.

PREDICTIVE VALUE THEORY

When *any* test is used to make a decision, there is some probability of drawing an erroneous conclu-

---

Table 18–13. Applications of monoclonal antibodies.

Diagnostic (Many achieved; some experimental.)
  Leukocyte identification
  Lymphocyte subset determination
  HLA antigen detection
    Individual specificities of A, B, C, DR loci
    Framework specificities
  Viral detection and subtyping, eg, influenza variants
  Parasite identification
  Other microorganism detection
  Polypeptide hormone detection
  Relatedness of hormones, eg, hGH, hCS, hPRL
  Detection of carcinoembryonic protein, eg, CEA, AFP
  Detection of cardiac myosin for myocardial injury
  Typing of leukemias and lymphomas
  Detection of tumor-related antigens
  Immunohistochemical application in tissue sections
Therapeutic (Experimental; can be coupled to a toxin or radioisotope to enhance in vivo effects.)
  Antitumor therapy
    Individual tumor antigen-specific
    Anti-idiotype to surface immunoglobulin on B cell lymphomas
  Immunosuppression
    Organ transplantation
    Autoimmune and hypersensitivity diseases
    Treatment of GVH disease
  Fertility control
    Anti-hCG or antitrophoblast antibodies
    Drug toxicity reversal, eg, digitalis intoxication

Table 18–14. Relative sensitivity of assays for antigens and antibodies.[1]

Technique	Approximate Sensitivity (per dL)
Total serum proteins (by biuret or refractometry)	100 mg
Serum protein electrophoresis (zone electrophoresis)	100 mg
Analytic ultracentrifugation	100 mg
Immunoelectrophoresis	5–10 mg
Immunofixation	5–10 mg
Single radial diffusion	< 1–2 mg
Double diffusion in agar (Ouchterlony)	< 1 mg
Electroimmunodiffusion (rocket electrophoresis)	< 0.5 mg
One-dimensional double electroimmunodiffusion (counterimmunoelectrophoresis)	< 0.1 mg
Nephelometry	0.1 mg
Complement fixation	1 μg
Agglutination	1 μg
Enzyme immunoassay (ELISA)	< 1 μg
Quantitative immunofluorescence	< 1 pg
Radioimmunoassay (RIA)	< 1 pg

[1]Modified and reproduced, with permission, from Ritzmann SE: *Behring Diagnostics Manual on Proteinology and Immunoassays,* 2nd ed. Behring Diagnostics (New Jersey), 1977.

sion. Predictive value theory can be used to deal with this problem. An example of its application in diagnosis of multiple sclerosis follows. This diagnosis is still made primarily by using the patient's history and physical findings. However, several laboratory tests are used as decision aids. One such test is the CSF IgG index, which is a ratio of ratios, [CSF IgG:albumin]:[serum IgG:albumin]. To simplify discussion, we have consolidated the patients into 2 groups, those with definite or probable multiple sclerosis, and all others. For every individual, 2 items of information are noted: (1) the diagnostic category (disease or no disease) and (2) the result of the laboratory test (normal or abnormal). This divides the results into 4 categories: **true positives** and **true negatives,** and **false positives** and **false negatives.** False-positive and false-negative results lead to erroneous conclusions. The results can be presented as a two-by-two contingency table as in Table 18–15.

Several basic terms are used in predictive value theory. **Diagnostic sensitivity** (not to be confused with analytic sensitivity, discussed in the context of ligand assay) is defined as the fraction of diseased subjects with abnormal test results. **Diagnostic specificity** is defined as the fraction of nondiseased subjects who have a normal laboratory test. The **positive predictive value** is the fraction of abnormal tests that represent disease, and **negative predictive value** is the fraction of normal tests that represent the absence of disease. Computing these values for the data in Table 18–15, we find

Diagnostic Sensitivity $= \dfrac{54}{64} = 0.84$

Diagnostic Specificity $= \dfrac{110}{129} = 0.85$

Positive predictive value $= \dfrac{54}{73} = 0.74$

Negative predictive value $= \dfrac{110}{120} = 0.92$

Note that diagnostic sensitivity and specificity reveal something about the test *given prior knowledge about the disease status,* whereas positive and negative predictive values estimate the *likelihood of disease given the test result.* Clearly, it is the latter case that is of interest when trying to make a diagnosis. In this context, it is vital to realize that although diagnostic sensitivity and specificity are qualities of a test, positive and negative predictive values are determined by both test performance and the prevalence of the disease in the patient population under study. Prevalence is defined as the proportion of the population afflicted by the disease in question. For the patient population in Table 18–15, the prevalence was ($^{64}/_{193} = 0.33$), or 33%. Table 18–16 illustrates the effect of prevalence by presenting data for the CSF index in which the sensitivity and specificity have remained the same as in Table 18–15, but the prevalence of disease has decreased 10-fold, to 3.3%.

The positive and negative predictive values are now

Positive predictive value $= \dfrac{54}{334} = 0.16$

Negative predictive value $= \dfrac{1586}{1596} = 0.99$

Note that although the negative predictive value has increased slightly, there has been a substantial drop in the positive predictive value. The latter effect is due to the presence of a large number of false positives. For the population studied in Table 18–15 we could say that a positive test indicated disease in 74% of cases. For the population studied in Table 18–16 a positive test is associated with disease in only 16% of cases.

Predictive value theory applies only to dichotomous tests, ie, tests that are classified as normal or abnormal. In the case of the CSF index, this requires the selection of some diagnostic cutoff for the test results that separates normal from abnormal values. The diagnostic sensitivity and specificity change as the cutoff is changed. More advanced decision theory provides more sophisticated tools for the analysis of tests reported as values from a continuous scale.

Table 18–15. A two-by-two contingency table.

| Test Status | Disease Status | | Totals |
	Present	Absent	
Positive	54 (True positives)	19 (False positives)	73
Negative	10 (False negatives)	110 (True negatives)	120
Totals	64	129	193

Table 18–16. The effect of prevalence upon predictive value.

| Test Status | Disease Status | | Totals |
	Present	Absent	
Positive	54 (True positives)	280 (False positives)	334
Negative	10 (False negatives)	1586 (True negatives)	1596
Totals	64	1866	1930

REFERENCES

General

Hudson L, Hay FC: *Practical Immunology,* 2nd ed. Blackwell, 1981.

Ritzmann SE (editor): Protein abnormalities. Vol 1. *Physiology of Immunoglobulins.* Vol 2. *Pathology of Immunoglobulins.* Liss, 1982.

Rose NR, Friedman H, Fahey J: *Manual of Clinical Immunology,* 3rd ed. American Society for Microbiology, 1986.

Use and abuse of laboratory tests in clinical immunology: Critical considerations of eight widely used diagnostic procedures. (Report of IUIS/WHO Working Group.) *Clin Exp Immunol* 1981:**46:**662.

Voller A, Bartlett A, Bidwell D: *Immunoassays for the '80s.* University Park Press, 1981.

Weir DM (editor): *Handbook of Experimental Immunology,* 4th ed. 4 vols. Blackwell, 1986.

Immunodiffusion

Crowle AJ: *Immunodiffusion,* 2nd ed. Academic Press, 1973.

Deverill I, Reeves WG: Light scattering and absorption developments in immunology. *J Immunol Methods* 1980;**38:**191.

Ouchterlony O, Nilsson LA: Immunodiffusion and immunoelectrophoresis. Chapter 32 in: *Handbook of Experimental Immunology.* Vol 1. Weir DM (editor). Blackwell, 1986.

Stiehm ER, Fudenberg HH: Serum levels of immune globulins in health and disease: A survey. *Pediatrics* 1966;**37:**715.

Electrophoresis

Cawley LP et al: *Basic Electrophoresis, Immunoelectrophoresis and Immunochemistry.* American Society of Clinical Pathologists Commission on Continuing Education, 1972.

Crowle AJ: *Immunodiffusion,* 2nd ed. Academic Press, 1973.

Gockman N, Burke MD: Electrophoretic techniques in today's clinical laboratory. *Clin Lab Med* 1986;**6:**403.

Jeppsson JO, Laurell CB, Franzen B: Agarose gel electrophoresis. *Clin Chem* 1979;**25:**629.

Ouchterlony O, Nilsson LA: Immunodiffusion and immunoelectrophoresis. Chapter 32 in: *Handbook of Experimental Immunology,* 4th ed. Vol 1. Weir DM (editor). Blackwell, 1986.

Roberts RT: Usefulness of immunofixation electrophoresis in the clinical laboratory. *Clin Lab Med* 1986;**6:**601.

Immunochemical & Physicochemical Methods

Brouet JC et al: Biological and clinical significance of cryoglobulins: A report of 86 cases. *Am J Med* 1974;**57:**775.

Lambert PH, Dixon FJ, Zubler RH: A collaborative study for the evaluation of eighteen methods for detecting immune complexes in serum. *J Lab Clin Immunol* 1978;**1:**1.

Somer T: Hyperviscosity syndrome in plasma cell dyscrasias. *Adv Microcirculation* 1975;**6:**1.

Williams RC: *Immune Complexes in Clinical and Experimental Medicine.* Harvard Univ Press, 1980.

Winfield JB: Cryoglobulinemia. *Hum Pathol* 1983; **14:**350.

Whicher JT, Warren C, Chambers RE: Immunochemical assays for immunoglobulins. *Ann Clin Biochem* 1984; **21:**78.

Binder-Ligand Assay

Butt WR (editor): Pages 71–101 in: *Practical Immunoassay: The State of the Art.* Dekker, 1984.

Dudley RA et al: Guidelines for immunoassay data processing. *Clin Chem* 1985;**31:**1264.

O'Sullivan MJ, Bridges JW, Marks V: Enzyme immunoassay: A review. *Ann Clin Biochem* 1979;**16:**221.

Rodgers RPC: Quality control and data analysis in binder-ligand assay. *Scientific Newsletters,* 1981.

Schall RF, Tenoso JH: Alternatives to radioimmunoassay: Labels and methods. *Clin Chem* 1981;**27:**157.

Immunohistochemical Techniques

Colvin RB, Bhan AK, McCluskey RT: *Diagnostic Immunopathology.* Raven Press, 1988.

Falini B, Taylor CR: New developments in immunoperoxidase techniques and their application. *Arch Pathol Lab Med* 1983;**107:**105.

Goldman M: *Fluorescent Antibody Methods.* Academic Press, 1968.

Guesdon JL, Ternynck T, Avrameas S: The use of avidin-biotin interaction in immunoenzymatic techniques. *J Histochem Cytochem* 1979;**27:**1131.

Kemery DM, Challacombe SJ: *ELISA and Other Solid Phase Immunoassays.* John Wiley, 1988.

Nairn RC: *Fluorescent Protein Tracing.* 4th ed. Longman, 1976.

Agglutination

Fudenberg HH: Hemagglutination inhibition. Pages 101–110 in: *A Seminar on Basic Immunology.* American Association of Blood Banks, 1971.

Herbert WJ: Passive hemagglutination with special reference to the tanned cell technique. Chapter 20 in: *Handbook of Experimental Immunology.* Weir DM (editor). Blackwell, 1978.

Complement Function

Fearon DT, Austen KF: The alternative pathway of complement: A system for host resistance to microbial infection. *N Engl J Med* 1980;**303:**259.

Harrison RA, Lachmann PJ: Complement technology. Chapter 39 in: *Handbook of Experimental Immunology,* 4th ed. Vol. 1. Weir DM (editor). Blackwell, 1986.

Müller-Eberhard HJ (editor): Complement. *Springer Semin Immunopathol* 1983;**6(No. 2/3).**

Osler AG: *Complement Mechanisms of Function.* Prentice Hall, 1976.

Monoclonal Antibodies

Diamond B, Yelton D, Scharff MD: Monoclonal antibodies: A new technology for producing serologic reagents. *N Engl J Med* 1981;**304:**1344.

Hurrell JGR (editor): *Monoclonal Hybridoma Antibodies: Techniques and Applications.* CRC Press, 1982.

McMichael AJ, Fabre JW: *Monoclonal Antibodies in Clinical Medicine.* Academic Press, 1982.

Milstein C: Overview: Monoclonal Antibodies and 4 following chapters in section on Monoclonal Antibodies in: *Handbook of Experimental Immunology,* 4th ed. Vol 4. Weir DM (editor). Blackwell, 1986.

Predictive Value Theory

Gottfried EL, Wagar EA: Laboratory testing: A practical guide. *Disease-a-Month* 1983;**29**:1.

Griner PF et al: Selection and interpretation of diagnostic tests and procedures. *Ann Intern Med* 1981;**4**:553.

Hershey LA, Trotter JL: The use and abuse of the cerebrospinal fluid CSF profile in the adult: A practical evaluation. *Ann Neurol* 1980;**8**:426.

Clinical Laboratory Methods for Detection of Cellular Immunity

19

Daniel P. Stites, MD

The immune system in humans can be divided into 2 major parts, one involving humoral immunity (antibody and complement) and the other cellular immunity. In many ways this separation is artificial, and many examples of the interdependence of cellular and humoral immunity exist. Nevertheless, dividing the immune system into parts in this way provides a conceptual and practical framework for the laboratory evaluation of immunity in clinical practice.

In the preceding chapter we reviewed methods of detecting antibodies and methods that employ antibodies for antigen detection. The role of a variety of distinct cell types (see Chapter 5) in immune mechanisms in normal and diseased persons has become measurable in the clinical laboratory. Immunocompetent cells, including lymphocytes, monocytemacrophages, and granulocytes, are all involved in the delayed hypersensitivity reactions that are so important in immunity to intracellular infection, tumor immunity, and transplant rejection. The clinical laboratory investigation of the number and function of these cells is still beset by difficulties in test standardization, biologic variability, the imprecise nature of many assays, and the complexity and expense of the procedures. Nevertheless, several tests that are of value in assessing cellular function have become available for clinical use. Many of these assays employ sophisticated immunochemical methods for detecting cellular antigens or markers. Of great importance is the advent of monoclonal antibodies to detect various leukocyte subsets. Molecular biologic techniques such as Southern blots have recently been employed to detect either immunoglobulin gene or T cell receptor gene rearrangements as markers of specific B and T cell lineages. Thus, we are witnessing an increasing fusion of biochemistry with cellular immunology.

The present chapter reviews the tests that have medical application in the detection of cell types and their corresponding functions. The intention is not to provide a comprehensive laboratory manual of all cellular immunologic procedures but to familiarize the reader with the principles, applications, and interpretation of assays with clinical applicability. Our understanding of cellular immunity continues to expand, and technologic advances in methods for its assessment have been developed. In Chapter 22 special application of these and other tests for evaluating immune competence is described.

The topics discussed include (1) delayed hypersensitivity skin tests, (2) assays for T and B lymphocytes, (3) lymphocyte activation, (4) monocytemacrophage assays, and (5) neutrophil function.

DELAYED HYPERSENSITIVITY SKIN TESTS

Despite the development of a multitude of complex procedures for the assessment of cellular immunity, the relatively simple intradermal test remains a useful tool, occasionally serving to establish a diagnosis. Delayed hypersensitivity skin testing detects cutaneous hypersensitivity to an antigen or group of antigens. However, when one is testing for an infectious disease, a positive test does not necessarily imply active infection with the agent being tested for. Delayed hypersensitivity skin tests are also of great value in the overall assessment of immunocompetence and in epidemiologic surveys. Inability to react to a battery of common skin antigens is termed **anergy,** and clinical conditions associated with this hyporeactive state are listed in Table 19–1.

Technique of Skin Testing

(1) Lyophilized antigens should be stored sterile at 4 °C, protected from light, and reconstituted shortly before use. The manufacturer's expiration date should be observed.

(2) Test solutions should not be stored in syringes for prolonged periods before use.

(3) A 25- or 27-gauge needle usually ensures intradermal rather than subcutaneous administration of antigen. Multiple test devices that deliver up to 8 antigens simultaneously are also available, but these devices utilize a prick test, which has not been fully evaluated for delayed hypersensitivity skin testing.

Table 19–1. Clinical conditions associated with anergy.[1]

I. Immunologic deficiency
Congenital
Combined deficiencies of cellular and humoral immunity
Ataxia-telangiectasia
Nezelof's syndrome
Severe combined immunodeficiency
Wiskott-Aldrich syndrome
Cellular immunodeficiency
Thymic and parathyroid aplasia (DiGeorge's syndrome)
Mucocutaneous candidiasis
Acquired
AIDS
Sarcoidosis
Chronic lymphocytic leukemia
Carcinoma
Immunosuppressive medication
Rheumatoid diseases
Uremia
Alcoholic cirrhosis
Biliary cirrhosis
Surgery
Hodgkin's disease and lymphomas
II. Infections
Influenza
Mumps
Measles
Viral vaccines
Typhus
Miliary and active tuberculosis
Disseminated mycotic infection
Lepromatous leprosy
Scarlet fever
III. Technical errors in skin testing
Improper antigen concentrations
Bacterial contamination
Exposure to heat or light
Adsorption of antigen on container walls
Faulty injection (too deep, leaking)
Improper reading of reaction

[1]Modified from Heiss LI, Palmer DL: Anergy in patients with leukocytosis. *Am J Med* 1974;**56:**323.

Subcutaneous injection leads to dilution of the antigen in tissues and can lead to a resultant false-negative test.

(4) The largest dimensions of both erythema and induration should be measured with a ruler and recorded at both 24 and 48 hours.

(5) Hyporeactivity to any given antigen or group of antigens should be confirmed by testing with higher concentrations of antigen or, in ambiguous circumstances, by a repeat test with the intermediate dose.

Contact Sensitivity

Direct application to the skin of chemically reactive compounds results in systemic sensitization to various metabolites of the sensitizing compound. The precise chemical fate of the sensitizing compound is not known, but sensitizing agents such as dinitrochlorobenzene (DNCB) probably form dinitrophenylprotein complexes with various skin proteins. Sensitization with DNCB has been used experimentally in skin testing for delayed hypersensitivity in selected patients with suspected anergy. It is not a routine procedure and should be reserved for instances in which thorough delayed hypersensitivity testing with other antigens is negative. Concern regarding its possible toxicity and cross-sensitizing properties exists. Furthermore, its use as a diagnostic reagent is not currently approved by the FDA. Following application of DNCB to the skin, a period of about 7–10 days elapses before contact sensitivity can be elicited by a challenge dose applied to the skin surface. This sensitivity persists for years. The ability of a subject to develop contact sensitivity is a measure of cellular immunity to a new antigen to which the subject has not been previously exposed. Thus, the establishment of a state of cutaneous anergy in various disease states may be confirmed and extended by testing with DNCB.

Interpretation of contact sensitivity reactions depends on development of a flare, papular, or vesicular reaction at the site of challenge. Induration rarely occurs, since the test dose is not applied intradermally. In some clinical situations, a nonspecific depression in the inflammatory response can result in apparent anergy.

Patch testing is commonly employed by allergists and dermatologists to detect cutaneous hypersensitivity to various substances thought to be responsible for contact dermatitis. The test substance is applied in a low concentration and the area covered with an occlusive dressing. After 48 hours, the dressing is removed and the site examined for presence of the inflammatory reaction described above. False-positive reactions can result from too high a concentration of the test substance, irritation rather than allergy, and allergy to the adhesive in the dressing. False-negative tests usually result from too low a concentration of the test substance or inadequate skin penetration. The results of patch testing must be carefully weighed with the clinical history and knowledge of the chemistry of the potential sensitizing agent. (See also Chapters 29 and 33).

Interpretation & Pitfalls

The inflammatory infiltrate that occurs 24–48 hours following intradermal injection of an antigen consists primarily of mononuclear cells. This cellular infiltrate and the accompanying edema result in induration of the skin, and the diameter of this reaction is an index of cutaneous hypersensitivity. A patient may also demonstrate immediate hypersensitivity to the same test antigen, ie, a coexistent area (wheal and flare) at 15–20 minutes and late-phase inflammation at 5–8 hours, but this usually fades by 12–18 hours (see Chapters 11 and 29). Induration of 5 mm or more in diameter is the generally accepted criterion of a positive delayed skin test. Smaller but definitely indurated reactions suggest sensitivity to a closely related or cross-reacting antigen. There is no definitive evidence that repeated skin testing can result in conversion of delayed hypersensitivity skin tests from negative to positive. However, with some antigens, intradermal testing can result in elevations of serum antibody titers and confuse a serologic diagnosis. For this reason, blood for serologic study should always be obtained before skin tests are performed.

False-negative results will be obtained in patients receiving systemic cortico-steroids because of the anti-inflammatory effect of these drugs.

Delayed hypersensitivity skin testing is of relatively little value in establishing the diagnosis of defective cellular immunity during the first year of life. Infants may fail to react owing to lack of antigen contact to the various test antigens. Consequently, in vitro assay for T cell numbers and function is much more useful in the diagnosis of congenital immunodeficiency disease (see Chapter 23). Recent evidence has also associated genetic markers in the HLA-DR region with failure to respond to various tuberculin antigens.

In late 1977, an FDA panel submitted a highly critical report to the Commissioner of the FDA on the safety and efficacy of several microbial skin test antigens. The evaluation considered various manufacturers' preparations of histoplasmin, tuberculin (PPD), coccidioidin, *Trichinella* extract, old tuberculin, diphtheria toxin for the Schick test, lymphogranuloma venereum antigen, and mumps skin test antigen. The Panel on Review of Skin Test Antigens found only 5 of the 23 tested products to be safe and effective. Immediate removal of 12 and temporary licensing of the remaining 6 were implemented by the Commissioner. The details of this report are published in *Federal Register* 1977;**42(Sept 30):**52, 674, which is published by the US Government Printing Office, Washington, DC.

Use of delayed and immediate hypersensitivity skin tests in diagnosis and management of allergies is discussed in Chapters 29–34.

Possible Adverse Reactions to Skin Tests

Occasional patients who are highly sensitive to various antigens will have marked local reactions to skin tests. If unusual sensitivity is suspected, a preliminary test should be performed with diluted antigen. Reactions include erythema, marked induration, and, rarely, local necrosis. Patch testing may rarely result in sensitization. Systemic side effects such as fever or anaphylaxis are uncommon. Injection of corticosteroids locally into hyperreactive indurated areas may modify the severity of the reaction. Similarly, the painful blistering and inflammation that sometimes occur following surface application of contact sensitizers can be reduced by topical corticosteroids.

ASSAYS FOR HUMAN LYMPHOCYTES & MONOCYTES

The era of modern cellular immunology began with the discovery that lymphocytes are divided into 2 major functionally distinct populations. Evidence for the existence of T (thymus-derived) and B (bone marrow-derived) lymphocytes in humans originated from studies of other mammalian and avian species and analysis of lymphocyte populations in immunodeficiency diseases (see Chapter 2). Extensive studies of cell surface molecules with monoclonal antibodies and in vitro functional assays have provided direct evidence for the existence of these major lymphocyte types and a third type called natural killer (NK) cells.

The terms T lymphocyte and B lymphocyte usually denote the 2 major classes of immunocompetent cells in peripheral blood. T lymphocytes arise in the thymus and migrate to peripheral lymphoid organs—lymph nodes, spleen, and circulate in the blood—during embryonic life. B lymphocytes mature during embryogenesis by a functional—but as yet anatomically undefined—equivalent of the avian bursa of Fabricius. T lymphocytes function as effector cells in cellular immune reactions, cooperate with B cells to form antibody (helper function), and suppress certain B cell functions (suppressor function). After appropriate antigenic stimulation, B lymphocytes differentiate into plasma cells that eventually secrete antibody. The notion that there is only one type of T cell or B cell has been found to be an oversimplification, since functionally distinct subclasses of T and B cells are now recognized.

Assays for T and B cells are currently in wide use in clinical immunology. Leukocytes are counted by microscopy or flow cytometry with specific antibodies to membrane antigens. The antibodies are conjugated either to fluorescent dyes or to enzymes that produce reactants. Such techniques can be applied either in tissue sections or in fresh suspensions of cells from blood, bone marrow, or other sites. Precise counting of T and B cells in human peripheral blood has made important contributions to our understanding of (1) immunodeficiency disorders, (2) autoimmune diseases, (3) tumor immunity, and (4) infectious disease immunity. It should be emphasized, however, that mere counting of T or B cells does not necessarily correlate with the functional capacity of these cells. At best, these assays provide a nosologic classification of immunocompetent cells; further evaluation of lymphocyte function usually should be performed to fully assess immunologic competence in clinical practice.

In 1983, the First International Workshop on Human Leukocyte Differentiation Antigens met and established a new nomenclature for immunologically defined cellular types and subtypes. They defined a series of **cluster of differentiation (CD)** types that define cellular antigens. In 1989, the fourth workshop refined and expanded this nomenclature. Definition of these CD types and relationship to other antigen or antibody designations are presented in Table 19–2. It should be emphasized that the CD nomenclature continues to replace the more familiar, often proprietary, antibody designations, eg, T4, Leu 3, or CD4, for example.

Separation of Peripheral Blood Mononuclear Cells for Lymphocyte & Monocyte Assays

Tests for human T and B cells are ordinarily performed on purified suspensions of mononuclear blood cells. An accepted procedure for obtaining mononuclear cell suspensions is density gradient centrifugation on Ficoll-Hypaque. This method results in a yield of 70–90% mononuclear cells with a high degree of purity but may selectively eliminate some lymphocyte subpopulations. Mononuclear preparations obtained by this method are relatively enriched in *monocytes*. These cells must be distinguished from lymphocytes by morphologic characteristics, phagocytic ability, endogenous enzymatic activity, or cell surface antigens (see below).

To avoid misinterpretation, results of tests for T and B cell markers on separated populations should generally be expressed as the number of cells per microliter of whole blood. Many published studies have indicated only the percentages of lymphocytes carrying a particular marker. Such a result could be due to an increase in the particular cell population or, alternatively, a decrease in other populations.

Thus, it is important that each laboratory establish standard absolute numbers of T and B cells per microliter of whole blood from normal individuals.

Methods for assessing cellular phenotypes utilizing whole unseparated blood have been developed. Cells are stained with fluorochrome-conjugated monoclonal antibodies, and erythrocytes are lysed. The residual washed leukocytes are counted by flow cytometry or fluorescence microscopy. The whole-blood method has the advantage of simplicity but has not yet been fully evaluated in many diseases. It is generally not useful for functional studies owing to potential interference by erythrocytes or plasma proteins.

T LYMPHOCYTE ASSAYS

Human T Cell-Specific Markers

Production of heteroantisera to normal and malignant human T cells created the potential for direct immunochemical detection of cellular subpopulations by immunofluorescence and other sensitive techniques. However, with few exceptions, conventional antisera raised in animals to T cell subsets have lacked sufficient specificity owing to extensive cross-reactivity and broad response to species-specific rather than lineage-specific antigens on the immunizing cells. Some degree of improvement in the quality of these reagents was achieved by use of naturally occurring human antibody derived from sera of patients with various autoimmune diseases or by use of purified or continuously cultured T cell subpopulations. However, with the advent of monoclonal antibodies produced by murine hybridomas (see Chapter 18), a major breakthrough was achieved in identification of human T cells.

Table 19–2. T cell differentiation antigens.

Cell Type Detected	CD Designation	Antibody Designation	Comments
Corticol thymocytes Langerhans cells	CD1	Leu 6 T6	Early T cell antigen also present on Langerhans cells, associated with β_2-microglobulin not present on peripheral T cells.
E rosette-forming cells T cells NK cells	CD2	Leu 5 T11	Pan-T cell antigen SRBC receptor on T cells.
Mature T cells T cell antigen receptor	CD3	Leu 4	Also present on T cell ALL and cutaneous T cell lymphoma.
Helper/inducer T cells Monocytes	CD4	Leu 3 T4	Can be further subdivided into helper and inducer subsets. Weakly expressed on monocytes.
Pan-T and -B cell subpopulation	CD5	Leu 1 T1 T101	B cell CLL. B cells following marrow transplant. B cells secrete autoantibodies.
Mature T cells	CD6	T12	Malignant T cells.
Pan-T cells, thymocytes NK cells	CD7	Leu 9 3A1	T cell leukemias.
Suppressor/cytotoxic T cells NK cells	CD8	Leu 2 T8	Can be further subdivided into cytotoxic and suppressor subsets.

Monoclonal antibodies have been produced in many laboratories to class-specific and subclass-specific T cell antigens. These antibodies are highly specific and sensitive reagents for detecting cells in suspensions or fixed tissue sections. An enormous proliferation of abbreviations for these sera has occurred simultaneously with their commercial availability. The use of CD terminology for some of these markers is compared with more common proprietary designations in Table 19–2. It is anticipated that new antigens defining specialized subsets of T cells will continue to emerge for the current groupings.

A. Performance of Test:

1. Production of T cell antibodies—T cells from various sources—especially thymocytes, purified peripheral blood T cells, T leukemia cells, or T cells from continuous culture—can be used for immunization of either goats or rabbits. The resulting antisera have both species-specific and T cell-specific antibodies. The former may be removed by absorption with B cells, liver, or kidney cells. Specificity must be shown by positive reaction with T cells and negative reaction with B cells. Monoclonal antibody is produced from murine hybridomas (see Chapter 18).

2. Detection of T cell antigens with specific antisera—Immunofluorescence of either live lymphocytes or frozen tissue sections is possible. Direct immunofluorescence is performed with fluorochrome-labeled γ-globulin fractions from anti-T cell serum or labeled hybridoma culture supernates or purified antibodies from the hybridomas.

In vitro cytotoxicity of human T cells by specific antisera may also be used to estimate T cell populations. Methods for assessing T cell killing include trypan blue vital staining or ^{51}Cr release assay.

B. Interpretation:

The percentage or absolute number of T cells or T cell subsets is determined by their binding to various specific antibodies. Cells are counted by direct observation using a fluorescence microscope or by flow cytometry (see below). The latter analysis has essentially replaced microscopy in clinical laboratories as simpler and less expensive instruments are developed. The overwhelming advantages of objectivity, sensitivity, and speed make flow-cytometric analysis preferable to the tedious process of counting cells by microscopic observation.

T Cell Subsets

Major subsets of T cells consist of helper and suppressor types. However, helper cells (CD4) consist of at least 2 phenotypically and functionally distinct subtypes: inducer cells (CD4$^+$, Leu 8$^+$, or TQ1$^+$), which influence induction of mature helper cells and suppressor cells; and helper cells (CD4$^+$, Leu 8$^-$, or TQ1$^-$), which influence antibody production of B cells. These 2 subtypes of the CD4 class are recognized phenotypically by the simultaneous expression of CD4 molecules and either Leu 8 or TQ1 (which have not yet received CD designations). So far, no single reagent has been developed that can identify these populations.

Suppressor cells (CD8) can similarly be subdivided into so-called true suppressor cells (CD8$^+$, CD11$^+$), which influence B cell antibody function, and cytotoxic T cells (CD8$^+$, CD11$^-$). Combinations of monoclonal antibodies are thus also used to detect these 2 important T cell subsets.

Helper:Suppressor Cell Ratios (T_H/Ts Ratio)

Largely because of the interest and concern generated by the current AIDS (acquired immunodeficiency syndrome) epidemic, many laboratories express results of helper/inducer and suppressor/cytotoxic T cell counts as a ratio or quotient. Caution must be exercised in using this approach, since the ratio may vary depending on changes in either numerator or denominator or both. Also, standardization of normal values and the clinical significance of slight deviations from the reference range are not well understood. Diseases or conditions that have been reported to be associated with high or low helper:suppressor ratios are presented in Table 19–3. Obviously, this laboratory test is not diagnostic of any particular condition and has to be interpreted cautiously based on the persistence or transience of the abnormality. In AIDS, for example, the reduction in the ratio seems to be permanent, whereas in some viral infections, eg, cytomegalovirus, it is reversible.

The use of absolute numbers or, in some instances, percentages of CD4 and CD8 cells is preferred. CD4 numbers are useful in AIDS prognosis and monitoring treatment. Levels of CD8 cells are transiently elevated in many viral infections.

Table 19–3. Helper:suppressor cell ratios in human peripheral blood.

Decreased in	Increased in
SLE with renal disease	Rheumatoid arthritis
Acute cytomegalovirus infection	Type I insulin-dependent diabetes mellitus
Burns	SLE without renal disease
GVH disease	Primary biliary cirrhosis
Sunburn or ultraviolet solarium exposure	Atopic dermatitis
Myelodysplasia syndromes	Sézary syndrome
Acute lymphocytic leukemia in remission	Psoriasis
Recovery from bone marrow transplant	Chronic autoimmune hepatitis
AIDS	
Herpes infections	
Infectious mononucleosis	
Measles	
Vigorous exercise	

E Rosette-Forming Cells

Human T cells were formerly identified by their ability to bind sheep erythrocytes (SRBC) to form rosettes (Fig 19–1). However, detection of this property has largely been replaced by more sensitive binding of monoclonal antibodies that identify the SRBC receptor. This receptor is now designated CD2.

B LYMPHOCYTE ASSAYS

B lymphocytes express a variety of cell surface molecules which can be detected with either monoclonal antibodies or polyclonal antisera. Mature B cells express CD19, CD20, and HLA-DR. Immature B cells may express additional molecules such as CD10 (CALLA) (Table 19–4). Some B cell tumors, particularly chronic lymphocytic leukemia, express CD5, and CD5-bearing B cells may produce autoantibodies in systemic lupus erythematosus and rheumatoid arthritis. The use of B cell surface markers in tumor diagnosis is discussed in detail in Chapter 48.

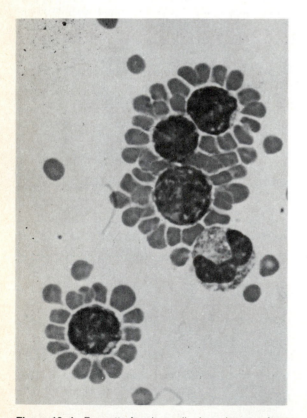

Figure 19–1. E rosette-forming cells. Lymphocytes from human peripheral blood that have formed rosettes with sheep erythrocytes. Such cells are T lymphocytes which bear the CD2 molecule. A granulocyte has failed to form a rosette. (Courtesy of M Kadin.)

Human B Cell-Specific Markers

A. Performance of Test: Monoclonal antibodies labeled with fluorochromes or enzymes are used to detect cells bearing the mature B cell markers CD19 and CD20. HLA-DR is also expressed on monocytes and activated on immature T cells. Fluorescence, or light microscopy in the case of enzyme-linked monoclonal antibodies, may be used, but flow cytometry is currently the preferred method. Additional markers for subsets of B cells are available (see Table 19–4) but have limited clinical utility. Plasma cells generally fail to express B cell markers, but have a set of their own (eg, PC1 + PCA − 1), which can be detected with monoclonal antibodies.

B. Interpretation: No functional information directly emerges from enumeration of B cells. Special problems exist with the use of non-murine polyspecific antisera and Fc receptor binding (see below).

Surface Immunoglobulin

B lymphocytes have readily demonstrable surface immunoglobulin. This surface immunoglobulin is synthesized by the lymphocyte and under ordinary conditions does not originate from serum; ie, it is not cytophilic antibody. Lymphocytes generally bear monoclonal surface immunoglobulin, ie, immunoglobulin of a single H chain class and L chain type.

A. Performance of Test: Polyspecific antisera against all immunoglobulin classes permit detection of total numbers of B cells in a blood sample. Alternatively, a mixture of anti-κ and anti-λ antisera will detect total numbers of B cells. Monospecific antisera are developed by immunization with purified paraproteins and appropriate absorptions.

Tests for surface immunoglobulin-bearing B cells are performed by direct immunofluorescence with fluorochrome-labeled γ-globulin fractions derived from heterologous anti-immunoglobulin antisera or monoclonal antibodies. A major difficulty is to ensure the absence of all aggregated immunoglobulin in these test reagents (see below).

Generally, small amounts of anti-immunoglobulin antisera are mixed with purified lymphocyte suspensions for 20–30 minutes at 4 °C. After removal of unbound immunoglobulin, the presence of surface immunoglobulin is determined by counting in a fluorescence microscope or by flow cytometry.

Table 19–5 summarizes data on the numbers of surface immunoglobulin-bearing B cells in normal subjects. In certain disease states, eg, systemic lupus erythematosus, antilymphocyte antibody may be bound to B or T cells in vivo. To prove that surface immunoglobulin is a metabolic product of that cell, enzymatic removal and resynthesis of surface immunoglobulin may be performed in vitro.

B. Interpretation: The percentages of IgG-bearing lymphocytes are in fact considerably lower than previously reported. Falsely high levels are detected owing to formation of IgG-anti-IgG com-

Table 19–4. B cell differentiation antigens.

Cell Type Detected	CD Designation	Antibody Designation	Comments
B cell subset T cells	CD5	Leu 1 T1 T101	B cell chronic lymphocytic leukemia B cell secretes autoantibodies
Immature B cells	CD10	CALLA J5	Pre B cells Granulocytes Antigen is neural endopeptidase (encephalinase)
Immature and mature B cells	CD19	Leu 12 B4	
B cell tumors	CD20	Leu 16 B1	
B cells in mantle and germinal centers	CD22	Leu 14	

plexes at the cell surface with binding to B cells via the Fc receptor. When $F(ab)'_2$ anti-IgG reagents were prepared, the percentage of IgG-bearing cells was reduced from 5% to less than 1%.

The problem of binding of anti-immunoglobulin reagents to Fc receptors on B cells and monocytes is particularly a problem with rabbit anti-human antisera. A recent study suggests that nonspecific binding is almost eliminated by use of goat or sheep antisera to human immunoglobulins. The use of monoclonal murine antibodies to H and L chains also avoids this problem. Most investigators agree that IgM and IgD are the predominant surface immunoglobulins on human peripheral B lymphocytes.

Cytoplasmic Immunoglobulins

In some lymphoid cancers, particularly Waldenström's macroglobulinemia, chronic lymphocytic leukemia, or B cell lymphomas with leukemia, circulating lymphocytes with monoclonal intracytoplasmic immunoglobulins are detected. This immunoglobulin is usually identical to the molecule found on the surface of these cells and is occasionally present as a paraprotein in serum. Rarely, the intracellular immunoglobulin forms distinct crystals that appear as spindles or spicules within cytoplasm.

A group of patients with acute lymphocytic leukemias have been described with pre-B cells that express only intracytoplasmic IgM and no surface immunoglobulins at all. It is important to test for intracellular IgM, particularly in so-called null cell acute lymphocytic leukemia patients, since the group with pre-B cell leukemia is probably a distinct clinical subgroup with a different course and prognosis. Most of these cells react with CD19 antisera as well.

Detection of intracellular immunoglobulins is done by direct immunofluorescence with specific antiheavy chain or light chain sera on acetone- or ethanol-fixed cytocentrifuged preparations of purified lymphocytes.

Functional B Cell Assays

In the clinical laboratory, B cell function has been traditionally measured by the assessment of immunoglobulin levels or antibody titers, since these are the end products of B cell differentiation. However, 2 additional in vitro approaches to assessing functional abnormalities in B cells are now available. These are B cell activation by mitogens and immunoglobulin synthesis and secretion.

A. B Cell Activation by Mitogens: B cells can be stimulated to proliferate by several mitogens. Pokeweed mitogen (PWM) functions with T cell cooperation and is not a direct B cell test. However, staphylococcal protein A (Cowan I strain) (SAC) directly stimulates B cell activation. Measurement of this B cell attribute is analogous to phytohemagglutinin (PHA) or concanavalin A (Con A) stimulation described later for T cells.

B. Immunoglobulin Biosynthesis: B cell activation by antigens or mitogens results in small but detectable quantities of polyclonal immunoglobulins. Following 7–10 days of culture, these products are measured by radioimmunoassay (RIA) or enzyme-linked immunosorbent assay (ELISA) methods. Al-

Table 19–5. Surface immunoglobulin-bearing B lymphocytes in normal adult blood.[1]

Surface Immunoglobulin	Mean % of Total Lymphocytes	Range
Total immunoglobulin	21	16–28
IgG	7.1	4–12.7
IgA	2.2	1–4.3
IgM	8.9	6.7–13
IgD[2]	6.2	5.2–8.2
IgE[3]	...	...
κ	13.9	10–18.6
λ	6.8	5–9.3

[1]From: WHO Workshop on Human T & B Cells. *Scand J Immunol* 1974;**3:**525.
[2]IgD and IgM are frequently expressed on the same cell.
[3]IgE B cells are extremely rare.

ternatively, B cells that produce immunoglobulins can be quantified by the reversed hemolytic plaque assay. In this assay, erythrocytes are coated with goat or rabbit anti-human immunoglobulins. They are mixed with putative immunoglobulin-producing lymphocytes and semisolid agar, and complement is added. The presence of hemolytic plaques indicates the presence of immunoglobulin-producing cells.

B cells that have differentiated into plasma cells during an in vitro assay can be enumerated by staining for intracellular immunoglobulins by direct immunofluorescence in fixed smears of cultured cells.

The advantage of these in vitro B cell function tests is that they allow for delineation of immunoregulatory defects involving T or B cells by substitution of various cell populations among healthy and diseased cell donors. These assays are not routinely available at present.

LEUKEMIA CELL-ASSOCIATED ANTIGENS

Terminal Deoxynucleotidyl Transferase (TdT)

Terminal deoxynucleotidyl transferase (TdT) is an enzyme that catalyzes the polymerization of deoxynucleoside triphosphates in the absence of a template. The enzyme is a marker for immature cells in the hematopoietic system. It is present in approximately 90% of cortical thymocytes and about 2% of bone marrow cells. Although transiently present in blood and other lymphoid organs during embryogenesis, it is not present in normal tissues (except marrow and thymus) in adult life.

TdT is a useful clinical marker for the presence of immature T cells in patients with leukemias and lymphomas. It can be detected by either enzyme assay or cellular homogenates or in fixed smears by immunofluorescence. There are increased numbers of TdT-containing cells in the marrow of nearly all patients with acute lymphocytic leukemia and in many cases of T cell lymphoma. Frequently the marker is present in the leukemic population that occurs in blast crisis of chronic myelogenous leukemia. It is not present in mature peripheral T cells and thus can best be considered a marker for pre-T cells and possibly other immature hematopoietic cells.

Common Acute Lymphoblastic Leukemia Antigen (CALLA)

This antigen, to which both monoclonal and conventional antisera have been prepared, is found on the tumor cells in approximately 80% of patients with acute lymphoblastic leukemia and 40–50% of patients with chronic myelogenous leukemia in blast crisis. It now has CD10 as an official designation. CALLA is an encephalinase with a molecular weight of 100,000 and is detected by the monoclonal antibodies J5, J13, and 24.1. Originally thought to be a tumor-specific antigen for acute lymphocytic leukemia, the antigen is also expressed on other cells including 2–6% of normal nucleated bone marrow cells, fibroblasts in tissue culture, and several nonhematopoietic tumor cell lines. It appears to detect early lineage of B cells and some other myeloid precursors.

TdT and CD10 (CALLA) are mainly used as markers of *bone marrow* cells in hematopoietic cancers. This contrasts with B cell markers described above for *blood* B cells in other disorders.

FLOW CYTOMETRY & CELL SORTING

Biochemical and biophysical measurements of single cells have been performed for years, primarily using visual analysis in various types of microscopes. Many of the immunohistochemical methods described in Chapter 18—and the cellular analysis methods discussed above—have become increasingly refined through the development of a new class of instruments called flow cytometers. A detailed description of the myriad applications of this general technique is beyond the scope of our discussion. In brief, flow cytometers are instruments capable of analyzing properties of single cells as they pass through an orifice at high velocity. Examples of measurements that can be made include physical characteristics such as size, volume, refractive index, and viscosity and chemical features such as content of DNA and RNA, proteins, and enzymes. These properties are detected by measuring light scatter, Coulter volume, and fluorescence. Instruments have been designed to analyze these properties and are combined with sophisticated electronics and computers. However, another class of even more sophisticated instruments—cell sorters—combine analytic capacity with the ability to sort cells based on various preselected properties. One type of sorter, the fluorescence-activated cell sorter, has found many applications in immunologic research. Since this type of machine is gradually being introduced into clinical laboratory immunology, particularly for analysis of T, B, and other lymphoid cells, a description of the principles of its operation is presented here.

Cell Analysis by Flow Cytometry

Counting individual cells in complex mixtures is a tedious and imprecise technique even with monoclonal fluorescent antibodies and sophisticated microscopes. With the aid of a flow cytometer used as an analytic instrument, a single cell suspension may be analyzed for various measurements simultaneously at the rate of nearly 5000 cells per second. By combining light scatter and Coulter volume measurements with the powerful tool of fluorescently labeled monoclonal antibodies, subpopulations can be easily identified. A typical histogram produced by analysis of human T cells is shown in Fig 19–2. The number of cells under the curves can be determined and thereby the percentage of positive and negative cells in relation to an arbitrary threshold of fluorescent signal.

The use of 2 differently colored fluorochromes each coupled to a particular antibody allows simultaneous 2-color immunofluorescence of individual cells. Recently, flow cytometers have been developed which can excite 2 different dyes that absorb light at similar wavelengths but emit light in orange and green. A "dot plot" graph of the results of simultaneous 2-color immunofluorescence in the analysis of activated DR antigen-positive suppressor/cytotoxin (CD8) cells in AIDS is shown in Fig 19–3.

Cells larger and smaller than lymphocytes can be "gated out" electronically so that the analysis concentrates solely on lymphocytes. With the addition of 90-degree-angle light scatter, granulocytes can also be identified and "gated out." This approach has allowed the development of whole-blood methods for lymphoid cell analysis.

Fluorescence-Activated Cell Sorters

A single cell suspension is isolated from blood or other tissues and labeled with either fluorescent antibody or another fluorochrome dye such as ethidium bromide, which specifically stains DNA (Fig 19–4). The cells are forced under pressure through a nozzle in a liquid jet surrounded by a sheath of saline or water. Vibration at the tip of the nozzle assembly causes the stream to break up into a series of droplets, and the size of the droplets can be regulated so that each will contain exactly one cell. The droplets are illuminated by the monochromatic laser beam and electronically monitored by fluorescence detectors. Droplets that emit appropriate fluorescent signals are electrically charged in a high-voltage field between deflection plates and are then sorted into collection tubes. Rapid, accurate, and highly reproducible separation of cells is thereby accomplished. Viability and sterility can be maintained, so that cells can be not only analyzed but also cultured or assayed functionally.

Clinical Applications of Flow Cytometry

The flow cytometer has had many applications in immunology. A partial list would include the following: (1) analysis and sorting of subpopulations of T cells by monoclonal fluorescent antibodies; (2) separation of various classes of lymphoid cells through sorting by size or antibody marker; (3) separation of live from dead cells; (4) cloning of individual cells by introducing microtiter plates in place of collection tubes; (5) analysis of cell cycle kinetics by various DNA stains; and (6) detection of rare cells such as monoclonal B cells in the blood of lymphoma patients. Clinical applications are listed in Table 19–6. Computers are used to analyze multiple parameters measured simultaneously by the flow cytometer, including 2-color fluorescence, forward-angle light scatter, and 90-degree-angle light scatter. Sophisticated data analysis and presentation software are available to produce clinically applicable information.

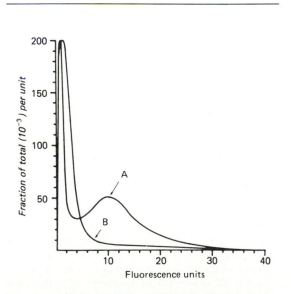

Figure 19–2. Single-color immunofluorescence histogram from flow cytometric analysis of human T cells. Human lymphocytes were stained with fluorescently labeled anti-T cell antibody **(A)** and control nonreactive FITC-labeled antiserum **(B)**. In both patterns, a high, sharp peak of autofluorescence from unstained cells is observed near the y-axis. However, in the curve labeled **(A)** stained with anti-T cell antibody, a significant peak appears at about 11 fluorescence units. No such increase in the number or intensity of fluorescent cells is observed in the control **(B)** peak. (Modified and reproduced, with permission, from: Melamed MR, Mullaney PF, Mendelsohn ML: *Flow Cytometry and Sorting.* Wiley, 1979.)

LYMPHOCYTE ACTIVATION

Lymphocyte activation or stimulation refers to an in vitro correlate of an in vivo process that regularly occurs when antigen interacts with specifically sensitized lymphocytes in the host. Lymphocyte transformation is a nearly synonymous term first used by Nowell in 1960 and later by Hirschhorn and others to describe the morphologic changes that resulted

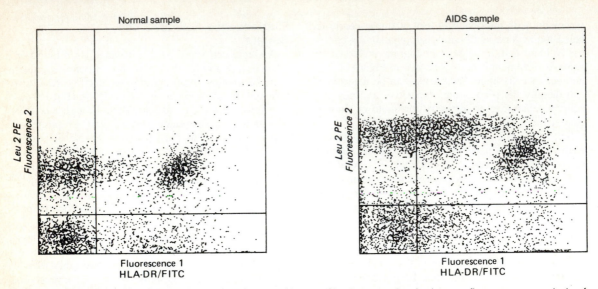

Figure 19–3. Presence of DR antigen on CD8+ (Leu 2+) cells. Simultaneous 2-color immunofluorescence analysis of human suppressor/cytotoxic T cells also bearing DR antigens. Human lymphocytes were stained with an FITC-labeled anti-DR antibody and a phycoerythrin-labeled anti-CD8 (Leu 2) antibody. The dot plot represents individual cells, with FITC-labeled cells on the x-axis and phycoerythrin-labeled cells on the y-axis. The coordinate of an individual dot thus indicates whether it is labeled with one or both antibodies. In addition, monocytes are labeled with antisera containing both fluorochromes and appear in both panels in the upper right quadrant. There is an increase in the number of doubly stained cells in AIDS versus the control panel.

when small, resting lymphocytes were transformed into lymphoblasts on exposure to the mitogen PHA. Blastogenesis refers to the process of formation of large pyroninophilic blastlike cells in cultures of lymphocytes stimulated by either nonspecific mitogens or antigens.

Lymphocyte activation is an in vitro technique commonly used to assess cellular immunity in patients with immunodeficiency, autoimmunity, infectious diseases, and cancer. A myriad of complex biochemical events occur in lymphocytes following incubation with mitogens. These are substances that stimulate large numbers of lymphocytes and do not require a sensitized host, as is the case with antigens. These biochemical events include early membrane-related phenomena such as increased synthesis of phospholipids, increased permeability to divalent cations, activation of adenylate cyclase, and resultant elevation of intracellular cAMP. Synthesis of protein, RNA, and finally DNA occurs shortly thereafter. It is this latter phenomenon, the increase in DNA synthesis, that eventually results in cell division and is the basis for most clinically relevant assays for lymphocyte activation. Convenience and custom have led clinical immunologists to use DNA synthesis rather than earlier events, eg, calcium influx or phospholipid metabolism, as a marker for lymphocyte activation.

Although the relationship between lymphocyte ac-

tivation and delayed hypersensitivity is not always absolute, the method has found widespread use in clinical immunology. The in vivo delayed hypersensitivity skin test is actually the result of a series of complex phenomena including antigen recognition, lymphocyte-macrophage interaction, release of lymphokines and monokines, and changes in vascular permeability. In vitro methods such as lymphocyte activation are useful for studying cellular hypersensitivity, since they permit analysis of specific stages in the immune response. In addition, they avoid challenge of the patient with potentially hazardous antigens such as drugs, transplantation antigens, or tumor antigens. Lymphocyte activation measures the *functional* capability of T or B lymphocytes to proliferate following antigenic challenge and is therefore a more direct test of immunocompetence than merely enumerating types of lymphocytes.

Lymphocyte responses can be suppressed or augmented by a variety of nonspecific factors present in human serum. This humoral modulation of responses to antigens or mitogens should be clearly differentiated from intrinsic suppression of cellular reactivity. Therefore, it is essential to avoid culture of lymphocytes in serum that may contain inhibitory substances. Their presence can usually be excluded by careful questioning of serum donors about their medications. If it is suspected that an individual's serum contains an inhibitor of lymphocyte activation, con-

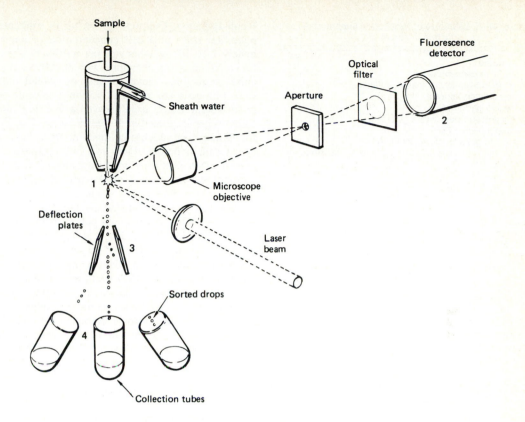

Figure 19–4. Cell purification by flow sorting. **1:** Fluorescently stained cells are forced out of a small nozzle in a liquid jet. **2:** Cellular fluorescence, measured immediately below the nozzle, is used to select the cells to be sorted. **3:** The jet is broken into droplets. Droplets containing selected cells are electrically charged in a high-voltage field between deflection plates. **4:** The charged droplets are electrically deflected into collection tubes. (Courtesy of Joseph Grey, PhD.)

Table 19–6. Clinical applications of flow cytometry.

Leukocyte phenotyping
 Diagnosis of congenital immunodeficiency diseases
 Assessment of prognosis of HIV-positive patients
 Monitoring of immunotherapy or chemotherapy in immun-
  odeficiency diseases
 Monitoring of immune reconstitution in bone marrow
  transplant recipients
Tumor cell phenotyping
 Diagnosis and classification of leukemias and lymphomas
 Determination of clonality of immunoglobulin-bearing cells
  from lymphomas and leukemias
 Differentiation of hematopoietic from nonhematopoietic
  tumors or cells
 Assessment of prognosis of cancers
DNA analysis
 Determination of aneuploidy
 Determination of cell cycle kinetics
Other applications
 Reticulocyte counting
 Platelet-associated immunoglobulin detection
 Leukocyte cross-matching in transplant recipients
 Cytogenetics

trols should be done utilizing carefully washed cells from that individual cultured in normal serum. A partial list of serum suppressive factors and drugs that may influence in vitro lymphocyte responses is presented in Table 19–7. A note of caution is warranted regarding the significance of this heterogeneous group of substances. Despite clear demonstration of substances with in vitro effects on lymphocyte responses, their in vivo action, particularly in view of the high concentrations often used in tissue culture, remains a matter of speculation.

METHODS & INTERPRETATIONS

Lymphocyte Activation by Mitogens

A number of plant lectins and other substances have been employed in assessing human lymphocyte function (Table 19–8). In contrast to studies in mice, there is no incontrovertible evidence that T or B

Table 19–7. Examples of lymphocyte suppressive factors in serum.

Serum proteins
Albumin (high concentration)
Specific antibodies to stimulating antigens
Immunoregulatory globulin
Alpha-1-acid glycoprotein
Pregnancy-associated serum globulins
C-reactive protein (CRP)
Serum alpha globulin of amyloid (SAA)
Alpha globulins in cancer, chronic infection, inflammatory diseases
Alpha-fetoprotein (AFP)
Low-density lipoprotein
Antigen-antibody complexes
HLA antibodies
T cell antibodies
Normal serum inhibitors (poorly characterized)
Hormones
Glucocorticoids
Progesterone
Estrogens
Androgens
Prostaglandins
Drugs
Aspirin
Cannabis
Chloroquine
Ouabain
Others
Interferon
Cyclic nucleotides

lymphocytes are selectively activated by nonspecific mitogens. PHA and Con A are predominantly T cell mitogens, whereas pokeweed mitogen stimulates B cells. Neither lipopolysaccharide nor anti-immunoglobulin antibody appears to be a potent B cell stimulant in humans. Staphylococcal protein A from *Staphylococcus aureus* cell walls may be a specific stimulant of human B cells, possibly by triggering cells into DNA synthesis via the Fc receptor for IgG.

Anti CD3 monoclonal antibody activates only those T cells that bear T cell receptor complex (see Chapter 6).

Lymphocyte Culture Technique for Mitogen Activation

Lymphocytes are purified from anticoagulated peripheral blood by density gradient centrifugation on Ficoll-Hypaque. Cultures are set up in triplicate in microtiter trays at a cell concentration of approximately 1×10^6 lymphocytes per milliliter. The culture medium is supplemented with 10–20% serum—either autologous, heterologous, or pooled human sera. Mitogens are added in varying concentrations on a weight basis, usually over a 2–3 log range. Cultures are incubated in a mixture of 5% CO_2 in air for 72 hours, at which time most mitogens have produced their maximal effect on DNA synthesis. The rate of DNA synthesis was originally estimated by morphologic assessment of the percentage of lymphoblasts present in the culture. However, this method has been supplanted by the more accurate measure of DNA synthesis by pulse-labeling the cultures with tritiated thymidine (^{3}H-Tdr), a nucleoside precursor that is incorporated into newly synthesized DNA. The amount of ^{3}H-Tdr incorporated—and therefore the rate of DNA synthesis—is determined by scintillation counting in a liquid scintillation spectrophotometer. Scintillation counting yields data in counts per minute (cpm) or corrected for quenching to disintegrations per minute (dpm), which are then used as a standard measure of lymphocyte responsiveness. The cpm in control cultures are either subtracted from or divided into stimulated cpm, which yields a ratio commonly referred to as the stimulation index.

Obviously there are a multitude of technical as well as conceptual variables that can affect the results of this sensitive assay system. These include the concentration of cells, the geometry of the culture vessel, contamination of cultures with nonlymphoid cells or microorganisms, the dose of mitogen, the incubation time of cultures, and the techniques of harvesting cells.

The degree of lymphocyte activation is also a function of the cellular regulatory influences present in the culture. Suppressor or helper T, B, and mononuclear cells are all capable of modifying the final degree of proliferation in the specifically stimulated cell population. Some mitogens, particularly Con A, are known to activate suppressor T cells, which may profoundly reduce the proliferative response in such cultures.

Of additional importance in lymphocyte activation are culture time and dose-response kinetics. Since

Table 19–8. "Nonspecific" mitogens that activate human lymphocytes

Mitogen	Abbreviation	Biologic Source	Relative Specificity
Phytohemagglutinin	PHA	*Phaseolus vulgaris* (kidney bean)	T cells
Concanavalin A	Con A	*Canavalia ensiformis* (jack bean)	T cells (different subset from PHA)
Antilymphocyte globulin	ALG	Heterologous antisera	T cells + B cells
Anti-CD3 (MAb)	CD3	Hybridoma supernate	T cell receptor-bearing cells
Staphylococcus protein A	SpA, SAC	*S aureus* (Cowan I strain)	B cells, T cell-independent
Pokeweed mitogen	PWM	*Phytolacca americana*	B cells, T cell-dependent
Streptolysin S	SLS	Group A streptococci	?(Probably T cells)

clinically important defects in cellular immunity are rarely absolute, quantitative relationships in lymphocyte activation are crucial. This is especially true when comparing the reduction of responsiveness of normal control subjects with a group of patients with altered lymphocyte function. With the use of microtiter culture systems and semiautomated harvesting devices, an attempt can be made to determine both dose- and time-response kinetics of either mitogen- or antigen-stimulated cultures (Figs 19–5 and 19–6).

Altered lymphocyte function can result in shifts in either time- or dose-response curves to the left or right. These shifts determine the optimal dose and optimal time of the lymphocyte response. Without such detailed analyses, it is usually impossible to accurately observe partial or subtle defects in lymphocyte responsiveness in various disease states. Cultures assayed at a single time with a single stimulant dose period are often grossly misleading.

Confusion may result from a nonstandardized format for presentation of data. Many laboratories present results of lymphocyte stimulation as a ratio of cpm in stimulated culture to those in control cultures—the so-called stimulation index. Others report "raw" cpm or dpm as illustrated in Figs 19–5 and 19–6. Neither method is entirely satisfactory. The stimulation index is a ratio, and marked changes can therefore result from changes in background or control cpm of the denominator. It is perhaps best to report data in both ways to permit better interpretations.

Antigen Stimulation

Whereas mitogens stimulate large numbers of lymphocytes, antigens stimulate far fewer cells that are specifically sensitized to the antigen in question. In most instances, only T cells respond to antigens in this test. A wide variety of antigens have been employed in lymphocyte activation, many of them also being used for delayed hypersensitivity skin testing (Table 19–9). In general, normal subjects show agreement between the results of skin tests and antigen-induced lymphocyte activation. However, in many conditions, the in vitro technique is apparently a more sensitive index of specific antigen-mediated cellular hypersensitivity. Furthermore, in vitro tests for T cell activation obviate the need for production of cytokines that produce dermal inflammation expressed as delayed hypersensitivity.

Lymphocyte Culture Technique for Antigen Stimulation

Culture methods are virtually identical to those described for mitogen stimulation. Additional factors to be considered include the possible presence in serum supplements of antibody directed against stimulating antigens. Antigen-antibody complexes may block or occasionally nonspecifically stimulate lymphocytes.

As in the case of mitogen-induced activation, time- and dose-response kinetics are crucial in generating reliable data. Representative examples of such curves are shown in Figs 19–7 and 19–8. In contrast to mitogen-induced lymphocyte activation, antigen stimulation results in lower total DNA synthesis. Furthermore, the time of maximal response does not occur until the culture has been allowed to

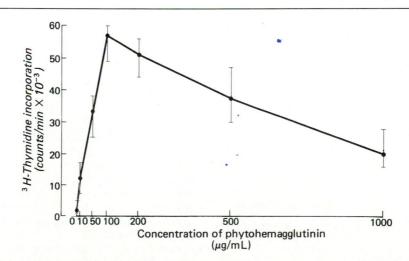

Figure 19–5. Dose-response curve for mitogen stimulation of 10^6 lymphocytes. Dose-response curve of a group of 10 normal adults whose peripheral blood lymphocytes were stimulated with varying concentrations of phytohemagglutinin for 72 hours. Lymphocytes were pulse-labeled with 2 μCi of tritiated thymidine 6 hours prior to harvesting. Counts per minute of ^{3}H-thymidine incorporation were determined by liquid scintillation spectrometry and are plotted as the mean of 10 individual determinations ± the range. A maximal response occurred at approximately 100–200 μg/mL of phytohemagglutinin.

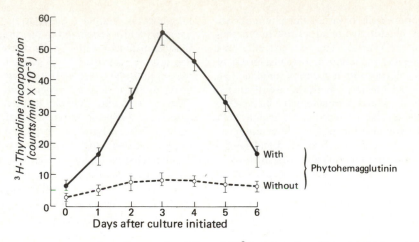

Figure 19–6. Time-response curve for mitogen stimulation of 10^6 lymphocytes. Time-response curve of peripheral blood lymphocytes from 10 normal adults stimulated in tissue culture for various lengths of time with an optimal concentration of phytohemagglutinin (100 μg/mL). Cultures were pulse-labeled with tritiated thymidine for 6 hours on the day of harvest. Maximal response occurred at 3 days after initiating the culture. Results are plotted as mean ± the range of counts per minute.

continue for 5–7 days. Fig 19–8 clearly illustrates both the usefulness of and the necessity for performing careful time- and dose-response kinetics in assessing human lymphocyte function.

MIXED LYMPHOCYTE CULTURE & CELL-MEDIATED LYMPHOLYSIS

Mixed lymphocyte culture (MLC) is a special case of antigen stimulation in which T lymphocytes respond to foreign histocompatibility antigen on unrelated lymphocytes or monocytes. This test is performed as either a "one-way" or "2-way" assay (Fig 19–9). In the one-way MLC, the stimulating cells are treated with either irradiation (~ 2000 R) or mitomycin to prevent DNA synthesis without killing the cell. The magnitude of the response is then entirely the result of DNA synthesis in the nonirradiated or nonmitomycin-treated cells. In the 2-way MLC, cells from both individuals are mutually stimulating and responding, and DNA synthesis represents the net response of both sets of cells, and the individual contributions cannot be discerned. The

Table 19–9. Antigens used to assess human cellular immunity in vitro.

PPD
Candida antigen
Streptokinase/streptodornase
Coccidioidin
Tetanus toxoid
Histoincompatible cells (MLC)
Trichophytin
Vaccinia virus
Herpes simplex virus

culture conditions, time of exposure, ^{3}H-Tdr pulse labeling, and harvesting procedures are usually identical to those for antigen stimulation. Controls include coculture of syngeneic irradiated and nonirradiated pairs and coculture of allogeneic irradiated pairs. The first control provides baseline DNA synthesis, and the second ensures adequate inactivation by irradiation (or mitomycin) of the stimulator cells.

In the use of MLC as a test for T cell function, difficulties in quantitation often arise owing to variations in stimulator cell antigens that determine the degree of genetic disparity between stimulator and responder cells. To overcome this difficulty and produce a more standardized test, frozen aliquots of viable pooled human allogeneic cells have been employed as stimulator cells.

There is interest in the identity of stimulating and responding cells as well as the responsible cell-associated antigens in the MLC. It appears that the stimulating antigens on human cells are class II MHC molecules encoded by the HLA-D locus (see Chapter 4). Responding cells are primarily T lymphocytes with obligate macrophage cooperation. B cells can also respond in MLC, since a marked increase in immunoglobulin synthesis can be detected. MLC may be used as a histocompatibility assay (Chapter 21) and as a test for immunocompetence of T cells, particularly in immunodeficiency disorders (Chapters 25 and 26).

Cell-mediated lympholysis (CML) is an extension of the MLC technique in which cytotoxic effector cells generated during MLC are detected (Fig 19–9). This test involves an initial one-way MLC culture followed by exposure of stimulated cells to ^{51}Cr-labeled target cells specifically lysed by sensitized killer lymphocytes. These target cells are HLA-

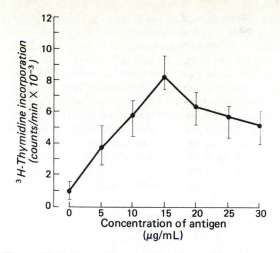

Figure 19–7. Dose-response curve for antigen stimulation of 10^6 lymphocytes. Dose-response curve of lymphocytes from 15 normal individuals with delayed hypersensitivity to the antigen. Cultures were harvested at 120 hours of culture after a 6-hour pulse with tritiated thymidine. Counts per minute were determined by scintillation spectrometry. Results are plotted as mean ± the range from 15 skin test-positive subjects at various antigen concentrations. Maximum response is at 15 µg/mL of antigen.

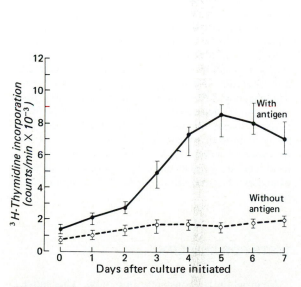

Figure 19–8. Time-response curve for antigen stimulation of 10^6 lymphocytes. Responses of peripheral blood lymphocytes from 15 normal adults with delayed hypersensitivity to the antigen. Cells were cultured as described in Fig 19–7. Antigen concentration for all cultures was 15 µg/mL. Maximal response occurred on days 5–7 of culture. Results plotted as mean ± the range for 15 individual determinations.

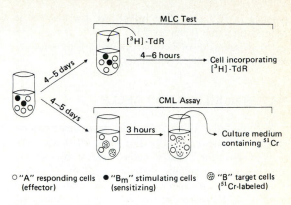

Figure 19–9. MLC and CML assays schematically represented. Cells (black and white balls) from separate individuals are cultured. In MLC, DNA synthesis in responding (noninactivated) cell is measured. In CML assay, the ability of "A" cells to kill ^{51}Cr-labeled "B" cells is measured. See text for further explanation. (Reproduced, with permission, from Bach FH, Van Rood JJ: The major histocompatibility complex: Genetics and biology. *N Engl J Med* 1976;**295**:806, 872.)

identical to the stimulator cells in MLC. Cytotoxicity is measured as percentage of ^{51}Cr released in specific target cells compared to percentage of ^{51}Cr released from control (nonspecific) target cells. Several lines of evidence indicate that cells which proliferate in MLC and killer cells which participate in CML assay are not identical. Killer cells are generated that have specificity for class I HLA-A, HLA-B, or HLA-C antigens on target cells, whereas in class II MLC, HLA-D antigen differences determine the reaction. CML assays provide an additional measure of T cell function and can be used to estimate presensitization and histocompatibility in clinical transplantation (see also Chapter 21).

CLINICAL APPLICATION OF B & T CELL ASSAYS

Counting of B and T cells in peripheral blood and tissue specimens has limited application in both the diagnosis and investigation of pathophysiologic mechanisms of many disease states. Current applications include the following:

(1) Diagnosis and classification of immunodeficiency diseases (Chapters 23–27, 55).

(2) Determination of origin of malignant lymphocytes in lymphocytic leukemia and lymphoma (Chapter 48).

(3) Evaluation of immunocompetence and mechanisms of tissue damage in autoimmune disease, eg, systemic lupus erythematosus and rheumatoid arthritis (Chapter 36).

(4) Detection of changes in cellular immune com-

petence in HIV and other infections that may be of prognostic value (Chapter 55).

(5) Monitoring of cellular changes following organ transplantation (Chapter 60).

NATURAL KILLER (NK) CELLS

Natural killer (NK) cells can be enumerated by specific monoclonal antibodies using methods identical to those for T and B cells. Several monoclonal antibodies are available that detect either Fc receptors (CD16) or specific differentiation antigens (CD56, CD57) present on these cells. Some NK cells also express antigens from the CD2 T cell family. Functional testing is done by measuring the ability of these nonimmune cells to kill special target cells such as erythroleukemia cell line K562. Cytotoxicity is usually performed by using the ^{51}Cr release assay (see below).

MONOCYTE-MACROPHAGE ASSAYS

The morphologic identification of normal peripheral blood monocytes in stained peripheral blood films ordinarily is quite simple. Monocytes are larger than granulocytes and most lymphocytes. They have round or kidney-shaped nuclei with fine, lightly stained granules. However, in suspension or even in tissue or blood specimens, additional markers may be required to differentiate monocytes from lymphocytes and primitive myeloid cells.

A reliable stain for monocytes is so-called nonspecific esterase, or α-naphthol esterase, which is present in monocytes but absent in most myeloid and lymphocytic cells. Monoclonal antibodies directed at specific differentiation antigens such as CD14 are available.

Functional attributes of monocytes are discussed in detail in Chapters 5 and 12. In the clinical laboratory, phagocytosis of particles or antibody-coated heat-killed microorganisms is a convenient test for functional identification of monocytes.

NEUTROPHIL FUNCTION

Polymorphonuclear neutrophils (PMN) are bone marrow-derived leukocytes with a finite life span which play a central role in defense of the host against infection. For many types of infections, the neutrophil plays the primary role as an effector or killer cell. However, in the bloodstream and extravascular spaces, neutrophils exert their antimicrobial effects through a complex interaction with antibody, complement, and chemotactic factors. Thus, in assessing neutrophil function, one cannot view the cell as an independent entity; its essential dependence on other immune processes, both cellular and humoral, must be taken into account.

Defects in neutrophil function can be classified as quantitative or qualitative. In quantitative disorders, the total number of normally functioning neutrophils is reduced below a critical level, allowing infection to ensue. Drug-induced and idiopathic neutropenia (see Chapter 38), with absolute circulating granulocyte counts of less than 1000/μL, are examples of this sort of defect. In these situations, granulocytes are functionally normal but are present in insufficient numbers to maintain an adequate defense against infection. In qualitative neutrophilic disorders, the total number of circulating PMN is either normal or sometimes actually elevated, but the cells fail to exert their normal microbicidal functions. Chronic granulomatous disease is an example of this type of disorder (see Chapter 27). In patients with chronic granulomatous disease the normal or increased numbers of circulating neutrophils are unable to kill certain types of intracellular organisms.

Phagocytosis by PMN can be divided into 5 distinct and temporally sequential stages: (1) motility, (2) recognition and adhesion, (3) ingestion, (4) degranulation, and (5) intracellular killing (Fig 19–10). The microbicidal activity of the neutrophil is the sum of the activity of these 5 phases. The clinical syndromes resulting from defects in many of the various stages in phagocytosis are discussed in Chapter 27. The laboratory tests used in clinical practice to evaluate phagocytic function in humans with various diseases will be discussed in terms of the 5 major steps in the process. It should be emphasized that for many neutrophil functions no standard assay exists; therefore, a variety of test choices depends on the local laboratory. The following sections will include examples of useful clinical tests of neutrophil function.

TESTS FOR MOTILITY

Neutrophils are constantly in motion. This movement can be either random or directed. Random or passive motion is the result of **brownian movement.** In **chemotactic movement** the cells are actively attracted to some chemotactic stimulus. Chemotaxins are produced by complement activation (C3a, C5a, C567; see Chapter 14), by fibronolysis (fibrinopeptide B), by microorganisms themselves (endotoxins),

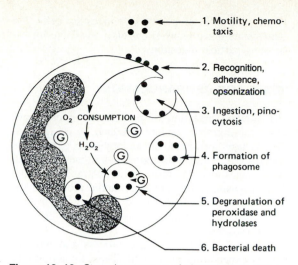

1. Motility, chemotaxis
2. Recognition, adherence, opsonization
3. Ingestion, pinocytosis
4. Formation of phagosome
5. Degranulation of peroxidase and hydrolases
6. Bacterial death

O_2 CONSUMPTION
H_2O_2

Figure 19–10. Steps in progress of phagocytosis. Schematic representation of phagocytosis by a granulocyte. **1:** Bacteria attract phagocytic cells by chemotactic stimulus. **2:** Presence of opsonins (immunoglobulin and complement) facilitates recognition and surface attachment. **3:** Invagination of cell membrane with enclosed opsonized bacteria. **4:** Intracellular organelle, the phagosome, forms. **5:** Granules fuse with phagosomes and release enzymes into the phagolysosome. **6:** Bacterial death and digestion result. (Modified from Baehner: Chronic granulomatous disease. Page 175 in: *The Phagocytic Cell in Host Resistance.* Bellanti JA, Dayton DH [editors]. Raven Press, 1975.)

and by other leukocytes (lymphocyte chemotactic factor). Products of lipoxygenation of arachidonic acid, particularly LTB_4, are also chemoattractants. Relatively simple assays have been designed to assess leukocyte movement in vitro. An in vivo technique, the Rebuck skin window, preceded the development of in vitro assays and was one of the earliest methods developed for assessing leukocyte function.

Test for Random Motility

Random motility is tested for by the **capillary tube method.** Purified neutrophils in 0.1% human albumin solution at a concentration of 5×10^6/mL are placed in a siliconized microhematocrit tube. The tube is enclosed in a chamber specially constructed from microscope slides and embedded in adhesive clay. After being filled with immersion oil, the entire chamber is placed on the stage of a microscope. Motility is assessed by observing the leading edge of the leukocyte column in the microscope at hourly intervals. Measurements are expressed in millimeters of movement from the starting boundary of the packed leukocyte layer.

Test for Chemotaxis

Directional locomotion of neutrophils toward various chemotactic stimuli is quantitated by use of a Boyden chamber. Cells to be tested are placed in the upper chamber and are separated from the lower chamber containing a chemotactic substance by a filter membrane of small pore size. Neutrophils can enter the filter membrane but are trapped in transit through the membrane. After a suitable incubation period, the filter is removed and stained and the underside is microscopically examined for the presence of neutrophils.

Although this method is theoretically simple, there are numerous technical difficulties. These include nonavailability of filters of standard pore size, observer bias in quantitation of migrating neutrophils in the microscope, loss of cells which fall off or completely traverse the filter, and failure of many workers to standardize cell numbers and serum supplements.

An additional method for measuring chemotaxis and random motility has been recently developed. This technique involves the radial migration of leukocytes from small wells cut into an agarose medium in a Petri dish. In many respects, the method is similar to single radial diffusion (see Chapter 18). Generally, 3 wells are cut into agarose. The cell population in question is placed in the center well. A chemoattractant is placed in an outer well, and a control nonattractant is placed in the remaining well. After several hours of migration, the distance from the center of the well originally containing cells to the leading edges of the migrating cells is measured. In this way, the directed motility and the random motion can be quantitated. This method has achieved widespread application and in many laboratories has supplanted the somewhat more cumbersome Boyden chamber technique.

TESTS FOR RECOGNITION & ADHESION

As the neutrophil in an immune host approaches its target, by either random or directed motility, it recognizes microorganisms by the presence of antibody and complement fixed to the surface of the microorganisms. Enhancement of phagocytosis (opsonization) occurs under these circumstances. Adherence and aggregation of neutrophils are promoted by a series of membrane glycoproteins.

The family of membrane glycoproteins that function as adherence molecules includes LFA-1 (lymphocyte function associated antigen type 1), Mac-1 (macrophage 1) and p 150,95. These molecules all contain a common β subunit (CD18) and a unique α subunit. Mac-1 functions as a receptor for C3bi. Deficiencies of the β subunit have been described (see Chapter 28). Monoclonal antibodies to CD18 (the β subunit) are available, as well as those to specific α subunits: CD11a = LFA-1, CD11b = Mac-1, and

CD11c = p 150,95. These molecules are present on granulocytes, monocytes, and some lymphocytes and can be readily measured by flow cytometry and immunofluorescence.

Tests to detect the presence of complement and antibody Fc receptors on neutrophils are rarely useful in clinical testing. The need for either antibody or complement (opsonins) coating of microorganisms for phagocytosis can be determined by employing sera devoid of either or both of these factors followed by an assay for ingestion and subsequent intracellular killing. Furthermore, IgG and complement receptors on neutrophils as well as mononuclear phagocytes can be readily detected by rosette formation with IgG-coated or complement-coated erythrocytes or by immunofluorescence with monoclonal antibodies.

TESTS FOR INGESTION

Ingestion of microorganisms by neutrophils is an active process that requires energy production by the phagocytic cell. Internalization of antibody-coated and complement-coated microorganisms occurs rapidly following their surface contact with neutrophils. Since subsequent intracellular events—ie, degranulation and killing—depend on the success of ingestion, tests for ingestion provide a rapid and relatively simple means of assessing the overall phagocytic process. Unfortunately, the term phagocytosis has often been used to denote *only* the ingestion phase of the process. Thus, terms such as phagocytic index which refer to the average number of particles ingested really should be considered measurements of ingestion rather than of phagocytosis.

All tests to measure the ability of neutrophils to ingest either native or opsonized particles employ 2 general approaches. Either a direct estimate is made of the cellular uptake of particles by assaying the cells themselves, or the removal of particles from the fluid or medium is taken as an indirect estimate of cellular uptake.

Methods for quantitation of the ingestion of particles by cellular assays include (1) direct counting by light microscopy; (2) estimation of cell-bound radioactivity after ingestion of a radiolabeled particle; and (3) measurement of an easily stained lipid, eg, oil red O, after extraction from cells.

One disadvantage of many of these assays is that particles adherent to the neutrophil membranes are included as ingested particles. Other elements that influence results in performing ingestion assays include the presence of humoral factors (opsonins) which enhance uptake, the presence of serum containing acute-phase reactants which depress uptake, the need for constant agitation or tumbling of cells and particles to maximize contact and subsequent uptake, the type or size of the test particle used, and,

finally, the ratio of particles to ingesting cells. No well-standardized assay is currently available for estimating particle ingestion.

TESTS FOR DEGRANULATION

Following ingestion of particles or microorganisms, the ingested element is bound by invaginated cell surface membrane in an organelle termed the **phagosome.** Shortly thereafter, lysosomes fuse with the phagosome to form a structure called the **phagolysosome.** Degranulation is the process of fusion of lysosomes and phagosomes with the subsequent discharge of intralysosomal contents into the phagolysosome.

Degranulation is an active process and requires energy expenditure by the cell. Thus, impairment of normal metabolic pathways of the neutrophil—especially oxygen consumption and the metabolism of glucose through the hexose monophosphate shunt—interferes with degranulation and subsequent intracellular killing.

A test for degranulation called frustrated phagocytosis has been developed and applied to the study of some neutrophil dysfunction syndromes. The frustrated phagocytosis system (Fig 19–11) allows for examination of degranulation independently of ingestion. Heat-aggregated γ-globulin or immune complexes are fixed to the plastic surface of a Petri dish so that they cannot be ingested. Neutrophils are placed in suspension in Petri dishes with and without attached aggregated γ-globulin. The cell membranes of the neutrophils are stimulated by contact between γ-globulin and appropriate cell membrane receptors. This process results in fusion of intraleukocyte granules (lysosomes) with the cell membrane. As a result, intralysosomal contents are discharged into the suspending medium. The rate of release of lysosomal enzymes, particularly β-glucuronidase and acid

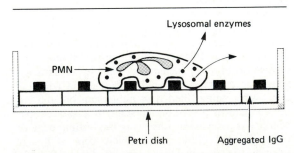

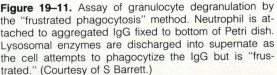

Figure 19–11. Assay of granulocyte degranulation by the "frustrated phagocytosis" method. Neutrophil is attached to aggregated IgG fixed to bottom of Petri dish. Lysosomal enzymes are discharged into supernate as the cell attempts to phagocytize the IgG but is "frustrated." (Courtesy of S Barrett.)

phosphatase, is taken as an estimate of the rate of degranulation. Nonspecific cell death or cytolysis can be estimated by measuring the discharge of lactate dehydrogenase (a nongranule enzyme) into the medium. This assay system has been used to demonstrate retardation in the degranulation rate by neutrophils from patients with chronic granulomatous disease.

TESTS FOR INTRACELLULAR KILLING

The primary function of the neutrophil in host resistance is intracellular killing of microorganisms. This final stage of phagocytosis is dependent on the successful completion of the preceding steps: motility, recognition, ingestion, and degranulation. A variety of intraleukocytic systems make up the antimicrobial armamentarium of the neutrophil (Table 19–10). Obviously, a defect in intracellular killing could be the result of any one or a combination of these functions. However, in clinical practice 2 assays have received widespread use, ie, the Nitro Blue Tetrazolium dye reduction test and the intraleukocytic killing test. It is hoped that specific metabolic and antimicrobial assays for other intraleukocytic events will also become available in the future.

Nitro Blue Tetrazolium Dye Reduction Test

Nitro Blue Tetrazolium (NBT) is a clear, yellow, water-soluble compound that forms formazan, a deep blue dye, on reduction. Neutrophils can reduce the dye following ingestion of latex or other particles subsequent to the metabolic burst generated through the hexose monophosphate shunt. The reduced dye can be easily measured photometrically after extraction from neutrophils with the organic solvent pyridine. The reduction of NBT to a blue color thus forms the basis of the quantitative NBT test. The precise mechanism of NBT reduction is not known, but the phenomenon is closely allied to metabolic

Table 19–10. Antimicrobial systems of neutrophils.[1]

Acid pH of phagolysosome
Lysozyme
Lactoferrin
Defensins
Cathepsin G
Myeloperoxidase-halogenation system
Hydrogen peroxide
Superoxide radical
Hydroxyl radical
Singlet oxygen

[1]For a further description of these systems, see Lehrer RI, et al: Neutrophils in host defense. *Ann Intern Med* 1988; **109:**127, and Boxer LA, Morganroth ML, Neutrophil function disorders. *Disease-a-Month* 1987;**33:**681.

events in the respiratory burst following ingestion, including increased hexose monophosphate shunt activity, increased oxygen consumption, and increased hydrogen peroxide and superoxide radical formation. Since the generation of reducing activity in intact neutrophils parallels the metabolic activities following ingestion, NBT reduction is a useful means of assaying overall metabolic integrity of phagocytizing neutrophils. Failure of NBT dye reduction is a consistent and diagnostically important laboratory abnormality in chronic granulomatous disease. Neutrophils from these patients fail to kill certain intracellular microbes and fail to generate H_2O_2 or the superoxide radical.

Quantitative NBT Test

Isolated neutrophils are incubated in a balanced salt solution with latex particles and NBT. After 15 minutes of incubation at 37 °C, the reduced dye (blue formazan) is extracted with pyridine and measured spectrophotometrically at 515 nm. The change in absorbance between cultures of cells that actively phagocytose latex particles and those that do not is taken as an index of neutrophil function. The test is strikingly abnormal in chronic granulomatous disease (see Chapter 27). Various modifications of the quantitative NBT test have been developed as screening tests for chronic granulomatous disease. Prominent among these are so-called slide tests in which neutrophils, latex, and NBT are placed in a drop on a glass slide and the reduction to blue formazan assayed under the microscope. It can be performed on a single drop of blood, but abnormal results should be confirmed with the more precise quantitative method described above.

Chemiluminescence

Neutrophils emit small amounts of electromagnetic radiation following ingestion of microorganisms. This energy can be detected as light by sensitive photomultiplier tubes, such as those in liquid scintillation counters. During the respiratory burst, H_2O_2, superoxide radicals, and singlet oxygen are generated. Singlet oxygen, a highly unstable and reactive species, combines with bacteria or other intralysosomal elements to form electronically unstable carboxyl groups. As these groups relax to ground state, light energy is emitted. This entire process has been termed **chemiluminescence** and forms the basis of an important assay of neutrophil function. Similar to NBT, it requires all steps prior to actual bacterial killing to be intact. Recent studies show a precise correlation between light emissions and microbicidal activity. The oxidative steps in the biochemical pathways present in the neutrophil generate the chemiluminescence, which is easily detected in a liquid scintillation spectrometer with the coincidence circuit excluded.

In the test, neutrophils are incubated in clear, colorless balanced salt solution in the presence of an ingestible particle, eg, latex or zymosan, in a scintillation vial. Luminol, an intermediate fluorescent compound, can be added to intensify the light emissions. The emission of photons of light is measured as cpm in a scintillation counter over the next 10 minutes at 2-minute intervals. Studies with this technique have revealed markedly reduced chemiluminescence in chronic granulomatous disease (patients and carriers) and in myeloperoxidase-deficient patients. This method appears to be somewhat more sensitive than the quantitative NBT test and can probably be performed on very small numbers of cells. Newer methods employ a whole-blood method that greatly simplifies the procedure by obviating the granulocyte separation steps. Many laboratories are substituting it for NBT reduction as a screening test for neutrophil dysfunction and in detection of carriers of chronic granulomatous disease.

Neutrophil Microbicidal Assay

Many strains of bacteria and fungi are effectively engulfed and killed by human neutrophils in vitro. Assuming that all of the stages of the phagocytic process that precede killing within the phagolysosome are intact, microbicidal assays are extremely useful tests for neutrophil function. As an example, the bactericidal capacity of neutrophils for the common test strain 502A of *S aureus* will be described in some detail.

Bacteria are cultured overnight in nutrient broth to make certain that they will be in a logarithmic growth phase. They are then diluted to give about 5 bacteria per neutrophil in the final test. Neutrophils are separated from whole heparinized blood by dextran sedimentation and lysis of erythrocytes with 0.84% NH_4Cl. Opsonin is provided as a 1:1 mixture of pooled frozen serum (-70 °C) and serum from freshly clotted blood. Bacteria, neutrophils, and opsonin are incubated in tightly capped test tubes and tumbled end over end at 37 °C. An aliquot of the entire mixture is sampled at zero time. After 30 minutes of incubation, antibiotics are added to kill extracellular bacteria. Aliquots of neutrophils with ingested organisms are sampled at 30, 60, and 120 minutes. Intracellular microorganisms are liberated by lysis of neutrophils by sterile water and the number of *viable* intracellular bacteria is estimated by serial dilutions and plating of lysed leukocytes. Results plotted as in Fig 19–12 show that normal neutrophils result in an almost 2-log reduction in viable intracellular *S aureus* 1 hour after incubation. Killing is virtually absent in cells from patients with chronic granulomatous disease and intermediate in heterozygous carriers of these inherited diseases.

By varying the test organism or the source of opsonin, this assay can be effectively used to measure a wide range of microbial activities and serum-related defects. Obviously, falsely "normal" killing

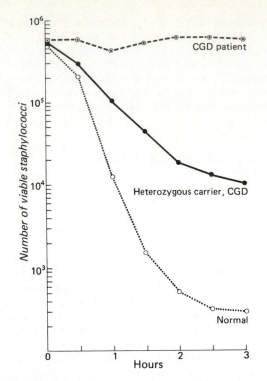

Figure 19–12. Bactericidal assay of granulocytes. Curves represent number of viable intracellular organisms that survive after being ingested by granulocytes. Note marked decline in bacterial survival in normal cells compared to reduced to absent killing by cells from patients and relatives with CGD (chronic granulomatous disease).

will be the interpretation of the results if cells fail to ingest organisms normally. Thus, an independent assay for microbial ingestion must be performed prior to the neutrophil microbicidal test.

Some diseases with defective microbicidal activity demonstrable with this assay are listed in Table 19–11. For further details, see Chapter 27.

Table 19–11. Disorders of neutrophil function.

Leukocyte adherence deficiency
Chronic granulomatous disease (X-linked or autosomal recessive)
Job's syndrome
Chédiak-Higashi syndrome
Myeloperoxidase deficiency
Glucose-6-phosphate dehydrogenase deficiency
Acute leukemia
Down's syndrome
Premature infants
Transient neutrophil dysfunction
    Acute infections
    Ataxia-telangiectasia
    Cryoglobulinemia

REFERENCES

General

Bloom BR, David JR (editors): *In Vitro Methods in Cell Mediated and Tumor Immunity.* Academic Press, 1976.

Mishell BB, Shiigi SM: *Selected Methods in Cellular Immunology.* Freeman, 1981.

Natvig JB, Perlmann P, Wigzell H: Lymphocytes: Isolation, fractionation and characterization. *Scand J Immunol* 1976;**Suppl 5.** [Entire issue.]

Rose NR, Friedman H, Fahey JL: *Manual of Clinical Immunology,* 3rd ed. American Society for Microbiology, 1986.

Weir DM et al (editors): *Handbook of Experimental Immunology,* 4th ed. 4 vols. Blackwell, 1986.

Delayed Hypersensitivity Skin Tests

Ahmed RA, Blose DA: Delayed hypersensitivity skin testing: A review. *Arch Dermatol* 1983;**119:**934.

Frazer IH et al: Assessment of delayed-type hypersensitivity in man. A comparison of the "multitest" and conventional intradermal injection of six antigens. *Clin Exp Immunol* 1985;**35:**182.

Heiss LI, Palmer DL: Anergy in patients with leukocytosis. *Am J Med* 1974;**56:**323.

Palmer DL, Reed WP: Delayed hypersensitivity skin testing: 1. Response rates in a hospitalized population. 2. Clinical correlates and anergy. *J Infect Dis* 1974;**130:**132, 138.

Assays for Human Lymphocytes & Monocytes

Adams DO, Edelson PJ, Koren HS (editors): *Methods for Studying Mononuclear Phagocytes.* Academic Press, 1981.

Bollum FJ: Terminal deoxynucleotidyl transferase: A hematopoietic cell marker. *Blood* 1979;**54:**1203.

Fauci AS et al: Activation and regulation of human immune responses: Implications in normal and disease states. *Ann Intern Med* 1983;**99:**61.

Knapp W: *Leukemia Markers.* Academic Press, 1981.

Bray RA, Landay AL: Identification and functional characterization of mononuclear cells by flow cytometry. *Arch Pathol Lab Med* 1989;**113:**579.

McMichael AJ, Fabre JW (editors): *Monoclonal Antibodies in Clinical Medicine.* Academic Press, 1982.

Reinherz EL et al: *Leukocyte Typing II.* 3 vols. Springer-Verlag, 1986.

Lymphocyte Activation

Ling NR: *Lymphocyte Stimulation.* North-Holland, 1968.

Oppenheim JJ et al: Use of lymphocyte transformation to assess clinical disorders. Page 87 in: *Laboratory Diagnosis of Immunologic Disorders.* Vyas GN, Stites DP, Brecher G (editors). Grune & Stratton, 1975.

Stobo JD: Mitogens. Page 55 in: *Clinical Immunobiology.* Vol. 4. Bach FH, Good RA (editors). Academic Press, 1980.

Wedner HJ, Parker CW: Lymphocyte activation. *Prog Allergy* 1976;**20:**195.

Flow Cytometry & Cell Sorting

Ault K: Clinical applications of fluorescence-activated cell sorting techniques. *Diagn Immunol* 1983;**1:**2.

Braylan RC, Benson NA: Flow cytometric analysis of lymphomas. *Arch Pathol Lab Med* 1989;**113:**627.

Fleisher TA, Hagengruber C, Marti GE: Immunophenotyping of normal lymphocytes. *Pathol Immunopathol Res* 1988;**7:**305.

Fulwyler MJ: Flow cytometry and cell sorting. *Blood Cells* 1980;**6:**173.

Herzenberg LA, Sweet RG, Herzenberg LA: Fluorescence-activated cell sorting. *Sci Am* (March) 1976;**234:**108.

McCarthy RC, Fetterhoff TJ: Issues of quality assurance in clinical flow cytometry. *Arch Pathol Lab Med* 1989;**113:**658.

Ryan DH, Fallon MA, Horan PK: Flow cytometry in the clinical laboratory. *Clin Chim Acta* 1988; **171:**125.

Proceedings of the Third Ortho Colloquium on Immunology. *Diagn Immunol* 1983;**1:**No. 3. [Entire issue.]

Neutrophil Function

Boxer LA, Morganroth ML: Neutrophil function disorders. *Disease-a-Month* 1987;**33:**681.

Douglas SD, Quie PG: Investigation of phagocytes in disease. In: *Practical Methods in Clinical Immunology Series.* Vol 3. Churchill Livingstone, 1981.

Gallin JI: Abnormal phagocyte chemotaxis: Pathophysiology, clinical manipulations and management of patients. *Rev Infect Dis* 1981;**3:**1196.

Horwitz MA: Phagocytosis of microorganisms. *Rev Infect Dis* 1982;**4:**104.

Lehrer RI et al: Neutrophils and host defense. *Ann Intern Med* 1988;**109:**127.

Root RK, Cohen MS: The microbicidal mechanisms of human neutrophils and eosinophils. *Rev Infect Dis* 1981;**3:**565.

Synderman R, Gaetze EJ: Molecular and cellular mechanisms of leukocyte chemotaxis. *Science* 1981; **213:**830.

Wade BH, Mandell GL: Polymorphonuclear leukocytes: Dedicated professional phagocytes. *Am J Med* 1983; **74:**686.

20

Blood Banking & Immunohematology

Elizabeth Donegan, MD, & Edith L. Bossom, SBB

The ability to successfully transfuse whole blood, or more specific blood components, has saved countless lives and supported the advance of modern surgery and cancer chemotherapy. The first lifesaving transfusion was performed less than 200 years ago by James Blundell in 1818. Today, 18 million blood components, prepared from 13 million blood donations, are transfused in the USA annually. Transfusion is increasingly safe because blood group systems and their relationship to the immune response have been defined; techniques have been developed to separate, store, preserve, and test blood prior to infusion; and improved transfusion methods have been developed.

Nevertheless, transfusion continues to require the removal of blood from one human being for infusion into another. This "living transplant" carries with it the complexities of its human source and thereby brings with it the potential of untoward reaction in the recipient. Some risks of transfusion are now known, and others have yet to be described. Consequently, the need for transfusion must be judged carefully in light of these risks.

BLOOD GROUPS

The first blood group system was described at the turn of the twentieth century by Karl Landsteiner. He observed that erythrocytes from some individuals clumped when mixed with the serum of others but not with their own. Using this agglutination technique, he classified an individual's erythrocytes into 4 types: A, B, AB, and O. It is now recognized that A and B represent carbohydrate antigens on the erythrocyte. Group O individuals have neither of these antigens on their erythrocytes, whereas erythrocytes from AB individuals have both A and B antigens. The ABO system remains the most important blood group system for transfusion purposes.

Knowledge about blood groups has expanded to include a diverse and numerous array of antigenic determinants on erythrocytes. Today, more than 400 erythrocyte antigens belonging to 24 systems are known. Each blood group system has members; each member may be composed of one or more different antigens. Each antigen is controlled by one gene. The antigenic determinants of a group are produced either directly (for proteins) or indirectly (for carbohydrates) by alleles at a single gene locus or at a gene locus so closely linked to another that crossing over is extremely rare. For any antigen of a group, a single allele is present at that locus and others are therefore excluded. Antigens on erythrocyte surfaces are usually detected by reacting erythrocytes with known antisera. Since the genotype cannot be directly determined by measuring erythrocyte antigens, these tests define a phenotype. The number of antigenic determinants per erythrocyte and their ability to elicit an immune response vary from antigen to antigen.

ERYTHROCYTE ANTIGENS

H & ABO

Antigenic determinants of these systems are carbohydrate moieties whose specificity resides in the terminal sugars of an oligosaccharide. On erythrocyte and endothelial surfaces, most of the antigens are bound to glycoprotein, although some carbohydrate is also bound to membrane lipid. Genetic control is via the production of transferase enzymes that conjugate terminal sugars to a stem carbohydrate. The H and ABO systems have separate gene loci and are independent of one another (Fig 20–1).

The H gene codes for a fucosyl transferase enzyme that effects the addition of fucose to precursor chains and completes the stem chain. The last 3 sugars of the stem chain are called H substance. The *H* gene (hh) is rarely absent; this phenotype is called O_h or Bombay type. In the absence of a complete stem chain, additional sugars cannot be added despite the presence of A or B transferase, and high-titer anti-H is produced.

The ABO blood groups are determined by allelic genes A, B, and O (Table 20–1). The A group transferase conjugates N-acetylglucosamine to the completed stem chain. The B group transferase conjugates a terminal galactose. The O gene produces no transferase to modify the blood group substance (Fig 20–1).

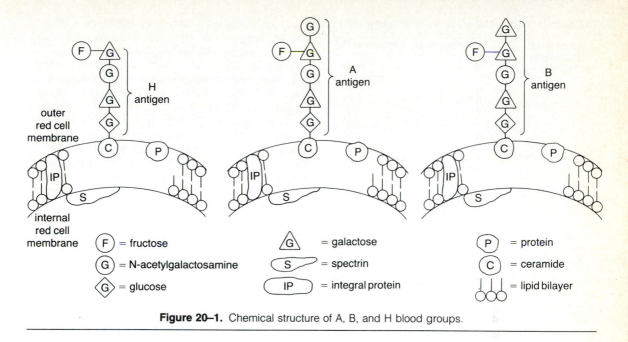

Figure 20–1. Chemical structure of A, B, and H blood groups.

Both groups A and B can be divided into subgroups. Eleven subgroups of A have been described, but most are rare. The most important are A_1 and A_2. Differences between subtypes of group A appear to be quantitative, ie, in the number of antigenic sites per erythrocyte surface. Of A blood, 78% is A_1, and 22% A_2. A_1 cells carry about one million copies of A antigen on their surface, and A_2 cells carry 250,000 copies. AB blood can also be divided into A_1B and A_2B types. To detect weak variants of A, which may go undetected in routine testing, blood grouping often includes the use of O serum that contains an anti-A capable of detecting these weaker forms, eg, A_4. Although less frequently detected, subgroups of group B can also be distinguished. Subgroups of group B, like those of group A, demonstrate a continuum in the number of antigenic sites per erythrocyte surface.

The naturally occurring antibodies to groups A and B are thought to be stimulated by very common substances. Intestinal bacteria are known to have substances chemically similar to and therefore anti-genically cross-reactive with A and B. These antibodies are first detected in children at 3–6 months of age, peaking at 5–10 years of age and falling with age and in some immunodeficiency states.

Two other systems directly interact with the ABO and H systems: Lewis and Secretor. Secretion of ABH substances in body fluids (saliva, sweat, milk, etc) is controlled by the allelic genes Se and se. These genes are independent of ABO and are inherited in a Mendelian dominant manner. Eighty percent of people are Se; they secrete Lewis and Sd antigens in addition to ABH substances. Typing of body fluids for these antigens has been useful in forensic investigations.

Rh

The Rhesus blood group system is second in importance only to the ABO system. Anti-Rh antibodies are the leading cause of hemolytic disease of the newborn and may also cause hemolytic transfusion reactions.

The mechanism of genetic control in this family of

Table 20–1. Routine ABO groupings.

			Frequency (%) in US Population			
Blood Group	Erythrocyte Antigens	Serum Antibody	White	Black	American Indian	Asian
O	H	Anti-A, Anti-B	45	49	79	40
A	A	Anti-B	40	27	16	28
B	B	Anti-A	11	20	4	27
AB	A and B	–	4	4	< 1	5

Table 20–2. Frequencies of common Rh haplotypes.[1]

Fisher-Race Terminology for Phenotypes		Frequency in US Population (%)		
		White	Black	Asian
CDe	Rh-positive	0.42	0.17	0.70
CDE		0.14	0.11	0.21
CDE		0.00	0.00	0.01
CDe		0.04	0.44	0.03
Cde	Rh-negative	0.37	0.26	0.03
Cde		0.02	0.02	0.02
CdE		0.01	0.00	0.00
CdE		0.00	0.00	0.00

[1]Adapted and reproduced, with permission, from Mourant et al, *The Distribution of Human Blood Groups and Other Polymorphisms,* 2nd ed. Oxford University Press, 1976.

more than 40 antigens is still unclear. It is recognized that each person inherits one codominant Rh gene or gene complex from each parent, which produces a complex erythrocyte membrane material. The absence of antigens produced by the Rh gene is called the Rh_{null} phenotype and is associated with an erythrocyte membrane defect and hemolytic anemia. It is not clear whether Rh is a single gene that produces a single product having multiple antigenic specificities or whether it represents the simultaneous inheritance of 3 closely linked genes that produce 3 separate allelic erythrocyte antigens.

These divergent theories have given rise to differing systems of nomenclature. In the Wiener nomenclature, multiple Rh alleles are designated as either R or r with one of many superscripts. R alleles produce the antigen Rh_o in a particular phenotype in addition to 2 other antigens; r alleles denote the absence of Rh_o in another phenotype. In the Fisher and Race system (see Table 20–2), 3 allelic gene pairs are thought to commonly produce 5 antigens (the remaining antigens are rare variants). Each antigen (D, C, c, E, and e) has a corresponding designation in the Wiener system (ie, D = Rh_o, C = rh′, etc). C and c, as well as E and e, function as alleles. No

d antigen is known; d describes the absence of D. The Rh antigens are inherited as 2 sets of 3, one from each parent (see below) (Table 20–3).

Clinically, Rh-positive (Rh^+) means the presence of D (Rh_o) and Rh-negative (Rh^-) indicates the absence of D (Rh_o). D is the most immunogenic of the Rh antigens. Slightly less than half of Rh^+ people are homozygous for D. Because there are no antisera to detect d, determination of zygosity depends on family studies. Roughly 15% of whites are Rh^-. Rh^- is less common in other races. Six weaker variants of D are described and are designated D^u. These weaker variants of D (D^u) can be missed in testing if blood is typed only with routine anti-D antisera but are detected if the indirect antiglobulin test is used. Although there is no harm in transfusing D^u individuals with Rh^- blood, Rh^- individuals can be sensitized with D^u-positive erythrocytes.

Other Erythrocyte Antigens

The majority of the remaining 20 blood group systems (representing more than 300 antigens) are rarely implicated in transfusion reactions. However, antibodies to the Kidd, Duffy, Kell, and MNS systems are known for their ability to cause hemolysis if antigen-positive blood is transfused into a sensitized recipient. The frequency of detecting shortened erythrocyte survival depends on the erythrocyte antigen and the antibody formed against it. The erythrocyte antigens more commonly involved in transfusion reactions are those that are both immunogenic and prevalent (high incidence). Low-incidence antigens, even if highly immunogenic, have a low likelihood of being transfused. In general, hemolytic antibodies are IgG and react at 37 °C (body temperature). IgM or cold-reacting antibodies rarely cause hemolysis.

Antibodies to Kidd antigens are a frequent cause of delayed hemolytic transfusion reaction. These antibodies are often difficult to identify in test systems because of poor reactivity. Four antigenic pheno-

Table 20–3. Inheritance of ABO types.[1]

Parents		Offspring	Parents		Offspring
O × O (OO) (OO)	→	**O** (OO)	**A × A** (AA) (AA) (AO) (AO)	→	**A or O** (AA) (OO) (AO)
O × A (OO) (AA) (AO)	→	**O or A** (OO) (AO)	**A × B** (AA) (BB) (AO) (BO)	→	**A, B, or O** (AO) (BO) (OO)
O × B (OO) (BB) (BO)	→	**O or B** (OO) (BO)	**A × AB** (AA) (AB) (AO)	→	**A, B, or AB** (AA) (BO) (AB)
O × AB (OO) (AB)	→	**A or B** (AO) (BO)	**B × B** (BB) (BB) (BO) (BO)	→	**B or O** (BB) (OO) (BO)
AB × AB (AB) (AB)	→	**A, B, or AB** (AA) (BB) (AB)	**B × AB** (BB) (AB) (BO)	→	**A, B, or AB** (AO) (BB) (AB)

[1]Phenotypes in bold; possible genotypes in italics below.

types have been described: JK (a+ b−), JK (a− b+), JK (a+ b+), and JK (a− b−). The JK (a− b−) phenotype is rare except in some Pacific island populations.

The antigens of the Duffy system (Fy^a and Fy^b) are controlled by codominant alleles. Antibodies to Fy^a are more commonly associated with delayed hemolytic transfusion reactions than are those to Fy^b. Many blacks have a third allele, which produces the Fy$^{(a- b-)}$ phenotype. Duffy antigens on erythrocytes serve as receptors for the entry of *Plasmodium vivax* into the erythrocytes. Fy$^{(a- b-)}$ individuals who lack Duffy antigens are resistant to *P vivax* infection but not to *P falciparium* infection.

The Kell system, as first described, included the allelic pair K and k, k antigen being the more frequent. The system now includes 2 additional allelic pairs and several variants. The K antigen is highly immunogenic, with one of 20 individuals transfused with K$^+$ cells developing antibody. Antibodies to Kell antigen cause hemolytic disease of the newborn, hemolytic transfusion reactions, and, occasionally, autoimmune hemolytic anemia. Individuals of the McLeod phenotype lack Kx antigen, which is a precursor in the synthesis of Kell antigens. Absence of Kx results in the depressed expression of k. These individuals have erythrocyte and neuromuscular system abnormalities. The McLeod phenotype is also associated with some cases of chronic granulomatous disease (see Chapter 27).

METHODS FOR DETECTION OF ANTIGEN & ANTIBODIES TO ERYTHROCYTES

Antiglobulin Tests

Antibody or complement adsorbed onto erythrocytes is detected by using antibodies to human serum globulins (AHG). AHG reagents are produced either in animals or in tissue culture by using monoclonal antibody techniques (see Chapter 18). These reagents may be polyspecific (a mixture of antibodies to IgG, complement, and heavy and light chains) or monospecific (antibodies to specific immunoglobulin or components of complement). The direct antiglobulin test (DAT) detects antibody or complement coating the surface of erythrocytes, whereas the indirect antiglobulin test (IDAT) identifies antibody in serum.

To perform the DAT (Fig 20–2), erythrocytes are washed with saline to remove unbound antibody or complement and then incubated with AHG. If antibody is present on the erythrocytes, the Fab portion of AHG attaches to the Fc portion of the erythrocyte-bound antibody. Bridging of AHG Fab molecules between erythrocytes results in visually detectable agglutination. A positive test requires a minimum of 500 antibodies per erythrocyte surface unless more

sensitive methods are used. The DAT is used in the investigation of autoimmune or drug-induced hemolytic anemia, hemolytic disease of the newborn, and suspected hemolytic transfusion reactions.

The IDAT detects **serum antibodies,** which can attach in vitro to erythrocytes (Fig 20–2). This test differs from the DAT in that before a DAT is performed, the serum to be tested is incubated with washed erythrocytes so that serum antibody, if present, binds to erythrocyte antigen. The erythrocytes are then washed to remove any unbound globulin, and AHG is added. If agglutination is observed, serum globulins to erythrocyte antigens are present. The IDAT is used by blood banks in 3 ways: (1) Recipient serum is tested by using panels of erythrocytes with known antigens on their surface to identify the presence and type of a recipient serum antibody. (2) Commercial serum reagents containing known erythrocyte antibodies are used to select blood donor cells that are free of specific erythrocyte antigens to transfuse recipients with identified erythrocyte antibodies. (3) Recipient serum is tested with blood donor cells to confirm the absence of an antigen-antibody reaction (cross-match).

Pretransfusion Testing

Blood is tested prior to transfusion to prevent clinically significant destruction of the recipient's erythrocytes. Clinically significant antibodies are those that are known to have caused unacceptably shortened erythrocyte survival in vivo or frank transfusion reaction. Generally, they are antibodies that react at 37 °C (body temperature) and that react in the antiglobulin test. Prior to transfusion, the recipient's erythrocytes and serum are tested for ABO and Rh$_o$ (D) types and for antibodies to erythrocyte antigens, respectively (type and screen). Additionally, the recipient's serum is tested for compatibility with the erythrocytes from the intended donor (cross-match).

Type & Screen

ABO and Rh$_o$ (D) **type** are determined by mixing the recipient's erythrocytes with anti-A, anti-B, and anti-D antisera. The ABO group is then confirmed by testing the recipient's serum against commercial A and B cells to detect isoagglutinins.

The recipient's serum is **screened** for alloantibodies that may not be demonstrated in the cross-match. In antibody screens, suspensions of O erythrocytes that contain known erythrocyte antigens on their surface are incubated with the recipient's serum. If antigen-antibody complexes are formed, hemolysis or agglutination of erythrocytes is observed. The screen is completed by the IDAT and again observed for agglutination.

In the **cross-match,** compatibility between donor and recipient is determined directly. Washed donor cells are combined with recipient serum, incubated, centrifuged, and observed for hemolysis or aggluti-

Coombs tests

A. **direct (DAT)**

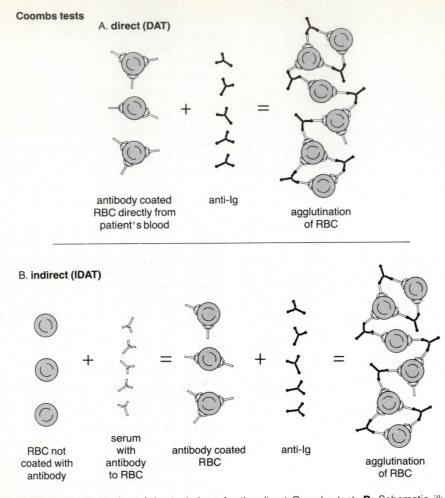

antibody coated   anti-Ig
RBC directly from
patient's blood

agglutination
of RBC

B. **indirect (IDAT)**

RBC not   serum   antibody coated   anti-Ig
coated with   with   RBC
antibody   antibody   agglutination
                to RBC   of RBC

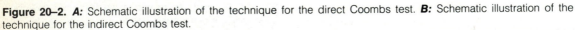

Figure 20–2. *A:* Schematic illustration of the technique for the direct Coombs test. *B:* Schematic illustration of the technique for the indirect Coombs test.

nation. If the recipient has either a history of previous erythrocyte antibody or has had antibody detected during the antibody screening procedure, the IDAT must be performed before a crossmatch may be considered compatible.

These tests that detect antigen-antibody reactions with erythrocytes are performed most simply in saline solution. It is recognized that this causes some loss in test sensitivity for IgG antibodies owing to ionic repulsion forces between erythrocytes generated by clustering of Na^+ and Cl^- ions near erythrocyte surfaces. A variety of methods to increase the sensitivity of these tests have been developed. These procedures add different reagents, such as albumin, LISS (low-ionic-strength solution), or polybrene, to the test system or utilize enzyme-treated erythrocytes, all of which generally increase sensitivity.

TRANSFUSION REACTIONS

Blood transfusion has become increasingly safe and effective, but a variety of adverse reactions, only some of which are preventable, continue to occur (Table 20–4). Transfusions must be monitored during infusion for immediate reactions and over time to detect delayed reactions.

Hemolytic Reactions

The transfusion of erythrocyte-incompatible blood may cause immediate hemolysis. Hemolytic reactions are fatal in 10% of ABO-incompatible transfusions, which generally occur when large amounts of ABO-incompatible blood are transfused as a result of human error. Incompatible transfusions involving other blood groups are usually less severe. Clini-

Table 20–4. Transfusion reactions.

Cause	Incidence	Manifestations	Treatment
Recipient erythrocyte antibodies Hemolytic (acute)	< 0.02%	Fever, chills, lowered blood pressure Pain in back or infusion site Hemoglobin in blood and urine	Stop transfusion; blood/urine to blood bank. Hydrate. Monitor hematocrit, liver, and renal function.
Hemolytic (delayed)		Lowered hematocrit, increased bilirubin; raised LDH days to weeks posttransfusion	Monitor hematocrit, also liver and renal function if severe.
Recipient leukocyte antibodies Febrile	< 2%	Temp raised ≥ 1 °C, chills	Stop transfusion: Rule out hemolytic reactions with patient's unit, blood/urine to blood bank; premedicate with antipyretics; give leukocyte-poor products if available.
Donor WBC antibodies		Noncardiac pulmonary edema, bronchospasm	Stop transfusion, treat symptoms; give leukocyte-poor products if available.
Plasma proteins Allergic	2–3%	Itching, urticaria, rarely asthma, bronchospasm, anaphylaxis	Stop transfusion; give antihistamines for urticaria; treat symptoms.

cally, reactions are often heralded by fever, chills, and burning at the injection site. Reaction may progress to dyspnea and hypotension, with joint or back pain. Shock, generalized bleeding, and renal failure may follow.

Delayed hemolytic transfusion reactions occur 3–10 days posttransfusion. Many of these reactions are clinically undetected but are thought to occur in about one in 6000 transfusions. They result either from primary immunization to transfused erythrocyte antigens or from an anamnestic response in a previously sensitized individual whose antibody titers are undetectable at the time of transfusion. They are characterized by fever and anemia with elevated levels of bilirubin and a positive DAT.

Febrile Reactions

Febrile nonhemolytic reactions are caused by cytotoxic or agglutinating antibodies in the recipient directed against donor leukocyte antigens. They are generally self-limiting and associated with fever of 38–39 °C and chills. They must be distinguished from fever associated with hemolytic transfusion reactions and from the high fever (> 40 °C) and rigors associated with bacterial contamination of blood components. Febrile transfusion reactions occur most frequently in multiply transfused recipients or in women sensitized to leukocytes from multiple pregnancies. Only one in 8 patients with a febrile reaction will have another reaction on subsequent transfusion. Recurrent febrile reactions are often controlled with antipyretics. Patients with uncontrolled febrile reactions may benefit from leukocyte-

poor components prepared in a variety of ways to decrease the number of leukocytes transfused by as much as 90%.

High-titer leukocyte antibodies in either recipient or donor plasma can cause pulmonary edema (see Chapter 45). Recipient antibody to donor granulocytes or donor antibody to recipient granulocytes can cause granulocyte aggregates, which are filtered by the lungs. Antibodies adherent to granulocyte aggregates will activate complement.

Allergic Reactions

Allergic reactions to transfusion are generally characterized by itching, hives, and local erythema and only rarely accompanied by cardiovascular instability. They are thought to be caused by infused plasma proteins and occur in 1–2% of transfusions. Patients with a history of allergy more frequently have allergic reactions to blood. Mild reactions can be treated with antihistamines, and the transfusion continued. Pretreatment with antihistamines often prevents these reactions if they are recurrent, but if they are severe, washed erythrocytes may be indicated. Anaphylactic reactions occur in some IgA-deficient recipients (see Chapter 24) after transfusion of as little as 10–15 mL of whole blood. Fortunately, these reactions are rare and are confined to individuals with high titers of anti-IgA. Reaction is due to the IgA present in transfused plasma and is prevented by transfusing washed erythrocytes.

Preventable transfusion reactions include those caused by bacterial contamination of blood components, congestive heart failure due to volume overload, and artificially produced donor erythrocyte destruction prior to infusion. Erythrocytes may be destroyed by inadvertent overheating or freezing of donor blood or mixing it with nonisotonic solutions.

Transfusion-Transmitted Infection

Transfusion may be complicated by a variety of infectious microorganisms, only some of which can be detected by current donor-screening methods (Table 20–5). The most frequently reported posttransfusion infections in developed countries are hepatitis and cytomegalovirus (CMV), HIV-1, and HTLV-I infections. In certain countries, posttransfusion malaria and Chagas' disease are significant problems. Elimination of potentially infected blood depends on successful donor screening by medical history, aseptic blood collection, and adequate laboratory testing of the donated blood. In the USA, all blood is tested for hepatitis by using HBsAg, anti-HBc, and alanine aminotransferase (ALT), and for syphilis, HIV-1, and HTLV-I by serologic means.

The incidence of posttransfusion hepatitis (PTH) is estimated to be 1–2%. PTH is caused by hepatitis B in 5% of cases and by the non-A, non-B hepatitis agent (hepatitis C virus) in 95% of cases. Of transfusion recipients who develop posttransfusion hepatitis, 50% develop chronic hepatitis; 10% of these develop cirrhosis. All blood components can transmit hepatitis, except those that can be pasteurized, such as albumin and other plasma proteins. It is hoped that specific testing for hepatitis C virus, now under development, will further decrease the frequency of PTH.

CMV is transmitted to CMV-seronegative transfusion recipients by leukocytes contaminating some blood components, particularly erythrocytes and platelets. Whether transfusion of CMV-seropositive blood to CMV-seropositive recipients causes superinfection or other complications is unknown. Roughly 50% of blood donors are infected with CMV, which limits the availability of CMV-negative blood. Posttransfusion CMV infection causes significant morbidity and mortality rates in severely immunocompromised patients. When possible, CMV-seronegative blood should be given to low-birth-weight infants (< 1250 g), CMV-seronegative pregnant women, and CMV-seronegative recipients of CMV-seronegative organ transplants.

HIV-1 infection due to transfusion has become increasingly infrequent with the initiation of donor HIV-1 antibody testing. HIV-1 can be transmitted by erythrocytes, platelets, cryoprecipitate, fresh-frozen plasma, and possibly other blood components. The risk of infection by transfusion is estimated to be between one in 40,000 and one in 100,000 transfusions since the institution of antibody-screening and other screening methods. The virus can be transmitted by blood collected from donors who have been recently infected but have not yet formed antibody to HIV-1 and who have not voluntary excluded themselves from donating blood. Another retrovirus, HTLV-I, has been recently recognized as being transmitted with 70% efficiency in cellular blood products. Prior to the availability of HTLV-I testing, one in 3500 to one in 5000 transfusion recipients were infected with HTLV-I. However, the extent to which HTLV-I causes transfusion-associated disease is unknown. HTLV-I is known to cause a form of T cell leukemia (see Chapter 48) and tropical spastic paraparesis in endemic populations.

Other Diseases Transmitted by Transfusion

Epstein-Barr virus may be transmitted by transfusion. In most cases it results in asymptomatic seroconversion, but it can cause a mononucleosis syndrome. Transfusion-acquired delta hepatitis requires the presence of both the hepatitis delta virus and hepatitis B virus in the blood donor for transmission to a recipient (see Chapter 51). Because effective donor screening for HBsAg eliminates almost all of these donors, the risk of transmitting this agent is low.

Posttransfusion syphilis is now rare. There is a low incidence of syphilitic infection in blood donors, and all donors are screened for antibody. Since the organism does not survive cold storage for more than 48–72 hours, it can be transmitted only by fresh blood or platelets.

Malaria remains a disease of major worldwide importance. The parasite is present in erythrocytes of carriers sometimes for years after infection. There are no laboratory tests that are simple and sensitive enough available for screening the blood donor population. Because of this, blood banks in the USA rely on histories taken at the time of donation. Donors who have traveled to endemic areas are deferred for 6 months (3 years if chemoprophylaxis is taken).

Other parasitic diseases reported to be transmitted by blood transfusion include the microfilariae *Wuchereria bancrofti, Acanthocheilonema persians, Mansonella ozzardi, Loa loa,* and *Brugia malayi.* Chagas' disease can be transmitted by *Trypanosoma cruzi. Toxoplasma gondii* can cause toxoplasmosis in transfusion recipients, and *Babesia microti* can cause babesiosis. Leishmaniasis is also reported as a posttransfusion infection.

Table 20–5. Transfusion-transmitted infection.

Infection[1]	Risk/Unit Transfused
CMV infection	1:20–1:100
Non-A, non-B hepatitis	1:100
Hepatitis B	1:200–1:300
HIV-1 infection	1:40,000–1:100,000

[1]Rare infections include syphilis, malaria, Epstein-Barr virus infection, delta hepatitis, brucellosis, Chagas' disease, babesiosis, and leishmaniasis.

Transfusion-transmitted bacterial infections are most frequently the result of inadequate decontamination of skin at the time of blood collection, but may be caused by contamination of the blood during storage and handling. Brucellosis may also be transmitted by an infected donor.

Immunologic Mechanisms of Transfusion Reactions

Hemolytic transfusion reactions are caused by antigen-antibody complexes on the erythrocyte membrane. These complexes activate Hageman factor (factor XIIa) and complement. Hageman factor, in turn, activates the kinin system (see Chapter 13). Bradykinins thus generated increase capillary permeability and dilate arterioles, causing hypotension. Complement is activated and leads to intravascular hemolysis as well as to histamine and serotonin release from mast cells. Hageman factor and free incompatible erythrocyte stroma activate the intrinsic clotting cascade, with consequent disseminated intravascular coagulation (DIC). Systemic hypotension with renal vasoconstriction and the formation of intravascular thrombi lead to renal failure. When complement activation is not complete, the reaction is less severe. Erythrocytes coated with C3b are cleared from the circulation by phagocytes, resulting in extravascular hemolysis, which takes place primarily in the liver.

Antileukocyte antibodies are either cytotoxic or agglutinating. These antibodies form complexes with antigens on leukocytes, activating complement. Activated complement generates vasoactive substances in the circulation. Endogenous pyrogens from destroyed granulocytes are also released into the circulation following cell lysis.

The mechanism of graft-versus-host disease depends upon the engraftment of donor lymphocytes in an immunoincompetent recipient. Donor lymphocytes recognize recipient tissue antigens as "foreign" and cause a clinical syndrome characterized by fever, skin rash, hepatitis, and diarrhea. Death may result. Engraftment can be prevented by irradiating lymphocyte-carrying components to preclude lymphocyte activation. Graft-versus-host disease occurs, rarely, in newborns undergoing exchange transfusion, patients with T cell immunodeficiencies, and patients severely immunosuppressed by intensive chemotherapy and irradiation (see Chapter 61).

Rh ISOIMMUNIZATION

The D antigen is a high-incidence, strongly immunogenic antigen, 50 times more immunogenic than the other Rh antigens. The prevalence of antibody formation to Rh^+ blood depends on the dose of Rh^+ cells: 1 mL of cells sensitizes 15% of individuals exposed; 250 mL sensitizes 60–70%. After the initial exposure to Rh^+ cells, weak IgM antibody can be detected as early as 4 weeks. This is followed by a rapid conversion to IgG antibody. A second exposure to as little as 0.03 mL of Rh^+ erythrocytes may result in the rapid formation of IgG antibodies.

The majority of potential transfusion reactions to Rh can be prevented by transfusing Rh^- individuals with Rh^- blood. Immunization and antibody formation to D antigen still occur owing to occasional Rh sensitization during pregnancy or to transfusion errors, particularly during emergencies. Immunization to other Rh antigens may occur because donor blood is typed routinely for D but not for other Rh antigens.

Hemolytic disease of the newborn occurs with the passage of Rh^+ cells from the fetus to the circulation of the Rh^- mother. Once anti-D antibody is formed in the mother, IgG but not IgM anti-D antibodies cross the placenta, causing hemolysis of fetal erythrocytes. Rh^- mothers become sensitized during pregnancy or at the time of delivery as a result of transplacental fetal hemorrhage. The size and number of fetal hemorrhages increase as pregnancy progresses. Following delivery, 75% of women will have had transplacental fetal hemorrhage. The risk of transplacental fetal hemorrhage increases as the pregnancy progresses (3% in the first trimester, 45% in the second trimester, 64% in the third trimester). Some obstetric complications increase the risk of transplacental fetal hemorrhage: antepartum hemorrhage, toxemia of pregnancy, cesarian section, external version, and manual removal of the placenta. Total transplacental fetal hemorrhage can also occur following spontaneous or therapeutic abortion or amniocentesis. Overall Rh immunization occurs in 8–9% of Rh^- women following the delivery of the first Rh^+ ABO-compatible baby and in 1.5–2.0% of Rh^- women who deliver Rh^+ ABO-incompatible babies.

Rh Prophylaxis

Rh immunization can now be suppressed almost entirely if high-titer anti-Rh immunoglobulin (RhIG) is administered by 72 hours after the potentially sensitizing dose of Rh^+ cells.

The protective mechanism of RhIG administration is not clear. RhIG does not effectively block Rh antigen from immunoresponsive cells by competitive inhibition, since effective doses of RhIG are known not to cover all Rh antigen sites. Intravascular hemolysis and rapid clearance of erythrocyte debris by the poorly immunoresponsive liver are also unlikely. Although this mechanism appears to explain the 90% protective effect of ABO incompatibility between mother and fetus, RhIG-induced erythrocyte hemolysis is extravascular. Rh^+ fetal cells are removed primarily by highly phagocytic cells in the spleen and, to a lesser extent, the lymph nodes. The most likely mechanism is a negative modulation of the primary immune response. Antigen-antibody complexes are bound to cells bearing Fc receptors in the lymph nodes and spleen. These cells presumably stimulate suppressor T cell responses, which prevent antigen-induced B cell proliferation and antibody formation.

A prophylactic dose of 300 μg of RhIG intramuscularly prevents Rh immunization following exposure to up to 30 mL of Rh⁺ erythrocytes. Initial recommendations were that 300 μg of RhIG be given to nonimmunized Rh⁻ mothers by 72 hours after delivery of an Rh⁺ infant. The recommended dose is different in some other countries. Doses may need to be increased in cases of massive transplacental fetal hemorrhage. These recommendations have been extended to include prophylaxis for nonimmunized Rh⁻ mothers following abortion and amniocentesis and, in some other countries, routinely during pregnancy. The administration of RhIG to pregnant women has not been shown to have a detrimental effect on the fetus.

Large doses of RhIG can effectively suppress immunization following inadvertent transfusion of Rh⁺ blood into Rh⁻ patients if given within 72 hours of transfusion. Once Rh immunization is demonstrated by the IDAT, administration of RhIG is ineffective.

BLOOD COMPONENT THERAPY

The transfusion of selective blood components has become increasingly important. More stringent screening and testing of blood donors has decreased the number of eligible donors at a time of increased need for blood. Increasing use of myelosuppressive chemotherapy for malignant diseases and organ transplantation requires more blood than ever before. The indications for transfusion are now assessed more critically. Blood transfusion is not entirely safe, and no transfusion should be given unless it is needed (Table 20–6).

Erythrocytes

The indications for erythrocyte transfusion and its effect depend on the clinical state of the recipient. One unit of erythrocytes is expected to increase the nonbleeding adult's hemoglobin by 1 g/dL and to increase the hematocrit by 3%. After senescent and damaged erythrocytes are cleared, 70–80% of transfused erythrocytes survive normally.

During acute blood loss, 1 hour or more is required for equilibration of intravascular and extravascular fluids and an accurate assessment of the fall in the hemoglobin level. Generally, a loss of 20% of blood volume can be corrected with crystalloid (electrolyte) solution alone, which can then be supplemented with colloid (protein) solution. Whole blood is indicated if blood loss exceeds one-third of blood volume. Operative blood loss of 1000–1200 mL rarely requires transfusion. If oxygen-carrying capacity is required in acute blood loss, packed erythrocytes are indicated.

A particular hemoglobin level is tolerated better in a patient with chronic anemia than in a patient with acute blood loss. Physiologic compensation by increased cardiac output and a shift of the oxyhemoglobin disassociation curve to the right for increased

Table 20–6. Guidelines for component therapy.

Component	Indications for Use
Red blood cells	Use to increase O_2-carrying capacity; 1 unit will increase hemoglobin 1 g/dL in a 70-kg patient. Consider the degree of anemia, intravascular volume, and presence of coexisting cardiac, pulmonary, or vascular conditions. 1. If hemoglobin > 10 g/dL, transfusion is rarely indicated. 2. If hemoglobin < 7 g/dL, transfusion is usually indicated. 3. If hemoglobin is 7–10 g/dL, assess clinical status, mixed venous pO_2, and O_2 extraction ratio.
Platelets	Use to control or prevent bleeding due to low platelet count or abnormal platelet function; 1 concentrate will increase platelet count by ca 5000 platelets/mL. 1. Generally, patients with platelet counts > 10,000–20,000 should not receive platelets to prevent bleeding. 2. Actively bleeding patients with platelet counts > 50,000 generally will not benefit from platelets. 3. Generally, platelets are not indicated in massive transfusion or cardiac surgery.
FFP	Used to increase clotting factors in patients with documented deficiencies (PT/PTT > 1.5 × normal)[1]; 1 unit will increase the level of any factor 2–3%. 1. FFP should not be used as a volume expander or nutritional source. 2. FFP is useful for treatment of factor II, V, VII, IX, X, and XI deficiencies when specific components are not available. 3. FFP is useful for patients with warfarin overdose who are actively bleeding or who require emergency surgery prior to vitamin K reversal. 4. FFP may be useful in massive blood transfusion (> 1 blood volume within a few hours). 5. FFP is useful as a source of antithrombin III in deficient patients undergoing surgery or heparin treatment, in infants with severe protein-losing enteropathy, and in patients with thrombotic thrombocytopenic purpura.

[1]PT, prothrombin time; PTT, partial thromboplastin time.

oxygen delivery to tissues allow for adequate oxygenation in these cases.

Exchange transfusion of neonates is a special circumstance in which whole blood less than 7 days old is required to ensure tolerable levels of plasma electrolytes and adequate levels of 2,3-diphosphoglycerate. Preferably, the blood should be irradiated to prevent the rare occurrence of graft-versus-host disease.

All erythrocyte components should be administered through blood filters. No medications of any kind, especially solutions containing calcium or glucose, should be infused with blood components.

Platelets

Platelets function to control bleeding by acting as hemostatic plugs on vascular endothelium. Platelet abnormalities that require transfusion may be either quantitative or qualitative. The vast majority of platelet transfusions are given to supplement small numbers of platelets due to decreased production, to pooling, or to dilution.

Platelets are available as either random donor concentrates (recovered from a blood donation) or as plateletpheresis (collected by using a cytopheresis machine). The transfusion of one concentrate is expected to increase the platelet count of a reasonably well 50-kg adult by 5000–10,000/μL. Plateletphereses are equivalent to 6 concentrates. The survival of transfused platelets is decreased in patients who are actively bleeding, who have splenomegaly, fever, infection, or disseminated intravascular coagulation, or who are sensitized to platelet antigens. The transfusion of ABO-incompatible platelets is associated with slightly decreased platelet survival.

Transient thrombocytopenias, which are the result of treatment regimens for malignancy, are responsible for most platelet transfusions. Prophylactic platelets are often transfused when the platelet count falls below 20,000/μL. Since there is little significant bleeding when platelet counts are above 10,000/μL, prophylactic platelets may be given to patients with counts of less than 10,000/μL, or therapeutic platelets may be transfused during bleeding episodes. The potential benefit of single-donor plateletpheresis over pooled random-donor concentrates in delaying alloimmunization and increasing platelet counts has yet to be adequately studied.

Platelets have a limited role in preventing bleeding in surgical patients. Platelet counts between 50,000 and 60,000/μL result in adequate hemostasis. In the event of massive transfusion (15–20 units), the dilutional effect on the platelet count by stored blood must be considered and corrected if necessary. Stored blood does not contain platelets. Although a functional platelet abnormality during cardiac surgery has been described, controlled trials do not demonstrate the need for platelet transfusion if counts are above 60,000/μL, regardless of a history of recent aspirin consumption.

Plasma Products

Fresh-frozen plasma (FFP), stored plasma, and cryoprecipitate are valuable sources of coagulation factors. Stored plasma and FFP can often be used interchangeably. Levels of factors V and VIII in stored plasma are half those in FFP, but levels of other factors are equivalent. Cryoprecipitate is used as a source of factor VIII, von Willebrand factor, and fibrinogen.

FFP is used for treating isolated congenital factor deficiencies, with the exception of factor IX (for which it is relatively ineffective) and for correcting warfarin overdoses. It is also used to treat thrombotic thrombocytopenic purpura and for bleeding patients with C1 esterase inhibitor or bleeding patients with heparin-dependent antithrombin III deficiency who are heparin-resistant. Massively transfused patients with a prothrombin time or partial thromboplastin time greater than 1.5 times normal and platelet counts above 50,000/μL should also receive plasma. Plasma should not be used for volume expansion.

Cryoprecipitate is used in young hemophiliacs or patients with mild hemophilia to decrease the number of donor exposures compared with the use of factor concentrates. Cryoprecipitate and deamino-8-arginine vasopressin have proved to be useful in managing bleeding uremic patients.

REFERENCES

Barton JC: Nonhemolytic, noninfectious transfusion reactions. *Semin Hematol* 1981;**18**:95.

Bowman JM: The prevention of Rh immunization. *Transfusion Med Rev* 1988;**2**:129.

Bowman JM, Pollock JM: Failures of intravenous Rh immune globulin prophylaxis: An analysis of the reasons for such failures. *Transfusion Med Rev* 1987;**1**:101.

Cohen ND et al: Transmission of retroviruses by transfusion of screened blood in patients undergoing cardiac surgery. *N Engl J Med* 1989;**320**:1172.

Gould SA: Blood components in surgery. *AABB News Briefs* (May) 1989;**12**:9.

Greenwalt TJ: Pathogenesis and management of hemolytic transfusion reactions. *Semin Hematol* 1981;**18**:84.

Huestis DW et al: *Practical Blood Transfusion*. Little, Brown, 1988.

Issitt PD: *Applied Blood Group Serology*, 3rd ed. Montgomery Scientific, 1985.

Mollison PL: *Blood Transfusion in Clinical Medicine*, 7th ed. Blackwell, 1983.

Mourant AE, Kopec AC, Domaniewska-Sobczak K: *The Distribution of Human Blood Groups and Other Polymorphisms,* 2nd ed. Oxford University Press, 1976.

NIH Consensus Conference: Platelet transfusion therapy. *JAMA* 1987;**257:**1777.

NIH Consensus Conference: Perioperative red blood cell transfusion. *JAMA* 1988;**260:**2700.

NIH Consensus Conference: Fresh-frozen plasma. *JAMA* 1985;**253:**551.

Pineda AA, Brzica SM, Taswell HF: Hemolytic transfusion reaction: Recent experience in a large blood bank. *Mayo Clin Proc* 1978;**53:**378.

Pittiglio DH, Baldwin AJ, Sohmer PR (editors): *Modern Blood Banking and Transfusion Practices*. FA Davis, 1983.

Tabor E et al: *Infectious Complications of Blood Transfusion*. Academic Press, 1982.

Widmann FK (editor): *Technical Manual for the American Association of Blood Banks*. American Association of Blood Banks, 1985.

Histocompatibility Testing

21

Beth W. Colombe, PhD

The human leukocyte antigen (HLA) system as we know it today has been defined largely by a single methodology, the complement-dependent lymphocytotoxicity test—a serologic assay. HLA antigens, encoded by the alleles of this genetic system, have been characterized through the reaction patterns of naturally occurring alloantibodies that bind to specific HLA antigens on target cells, fix complement, and then kill the cells. Through the discovery and testing of numerous alloantisera with lymphocytotoxic activity, the extensive polymorphism of the HLA system has been revealed (see Chapter 4).

When examined by methods other than lymphocytotoxicity, the extent of HLA antigen polymorphism appears quite different from the classic system. Few if any antigen "splits" (antigen subtypes or variants) would have been defined if alloantibody binding alone had been used. For example, a cytotoxic antibody to B49, or Bw50 (the 2 splits of B21) will bind equally well to the opposite split, presumably reacting to some common determinant that characterizes "B21" from other antigens. Binding studies with monoclonal antibodies generated against HLA determinants often react with several HLA alleles not previously thought to be cross-reactive, blurring the apparent antigen diversity even further. In contrast with alloantisera, some monoclonal antibodies bind to antigens encoded by more than one genetic locus. Conversely, by their exquisite specificity, monoclonal antibodies are able to enlarge the number of identifiable HLA alleles.

Speculation on the amount of HLA polymorphism is now becoming resolved by applying the new techniques of molecular biology to HLA. Now the serologically defined polymorphisms of the HLA system have a molecular basis in the variations that exist in the exact sequences of nucleotides of genomic DNA and the amino acid sequences of the HLA antigens themselves. As more alleles are being sequenced, a new image of increasing complexity and allelic variation is emerging. For example, there are now 7 variants of HLA B27, 5 of A2, 3 of A30, 3 of DQW3, etc. Whether such sequence differences have clinical significance remains to be determined (see Chapter 4 for a discussion of the new HLA polymorphisms and disease). Despite these new advances, the majority of histocompatibility testing is currently focused upon the "classic" HLA specificities as defined serologically.

During the past 25 years, genetic and clinical studies have shown that HLA antigens are the major "transplantation antigens" that determine the compatibility of transplanted tissues and organs. Histocompatibility between individuals is based upon the extent of matching of inherited HLA antigens and the degree of immunologic reactivity to these antigens in cellular and serologic cross-match testing. HLA matching has an enormous practical influence upon contemporary organ transplantation practices in clinical medicine.

HISTOCOMPATIBILITY TESTING & TRANSPLANTATION

The practice of testing for histocompatibility between an organ donor and the selected recipient is based on the presumption that tissue compatibility will promote graft acceptance and avoid immune rejection (see Chapter 6). The foundation for this assumption is the evidence that identical twins can accept and retain grafts from one another indefinitely, whereas grafts from all others are ultimately rejected in the absence of immunosuppressive therapy. Efforts to define the inherited basis for tissue compatibility have focused mainly upon the HLA antigen system. It follows that the greater the identity of HLA antigens, the greater the histocompatibility of the graft with the recipient. Identification of HLA antigens is known as **tissue typing.** Cellular methods for tissue typing include the use of homozygous typing cells (HTC testing) and the mixed-lymphocyte culture (MLC) test for HLA compatibility. A state of histocompatibility between donor and recipient may also be inferred from absence of preformed antibodies and cytotoxic lymphocytes directed against the donor HLA antigens. Serologic testing for anti-donor antibodies is called cross-matching; cellular testing is done by the direct cell-mediated lympholysis (CML) assay.

Table 21–1 shows a flowchart that outlines a typical course of histocompatibility testing for a prospective kidney graft recipient. In the following sections, these various tests will be described, including the interpretation of results and rationale for use.

Table 21–1. Flowchart of histocompatibility testing for the renal transplant patient.

A. Perform preliminary immunologic evaluation
1. Patient
   HLA typing
   ABO/Rh typing
   Screening of serum for antibodies reactive with HLA antigens
   Testing of serum for autoantibodies
2. Living related donors
   HLA typing
   ABO/Rh typing
   Cross-match with serum of patient to detect anti-donor antibodies
   MLC test with patient
B. Select living related donor
This is based on:
   ABO compatibility
   Best match for HLA antigens
   Low stimulation of patient's cells in MLC test
   Negative preliminary cross-match
   If there is no appropriate living related donor, then
C. Place patient on waiting list for cadaver kidney
   Register patient with UNOS
   Screen serum sample monthly for antibodies reactive to HLA antigens
D. Select appropriate recipient for cadaver kidney
   HLA and ABO type cadaver donor
   Cross-match cadaver with ABO-compatible recipients
   Select candidates having no antibodies to donor's HLA antigens
E. Transplant: living-related and cadaver donors
   Cross-match with most recent patient sample drawn immediately pretransplant

RATIONALE FOR TISSUE TYPING FOR TRANSPLANTATION

Comparison of the tissue types of a donor and the potential (unrelated) recipient usually reveals some degree of antigen mismatching because of the extensive polymorphism of the HLA antigen system. When nuclear family members are tissue typed for a living-related transplant, only 25% of full siblings will be HLA identical to the transplant recipient, and parents and 50% of siblings will be matched at one haplotype. Cadaver donors will be genotypically complete mismatches to the random recipient, although there is a finite probability of complete or partial phenotypic identity. If the phenotypes of the patient and the cadaver are composed of the more common antigens, such as HLA-A1, -A2, -B8, etc, the likelihood of HLA antigen matching increases.

A positive effect of HLA matching on kidney graft outcome has been clearly documented in reports from the two largest studies of renal transplant data: the UCLA Transplant Registry, Los Angeles, Calif, which has collected data on 70,000 transplants since 1970, and the Collaborative Transplant Study (CTS), Heidelberg, West Germany, with data on 60,000 renal transplants since 1982. Both of these studies agree that the main factor that improves long-term (up to 10-year) renal allograft survival is donor-recipient matching for HLA antigens (Table 21–2).

Beneficial effects of HLA matching on short-term graft survival (1 year) are no longer apparent in the results from many individual transplant centers. Immunosuppression with cyclosporine has improved first-transplant graft survival of cadaver and one-haplotype-matched living-related transplants to near that of HLA-identical transplants: approximately 80% after 1 year. For short-term (1–3 years) graft outcome, reports from single centers offer conflicting statistics, with some centers seeing no difference in graft outcome from unmatched transplants and others reporting clear advantages for HLA-matching in specific patient groups. For example, whites but not blacks benefit from HLA-matched cadaver kidneys, whereas blacks do benefit from receiving matched living-related grafts.

Statistics from single centers are limited by small numbers of cases and can be influenced by other factors, including patient selection, patient compliance, regimens of pre- and posttransplant care, extent of patient follow-up, the quality of histocompatibility testing, and even the methods for calculation of the survival statistics. From the CTS database of 10,000 first transplants in the cyclosporin era, matching for HLA-B and -DR antigens does show a stepwise improvement in 3-year graft outcome from 55% survival with 4 mismatches to 80% survival with no mismatches (Table 21–3). For second transplants, HLA-A locus matching becomes an additional significant factor.

Matching for the splits (subtypes) of HLA antigens may be even more significant for graft outcome than simple matching of the "generic" HLA antigens (for example, matching for B51 or Bw52 rather than for the broad B5 antigen). As shown in Table 21–3, from a recent CTS review of 30,000 first transplants, matching for A and B locus antigen splits in conjunction with HLA-DR shows a striking correlation with 3-year graft survival.

Despite the dramatic improvement in 1-year survival, however, the ensuing rate of graft loss due to chronic rejection remains essentially unchanged; ie, half of cadaver grafts are still lost by 8.5 years, compared with 7.5 years in 1978. Thus, the use of cyclosporine has not established an operational state of long-term organ tolerance. Overall, the 10-year renal

Table 21–2. Effect of HLA matching on long-term renal allograft survival[1]

Organ Donor	No. of Haplotypes Matched	% Graft Survival	
		4 year	10 year
HLA-identical sibling	2	80	67
Parent	1	70	42
Cadaver[2]	0	58	24

[1]Data from Terasaki PI (editor). *Clinical Transplantation 1987*, p 469. UCLA Tissue Typing Laboratory, 1987.
[2]Recipient treated with cyclosporine.

Table 21–3. Effect of HLA antigen matching on 3-year renal allograft survival[1]

HLA Antigens Considered	No. of Antigens Mismatched	% Graft Survival
HLA-B, HLA-DR	0	80
	2	68
	4	55
HLA-A,B (splits) + HLA-DR	0	80
	6	49
HLA-A,B (broad) + HLA-DR	0	68
	6	56

[1]Data from Opelz, G: Importance of HLA antigen splits for kidney transplant matching. *Lancet* 1988;**8602**:61.

graft survival percentages are as follows: cadaver transplants, 24%; parental (one haplotype matched) grafts, 42%; and HLA-identical sibling transplants, 67%. It is estimated that if all kidneys were shared nationally, 25% of all waiting patients could be transplanted with kidneys with no HLA-A, -B, or -DR mismatches. These statistics argue in favor of sharing organs on a regional and national scale to promote the most beneficial usage of scarce organ resources. To achieve this end, the National Organ Transplant Act of 1987 has established the United Network for Organ Sharing (UNOS). UNOS links local and regional transplant procurement centers with a national registry of waiting recipients and establishes mandatory criteria for selection of recipients based on a point system for the following attributes: quality of HLA matching, degree of sensitization (panel-reactive antibody; PRA), time on the waiting list, medical emergency status, and geographic factors.

In heart transplantation, distribution of hearts based on HLA matching is impractical because of the lack of availability of the organ. Retrospective analysis indicates a 15% improvement in 3-year graft survival when there were less than 2 HLA-B and -DR mismatches compared with 2 or more mismatches (80% and 65% survival, respectively). For liver transplantation, better HLA-matched livers are associated with fewer rejection episodes, but, paradoxically, liver graft survival results show no advantage from HLA matching and, possibly, a detrimental effect. The value of HLA matching for liver transplantation and for other organs, such as the pancreas, must await the collection of more data. Preliminary data for cornea transplantation do show that patients with previously rejected transplants will benefit from a well-matched transplant.

ANTIBODIES TO DETECT SENSITIZATION TO HLA ANTIGENS

Exposure to HLA antigens can occur as a consequence of blood transfusions, prior organ grafts, or pregnancy. The resultant formation of specific antibodies to those antigens is termed "sensitization." Reexposure to the previously immunizing antigens on a new allograft can produce rapid humoral and cellular immune responses, leading to hyperacute or accelerated rejection. Detection of such preformed specific antibodies is of paramount importance in evaluating the state of initial histocompatibility between recipient and donor, especially in the face of known HLA antigen mismatches. Two standard procedures have been developed, both of which involve the exposure of lymphocytes to the patient's serum. Antibody screening tests a serum sample against a panel of HLA-typed lymphocytes for anti-lymphocyte reactivity; cross-matching tests the patient's serum against the lymphocytes of a selected prospective organ donor to detect donor-specific antibodies.

SEROLOGIC METHODS IN HISTOCOMPATIBILITY TESTING

The simplest and fastest methods for histocompatibility testing are serologic; that is, they utilize blood serum that contains antibodies to HLA antigens. Anti-HLA antibodies are highly specific for the individual structural determinants that characterize the different antigens of the HLA system. Thus, when sera containing HLA antibodies are mixed with lymphocytes, the antibodies will bind only to their specific target antigens.

When the antigen-antibody complex is formed on the cell surface in the presence of complement, complement activation leads to cell lysis. Thus, cell death is an indicator of the common specificity of antigen and antibody and is a "positive" test result. Detection of this identity between antibody and antigen provides the answer to most basic questions in histocompatibility testing: (1) What are the HLA antigens of a particular cell? When the antibody specificity is known, as for the HLA typing reagents, and the cell is of unknown phenotype, the positive test results with specific antisera will identify the antigens of the cell. (2) Are there anti-HLA antibodies in a particular serum? When the serum is being tested for the presence of HLA antibodies, and when the HLA phenotype of the test cell is known, a positive test indicates anti-lymphocyte activity in the serum. From the pattern of reactions with a panel of HLA-typed cells, the specificity of the antibodies may be inferred. If the patient's serum reacts with the donor cell, the 2 individuals are incompatible.

Thus, through an iterative process of testing serum and typing cells, HLA antigens are defined, panels of typed lymphocytes are generated, and collections of HLA typing sera of known specificity are created.

TISSUE TYPING BY THE LYMPHOCYTOTOXICITY TEST

Tissue typing is accomplished by exposing the unknown cell to a battery of antisera of known HLA specificity. The typing sera are selected to give unequivocally strong positive scores to ensure reproducibility. When the cells are killed by the antiserum and complement, the cell is presumed to have the same HLA antigen as the specificity of the antibody.

Cell Isolation

Lymphocytes are the preferred cell type for HLA typing, antibody screening, and cross-matching. They are normally isolated from whole peripheral blood by buoyant density gradient separation (see Chapter 19), from buffy coat, or, in cadaveric testing, from lymph nodes and spleen. Care must be taken to prepare a cell suspension of excellent viability as well as one that is free of erythrocyte and platelet contamination. Although other cell types that bear HLA antigens, such as platelets, amniocytes, and fibroblasts, can be used for HLA typing in spe-

cial circumstances, lymphocytes are the most responsive and reproducible target for the standard cytotoxicity assay.

The Complement-Dependent Lymphocytotoxicity Test: NIH Standard Method

Individual HLA antisera are predispensed in 1-μL quantities into the microtest wells of specifically designed plastic trays composed of 60 or 72 wells. Replicates of the test tray are stored frozen for later use. Into a thawed test tray, 2000 isolated lymphocytes are dispensed per well, and the tray is incubated for 30 minutes at room temperature to allow anti-HLA antibodies to bind to their specific target HLA antigens. Complement (5 μL) is added, usually as rabbit serum, and the tray is incubated for another 60 minutes. To visualize the dead and live cells under phase contrast microscopy, a vital dye, eosin Y, is added, followed by formalin to fix the reaction. Live cells exclude the dye and appear bright and refractile, while dead cells take up the dye and are swollen and dark (Fig 21–1). In an alternative

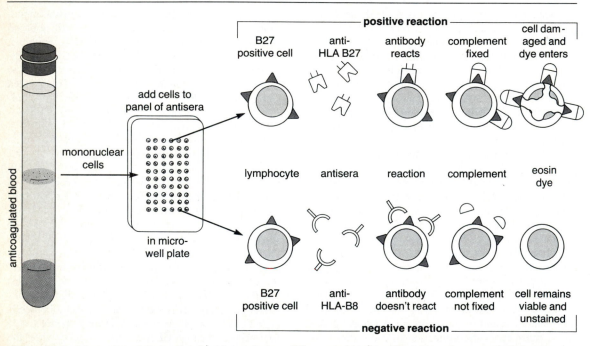

Figure 21–1. Microcytotoxicity testing for HLA antigens. PBL are isolated by Ficoll-Hypaque centrifugation and adjusted to 2 × 10⁶ cells/mL. Then 1 μL of cells is added to each well of a tissue-typing plate that has been predispensed with a panel of HLA typing sera, each containing alloantibodies to specific HLA antigens. Illustrated are the reactions of HLA B27 cells with antisera specific for B27 (**upper**) and B8 (**lower**). B27 antibodies bind to B27 antigens on the cell surface, the antigen-antibody complex activates and fixes serum complement, the cell membrane is damaged, and the cell dies. Eosin dye penetrates the dead cells, staining them dark red under phase contrast microscopy, giving a positive test result. In contrast, the anti-B8 antibodies do not complex with the B27 antigen, the complement components are not activated, the cells remains undamaged, and eosin dye is excluded, resulting in a negative test. The cell is thus typed as B27-positive and B8-negative. Each test well is scored as percent dead cells (see Table 21–4), and the overall reaction pattern of the typing sera is interpreted to give the HLA antigen phenotype of the individual (see Table 21–5).

method known as fluorochromasia, the cells are pre-labeled with a fluorochrome such as fluorescein diacetate (green) prior to plating. When the cells are killed in the positive test, the fluorescein leaks out and the cells "disappear." Positive results are compared with a negative well where all the cells are visible. A second fluorochrome of contrasting color such as ethidium bromide (red) may be added to visualize the dead cells.

Each test well is scored individually by inspection, with the percentage of dead cells per well being noted. The test is unequivocally positive when at least half of the cells are killed. (Table 21–4).

Interpretation of the Tissue-Typing Test

An antigen is assigned by noting the patterns of reactivity of the individual sera and their specificities. The typing sera that reacted positively with the test cells should have antibody specificities in common. For an antigen to be assigned, the majority of sera of that specificity must be unequivocally positive. In phenotyping an individual for class I HLA, one expects to find patterns with 2 antigens each from the A, B, and C loci. When only a single antigen is identified at a locus, the individual may be homozygous for that allele or the laboratory has failed to identify the second antigen, usually owing to inadequacies in the array of typing sera. Table 21–5 shows a representation of HLA-typing test results.

TISSUE-TYPING REAGENTS: HLA ALLOANTISERA

Sources of HLA Typing Sera

The majority of HLA antisera are complex sera obtained from multiparous women. Maternal exposure to the mismatched paternal HLA antigens in the fetus gives rise to a polyclonal antibody response that frequently results in sera with multiple specificities. Consequently, several different antisera are used to type for a specific antigen. It is not unusual for a laboratory to use typing trays composed of more than 200 different sera to type a single individual for HLA-A, -B, -C, and -DR antigens.

Placental fluid, a mixture of serum and tissue flu-

Table 21–5. An example of HLA typing test results.[1]

Serum Name	Specificities	Score
A-001	A1	1
A-002	A1, Aw36	1
A-003	A1, A11	1
A-004	A2	1
A-005	A2, A28	6
A-006	A2, A28, B7	8
A-007	A3	8
A-008	A3	6
A-009	A3, A10, A11, Aw19	8
A-010	A11	1
A-011	A10, A11	1
A-012	A11, A1, A3 (weak)	4
B-001	B51, Bw52, B35	1
B-002	B51, Bw52	1
B-003	B51, Bw52, Bw53	1
B-004	B7, Bw42	8
B-005	B7, B27	8
B-006	B7, Bw55	8
B-007	B8	1
B-008	B8, Bw59	2
B-009	B44, B45, B21	6
B-010	B44, B45	8
B-011	B44	8
B-012	B45	1

[1]Interpretation: HLA phenotype is: A28, A3, B7, B44 (see Table 21–6).

ids, has proved to be a valuable second source of alloantisera for tissue typing. Antibodies of high titer can be recovered from the fluid shed from fresh placentae that have been refrigerated for 24 hours post-delivery. Attempts to immunize other animals, such as rabbits, for production of HLA antisera have largely failed. The xenoantisera reacted primarily with antigens broadly representative in humans, such as the HLA-DR constant region. Thus, currently, the majority of HLA reagents are found among human sources by means of extensive serum-screening programs, a task undertaken by many tissue-typing laboratories. Through voluntary national and worldwide serum exchange programs, these reagents are distributed within the tissue-typing community for mutual benefit.

HLA antibodies are also found in the sera of patients exposed to HLA antigens through transfusions of blood and organ grafts. Generally, patients are not used as sources of HLA typing sera, since the quantities obtainable would be limited by their medical conditions.

MONOCLONAL ANTIBODIES TO HLA ANTIGENS

Recent efforts in numerous laboratories have resulted in a limited production of monoclonal antibodies to HLA specificities. It was hoped that hybridoma cell lines (see Chapter 18) would produce inexhaustible quantities of monospecific antibodies to HLA antigens. In reality, many murine mono-

Table 21–4. Scoring the lymphocytotoxicity test for HLA typing.

% Dead Lymphocytes in Test Well	Score	Interpretation
0–10	1	Negative
11–20	2	Doubtful positive
21–50	4	Weak positive
51–80	6	Positive
81–100	8	Strong positive

clonal antibodies have been directed against human monomorphic framework determinants or to common epitopes rather than to the private polymorphic determinants of the individual HLA antigens. Unfortunately, most murine monoclonal antibodies do not fix complement. Non-complement-fixing antibodies can be used in assays that require only antigen binding, such as enzyme-linked immunosorbent assay (ELISA) and flow cytometry, but these are not in standard usage currently (see Chapters 18 and 19). Some monoclonal antibodies are reactive with more than one HLA specificity, indicating the existence of common antigenic determinants on HLA molecules.

SPECIFICITY OF HLA ANTIBODIES: PRIVATE & PUBLIC

An ideal HLA typing serum would be monospecific, that is, would have specificity for a single HLA antigen; however, in reality, the observed alloantibodies in a single serum are usually polyspecific. An alloantiserum can contain antibodies to multiple determinants on the immunizing antigen(s). Some determinants are the classic HLA **private** specificities that characterize each HLA allele. Others are **public,** that is, are shared by several antigens that collectively constitute a cross-reacting antigen group. Some complex sera can be rendered monospecific by dilution, whereas others lose all activity for all specificities simultaneously.

To determine the specificities of HLA antibodies, sera are tested against panels of cells of known HLA phenotype, a process termed "screening." The cell panel, usually from 40 to 60 cells, is preselected to provide a minimum of 2–3 representations of the most frequent HLA antigens. The antigens must be distributed among the cells so that the reaction pattern for one antigen will not be entirely included within the pattern for a second antigen; for example, all of the HLA-A1 cells must not be the only HLA-B8 cells as well. If they were, the reaction patterns for both antibodies would be identical and the determination of A1 or B8, or both, could not be made with certainty. When the sera react with a subset of the panel, the specificity of the antibody is deduced by inspecting the HLA phenotypes of the positive cells. Table 21–6 illustrates the type of reaction patterns obtained on reagent or patient serum screens. The percent panel reactive antibody (PRA) is calculated as the ratio of the number of positive cells to the number of total panel cells multiplied by 100. PRA is indicative of the extent of sensitization of the patient to HLA. Note that the antibody specificities of sera with high PRA cannot be determined from these results. Special procedures must be used, such as dilution or treatment of the sera, or both, to determine antibody specificities.

Table 21–6. An example of results of serum screening for class I HLA antibodies.[1]

Panel Cell HLA Antigens	Cytotoxicity Test Score for Patient Serum No:				
	1	2	3	4	5
A, A, B, B (locus)					
1, 2, 7, w60	1	1	8	1	8
2, 3, 8, 51	1	8	8	8	8
3, 29, 35, 44	1	8	1	6	8
30, w33, w55, w60	1	1	1	1	8
1, 30, 13, 51	1	1	1	8	8
24, 28, 35, w55	1	1	4	6	4
3, 28, 7, 44	1	8	4	1	6
2, 28, 35, 38	1	1	8	8	8

[1]PRA (panel reactive antibody) was 0%, 38%, 50%, 63%, and 100%, for patient sera 1 through 5, respectively. PRA is calculated as the number of positive tests/number of cells tested × 100. Analyzed antibodies were as follows (patient sera 1 through 5, respectively): None; A3; A2, weak A28; B51, B35; and Unknown (auto-antibody?).

TISSUE TYPING FOR CLASS II HLA ANTIGENS BY SEROLOGIC METHODS

Tissue typing for class II HLA antigens, HLA-DR and -DQ, is performed on lymphocyte preparations that are enriched for B lymphocytes. Special isolation procedures are required since approximately 80% of normal peripheral blood lymphocytes (PBL) are resting T cells that lack class II HLA antigens on their surface. The most widely used separation technique is adherence of B cells to nylon wool fibers. The PBL are passed through nylon-wool-packed columns made from plastic drinking straws or small syringes. The columns are filled with warm culture medium, and the cells are incubated in the wool for 30 minutes at 37 °C, allowing the B lymphocytes and macrophages to adhere to the fibers. The nonadherent T cells are then flushed out and saved for other tests. The B cells remaining are removed from the column by mechanical agitation of the wool and exposure to cooled medium. A minimum enrichment of 80% B cells is necessary for successful class II typing. Other techniques for B cell isolation employ beads coated with antibodies to B cell antigens, which adsorb B cells. Large plastic surface can be used for adherence and subsequent release of B cells, too.

Because B cell separation methods are laborious and time-consuming, alternative strategies have been developed that allow the use of unseparated PBL in the standard cytotoxicity test. These require that the B cells be distinguished from the predominant T cells. The Van Rood 2-color method marks the B cells with a fluorescein-labeled anti-human immunoglobulin that binds to the surface immunoglobulin of B cells, surrounding them with a green halo. The red fluorochrome ethidium bromide is then added to visualize the dead cells. A positive test appears as numerous red (dead), green-rimmed B cells. Any dead T cells will also appear as red-stained cells, which can create a visually confusing picture if the overall cell viability is poor.

In a variation of the fluorochromasia method, it is possible to make the T component of PBL disappear by killing them with an anti-CD11 antibody that can fix complement. CD11 is the classic sheep erythrocyte receptor specific for T cells. At the outset of the assay, all cells are exposed to the anti-CD11 antibody and labeled with carboxyfluorescein diacetate, which is retained by living cells. The cells are then plated into standard DR typing trays, and the HLA-DR antibodies are allowed to bind to the cells. Following the addition of complement, all T cells and B cells with bound HLA-DR antibody are killed and disappear from view as the fluorescein leaks out. Negative test wells have visible, living B cells, whereas positive wells are devoid of any cells. When the anti-CD11 antibody is strong and the appropriate complement is used, this assay is reproducible and rapid.

Antisera for Class II HLA Typing

Antisera for class II HLA tissue typing must be free of antibodies to class I HLA antigens. Unfortunately, the majority of HLA alloantisera contain mixtures of antibodies to class I and class II HLA antigens. Because their membranes have no class II antigens, pooled platelets are used as absorbents to clear HLA sera of any contaminating class I antibodies. Such manipulation of these sera can leave them diluted and operationally less reliable. Because B lymphocytes have more class I HLA antigens on their surface than do T cells, false-positive reactions from residual class I antibodies are possible. It is necessary that all absorbed class II antisera be thoroughly screened on T and B cells to ensure that absorption is complete. Overall, HLA typing sera for class II antigens are of poorer quality and in shorter supply than are reagents for class I typing. Currently, very few sera for HLA-DP typing are available. The antigens of the DP locus have been defined mainly by cellular assays (see below). Because of the paucity of good DR and DQ typing sera, serologic methods have had limited success in defining class II polymorphisms. Biochemical and molecular-biologic methods have provided significant new information.

The complement-dependent cytotoxicity assay for class II HLA DR and DQ typing is performed with appropriate class II typing sera but is modified as follows: Initial incubation of cells and serum is performed at 37 °C for 60 minutes; after addition of complement, the mixture is incubated for 120 minutes at room temperature. The extended incubation times are used to promote binding of antibodies and complement. The temperature increase is used to avoid the false-positive reactions that can result from the binding of cold reactive nonspecific antibodies.

Variability in Tissue-Typing Results

HLA typing sera are not standardized by the usual practices of regulated quality control and licensure. The multiplicity of HLA antigens and the scarcity of the defining antisera make it impossible to license a standard reagent for each specificity. Each tissue-typing laboratory has the responsibility of obtaining the appropriate antisera and monitoring their performance. Typing sera are collected through serum exchange programs between laboratories, and new sera are discovered by means of extensive testing of sera from pregnant women, fluids recovered from placentae, and, occasionally, patient sera. Commercial typing trays are also available. Results with the laboratory's own serum trays may be compared with those of other collections of sera for confirmation of an HLA phenotype. All tissue-typing laboratories are required by the standards set by the American Society for Histocompatibility and Immunogenetics (ASHI) to control the quality of serologic and cellular reagents used for clinical testing. International and national quality control programs are available for typing, cross-matching, and serum analysis, and satisfactory performance is mandatory for ASHI accreditation of the laboratory.

A second variable in tissue typing is the serum complement, a reagent commercially available as the pooled serum from several hundred rabbits. Rabbit serum contains heterophile antibodies with anti-human lymphocyte activity that enhances its effectiveness in the cytotoxicity assay. Overabundance of these anti-human antibodies will render the complement innately cytotoxic and therefore produces false-positive results. As with typing sera, the individual laboratory must screen its source of complement to find one that promotes strong serum reactions without causing nonspecific toxicity. Because there is no standard complement source, it follows that the same serum tested in different laboratories has the potential of giving different results.

A third variable is the choice of method used to visualize the live and dead cells. Among these methods there are variations in incubation times and also in the definition of the end of the test period. Thus, in the exchange of typing sera between laboratories, it is important to note the method by which the serum was characterized.

CROSS-MATCHING

The purpose of the cross-match test is to detect the presence of antibodies in the patient's serum that are directed against the potential donor HLA antigens. If present, the antibodies signal that the immune system of the recipient has been sensitized to those donor antigens and is therefore primed to vigorously reject any graft bearing them. In the transplanted kidney, the main target of these antibodies is probably the HLA antigens on vascular endothelium of capillaries and arterioles. HLA antigen-antibody complexes on endothelium activate complement and lead to cell damage. Platelets then aggregate, eventually producing fibrin clots, which clog the vessels. This causes ischemic necrosis. Even weak, low-titer antibodies, particularly those directed against class I antigens, can contribute to graft rejection. Therefore, the ultimate goal of the cross-match is a test of both great sensitivity and specificity for HLA antigens.

Cross-Matching by Lymphocytotoxicity

A simple cross-match by the standard cytotoxicity method (see above) may be performed with donor PBL as targets. PBL cross-matches are usually included in the preliminary evaluation of potential living-related donors for renal graft recipients. PBL are normally about 80% T cells, which carry class I HLA antigens only, and 20% B cells and monocytes, which bear both class I and class II antigens. A strongly positive cross-match by cytotoxicity (50% or more cell death per well) clearly indicates the presence of antibodies to class I antigens. However, 10–20% cell killing could result from an antibody specific for class II or could be due to a weak anti-class I antibody. To resolve the specificity of the antibody, cross-matching is then performed on cell preparations enriched for either T or B lymphocytes.

Cross-Matching with Separated T & B Lymphocytes

A. T Cell Cross-Matches: T cell cross-matches are performed at room temperature and also at 37 °C in some laboratories to avoid the binding of cold-reactive antibodies, presumed to be autoreactive. A positive T cell cross-match by any method contraindicates transplantation, no matter how weak the reaction level; ie, a reaction of 4+ (20–50% dead cells per well above background) is considered just as positive a result as 6+ or 8+ (51% dead cells or greater).

Several methods to improve the sensitivity of T cell cross-matches by complement-dependent cytotoxicity have been developed. These include the following.

1. Extended incubation–The simplest modification in the cytotoxicity assay to increase sensitivity is to extend the incubation time of cells, serum, and complement.

2. The Amos wash step–This method interjects a wash step after the incubation of cells and serum and prior to the addition of complement to remove anti-complementary factors in the serum.

3. Anti-human globulin (AHG)–The cytotoxicity of some antibodies may be enhanced by the addition of a second-step antibody, usually a polyclonal anti-human immunoglobulin reagent.

B. B Cell Cross-Matches: Cross-matching for antibodies to class II HLA antigens requires the use of B lymphocytes as targets and the same extended incubation times as HLA-DR and -DQ serologic typing. A positive B cell cross-match may result from antibodies binding to class I or class II HLA antigens. Moreover, B cells are a more sensitive indicator for weak class I antibodies, since they carry class I molecules in greater density than T cells do. Cross-matching by flow cytometry can readily distinguish between "true B" antibodies and weak class I antibodies of a positive B cell cross-match. The significance for transplant outcome of preformed antibodies to class II antigens is not yet clear. Successful transplantation into patients with low-titer anti-class II antibodies (titer of 1:1 or 1:2) has been reported, as has the acute rejection of grafts transplanted in the face of high-titer (1:8) antibodies. It is possible that the loss of grafts transplanted in the face of T-negative, B-positive cross-matches is due to the anti-class I component of these alloreactive sera.

C. Flow Cytometry Cross-Matching (See Chapter 19): Cross-matching by flow cytometry (FCC) has been shown to be up to 100 times more sensitive than visual serologic methods for the detection of HLA antibodies on lymphocytes. In this cross-matching application, T cells can be separated from B cells electronically through the use of a fluoresceinated anti-human IgG reagent (Fig 21–2). Following incubation of donor lymphocytes with patient serum, a fluorescein isothiocyanate (FITC)-labeled goat-anti-human IgG is added. The fluorescent anti-immunoglobulin reagent will bind to the surface immunoglobulin of all B cells and also to any T cell that has bound patient antibody. The B cells become highly fluorescent, and the B cell peak of the histogram moves to the right, away from the T cell peak (Fig 21–2). A shift to the right of the T cell peak in the experimental test compared with the control indicates that anti-class I HLA antibody from the patient serum has bound to the donor T cells.

FCC is generally performed with the most recent and selected previously obtained sera for all cadaver waiting list patients who have rejected prior transplants or who have high PRAs and for patients with living related donors in the event of a negative T cell and positive B cell serologic cross-match.

Occasionally, positive FCC cross-matches occur when both the serologic T and B cell cross-matches are negative. The nature of these antibodies is unknown and has been considered by some to be irrelevant to transplantation. For the unsensitized patient, such conclusions may be correct. However, for patients with high PRAs, caution (and further testing) is justified before the transplant is performed.

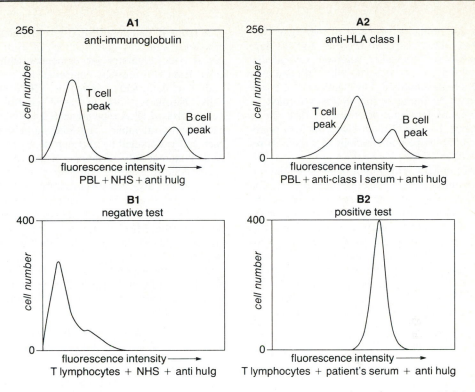

Figure 21–2. Flow cytometry cross-matching (FCC) with PBL and T cells. **A1:** Schematic tracing of a FCC fluorescence histogram illustrating the formation of the T and B cell peaks. PBL are incubated with normal human serum (NHS), and then fluoresceinated goat anti-human immunoglobulin (FITC-IgG) is added. The FITC binds to the surface immunoglobulin of B cells, causing the intensely fluorescent B cell peak to move to the right, away from the T cells. The T cells remain unlabeled. **A2:** In the positive control serum (anti-HLA class I) the T cells have bound anti-class I antibody and subsequently become labeled with FITC-IgG, resulting in a shift of the T cell peak toward higher intensity. **B1:** FCC tracings illustrating the position of the T cell peak in the presence of a negative patient serum (**B2** shows a positive anti-class I antibody-containing patient serum). The mean channel of the T cell peak has shifted more than 100 channels from the normal (negative) serum control, indicating the presence of a very strong anti-class I antibody.

Cross-Matching for Autoantibodies

In cross-matching patient serum for donor compatibility, it is most important to distinguish nonspecific anti-lymphocyte antibodies, referred to as autoantibodies, from the specific anti-donor antibodies. The presence of autoantibodies is detected by the auto-cross-match, in which the patient's own serum and cells are combined in the standard cytotoxicity test. Autoantibodies can give a false-positive result in a donor cross-match, leading to the erroneous disqualification of that donor. Alternatively, preexisting autoantibodies can mask the presence of specific anti-donor antibodies. Autoantibody cross-matches are routinely performed in conjunction with all living-donor cross-matches for each serum that is tested.

CELLULAR ASSAYS FOR HISTOCOMPATIBILITY

In vivo, recognition of nonself antigens and destruction of cells bearing such markers is accomplished by cells of the immune system. Some of the clinically relevant class II HLA antigens that can trigger the immune response are not readily detected by the serologic methods discussed above. Instead, lymphocytes are used as discriminatory reagents for the HLA-Dw and -DP antigens and as indicators of histoincompatibility between donor and recipient. The functions of cellular recognition are utilized in the MLC, HTC, and primed lymphocyte typing (PLT) tests, and the dual functions of recognition and effector cell killing are used in the CML test.

MLC Test (See Chapter 19)

This is also known as the mixed-lymphocyte reaction (MLR). When the lymphocytes of 2 HLA-disparate individuals are combined in tissue culture, the cells enlarge, synthesize DNA, and proliferate, whereas HLA-identical cells remain quiescent. The proliferation is driven primarily by differences in the class II HLA antigens between the 2 test cells.

On the basis of MLC testing, class II antigens were originally described as a series of lymphocyte-activating determinants, products of the HLA-"D" locus (-Dw1, -Dw2, etc). No D locus products have ever been isolated, however, although several distinct "D region" loci (-DR, -DQ, and -DP) and their alleles have been identified. Dw "antigens" are now considered to be immunogenic epitopes formed by combinations of D region determinants that can be recognized by T cells. Distinct Dw types may represent unique haplotype combinations of various D region products.

Reactivity in MLC probably reflects the initial immune recognition step of graft rejection in vivo. The more immunogenic the D locus difference, the greater the cellular response in MLC and the more likely the rejection of the graft. Normally, both cells will proliferate, forming the 2-way MLC. To monitor the response of a single responder cell (the one-way MLC), the partner cell (stimulator) is inactivated by radiation or drugs (such as mitomycin C) that inhibit DNA synthesis (Fig 21–3). A maximum proliferative response usually occurs after incubation at 37 °C for 5–6 days. The culture is then pulsed with [³H]thymidine for 5–12 hours to label the newly synthesized DNA. Finally, the cells are harvested, washed free of unbound radioactivity, and counted in a beta counter.

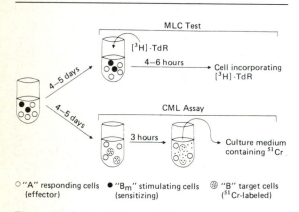

Figure 21–3. The MLC and CML tests. In the one-way MLC, responder PBLs are mixed 1:1 with irradiated stimulator cells and incubated at 37 °C in a humidified atmosphere with 5% CO₂. After 5 days, the culture is pulsed with [³H]thymidine to label the nucleic acid in the responder cells. After 18 hours, cells are harvested and counted for internalized radioactivity. If the class II HLA antigens of the stimulator cells differ from those of the responder cells, the responder cells undergo blastogenesis, synthesize DNA, and proliferate. Increased sample radioactivity signals recognition of class II HLA differences. When responder and stimulator cells are class II identical, the proliferative responses are less than 20% of the maximum response to the mismatched controls and less than 2% over autologous (background) controls. (Reproduced, with permission, from Bach FH, Van Rood JJ: The major histocompatibility complex: Genetics and biology. *N Engl J Med* 1976;**295**:806, 872.)

A properly composed MLC test includes a checkerboard of one-way combinations of each cell serving as both stimulator and responder with all other cells. Each cell must be controlled for its ability to both stimulate and respond to HLA-mismatched cells. Normally, 2–4 unrelated control cells of known class II HLA type are tested individually with each family member. The maximum response of each cell is obtained by exposure to a pool of irradiated stimulator cells of diverse HLA types.

Autologous controls combining self with irradiated self are also run to normalize the response of each cell to stimulators. Each test should be run in triplicate. It is absolutely necessary to perform the entire familial MLC at one time owing to the inherent variability of individual cellular responses from day to day.

Results are expressed as a stimulation index (SI) or relative response (RR). The SI is the ratio of counts per minute of the test over the autologous test for that cell:

$$SI = cpm \text{ of } \frac{\text{Responder vs Stimulator (irradiated)}}{\text{Responder vs Responder (irradiated)}}$$

A value of SI ≤ 2 or less is interpreted as HLA identity at HLA-D. The RR calculates the response in the experimental MLC relative to the maximum response of that cell elicited by the pool. Counts per minute of both are corrected by subtraction of the autologous control for the responder cell.

$$RR = cpm \text{ of } \frac{\text{Responder vs Stimulator (irradiated)} - \text{Autologous control}}{\text{Responder vs Pool (irradiated)} - \text{Autologous control}} \times 100$$

MLC testing can be useful in selecting the most compatible (least stimulatory) organ donor if several nonidentical family members (matched for zero or one haplotype) are available. The donor who is the least stimulatory to the patient is the preferred organ donor. The results of an intrafamilial MLC can address such questions as (1) Are 2 serologically identical DR antigens also functionally identical? (2) Is the individual with only one identifiable DR antigen a homozygote, or is the DR "blank" really a second DR antigen that was missed in the serologic testing? (3) Are the serologically assigned class II antigens consistent with the MLC results? If apparently HLA-identical individuals are reactive, there may have been a genetic recombination event.

The MLC test is frequently used to confirm apparent HLA identity in the living-related transplant situation and is especially useful if haplotyping could not be accomplished. When the HLA-identical recipient and donor are unrelated, as in voluntary bone marrow donation, MLC testing is extremely important in revealing hidden class II incompatibilities that could affect recipient tolerance to the graft and promote graft-versus-host disease.

HTC Test

MLC nonreactivity indicates HLA-Dw identity, and therefore the MLC test can be used to type for specific Dw alleles. Since most individuals to be tested are heterozygous at the D region, it follows that the stimulator cell must be homozygous for a given Dw antigen to result in MLC nonresponsiveness. Such HTCs have been identified in the random population, but the best source for HTCs is among the progeny of first-cousin marriages. True HTCs are rare and precious reagents, and few laboratories can afford to maintain the large cell panel necessary for complete and accurate testing.

The lymphocytes to be Dw typed are set up as responders in multiple MLC tests, each test with a different inactivated stimulator HTC. HTC testing can discriminate among the various subtypes of serologically identified DR antigens and thus can provide a finer definition of true class II HLA compatibility.

PLT Test

Lymphocytes already exposed (primed) to a specific antigen in a primary MLC will proliferate rapidly upon reexposure to the same antigen. Thus, a primed cell can be used to test an unknown cell for the presence of the original stimulating antigen. With cells primed to class II HLA antigens, this assay can be used as an HLA typing test for D region antigens. As in HTC typing, an extensive panel of specifically primed cells must be maintained for PLT testing.

PLT currently has a very special application in histocompatibility testing: to type for HLA-DP antigens. Antigens of the -DP locus (originally called SB antigens) do not stimulate in the primary MLC test but can prime cells for a secondary response. Through PLT testing, 6 DP antigens have been officially recognized, and several more identified. Until serologic reagents become available, DP typing will remain a specialized histocompatibility testing procedure performed in only a few laboratories.

CML Test

In primary MLC, exposure to nonself class I and class MHC II antigens can result in the generation of cytotoxic T lymphocytes (CTL). CTL kill their targets through direct contact, probably by the release of toxic mediators that lead to cell lysis. CD4 and CD8 CTL can be found infiltrating kidney allografts during rejection and are considered to be important effector cells in graft loss (see Chapter 60). To test for the capacity to generate CTL, a primary MLC is run with the patient as the responder and prospective donor cells as inactivated stimulators. After the MLC, the patient's cells are harvested and then reexposed in culture to fresh donor target cells that have been loaded with ^{51}Cr (Fig 21–3). Usually, the targets are preincubated with the mitogen phytohemagglutinin (PHA) for 6 days, since PHA-activated

blast cells can incorporate more ^{51}Cr than resting lymphocytes can. CTL and targets are plated in effector:target-cell ratios of 100:1, 50:1, and 10:1. Control wells include targets alone to measure the spontaneous release of label and test wells containing target cells that are treated with detergent to release the maximum incorporated label. The test requires 4 hours of incubation in a humidified CO_2 atmosphere at 37 °C. At the conclusion, the supernatant of each test well is sampled and counted. In the experimental wells, the amount of ^{51}Cr released is corrected for the background level of spontaneously released label and compared with the maximum amount of label released:

$$\% \text{ Specific Release} = \frac{\text{cpm (Experimental)} - \text{cpm (Spontaneous)}}{\text{cpm (Maximum)} - \text{cpm (Spontaneous)}} \times 100$$

Elevated counts of 30–50% above spontaneous background are indicative of CTL activity.

Direct CML testing can be used to monitor posttransplant rejection by testing for the presence of activated circulating anti-donor CTL. The patient's PBL are placed directly in culture with ^{51}Cr-labeled donor cells as targets. An elevated donor cell lysis compared with pretransplant levels is considered evidence of circulating CTL, which are particularly prevalent during rejection.

CML testing has applications in living-related renal and bone marrow transplantation. The preferred kidney donor will be the one who fails to stimulate the recipient to form CTL. In bone marrow transplantation, the recipient is at risk for immune attack by the marrow donor (graft-versus-host disease). The capacity of the prospective donors to form CTL against the recipient may be assessed through MLC plus CML testing.

A summary of the serologic and cellular methods for histocompatibility testing is presented in Table 21–7. All of these methods are in current use and are accepted as appropriate (in some instances mandatory) procedures for clinical histocompatibility testing.

HISTOCOMPATIBILITY TESTING BY MOLECULAR-BIOLOGIC METHODS

Until recently, the structure of HLA antigens has been inferred from antibodies or cells used for HLA typing. Now, the biochemical and gene-cloning techniques of molecular biology have begun to reveal the primary structure of HLA antigens (see Chapter 4). Once the common and specific antigenic sequences are known, several new methods for histocompatibility testing become feasible.

HLA Typing by Restriction Length Fragment Polymorphism (RFLP)

The technique of RFLP typing is based upon de-

Table 21–7. Methods used in histocompatibility testing.

Test	Test Type and Components	Time	Application
Tissue typing			
Complement-dependent lymphocytotoxicity	Serologic (HLA antisera; complement; test cells)	3 h	Identification of class I and II HLA antigens.
MLC test	Cellular (donor and recipient cells combined in tissue culture)	6 d	Class II HLA antigen compatibility.
HTC test	Cellular (test cell and HTC combined in tissue culture)	6 d	Identification of HLA-D locus (Dw) antigens.
PLT	Cellular (lymphocytes primed to specific DP antigen; test cells)	2 d	Identification of HLA-DP antigens.
Cross-matching			
PBL cross-match	Serologic (recipient serum; donor cells; complement; AHG optional)	3 h	Detection of preformed anti-donor antibodies in patient serum.
T/B cell cross-match	Serologic (purified donor T or B cells; recipient serum; AHG optional with T cells)	3–6 h	T cells: detection of anti-donor class I HLA antibodies; B cells: detection of antibodies to class I and II HLA.
CML test	Cellular (patient cells from primary MLC; fresh donor stimulators as targets)	4 h	Detection of anti-donor CTL.
FCC	Serologic (patient serum; donor cells; fluorescent anti-human immunoglobulin)	3–4 h	Detection of very weak and noncytotoxic anti-donor antibodies.
Auto–cross-match	Serologic (patient PBL, T and B cells, and serum)	3–4 h	Detection of nonspecific anti-lymphocyte antibodies (autoantibodies).
Screening			
Screening for class I HLA antibodies	Serologic (patient serum; panel of HLA-typed T cells or PBL	3 h × 40 cells	Detection of class I HLA antibodies; identification of antibody specificity.
Screening for class II HLA antibodies	Serologic (patient serum absorbed; B cell panel typed for HLA-DR, -DQ)	4 h × no. of cells plus absorption time	Detection of class II HLA antibodies; identification of antibody specificity.

tecting the nucleotide sequences that encode HLA antigens and that are either common among HLA alleles or unique to particular HLA alleles.

A high degree of homology exists in the nucleotide sequences specifying the genes of class I heavy chains of HLA-A, -B, and -C loci. Pieces of the gene that include these consensus sequences are cloned, thereby producing a DNA probe that can serve as a marker for any class I HLA antigen sequence. Locus-specific patterns are also found in class II alleles, and specific probes for DR-α, DR-β, DQ-α, etc, chains have been produced. The cloned DNA probes are the complementary strands to the mRNA transcript of the HLA gene and are thus called complementary DNA (cDNA).

Polymorphism of HLA alleles is apparent in deviations from consensus sequences. These deviations occur at certain variable and hypervariable regions of the molecules, thereby creating unique nucleotide sequences, which define specific HLA alleles. These points of variation serve as target sites for cleavage by bacterial restriction endonucleases. Such restriction sites are usually 4 or 6 bases in length. More than 90 enzymes are known, each recognizing a restriction site of a unique nucleotide sequence. Thus, each HLA haplotype will be cut into fragments of different lengths depending on the locations of the restriction cut sites, transforming the familiar polymorphism of HLA system into RFLP of the actual gene. Genomic DNA polymorphisms are more numerous than actual antigen polymorphisms. This is because sequence differences in the introns (nontranscribed gene products) as well as in the exons (transcribed and translated gene products) of the genes are included in the restriction fragments.

Generation and visualization of the genomic DNA fragments are accomplished by a 4-step process called Southern blotting. This involves restriction endonuclease digestion of cellular DNA, gel electrophoresis of the fragment mixture, transfer of the protein fragments by blotting onto a membrane, and exposure of the blot to particular cDNA probes to locate the position of the DNA sequence of interest. A pattern of bands results that is characteristic of the enzyme-probe combination used (Fig 21–4).

A. Uses of RFLP Typing: In instances in which serologic HLA typing fails owing to lack of HLA expression (as in bare lymphocyte syndrome), cell fragility, or lymphopenia, HLA typing by RFLP is possible. Because RFLP can reveal mutations, genetic recombinations, and allelic variations that serology cannot, RFLP can supply another dimension to histocompatibility testing. For transplantation purposes, it may be sufficient simply to compare RFLP

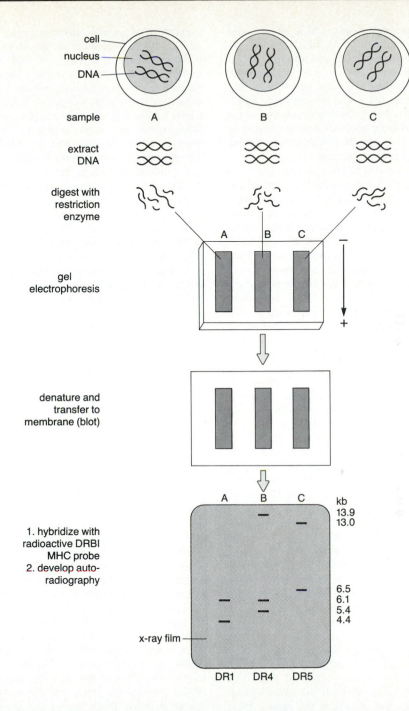

Figure 21–4. Tissue typing by RFLP. A comparison of RFLP tissue typing of 3 samples, A, B, and C, is shown. Genomic DNA is extracted from the cells and digested with selected restriction endonucleases. Digests are dispersed by agarose gel electrophoresis, the DNA is denatured into single strands, and the gel pattern of fragments is transferred to a support membrane by blotting (Southern blot). The DNA fragments are hybridized with a radiolabeled HLA locus-specific probe (eg, DRB1) that will complex with DNA nucleotide sequences. After autoradiography, the restriction fragments that have hybridized with the probe appear as patterns of isolated bands of specific size (kilobases; kb). Control digests containing fragments of known size permit sizing of the bands. Many HLA alleles have characteristic band patterns (fragment length polymorphism) when digested with specific endonucleases. HLA antigens can be assigned from these patterns, as illustrated here for DR1, DR4 and DR5. (Reproduced, with permission, from Bidwell JL et al: A DNA RFLP typing system that positively identifies serologically well-defined and ill-defined HLA-DR and DQ alleles, including DRw10. *Transplantation* 1988;**45**:640.)

patterns to confirm the putative HLA identity between siblings or unrelated individuals. New programs in transplantation of bone marrow from HLA-identical but unrelated donors can apply RFLP testing to select the potential donor who most nearly matches the patient. Once the pretransplant RFLP has been performed, posttransplant monitoring of the recipient for engraftment becomes a simple matter of using the same enzyme-probe combination that revealed the original polymorphisms.

In the area of forensics, HLA typing has been applied to parentage testing and the matching of tissue and blood samples in criminal cases. The HLA system is one of several genetic systems that can be probed for similarities between individuals. Others include tandem-repetitive "minisatellite" regions of DNA that are highly polymorphic owing to the variability in the number of repetitions of core sequences of 10–15 base pairs. Many such hypervariable regions have been located in human DNA. Data from family studies indicate that there are multiple loci within minisatellite sequences that are inherited in Mendelian fashion. In a single individual, as many as 8 different nonallelic fragments have been shown to be inherited from the parents, producing a unique genetic "fingerprint." It has been calculated that through the combined use of two different minisatellite cDNA probes, the probability of a chance association (identity) between 2 fingerprints is less than 5×10^{-19}. RFLP fingerprinting can powerfully augment histocompatability testing for bone marrow engraftment, disease association, and aid in the the confirmation of monozygosity of identical twins. Forensic applications of DNA fingerprinting include parentage testing and criminal and civil cases.

Typing: for Class II Antigens With Oligonucleotide Probes

The method of HLA typing by RFLP and Southern blotting has several limitations: at least 5–10 μg of DNA is required, the RFLPs revealed by the enzymes of choice may be noninformative for some antigens (particularly class I), and the procedure can take several weeks. The ultimate solution would be to have a separate probe for the specific DNA sequence unique to each HLA antigen, assuming one had sufficient quantity of the portion of DNA that codes for the HLA locus probe. If the probe hybridizes to the sample, the subject is the same "HLA type" as the probe; if the 2 sequences are not exactly complementary, the test result is negative for that antigen. Two recent technical developments, oligonucleotide probes and amplification of DNA by the polymerase chain reaction (PCR), provide such a direct molecular typing approach.

A. Oligonucleotide Probes: These are small segments of single-stranded DNA commonly 19–24 nucleotides long. A sequence of this length is likely to be unique in the human genome and technically capable of detecting differences in single nucleotides. Single-nucleotide differences in certain hypervariable regions of HLA-DR and -DQ genes determine alleles. For example, sequence-specific nucleotide probes have been prepared for the unique sequences in the region of amino acids 27–32 on the DRB1 chain for all DR antigens except DRw6. Some probes are unique to private DR specificities, whereas others are directed to shared sequences, which suggests that oligonucleotide typing will utilize combinations of probes for tissue typing. For example, by using combinations of 9 different probes, it is possible to distinguish the 5 different Dw types that are associated with DR4.

Because of their specificity, the oligonucleotide probes circumvent the need to disperse genomic DNA by electrophoresis and can be applied directly to extracted and enzymatically digested cellular DNA. A "slot blot" is prepared; the samples of DNA from several individuals are dotted onto a support membrane with as many dots as there are probes and controls to be tested (Fig 21–5). The blots are then cut into strips, and each strip exposed to a different isotope-labeled probe. After hybridization and development by autoradiography, the strips are reassembled and the patterns for each cell sample are compared with the expected patterns for the known HLA phenotypes. As in serologic typing, any deviation from the expected patterns indicates the presence of a new allele.

B. Polymerase Chain Reaction (PCR): PCR is an automated method for the amplification of a specific known DNA sequence which can be applied to genes of the HLA system. A segment of DNA containing the gene of interest is sequenced. Two oligonucleotide primers are then synthesized that are complementary to the two flanking regions of the DNA segment to be amplified. The upstream and downstream primers are usually different from one another, and can range from 20 to 30 base pairs in length. The oligonucleotides will hybridize to the flanking regions of the gene and serve as primers for the replication of the selected gene. The PCR procedure involves the repetition of 3 steps: (1) denaturation of the sample DNA to single strands, (2) annealing of sequence-specific oligonucleotide primers to the boundaries of the segment, and (3) extension of the primers by DNA polymerase to form new double-stranded DNA across the segment. It is a chain reaction, since the reaction products become the templates for the next cycle of the process (Fig 21–6). Repetition of the PCR will rapidly lead to the exponential accumulation of thousands of copies of the gene segment encompassed by the 5' ends of the two primers. In a few hours, over approximately 25–30 cycles, more than one million copies of the chosen sequence are produced by PCR.

The reaction mixture includes template DNA, a mixture of nucleotides (deoxyribonucleoside triphosphates), the 2 PCR primers, Taq polymerase, and buffer.

Through amplification by PCR, sequences present in picogram quantities become available for identification by molecular methods for histocompatibility testing and other diagnostic and research purposes. In bone marrow transplantation, in which patient material may be very scarce or peripheral cells may be abnormal, PCR has the potential to provide sufficient sample for HLA typing and testing for engraftment. The research in the association between HLA and disease can be focused on discrete sequences in the major histocompatibility complex and detected in amplified material derived from amniotic and chorionic villus fetal samples. For example, cDNA probes for 21-hydroxylase deficiency are already available for genotyping. Oligomer primers used in conjunction with restriction site analysis with PCR-generated material can detect the gene for sickle cell anemia. It should be emphasized that at present, histocompatibility testing by molecular methods is available in only a few laboratories. However, it is a powerful tool that will undoubtedly be more widely applied in the future.

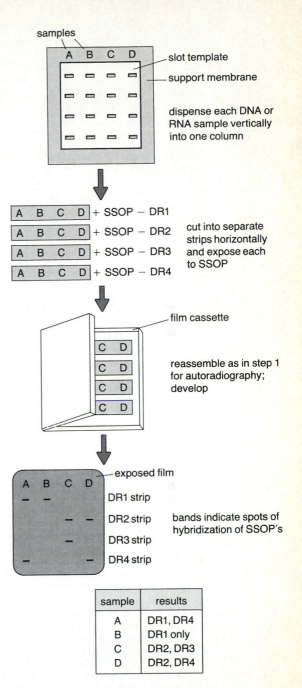

Figure 21–5. HLA typing By sequence-specific oligonucleotide probes. Samples of DNA (or RNA) (A, B, C, or D) are dotted directly onto a support membrane by using a slotted template (the slot blot). Replicates of a single sample are placed into a single column of slots. After all samples have been dispersed, the membrane is cut horizontally into strips. Individual probes are prepared that are specific and diagnostic for individual HLA alleles, such as DR1 and DR2. Each strip is hybridized with a different radiolabeled sequence-specific oligonucleotide probe (SSOP). The probes hybridize only to an exactly complementary nucleotide sequence in the sample. The membrane is reassembled and developed by autoradiography. A band indicates the presence in the sample of the sequence of the corresponding HLA allele, and the antigen can be assigned, as illustrated here.

sample	results
A	DR1, DR4
B	DR1 only
C	DR2, DR3
D	DR2, DR4

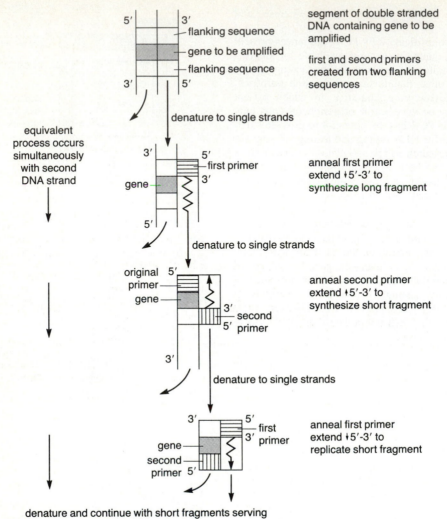

Figure 21–6. Amplification of DNA by the PCR. The segment of DNA that contains the gene of interest is sequenced, including upstream and downstream flanking regions. Primers are prepared with complementary sequences to the 2 flanking regions. The PCR amplification process has 3 steps: denaturation of the DNA to single strands; annealing of the primer to the flanking region of the gene; and extension of the primer across the gene segment, resulting in synthesis of a new copy of the gene. The new copies serve as templates for the subsequent cycles. As illustrated here, the original DNA sample is denatured into single strands and is mixed with the primers, nucleotides (deoxynucleoside triphosphates), and Taq polymerase. The first primer anneals to a flanking sequence. The polymerase extends 5′ to 3′ across the gene, creating a fragment of indeterminant length (the long fragment). The new DNA is denatured to 2 single strands. The second primer anneals to the long fragment (which contains the first primer) at the opposite flanking sequence. The polymerase extends the primer 5′ to 3′ across the gene, ending at the sequence of the first primer, creating the short fragment. From this point, subsequent cycles will amplify the short fragment geometrically, leading to a 10^6-fold replication at 30 cycles.

REFERENCES

General

Albert ED, Baur MP, Mayr WR: *Histocompatibility Testing 1984*. Springer-Verlag, 1984.

Ferrone S, Solheim BG (editors): *HLA Typing: Methodology and Clinical Aspects*. Vols. I and II. CRC Press, 1982.

Miller WV, Rodney G: *HLA Without Tears*. American Society of Clinical Pathologists, 1981.

Ray, JG Jr (editor): *Manual of Tissue Typing Techniques*. NIH Publication 80-545, US Department of Health, Education and Welfare, 1979.

Zachary AA, Braun W (editors): *AACHT Laboratory Manual*. American Association for Histocompatibility Testing, 1981.

Special Methods

Bodmer WF, Bodmer JG: Cytofluorochromasia for HLA-A, -B, -C and DR typing. Page 46 in: *Manual of Tissue Typing Techniques*. Ray JG (editor). NIH publication 80-545. US Department of Health, Education and Welfare, 1979.

Böyum A: Separation of leukocytes from blood and bone marrow. *Scand J Clin Lab Invest* 1968; **21(Suppl):**97.

Garovoy MR et al: Flow cytometry analysis: A high technology crossmatch technique facilitating transplantation. *Transplant Proc* 1983;**15:**1939.

Hirschberg H, Skare H, Thorsby E: Cell mediated lymphocytes: CML. A microplate technique requiring few target cells and employing a new method of supernatant collection. *J Immunol Methods* 1977; **16:**131.

Rudy T, Opelz G. Dithiothreitol treatment of crossmatch sera in highly immunized transplant recipients. *Transplant Proc* 1987;**19:**800.

Sheeky MJ, Bach FH: Primed LD typing (PLT)—technical considerations. *Tissue Antigens* 1976; **8:**157.

Terasaki PI et al: Microdroplet testing for HLA-A, -B, -C and -D antigens. *Am J Clin Pathol* 1978;**69:**103.

HLA & Transplantation

Cook DJ et al. The flow cytometry crossmatching kidney transplantation. Page 409 in: *Clinical Transplants 1987*. Terasaki PI (editor). UCLA Tissue Typing Laboratory, 1987.

Delmonico FL et al. New approaches to donor crossmatching and successful transplantation of highly sensitized patients. *Transplantation* 1983;**36:**629.

Oplez G: Importance of HLA antigen splits for kidney transplant matching. *Lancet* 1988;**8602:**61.

Terasaki PI (editor): *Clinical Transplantation 1987*. UCLA Tissue Typing Laboratory, 1987.

Molecular-Biologic Techniques

Bidwell JL et al: A DNA RFLP typing system that positively identifies serologically well-defined and ill-defined HLA-DR and DQ alleles, including DRw10. *Transplantation* 1988;**45:**640.

Cohen D et al: Analysis of HLA class I genes with restriction endonuclease fragments: Implications for polymorphism of the human major histocompatibility complex. *Proc Natl Acad Sci USA* 1983;**80:**6289.

Erlich HA, Gelfand DH, Saiki RS: Specific DNA fragments separated by gel electrophoresis. *J Mol Biol* 1975;**98:**503.

Erlich HA et al: Segregation and mapping analysis of polymorphic HLA class I restriction fragments: Detection of a novel fragment. *Science* 1983;**222:**72.

Freeman SM, Noreen HJ, Bach FH: Oligonucleotide probing. *Arch Pathol Lab Med* 1988;**112:**22.

Jeffreys AJ, Wilson V, Swee LT: Hypervariable 'mini-satellite' regions in human DNA. *Nature* 1985;**314:**67.

Jeffreys AJ, Wilson V, Thein SL: Individual specific fingerprints of human DNA. *Nature* 1985;**316:**76.

Oste C: Polymerase chain reaction. *Biotechniques* 1988;**6:**162.

22 Laboratory Evaluation of Immune Competence

Daniel P. Stites, MD

The integrity of the human immune system depends on the presence of adequate numbers of functionally competent cells. These cells and their many secreted products interact in a complex manner to protect the host from invading microorganisms (for a summary, see Chapter 5). The several cardinal clinical manifestations of a failure in immune competence include (1) increased frequency of infections, (2) failure to clear infections rapidly despite adequate therapy, (3) dissemination of local infections to distant sites, and (4) occurrence of opportunistic infections. An increased risk of developing certain types of cancer may be a long-term consequence of immunodeficiency; however, the susceptibility to cancer in general and, particularly, the responsible mechanisms are still controversial (see Chapters 47 and 48). Similarly, development of autoimmunity may theoretically follow the loss of key suppressive regulatory influences within the immune system. Loss of such regulatory control can result in hypersensitivity or immune hyperfunction as a consequence of immunodeficiency (see Chapter 35).

UTILITY OF LABORATORY TESTS

A seemingly bewildering array of laboratory tests are now available to finely dissect nearly every component of the immune response. Most assays have emerged from applications in basic or clinical immunology research. Relatively few such laboratory tests have developed established clinical reliability for diagnosis. To define a practical approach to clinical laboratory testing for immune competence, 2 key features of tests need to be established: (1) sensitivity and specificity of test for disease, and (2) technical accuracy of the testing procedure. One needs to know predictive values that emerge from the sensitivities and specificities of the various tests in question (see Chapter 18). This usually requires extensive clinical investigation of large numbers of diseased patients and normal subjects for each test. Unfortunately, this information is often lacking or difficult to obtain (see Chapter 18). Applications of quality control procedures, internationally accepted reagent standards, and uniformly accepted laboratory

techniques are, for the most part, also lacking. Nevertheless, a variety of relatively useful and technically reproducible laboratory tests are available in many clinical immunology laboratories. Appropriate use of these tests can lead to a very complete profile of a patient's immune competence. However, several important limitations regarding the application of laboratory tests in a clinical context must be kept in mind.

VARIABILITY OF TESTS

In contrast to its use for immunologic, epidemiologic, or other types of research, laboratory testing for immunologic competence must always be interpreted in the context of a particular patient's history and physical examination. Ordinarily, the purpose of performing any laboratory test is to aid in a patient's diagnosis or management. Statistically speaking, abnormalities outside accepted reference ranges in laboratory tests in otherwise healthy individuals are to be expected. Many currently available tests have high inherent biologic and technical variability. The sources of biologic variability in test results include age, sex, race, diurnal variations, medications, nutritional status, and other less well-defined environmental factors. Technical variability is largely a function of instrumentation, reagents, and, especially, human error in sample labeling, preparation, and actual test performance. The presence of active disease, particularly of an infectious nature, can greatly influence immune-system test results. In general, then, immune-competence testing should be done during relatively disease-free intervals.

LIMITATIONS OF TESTING

Nearly all assays currently in clinical use are performed on blood cells or serum, even though blood is rarely, if ever, the site of functional immunologic activity. Obviously, the ensuing results must be interpreted somewhat narrowly with respect to the circulating blood compartment as the source of test materials. For freely diffusible humoral proteins, such as most antibodies that are in equilibrium with extracellular fluid, blood levels directly reflect tissue levels, and do not present a problem. However, lymphocytes and monocytes may be sequestered extravascularly or not distributed in blood in the same proportions as in other organs. IgM antibodies are generally restricted to the intravascular and intralymphatic spaces as a result of their molecular size. The additional limitation of in vitro artifacts and the relatively crude nature of currently available in vivo tests must also be considered. Thus, new, relatively noninvasive techniques to measure immune-cell function and turnover in vivo are needed. Sampling cells or fluids from other sites such as bronchoalveolar lavage fluid, cerebrospinal fluid, lymph nodes, mucosal sites and secretions, and skin can give specialized insights into local immune competence in these organs. However, obtaining such specimens is often difficult. Special problems of technical standardization, in homogeneity of samples (eg, bronchoalveolar lavage), lack of reference ranges, and continuous migration to and from these nonvascular sites make interpretation and measurement even more difficult. Serum versus cerebrospinal fluid ratios for albumin and IgG, for example, have been used to address the problem of compartmentalization and local antibody synthesis in the central nervous system (see Chapter 43).

In testing for immune competence, the clinical laboratory provides 2 types of quantitative information regarding various components of the immune system. These are (1) enumeration of various elements (eg, lymphocytes) and (2) functional competence of these elements, ie, the ability of T cells to proliferate in response to a particular recall antigen. A common pitfall in test interpretation is to confuse the mere *presence* of normal numbers or levels of a given immunologic element with *functional competence*. Thus, even though an individual's CD4 T cell counts are within the laboratory's reference range, their normality is moot unless functional studies are performed. In addition, most currently used laboratory tests for immune competence are not antigen- or epitope-specific. Thus, finding a normal serum concentration of IgG, for example, provides no information about specific antibodies to particular bacterial antigens. In practice it is, of course, not possible to assess immune competence to a specific antigen if the antigen is not available in a form that can be used in the test.

CLINICAL UTILITY OF TESTING

What are clinical situations in which performance of laboratory tests for evaluation of immune competence is indicated? Specific details of laboratory tests that are used for various diseases are included in the clinical chapters later in this volume. In general,

these tests are useful in diagnosis, monitoring of treatment, and, occasionally, assessing prognosis in a limited group of clinical situations (Table 22–1). Most probably, additional applications will be defined in the future. Also, many additional tests and many other applications of the limited group of tests described below can be found in the scientific investigation of immune disorders in contrast to clinical laboratory testing.

SPECIFIC TESTING FOR IMMUNE COMPETENCE

A brief summary of one approach to testing basic elements of immune competence, including T cells, B cells, NK cells, complement, and phagocytes, is described. These are summarized in Table 22–2. There are obviously other tests available, and in some cases additional uses for the tests are described (see Table 22–4). The specific details of methods for detecting these elements and their functional states are presented in Chapters 18 and 19. "Normal" values or reference ranges for these tests are not given here because they need to be determined in individual laboratories.

T CELLS (see Table 22–3)

Enumeration

The numbers and percentages of circulating T lymphocytes are maintained within fairly narrow limits by homeostatic mechanisms. Since T cells have no morphologically distinguishing features, they can be counted only by detection of lineage-specific molecules or antigenic markers. For all T cells, the most universal among these markers is CD3, a major structural component of the T cell receptor for antigens. Other cell surface markers are

Table 22–1. Indications for laboratory testing for immune competence.

Clinical diagnosis, therapeutic monitoring, or prognosis of[1]:
1. Congenital and acquired immunodeficiency diseases (see Chapters 24, 25, 26, 27, 28, 48 and 55)
2. Immune reconstitution following bone marrow or other lymphoid tissue grafts (see Chapter 60)
3. Immunosuppression induced by drugs, radiation or other means (see Chapter 61) for transplant rejection or cancer treatment
4. Autoimmune disorders (see Chapter 35), as a possible adjunct to diagnosis (rarely useful)
5. Immunization (see Chapter 58) to monitor efficacy or immune status
6. Clinical or Basic Research

[1]Tests must be interpreted in the clinical context, particularly in conjunction with a thorough history and physical examination.

Table 22–2. Summary of immune competence testing.

Immune Cells	Detection or Enumeration	Function
T Cells	FCM[1] with MAbs[2] for CD2, 3, or 5	Lymphocyte proliferation to mitogens or antigens, DHS[3] skin test
T Cell Subsets	FCM with MAbs for CD4 (helper inducer) and CD8 (suppressor cytotoxic)	Functional assays for help, suppression, cytotoxicity
B Cells	FCM with MAbs for CD19, 20, anti-H and anti-L chains	Serum immunoglobulins or subclasses, antibodies especially postimmunization
NK Cells	FCM with MAbs for CD16 or 56	K562 cellular cytotoxicity, ADCC
Complement	Immunochemical component detection	CH_{50} or specific hemolytic assay for components
Neutrophils	Morphologic or histochemical features by cell counter	Biochemical and microbicidal
Monocyte-Macrophages	Morphologic histochemical or features MAb to CD14	Biochemical and microbicidal

[1]FCM, Flow cytometry.
[2]MAbs, monoclonal antibodies.
[3]DHS, Delayed hypersensitivity.

either incompletely expressed or specific for subsets of T cells. CD5 is also present on a subpopulation of B cells; CD2 can also be found on some natural killer (NK) cells; and CD7 is only weakly expressed on some mature T cells.

Technical Considerations

For accurate enumeration, flow cytometry is clearly the method of choice. Monoclonal antibodies directed at all known CD molecules on T cells are commercially available. Accurate determination of percentages of T cells in whole lysed blood is generally made by counting 10,000 cells per sample. Clearly, the accuracy of this technique is highly dependent on gating techniques to distinguish lymphocytes from other blood leukocytes. Manual counts of T cells by fluorescence microscopy are less desirable than flow cytometry, owing to the imprecision and laboriousness of cell-counting in a microscope. For calculation of absolute numbers of T cells, the percentage determined by immunofluorescence in a flow cytometer must be multiplied by the absolute lymphocyte count, usually determined by Coulter counting or manually in a hemacytometer. Lack of precision or accuracy in determining the absolute lymphocyte count from the leukocyte and differential count is a major source of technical variability in determining T cell counts.

T Cell Subsets

The 2 major T cell subsets, CD4- and CD8-bearing cells, are most appropriately enumerated by using fluorochrome-linked monoclonal antibodies and flow cytometry with lymphocyte gating (some monocytes also express low levels of CD4). Simultaneous 2-color analysis with additional monoclonal antibodies paired with anti-CD4 and anti-CD8 resolve CD4 and CD8 into further subpopulations (see Chapter 19), but these finer distinctions are rarely of clinical value in assessing immune competence. One such example is the use of CD4 subsets in determining disease activity in multiple sclerosis.

Functional Assays

A. All T Cells: Activation of T cells with nonspecific plant lectins or anti-CD3 monoclonal antibodies results in a complex series of biochemical

Table 22–3. Summary of major tests for T cell immune competence.

Test	Technique	Parameters Measured	Limitations and Comments
Total T cells (numbers or percentages)	Flow cytometry with MAbs to CD2, CD3, or CD5	Percentage of cells bearing these epitopes in a particular gated mononuclear cell population	Need absolute lymphocyte count to convert to T cell numbers; no functional or cloned antigen specific information.
T cell subsets (numbers and percentages) Helper-inducer cells Suppressor-cytotoxic cells	Flow cytometry with MAbs to CD4 CD8	Percentage of cells in mononuclear cell gate that bear these surface molecules	CD4 also expressed on some monocytes; both subsets are functionally heterogeneous (eg, CD8 contains suppressor and cytotoxic T cells).
Lymphocyte proliferation Mitogens and allogeneic cells	Lymphocyte culture with DNA synthesis detected by radioactive thymidine incorporation	Ability of polyclonal T cells to undergo activation to DNA synthesis	Does not define multiple possible defects in cellular physiology.
Antigens	Same	Clonal proliferation to epitopes	Avoids the need to perform skin test for DHS; relevant antigens may be unknown or unavailable for testing.

events culminating in cellular DNA synthesis. Phytomitogens such as phytohemagglutinin, concanavalin A, and pokeweed mitogen are used for this purpose. Also, allogeneic cells can be used as relatively nonspecific stimulants in a mixed-lymphocyte culture (MLC). Anti-CD3, which directly interacts with membrane T cell receptors, can provide a particularly strong activation signal. Cellular responses are usually assessed by measuring radioactive thymidine uptake (see Chapter 20). Response to mitogen stimulation by these agents is macrophage-dependent but much less so than is the response to specific antigens.

B. T Cell Subsets: CD4 and CD8 cells do not proliferate in response to monoclonal antibodies to these epitopes. Complex functional tests to assess helper, suppressor, or cytotoxic functions of these cells are still predominantly in the realm of research laboratories, but are occasionally useful in clinical situations (see below).

Antigen-specific T cells will proliferate in response to soluble or cell-bound antigens in vitro (see Chapter 19). This test is particularly useful when one wants to avoid direct in vivo contact with potentially toxic antigens by patch testing or delayed hypersensitivity intradermal tests.

C. Delayed Hypersensitivity Skin Tests: The ability to mount cutaneous delayed hypersensitivity to intradermal or epidermally applied antigens (patch testing) is dependent on both specific antigen-reactive and other relatively noncommitted T cells. Antigen-stimulated T cells release mediators that affect vascular permeability, monocyte function and movement, and proliferation of other noncommitted T cells. These cytokines and cells all contribute to local erythema and induration characteristic of this response. Thus, the delayed hypersensitivity skin test is not a measure solely of T cells. However, positive reactions to delayed hypersensitivity skin tests of one or more antigens mean that broadly reactive T cell immune competence is likely to be largely intact (see Chapter 19).

Additional tests for T cell function, which are not regularly available clinically, are listed in Table 22–4.

B CELLS

In contrast to assessing T cell competence, tests for B cell competence rely heavily on detecting the products of the B cell-plasma cell series, ie, immunoglobulins. Specific assays for antibody directed at selected epitopes of microorganisms are also available (Table 22–5).

Enumeration

A variety of specific B cell surface markers (CD antigens) that can be detected by monoclonal anti-

Table 22–4. Additional tests for T cell competence not regularly available clinically.

Lymphokine production
  IL-2, IL-3, IL-5
  Gamma interferon
  IL-4
  TNF
Receptors for lymphokines
  IL-1
  IL-2
Responsiveness to lymphokines
  IL-1
  IL-2
  IL-4
  Interferon-γ
Lymphocyte cytotoxicity
  MHC restricted
  MHC nonrestricted
  Antigen-specific
  Lectin-dependent (PHA)
Helper and suppressor T cell assays
  Polyclonal immunoglobulin synthesis (pokeweed mitogen induced)
  Mitogen or antigen proliferation
  T cell cytotoxicity
  Lymphokine release or effect

bodies have been described. Initially, surface immunoglobulins using either H- or L-chain-specific antisera were used. More recently, monoclonal antisera that detect CD19 (Leu 12, B4) or CD20 (Leu 16, B1) have also been used relatively interchangeably as pan-B cell markers. Additional antibodies that detect B cells from earlier stages of maturation or from other subsets are available (eg, CD22 [Leu 14] and CD10 [CALLA or J5]) but are rarely useful in assessing B cell competence in peripheral blood of adults or even children. The coexpression of CD5 on T cells and CD1 on dendritic cells and thymocytes restricts the usefulness of these markers for B cell enumeration. Since plasma cells rarely circulate, antibodies directed at their special differentiation antigens, eg, PC-1 or PCA-1, are of use only in examining lymph nodes, spleen, bone marrow, or other lymphoid tissues. The typical morphologic features of plasma cells render them easily recognizable without immunohistochemical staining.

Technical Considerations

These are essentially the same as those discussed for T cells. Flow cytometry is the preferred method.

B Cell Subsets

B cells at early stages of maturation, eg, pre-B cells, do express unique surface markers and cytoplasmic μ chains. Detecting these cells is primarily of use in phenotyping B cell cancers or investigating the detailed pathogenic cellular mechanisms of B cell immunodeficiency diseases. Markers for other B cell subsets can be detected, but their clinical utility is unknown. Clonal or antigen-specific B cell detec-

Table 22–5. Summary of major tests for B cell immune competence.

Test	Technique	Parameters Measured	Limitations and Comments
Total B cells (numbers or percentages)	Flow cytometry with MAbs to CD19 or CD20 or antibodies to H or L chains	Percentage of cells that express these epitopes in a particular gated mononuclear cell population	Need absolute count to convert to B cell numbers; no functional or antigen-specific information.
Immunoglobulin concentrations (IgG, IgA, IgM)	Radial immunodiffusion or rate nephelometry with specific anti-H and anti-L chain antisera	Concentration of polyclonal immunoglobulin present in particular body fluid, eg, serum, cerebrospinal fluid, saliva	No clonal or antigen-specific information; results are highly age-dependent.
Antibody to specific epitopes or microorganisms	ELISA, radioimmunoassay, agglutination, precipitation, etc (see Chapter 18)	Titers of antibody to a specific epitope or group of epitopes on antigen from microorganisms	Deliberate immunization with pre- and postantibody titers useful; anti A and anti B are IgM isohemagglutinins.

tion has generally not been applied to assessment of clinical immunocompetence.

Functional Assays

The primary product of the B cell-plasma cell series is antibody, and, as such, measurement of immunoglobulins or specific antibodies provides the major route for assessing the function of B cell competence (see Chapter 18).

Immunoglobulin levels should be measured if a state of humoral immunodeficiency or B cell failure is suspected. The use of less specific tests such as protein electrophoresis or immunoelectrophoresis, which are only semiquantitative, is not recommended. These tests are used primarily in paraprotein diagnosis. Consideration of the patient's age is critical in interpreting immunoglobulin levels, since these levels are particularly susceptible to variation with age (see Chapter 18). Generally, IgG, IgA, and IgM levels are sufficient. Serum IgD levels are not useful in assessing immune competence, and, with the rare exception of the hyper-IgE syndrome with recurrent infections (see Chapter 27), IgE levels are also not helpful in diagnosis of immune deficiencies.

In some instances, particularly following deliberate immunization to test B cell competence, specific antibody is measured. Sera should be collected and kept frozen prior to administration of antigen and then subsequently some days or weeks later when serum antibody responses to the antigen in question are known to be elevated in the blood. Antibody should then be measured in both preimmunization and postimmunization specimens simultaneously. This approach can be used to detect primary antibody responses to antigens such as keyhole limpet hemocyanin or recall antigens such as *Streptococcus pneumoniae* with polyvalent pneumococcal antigens, tetanus toxoid, or influenza virus vaccine. One should never expose a suspected or known immunodeficient patient to live or attenuated viral vaccine, since this may result in dissemination followed by disease and possibly death.

Isohemagglutinins, anti-A and anti-B, are IgM an-

tibodies directed at naturally occurring microbial polysaccharides that cross-react with antigens of the human ABH blood groups (see Chapter 20). In individuals older than 1 year, their titer is approximately 1:4. In incompatibly transfused or in utero-sensitized individuals, ABH antibodies may also be of IgG or other classes besides IgM. Rarely, the Schick test in diphtheria-immunized individuals can be used to measure specific IgG anti-diphtheria antibodies.

In vitro tests for immunoglobulin synthesis by mixed cultures of blood monocytes, T cells, and B cells have been extensively utilized in immunologic research. These tests depend on polyclonal immunoglobulin production induced by B cell mitogens such as pokeweed mitogen or staphylococcal protein A. By varying or eliminating selective T cell subsets or monocytes, suppression, helper, or antigen-presenting functions can be assessed. Currently, such intricate B cell functional assays have not achieved demonstrable routine clinical application.

IgG Subclasses

In some individuals with normal, reduced, or even elevated IgG levels, the level of one or more of the 4 IgG subclasses may be reduced (see Chapter 24). Since deficiency in some of these IgG subclasses, particularly IgG2, may be associated with recurrent infections, determination of their serum level is useful. Other possible indications and disease associations of IgG subclass deficiency are discussed in Chapter 24.

NK CELLS

NK cells represent a minor or third subpopulation (10–15%) of circulating peripheral-blood mononuclear cells. They appear as large granular lymphocytes. Functionally, these cells kill a variety of autologous and allogeneic target cells, but without prior sensitization or known restriction by human leukocyte antigens (HLA antigens). They are thought to provide defense against viral infections and possibly some tumors. Recently, a few patients with selective absence of NK cells and recurrent infections (particularly herpesvirus infections) have been described. Chédiak-Higashi syndrome patients also have defective NK cells (see Chapter 27). Research is under way to elucidate possible antitumor effects of NK cells stimulated by interleukin-2 (IL-2) or other lymphokines, as well as their modulation within the neuroimmunologic axis.

Enumeration

Monoclonal antibodies to specific cell surface CD antigens of NK cells include CD56 (NKH1) and CD16 (FcIgG). These are used to count NK cells by microscopy or flow cytometry.

Functional Assays

NK cells kill ''NK-sensitive'' target cells in vitro. An example of such a target cell is the erythroleukemia cell line K562. Cytolysis by measurement of ^{51}Cr lysis is the most common test to detect NK cell function (see Chapter 19). NK cells also mediate antibody-dependent cellular cytotoxicity (ADCC). Assays for ADCC employ cytolysis of ^{51}Cr-labeled target cells (eg, erythrocytes) that are coated with either human or rabbit antibodies which contain γ-Fc regions which bind FcIgG receptors present on NK cells.

NK cell enumeration and functional assays have not yet achieved widespread application in clinical laboratories.

COMPLEMENT

Genetic and some acquired deficiencies of complement are associated with a breakdown in host resistance to microorganisms (see Chapter 28). Complement is involved in host defense mechanisms in several ways, including (1) as an opsonin (C3a), (2) in lysing microorganisms (C1–C9), (3) in chemotaxis (C5a), and (4) in altering vascular permeability (C3a, C4a, C5a). Thus, any evaluation of host defense failure clearly should include measurement of complement.

Screening for Complement Deficiencies

Defects in C1–C9, properdin, and complement-regulatory factors have all been described. For components C3–C9 (inclusive), determination of hemolytic complement activity (CH_{50}) (see Chapter 18) will generally adequately screen for congenital lack of one of these components. In genetic defects of complement, eg, C6 deficiency, the entire activity of the protein is lost and hence the lytic function of the entire sequence is blocked. Thus, CH_{50} values approach zero. In acquired deficiency, variable reductions in CH_{50} occur depending on selective loss of the critical components of the lytic pathway. Defects in the alternative pathway proximal to C3 must be tested immunochemically or with specialized functional assays not ordinarily available in most clinical laboratories.

Identification of Specific Component Defects

Genetic or acquired reductions in specific components of either the classic or alternative pathway can be measured by either specific functional or immunochemical assays for these components (see Chapters 14 and 18). Generally, specific antisera are used in the clinical laboratory in either radial diffusion or nephelometric tests. Reduction in the CH_{50} or specific components can be the result of hypercatabolism or underproduction, or both, depending on the disease state. Functional assays such as chemotaxis or opsonization are usually performed in conjunction with the evaluation of phagocytic function.

PHAGOCYTIC CELLS

Polymorphonuclear leukocytes, particularly neutrophils (PMN) and monocyte-macrophages, play a crucial role in host defense against nearly all microorganisms. From an evolutionary standpoint, this is the oldest and most primitive form of immunity (see Chapter 2), predating antibody or T cell immunity by a considerable stretch of evolutionary development.

Enumeration

A. PMN: Peripheral-blood neutrophils are most readily counted by a routine leukocyte count and leukocyte differential. Although such counts can be made with a microscope, the use of automatic cell or Coulter counters provides much more accurate information. Morphologic assessments of neutrophils, particularly to assess maturity and granule content, also constitute an essential step in immune competence evaluation. In cases of very low or high neutrophil counts, a bone marrow examination may be required to evaluate the integrity of granulocytopoesis.

B. Monocyte-Macrophages: Circulating monocytes can be counted by leukocyte counting and leukocyte differential similar to PMN. Histochemical stains, especially for nonspecific or α-naphthol esterase, are useful for identification. Monoclonal antibodies directed at CD14 (Leu M3, MO2) or volume and light-scattering characteristics can be used to identify and count relative numbers of monocytes by flow cytometry.

Functional Assays

Granulocyte function includes a variety of stages outlined in Chapter 19. Screening for granulocytic function related to immune competence involves at least a biochemical assay for the hexose monophosphate shunt such as nitro blue tetrazolium dye reduction, chemiluminescence, or dichlorofluorescein fluorescence by flow cytometry.

More extensive microbicidal assays can be used to confirm defects in neutrophil function or to detect specific lesions related to particular microorganisms. The principles and examples of these assays are discussed in Chapter 19. Monocyte function can be assessed by similar biochemical or microbicidal tests with isolated enriched monocytes (See Chapter 19).

REFERENCES

General

Good PA, Pahwa RN: The recognition and management of immunodeficient disorders. *Pediatr Infect Dis J* 1988; **7(part 5):**S2–S125. [entire volume.]

Van der valk P, Herman C: Biology of disease: Leukocyte functions. *Lab Invest* 1987;**57:**127.

T and B Cell Assessment

Marti GE, Fleisher TA: Application of lymphocyte immunophenotyping in selected diseases. *Pathol Immunopathol Res* 1988;**7:**319.

Nicholson JKA: Using flow cytometry in the evaluation and diagnosis of primary and secondary immunodeficiency diseases. *Arch Pathol Lab Med* 1989; **113:**598.

Delayed Hypersensitivity Skin Tests

Ahmed AR, Blose DA: Delayed hypersensitivity skin testing: A review. *Arch Dermatol* 1983;**119:**934.

NK Cells

Biron CA, Byron KS, Sullivan JL: Severe herpes infections in an adolescent without natural killer cells. *N Engl J Med* 1989;**320:**1731.

Jondal M: The human NK cell. *Clin Exp Immunol* 1987;**70:**255.

Ritz J: The role of natural killer cells in immune surveillance. *N Engl J Med* 1989;**320:**1748.

Immunoglobulins

French MAH: *Immunoglobulins in Health and Disease. Immunology and Medicine Series.* MTP Press, 1986.

Hamilton, RG: Human IgG subclass measurements in the clinical laboratory. *Clin Chem* 1987;**33:**1707.

Complement

Fries LF, Frank MM: Complement and relative proteins: Inherited deficiencies. Page 89 in: *Inflammation: Basic Principles and Clinical Correlates.* Gallin JI, Goldstein IM, Snyderman R (editors). Raven Press, 1988.

Ross SC, Denson P: Complement deficiency states and infections. *Medicine* 1984;**63:**243.

Phagocytic Cells

Borregaard N: The human neutrophil: Function and dysfunction. *Eur J Hematol* 1988;**41:**401.

Boxer LA, Morganroth ML: Neutrophil function disorders. *Disease-a-Month* 1987;**33:**681.

Section III.
Clinical Immunology

Mechanisms of Immunodeficiency

23

Arthur J. Ammann, MD

Four major components of the immune system assist the individual in defending against a constant assault by viral, bacterial, fungal, protozoal, and nonreplicating agents that have the potential to produce infection and disease. These systems consist of antibody-mediated (B cell) immunity, cell-mediated (T cell) immunity, phagocytosis, and complement. Each system may act independently or in concert with one or more of the others.

Deficiency of one or more of these systems may be congenital (eg, X-linked infantile hypogammaglobulinemia) or acquired (eg, acquired hypogammaglobulinemia). Deficiencies of the immune system may be secondary to an embryologic abnormality (eg, DiGeorge's syndrome), may be due to an enzymatic defect (eg, chronic granulomatous disease), or may be of unknown cause (eg, chronic mucocutaneous candidiasis). The multiple causes of immunodeficiency are listed in Table 23–1.

In general, the symptoms and the physical findings of immunodeficiency are related to the degree of deficiency and the particular system that is deficient in function. General features are listed in Table 23–2. Features associated with specific immunodeficiency disorders are also listed in Table 23–2. The types of infections that occur often provide an important clue to the type of immunodeficiency disease present. Recurrent bacterial otitis media and pneumonia are common in hypogammaglobulinemia. Patients with defective cell-mediated immunity are susceptible to fungal, protozoal, and viral infections that may present as pneumonia or chronic infection of the skin and mucous membranes or other organs. Systemic infection with uncommon bacterial organisms, normally of low virulence, is characteristic of chronic granulomatous disease. Other phagocytic disorders are associated with superficial skin infections or systemic infections with pyogenic organisms.

Numerous advances have recently been made in the diagnosis of specific immunodeficiency disorders

(Table 23–3). Screening tests are available for each component of the immune system (Table 23–4). These tests enable the physician to diagnose more than 75% of immunodeficiency disorders. The remainder can be diagnosed by means of more complicated studies (see Chapters 18 and 19), which may not be available in all hospital laboratories. There are still a number of individuals with an immunodeficiency disorder in whom the precise etiology or mechanism of immunodeficiency is unknown.

Table 23–1. Causes of immunodeficiency.

Genetic patterns
Autosomal recessive
Autosomal dominant
X-linked
Gene deletions and rearrangements

Biochemical and metabolic deficiency
Adenosine deaminase deficiency
Purine nucleoside phosphorylase deficiency
Biotin dependent multiple carboxylase deficiency
Deficient membrane glycoproteins

Vitamin or mineral deficiency
Biotin
B_{12}
Zinc

Arrest in embryogenesis

Autoimmune diseases
Passive antibody (maternal to fetus)
Active antibody (antibody to T cells)
Active T cell (anti B cell)

Acquired immunodeficiency
Post-viral infection
Posttransfusion
Multiple transfusions
Chronic infection
Nutritional deficiency
Drug abuse
Maternal alcoholism
Radiation therapy
Immunosuppressive therapy
Cancer
Chronic renal disease

Table 23–2. Clinical features associated with immunodeficiency.

Features frequently present and highly suspicious
Chronic infection
Recurrent infection (more than expected)
Unusual infecting agents
Incomplete clearing between episodes of infection or incomplete response to treatment

Features frequently present and moderately suspicious
Skin rash (eczema, cutaneous candidiasis, etc)
Diarrhea (chronic)
Growth failure
Hepatosplenomegaly
Recurrent abscesses
Recurrent osteomyelitis
Evidence of autoimmunity

Features associated with specific immunodeficiency disorders
Ataxia
Telangiectasia
Short-limbed dwarfism
Cartilage-hair hypoplasia
Idiopathic endocrinopathy
Partial albinism
Thrombocytopenia
Eczema
Tetany

Table 23–3. Classification of immunodeficiency disorders.

Antibody (B cell) immunodeficiency disorders
X-linked hypogammaglobulinemia (congenital hypogammaglobulinemia)
Transient hypogammaglobulinemia of infancy
Common, variable, unclassifiable immunodeficiency (acquired hypogammaglobulinemia)
Immunodeficiency with hyper-IgM
Selective IgA deficiency
Selective IgM deficiency
Selective deficiency of IgG subclasses
Secondary B cell immunodeficiency associated with drugs, protein-losing states
X-linked lymphoproliferative disease

Cellular (T cell) immunodeficiency disorders
Congenital thymic aplasia (DiGeorge's syndrome)
Chronic mucocutaneous candidiasis (with or without endocrinopathy)
T cell deficiency associated with purine nucleoside phosphorylase deficiency
T cell deficiency associated with absent membrane glycoprotein
T cell deficiency associated with absent class I or II MHC antigens or both (bare lymphocyte syndrome)

Combined antibody-mediated (B cell) and cell-mediated (T cell) immunodeficiency disorders
Severe combined immunodeficiency disease (autosomal recessive, X-linked, sporadic)
Cellular immunodeficiency with abnormal immunoglobulin synthesis (Nezelof's syndrome)
Immunodeficiency with ataxia-telangiectasia
Immunodeficiency with eczema and thrombocytopenia (Wiskott-Aldrich syndrome)
Immunodeficiency with thymoma
Immunodeficiency with short-limbed dwarfism
Immunodeficiency with adenosine deaminase deficiency
Immunodeficiency with nucleoside phosphorylase deficiency

(continued)

Table 23–3 (cont'd.). Classification of immunodeficiency disorders.

Biotin dependent multiple carboxylase deficiency
Graft-versus-host (GVH) disease
Acquired immunodeficiency syndrome (AIDS)

Phagocytic dysfunction
Chronic granulomatous disease
Glucose-6-phosphate dehydrogenase deficiency
Myeloperoxidase deficiency
Chédiak-Higashi syndrome
Job's syndrome
Tuftsin deficiency
Lazy leukocyte syndrome
Elevated IgE, defective chemotaxis, and recurrent infections

In addition to antimicrobial agents for the treatment of specific infections, new forms of immunotherapy are available to assist in the control of immunodeficiency or perhaps even to cure the underlying disease (Table 23–5). The usefulness of some of these treatment methods, such as bone marrow transplantation, is limited by the availability of suitable donors. The discovery of enzyme deficiencies (eg, adenosine deaminase deficiency) in association with immunodeficiency offers a potential new avenue of therapy by means of enzyme replacement.

Immunodeficiency disorders are discussed in the next 4 chapters under the following categories: antibody (B cell) deficiency, cellular (T cell) deficiency, combined T cell and B cell deficiency, and phagocytic dysfunction. Complement factor deficiencies are discussed in Chapter 28. AIDS is discussed in Chapter 55. In general, the terminology used for specific deficiencies is based on the classification recently proposed by a committee of the World Health Organization (Table 23–3).

Table 23–4. Initial screening evaluation.

Antibody-mediated immunity
Quantitative immunoglobulin levels: IgG, IgM, IgA
Schick test: measures specific IgG antibody response
Isohemagglutinin titer (anti-A and anti-B): measures IgM antibody function primarily
Specific antibody levels following immunization

Cell-mediated immunity
Leukocyte count with differential: measures total lymphocytes
Total T cells and T cell subsets: measures total T cells, helper T cells, and suppressor T cells
Delayed hypersensitivity skin tests: measures specific T cell and inflammatory response to antigens

Phagocytosis
Leukocyte count with differential: measures total neutrophils
Nitro Blue Tetrazolium (NBT), chemiluminescence: measures neutrophil metabolic function

Table 23–5. Treatment of immunodeficiency.

Treatment	B Cell Disorders	T Cell Disorders	Phagocytic Disorders
γ-Globulin.	X-linked hypogammaglobulinemia; acquired hypogammaglobulinemia; secondary hypogammaglobulinemia when associated with infection. Do not use in selective IgA deficiency.	Use only when absent antibody response is demonstrated. Not recommended for intramuscular use in Wiskott-Aldrich syndrome. γ-globulin does not transmit virus, eg, hepatitis, retrovirus.	Not recommended.
Hyperimmune γ-globulin.	Use in above disorders when specific exposure has occurred.	May be used when specific exposure has occurred.	May be used when specific exposure has occurred.
Frozen plasma by intravenous infusion. Largely replaced by intravenous γ-globulin. Risk of transmitting viral infections.	X-linked hypogammaglobulinemia and acquired hypogammaglobulinemia when intramuscular administration is not tolerated or is ineffective. Screen for HIV and HBV.	Use only when absent antibody response is demonstrated. Irradiate to prevent GVH disease.	Not recommended.
Infusions of leukocytes.	Not recommended.	Not recommended.	Questionable value.
Infusion of erythrocytes.	Not recommended.	May be of benefit in certain enzyme deficiencies associated with immunodeficiency (adenosine deaminase, purine nucleoside phosphorylase). Irradiate to prevent GVH disease.	Not recommended.
Bone marrow transplant.	Not recommended.	Use only when T cell function is impaired. Histocompatible donor preferred.	Not recommended.
Fetal thymus transplantation.	Not recommended.	DiGeorge's syndrome.	Not recommended.
Cultured thymus epithelium.	Not recommended.	Selected cases of T cell disorders in which no suitable bone marrow donor is available.	Not recommended.
Fetal liver transplantation. (Primarily of historic interest.)	Not recommended.	Used in past in severe combined immunodeficiency in absence of suitable bone marrow donor.	Not recommended.
Thymosin, thymopentin, α_1 facteur thymique serique. (Investigational.)	Not recommended.	Limited evaluation to date. May enhance T cell function in a variety of T cell disorders, including DiGeorge's syndrome. No effect in chronic candidiasis or severe combined immunodeficiency.	Not recommended.
Adenosine deaminase polyethylene glycol.	Not recommended.	Specific for adenosine deaminase deficiency.	Not recommended.

REFERENCES

Good RA, Pahwa RN (editors): The recognition of immunodeficient disorders. (Symposium.) *Pediatr Infect Dis J* 1988;**7(Suppl):**S2.

Stiehm ER: *Immunologic Disorders in Infants and Children,* 3rd ed. Saunders, 1989.

Symposium: Childhood immunodeficiency disorders: Diagnosis, prevention, and management. *Clin Immunol Immunopathol* 1986;**40:**1.

Antibody (B Cell) Immunodeficiency Disorders

Arthur J. Ammann, MD

Antibody immunodeficiency disorders comprise a spectrum of diseases characterized by decreased immunoglobulin levels ranging from complete absence of all classes to selective deficiency of a single class or subclass. There are also cases of specific antibody deficiency, particularly the inability to form antibody to polysaccharide antigens. The morbidity found in patients with antibody immunodeficiency disorders is dependent chiefly on the degree of antibody deficiency. Patients with hypogammaglobulinemia become symptomatic earlier and experience more severe disease than do patients with selective immunoglobulin deficiency. Screening tests for the specific diagnosis of antibody deficiency disorders are readily available in most hospital laboratories (see Table 23–4 and Chapter 18). They permit early diagnosis and prompt institution of appropriate treatment. Other procedures, such as quantitation of B cells in peripheral blood, determination of in vitro immunoglobulin production, and suppressor cell assays, may yield more precise diagnosis and insight into the cause or mechanism of the observed deficiency (Table 24–1). The exact role of these and other tests of B cell function has not been established for most clinical conditions.

X-LINKED INFANTILE HYPOGAMMAGLOBULINEMIA

Major Immunologic Features

- Symptoms of recurrent pyogenic infections usually begin by 5–6 months of age.
- IgG is less than 200 mg/dL, with absence of IgM, IgA, IgD, and IgE.
- B cells are absent in peripheral blood.
- Patients respond well to treatment with gamma globulin.

General Considerations

In 1952 Bruton described a male child with hypogammaglobulinemia, and this is now recognized as the first clinical description and precise diagnosis of an immunodeficiency disorder. The disorder is easily diagnosed by using standard laboratory tests that demonstrate marked deficiency or complete absence of all 5 immunoglobulin classes. Male infants with this disorder usually become symptomatic following the natural decay of transplacentally acquired maternal immunoglobulin at about 5–6 months of age. They suffer from severe chronic bacterial infections, which can be controlled readily with gamma globulin and antibiotic treatment. The prevalence of this disorder in the USA is not precisely known, but estimates in the United Kingdom suggest that it is one case per 100,000 population. Recently, 2 female siblings with congenital hypogammaglobulinemia have been reported.

Table 24–1. Evaluation of antibody-mediated immunity.

Test	Comment
Protein electrophoresis	For presumptive diagnosis of hypogammaglobulinemia or to evaluate for paraproteins.
Radial immunodiffusion or rate nephelometry	Best procedure for quantitation of IgG, IgM, IgA, and IgD.
Enzyme-linked immunosorbent assay (ELISA)	IgE quantitation.
Schick test	Diphtheria immunization must be complete. Formerly used to evaluate IgG function, but now largely supplanted by specific antibody tests.
Isohemagglutinins	For evaluation of IgM function. Expected titer of >1:4 after 1 year of age.
Specific antibody response	For evaluation of immunoglobulin function. Immunize with tetanus or diphtheria toxoid or typhoid. Do not immunize with live virus if immunodeficiency is suspected.
B cell quantitation with monoclonal antibody	Normally 10–25% (total IgG-, IgM-, IgD-, and IgA-bearing cells) of total circulation lymphocytes.
In vitro immunoglobulin synthesis with T cell subsets	Determines helper/suppressor T cell function in hypogammaglobulinemia.

Immunologic Pathogenesis

Extirpation of the bursa of Fabricius in birds results in complete hypogammaglobulinemia. Several investigators think that the human equivalent of the bursa, the source of B cell precursors, is the gastrointestinal tract-associated lymphoid tissue (tonsils, adenoids, Peyer's patches, and appendix), whereas others assign this role to stem cells in fetal liver and bone marrow. In X-linked infantile hypogammaglobulinemia, a stem cell population is presumed to be absent, resulting in the complete absence of B lymphocytes and plasma cells. However, recent investigations have provided some evidence of pre-B cells in the marrow and peripheral blood of patients, suggesting that the defect may be at a later stage of B cell differentiation. These pre-B cells do not secrete immunoglobulin.

The individual immunoglobulin isotypes are a result of immunoglobulin heavy (H)-chain diversity. The formation of individual H chains is a result of somatic rearrangement of variable (V), diversity (D), and joining (J) segment genes, as described in Chapter 10. In some forms of X-linked infantile hypogammaglobulinemia, a truncated μ chain is produced as a consequence of premature transcription prior to D-J segment rearrangement. A second form has been shown to be a result of failure of V_H gene rearrangement, resulting in the production of truncated μ and α H chains.

Clinical Features

A. Symptoms and Signs: Patients with X-linked infantile hypogammaglobulinemia usually remain asymptomatic until 5–6 months of age, at which time the passively transferred maternal IgG reaches its lowest level. The loss of protection from maternal antibodies usually coincides with the age at which these children are increasingly exposed to pathogens. Initial symptoms consist of recurrent bacterial otitis media, bronchitis, pneumonia, meningitis, dermatitis, and, occasionally, arthritis or malabsorption. Many infections respond promptly to antibiotic therapy, and this response occasionally will delay the diagnosis of hypogammaglobulinemia. The most common organisms responsible for infection are *Streptococcus pneumoniae* and *Haemophilus influenzae;* other streptococci and certain gram-negative bacteria are occasionally responsible. Although patients normally have intact T cell immunity and respond normally to viral infections such as varicella and measles, there have been reports of paralytic poliomyelitis and progressive encephalitis following immunization with live vaccines or exposure to wild virus. Fatal echovirus infection has been reported in patients with congenital hypogammaglobulinemia. The encephalitis in a few patients has responded to treatment with intravenous gamma globulin or plasma. A relationship of echovirus infection, dermatomyositis, and hypogammaglobulin-

emia has been proposed. These observations suggest that some patients with hypogammaglobulinemia may also be unusually susceptible to some viral illnesses.

An important clue to the diagnosis of hypogammaglobulinemia is the failure of infections to respond completely or promptly to appropriate antibiotic therapy. In addition, many patients with hypogammaglobulinemia have a history of continuous illness; ie, they do not have periods of well-being between bouts of illness.

Occasionally, patients with hypogammaglobulinemia may not become symptomatic until early childhood. Some of these patients may present with other complaints, such as chronic conjunctivitis, abnormal dental decay, or malabsorption. The malabsorption may be severe and may cause retardation of both height and weight. Frequently, the malabsorption is associated with *Giardia lamblia* infestation. A disease resembling rheumatoid arthritis has been reported in association with hypogammaglobulinemia. This occurs principally in untreated infants or is an indication for more intensive therapy with gamma globulin.

Physical findings usually relate to recurrent pyogenic infections. Chronic otitis media and externa, serous otitis, conjunctivitis, abnormal dental decay (Fig 24–1), and eczematoid skin infections are frequently present. Despite the repeated infections, lymphadenopathy and splenomegaly are absent.

B. Laboratory Findings: The diagnosis of X-linked infantile hypogammaglobulinemia is based on the demonstration of absence or marked deficiency of all 5 immunoglobulin classes. Although the diag-

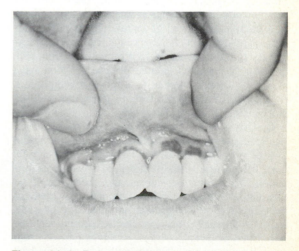

Figure 24–1. Early periodontal disease in a child with hypogammaglobulinemia. Recurrent ear infections and dental disease were the first manifestations of susceptibility to infection.

nosis is suspected from serum protein electrophoresis and established by immunoelectrophoresis (see Chapter 18), specific quantitation of immunoglobulins is necessary, especially during early infancy. Total immunoglobulin levels are usually below 250 mg/dL. The IgG level is usually below 200 mg/dL, while IgM, IgA, IgD, and IgE levels are extremely low or undetectable. Rarely, patients have complete absence of IgG, IgA, IgM, and IgD, but normal amounts of IgE. It is unusual for patients with hypogammaglobulinemia to have depressed levels of IgG and normal levels of IgM or IgA. Before a diagnosis of immunodeficiency is established in a patient with hypogammaglobulinemia, failure to make antibody following antigenic stimulation should be demonstrated. The diagnosis is difficult in infants under 6 months of age because of maternal IgG in the serum.

Isohemagglutinins that result from natural immunization are normally present in infants of the appropriate blood group by 1 year of age. Titers of anti-A and anti-B should be greater than 1:4 in normal individuals. Those who have received the complete series of DPT immunizations should react negatively to the Schick test. Within a period of 1 month following gamma globulin therapy the Schick test may be nonreactive in a patient with hypogammaglobulinemia. Antibody to a specific antigen may be measured following immunization, but a patient suspected of having an immunodeficiency disorder should never be immunized with live attenuated viral vaccine. Although lymph node biopsies have been recommended in the past, this is probably unnecessary with currently available diagnostic studies. Rarely, an intestinal biopsy to determine the presence or absence of plasma cells may be necessary to assist in the diagnosis in difficult cases. In X-linked infantile hypogammaglobulinemia, there are no plasma cells in the lamina propria of the gut. There is a complete absence of circulating B cells, with normal to increased numbers of T cells. T cell immunity is intact. Delayed hypersensitivity skin tests are usually positive; isolated peripheral blood lymphocytes respond normally to phytohemagglutinin (PHA) and to allogeneic cells in mixed-lymphocyte culture (MLC).

C. Other Tests: X-ray of the lateral nasopharynx has been suggested as a method of demonstrating the lack of lymphoid tissue, but this rarely adds significant information to the findings on physical examination. X-rays of the sinuses and chest should be obtained at regular intervals to monitor the course of the patient and to determine the adequacy of treatment. Pulmonary function studies should also be performed on a regular basis, when the patient is old enough to cooperate. Patients with hypogammaglobulinemia who have gastrointestinal tract symptoms should be investigated for the presence of *G. lamblia* and other causes of malabsorption.

Immunologic Diagnosis

Total immunoglobulin levels are below 250 mg/dL; the IgG level is below 200 mg/dL, and IgM, IgA, IgD, and IgE levels are markedly reduced or absent. B cells are absent in peripheral blood, and there are no plasma cells containing immunoglobulins in tissue and lymph nodes. Lymph nodes are markedly depleted in B-cell-dependent areas. No antibodies are formed following specific immunization. T cell numbers and functions are intact. Natural killer (NK) cell activity is normal.

Differential Diagnosis

A diagnosis of X-linked infantile hypogammaglobulinemia may be difficult to establish in the age range of 5–9 months. By this time most infants have lost their maternal immunoglobulins and are susceptible to recurrent infections. The majority of normal infants during this time have IgG levels below 350 mg/dL but usually show some evidence of IgM and IgA production (usually >20 mg/dL). If the diagnosis appears uncertain, several approaches may be taken. Immunoglobulin levels may be determined again 3 months after the initial values. If there is an increase in IgG, IgM, or IgA, it is highly unlikely that the patient has hypogammaglobulinemia. Alternatively, the patient may be immunized with killed vaccines, and specific antibody levels determined. The most difficult diagnostic problem is the differentiation of prolonged physiologic hypogammaglobulinemia from X-linked infantile hypogammaglobulinemia. In the former, the hypogammaglobulinemia may sometimes be severe enough to require treatment, and immunoglobulin levels may be as low as those of patients with congenital hypogammaglobulinemia. Normal production of immunoglobulins may not occur until as late as 18 months of age in patients with physiologic hypogammaglobulinemia. In most instances these patients will begin to produce their own immunoglobulin despite concurrent gamma globulin administration. This is manifested by increasing levels of IgG as well as IgM and IgA. Since IgM and IgA make up less than 10% of commercial gamma globulin, a gradual increase in these levels argues strongly against a diagnosis of congenital hypogammaglobulinemia. The best way to avoid mistaking congenital hypogammaglobulinemia for prolonged physiologic hypogammaglobulinemia in infants is to compare immunoglobulin levels with those in age-matched controls and to obtain sequential measurements of immunoglobulins at 3-month intervals during the first year of diagnostic uncertainty. Rarely, patients with human immunodeficiency virus (HIV) infection have hypogammaglobulinemia.

Patients with severe malabsorption—particularly protein-losing enteropathy—may have severely depressed levels of immunoglobulins because of enteric loss. In most instances, a diagnosis of protein-losing enteropathy can be established by the demonstration of a concomitant deficiency of serum albumin. Occasionally, however, patients with severe malabsorption and primary hypogammaglobulinemia may also lose albumin through the intestinal tract. Under these circumstances, a diagnosis can best be made by obtaining an intestinal biopsy. Patients with protein-losing enteropathy have normal numbers of plasma cells containing intracellular immunoglobulins in the gut and in other lymphoid tissues. These patients also have normal numbers of circulating B cells.

Polyarthritis may be a presenting feature in patients with hypogammaglobulinemia. Most patients with juvenile rheumatoid arthritis have elevated levels of immunoglobulins. Patients with arthritis and hypogammaglobulinemia usually respond promptly to gamma globulin therapy. Patients with chronic lung disease should also be suspected of having cystic fibrosis, asthma, α-antitrypsin deficiency, or immotile cilia syndrome.

Treatment

Replacement gamma globulin therapy consists primarily of the use of intravenous gamma globulin. Although manufacturing techniques may vary for the different preparations that have been approved for clinical use, their compositions are similar. All contain almost exclusively IgG, with only trace amounts of IgM or IgA. Some preparations contain a more physiologic representation of the IgG subclasses and therefore may be useful in the treatment of IgG subclass deficiencies. All of the preparations may contain small amounts of other nonantibody proteins. Intramuscular gamma globulin is prepared in a manner similar to that of intravenous gamma globulin, but with the omission of chemical treatment steps that prevent it from aggregating or stimulating the complement pathway in vivo. Although intramuscular gamma globulin is safe to use by local injection, it will cause severe anaphylactoid reactions if given intravenously. Even though it is inexpensive to use and easy to administer, it has been largely replaced by intravenous gamma globulin, as larger amounts of the latter can be safely given to patients. The use of intramuscular gamma globulin has been largely relegated to preventing hepatitis and other infectious diseases in normal individuals.

Starting doses of intravenous gamma globulin range from 100 to 200 mg/kg given intravenously once each month. The total amount given is dependent on the control of symptoms. Patients whose symptoms are not controlled on lower doses may have the total dose increased to as much as 400 mg/kg given on a monthly basis or even as frequently as every week. During an acute illness, such as meningitis or pneumonia, gamma globulin may be given as frequently as every day if the patient fails to respond appropriately to antibiotics plus standard doses of gamma globulin. If a patient with an acute illness has not received gamma globulin for 2 weeks, it is advisable to provide a repeat maintenance dose. The maximum dose of intravenous gamma globulin has not been defined, but certain factors should be considered when doses larger than 400 mg/kg are used or the frequency of administration is greater than once a week. Pulmonary function may be acutely impaired when large amounts of intravenous gamma globulin have been administered to children with pulmonary disease. Also, there are no data to suggest that giving excess amounts of passive antibody is therapeutically advantageous.

The half-life of intravenous gamma globulin is between 15 and 25 days. Serum levels of IgG approaching normal can be achieved for the first 2–4 days following intravenous administration, but they return to abnormal values after 2–3 weeks. Weekly administration results in stabilization of levels, but this has not been shown to be of clinical benefit. Because there are limitations in the amount of gamma globulin that can be given intramuscularly, this method of administration does not result in an increase in serum IgG levels.

Reactions to intravenous gamma globulin are rare. Patients may occasionally experience dyspnea, sweating, increased heart rate, or abdominal pain. In most instances these symptoms will subside when the infusion rate is temporarily slowed.

Anaphylactoid reactions to gamma globulin administration have been observed. These are not mediated through the IgE allergic pathway, since most patients with hypogammaglobulinemia do not form IgE antibodies. The chief causes of these reactions are aggregate formation in the gamma globulin preparation and inadvertent intravenous administration of intramuscular preparations. Patients who have repeated reactions to gamma globulin should first be treated with an alternative preparation obtained from a different commercial source. If reactions continue, it may be necessary to centrifuge the preparation to remove aggregates prior to administration.

Therapeutic gamma globulin is prepared from pools of serum obtained from donors screened for absence of viruses causing hepatitis or acquired immunodeficiency syndrome (AIDS).

Additional therapy may be necessary in patients who fail to respond to maximum doses of gamma globulin. Continuous use of antibiotics may be necessary. Prophylactic broad-spectrum antibiotics such as ampicillin in low to moderate doses may be effective in controlling recurrent infection. Physical therapy with postural drainage should be used for patients with chronic lung disease or bronchiectasis.

Occasionally, a patient with hypogammaglobulinemia may be discovered who has minimal or no symptoms. These patients should receive gamma globulin therapy, even though they have not experienced repeated infection, to avoid future infections that may subsequently cause permanent complications.

Malabsorption, occasionally found in patients with hypogammaglobulinemia, usually responds to treatment with gamma globulin, intravenous fresh-frozen plasma, or both. If *G. lamblia* is found, the patient should be treated with metronidazole in doses of 35–50 mg/kg/d in 3 divided doses for 10 days (for children) or 750 mg orally 3 times a day for 10 days (for adults).

Complications & Prognosis

Although patients with congenital hypogammaglobulinemia have survived to the second and third decades, the prognosis must be guarded. Despite what may appear to be adequate gamma globulin replacement therapy, many patients develop chronic lung disease. The presence of severe infection early in infancy may result in irreversible lung damage. Patients who recover from meningitis may have severe neurologic handicaps. Patients with severe pulmonary infection frequently develop bronchiectasis and chronic lung disease. Regular examinations and prompt institution of therapy are necessary to control infections and to prevent complications. Fatal echovirus infections of the central nervous system have been reported even in patients receiving gamma globulin therapy. Some of these infections have been associated with dermatomyositis. Some patients may develop leukemia or lymphoma.

TRANSIENT HYPOGAMMAGLOBULINEMIA OF INFANCY

Under normal circumstances, maternal IgG is passively transferred to the infant beginning at week 16 of gestational life. At the time of birth, the serum IgG level in the infant is usually higher than that in the mother. IgA, IgM, IgD, and IgE are not placentally transferred under normal circumstances. In fact, the presence of elevated levels of IgM or IgA in cord blood suggests premature antibody synthesis, usually a sign of intrauterine infection. Over the first 4–5 months of life, there is a gradual decrease in the serum IgG level and a gradual increase in the serum IgM and IgA levels (Fig 24–2). The IgM level usually rises more rapidly than the IgA level. Almost all infants go through a period of hypogammaglobulinemia at approximately 5–6 months of age. At this time, the serum IgG level reaches its lowest point (approximately 350 mg/dL), and many normal infants begin to experience recurrent respiratory tract infections. Occasionally, an infant may fail to produce normal amounts of IgG at this time, resulting in transient hypogammaglobulinemia, or so-called physiologic hypogammaglobulinemia. The presence of normal serum levels of IgM or IgA argues

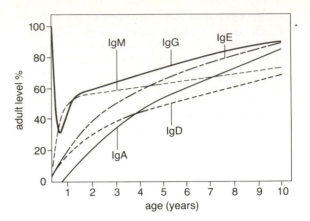

Figure 24–2. Development of serum immunoglobulins with increasing age. Levels are expressed as percentages of adult levels. Maternally acquired IgG levels decrease rapidly over the first 6 months of age. IgM levels increase more rapidly than IgA, IgD, and IgE levels.

strongly against a diagnosis of X-linked hypogammaglobulinemia. However, some infants with transient hypogammaglobulinemia may also fail to produce normal amounts of IgM or IgA.

Additional studies may be of no diagnostic usefulness, since many infants fail to respond to immunization at this age and isohemagglutinin titers may be low. Under these circumstances, a lymph node or intestinal biopsy may assist in establishing the diagnosis. Patients with congenital hypogammaglobulinemia lack plasma cells containing immunoglobulins in the intestinal tract and in peripheral lymph nodes. In addition, patients with congenital hypogammaglobulinemia lack circulating B cells, whereas children with physiologic hypogammaglobulinemia do not. If the patient is not experiencing severe recurrent infection, it is best to wait 3–5 months and repeat immunoglobulin measurements rather than to perform invasive procedures. In the presence of an increasing IgG, IgM, or IgA level, congenital hypogammaglobulinemia is unlikely. If the patient has been treated with gamma globulin to prevent severe or recurrent infection, measurement of IgM and IgA levels assumes greater importance. Because commercial gamma globulin contains primarily IgG, the administration of gamma globulin will not affect serum levels of IgM and IgA. Increasing levels of these immunoglobulin classes indicate that the patient had transient hypogammaglobulinemia. Hypogammaglobulinemia may persist for as long as 2 years.

The cause of transient hypogammaglobulinemia is not known. In some cases, IgG anti-Gm antibodies have been demonstrated during the last trimester of pregnancy in women who have previously had infants with transient hypogammaglobulinemia. It is postulated that these antibodies cause suppression of the infant's endogenous immunoglobulin production in a manner similar to the suppression of normal erythrocyte production from placental transfer of antibody against Rh factors. Recent studies indicate that patients with transient hypogammaglobulinemia have normal numbers of B cells but a transient deficiency in the number and function of helper T cells.

Occasionally, these infants become sufficiently symptomatic that they must be treated just like those with X-linked infantile hypogammaglobulinemia. Gamma globulin therapy may be required for as long as 18 months. Routine immunization should not be given during the period of transient hypogammaglobulinemia. The continued administration of gamma globulin will not delay the development of normal IgG. Once a normal immune system has been established, the complete series of pediatric immunizations should be administered.

COMMON, VARIABLE, UNCLASSIFIABLE IMMUNODEFICIENCY (Acquired Hypogammaglobulinemia)

Major Immunologic Features
- Recurrent pyogenic infections occur, with onset at any age.
- There is increased incidence of autoimmune disease.
- The total immunoglobulin level is less than 300 mg/dL, with the IgG level below 250 mg/dL.
- B cell numbers are usually normal.

General Considerations
Patients with acquired hypogammaglobulinemia present clinically like patients with X-linked infantile hypogammaglobulinemia, except that they usually do not become symptomatic until 15–35 years of age. In addition to increased susceptibility to pyogenic infections, they have a high prevalence of autoimmune disease. These patients also differ from those with congenital hypogammaglobulinemia in that they have a higher than normal prevalence of abnormalities in T cell immunity, which in most instances progressively deteriorates with time. Acquired hypogammaglobulinemia affects both males and females and may occur at any age.

Immunologic Pathogenesis
The cause of acquired hypogammaglobulinemia is unknown. Most patients have an intrinsic defect in B cells. Peripheral blood lymphocytes from some patients with acquired hypogammaglobulinemia have an inhibiting effect on the immunoglobulin synthesis in cells from normal patients, suggesting that the course of this disorder may reside at the level of suppressor T cells. Other patients have diminished

numbers of helper T cells. Some studies have shown a heterogeneity of arrested B cell development ranging from normal proliferative B cell responses and IgM-secreting cells to absent proliferative responses. Two enzymatic abnormalities have been described. In some patients there is a failure of glycosylation of the heavy-chain IgG. In others, a deficiency of 5′-nucleotidase has been found. The latter abnormality is most probably secondary to alterations in T cell:B cell ratios rather than being a primary defect. An X-linked lymphoproliferative disorder associated with acquired hypogammaglobulinemia has been described following Epstein-Barr virus (EBV) infection. Genetic studies of acquired hypogammaglobulinemia have demonstrated an autosomal recessive mode of inheritance in certain families in which abnormal lymphocyte metabolism has been shown to be inherited. In most instances, however, there is no clear-cut evidence of genetic transmission. An increased prevalence of other immunologic disorders, including autoimmune disease, has been observed in families of patients with acquired hypogammaglobulinemia. The presence of normal numbers of circulating peripheral blood B cells in most of these patients suggests that the disorder is a result of diminished synthesis or release of immunoglobulin rather than production of fewer cells synthesizing immunoglobulin.

Clinical Features
A. Symptoms and Signs: Recurrent sinopulmonary infection is the initial presentation of acquired hypogammaglobulinemia in most cases. These may be chronic rather than acute and overwhelming, as in X-linked infantile hypogammaglobulinemia. Infections may be caused by pneumococci, *H influenzae,* or other pyogenic organisms. Chronic bacterial conjunctivitis may be an additional presenting complaint. Some patients develop severe malabsorption prior to the diagnosis of hypogammaglobulinemia. The malabsorption may be severe enough to cause protein loss sufficient to produce edema. Giardiasis, cholelithiasis, and achlorhydria are additional findings.

Autoimmune disease has been a presenting complaint in some patients with acquired hypogammaglobulinemia. A rheumatoid arthritis-like disorder, systemic lupus erythematosus (SLE), idiopathic thrombocytopenic purpura, dermatomyositis, hemolytic anemia, hypothyroidism, Graves' disease, and pernicious anemia have been reported in association with acquired hypogammaglobulinemia.

In contrast to patients with X-linked infantile hypogammaglobulinemia, those with acquired hypogammaglobulinemia may have marked lymphadenopathy and splenomegaly. Intestinal lymphoid nodular hyperplasia has been described in association with malabsorption. Other abnormal physical findings relate to the presence of chronic lung disease or intestinal malabsorption. Leukemia, lymphoma, and gastric carcinoma occur with increased frequency.

B. Laboratory Findings: Immunoglobulin measurements may show slightly higher IgG levels than are reported in X-linked infantile hypogammaglobulinemia. Total immunoglobulin levels are usually below 300 mg/dL, and the IgG level is usually below 250 mg/dL. IgM and IgA may be absent or present in significant amounts. The Schick test is useful to demonstrate a lack of normal antibody response, but it should be performed following booster immunization with diphtheria antigen. Blood group isohemagglutinins are absent or present in low titers (<1:10). The failure to produce antibody following specific immunization establishes the diagnosis in patients who have borderline immunoglobulin values. Live attenuated vaccines should not be used for immunization. Peripheral blood B lymphocytes are usually present in normal numbers in patients with acquired hypogammaglobulinemia, in contrast to their absence in patients with X-linked infantile hypogammaglobulinemia.

Although most patients with acquired hypogammaglobulinemia have intact cell-mediated immunity, a significant number demonstrate abnormalities as evidenced by absent delayed hypersensitivity skin test responses, depressed responses of isolated peripheral blood lymphocytes to PHA and allogeneic cells, and decreased numbers of T cell rosettes. NK cell activity is normal. A few patients have been found to have abnormal macrophage–T cell interaction. Repetition of these tests is important, because the immunodeficiency appears to progressively involve cell-mediated immunity, resulting in additional immunologic deficiencies.

Biopsy of lymphoid tissue demonstrates a lack of plasma cells. Although some lymph node biopsies may reveal lymphoid hyperplasia, there is a striking absence of cells in the B cell-dependent areas similar to that seen in congenital hypogammaglobulinemia.

C. Other Tests: Other tests that may be abnormal in these patients relate to associated disorders. The chest x-ray usually shows evidence of chronic lung disease, and sinus films show chronic sinusitis. Pulmonary function studies are abnormal. Patients with malabsorption may have abnormal gastrointestinal tract biopsies, with blunting of the villi similar to that seen in celiac disease. Studies for malabsorption may indicate a lack of normal intestinal enzymes and an abnormal D-xylose absorption test. Occasionally, autoantibodies may be found in patients who have an associated autoimmune hemolytic anemia or SLE. Autoantibodies are not found in those with an associated pernicious anemia, but biopsies of the stomach demonstrate marked lymphoid cell infiltration. Lymphoreticular cancers and thymomas have occurred in some patients.

Immunologic Diagnosis

The total immunoglobulin level is below 300 mg/dL, with the IgG level below 250 mg/dL. IgM and IgA may be absent or present in normal amounts. The antibody response following specific immunization is absent. Isohemagglutinins are depressed, and the Schick test is reactive. The number of circulating peripheral blood B cells is usually normal but may be decreased.

Cell-mediated immunity may be intact or may be depressed, with negative hypersensitivity skin tests, depressed responses of peripheral blood lymphocytes to PHA and allogeneic cells, and decreased numbers of circulating peripheral blood T cells. The number of B cells in the peripheral blood may be normal or diminished. There is occasionally an increased number of null cells, ie, lymphocytes lacking surface markers for either T or B cells.

Differential Diagnosis

The clinical presentation of patients with X-linked infantile hypogammaglobulinemia and those with acquired hypogammaglobulinemia may be similar. This does not present a major clinical problem. Severe malabsorption in protein-losing enteropathy may cause hypogammaglobulinemia, but these patients always have a concomitant deficiency of serum albumin. Differentiating between protein-losing enteropathy and acquired hypogammaglobulinemia may be difficult under circumstances where protein-losing enteropathy is accompanied by gastrointestinal loss of lymphoid cells. In both groups of patients, antibody responses and cell-mediated immunity may be impaired. When the presenting feature of acquired hypogammaglobulinemia is an autoimmune disease, there may be a delay in recognizing and treating the immune deficiency. In most instances, however, patients with autoimmune disease have normal or elevated immunoglobulin levels. Patients with chronic lung disease should also be investigated for cystic fibrosis, chronic allergy, α_1-antitrypsin deficiency, or immotile cilia syndrome. Patients with HIV infection may occasionally develop hypogammaglobulinemia.

Treatment

The treatment of acquired hypogammaglobulinemia is identical to that of X-linked infantile hypogammaglobulinemia (Table 23–5). Gamma globulin and continuous administration of antibiotics are usually required. Intravenous gamma globulin at doses of 100–200 mg/kg is given once each month. During acute illnesses, gamma globulin can be given weekly or daily. Patients should be monitored at regular intervals with chest x-rays and pulmonary function tests to determine the adequacy of therapy. Pulmonary physical therapy is an essential part of treatment in patients with chronic lung disease.

Specific treatment of malabsorption problems may be required. Some patients respond to treatment with gamma globulin. In others, the malabsorption may be associated with secondary enzymatic deficiencies that resemble celiac disease. These patients may respond to dietary restrictions. If the malabsorption is associated with *G lamblia* infection, metronidazole therapy should be used.

Caution should be exercised in the treatment of associated autoimmune disorders. The use of corticosteroids and immunosuppressive agents in a patient with immunodeficiency may result in markedly increased susceptibility to infection. Splenectomy has been used in the treatment of hypogammaglobulinemia and hemolytic anemia, but the mortality rate from overwhelming infection is high.

Complications & Prognosis

Patients with acquired hypogammaglobulinemia may survive to the seventh or eighth decade. Women with this disorder have had normal pregnancies and delivered normal infants (albeit hypogammaglobulinemic until 6 months of age). The major complication is chronic lung disease, which may develop despite adequate gamma globulin replacement therapy. An increased prevalence of malignant disease, including leukemia, lymphoma, and gastric carcinoma, has been observed. Patients who develop acquired T cell deficiencies have increasing difficulty with infection characteristic of both T and B cell deficiencies.

IMMUNODEFICIENCY WITH HYPER-IgM

This syndrome, characterized by an increased level of IgM (ranging from 150 to 1000 mg/dL) associated with a deficiency of IgG and IgA, is relatively rare and in most instances appears to be inherited in a X-linked manner. However, several cases have been reported of an acquired form that affects both sexes. The cause is not known. It has been postulated that in the normal individual there is a sequential development of immunoglobulins, initiated by IgM production and subsequently resulting in the production of IgG and IgA. Arrest in the development of immunoglobulin-producing cells after the formation of IgM-producing cells would be a possible cause. The disorder may be congenital, acquired, or a complication of EBV infection. Inheritance may be X-linked or autosomal dominant or recessive.

Patients present with recurrent pyogenic infections, including otitis media, pneumonia, and septicemia. Some have recurrent neutropenia, hemolytic anemia, or aplastic anemia.

Laboratory evaluation reveals a marked increase in the serum IgM level, with absence of IgG and IgA. Isohemagglutinin titers may be elevated, and the patient may form antibodies following specific immunization. Detailed studies of cell-mediated immunity have not been performed, but some reports indicate that it is intact. Patients with this disorder may develop an infiltrating neoplasm of IgM-producing plasma cells.

Treatment is similar to that of X-linked infantile hypogammaglobulinemia (Table 23–5). Because so few cases have been reported, it is difficult to determine the prognosis.

SELECTIVE IgA DEFICIENCY

Major Immunologic Features

■ IgA level is below 5 mg/dL, with other immunoglobulin levels normal or increased.

■ Cell-mediated immunity is usually normal.

■ There is increased association with allergies, recurrent sinopulmonary infection, gastrointestinal tract disease, and autoimmune disease.

General Considerations

Selective IgA deficiency is the most common immunodeficiency disorder. The prevalence in the normal population has been estimated to vary between 1:800 and 1:600. Considerable debate exists about whether individuals with selective IgA deficiency are "normal" or have significant associated diseases. Studies of individual patients and extensive studies of large numbers of patients suggest that absence of IgA predisposes to a variety of diseases. The diagnosis of selective IgA deficiency is established by finding a serum IgA level of less than 5 mg/dL.

Immunologic Pathogenesis

The cause of selective IgA deficiency is not known. An arrest in the development of B cells has been suggested on the basis of the observation that these patients have increased numbers of B cells with both surface IgA and IgM or surface IgA and IgD. An associated IgG2 subclass deficiency has been found in some patients, and this has been used to explain the varied clinical manifestations related to antibody deficiency. The presence of normal numbers of circulating IgA-bearing B cells suggests that this disorder is associated with decreased synthesis or release of IgA or impaired differentiation to IgA plasma cells rather than with the absence of IgA B lymphocytes. Utilizing the concept of sequential immunoglobulin production (IgM to IgG to IgA), selective IgA deficiency could result from an arrest in the development of immunoglobulin-producing cells following the normal sequential development of IgM to IgG. The variety of diseases associated with selective IgA deficiency may be the result of enhanced or prolonged exposure to a spectrum of microbial agents and nonreplicating antigens as a consequence of deficient secretory IgA. The continuous assault by these agents on a compromised mucosal immune system could result in an increased incidence of infection, autoantibodies, autoimmune disease, and cancer. Recently, an increased prevalence of HLA-A1, -B8, and -Dw3 has been found in patients with IgA deficiency and autoimmune disease.

Lymphocyte culture studies in IgA-deficient patients have demonstrated that IgA cells synthesize but fail to secrete IgA. Some individuals have suppressor T cells that selectively inhibit IgA production by normal lymphocytes.

Acquired IgA deficiency and susceptibility to sinopulmonary tract infections occur frequently in patients treated with phenytoin or penicillamine. In at least some instances, the IgA level returns to normal when the drug therapy is stopped.

Clinical Features

A. Symptoms and Signs:

1. Recurrent sinopulmonary infection–The most frequent presenting symptoms are recurrent sinopulmonary viral or bacterial infections. Patients may occasionally present with recurrent or chronic right middle lobe pneumonia. Pulmonary hemosiderosis occurs with increased frequency and may be erroneously diagnosed as chronic lung infection.

2. Allergy–In surveys of selected atopic populations the prevalence of selective IgA deficiency is 1:400–1:200, compared with a prevalence of 1:800–1:600 in the normal population. Although the reasons for this association are not known, the absence of serum IgA may result in a significant reduction in the amount of antibody competing for antigens capable of combining with IgE. Alternatively, patients who lack IgA in their secretions may more readily absorb allergenic proteins, thereby enhancing the formation of IgE antibodies. Allergic diseases in patients with selective IgA deficiency are often more difficult to control than the same allergies in other patients. Allergic symptoms in these patients may be "triggered" by infection as well as by other environmental agents.

An increase in circulating antibody to bovine proteins, sometimes associated with circulating immune complexes, including complexes with human antibody to bovine immunoglobulin, has been found in patients with selective IgA deficiency. This has been interpreted as providing additional evidence for abnormal gastrointestinal tract absorption. However, removal of cow's milk from the diet is usually not effective in ameliorating symptoms.

A unique form of allergy exists in these patients. Certain patients with selective IgA deficiency develop high titers of antibody directed against IgA. Anaphylactic reactions from infusion of blood products containing IgA occur in some of these patients. The prevalence of antibodies directed against IgA in patients, however, is much higher (30–40%) than the prevalence of such anaphylactic transfusion reactions. Most patients who have anti-IgA antibodies have not had a history of gamma globulin or blood administration, suggesting that these antibodies are "autoantibodies" or that they arise from sensitization to breast milk, passive transfer of maternal IgA, or cross-reaction with bovine immunoglobulin from ingestion of cow's milk.

3. Gastrointestinal tract disease–An increased prevalence of celiac disease has been noted in patients with selective IgA deficiency. The disease may present at any time and is similar to celiac disease unassociated with IgA deficiency. Intestinal biopsies show an increase in the number of IgM-producing cells. An anti-basement membrane antibody has also been found with increased incidence. Ulcerative colitis and regional enteritis have also been reported in association with selective IgA deficiency. Pernicious anemia has been found in a significant number of patients who also have antibodies to both intrinsic factor and gastric parietal cells.

4. Autoimmune disease–A number of autoimmune disorders are associated with selective IgA deficiency. They include SLE, rheumatoid arthritis, dermatomyositis, pernicious anemia, thyroiditis, Coombs-positive hemolytic anemia, Sjögren's syndrome, and chronic active hepatitis. Although the association of IgA deficiency and certain autoimmune disorders may be fortuitous, the increased prevalence of IgA deficiency in patients with SLE and rheumatoid arthritis (1:200–1:100) is statistically significant.

The clinical presentation of patients with autoimmune disease associated with selective IgA deficiency does not appear to differ significantly from that of individuals with the identical disorder and normal or elevated levels of IgA. Because patients with selective IgA deficiency are capable of making normal amounts of antibody in the other immunoglobulin classes, they usually have the autoantibodies that characterize the specific autoimmune disease (antinuclear antibody, anti-DNA antibody, antiparietal cell antibody, etc).

5. Selective IgA deficiency in apparently healthy adults–Patients with selective IgA deficiency are capable of making normal amounts of antibody of the IgG and IgM classes. Many are entirely asymptomatic, although long-term follow-up of some of these patients indicates that they may develop significant disease with time. There are several reasons why some patients remain asymptomatic. A small percentage of patients with selective IgA deficiency have normal amounts of secretory IgA and normal numbers of plasma cells containing IgA along the gastrointestinal tract. IgA-deficient patients have increased amounts of low-molecular-weight (7S) IgM in their secretions, which may subserve the secretory antibody function in place of IgA antibodies. Finally, patients with selective IgA deficiency may have different exposures to pathogens and noxious agents in the environment.

6. Selective IgA deficiency and genetic factors—Both an autosomal recessive and an autosomal dominant mode of inheritance of IgA deficiency have been postulated. IgA deficiency appears with greater than normal frequency in families with other immunodeficiency disorders such as hypogammaglobulinemia. Partial deletion of the long or short arm of chromosome 18 (18q syndrome) or ring chromosome 18 has been described in selective IgA deficiency. However, many patients with abnormalities of chromosome 18 have normal levels of IgA in their serum. Selective IgA deficiency has been reported in one identical twin but not the other. In a study of familial IgA deficiency, an association with HLA-A2, -B8, and -Dw3 was described. Other studies have shown an increase in association with HLA-A1 and -B8.

7. Selective IgA deficiency and cancer—Selective IgA deficiency has been reported in association with thymoma, reticulum cell sarcoma, and squamous cell carcinoma of the esophagus and lungs. Several patients with IgA deficiency and cancer also had concomitant autoimmune disease and recurrent infection.

8. Selective IgA deficiency and drugs—Phenytoin and other anticonvulsants have been implicated as a possible cause of some cases of selective IgA deficiency or hypogammaglobulinemia, and these patients are frequently symptomatic with recurrent sinopulmonary infections. Withdrawal of the drug does not always result in a return to normal IgA levels. In vitro production of IgA by peripheral blood lymphocytes in these patients may be normal or deficient. Deficient T-cell/B-cell interaction is found in some patients.

B. Laboratory Findings: Selective IgA deficiency is defined as a serum level of IgA below 5 mg/dL, with normal or increased levels of IgG, IgM, IgD, and IgE. Some patients with IgA deficiency may also have IgG2 subclass deficiency. Because there are a number of methods for measuring immunoglobulin levels, each laboratory should establish standards for detection of low IgA levels. B cells from these patients are capable of forming normal amounts of antibody following immunization. In most instances, absence of IgA in the serum is associated with absence of IgA in the secretions and with the presence of normal secretory component. Increased amounts of 7S IgM may be found in the serum and secretions. As discussed above, some patients have autoantibodies including antibodies directed against IgG, IgM, and IgA. The number of circulating peripheral blood B cells (including IgA-bearing B cells) is normal. Increased numbers of suppressor T cells have been found in some patients.

Cell-mediated immunity is normal in most patients. Delayed hypersensitivity skin tests, the response of isolated peripheral blood lymphocytes to PHA and allogeneic cells, and the number of circulating T cells are normal. A few patients have low levels of T cells, diminished production of T cell interferon, and decreased lymphocyte mitogenic responses.

Other laboratory abnormalities are those typical of the associated diseases. Individuals who have chronic sinopulmonary infection may have abnormal x-rays and abnormal pulmonary functions. Patients with IgA deficiency and celiac disease show appropriate pathology on gastrointestinal tract biopsies, impaired D-xylose absorption, and antibody directed against basement membrane in some cases. Patients with IgA deficiency and autoimmune disease have characteristic autoantibodies, eg, anti-DNA, antinuclear, antiparietal cell, and a positive Coombs test. An increase in circulating immune complexes has been described.

Differential Diagnosis

Selective IgA deficiency must be distinguished from other more severe immunodeficiency disorders with a concomitant deficiency of IgA. Forty percent of patients with ataxia-telangiectasia have IgA deficiency. These patients usually have cellular immunodeficiency as well. If IgA deficiency is found during the first years of life, a definitive diagnosis may not be possible because the complete ataxia-telangiectasia syndrome may not be present until the patient is 4–5 years old. Other immunodeficiency disorders that have been associated with selective IgA deficiency are chromatic mucocutaneous candidiasis and cellular immunodeficiency with abnormal immunoglobulin synthesis (Nezelof's syndrome) and selective deficiency of IgG2. A careful history should be obtained to rule out IgA deficiency secondary to drugs, especially anticonvulsants or penicillamine.

Treatment

Patients with selective IgA deficiency should not be treated with gamma globulin. Therapeutic gamma globulin contains only a small quantity of IgA, and this is not likely to reach mucosal secretions through parenteral administration. Furthermore, IgA-deficient patients are capable of forming normal amounts of antibody of other immunoglobulin classes. Finally, they recognize injected IgA as foreign, so that gamma globulin infusions in these patients enhance the risk of development of anti-IgA antibodies and subsequent anaphylactic transfusion reactions. There is as yet no means by which the deficient IgA can be safely replaced. Patients with combined IgA and IgG subclass deficiency with documented impaired antibody formation have been treated with gamma globulin, but its efficacy has yet to be documented. Patients with recurrent sinopulmonary infection should be treated aggressively with broad-spectrum antibiotics to avoid permanent pulmonary complications. Patients with SLE, rheumatoid arthritis, celiac disease, etc, are treated in the same fashion as patients with the same diseases without IgA deficiency.

Transfusion reactions in patients with selective IgA deficiency may be minimized by several means. Packed washed (3 times) erythrocytes should be used to treat anemia. Although this does not completely eliminate the possibility of a transfusion reaction, it will decrease the risk. Alternatively, patients may be given blood from an IgA-deficient donor whose blood type matches the recipient's. Preserving the patient's own plasma and erythrocytes for future use is recommended if possible.

Complications & Prognosis

IgA-deficient patients have survived to the sixth or seventh decade without severe disease. Most individuals, however, become symptomatic during the first decade of life. Recognition of the potential complications and prompt therapy for associated diseases will increase longevity and reduce the morbidity rate. Regular follow-up examinations are necessary for early detection of associated disorders and complications. A very few patients have developed normal IgA levels after years of IgA deficiency.

SELECTIVE IgM DEFICIENCY

Selective IgM deficiency is a rare disorder associated with the absence of IgM and normal levels of other immunoglobulin classes. IgM-bearing B cells are present in normal numbers. Some patients have decreased helper T cell activity. Some patients are capable of normal antibody responses in the other immunoglobulin classes following specific immunization, whereas others respond poorly. Cell-mediated immunity appears to be intact, but there has been an insufficient number of detailed studies to confirm this.

The cause of selective IgM deficiency is unknown. Increased suppressor T cell activity specific for IgM has been described. The absence of IgM in the presence of IgG and IgA has yet to be explained, since it appears to contradict the theory of sequential immunoglobulin development. The disorder has been found in both males and females.

Patients with selective IgM deficiency are susceptible to autoimmune disease and to overwhelming infection with polysaccharide-containing organisms (eg, pneumococci, *H influenzae*). They may also have chronic dermatitis, diarrhea, and recurrent respiratory infections. Insufficient data are available to determine appropriate therapy. It would appear logical to manage these patients in a manner similar to the way an infant is managed following splenectomy, ie, either immediate antibiotic (penicillin or

ampicillin) treatment of all infections or continuous antibiotic treatment. If patients are unable to form antibody to specific antigens, gamma globulin therapy should be given.

SELECTIVE DEFICIENCY OF IgG SUBCLASSES

Major Immunologic Features

- One or more IgG subclasses are deficient.
- T cell immunity is normal.
- Patients have recurrent bacterial infections.
- The condition is sometimes associated with other immunodeficiencies such as selective IgA deficiency or ataxia-telangiectasia.

General Considerations

IgG antibodies exist in 4 isotypic variants identified by antigenic differences of the Fc portion of the immunoglobulin molecule. These are termed IgG1, IgG2, IgG3, and IgG4 and make up approximately 65%, 20%, 10%, and 5% of the total serum immunoglobulin levels, respectively (Fig 24–3). IgG subclasses develop independently, with IgG1 and IgG3 maturing more rapidly than IgG2 or IgG4. Deletion of constant heavy-chain genes or abnormalities of

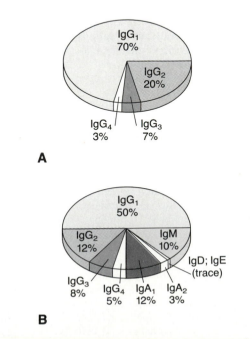

Figure 24–3. Normal distribution of serum immunoglobulins. **A:** Percentages of IgG subclasses relative to total IgG. **B:** Percentages of immunoglobulin classes and subclasses relative to total immunoglobulin.

isotype switching may result in deficiencies of one or more of the IgG subclasses.

Clinically, patients have recurrent respiratory tract infections and repeated pyogenic sinopulmonary infections with *S pneumoniae, H influenzae,* and *Staphylococcus aureus*. Some patients develop or present with evidence of autoimmune diseases such as SLE or pulmonary hemosiderosis. As selective deficiency of IgG subclasses may be found in other immunodeficiency disorders such as ataxia-telangiectasia or selective IgA deficiency, other features of immunodeficiency may predominate.

IgG2-IgG4 deficiency is usually found in individuals with recurrent infections or autoimmune disease who are either normoglobulinemic or hypergammaglobulinemic. A few healthy individuals with this deficiency have been described. It is also found in some patients with ataxia-telangiectasia.

IgG2 deficiency is associated with recurrent sinopulmonary infections and an inability to respond to polysaccharide antigens (such as pneumococcal or *H influenzae* polysaccharide). However, the patient does respond normally to protein antigens such as tetanus or diphtheria toxoid.

IgG3 deficiency is found in a small percentage of individuals with recurrent infections who are screened by specific IgG subclass determinations for antibody deficiency. Familial occurrence of IgG3 deficiency has been reported.

IgG4 deficiency is also associated with recurrent respiratory infections and/or manifestations of autoimmune disease. It occurs with approximately the same frequency in individuals with recurrent respiratory tract infections as does IgG3 deficiency.

A diagnosis of one or more IgG subclass deficiencies is made by the finding of significantly low levels of one or more IgG subclasses compared with those in age-matched normal controls. The total IgG concentration may be normal, low, or elevated. The response to immunization may be variable, ranging from normal to a selective inability to respond to polysaccharide antigens. T cell immunity is usually intact.

Most patients with selective IgG subclass deficiency respond to treatment with gamma globulin administered in a manner similar to that used in the treatment of hypogammaglobulinemia.

X-LINKED LYMPHOPROLIFERATIVE SYNDROME
(Duncan's Syndrome)

Major Immunologic Features

- Patients are susceptible to fatal EBV infection.
- Hypogammaglobulinemia develops.
- Lymphoma develops.

General Considerations

The X-linked lymphoproliferative syndrome is associated with EBV infection. Following infection with EBV, several outcomes are possible: (1) fatal infectious mononucleosis, with severe liver disease and hepatitis accounting for most of the deaths; (2) fatal infectious mononucleosis with lymphoma; (3) infectious mononucleosis with immunodeficiency; and (4) lymphoma. Approximately 63% of patients develop fatal infectious mononucleosis, 29% develop immunodeficiency, and 24% develop lymphoma. The mortality rate associated with this syndrome is 85% by 10 years of age and 100% by 40 years of age.

Immunologic abnormalities include inverted helper/suppressor T cell ratios, deficient proliferative responses of mononuclear cells to mitogenic stimulation, defective gamma interferon production, and decreased NK cell activity. Abnormalities of B cell immunity include hypogammaglobulinemia, failure to switch from IgM- to IgG-specific antibody following immunization with bacteriophage, and lack of antibody to EBV, especially to EBV nuclear antigen (EBNA). These abnormalities are found primarily in long-term survivors. In contrast, patients who die early as a result of EBV infection may have normal T cell and B cell immunity prior to infection, suggesting that the immune defect in X-linked lymphoproliferative syndrome is probably a progressive one.

There is no effective treatment to prevent the progression of the immunodeficiency in this syndrome. If hypogammaglobulinemia develops, gamma globulin therapy should be given. Recently, the genetic defect has been located by restriction fragment length polymorphism mapping. In the future it should be possible to identify carriers of the genetic defect, provide appropriate genetic counseling, and diagnose the disease in utero.

REFERENCES

X-Linked Infantile Hypogammaglobulinemia

Rosen FS, Janeway CA: The gamma globulins. 3. The antibody deficiency syndromes. *N Engl J Med* 1966; **275:**709.

Siegel RL et al: Deficiency of T helper cells in transient hypogammaglobulinemia of infancy. *N Engl J Med* 1981;**305:**1307.

Van Maldergem L et al: Echovirus meningoencephalitis in X-linked hypogammaglobulinemia. *Acta Paediatr Scand* 1989;**78:**325.

Common Variable Hypogammaglobulinemia

Cunningham-Rundles C: Clinical and immunologic analyses of 103 patients with common variable immunodeficiency. *J Clin Immunol* 1989;**9:**22.

Hermans PE, Diaz-Buxo JA, Stobo JD: Idiopathic late-onset immunoglobulin deficiency: Clinical observations in 50 patients. *Am J Med* 1976;**61:**221.

Ochs H: Intravenous immunoglobulin therapy of patients with primary immunodeficiency syndromes. Pages 9–14 in: *Immunoglobulins: Characteristics and Uses of Intravenous Preparations.* US Department of Health and Human Services, 1981.

Saiki O et al: Three distinct stages of B cell defects in common varied immunodeficiency. *Proc Natl Acad Sci USA* 1982;**79:**6008.

White WB et al: Immunoregulatory effects of intravenous immune serum globulin therapy in common variable hypogammaglobulinemia. *Am J Med* 1987;**83:**431.

X-Linked Immunodeficiency with Hyper-IgM

Eskola J et al: Regulatory T-cell function in primary humoral immunodeficiency states. *J Clin Lab Immunol* 1989;**28:**55.

Ohno T et al: Selective deficiency in IL-2 production and refractoriness to extrinsic IL-2 in immunodeficiency with hyper-IgM. *Clin Immunol Immunopathol* 1987;**45:**471.

Stiehm ER, Fudenberg HH: Clinical and immunologic features of dysgammaglobulinemia type 1. *Am J Med* 1966;**40:**895.

Selective IgA Deficiency

Ammann AJ, Hong R: Selective IgA deficiency: Presentation of 30 cases and a review of the literature. *Medicine* 1971;**50:**223.

Ferreira A et al: Anti-IgA antibodies in selective IgA deficiency and in primary immunodeficient patients treated with gamma-globulin. *Clin Immunol Immunopathol* 1988;**47:**199.

Oxelius VA et al: IgG subclass deficiency in selective IgA deficiency. *N Engl J Med* 1981;**305:**1476.

Selective IgM Deficiency

Guill MF et al: IgM deficiency: Clinical spectrum and immunologic assessment. *Ann Allergy* 1989;**62:**547.

IgG Subclass Deficiency

Heiner DC: Recognition and management of IgG subclass deficiencies. *Pediatr Infect Dis J* 1987;**6:**235.

Ochs HD, Wedgwood RJ: Disorders of the B-cell system. Pages 226–256 in: *Immunologic Disorders in Infants and Children.* Stiehm ER (editor). Saunders, 1989.

Ochs HD, Wedgwood RJ: IgG subclass deficiencies. *Annu Rev Med* 1987;**38:**325.

Schur PH et al: Selective gamma-G globulin deficiencies in patients with recurrent pyogenic infections. *N Engl J Med* 1970;**283:**631.

X-Linked Lymphoproliferative Syndrome

Grierson H, Putillo DT: Epstein-barr virus infections in males with X-linked lymphoproliferative syndrome. *Ann Intern Med* 1987;**106:**538.

Webster AD et al: Viruses and antibody deficiency syndromes. *Immunol Invest* 1988;**17:**93.

T Cell Immunodeficiency Disorders 25

Arthur J. Ammann, MD

Immunodeficiency disorders associated with isolated defective T cell immunity are rare. These diseases were formerly called cellular immunodeficiencies. In most patients, defective T cell immunity is accompanied by abnormalities of B cell immunity. This reflects the collaboration between T cells and B cells in the process of antibody formation. Thus, almost all patients with complete T cell deficiency have some impairment of antibody formation. Some patients with T cell deficiency have normal levels of immunoglobulin but fail to produce specific antibody following immunization. These patients are considered to have a qualitative defective in antibody production.

Patients with cellular immunodeficiency disorders are susceptible to a variety of viral, fungal, and protozoal infections. These infections may be acute or chronic.

Screening tests utilized to evaluate T cell immunity are listed in Table 23–4. The availability of additional tests for the evaluation of T cell immunity (Table 25–1) permits more precise diagnosis in many instances.

CONGENITAL THYMIC APLASIA (DiGeorge's Syndrome, Immunodeficiency With Hypoparathyroidism)

Major Immunologic Features
- There is congenital aplasia or hypoplasia of the thymus.
- Lymphopenia reflects a decreased number of T cells.
- T cell function in peripheral blood is absent.
- Antibody levels and function are variable.
- Treatment with thymus graft is successful.

General Considerations
DiGeorge's syndrome is one of the few immunodeficiency disorders associated with symptoms immediately following birth. The complete syndrome consists of the following features: (1) abnormal facies consisting of low-set ears, "fish-shaped" mouth, hypertelorism, notched ear pinnae, micrognathia, and an antimongoloid slant of eyes (Fig 25–1); (2) hypoparathyroidism; (3) congenital heart disease; and (4) cellular immunodeficiency. Initial symptoms are related to associated abnormalities of the parathyroids and heart and may result in hypocalcemia and congestive heart failure, respectively. If the diagnosis of DiGeorge's syndrome is suspected because of these early clinical findings, confirmation may be obtained by demonstrating defective T cell immunity. The importance of early diagnosis is related to the complete reconstitution of T cell immunity that can be achieved following a fetal thymus transplant or thymic factor therapy (Table 23–5).

Immunologic Pathogenesis
During weeks 6–8 of intrauterine life, the thymus and parathyroid glands develop from epithelial evaginations of the third and fourth pharyngeal pouches (Fig 25–2). The thymus begins to migrate caudally during week 12 of gestation. At the same

Table 25–1. Evaluation of cell-mediated immunity.

Test	Comment
Total lymphocyte count	Normal at any age: >1200/ μL.
Delayed hypersensitivity skin test	Used to evaluate specific immunity to antigens. Suggested antigens are *Candida,* mumps, purified protein derivative, and streptokinase-streptodornase (4 units per 0.1 mL).
Lymphocyte response to mitogens (PHA), antigens, and allogeneic cells (mixed-lymphocyte culture)	Used to evaluate T cell function. Results are expressed as stimulated counts divided by resting counts (stimulated index).
Total T cells using monoclonal antibodies to CD3, CD2, or CD4 plus CD8	Used to quantitate the number of circulating T cells. Normal: >60% of total lymphocytes.
Monoclonal antibody to T cells and T cell subsets (CD4 and CD8)	Determines total number of T cells as well as T cell subsets, eg, helper/ suppressor.
Cytokine production (IL-1, IL-2, lymphotoxin, tumor necrosis factor, etc)	Used to detect specific cytokine production from subsets of mononuclear cells as an index of function.
Helper/suppressor T cell function	Provides information on T cell regulation of immunity.

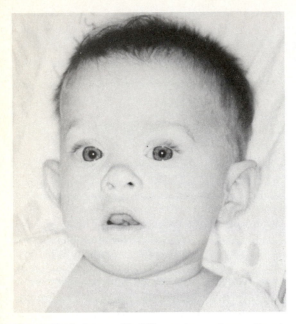

Figure 25–1. Infant with DiGeorge's syndrome. Prominent are low-set and malformed ears, hypertelorism, fish-shaped mouth. Also note the surgical scar from cardiac surgery.

time, the philtrum of the lip and the ear tubercle become differentiated along with other aortic arch structures. It is likely that DiGeorge's syndrome is the result of interference with normal embryologic development at approximately 12 weeks of gestation. In some patients, the thymus is not absent but is in an abnormal location or is extremely small, though the histologic appearance is normal. It is possible that such patients have "partial" DiGeorge's syndrome, in which hypertrophy of the thymus may take place with subsequent development of normal immunity. Following thymic transplantation, there is rapid T cell reconstitution, lack of graft-versus-host (GVH) reaction, and lack of cellular chimerism, suggesting that patients lack a thymic humoral factor capable of expanding their own T cell immunity.

Clinical Features

A. Symptoms and Signs: The most frequent presenting sign in patients with DiGeorge's syndrome occurs in the first 24 hours of life with hypocalcemia that is resistant to standard therapy. Various types of congenital heart disease have been described, including interrupted aortic arch, septal defects, patent ductus arteriosus, and truncus arteriosus. Renal abnormalities may also be present. Some

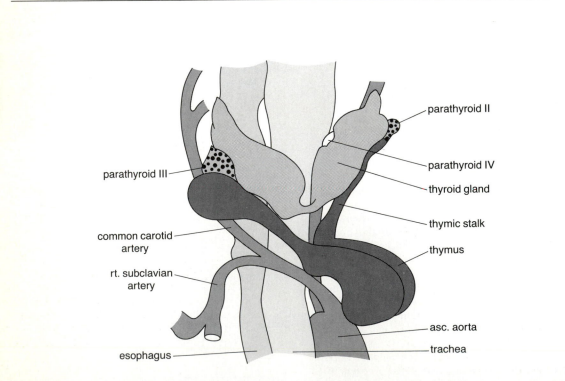

Figure 25–2. Embryologic development of the thymus and parathyroid glands from the third and fourth pharyngeal pouches.

patients have the characteristic facial appearance described above. Patients who survive the immediate neonatal period may then develop recurrent or chronic infection with various viral, bacterial, fungal, or protozoal organisms. Pneumonia, chronic infection of the mucous membranes with *Candida,* diarrhea, and failure to thrive may be present.

Spontaneous improvement of T cell immunity occasionally occurs. These patients are considered to have "partial" DiGeorge's syndrome, but the reason for the spontaneous improvement in T cell immunity is not known. Patients have also been suspected of having DiGeorge's syndrome on the basis of hypocalcemia and congenital heart disease with or without the abnormal facies, but have been found to have normal T cell immunity. Subsequently, these patients may develop severe T cell deficiency.

B. Laboratory Findings: Evaluation of T cell immunity can be performed immediately after birth in a patient suspected of having DiGeorge's syndrome. The lymphocyte count is usually low ($<1200/\mu L$) but may be normal or elevated. In the absence of stress during the newborn period, a lateral view x-ray of the anterior mediastinum may reveal absence of the thymic shadow, indicating failure of normal development. Delayed hypersensitivity skin tests to recall antigens are of little value during early infancy, because sufficient time has not elapsed for sensitization to occur. T cells are markedly diminished in number, and the peripheral blood lymphocytes fail to respond to phytohemagglutinin (PHA) and allogeneic cells.

Studies of antibody-mediated immunity in early infancy are not helpful, because immunoglobulins consist primarily of passively transferred maternal IgG. Although it is believed that some of these patients have a normal ability to produce specific antibody, the majority have some impairment of antibody formation. Sequential studies of both T cell and B cell immunity are necessary, since spontaneous remissions and spontaneous deterioration of immunity with time have been described.

A diagnosis of hypoparathyroidism is established by the demonstration of low serum calcium levels, elevated serum phosphorus levels, and an absence of parathyroid hormone. Congenital heart disease may be diagnosed immediately following birth and may be mild or severe. Other congenital abnormalities include esophageal atresia, bifid uvula, and urinary tract abnormalities.

Immunologic Diagnosis

T cell immunity is usually absent at birth as indicated by lymphocytopenia, depressed numbers of circulating T cells, and no response of peripheral blood lymphocytes to PHA and allogeneic cells. Rarely, normal T cell immunity may develop with time or previously normal T cell immunity may become deficient. In some patients, studies of T cell functions are variable and range from diminished T cell numbers with normal function to a complete absence of T cell immunity.

Some patients with DiGeorge's syndrome have normal B cell immunity as indicated by normal levels of immunoglobulins and a normal antibody response following immunization. However, some patients have low immunoglobulin levels and fail to make specific antibody following immunization. Live attenuated viral vaccines should not be used for immunization. Natural killer (NK) cell activity is normal.

Rarely, a patient may present with the immunologic features of severe combined immunodeficiency, ie, absent T cell and B cell immunity. The presence of hypocalcemia or congenital abnormalities of the third and fourth aortic arch establishes the diagnosis.

Differential Diagnosis

Many infants with severe congenital heart disease and subsequent congestive heart failure develop transient hypocalcemia. These infants should be suspected of having DiGeorge's syndrome. When the characteristic facial features are found, in addition to the hypocalcemia and congenital heart disease, an even stronger suspicion is present. Studies of T cell immunity will usually establish a diagnosis, except in infants with DiGeorge's syndrome who have developed effective T cell immunity with time. It is essential that all infants with congenital heart disease and hypocalcemia be monitored until they are at least 1 year old. The hypocalcemia associated with DiGeorge's syndrome is usually permanent, in contrast to that seen in congenital heart disease with congestive heart failure. Congenital hypoparathyroidism is usually not associated with congenital heart disease. However, both in this disorder and in DiGeorge's syndrome, levels of parathyroid hormone are low to absent and the patients are resistant to the standard treatment for hypocalcemia. Low parathyroid hormone levels may also be found in transient hypocalcemia in infancy. Two patients with DiGeorge's syndrome are known to have had spontaneous remissions of their hypoparathyroidism.

Immunologic studies in DiGeorge's syndrome and in severe combined immunodeficiency disease may be identical in the newborn period. The presence of hypocalcemia, congenital heart disease, and an abnormal facies differentiate DiGeorge's syndrome from severe combined immunodeficiency disease.

Patients with the fetal alcohol syndrome may have similar facial and cardiac abnormalities to those in patients with DiGeorge's syndrome, as well as recurrent infections associated with decreased T cell immunity.

Treatment

A fetal thymus transplant should be given as soon

as possible following diagnosis. This can result in permanent reconstitution of T cell immunity. The technique of thymus transplantation varies from local implantation in the rectus abdominis muscle to implantation of a thymus in a Millipore chamber. The thymus may also be minced and injected intraperitoneally. Because patients with DiGeorge's syndrome have been observed to develop a GVH reaction following administration of viable immunocompetent lymphocytes, fetal thymus glands older than 14 weeks of gestation should not be used. Thymocytes from glands younger than 14 weeks of gestation lack cells capable of GVH reaction but can provide needed stem cells or thymic epithelial cells for further T cell development. Patients have been successfully treated with thymosin and thymus epithelial transplants.

The hypocalcemia is rarely controlled by calcium supplementation alone. Calcium should be administered orally in conjunction with vitamin D or parathyroid hormone.

Congenital heart disease frequently results in congestive heart failure and may require immediate surgical correction. If surgery is performed prior to the availability of a fetal thymus transplant, any blood given should be irradiated with 3000 R to prevent a GVH reaction.

Complications & Prognosis

Prolonged survivals have been reported following successful thymus transplantation or spontaneous remission of immunodeficiency. Sudden death may occur in untreated patients or in patients initially found to have normal T cell immunity. Congenital heart disease may be severe, and the infant may not survive surgical correction. Death from GVH disease following blood transfusions has been observed in patients in whom a diagnosis of DiGeorge's syndrome was not suspected.

CHRONIC MUCOCUTANEOUS CANDIDIASIS
(With & Without Endocrinopathy)

Major Immunologic Features
■ Onset may be either with chronic candidial infection of the skin and mucous membranes or with endocrinopathy.
■ Delayed hypersensitivity skin tests to *Candida* antigen are negative despite chronic candidal infection.

General Considerations

Chronic mucocutaneous candidiasis affects both males and females. A familial occurrence has been reported, suggesting an autosomal recessive inheritance. The disorder is associated with a selective defect in T cell immunity, resulting in susceptibility to chronic candidal infection. B cell immunity is intact,

resulting in a normal antibody response to *Candida* and, in some patients, the development of autoantibodies associated with idiopathic endocrinopathies. The disorder may appear as early as 1 year of age or may be delayed until the second decade.

Various theories have been proposed to explain the association of chronic candidal infection and the development of endocrinopathy. Initially it was believed that hypoparathyroidism predisposed to candidal infection. Subsequently it was found that many patients developed severe candidal infection without evidence of hypoparathyroidism. A basic autoimmune disorder has been postulated, with the suggestion that the thymus also functions as an endocrine organ and that the thymus and other endocrine glands are involved in an autoimmune destructive process.

Clinical Features
A. Symptoms and Signs: The initial presentation of chronic mucocutaneous candidiasis may be either chronic candidal infection or the appearance of an idiopathic endocrinopathy. If candidal infection appears first, several years to several decades may elapse before endocrinopathy occurs. Other patients may present with the endocrinopathy first and subsequently develop the infection. Candidal infection may involve the mucous membranes, skin, nails, and, in older patients, the vagina. In severe forms, infection of the skin occurs in a "stocking-glove" distribution and is associated with the formation of granulomatous lesions (Fig 25–3). Patients are usually not susceptible to systemic candidiasis. Rarely, they may develop infection with other fungal agents.

Other symptoms are related to the specific endocrinopathy. Hypoparathyroidism is the most common and is associated with hypocalcemia and tetany. Addison's disease is the next most common. A variety of other endocrinopathies have been reported, including hypothyroidism, diabetes mellitus, and pernicious anemia. Occasionally, there is a history of acute or chronic hepatitis preceding the onset of endocrinopathy. Additional disorders include pulmonary fibrosis, ovarian failure, adrenocorticotropic hormone (ACTH) deficiency, and keratoconjunctivitis.

B. Laboratory Findings: Studies of T cell immunity reveal a specific although variable defect. Patients usually have a normal total lymphocyte count. Peripheral blood lymphocytes respond normally to PHA, allogeneic cells, and antigens other than *Candida* antigens. The least severe T cell defect is an absent delayed hypersensitivity skin test response to *Candida* antigen in the presence of documented chronic candidiasis. Other patients may have additional defects, including the inability to form migration inhibitory factor (MIF) in response to *Candida* antigens or inability of lymphocytes to be activated by *Candida* antigens and decreased suppressor

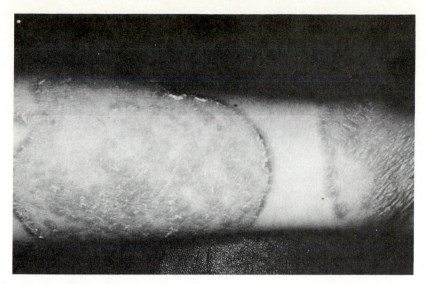

Figure 25–3. Chronic *Candida* infection in a patient with mucocutaneous candidiasis. Note the well-demarcated areas of involvement.

T cell activity. B cell immunity is intact, as demonstrated by the presence of normal or elevated levels of immunoglobulins, increased amounts of antibody directed against *Candida,* and autoantibody formation. Occasionally, selective absence of IgA or elevated levels of immunoglobulins may be observed. Plasma inhibitors of T cell function and increased numbers of suppressor T cells have been reported in some cases. Isolated cases have been described with neutrophil chemotaxis or macrophage abnormalities.

Other laboratory abnormalities are related to the presence of endocrinopathies. Hypoparathyroidism is associated with decreased serum calcium levels, elevated serum phosphorus levels, and low or absent parathyroid hormone levels. Increased skin pigmentation may herald the onset of Addison's disease prior to disturbances in serum electrolytes. An ACTH stimulation test is useful to document the presence of Addison's disease. Other abnormalities of endocrine function include hypothyroidism, abnormal vitamin B_{12} absorption, and diabetes mellitus. Abnormal liver function studies may indicate chronic hepatitis. Occasionally, iron deficiency is present, which, when treated, results in improvement in the candidal infection. Autoantibodies associated with specific endocrinopathy are usually present before and during the development of endocrine dysfunction. They may be absent when complete endocrine deficiency is present. Patients should be evaluated on a yearly basis for endocrine function because the endocrinopathies are progressive.

Immunologic Diagnosis

Major aspects of T cell immunity are normal, as indicated by a normal response of peripheral blood lymphocytes to PHA and allogeneic cells. Activation of lymphocytes and MIF production in response to antigens other than *Candida* antigens is normal. T cell numbers are normal. In some patients, only the delayed hypersensitivity skin test response to *Candida* antigens is absent. Other patients have absent MIF production or an absence of lymphocyte activation by *Candida* antigens. Plasma inhibitors of cellular immunity may also occur. B cell immunity is intact with normal production of antibody to *Candida.*

Differential Diagnosis

Children with chronic candidal infection of the mucous membranes may have a variety of immunodeficiency disorders. Detailed studies of B cell and T cell immunity differentiate between chronic mucocutaneous candidiasis, in which there is a selective deficiency of T cell immunity to *Candida* antigens, and other disorders in which T cell immunity may be completely deficient. Patients with DiGeorge's syndrome (thymic aplasia and hypoparathyroidism) present early in infancy, whereas chronic mucocutaneous candidiasis with hypoparathyroidism is a disorder of later onset and progressive nature. Patients with late-onset idiopathic endocrinopathies should be considered to have chronic mucocutaneous candidiasis, even though candidal infection is not present at the time of diagnosis. These patients may develop chronic candidal infection as late as 10–15 years after the onset of endocrinopathy.

Treatment

There is no treatment to prevent the development of idiopathic endocrinopathy. The physician must be alert to the gradual development of endocrine dysfunction—particularly Addison's disease, which is the major cause of death. Chronic skin and mucous membrane candidal infection is difficult to treat. Topical treatment with a variety of antifungal agents has been attempted but has usually been unsuccessful. Local miconazole therapy has provided control in some patients in recent trials. Courses of intravenous amphotericin B have resulted in improvement in a significant number of patients, but this form of treatment is limited by the renal toxicity of the drug. Oral clotrimazole is occasionally beneficial. Oral ketoconazole, an antifungal agent, has been successfully used. The efficacy of transfer factor therapy with or without amphotericin B is unproven. Two patients refractory to all other forms of therapy were successfully treated with fetal thymus transplants.

Complications & Prognosis

Patients may survive to the second or third decade but usually experience extensive morbidity. Individuals with severe candidal infection of the mucous membranes and skin develop serious psychologic difficulties. Systemic infection with *Candida* usually does not occur. Rarely, patients may develop systemic infection with other fungal agents. Hypoparathyroidism is difficult to manage, and complications are frequent. Addison's disease is the major cause of death and may develop suddenly without previous symptoms.

IMMUNODEFICIENCY ASSOCIATED WITH NATURAL KILLER (NK) CELL DEFICIENCY

NK cells are negative for the T cell receptor-CD3 complex, but have receptors for the Fc portion of the immunoglobulin molecule (CD16) and a member of the complement/lymphocyte adhesion molecule (CD11b). In addition, they have the NKH-1 (CD56) determinant, which identifies the large granular lymphocyte population that NK cells resemble morphologically. NK cells spontaneously lyse a number of target cells, including tumor cells, but when activated by interleukin-2 (IL-2) or gamma interferon, they will lyse a broad range of virus-infected cells. It is therefore believed that these cells play a role in host defense against cancer and microbial infection.

Deficiency of NK cells is not confined to a single defined immunodeficiency disorder, although there are isolated case reports of what appear to be selective NK deficiencies. NK cell deficiency has been documented in the Chédiak-Higashi syndrome, the X-linked lymphoproliferative syndrome, the chronic fatigue syndrome, and leukocyte adhesion molecule (CD11/CD18) deficiency. NK cell deficiency has also been detected in primary immunodeficiency diseases, primarily in severe combined immunodeficiency disease and other T cell disorders, suggesting an association between NK and T cell defects.

Although NK cell deficiency has been detected most consistently in the X-linked lymphoproliferative syndrome, which is associated with fatal Epstein-Barr virus infection, cancer, and hypogammaglobulinemia, there has been a report of a female child who had recurrent severe infections with herpesviruses, including varicella, cytomegalovirus infection, and herpes simplex. Immunologic evaluation was normal, except for deficient NK cell numbers and function. The peripheral blood mononuclear cells were unable to mediate spontaneous or IL-2-induced NK cell functions. This case suggests that isolated defects in NK cell function exist. No specific treatment to correct the NK cell defect was attempted. Acyclovir was used to treat the acute infections, and the patient was maintained on intravenous gamma globulin.

REFERENCES

Thymic Aplasia with Hypoparathyroidism

Barrett DJ et al: Clinical and immunologic spectrum of the Di-George syndrome. *J Clin Lab Immunol* 1981;**6**:1.

DiGeorge AM: Congenital absence of the thymus and its immunologic consequences: Concurrence with congenital hypoparathyroidism. In: *Immunologic Deficiency Diseases in Man.* Bergsma D, McKusick FA (editors). National Foundation–March of Dimes Original Article Series. Williams & Wilkins, 1968.

Radford DJ et al: Spectrum of Di George syndrome in patients with truncus arteriosis: Expanded Di George syndrome. *Pediatr Cardiol* 1988;**9**:95.

Chronic Mucocutaneous Candidiasis

Arulanantham K, Dwyer JM, Genel M: Evidence for defective immunoregulation in the syndrome of familial candidiasis endocrinopathy. *N Engl J Med* 1979; **300**:164.

Kirkpatrick CH: Chronic mucocutaneous candidiasis. Antibiotic and immunologic therapy. *Ann NY Acad Sci* 1988;**544**:471.

Kirkpatrick CH, Rich RR, Bennett JE: Chronic mucocutaneous candidiasis: Model building in cellular immunity. *Ann Intern Med* 1971;**74**:955.

Mobacken H, Moberg S: Ketoconazole treatment of 13 patients with chronic mucocutaneous candidiasis: A prospective three year trial. *Dermatologica* 1986; **173**:229.

Natural Killer Cell Deficiency

Biron CA, Byron KS, Sullivan JL: Severe herpes virus infections in an adolescent without natural killer cells. *N Engl J Med* 1989;**320**:1731.

Ritz J: The role of natural killer cells in immune surveillance. *N Engl J Med* 1989;**320**:1789.

Combined Antibody (B Cell) & Cellular (T Cell) Immunodeficiency Disorders

26

Arthur J. Ammann, MD

Combined immunodeficiency diseases are variable in cause and severity. Defective T cell and B cell immunity may be complete, as in severe combined immunodeficiency disease, or partial, as in ataxia-telangiectasia. The distinct clinical features of ataxia-telangiectasia serve to further differentiate the disorder from severe combined immunodeficiency disease and also suggest that these disorders do not have the same cause. Enzymatic deficiencies in the purine pathway have been described in association with combined immunodeficiency. This discovery has provided additional evidence for a diverse origin of combined immunodeficiency disease.

Studies of both T cell and B cell immunity are necessary to completely evaluate patients with combined immunodeficiency disorders (see Tables 23–4, 24–1, and 25–1). In addition, analysis of erythrocyte and leukocyte enzymes (adenosine deaminase and nucleoside phosphorylase, respectively) can assist appropriate classification.

The onset of symptoms in patients with combined immunodeficiency diseases is usually early in infancy. These patients are susceptible to a very wide spectrum of microorganisms. Immunotherapy is frequently difficult and often not available.

SEVERE COMBINED IMMUNODEFICIENCY DISEASE

Major Immunologic Features
- The onset of symptoms occurs by 6 months of age, with recurrent viral, bacterial, fungal, and protozoal infections.
- X-linked, autosomal, and sporadic forms occur.
- Both T cell and B cell immunity are absent.

General Considerations
The immunologic deficiency includes the absence of T cell and B cell immunity, resulting early in susceptibility to infection by virtually all types of microorganisms. Patients rarely survive beyond 1 year of age before succumbing to one or more opportunistic infections. The disease is inherited in 2 forms: an X-linked recessive form (X-linked lymphopenic agammaglobulinemia) and an autosomal recessive form (Swiss-type lymphopenic agammaglobulinemia). The exact prevalence of this disorder is not known, and many patients die before the diagnosis is made. Because the immune system of patients with this disorder may be made completely normal by bone marrow transplantation, early diagnosis is crucial to prevent irreversible complications.

Immunologic Pathogenesis
The basic defect is not known, but it has been postulated that severe combined immunodeficiency disease is a result of failure of differentiation of stem cells into T cells and B cells. The successful use of histocompatible bone marrow transplantation has provided support for the concept of a basic stem cell defect. However, the defect may reside in the failure of the thymus and bursa equivalent to develop normally. Under these circumstances, normal stem cells would not be processed into T cells and B cells. Others argue for an intrinsic defect within the thymus, since the excess immature T cells from the patients mature when cultured in the presence of thymus epithelium.

Clinical Features
A. Symptoms and Signs: Patients with severe combined immunodeficiency disease usually succumb to overwhelming infection within the first year of life. Early findings include failure to thrive, chronic diarrhea, persistent thrush (oral candidiasis), pneumonia, chronic otitis media, and sepsis. The microorganisms that result in acute and chronic infection include viruses, bacteria, fungi, and protozoa. Infants with this disease are particularly susceptible to *Candida,* cytomegalovirus, and *Pneumocystis carinii* infection. When smallpox immunization was routinely administered, many of these infants developed progressive vaccinia. Death from progressive poliomyelitis following attenuated-virus immunization has been documented. During the first several months of life, patients may be partially protected from bacterial infections by the transplacental passive transfer of maternal IgG antibod-

ies. They subsequently develop susceptibility to a wide variety of gram-positive and gram-negative organisms.

As these patients lack T cell immunity entirely, they are susceptible to graft-versus-host (GVH) reactions that may develop following maternal infusion of cells during gestation or delivery, infusion of viable cells in the form of blood transfusions, or attempts at immunotherapy (see the discussion of GVH disease below). The presence of an acute or chronic GVH reaction, as a consequence of blood transfusion or engraftment of maternal cells, may complicate the diagnosis of severe combined immunodeficiency disease. Some of these patients have been misdiagnosed as having an acute viral illness, histiocytosis X, or other chronic disorders.

Physical findings relate to the degree and type of infections present. Pneumonia, otitis media, thrush, dehydration, skin infections, and developmental retardation may be present. Lymphoid tissue and hepatosplenomegaly are absent unless the disease is complicated by GVH reaction.

B. Laboratory Findings: All tests of T cell immunity are abnormal. The thymus is absent roentgenographically, lymphopenia is usually present, T cell numbers are markedly depressed, and the response of isolated peripheral blood lymphocytes to phytohemagglutinin (PHA) and allogeneic cells is absent. Rarely, there is a proliferative response to allogeneic cells. T cell subset analysis varies considerably. Specific antigens on T cells are absent in some patients, whereas in others they show developmental arrest at the prothymocyte level. Delayed hypersensitivity skin tests are not useful for diagnosis, because in most cases the patient is too young for sufficient time to have elapsed for antigen exposure and sensitization to occur. During the first 5–6 months of life, a diagnosis of severe combined immunodeficiency disease may be difficult to establish because of the presence of maternal IgG. However, most normal infants who have had repeated infection will develop significant amounts of serum IgM, IgA, or both. If the diagnosis is doubtful, it may be necessary to immunize the patient to determine specific antibody responses. Patients suspected of having immunodeficiency diseases should never be immunized with attenuated live virus vaccines. In the majority of patients with severe combined immunodeficiency, B cells are absent or markedly reduced from birth. A subgroup of patients exists in whom B cell numbers may be elevated. Natural killer (NK) cell activity may be normal or deficient. Adenosine deaminase activity is normal.

Biopsy of lymphoid tissue is rarely necessary to establish a diagnosis. If biopsies are obtained, they should be performed with strict antiseptic measures because secondary infection is frequent. Biopsy of lymph nodes (if they can be found) demonstrates severe depletion of lymphocytes, without cortico-medullary differentiation and without follicle formation. Biopsy of the intestinal tract shows a complete absence of plasma cells.

Patients who have pulmonary infiltrates that do not respond to antibiotic therapy or who have rapid respiration and low arterial blood P_{O2} should be suspected of having *P carinii* infection regardless of whether the x-ray is abnormal. Because this disorder can be treated, it is important to establish an early diagnosis. Some debate exists about whether the diagnosis is best made by means of concentrated-sputum examination, bronchoscopy, needle biopsy, or open-lung biopsy. In some instances, open-lung biopsy provides the most complete information. Cytomegalovirus infection should be considered in all patients. Cultures of blood, mucous membranes, and stools for predominant bacteria may be important in determining subsequent treatment. Individuals who have been inadvertently immunized with live poliovirus vaccine should have stools cultured for poliovirus.

Patients frequently have anemia and lymphopenia. Complications such as chronic systemic infection and GVH reaction may result in multiple abnormalities, including elevation of liver enzyme levels, jaundice, chronic diarrhea with subsequent electrolyte abnormalities and dehydration, pulmonary infiltrates, cardiac irregularities, and abnormal cerebrospinal fluid analysis.

Immunologic Diagnosis

Severe combined immunodeficiency disease is associated with complete absence of T cell and B cell immunity. Evaluation of T cell immunity reveals lymphopenia; absence of thymus shadow; depressed T cell numbers; absence of peripheral blood lymphocyte responses to PHA, allogeneic cells, and antigens; and absence of response to delayed hypersensitivity skin tests. Evaluation of B cell immunity reveals hypogammaglobulinemia, absence of antibody response following immunization, and few or no circulating B cells (rarely, elevated B cell numbers are found).

Differential Diagnosis

Severe combined immunodeficiency disease must be differentiated from other immunodeficiency disorders with defects in T cell and B cell immunity. The early onset of symptoms and the complete absence of both T cell and B cell immunity found in severe combined immunodeficiency disease usually result in a specific diagnosis. Combined immunodeficiency associated with the absence of an enzyme (adenosine deaminase) in the purine pathway may be differentiated from severe combined immunodeficiency disease by specific determination of adenosine deaminase activity. This disorder initially is usually less severe clinically and immunologically. The presence of a GVH reaction in a patient with severe combined immunodeficiency disease may complicate the diagnosis. If chronic dermatitis is present in association with hepatosplenomegaly and histiocytic infiltration, the condition may be mistaken for Letterer-Siwe syndrome. Some patients may present with chronic diarrhea and pigmentary skin changes, resulting in an erroneous diagnosis of acrodermatitis enteropathica (see the discussion of GVH disease below). Omenn's syndrome closely resembles severe combined immunodeficiency with GVH disease and is believed by some not to be a distinct syndrome.

Treatment

Aggressive diagnostic measures are necessary to establish the cause of chronic infection before treatment can be instituted. Open-lung biopsy should be performed if *P carinii* infection is suspected. The treatment of choice for *P carinii* infection consists of pentamidine and trimethoprim-sulfamethoxazole given simultaneously. Specific antibiotic treatment is necessary for suspected bacterial infection. Superficial candidal infection is treated with topical antifungal drugs, but systemic infection requires intravenous amphotericin B or ketoconazole therapy.

Complications must be avoided. Immunization with live attenuated virus should not be performed. Blood products containing potentially viable lymphocytes should be irradiated with 3000–6000 R prior to administration (see the discussion of GVH disease below). Prophylactic trimethoprim-sulfamethoxazole should be used to prevent *P carinii* infection.

During the initial period of evaluation, gamma globulin may be administered in doses of 0.2–0.4 mL/kg intramuscularly once a month or as frequently as once a week. Severely ill patients appear to improve with the use of intravenous gamma globulin in doses of 100–400 mg/kg every 1–4 weeks. Definitive treatment consists of transplantation of histocompatible bone marrow. Because of the inheritance of the histocompatibility antigens, the usual donor for a bone marrow transplant is a histocompatible sibling. The bone marrow must be matched for human leukocyte antigens (HLA) A, B, C, and D by the mixed leukocyte reaction (MLR). Despite careful matching, a GVH reaction may develop. Several techniques have been used in performing bone marrow transplantation, including intraperitoneal injection and intravenous infusion of filtered bone marrow. The dose of bone marrow cells administered has varied, but injection of as few as 1000 nucleated cells per kilogram has resulted in successful immunologic reconstitution. Transplantation of unmatched marrow has previously resulted in a fatal GVH reaction. Recently, however, some investigators have used unmatched marrow from nonsibling donors, which was prepared by lectin separation of cells or marrow treated with monoclonal antibody to reduce the GVH potential. The results are promising.

In the absence of a histocompatible bone marrow donor, other forms of therapy have been used. Long-term survivors of fetal liver (<9 weeks' gestation) transplants and of fetal thymus (<14 weeks' gestation) transplantation have been observed. In both of these techniques, the use of older fetal liver or thymus will result in a fatal GVH reaction, probably because of the presence of mature immunocompetent cells. Thymus epithelial transplants and combined fetal liver and thymus transplants have also been used. In most instances these approaches have been replaced by bone marrow transplantation.

Complications & Prognosis

Patients with severe combined immunodeficiency disease are unusually susceptible to infection with many microorganisms and will die before 1 year of age if untreated. If the diagnosis is not made immediately, the patient may receive live attenuated poliovirus immunization and succumb to progressive poliomyelitis. In other instances, patients may receive unirradiated blood products and die from complications of GVH disease. Following successful bone marrow transplantation, 10-year survivals with maintenance of normal T cell and B cell function have been recorded. Patients have survived as long as 1 year following fetal liver transplantation and as long as 6 years following fetal thymus transplantation. Complete reconstitution of immunity in patients receiving fetal organ transplantation has not yet been achieved.

CELLULAR IMMUNODEFICIENCY WITH ABNORMAL IMMUNOGLOBULIN SYNTHESIS (Nezelof's Syndrome)

Major Immunologic Features

- Patients are susceptible to viral, bacterial, fungal, and protozoal infection.
- T cell immunity is depressed or absent.
- There are various degrees of B cell immunodeficiency associated with various combinations of increased, normal, or decreased immunoglobulin levels.

General Considerations

The disorders included in this classification are diverse and probably do not all have the same cause. Consistent features include marked deficiency of T cell immunity and various degrees of deficiency of B cell immunity. Disorders with specific clinical symptomatology or laboratory abnormalities, such as ataxia-telangiectasia and Wiskott-Aldrich syndrome, and those associated with enzyme deficiency, such as adenosine deaminase deficiency, are excluded here. Part of the difficulty in defining disorders in this category relates to recent developments in the diagnosis of T cell immunity that were not available when some of these cases were first reported. Most of the cases included in this category are sporadic and do not have a defined inheritance pattern.

Immunologic Pathogenesis

The cause is not known. There appears to be no specific genetic pattern. The syndrome is sporadic in distribution and occurs in both males and females. The presence of moderate to severe deficiencies of T cell immunity with various degrees of B cell immunodeficiency suggests that the primary defect is within the thymus. It is possible that this disorder is the result of thymic hypoplasia with deficient interaction of T cells and B cells and subsequent abnormal antibody formation.

Clinical Features

A. Symptoms and Signs: Patients are susceptible to recurrent fungal, protozoal, viral, and bacterial infections. The spectrum of infection is similar to that found in patients with congenital hypogammaglobulinemia and other forms of combined immunodeficiency. Patients frequently have marked lymphadenopathy and hepatosplenomegaly, in contrast to patients with congenital hypogammaglobulinemia and severe combined immunodeficiency disease.

B. Laboratory Findings: T cell immunity is abnormal, but the degree of deficiency may vary. Lymphopenia may be present, but occasionally a normal lymphocyte count is obtained. T cell numbers are moderately to markedly decreased. The lymphocyte response to PHA and specific antigens may be absent or slightly depressed, and the lymphocyte response to allogeneic cells may vary from zero to normal. B cell immunity is abnormal. The 5 immunoglobulin classes may be present in various combinations of increased, normal, or decreased amounts. Total circulating B cells are usually present in normal numbers, although the distribution among various types of surface immunoglobulin-bearing B cells may vary. Despite the presence of normal or elevated levels of immunoglobulin, there is no antibody response following specific immunization. Antibodies to specific antigens may be present, however, indicating that at one time some of these patients may have been able to form antibody. Isohemagglutinins may be absent or normal, and the Schick test may be either reactive or nonreactive.

Biopsy of lymphoid tissue in these patients may reveal the presence of plasma cells. The lymph nodes may be large and may contain numerous histiocytes and macrophages with granuloma formation.

Immunologic Diagnosis

The principal immunologic features in this group of disorders are moderate to marked reductions in the number of total lymphocytes and T cells and a diminished response of peripheral blood lymphocytes to PHA, allogeneic cells, and specific antigens. There is usually no response to delayed hypersensitivity skin tests. Variable degrees of B cell deficiency are present, consisting of various combinations of elevated, normal, or low levels of specific immunoglobulin classes. The antibody response to specific antigens is usually absent. Some evidence of prior antibody formation may be found, eg, a nonreactive Schick test and the presence of isohemagglutinins. The number of total circulating B cells is usually normal.

Differential Diagnosis

Because there is a lack of uniformity in the clinical and laboratory presentation of these patients, it is necessary to rule out other disorders with definite clinical or laboratory associations. The clinical features of ataxia-telangiectasia are usually present by 3–4 years of age, and an elevated level of alpha-fetoprotein is usually present by 1 year of age. Patients with Wiskott-Aldrich syndrome have thrombocytopenia from birth and can be excluded on this basis. Patients with severe combined immunodeficiency disease have complete absence of T cell and B cell immunity. Immunodeficiency disorders with associated enzyme deficiencies may have a similar presentation and are excluded on the basis of enzyme analysis of erythrocytes or leukocytes. Patients with short-limbed dwarfism are excluded on the basis of characteristic clinical and radiologic features. Patients with cellular immunodeficiency and abnormal immunoglobulin synthesis do not develop endocrine abnormalities and can therefore be distinguished from patients with DiGeorge's syndrome and chronic mucocutaneous candidiasis, who are capable of normal antibody synthesis. Culture of human immunodeficiency virus (HIV) or antibody to HIV is necessary to distinguish a child with acquired immunodeficiency syndrome (AIDS) from one with this disorder.

Treatment

Aggressive treatment of infection is necessary. Patients failing to show an antibody response after immunization (even if immunoglobulin levels are normal) should receive gamma globulin once a month (see the discussion of the treatment of hypogammaglobulinemia above). Continuous broad-spectrum antibiotic coverage may be useful. Postural drainage is important to prevent chronic lung disease.

Although histocompatible bone marrow transplantation would appear to be curative in these patients, few successes have been reported. This appears to be due to a lack of histocompatible donors rather than the complications of transplantation. Thymus transplantation and the use of several thymus factors have been reported to provide reconstitution of T cell immunity and partial reconstitution of B cell immunity.

Patients should not be immunized with attenuated live viral vaccines. All blood products should be irradiated with 3000 R.

Complications & Prognosis

Patients do not develop the severe complications observed in severe combined immunodeficiency disease. A GVH reaction is possible, but none has been reported. Some of these patients, however, may develop progressive encephalitis following immunization with live attenuated virus. Chronic lung disease, chronic fungal infection, and later development of cancer are long-term complications. Survival until the age of 18 years has been recorded.

IMMUNODEFICIENCY WITH ATAXIA-TELANGIECTASIA

Major Immunologic Features

- Clinical onset occurs by 2 years of age.
- Complete syndrome consists of ataxia, telangiectasia, and recurrent sinopulmonary infection.
- Selective IgA deficiency is present in 40% of patients.

General Considerations

Ataxia-telangiectasia is inherited in an autosomal recessive manner. It is associated with characteristic features, including ataxia, telangiectasia, recurrent sinopulmonary infection, and abnormalities in both T cell and B cell immunity. The disorder was first considered to be primarily a neurologic disease; it is now known to involve the neurologic, vascular, endocrine, and immune systems.

Immunologic Pathogenesis

There is no unifying theory that explains the multisystem abnormalities present in ataxia-telangiectasia. A defect in the development of mesoderm has been postulated but not confirmed. Other abnormalities that may account for some of the multisystem disorders are abnormal collagen (deficient in hydroxylysine); elevated alpha-fetoprotein level, indicative of a defect in organ maturation; enhanced susceptibility of cells to radiation damage; and defective DNA repair. Clones of lymphocytes with structural rearrangements of band q11 of chromosome 14 and bands q32-35 and p13-15 of chromosome 7 have been consistently found. These chromosome markers may be found in malignant cell lines isolated from ataxia-telangiectasia patients. It is of interest that the structural rearrangements are at the locations that bear the T cell receptor genes. The disorder is progressive, with both the neurologic abnormalities and the immunologic deficiency becoming more severe over time.

Clinical Features

A. Symptoms and Signs: The onset of ataxia may occur at 9 months to 1 year of age or may be delayed as long as age 4–6 years. Telangiectasia is usually present by 2 years of age but has been delayed until 8–9 years of age (Fig 26–1). As patients become older, additional neurologic symptoms develop, consisting of choreoathetoid movements, dysconjugate gaze, and extrapyramidal and posterior column signs. Telangiectasia may develop first in the bulbar conjunctiva and subsequently appear on the bridge of the nose, on the ears, or in the antecubital fossae. Recurrent sinopulmonary infections may begin early in life, or patients may remain relatively symptom-free for 10 years or more. There is increased susceptibility to both viral and bacterial infections. Secondary sexual characteristics rarely develop in patients at puberty, and most patients appear to develop mental retardation with time.

B. Laboratory Findings: Various degrees of abnormalities in T and B cell immunity have been described. Lymphopenia may be present, T cell numbers may be normal or decreased, and the response of lymphocytes to PHA and allogeneic cells may be normal or decreased. There may be no response to delayed hypersensitivity skin tests. IgG2, IgG4, or IgA2 subclass deficiency is present in some patients. In still other patients, IgE may be absent. Antibody responses to specific antigens may be depressed. The number of circulating B cells is usually normal. NK cell activity is normal.

Other laboratory abnormalities relate to associated findings. Abnormalities have been shown on pneumoencephalography. Endocrine studies have shown decreased 17-ketosteroids and increased follicle-stimulating hormone (FSH) excretion. An insulin-resistant form of diabetes has been found. Cytotoxic antibodies to brain and thymus have been found. Increased levels of alpha-fetoprotein have been found in all patients tested, but may not be specific for the disease, as increased levels have also been found in other immunodeficiency disorders. Alpha-feto-

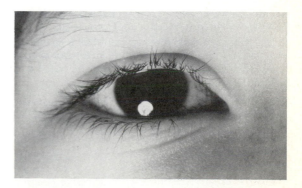

Figure 26–1. Telangiectasis of the conjunctivae and over the bridge of the nose in a child with ataxia-telangiectasia.

protein levels are also high in normal infants until 1 year of age. Many patients have elevated titers to Epstein-Barr virus (EBV) antigens.

Immunologic Diagnosis

Selective IgA deficiency is found in 40% of patients. IgA2, IgG2, or IgG4 subclass deficiency has also been described. IgE deficiency and variable deficiencies of other immunoglobulins may also be found. The antibody response to specific antigens may be depressed. Variable degrees of T cell deficiency are observed; these usually become more severe with advancing age.

Differential Diagnosis

If the onset of recurrent infection occurs before the development of ataxia or telangiectasia, it may be difficult to differentiate this disorder from cellular immunodeficiency with abnormal immunoglobulin synthesis. If a patient has a gradual onset of cerebellar ataxia unassociated with telangiectasia and immunologic abnormalities, it may take years before a diagnosis can be established with certainty. Usually, by the age of 4 years, the characteristic recurrent sinopulmonary infections, immunologic abnormalities, ataxia, and telangiectasia are present simultaneously. Because selective IgA deficiency is the most common immunodeficiency disorder detected and many patients with selective IgA deficiency have no associated symptomatology, it may take several years before a diagnosis of ataxia-telangiectasia can be excluded. Alpha-fetoprotein levels are normal in patients with IgA deficiency.

Treatment

Early treatment of recurrent sinopulmonary infections is essential to avoid permanent complications. Some patients may benefit from continuous broad-spectrum antibiotic therapy. In patients who develop chronic lung disease, physical therapy with postural drainage is beneficial. Successful bone marrow transplantation has not been performed, but this is probably related to the lack of histocompatible bone marrow donors. Fetal thymus transplantation has provided some benefit in a limited number of patients. Thymic factor therapy has been used on an experimental basis to treat a limited number of patients. The use of intravenous gamma globulin in a patient unable to form antibody may result in a reduced number of infections (see Chapter 24).

Attenuated viral vaccines should not be given. All blood products should be irradiated with 3000 R prior to administration.

Complications & Prognosis

Long-term survivors develop progressive deterioration of neurologic and immunologic functions. The oldest patients have reached the fifth decade of life. The chief causes of death are overwhelming infec-

tion and lymphoreticular or epithelial cell cancer. Leukemias, some with associated abnormalities of chromosome 14, have been reported in 24% of patients (Fig 26–2) and non-Hodgkin lymphomas have been reported in 45% of patients. As these patients reach the second decade, morbidity becomes severe, with chronic lung disease, mental retardation, and physical debility being the principal problems. Heterozygote carriers as well as family members have an increased incidence of cancer.

IMMUNODEFICIENCY WITH THROMBOCYTOPENIA, ECZEMA, & RECURRENT INFECTION (Wiskott-Aldrich Syndrome)

Major Immunologic Features

- Complete syndrome consists of eczema, recurrent pyogenic infection, and thrombocytopenia.
- It can be diagnosed at birth by demonstration of thrombocytopenia in a male infant with a positive family history.
- The serum IgM level is usually low, with elevated serum IgA and IgE levels.
- Thrombocytopenia is characterized by small platelets.

General Considerations

Patients may become symptomatic early in life, with bleeding secondary to thrombocytopenia. Subsequently they develop recurrent bacterial infection in the form of otitis media, pneumonia, and meningitis. Eczema usually appears by 1 year of age. The disease is progressive, with increasing susceptibility to infection and cancer. It is inherited in an X-linked manner. At autopsy, the thymus and lymph nodes have an abnormal architecture, with depletion of T cells, poor follicle formation, and poor corticomedullary differentiation.

Immunologic Pathogenesis

Two of the earliest abnormalities are thrombocytopenia and hypercatabolism of immunoglobulin.

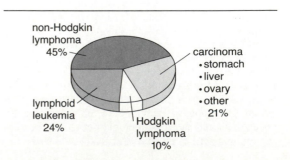

Figure 26–2. Relative percentages of cancers reported in patients with ataxia-telangiectasia.

There are several hypotheses linking thrombocytopenia, eczema, and recurrent infection. It has been suggested that there are abnormal α granules of platelets and macrophages in patients and carriers. Another suggestion is that the inability of patients to respond to polysaccharide antigens results in immunologic attrition. This, however, does not explain the thrombocytopenia or eczema. An MW 115,000 surface glycoprotein termed sialophorin is absent, present at reduced levels, or abnormal in lymphocytes from patients. Normally this glycoprotein is present in lymphocytes, monocytes, and platelets, and its absence is believed to result in early senescence of cells.

Clinical Features

A. Symptoms and Signs: Recurrent infection usually does not start until after 6 months of age. Patients are susceptible to infection with capsular polysaccharide-type organisms (eg, *Pneumococcus, Meningococcus,* and *Haemophilus influenzae*), which cause meningitis, otitis media, pneumonia, and sepsis. As the patients become older, they become susceptible to infection with other types of organisms and may have recurrent viral infection. Eczema is usually present by 1 year of age and is typical in distribution (Fig 26–3). It may be associated with other allergic manifestations. Frequently, it is secondarily infected. Thrombocytopenia is present at birth and may result in early manifestations of bleeding. Bleeding is usually increased during episodes of infection and is associated with a decrease in the platelet count. The bleeding tendency becomes less severe as the child becomes older.

B. Laboratory Findings: Thrombocytopenia is present at birth, and this fact is helpful in diagnosis. The platelet count may range from 5000 to 100,000/μL. Platelets are small in Wiskott-Aldrich syndrome, in contrast to those in other disorders associated with thrombocytopenia, eg, idiopathic

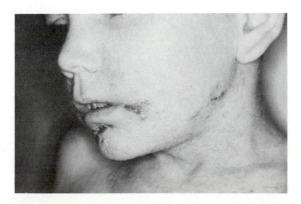

Figure 26–3. Chronic facial eczema in a child with Wiskott-Aldrich syndrome.

thrombocytopenia, in which they are larger than normal. Anemia is frequently present and may be Coombs-positive. An increased incidence of chronic renal disease has been reported.

Immunologic Diagnosis

The earliest detected immunologic abnormality consists of hypercatabolism of immunoglobulins. Studies of B cell immunity demonstrate normal IgG levels, decreased IgM levels, increased IgA and IgE levels, few or absent isohemagglutinins, normal numbers of B cells, and an inability to respond to immunization with polysaccharide antigen. Paraproteins are frequently observed. T cell immunity is usually intact early in the disease but may decline with advancing years.

Differential Diagnosis

When the complete syndrome is present, there is little doubt about the diagnosis. Idiopathic thrombocytopenia in a male child may be difficult to differentiate from Wiskott-Aldrich syndrome. In idiopathic thrombocytopenia, the immunoglobulins, isohemagglutinins, and response to polysaccharide antigens are normal. Small platelets favor the diagnosis of Wiskott-Aldrich syndrome. Male patients with eczema and recurrent infection have normal immunologic studies and normal platelet counts, although they may have elevated levels of serum IgA and IgE.

Treatment

Infections should be treated promptly and aggressively with antibiotics effective against the most common organisms. Corticosteroids should not be used to treat the thrombocytopenia, since they will enhance the susceptibility to infection. Splenectomy has been fatal in this disease, but there have been recent attempts to use splenectomy and continuous antibiotic prophylaxis to prevent both bleeding and infectious complications. Treatment of immunodeficiency is difficult. Intramuscular gamma globulin is not used, because of the thrombocytopenia and potential bleeding at injection sites, but intravenous gamma globulin can be given (see Chapter 24). Successful bone marrow transplantation has been achieved.

Complications & Prognosis

With aggressive therapy, the long-term prognosis has improved. Immediate complications are related to bleeding episodes and acute infection. As patients become older, they become susceptible to a wider spectrum of microorganisms. Chronic keratitis secondary to viral infection is frequent. Lymphoreticular cancers, especially of the central nervous system, occur in older patients. Myelogenous leukemia occurs more frequently in this disorder than in other immunodeficiency disorders.

IMMUNODEFICIENCY WITH THYMOMA

Major Immunologic Features
- Recurrent infections occur.
- Acquired hypogammaglobulinemia may precede or follow thymoma.

General Considerations

Recurrent infection may be the presenting sign if the thymoma is associated with immunodeficiency. This takes the form of sinopulmonary infection, chronic diarrhea, dermatitis, septicemia, stomatitis, and urinary tract infection. Thymoma has also been associated with muscle weakness (when found in conjunction with myasthenia gravis), aregenerative anemia, thrombocytopenia, diabetes, amyloidosis, chronic hepatitis, and the development of nonthymic cancer.

Patients with acquired hypogammaglobulinemia should be observed at regular intervals for the development of thymoma, which is usually detected on routine chest x-rays. Occasionally, the thymoma may be detected prior to the development of immunodeficiency. Marked hypogammaglobulinemia is usually present. The antibody response following immunization may be abnormal. Some patients have deficient T cell immunity as assayed by delayed hypersensitivity skin tests and response of peripheral blood lymphocytes to PHA. Increased activity of suppressor cells has been found in some patients. In patients who have aregenerative anemia, pure erythrocyte aplasia is seen on marrow aspiration. Thrombocytopenia, granulocytopenia, and autoantibody formation are occasionally observed. In 75% of cases, the thymoma is of the spindle cell type. Some tumors may be malignant.

In no instance has the removal of the thymoma resulted in improvement of immunodeficiency. This is in contrast to pure erythrocyte aplasia and myasthenia gravis, which may improve following removal of the thymoma. Gamma globulin is beneficial in controlling recurrent infections and chronic diarrhea (see Chapter 24).

The overall prognosis is poor, and death secondary to infection is common. Death may also be related to associated abnormalities such as thrombocytopenia and aregenerative anemia.

IMMUNODEFICIENCY WITH SHORT-LIMBED DWARFISM

Major Immunologic Features
- Both T and B cell immunodeficiency may be found.
- Recurrent systemic infections occur.
- Prognosis is variable.

General Considerations

Three forms of immunodeficiency with short-limbed dwarfism exist. Type I is associated with combined immunodeficiency, type II with T cell immunodeficiency, and type III with B cell immunodeficiency.

The clinical features of each type vary with the degree of immunodeficiency. In short-limbed dwarfism associated with combined immunodeficiency, symptoms of infection are identical to those seen in severe combined immunodeficiency disease. Susceptibility to viral, bacterial, fungal, and protozoal infection is observed. Patients usually die in the first year of life. Patients with short-limbed dwarfism and T cell immunodeficiency are susceptible to recurrent sinopulmonary infection, fatal varicella, and progressive vaccinia, and they may develop a malabsorptionlike syndrome. Patients with short-limbed dwarfism and B cell immunodeficiency experience recurrent pyogenic infections in the form of pneumonia, sepsis, otitis media, and meningitis. In all patients, short-limbed dwarfism is characterized by short, pudgy hands and extremities (Fig 26–4). The head is normal in size, which distinguishes this dis-

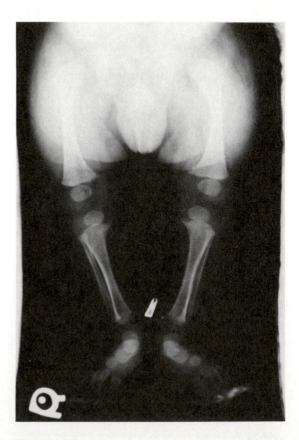

Figure 26–4. X-ray of extremities in a child with cartilage-hair hypoplasia and immunodeficiency. Note the redundant skin folds.

order from achondroplasia. During infancy, redundant skin folds are often seen around the neck and large joints of the extremities. Patients with short-limbed dwarfism and T cell immunodeficiency may also have cartilage-hair hypoplasia, manifested by light, thin, and sparse hair.

Immunologic abnormalities vary with the degree of immunodeficiency. In short-limbed dwarfism associated with combined immunodeficiency, T cell and B cell immunity are absent. In short-limbed dwarfism associated with T cell immunodeficiency, T cell immunity is deficient as measured by delayed hypersensitivity skin tests and responsiveness of peripheral blood lymphocytes to PHA, allogeneic cells, and varicella antigens, whereas B cell immunity is intact. In short-limbed dwarfism associated with B cell immunodeficiency, B cell immunity is absent and T cell immunity is intact.

Radiologic abnormalities consist of scalloping, irregular sclerosis, and cystic changes in the metaphyseal portions of long bones (Fig 26–4). Aganglionic megacolon has been reported. Patients with cartilage-hair hypoplasia have reduced hair diameters and lack the pigmented central core.

Treatment of these disorders is individualized to the associated immunodeficiency (eg, severe combined immunodeficiency, cellular immunodeficiency, and antibody immunodeficiency).

The prognosis varies with the degree of immunodeficiency. There have been no survivors with severe combined immunodeficiency disease. Patients with T cell immunodeficiency may survive to the fourth or fifth decade only to succumb to overwhelming varicella infection. The prognosis in patients with antibody immunodeficiency is similar to that of patients with X-linked hypogammaglobulinemia, but loss of T cell function may occur over time.

IMMUNODEFICIENCY WITH ENZYME DEFICIENCY

1. ADENOSINE DEAMINASE & NUCLEOSIDE PHOSPHORYLASE DEFICIENCY

Major Immunologic Features

- Recurrent and severe viral, bacterial, fungal, and protozoal infections occur.
- There are varied degrees of T and B cell immunodeficiency.
- Purine enzyme activity is absent or reduced.

General Considerations

Patients with enzyme deficiency and immunodeficiency may have clinical and laboratory abnormalities identical to those of patients with immunodeficiency and normal enzyme activity. Enzyme deficiency as a cause of immunodeficiency probably accounts for fewer than 15% of immunodeficiency disorders at present. It is almost certain that additional enzyme deficiencies will be discovered.

Adenosine deaminase and purine nucleoside phosphorylase are necessary for the normal catabolism of purines (Fig 26–5). Adenosine deaminase catalyzes the conversion of adenosine and deoxyadenosine to inosine and deoxyinosine. Nucleoside phosphorylase catalyzes the conversion of inosine, deoxyinosine, guanosine, and deoxyguanosine to hypoxanthine and guanine. Several mechanisms have been postulated to explain the means whereby these enzyme deficiencies result in immunodeficiency. Experimental evidence indicates that adenosine, in increased amounts, may result in increased cyclic AMP (cAMP) activity, which is known to be associated with inhibition of lymphocyte function. Adenosine has also been shown to be toxic to cells in culture as a result of pyrimidine starvation. There is also evidence that exogenous adenosine can lead to the intracellular accumulation of S-adenosylhomocysteine, which acts as a potent inhibitor of DNA methylation. However, the most likely mechanism of inhibition of lymphocyte function is a result of the accumulation of deoxyadenosine and subsequently deoxy-ATP, which results in inhibition of ribonucleotide reductase and subsequent depletion of deoxyribonucleoside triphosphates. In purine nucleoside phosphorylase deficiency, deoxyguanosine has been shown to result in the accumulation of deoxy-GTP. Again, this most probably results in inhibition of ribonucleotide reductase. These mechanisms have great importance in devising potential biochemical treatment for these disorders.

The degree of combined immunodeficiency is variable. The spectrum of immunologic aberrations varies from complete absence of T cell and B cell immunity, as observed in patients with severe combined immunodeficiency disease, to mild abnormalities of T cell and B cell function. Patients with enzyme deficiencies should be evaluated completely to determine the extent of the immunologic deficiency. As a result of the marked variability in immunodeficiency, there is considerable variation in the age at onset, severity of symptoms, and eventual outcome. Patients with adenosine deaminase deficiency and severe combined immunodeficiency may have radiologic abnormalities that include concavity and flaring of the anterior ribs, abnormal contour and articulation of posterior ribs and transverse processes, platyspondylisis, thick growth arrest lines, and an abnormal bony pelvis. Patients with nucleoside phosphorylase deficiency and T cell immunodeficiency have normal bone x-rays, absent T cell immunity, normal B cell immunity, a history of recurrent infection, and autoantibody formation. They are susceptible to fatal varicella and vaccinia infections.

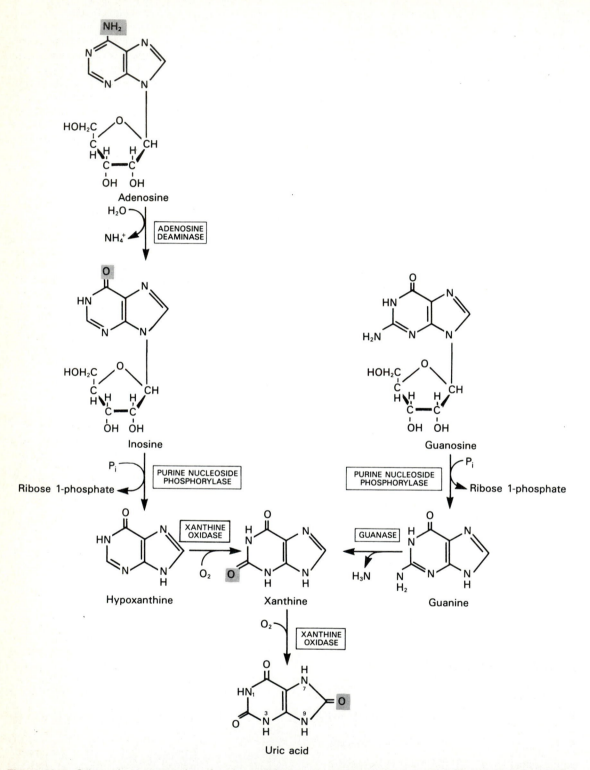

Figure 26–5. Schematic representation of purine metabolic pathway illustrating the critical role of adenosine deaminase and purine nucleoside phosphorylase. (Reproduced, with permission, from Murray RK et al: *Harper's Review of Biochemistry,* 22nd ed. Appleton & Lange, 1990.)

The mode of inheritance of these enzyme defects appears to be autosomal recessive. The carrier state can be demonstrated in both sexes by diminished adenosine deaminase or nucleoside phosphorylase activity. The enzymes are absent in erythrocytes, leukocytes, tissue, and cultured fibroblasts in these patients. An intrauterine diagnosis of adenosine deaminase deficiency has been made. Patients may not be immunodeficient at birth.

Treatment of this disorder is similar to that of severe combined immunodeficiency or combined immunodeficiency. Several successful bone marrow transplants have been performed, with subsequent return of immunologic function. The patients' cells continue to have absent enzyme activity following transplantation.

Some patients with adenosine deaminase deficiency have been successfully treated by monthly infusions of irradiated erythrocytes as a source of enzyme. Other patients have responded partially or not at all. Biochemical treatment of a single nucleoside phosphorylase-deficient patient with oral uridine was unsuccessful. Deoxycytidine therapy was evaluated in a single patient without any evidence of success. Others have responded partially to thymosin, thymus transplantation, or both. Additional patients have been successfully treated with bovine adenosine deaminase plus polyethylene glycol to prolong the enzyme half-life and reduce immunogenicity of the enzyme.

2. 5′-NUCLEOTIDASE DEFICIENCY

There have been several reports of decreased activity of 5′-nucleotidase and immunodeficiency. This enzyme deficiency has been described in association with acquired hypogammaglobulinemia, X-linked hypogammaglobulinemia, Wiskott-Aldrich syndrome, AIDS, and selective IgA deficiency. However, 5′-nucleotidase may be a differentiation marker of lymphocytes—in particular B lymphocytes—and the deficiency may therefore reflect a diminished number of B cells or an abnormality of maturation in the peripheral circulation of these patients.

3. TRANSCOBALAMIN II DEFICIENCY

Several patients have been described with a deficiency of transcobalamin II, a vitamin B_{12}-binding protein necessary for the transport of vitamin B_{12} into cells. These patients were found to have hypogammaglobulinemia, macrocytic anemia, lymphopenia, granulocytopenia, thrombocytopenia, and severe intestinal malabsorption. Vitamin B_{12} treatment resulted in the reversal of all of the manifestations of the disorder. Specific antibody synthesis occurred following administration of vitamin B_{12}.

4. BIOTIN-DEPENDENT CARBOXYLASE DEFICIENCIES

Patients with infantile chronic mucocutaneous candidiasis, ataxia, alopecia, intermittent lactic acidosis, and increased excretion of β-hydroxypropionate, methylcitrate, β-methylcrotonylglycine, and 3-β-hydroxyisovalerate in the urine have been described. Immunologic abnormalities in both B cell and T cell function were found. A second (neonatal) form has been described that is associated with severe acidosis and multiple episodes of sepsis. An intrauterine diagnosis has been made, and intrauterine therapy with biotin has been given. Treatment with biotin, 10 mg/d, reduced the abnormal metabolites in the urine and reversed the alopecia, ataxia, and chronic candidiasis. Multiple biotin-dependent carboxylase deficiencies may be one of several causes of the chronic mucocutaneous candidiasis syndrome with abnormal T cell function or severe recurrent sepsis. Biotin deficiency and immunodeficiency may also be a result of nutritional deficiencies and has been found in patients receiving hyperalimentation without biotin supplementation and in individuals on diets high in avidin (raw eggs), which binds biotin and prevents absorption.

GRAFT-VERSUS-HOST (GVH) DISEASE

GVH disease occurs when there is an unopposed attack of histoincompatible cells on an individual who is unable to reject foreign cells. The requirements for the GVH reaction are (1) histocompatibility differences between the graft (donor) and host (recipient), (2) immunocompetent graft cells, and (3) immunodeficient host cells. A GVH reaction may result from the infusion of any blood product containing viable lymphocytes, as may occur in maternal-fetal blood transfusion, intrauterine transfusion, therapeutic whole-blood transfusions or transfusions of packed erythrocytes, frozen cells, platelets, fresh plasma, or leukocyte-poor erythrocytes, or from transplantation of fetal thymus, fetal liver, or bone marrow. The onset of the GVH reaction occurs 7–30 days following infusion of viable lymphocytes. Once the reaction is established, little can be done to modify its course. In the majority of immunodeficient patients a GVH reaction is fatal. The exact mechanism by which a GVH reaction is produced is not known. Biopsy of active GVH lesions usually demonstrates infiltration by mononuclear cells and eosinophils as well as phagocytic and histiocytic cells. The GVH reaction may appear in 3 distinct forms: acute, hyperacute, and chronic.

In the acute form of GVH reaction, the initial manifestation is a maculopapular rash, which is frequently mistaken for a viral or allergic rash (Fig 26–6). Initially, it blanches with pressure and then be-

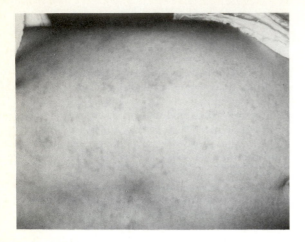

Figure 26–6. Maculopapular rash in early GVH disease in an infant with severe combined immunodeficiency disease.

comes diffuse. If the rash is persistent, it will begin to scale. Diarrhea, hepatosplenomegaly, jaundice, cardiac irregularity, central nervous system irritability, and pulmonary infiltrates may occur during the height of the reaction. Enhanced susceptibility to infection is also present and may result in death from sepsis.

In the hyperacute form of GVH reaction, the rash may also begin as a maculopapular lesion, but then it rapidly progresses to a form resembling toxic epidermal necrolysis, usually associated with severe diarrhea. This has not been associated with staphylococcal infection. Clinical and laboratory abnormalities similar to those found in the acute form may be observed. Death occurs shortly after the onset of the reaction.

The chronic form of GVH reaction may be a result of maternal-fetal transfusion or attempts at immunotherapy with histocompatible bone marrow transplantation. The clinical and laboratory features may be markedly abnormal or only slightly so. Interference with normal nail growth results in a dysplastic appearance. Chronic desquamation of the skin is usually present. Hepatosplenomegaly may be prominent, along with lymphadenopathy. Chronic diarrhea and failure to thrive are common. Secondary infection is a frequent complication. On biopsy of skin or lymph nodes, histiocytic infiltration may be found, leading to an erroneous diagnosis of Letterer-Siwe disease. Patients with Letterer-Siwe disease have normal immunoglobulin levels and normal T cell immunity, but patients with chronic GVH disease have severe immunodeficiency. Chronic GVH disease has also been confused with acrodermatitis enteropathica.

The diagnosis is suggested by the diffuse clinical abnormalities present in a patient who is known to have cellular immunodeficiency and who has received a transfusion of potentially immunocompetent cells in the preceding 5–30 days. The diagnosis is established by the demonstration of sex chromosome or HLA chimerism (Fig 26–7). On occasion, patients with known GVH disease fail to have detectable chimerism. Incubation of peripheral blood mononuclear cells with interleukin-2 may result in detectable chimerism.

There is no adequate treatment of GVH disease once it is established. Corticosteroids merely serve to enhance the susceptibility to infection. Antilymphocyte globulin also results in further suppression of immunity. Cyclosporine, a more specific immunosuppressive agent, may be useful. As treatment is inadequate, prevention is essential. Any patient who is suspected of having cellular immunodeficiency and who requires the administration of a blood product should receive cells that have been subjected to 3000–6000 R of radiation to destroy viable lymphocytes and thus prevent GVH disease. Blood products to be irradiated include whole blood, packed erythrocytes, lymphocyte-poor erythrocytes, platelets, and fresh plasma.

IMMUNODEFICIENCY WITH CELL MEMBRANE ABNORMALITIES

A number of immunodeficiency disorders have now been linked to deficiencies of an essential cell membrane component. Undoubtedly, more of these abnormalities will be discovered. The 3 primary syndromes that have been described include the bare

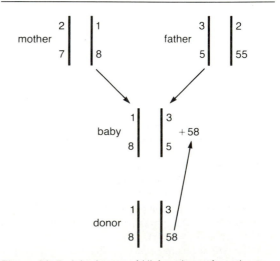

Figure 26–7. Inheritance of HLA antigens from the parents of a child with GVH disease and detection of additional antigen from the blood donor.

lymphocyte syndrome, LFA-1/Mac-1 glycoprotein deficiency, and gpL-115 glycoprotein deficiency.

1. BARE LYMPHOCYTE SYNDROME

Major Immunologic Features
- Susceptibility to viral infections occurs.
- Class I or class II HLA antigens, or both, are absent.
- Immunologic features are similar to those of combined immunodeficiency disease.

General Considerations
Patients with the bare lymphocyte syndrome have deficient expression of HLA molecules associated with immunodeficiency. A description of the HLA genes of the major histocompatibility complex (MHC) on the short arm of chromosome 6, the families of cell surface proteins encoded by these genes, their expression on cells of the immune system, and their role in the immune response is found in Chapter 4. Absence or low-level expression of class I or class II antigens, or both, occurs in the bare lymphocyte syndrome and is thought to be the primary reason for the impaired immunity observed in these patients.

Immunologic Pathogenesis
The bare lymphocyte syndrome is a rare disorder, occurring primarily in families from the Mediterranean area, and is often the product of a consanguineous union. It is inherited in an autosomal recessive manner. The first case was discovered by an inability to HLA type the patient's cells. From detailed investigations of subsequent patients, it is unlikely that the bare lymphocyte syndrome represents a single disorder; rather, it is a collection of genotypic abnormalities with various phenotypic expressions. The defect in patients is a result of abnormally low or absent expression of class I or class II HLA antigens, or both. In patients with deficient cell surface class II antigen expression, both the presence and absence of the class II gene has been found. In some instances, when the gene is present, class II antigens can be induced following stimulation of cells in vitro with antigens or gamma interferon. In other studies, it has been shown that there is an abnormality of the *trans*-activating class II regulatory gene that lies outside the major histocompatibility locus. Other investigators have shown that the class II deficient variant is a deficiency in a DNA-binding protein referred to as the X-box-binding protein (RF-X), which may play an important role in the regulation of class II gene transcription.

Clinical Features
A. Symptoms and Signs: Individuals may be entirely healthy or symptomatic with features similar to those observed in patients with combined immunodeficiency. The symptoms include opportunistic infections, chronic diarrhea, recurrent viral infections, oral candidiasis, central nervous system viral infection, aplastic anemia, and growth failure.

B. Laboratory Findings: Lymphopenia with diminished T cell numbers and function is found in severe cases. The response of peripheral blood lymphocytes to antigens is usually reduced, while the response to mitogens may be normal. B cell numbers are normal or elevated.

Immunologic Diagnosis
Routine typing for histocompatibility antigens will reveal the absence or decreased expression of HLA class I or class II antigens, or both. An intrauterine diagnosis can be established in the presence of a family history of the syndrome by analyzing fetal blood cells or chorionic villus biopsy material. To assist in bone marrow transplantation and matching, HLA genotyping was performed in several patients by using restriction enzyme fragments and specific HLA probes.

Differential Diagnosis
The bare lymphocyte syndrome should not be confused with other combined immunodeficiency diseases. In rare instances, severe leukopenia associated with another form of immunodeficiency may make HLA typing difficult.

Treatment
Severe forms of the bare lymphocyte syndrome require bone marrow transplantation. Determining an appropriate match for transplantation may be difficult and may require special techniques such as DNA hybridization. Supportive therapy is similar to that for severe combined immunodeficiency, with the use of intravenous gamma globulin and prophylactic trimethoprim-sulfamethoxazole. Immunotherapy with delta interferon may be of use in selected patients, as delta interferon results in the expression of HLA antigens following incubation of cells in vitro in certain forms of the syndrome.

Complications & Prognosis
Without appropriate treatment, patients may succumb to overwhelming infection, opportunistic infection, or progressive viral infection. Some individuals remain asymptomatic throughout their lives and have normal immunologic function.

2. LFA-1/MAC-1 GLYCOPROTEIN DEFICIENCY

Major Immunologic Features
- Recurrent bacterial infections occur.
- There is an abnormal inflammatory response with an inability to form pus.

■ Cell surface glycoproteins LFA-1/Mac-1 are absent.

General Considerations

Patients with LFA-1/Mac-1 deficiency have recurrent pyogenic infections, with onset in the first weeks of life. Common microbial agents of these infections include *Staphylococcus aureus, Pseudomonas aeruginosa, Klebsiella, Proteus,* and enterococci. Delayed separation of the umbilical cord is common. As patients become older, they develop recurrent skin infections, sinusitis, vaginitis, perianal abscesses, periodontal disease, tracheobronchitis, pneumonia, and septicemia. The disease may be fatal in the first years of life, or it may follow a more protracted course. The inheritance pattern is autosomal recessive.

The cause of the immunologic and clinical abnormalities is a deficiency of the LFA-1/Mac-1 family of glycoproteins. LFA-1 (lymphocyte function-associated antigen 1) and Mac-1 (macrophage 1) glycoproteins are found on the surface of cells, along with a third glycoprotein referred to as p150,95 (molecular weight designations). They function as adhesion molecules and are present on lymphocytes, monocytes, granulocytes, and large granular lymphocytes. Mac-1 functions as a complement receptor (CR3) for a cleaved form of complement (C3bi). It has been identified with monoclonal antibodies termed OKM-1 OKM-10, and Leu 15.

LFA-1, Mac-1, and p150,95 have a common β chain but have distinct α chains termed L1 (LFA-1 molecule), M1 (Mac-1 molecule), and X1 (p150,95 molecules) (Fig 26–8). It is believed that a deficiency in the β subunit is responsible for the decreased expression of LFA-1/Mac-1 glycoproteins. The genetic defect is on chromosome 21.

Deficiency of the adherence glycoproteins LFA-1/Mac-1 results in several immunologic abnormalities. In vivo and in vitro chemotaxis of granulocytes and in vitro cell spreading are abnormal. Zymosan-induced chemiluminescence, but not phorbol myristate acetate-induced chemiluminescence, is abnormal. Antibody-dependent cellular cytotoxicity and natural killer (NK) cell functions are also abnormal in some patients. Lymphocytes do not respond

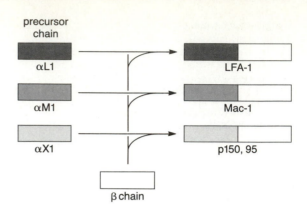

Figure 26–8. Comparative structures of leukocyte adhesion glycoproteins.

well to the mitogens PHA and concanavalin A. Following immunization, impaired antibody responses are observed.

Treatment of LFA-1/Mac-1 deficiency is directed toward the specific infectious agents involved. As patients are infected with common pathogenic organisms but not with the opportunistic ones, they should respond to appropriate antibiotic therapy. Early aggressive treatment should be used, and prophylactic therapy should be given under certain circumstances, such as dental procedures.

3. DEFICIENT GPL-115 MEMBRANE GLYCOPROTEIN

Patients have been described who had a clinical syndrome of recurrent viral, protozoal, and bacterial infections. These patients had normal levels of serum immunoglobulins. A decreased response of lymphocytes to mitogens and specific antigens was described. Lymphocytes were also characterized as having a reduced cell volume. The disorders are X-linked immunodeficiencies. There is considerable molecular heterogeneity in gpL-115. Similar abnormalities, affecting both lymphocytes and platelets, are found in patients with Wiskott-Aldrich syndrome.

REFERENCES

Severe Combined Immunodeficiency Disease

Hitzig WH: Congenital thymic and lymphocytic deficiency disorders. In: *Immunologic Disorders in Infants and Children.* Stiehm ER, Fulginiti V (editors). Saunders, 1973.

Pahwa R et al: Recombinant interleukin 2 therapy in severe combined immunodeficiency disease. *Proc Natl Acad Sci USA* 1989;**86**:5069.

Pahwa SG, Pahwa RN, Good RA: Heterogeneity of B lymphocyte differentiation in severe combined immunodeficiency disease. *J Clin Invest* 1980;**66**:543.

Cellular Immunodeficiency With Abnormal Immunoglobulin Synthesis

Lawlor EJ et al: The syndrome of cellular immunodeficiency with immunoglobulins. *J Pediatr* 1974; **84**:183.

Ataxia-Telangiectasia

Baxter GD, Kumar S, Lavin MF: T cell receptor gene rearrangement and expression in ataxia-telangiectasia B lymphoblastoid cells. *Immunol Cell Biol* 1989;**67**:57.

Boder E, Sedgwick RP: Ataxia-telangiectasia: A familial syndrome and progressive cerebellar ataxia, oculocutaneous telangiectasia and frequent pulmonary infection. *Univ South Cal Med Bull* 1957;**9**:15.

Bridges BA, Harnden DG: Untangling ataxia-telangiectasia. *Nature* 1981;**289**:222.

Swift M et al: Breast and other cancers in families with ataxia-telangiectasia. *N Engl J Med* 1987;**316**:1289.

Wiskott-Aldrich Syndrome

Cooper MD et al: Wiskott-Aldrich syndrome: Immunologic deficiency disease involving the afferent limb of immunity. *Am J Med* 1968;**44**:489.

Parkman R et al: Complete correction of the Wiskott-Aldrich syndrome by allogeneic bone marrow transplantation. *N Engl J Med* 1978;**298**:921.

Parkman R et al: Surface protein abnormalities in lymphocytes and platelets from patients with Wiskott-Aldrich syndrome. *Lancet* 1981;**2**:1387.

Reisinger D, Parkman R: Molecular heterogeneity of a lymphocyte glycoprotein in immunodeficient patients. *J Clin Invest* 1986;**79**:595.

Shelley CS et al: Molecular characterization of sialophorin (CD43), the lymphocyte surface sialoglycoprotein defective in Wiskott-Aldrich syndrome. *Proc Natl Acad Sci USA* 1989;**86**:2819.

Immunodeficiency with Thymoma

Soppi E et al: Thymoma with immunodeficiency (Good's syndrome) associated with myasthenia gravis and benign IgG gammopathy. *Arch Intern Med* 1985; **145**:1704.

Waldmann TA et al: Thymoma, hypogammaglobulinemia and absence of eosinophils. *J Clin Invest* 1967; **46**:1127.

Immunodeficiency with Short-Limbed Dwarfism

Ammann AJ, Sutliff W, Millinchick E: Antibody mediated immunodeficiency in short-limbed dwarfism. *J Pediatr* 1974;**84**:200.

Lux SE et al: Chronic neutropenia and abnormal cellular immunity in cartilage-hair hypoplasia. *N Engl J Med* 1970;**282**:234.

Polmar SH, Pierce GF: Cartilage hair hypoplasia: Immunological aspects and their clinical implications. *Clin Immunol Immunopathol* 1986;**40**:87.

Combined Immunodeficiency with Enzyme Deficiency

Cowan MJ, Ammann AJ: Immunodeficiency associated with inherited metabolic disorders. *Clin Haematol* 1981; **10**:139.

Cowan MJ et al: Multiple biotin-dependent carboxylase

deficiencies associated with defects in T cell and B cell immunity. *Lancet* 1979;**1**:115.

Giblet ER et al: Nucleoside phosphorylase deficiency in a child with severely defective T cell immunity and normal B cell immunity. *Lancet* 1975;**1**:1010.

Hershfield MS et al: Treatment of adenosine deaminase deficiency with polyethylene glycol-modified adenosine deaminase. *N Engl J Med* 1987;**316**:589.

Hirschhorn R, Martin DW: Enzyme defects in immunodeficiency diseases. *Semin Immunopathol* 1978; **1**:299.

Levy Y et al: Adenosine deaminase deficiency with late onset of recurrent infections: Response to treatment with polyethylene glycol-modified adenosine deaminase. *J Pediatr* 1988;**113**:312.

Meuwissen HJ, Pollara B, Pickering RJ: Combined immunodeficiency disease associated with adenosine deaminase deficiency. *J Pediatr* 1975;**86**:169.

Morgan G et al: Heterogeneity of biochemical, clinical and immunologic parameters in severe combined immunodeficiency due to adenosine deaminase deficiency. *Clin Exp Immunol* 1987;**70**:491.

Shanon A et al: Combined familial adenosine deaminase and purine nucleoside phosphorylase deficiencies. *Arch Dis Child* 1988;**63**:931.

Bare Lymphocyte Syndrome

Marcadet A et al: Genotyping with DNA probes in combined immunodeficiency syndrome with defective expression of HLA. *N Engl J Med* 1985;**312**:1287.

Reith W et al: Congenital immunodeficiency with a regulatory defect in MHC class II gene expression lacks a specific HLA-DR promoter binding protein, RF-X. *Cell* 1988;**53**:897.

LFA-1/Mac-1 Glycoprotein Deficiency

Kishimoto TK et al: Heterogeneous mutations in the beta subunit common to the LFA-1, Mac-1, and p150,95 glycoproteins cause leukocyte adhesion deficiency. *Cell* 1987;**50**:193.

Marlin SD et al: LFA-1 immunodeficiency disease. *J Exp Med* 1986;**164**:855.

Springer TA: The LFA-1, Mac-1 glycoprotein family and its deficiency in an inherited disease. *Fed Proc* 1985; **44**:2660.

Sullivan KE, Stobo JD, Peterlin P: Molecular analysis of the bare lymphocyte syndrome. *J Clin Invest* 1985; **76**:75.

Wacholtz MC, Patel SS, Lipsky PE: Leukocyte function-associated antigen 1 is an activation molecule for human T cells. *J Exp Med* 1989;**170**:431.

Deficient gpL-115 Membrane Glycoprotein

Parkman R et al: Immune abnormalities in patients lacking a lymphocyte surface glycoprotein. *Clin Immunol Immunopathol* 1984;**33**:363.

Phagocytic Dysfunction Diseases

Arthur J. Ammann, MD

Phagocytic disorders may be divided into extrinsic and intrinsic defects. The extrinsic category includes deficiencies of opsonins secondary to deficiencies of antibody and complement factors, suppression of the total number of phagocytic cells by immunosuppressive agents, interference of phagocytic function by corticosteroids, and suppression of the number of circulating neutrophils by autoantibody directed specifically against neutrophil antigens. Other extrinsic disorders may be related to abnormal neutrophil chemotaxis secondary to complement deficiency or abnormal complement components. The intrinsic phagocytic disorders are the result of enzymatic deficiencies within the metabolic pathway necessary for killing of bacteria. These include chronic granulomatous disease with abnormalities in the respiratory burst pathway, myeloperoxidase deficiency, and glucose-6-phosphate dehydrogenase deficiency.

Susceptibility to infection in phagocytic dysfunction syndromes may range from mild recurrent skin infections to severe, overwhelming, fatal systemic infection. Characteristically, all of these patients are susceptible to bacterial infection and do not have difficulty with viral or protozoal infections. Some of the more severe disorders may be associated with overwhelming fungal infections.

Numerous tests can now be performed to evaluate phagocytic dysfunction (see Chapter 19). Screening tests are listed in Table 23–4, and definitive studies are listed in Table 27–1.

CHRONIC GRANULOMATOUS DISEASE

Major Immunologic Features
- There is susceptibility to infection with organisms normally of low virulence, eg, *Staphylococcus epidermidis, Serratia marcescens, Aspergillus.*
- Inheritance is X-linked (autosomal variant occurs).
- Onset of symptoms occurs by 2 years of age: draining lymphadenitis, hepatosplenomegaly, pneumonia, osteomyelitis, and abscesses.
- Diagnosis is established by quantitative Nitro Blue Tetrazolium test, quantitative killing curve, or chemiluminescence.

General Considerations

Chronic granulomatous disease is inherited as an X-linked disorder, with clinical manifestations appearing during the first 2 years of life. An autosomal variant of the disease has been described. Patients are susceptible to infection with a variety of normally nonpathogenic and unusual organisms. Characteristic abnormal laboratory studies will detect both patients and female carriers of the disease. Female carriers are usually asymptomatic. Early diagnosis and aggressive therapy have improved the prognosis for these patients.

Immunologic Pathogenesis

There are several different genetic forms of chronic granulomatous disease based on different biochemical abnormalities and patterns of inheritance. However, the functional defect, which occurs

Table 27–1. Evaluation of phagocytosis.

Test	Comment
Quantitative Nitro Blue Tetrazolium (NBT)	Used for diagnosis and screening of chronic granulomatous disease and for detection of carrier state.
Quantitative intracellular killing curve	Used for diagnosis of chronic granulomatous disease. Can be performed with organisms isolated from the individual patient.
Chemotaxis	Abnormal in a variety of disorders associated with frequent bacterial infection. Does not provide a specific diagnosis. Performed by using a Boyden chamber and a microscopic or radioactive technique to determine cell migration. Rebuck skin window provides a qualitative result in vivo.
Random migration	Abnormal in lazy leukocyte syndrome. Tests nonchemotactic migration of leukocytes.
Chemiluminescence	Abnormal in chronic granulomatous disease and myeloperoxidase deficiency.
Enzyme tests	Deficiencies of specific enzymes: glucose-6-phosphate dehydrogenase, alkaline phosphatase, myeloperoxidase.
Membrane glycoproteins	Deficient in LFA-1/Mac-1 syndrome associated with abnormal leukocyte adherence.

in the respiratory burst, is similarly abnormal in the various forms and results in characteristic clinical abnormalities. The respiratory burst in neutrophils and monocytes is triggered by opsonized microorganisms or other appropriate stimuli, resulting in an increase in intracellular oxygen consumption with conversion of oxygen to hydrogen peroxide, oxidized halogens, and superoxide and hydroxyl radicals (Fig 27–1). Patients with the various forms of chronic granulomatous disease are unable to generate a respiratory burst after stimulation of neutrophils and monocytes and are therefore unable to kill certain microorganisms.

The central enzyme in the respiratory burst is NADPH oxidase. Certain classes of redox groups participate in election transport by the respiratory burst oxidase. Two of these—flavin and cytochrome b558—have been shown to be deficient in some forms of chronic granulomatous disease. Cytochrome b is deficient in the X-linked form of the disease (about 60% of the cases) but is present in what appears to be the autosomal form of the disease (about 30% of the cases). However, a number of additional biochemical variants have been described, including a low-affinity NADPH oxidase. Additional defects include deficiency of the flavoprotein component of the NADPH-dependent superoxide-generating oxidase and lack of neutrophil cytosolic factors required for activation of oxidative metabolism. Because the various abnormalities overlap, it is difficult to determine the inheritance of chronic granulomatous disease in the absence of a strong family history. Genetic and biochemical studies suggest that there are 3 major forms of chronic granulomatous disease: (1) X-linked with deficiency of cytochrome b588, (2) autosomal recessive with normal cytochrome b588, and (3) autosomal recessive with deficient cytochrome b588.

Clinical Features

A. Symptoms and Signs: In the majority of patients, the diagnosis can be established before 2 years of age. The most frequent abnormalities consist of marked lymphadenopathy, chronic infected ulcerations, hepatosplenomegaly, chronic draining lymph nodes, and at least one episode of pneumonia. Other manifestations include rhinitis, conjunctivitis, dermatitis, ulcerative stomatitis, perianal abscess, osteomyelitis, chronic diarrhea with intermittent abdominal pains, esophageal stenosis, and intestinal obstruction. Chronic and acute infection occurs in lymph nodes, skin, lungs, intestinal tract, liver, and bone. A major clue to early diagnosis is the finding of normally nonpathogenic or unusual organisms. Organisms responsible for infection include *S aureus, S epidermidis, Serratia marcescens, Pseudomonas, Escherichia coli, Candida* and *Aspergillus.*

B. Laboratory Findings: The most widely available test for diagnosis is the quantitative Nitro Blue Tetrazolium (NBT) test. Patients have absent NBT dye reduction, whereas carriers may have normal or reduced NBT reduction. Patients with chronic granulomatous disease are unable to kill certain intracellular bacteria at a normal rate. The leukocyte-killing curves for organisms to which these individuals are susceptible usually indicate little or no killing over a period of 2 hours (Fig 27–2). Other abnormal findings include decreased oxygen uptake during phagocytosis and abnormal bacterial iodination. Natural killer (NK) cell activity is normal.

The blood leukocyte count is usually elevated even if the patient does not have active infection. Hypergammaglobulinemia is present, and antibody function is normal. T cell immunity is normal. Complement factors may be elevated. During episodes of pneumonia, the chest x-ray is frequently severely abnormal. Liver function tests may be abnormal as a

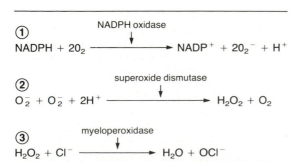

Figure 27–1. Respiratory burst resulting in the generation of superoxide (O_2^-), hydrogen peroxide (H_2O_2), and hypochlorite (OCl^-).

①
$$NADPH + 2O_2 \xrightarrow{\text{NADPH oxidase}} NADP^+ + 2O_2^- + H^+$$

②
$$O_2^- + O_2^- + 2H^+ \xrightarrow{\text{superoxide dismutase}} H_2O_2 + O_2$$

③
$$H_2O_2 + Cl^- \xrightarrow{\text{myeloperoxidase}} H_2O + OCl^-$$

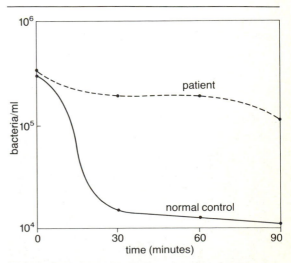

Figure 27–2. Bacterial killing curves in normal control and in patient with chronic granulomatous disease. The patient's phagocyte cells are unable to kill significant numbers of bacteria following an in vitro incubation period of 90 minutes.

result of chronic infection. Pulmonary function tests are usually abnormal following episodes of pneumonia and may not return to normal for several months. Several patients have been reported to have a rare Kell blood group, the "McLeod" phenotype. Histologic examination of the infected area often reveals an accumulation of pigmented histiocytes.

Immunologic Diagnosis

A diagnosis can be established by using the quantitative NBT dye reduction assay or quantitative chemiluminescence and confirmed by using specific bactericidal assays (see Chapter 19). These assays may also be used to identify the carrier state and to establish an intrauterine diagnosis. Both male and autosomal variants of chronic granulomatous disease have abnormal test results. B cell immunity, T cell immunity, and complement are normal. Chemiluminescence is the best method for detecting the carrier state. Several instances of an intrauterine diagnosis have been reported by using fetal blood and NBT or chemiluminescence test.

Differential Diagnosis

Few clinical disorders are confused with chronic granulomatous disease. Two other disorders with abnormal enzymatic function are associated with clinical symptoms and laboratory features similar to those of chronic granulomatous disease. One of these is the autosomal variant of chronic granulomatous disease associated with deficient glucose-6-phosphate dehydrogenase. Myeloperoxidase deficiency may have some similar clinical features. Any child presenting with osteomyelitis, pneumonia, liver abscess, or chronic draining lymphadenopathy associated with a normally nonpathogenic or unusual organism should be suspected of having chronic granulomatous disease.

Treatment

Aggressive diagnostic measures and therapy are necessary for long-term survival and diminished morbidity. Blood cultures, aspiration of draining lymph nodes, liver biopsy, and open-lung biopsy should be used to obtain a specific bacterial diagnosis. Therapy should be instituted immediately, while results of cultures are pending. The choice of antibiotics should be appropriate for the spectrum of bacterial infections, such as a combination of penicillin and gentamicin or penicillin and chloramphenicol. These would cover the majority of organisms, but not *Candida* or *Aspergillus,* for which amphotericin B is the treatment of choice. Amphotericin B therapy should be given intravenously, starting with high doses in the range of 1 mg/kg/d. The ultimate survival of the patient is dependent upon early and intensive therapy. Treatment with antibiotics may be prolonged, requiring 5–6 weeks of total therapy. Additional therapy has included the use of leukocyte

infusions, but experience has been extremely limited. Several investigators have used continuous anti-infective therapy with sulfisoxazole. A single successful bone marrow transplant has been performed. Recently, patients have been treated with delta interferon, which increases the respiratory burst activity of neutrophils and monocytes.

Complications & Prognosis

Chronic organ dysfunction may result from severe or chronic infection. Examples are abnormal pulmonary function, chronic liver disease, chronic osteomyelitis, and malabsorption secondary to gastrointestinal tract involvement. The mortality rate in chronic granulomatous disease has been considerably reduced by early diagnosis and aggressive therapy. Survival into the second decade and beyond has been recorded. Female carriers have an increased incidence of systemic and discoid lupus erythematosus.

GLUCOSE-6-PHOSPHATE DEHYDROGENASE DEFICIENCY

Glucose-6-phosphate dehydrogenase deficiency is inherited in an X-linked manner. Complete absence of leukocyte glucose-6-phosphate dehydrogenase activity has been associated with a clinical picture similar to that of chronic granulomatous disease. The defect in leukocytes is believed to be a result of deficient generation of NADPH needed as a reducing equivalent for the oxidase. Some investigators have demonstrated decreased hexose monophosphate shunt activity and decreased hydrogen peroxide production in the leukocytes. Leukocytes are unable to kill certain organisms at a normal rate, similar to the situation in chronic granulomatous disease. The susceptibility of these patients to microorganisms is similar to that of patients with chronic granulomatous disease. Glucose-6-phosphate dehydrogenase deficiency differs in that the onset is later, both males and females are affected, and hemolytic anemia is present. The laboratory diagnosis is based on the demonstration of deficient leukocyte glucose-6-phosphate dehydrogenase. The NBT test, the leukocyte intracellular killing curve, the production of hydrogen peroxide, and the consumption of oxygen are all abnormal. Treatment and prognosis are similar to those of chronic granulomatous disease. This disorder should be distinguished from the more common erythrocyte deficiency of this enzyme, which is associated with hemolytic anemia but without recurrent infections.

MYELOPEROXIDASE DEFICIENCY

Several patients with complete deficiency of leukocyte myeloperoxidase have been described. Myeloperoxidase is one of the enzymes necessary for normal intracellular killing of certain organisms. It catalyzes the oxidation of microorganisms by intracellular H_2O_2 in the presence of halides (Fig 27–1). The leukocytes of these patients have normal oxygen consumption, hexose monophosphate shunt activity, and superoxide and hydrogen peroxide production. The intracellular killing of organisms is delayed, but may reach normal levels with increased in vitro incubation times. Chemiluminescence of leukocytes is decreased. Susceptibility to candidal and staphylococcal infections has been the chief problem. The diagnosis can be established by using a peroxidase stain of peripheral blood. No specific treatment is available other than appropriate antibiotic therapy.

ALKALINE PHOSPHATASE DEFICIENCY

Several patients have been reported who have recurrent bacterial infection associated with absent leukocyte alkaline phosphatase activity. There is a modest reduction in bactericidal activity.

CHÉDIAK-HIGASHI SYNDROME

Chédiak-Higashi syndrome is a multisystem autosomal recessive disorder. Symptoms include recurrent bacterial infections with a variety of organisms, hepatosplenomegaly, partial albinism, central nervous system abnormalities, and a high incidence of lymphoreticular cancers.

The characteristic abnormality of giant cytoplasmic granular inclusions in leukocytes and platelets is observed on routine peripheral blood smears under ordinary light microscopy. Additional abnormalities include elevated Epstein-Barr virus (EBV) antibody titers, abnormal neutrophil chemotaxis, decreased NK cell activity, and abnormal intracellular killing of organisms (including streptococci and pneumococci as well as the organisms found in chronic granulomatous disease). The killing defect is manifested in vitro by delayed intracellular killing. Oxygen consumption, hydrogen peroxide formation, and hexose monophosphate shunt activity are normal. Abnormal microtubule function, abnormal lysosomal enzyme levels in granulocytes, and protease deficiency in granulocytes have been described and are associated with increased levels of leukocyte cyclic AMP (cAMP). Abnormal leukocyte function in vitro has been corrected by ascorbate, but the results of treatment in vivo are contradictory. Improved granulocyte function in vitro has also been observed after treatment with anticholinergic drugs.

There is no definitive treatment other than specific antibiotic therapy against infecting organisms. The prognosis is poor because of progressive increased susceptibility to infection and neurologic deterioration. Most patients die during childhood, but survivors to the second and third decades have been reported.

JOB'S SYNDROME

Job's syndrome was originally described as a disorder of recurrent cold staphylococcal abscesses of the skin, lymph nodes, or subcutaneous tissue (Fig 27–3). The first patients were fair-skinned, red-haired girls of Italian descent. Initial descriptions also included eczematoid skin lesions, otitis media, and chronic nasal discharge. Few signs of systemic infection or inflammatory response occurred in association with the infection. Additional reports of Job's syndrome indicated that the disorder might be a variant of chronic granulomatous disease. However, most of the patients do not have abnormal immunologic tests. Patients with hyper-IgE syndrome have clinical and laboratory features similar to those of

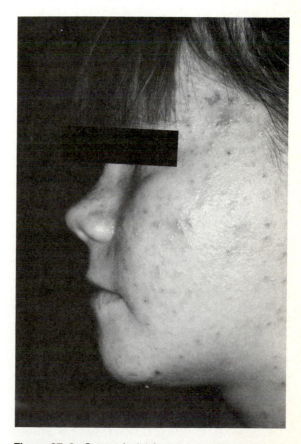

Figure 27–3. Coarse facial features, multiple small abscesses, and "saddle" nose in a female with Job's syndrome.

Job's syndrome; in fact, these may be the same disorder (see below). Treatment consists of appropriate antibiotic therapy. The prognosis is uncertain.

TUFTSIN DEFICIENCY

Tuftsin disease has been reported as a familial deficiency of a phagocytosis-stimulating tetrapeptide that is cleaved from a parent immunoglobulinlike molecule (termed leukokinin) in the spleen. Tuftsin also appears to be absent in patients who have been splenectomized. Local and severe systemic infections occur with *Candida, S aureus,* and *Streptococcus pneumoniae.* Tuftsin levels are determined only in a few specialized laboratories. There is no treatment, and the prognosis is uncertain. Gamma globulin therapy appeared to be beneficial in the 2 families in which it was tried.

LAZY LEUKOCYTE SYNDROME

Patients have been described who have a defective chemotactic response of neutrophils in association with neutropenia. These individuals also have an abnormal in vivo inflammatory response as determined by the ''Rebuck skin window'' technique, and they fail to demonstrate an increased number of peripheral blood neutrophils following epinephrine or endotoxin stimulation. The random migration of peripheral leukocytes is abnormal as determined by the vertical migration of leukocytes in a capillary tube. Patients are susceptible to severe bacterial infections. Treatment with antibiotics specific for the infections is indicated. The prognosis is unknown.

ELEVATED IGE, DEFECTIVE CHEMOTAXIS, ECZEMA, & RECURRENT INFECTION (Hyper-IgE Syndrome)

These patients—both males and females—have an early onset of eczema and recurrent bacterial infections in the form of abscesses involving the skin, lungs, ears, sinuses, and eyes. Systemic infection may involve other areas. Organisms causing infection include *S aureus, Candida, H influenzae, Streptococcus pneumoniae* and group A streptococci.

Laboratory findings consist of eosinophilia, IgE concentrations in excess of 5000 IU/mL, diminished antibody response following immunization, and normal lymphocyte response to phytohemagglutinin (PHA) and concanavalin but reduced response to antigens and allogeneic cells by mixed lymphocyte culture (MLC). Abnormalities of chemotaxis are present in some but not all patients. Patients have been shown to have decreased numbers of suppressor T cells with increased spontaneous IgE production in vitro. Increased amounts of IgE antibody and decreased amounts of IgA antibody to *Staphylococcus* antigens are found. Antibiotic therapy is indicated for specific infections. The prognosis is unknown, although patients have survived to adulthood.

LEUKOCYTE MOVEMENT DISORDERS

A number of patients have been described who have decreased leukocyte chemotaxis and recurrent infections (usually bacterial). In some cases, there is a deficiency of IgG and an IgG inhibitor of chemotaxis. Defective actin polymerization was found in association with defective neutrophil phagocytosis and locomotion. Abnormal chemotaxis has been found in congenital ichthyosis. Mannosidosis, a storage disease manifested by mental retardation and recurrent infections, in associated with abnormal chemotaxis and delayed phagocytosis. Mannose, which accumulates within leukocytes, may interfere with cell function. Similar abnormalities have been described in type IB glycogen storage disease.

MISCELLANEOUS PHAGOCYTIC DISORDERS

A variety of rare phagocytic disorders have also been described. They are usually associated with recurrent skin infections and systemic bacterial infections. Diagnosis of these rare disorders is usually made by sophisticated tests, which are not available in most medical centers. Abnormalities that have been described include decreased lactoferrin granules, abnormal polymerization of actin, and deficiency of specific granules. Because of the rarity of these disorders, there is insufficient information on which to base recommendations regarding treatment and prognosis.

REFERENCES

Chronic Granulomatous Disease
  Cheson BD, Curnutte JT, Babior BM: The oxidative killing mechanism of the neutrophil. *Prog Clin Immunol* 1977;**3**:1.
  Curnutte JT, Babior BM: Chronic granulomatous dis-
ease in advances. *Hum Genet* 1987;**16**:229.
  Johnston RB, Baehner RL: Chronic granulomatous disease: Correlation between pathogenesis and clinical findings. *Pediatrics* 1971;**48**:730.
  Lomax KJ et al: Recombinant 47-kilodalton cytosol fac-

tor restores NADPH oxidase in chronic granulomatous disease. *Science* 1989;**245**:409.

Orkin SH: Molecular genetics of chronic granulomatous disease. *Annu Rev Immunol* 1989;**7**:277.

Glucose-6-Phosphate Dehydrogenase Deficiency

Cooper MR et al: Complete deficiency of leukocyte glucose-6-phosphate dehydrogenase with defective bactericidal activity. *J Clin Invest* 1972;**51**:769.

Quie PG, Abramson JS: Disorders of the polymorphonuclear phagocytic system. Pages 343–383 in: *Immunologic Disorders in Infants and Children.* Stiehm ER (editor). Saunders, 1989.

Myeloperoxidase Deficiency

Lehrer RI, Cline MJ: Leukocyte myeloperoxidase deficiency and disseminated candidiasis: The role of myeloperoxidase in resistance to *Candida* infection. *J Clin Invest* 1969;**48**:1478.

Nauseef WM: Myeloperoxidase deficiency. *Hematol Oncol Clin North Am* 1988;**2**:577.

Czarnetzki BM: Disorders of phagocyte killing and digestion (CGD, G-6-PD and myeloperoxidase deficiencies). *Curr Probl Dermatol* 1989;**18**:101.

Chédiak-Higashi Syndrome

Ganz T et al: Microbicidal/cytotoxic proteins of neutrophils are deficient in two disorders: Chédiak-Higashi syndrome and specific granule deficiency. *J Clin Invest* 1988;**82**:552.

Haliotis T et al: Chédiak-Higashi gene in humans. 1. Impairment of natural-killer function. *J Exp Med* 1980; **151**:1039.

Stolz W et al: Chédiak-Higashi syndrome: Approaches in diagnosis and treatment. *Curr Probl Dermatol* 1989;**18**:93.

Stossel TP, Root RK, Vaughn M: Phagocytosis in chronic granulomatous disease and the Chédiak-Higashi syndrome. *N Engl J Med* 1972;**286**:120.

Tuftsin Deficiency

Constantopoulos A: Congenital tuftsin deficiency. *Ann NY Acad Sci* 1983;**419**:214.

Phillips JH, Babcock GF, Nishioka K: Tuftsin, a naturally occurring immunopotentiating factor. 1. In vitro enhancement of murine natural cell-mediated cytotoxicity. *J Immunol* 1981;**126**:915.

Spirer Z et al: Tuftsin stimulates IL-1 production by human mononuclear cells, human spleen cells and mouse spleen cells in vitro. *J Lab Clin Immunol* 1989;**28**:27.

Lazy Leukocyte Syndrome

Miller ME, Oski FA, Harris BM: Lazy-leukocyte syndrome: A new disorder of neutrophil function. *Lancet* 1971;**1**:665.

Increased IgE, Defective Chemotaxis, & Recurrent Infections

Durkin HG et al: Control of IgE responses. *Clin Immunol Immunopathol.* 1989;**50**:S52.

Hill HR, Quie PG: Raised serum IgE levels and defective neutrophil chemotaxis in three children with eczema and recurrent bacterial infections. *Lancet* 1974;**1**:183.

Kraemer MJ et al: In vitro studies of the hyper-IgE disorders: Suppression of spontaneous IgE synthesis by allogeneic suppressor T lymphocytes. *Clin Immunol Immunopathol* 1982;**25**:157.

Leung DY, Geha RS: Regulation of the human IgE antibody response. *Int Rev Immunol* 1987;**2**:75.

Matter L et al: Abnormal immune response to *Staphylococcus aureus* in patients with *Staphylococcus aureus* hyper IgE syndrome. *Clin Exp Immunol* 1986;**66**:450.

Leukocyte Movement Disorders

Boxer LA, Henley-Whyte ET, Stossel TP: Neutrophil action dysfunction and abnormal neutrophil behavior. *N Engl J Med* 1974;**291**:1093.

Quie PG, Abramson JS: Disorders of the polymorphonuclear phagocytic system. Pages 343–383 in: *Immunologic Disorders in Infants and Children.* Stiehm ER (editor). Saunders, 1989.

Complement Deficiencies

Michael M. Frank, MD

As discussed in detail in Chapter 14, there are 2 major pathways of complement activation. In each pathway, peptides derived from several complement components assemble to form a complex enzyme capable of binding and cleaving C3, the principal component formed by complement activation. Once these pathways have joined at the level of the component C3, they proceed together to interact with C5, C6, C7, C8, and C9 to produce a lytic lesion when activated at a cell surface. These later-acting components have together been termed the membrane attack complex, since they form the C5b–9 complex that inserts into biologic membranes to cause lysis. There are a limited number of patients with a genetically controlled deficiency of one of the components of the classic, alternative, or terminal attack pathways. In addition, there are patients who are known to have defects in control proteins that regulate a number of steps in the cascade. The major clinical features of each are shown in Table 28–1. For the most part, the consequences of these defects can be predicted from a knowledge of the mechanisms of activation and the biologic activities of the various complement components.

In general, defects of components of the 2 pathways behave as autosomal recessive traits. Individuals with one normal gene have about half-normal levels of the deficient proteins. Affected individuals are those with little or no gene product; they are the product of 2 heterozygous deficient parents. A few complement components composed of subunits are encoded by multiple genes. Individual independently inherited genes code for C1q, C1r, and possibly C1s as well as C8 α-γ chain and C8 β chain. Inheritance of these also follows an autosomal recessive pattern. Since there is a broad range of plasma concentrations for many of the components in normal individuals, it is not always possible to distinguish heterozygous individuals from normal individuals on the basis of their plasma complement component levels. In most cases, heterozygous individuals are phenotypically normal, except as noted below. When an individual with the homozygous phenotype is totally deficient in one of the proteins of the classic pathway or one of the terminal components, the lytic pathway is interrupted at the point at which that component must function and the complement titer (CH50) is zero; ie,

the quantity of serum required to lyse an antibody-sensitized sheep erythrocyte is infinite. Similarly, with a defect in the alternative-pathway components or terminal components, the alternative-pathway titer is zero.

ALTERNATIVE PATHWAY COMPONENT DEFICIENCIES

The alternative complement pathway is believed to be the older pathway phyogenetically and to provide the first line of host defense to bacterial attack, before the host has had sufficient time to respond to the infection by developing antibody. For that reason it might be expected that defects in the early steps of the alternative pathway might predispose individuals toward serious infection. The individual's ability to bind and activate C3 to provide adequate opsonic and other complement functions is compromised, and such patients have frequent infections with high-grade pathogens (eg, pneumococci, *Haemophilus influenzae,* and staphylococci). Relatively few such individuals have been reported. An increased incidence of neisserial infection, in addition to infections with high-grade pathogens, has been reported in properdin deficiency.

CLASSIC PATHWAY COMPONENT DEFICIENCIES

Since the alternative pathway provides a first line of defense against bacterial infection, one might expect that the deficiencies in the early steps of the classic pathway would not be associated with frequent severe infections, and this is the case. Nevertheless, it has become increasingly clear, as the relatively few patients with defects in this portion of the cascade have been observed for more prolonged periods, that these individuals do not have normal host resistance. Patients with deficiency of early classic-pathway components generally recover from infections well, but they are at a clear disadvantage when other defense mechanisms are inadequate. They are more likely to die from overwhelming in-

Table 28–1. Inherited complement and complement-related protein deficiency states.

Deficient Protein	Observed Pattern of Inheritance at Clinical Level	Reported Major Clinical Correlates[1]
C1q	Autosomal recessive	Glomerulonephritis, SLE
C1r	Probably autosomal recessive	SLE-like syndrome
C1s	Found in combination with C1r deficiency	SLE
C4	Probably autosomal recessive (2 separate loci C4A and C4B)[2]	SLE-like syndrome
C2	Autosomal recessive, HLA-linked	SLE, discoid lupus erythematosus, juvenile rheumatoid arthritis, glomerulonephritis
C3	Autosomal recessive	Recurrent pyogenic infections, glomerulonephritis
C5	Autosomal recessive	Recurrent disseminated neisserial infections, SLE
C6	Autosomal recessive	Recurrent disseminated neisserial infections
C7	Autosomal recessive	Recurrent disseminated neisserial infections, Raynaud's phenomenon
C8 (β chain or α-γ chains)	?Autosomal recessive	Recurrent disseminated neisserial infections
C9	Autosomal recessive	None identified
Properdin	X-linked recessive	Recurrent pyogenic infections, fulminant meningococcemia
Factor D	?	Recurrent pyogenic infections
C1 inhibitor	Autosomal recessive	Hereditary angioedema, increased incidence of several autoimmune diseases[3]
Factor H	Autosomal recessive	Glomerulonephritis
Factor I	Autosomal recessive	Recurrent pyogenic infections
CR1	Autosomal recessive[4]	Association between small erythrocyte CR1 numbers and SLE
CR3	Autosomal recessive[5]	Leukocytosis, recurrent pyogenic infections, delayed umbilical cord separation

[1]A significant number of individuals with complement deficiencies, especially C2 and the terminal components, are clinically well. A significant number of patients with defects in C5–9 have had autoimmune disease.

[2]Individuals lacking C4A or C4B are designated "q0" (quantity 0). Thus, individuals can be C4Aq0 or C4Bq0. Such individuals are reported to have a higher than normal incidence of autoimmune diseases. Similarly, heterozygous C2 deficient individuals are reported to have an increased incidence of autoimmune disease.

[3]Includes approximately 85% of cases with silent alleles and 15% with alleles encoding for dysfunctional variant C1 inhibitor protein.

[4]Homozygosity for low (not absent) numerical expression of CR1 on erythrocytes is detectable in vitro and appears to be associated with SLE. An acquired defect in CR1 numbers may also be operative.

[5]Low but not absent leukocyte CR3 is detectable in both parents of most CR3-deficient children.

fection than are persons with normal levels of all complement components.

C3 & TERMINAL COMPONENT DEFICIENCIES

C3 is critical to both the classic and alternative pathways, and, as might be expected, patients with C3 deficiency are prone to develop overwhelming sepsis with high-grade pathogens. Patients with defects in the later-acting terminal components respond quite well to most infectious agents. Their opsonic function, mediated by both the classic and alternative pathways, is intact. However, they have a much higher than normal frequency of disseminated meningococcal and gonococcal (neisserial) infections. Presumably, the lytic function of the late-acting components is required to defend adequately against these highly encapsulated organisms. It is interesting that neisserial infections in individuals with deficiencies in late-acting components follow a quite different course from those in noncomplementemic individuals. These infections tend to occur in older individuals, involve different groups of neisserial organisms (untypable and Y type organisms), and are less likely to be lethal than infections that occur in normal individuals. Presumably, such complement-deficient patients synthesize antibody to the organisms, and this antibody provides partial but not complete protection. Individuals with no antibody to the organisms are far more likely to die from overwhelming sepsis than are individuals with antibody.

A large group of C9-deficient individuals has been discovered by mass screening in Japan. The consequences of this defect in the Japanese population are still being evaluated, but it is striking that no major medical illnesses have been reported. It should be recalled that lytic lesions often can be formed in target cells by the action of the C5–C8 component. The function of C9 is to enlarge and stabilize the C5678 lytic lesion, but the action of C5–C8 on the infecting organism may be sufficient to protect against disease.

COMPLEMENT DEFICIENCIES & AUTOIMMUNITY

Patients missing proteins of the classic or alternative pathway, as well as some individuals with late-component defects, have an unexpectedly high incidence of autoimmune disease, particularly systemic lupus erythematosus (SLE) and glomerulonephritis. It is currently believed that one of the biologic consequences of complement activation is to cause antigen–antibody complexes to adhere to circulating erythrocytes via the erythrocyte complement receptor CR1. Presumably, such complexes, adherent to the erythrocyte surface, are less likely to escape from the circulation into the tissues, where they can cause tissue damage.

The genes for at least 3 complement proteins, C4, C2, and factor B, are located within the major histocompatibility locus on chromosome 6 in humans (class 3 histocompatibility genes). One of these genes, C4, normally exists in 2 copies on each chromosome, coding for 2 different gene products, C4A and C4B. These 2 proteins have biochemical differences, and they differ in their efficiency in mediating complement attack. It is quite common to find individuals missing one or more of the C4 alleles and others deficient in one of the C2 genes. Many investigators have found that such individuals who are heterozygous for the deficiency are more prone to develop the signs and symptoms of autoimmune disease than are normal controls. In particular, individuals missing the C4A alleles and designated C4AqO (for C4A quantity 0) are far more likely to develop systemic lupus erythematosus. Because the C4B allele is much more active hemolytically and because the range of normal values is wide, these individuals can be identified only by specific characterization of the circulating protein by methods not available in most hospital laboratories.

COMPLEMENT REGULATORY FACTOR DEFICIENCIES

Regulatory proteins that control complement activation may also be deficient. The best-studied and most common of these deficiencies is the partial deficiency of the control protein C1 inhibitor (C1INH). This protein functions to inactivate the subcomponents of C1, C1r, and C1s following their activation by stoichiometrically binding to the enzymatic sites on these proteins. The C1 inhibitor also acts to inactivate activated Hageman factor and its enzymatically active fragments, as well as those pathways activated by Hageman factor, the intrinsic clotting pathway (factor XI), the kinin-generating pathway (kallikrein), and the fibrolytic pathways (plasmin).

HEREDITARY ANGIOEDEMA

The disease of C1INH deficiency, hereditary angioedema, is characterized by recurrent attacks of edema of subcutaneous and submucosal tissues. It particularly affects the extremities and the mucosa of the gastrointestinal tract. Typically, attacks last for 1–4 days and are harmless, although when they involve the bowel wall they usually induce severe abdominal pain. Occasionally, attacks affect subcutaneous and submucosal tissue in the region of the upper airway. In this case they may be associated with respiratory obstruction and asphyxiation. Attacks are sporadic, but in some patients they may be induced by emotional stress or physical trauma. Although attacks usually begin in childhood, they seldom become severe until puberty.

Diagnosis is important, because patients respond poorly to the drugs usually used to treat episodic angioedema: epinephrine, antihistamines, and glucocorticoids. Diagnosis is established by the demonstration of low antigenic or functional levels of C1 esterase inhibitor. Such patients usually have normal levels of C1, low levels of C4 and C2, and normal levels of C3. The actual mechanism of angioedema formation is unknown; investigators have implicated both the complement- and kinin-generating systems in the production of attacks.

Two classes of drugs provide effective therapy. Plasmin inhibitors are fairly effective, although they do not correct the biochemical abnormality (low C4 and C2 levels), suggesting that their principal action is not the inhibition of enzymatic C1. Their mode of action is unknown. The second class of drugs that has proved useful is the group of anabolic steroids or impeded androgens. Investigators at the National Institutes of Health have had the most experience with danazol, which causes a striking increase in C1 inhibitor, presumably owing to increased synthesis. This leads to a rise in C4 and C2 levels toward normal, and in most patients the drug completely alleviates symptoms. All the useful oral androgens appear to have similar clinical activity, although the effect on levels of C1 inhibitor, C4, and C2 is much less striking with some.

Hereditary angioedema is different from most hereditary complement deficiency diseases in that it results from autosomal dominant rather than recessive inheritance. Individuals with this disease have defective production of C1INH by one of the 2 genes present on chromosome 11. Approximately 85% of patients have one nonproductive gene and have ⅓ to ½ normal levels of C1INH. The other 15% of patients have a gene mutation that leads to production of an abnormal C1INH product with no functional activity of the abnormal gene product. The product of one normal gene does not appear to be sufficient to control activation of the various mediator pathways. Hereditary angioedema is treated effectively in most patients by administration of androgens or anabolic steroids. Although the mechanism of action of these drugs is not formally proven, they appear to act by inducing synthesis of the C1INH protein by hepatocytes, thereby correcting the defect. These drugs markedly diminish the frequency and severity of angioedema attacks. For unknown reasons, drugs that inhibit active plasmin are also therapeutically useful. They improve the clinical manifestations but do not correct the C1INH deficiency.

There are rare patients with an acquired form of C1 esterase inhibitor deficiency who present with clinical findings of recurrent angioedema similar to the patients with the inherited form of the disease. In most cases, this is due either to the formation of a monoclonal autoantibody to the C1INH protein that blocks normal C1 inhibitor function or to excessive activation of C1 with utilization of C1INH at a higher rate than the rate of resynthesis. The latter may occur during the course of an autoimmune disease such as SLE or may occur in the setting of a cancer, where it appears that the malignant cell synthesizes molecules that activate C1 and deplete C1 inhibitor. Interestingly, diseases associated with depletion of C1 inhibitor also often respond to treatment with anabolic steroids. Whereas patients with the inherited form of C1 esterase inhibitor deficiency have normal plasma levels of C1 and C3 and markedly depressed levels of C4 and C2, patients with the acquired form have profoundly depressed C1 titers, reflecting the marked activation and utilization of C1 that, in turn, depletes C1 inhibitor.

Patients have also been described who are deficient in the C3 regulatory factors H and I. These individuals also have a higher than expected incidence of infections, reflecting the fact that normal degradation of C3b does not occur, alternative-pathway activation is poorly regulated, and C3 is abnormally consumed. Thus, these individuals act as if they were partially deficient in C3 and other alternative-pathway regulatory factors. They also would be expected to have an abnormally high incidence of autoimmune disease.

COMPLEMENT RECEPTOR DEFICIENCIES

There are many cell membrane-bound complement-regulatory factors. In general, inherited deficiencies of these proteins are rare. A group of children has been identified who fail to express the iC3b receptor (CR3) on their cell surface. These children fail to express the 3 CD11 membrane proteins. These 3 proteins have different α chains (CD11a, b, and c) and the same β chain (CD18) and are members of an adhesion-promoting group of molecules termed **integrens.** Presumably, the β chain is important in protein transport and this inherited defect causes a failure to transport synthesized CD11/18 proteins to the cell surface. All of these children have phagocytes with defective cell–cell adhesion properties and defective adhesion to glass and other surfaces. The children show abnormal separation of the umbilical cord after birth and have frequent infections, often of the skin.

It has been reported that individuals with SLE have decreased numbers of CR1 on their cell surfaces as an inherited defect, but this point remains controversial. Clearly, the expression of CR1 on erythrocytes is an inherited trait, with some individuals showing higher numbers of receptors than others.

COMPLEMENT ALLOTYPE VARIANTS

Many of the complement proteins exist in allotypic forms, with many inherited variants that can be detected by difference in their electrophoretic mobility. Some of these electrophoretic variants show a predilection for certain disease states, especially autoimmune disease. Whether this reflects a change in function of the complement protein caused by a mutation that leads to the electrophoretic variant or a linkage of the gene for one complement variant to other nearby disease-causing genes on the same chromosome that segregate together is not clear. Nevertheless, these cases of linkage disequilibrium have been well documented in population studies.

REFERENCES

General Reviews

Agnello V: Complement deficiency states. *Medicine* 1978;**57**:1.

Ross SC, Densen P: Complement deficiency states and infection: Epidemiology, pathogenesis and consequences of neisserial and other infections in an immune deficiency. *Medicine* 1984;**63**:243.

Complement Deficiency & Infection

Alper CA et al: Increased susceptibility to infection associated with abnormalities of complement-mediated functions and of the third component of complement (C3). *N Engl J Med* 1970;**282**:349.

Densen P et al: Familial properdin deficiency and fatal meningococcemia correction of the bactericidal defect by vaccination. *N Engl J Med* 1987;**316**:922.

Ellison RT et al: Prevalence of congenital or acquired complement deficiency in patients with sporadic meningococcal disease. *N Engl J Med* 1983;**308**:913.

Ellison RT et al: Underlying complement deficiency in patients with disseminated gonococcal infection. *Sex Transm Dis* 1987;**14**:201.

Fine DP et al: Meningococcal meningitis in a woman with inherited deficiency of the ninth component of complement. *Clin Immunol Immunopathol* 1983;**28**:413.

C9 Deficiency in Population Studies

Inai S et al: Deficiency of the ninth C1 component of complement in man. *J Clin Lab Immunol* 1979;**2**:85.

Complement Deficiency & Autoimmunity

Berger M et al: Circulating immune complexes and glomerulonephritis in a patient with congenital absence of the third component of complement. *N Engl J Med* 1983;**308**:1009.

Berliner S et al: Familial systemic lupus erythematosus and C4 deficiency. *Scand J Rheumatol* 1981;**10**:280.

Glass D et al: Inherited deficiency of the second component-complement rheumatic disease association. *J Clin Invest* 1976;**58**:853.

Genetics & HLA Linkage

Colten HR: Genetics and synthesis of components of the complement system. Page 163 in: *Immunobiology of the Complement System*. Ross GD (editor). Academic Press, 1986.

Dawkins RL et al: Disease associations with complotypes, supratypes and haplotypes. *Immunol Rev* 1983;**70**:1.

Howard PF et al: Relationship between C4 null genes, HLA-D region antigens, and genetic susceptibility to systemic lupus erythematosus in Caucasian and black Americans. *Am J Med* 1986;**81**:187.

Rich S et al: Complement and HLA: Further definition of high-risk haplotypes in insulin dependent diabetes. *Diabetes* 1985;**34**:504.

Hereditary Angioedema & Acquired C1 Inhibitor

Alsenz J, Bork K, Loos M: Autoantibody-mediated acquired deficiency of C1 inhibitor. *N Engl J Med* 1987;**316**:1360.

Frank MM, Gelfand JA, Atkinson JP: Hereditary angioedema: The clinical syndrome and its management. *Ann Intern Med* 1976;**84**:580.

Frank MM et al: Epsilon aminocaproic acid therapy of hereditary angioneurotic edema: A double-blind study. *N Engl J Med* 1972;**286**:808.

Gelfand JA et al: Acquired C1 esterase inhibitor deficiency and angioedema: A review. *Medicine* 1979;**58**:321.

Gelfand JA et al: Treatment of hereditary angioedema with danazol: Reversal of clinical and biochemical abnormalities. *N Engl J Med* 1976;**295**:1444.

Rosen FS et al: Genetically determined heterogeneity of the C1 esterase inhibitor in patients with hereditary angioneurotic edema. *J Clin Invest* 1971;**50**:2143.

Schapira M et al: Biochemistry and pathophysiology of human C1 inhibitor: Current issues. *Complement* 1985;**2**:111.

CD11/CD18 Deficiency

Anderson DC et al: The severe and moderate phenotypes of heritable Mac-1, LFA-1 deficiency: Their quantitative definition and relation to leukocyte dysfunction and clinical features. *J Infect Dis* 1985;**152**:668.

Mechanisms of Hypersensitivity

29

Abba I. Terr, MD

Allergy refers to certain diseases in which immune responses to environmental antigens cause tissue inflammation and organ dysfunction. The clinical features of each allergic disease reflect the immunologically induced inflammatory response in the organ or tissue involved. These features are generally independent of the chemical or physical properties of the antigen. The diversity of allergic responses arises from the involvement of different immunologic effector pathways, each of which generates a unique pattern of inflammation. The classification of allergic diseases is based on the type of immunologic mechanism involved. This chapter will cover mechanisms, classification, and clinical evaluation of the allergic diseases.

DEFINITIONS

An **allergen** is any antigen that causes allergy. The term is used to denote either the antigenic molecule itself or its source, such as pollen grain, animal dander, insect venom, or food product. **Hypersensitivity** and **sensitivity** are often used as synonyms for allergy. **Immediate hypersensitivity** and **delayed hypersensitivity** are the terms formerly used to define antibody-mediated allergy and T lymphocyte-mediated allergy, respectively.

PREVALENCE

Allergy is common throughout the world. The predilection for specific allergic diseases, however, varies among different age groups, sexes, and races. The prevalence of sensitivity to specific allergens is determined both by genetic predilection and by geographic and cultural factors responsible for exposure to the allergen.

ALLERGENS

Any foreign substance capable of inducing an immune response is a potential allergen. Many different chemicals of both natural and synthetic origin are known to be allergenic. Complex natural organic chemicals, especially proteins, are likely to cause antibody-mediated allergy, whereas simple organic compounds, inorganic chemicals, and metals more frequently cause T cell-mediated allergy. In some cases the same allergen may be responsible for more than one type of allergy. Exposure to the allergen may be through inhalation, ingestion, injection, or skin contact.

Allergies caused by certain allergens are encountered frequently in clinical practice, whereas others are rare. Examples of common allergens are antigen E in ragweed pollen and pentadecylcatechol in poison ivy. Sensitization of a specific individual to a particular environmental allergen is the result of a complex interplay of the chemical and physical properties of the allergen, the mode and quantity of exposure, and the unique genetic makeup of the individual.

SUSCEPTIBILITY TO ALLERGY

A clinical state of allergy affects only some of the individuals who encounter each allergen. The occurrence of allergic disease on exposure to an allergen requires not only prior sensitization but also other factors that determine the localization of the reaction to a particular organ (Table 29–1). This is particu-

Table 29–1. Factors that determine expression of disease in allergy.

Allergen Exposure	Allergic Sensitization	Target Organ Susceptibility	Clinical Disease	Type of Disease
− or +	−	−	−	No disease
+	+	−	−	Asymptomatic sensitivity
+	+	+	+	Allergic disease
− or +	−	+	+	Nonallergic disease

larly evident in atopic allergy, where sensitization may cause disease localized to the nasal mucosa, the bronchial mucosa, the skin, the gastrointestinal tract, or a combination of 2 or more of these sites (see Fig 30–1). The nonimmunologic factors involved in the expression of clinical atopic disease are not yet known, although a disturbance in autonomic control, such as β-adrenergic blockade or cholinergic hyperreactivity in the target tissue, has been postulated.

Most of the diseases in which allergy is expressed, eg, asthma, rhinitis, atopic dermatitis, contact dermatitis, anaphylaxis, and urticaria-angioedema, can occur in the absence of allergy. Recognition of these nonimmunologic diseases is important in differential diagnosis. In some cases, environmental triggers are nonspecific or cannot be identified. In other cases a specific environmental agent activates inflammatory mediators nonimmunologically. Examples of the latter phenomenon include direct mast cell release of histamine by opiate drugs, aspirin-induced asthma (possibly an aberrant metabolism of arachidonic acid), anaphylactoid reactions from radioiodinated contrast media, urticaria from eating shellfish and berries, and occupational isocyanate asthma. In these examples, no allergen-specific immunologic sensitivity has been shown to be responsible for the reaction, even though the reaction occurs in only a limited percentage of the exposed population.

MECHANISMS & CLASSIFICATION OF ALLERGIC DISEASE

Allergy is an immunologic phenomenon. The disease occurs when an exposure to the allergen induces an immune response, referred to as "sensitization" rather than immunization (Fig 29–1A). Once sensitization occurs, an individual will be asymptomatic until there is an exposure to the allergen. Then the reaction of allergen with specific antibody or sensitized effector T lymphocyte induces an inflammatory response, producing the symptoms and signs of the allergic reaction (Fig 29–1B).

Among the currently recognized pathways of immunologically induced inflammation (see Chapter 11), 3 different ones are responsible for the known allergic diseases: (1) the IgE-mast cell-mediator pathway, (2) the IgG or IgM immune complex-complement-neutrophil pathway, and (3) the effector T lymphocyte-lymphokine pathway. Specific diseases associated with each of these processes are shown in Table 29–2 and are discussed in the following 3 chapters. A brief description of the immunologic mechanisms is given here. More detailed information can be found in the first section of this book.

THE IGE-MAST CELL-MEDIATOR PATHWAY

IgE antibodies have a unique configuration on the Fc portion of the molecule for fixation to mast cells (Fig 29–2). Fixation occurs at a high-affinity mast cell surface receptor, **FcεRI.** The allergic reaction is initiated when the polyvalent allergen molecule reacts with antibodies occupying these receptors. The result is a bridging of FcεRI, thereby altering the cell surface membrane. This, in turn, signals intracellular events causing release and activation of mediators of inflammation: histamine, leukotrienes, chemotactic factors, platelet-activating factor, and proteases. Mast cell activation is modulated by intracellular cyclic nucleotides and is accompanied by cell degranulation. The released activated mediators act locally and cause increased vascular permeability, vasodilatation, smooth muscle contraction, and mucous gland secretion. These biologic events account for the salient clinical features of the **immediate phase,** occurring in the first 15–30 minutes following allergen exposure. Over the succeeding 12 hours there is a progressive tissue infiltration of inflammatory cells, proceeding from neutrophils to eosinophils to mononuclear cells in response to other chemical mediators and biochemical events not yet fully delineated. The period of 6–12 hours after allergen exposure is designated the **late phase** of the IgE response and is characterized by clinical manifestations of cellular inflammation.

This mechanism is responsible for the atopic diseases, anaphylaxis, and urticaria. The reaction can be triggered by extremely small amounts of allergen.

THE IGG OR IGM-COMPLEMENT-NEUTROPHIL PATHWAY

IgG or IgM antibodies form complexes with antigen, and such complexes cause tissue inflammation. This pathway contributes to the pathogenesis of many human diseases, including allergic diseases. Allergen-antibody complexes activate the complement system through the classic pathway via receptors on C1q for the Fc portion of the IgG or IgM antibody molecule. Complement activation generates anaphylatoxins and chemotactic peptides, which cause increased vascular permeability and infiltration of neutrophils. Activated neutrophils generate additional inflammatory and toxic products. Macrophages are also recruited and become activated, contributing further to tissue inflammation and injury.

This mechanism is responsible for the cutaneous Arthus reaction, serum sickness, and the acute phase of hypersensitivity pneumonitis (extrinsic allergic alveolitis). Because immune complexes in moderate antigen excess are the most efficient for activating C1q, relatively large quantities of allergen are required to initiate the reaction.

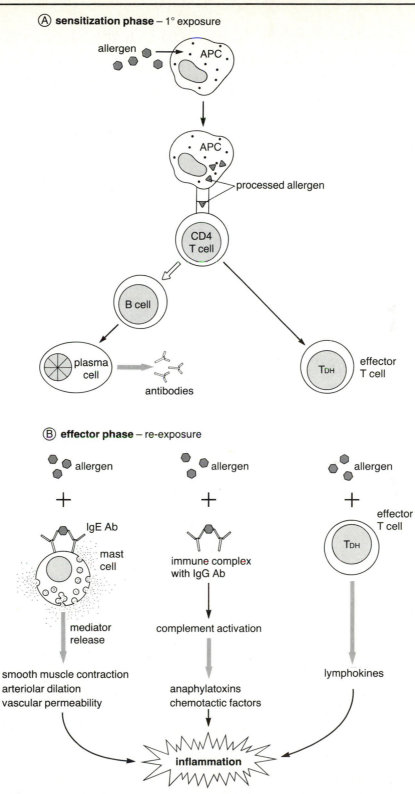

Figure 29–1. Role of the immune system in allergy. **A:** Sensitization phase, showing immunologic response to allergen from unsensitized (nonallergic) state to sensitized (allergic) state. **B:** Effector phase, showing reaction on reexposure of allergen to specific antibody or to specifically sensitized effector T cell.

Table 29–2. Classification of allergic diseases based on immunologic mechanisms.

1. **Allergic disease caused by IgE antibodies and mast cell mediators**
   a. Atopic diseases
      1. Allergic rhinitis
      2. Allergic asthma
      3. Atopic dermatitis
      4. Allergic gastroenteropathy
   b. Anaphylactic diseases
      1. Systemic anaphylaxis
      2. Urticaria-angioedema
2. **Allergic disease caused by IgG or IgM antibodies and complement activation**
   a. Serum sickness
   b. Acute hypersensitivity pneumonitis
3. **Allergic disease caused by sensitized T lymphocytes**
   a. Allergic contact dermatitis
   b. Chronic hypersensitivity pneumonitis

Table 29–3. Immunologic pathways potentially capable of allergen-antibody activation.

1. Alternative complement pathway activation via IgA antibodies
2. Anaphylatoxins (C3a, C5a, C4a) generated by classic or alternative pathway complement activation
3. IgG4 antibody activation of mast cells for mediator release
4. Complement activation of the kininogen-kallikrein-kinin system

THE EFFECTOR T LYMPHOCYTE-LYMPHOKINE PATHWAY

Some allergic diseases are not mediated by antibody but, rather, by reaction of allergen with the effector T lymphocyte sensitized to the specific allergen from a prior exposure. The effector T cell has the CD4 phenotype, and when it encounters the allergen it is activated to generate lymphokines; this results in the accumulation over several days of a mononuclear cell infiltrate.

Other immunologic pathways leading to inflammation have been studied so far only at an in vitro level but have not yet been clearly identified as the primary pathogenetic mechanism of human disease. These potential mechanisms for allergy are listed in Table 29–3. They may play a secondary role in diseases caused by the 3 primary pathways described above.

CLINICAL EVALUATION

GENERAL CONSIDERATIONS

When allergy is suspected, the diagnostic process is aimed at determining whether the disease is caused by allergy and, if so, to identify the type of allergy and each of the responsible allergens. Many straightforward cases of seasonal hay fever caused by pollen or contact dermatitis caused by poison ivy can be diagnosed easily and quickly, but more complex or obscure allergic diseases require considerable detective work. History, physical examination, and appropriate laboratory tests are required, as in the diagnosis of any medical condition.

HISTORY

The history is essential. It is critically important to correlate results of specific allergy testing to the patient's history. Whenever allergy is suspected, the physician should be prepared first to obtain a detailed description of the symptoms and the timing and environmental locations associated with appearance and disappearance of those symptoms. Allergen exposure may occur through inhalation, ingestion, injection, or skin or mucous membrane contact. Variations in symptoms during the course of a day, week, month, and year and the association with home, work, school, or vacation trips are useful clues in diagnosis of the common inhalant and occupational allergies. When inhalant allergy is suspected, an environmental history should include details of work, hobbies, pets, and the influence of weather and climate on respiratory symptoms. A history of medication usage and dietary habits is relevant for possible ingested allergens. Drugs and insect bites and stings may cause allergy by injection.

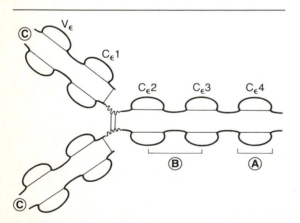

Figure 29–2. Schematic diagram of the IgE antibody molecule. The structure is similar to that of IgG, but there is an additional H chain domain (**A**), accounting for its higher molecular weight. The regions of the molecule containing the site for fixation to mast cell FcεRI (**B**) and the allergen-binding sites (**C**) are indicated.

When allergic contact dermatitis is suspected, the physician should inquire especially about exposure to plants, perfumes, cosmetics, clothing, topical medications, work, and hobbies.

Other important historical data are the age of onset, the course of the illness, and the effect of hormonal factors such as puberty, menstrual-cycle variations, and pregnancy. The influence of prior treatments such as antihistamine drugs, antibiotics, and corticosteroids may help to distinguish allergic from nonallergic conditions. The presence of other known allergies and results of prior allergy evaluations in the patient, as well as family history of allergy, may also be helpful.

Many allergists use standard questionnaires for part or all of the history. If the questionnaire is self-administered, the patient's answers should be reviewed by the physician.

PHYSICAL EXAMINATION

Allergic diseases are often episodic, because signs and symptoms are dependent upon exposure to the allergen. Objective signs of allergy are therefore present when the physical examination is performed during the period of allergen exposure. A negative physical examination performed during a period of allergen avoidance does not mean that the patient does not have allergy. The examination should be thorough enough to rule out other causes for the patient's symptoms. In allergic dermatoses the appearance, distribution, and extent of the skin lesions will direct the questioning to likely sources of the allergen.

LABORATORY TESTING

A variety of laboratory tests are available to supplement the history and physical examination. There are procedures for quantitating the extent of functional and anatomic effects on a particular organ, for sampling fluids or tissues for evidence of disease, and for establishing the presence of specific immune responses.

1. TESTS OF AIRWAY FUNCTION

The standard pulmonary-function tests quantitate the amount of obstructive airway and restrictive lung disease in patients with respiratory allergy. Reversible airway obstruction can be shown by bronchodilator response in a patient with current airway obstruction or by bronchoconstrictor response in a patient without baseline airway obstruction. Tests of nasal airway resistance are available but are not suitable for routine use. Tympanometry may aid in diagnosis of otitis media complicating allergic rhinosinusitis.

Airway hyperirritability in patients with asthma can be quantitated by bronchoprovocation tests with inhalation of certain chemicals (histamine, methacholine) or with physical stimuli (exercise). The former are more sensitive but may be positive in nonasthmatics under certain conditions, whereas the latter are more specific to asthma but less sensitive.

The usual measurement used for the various bronchoprovocation tests is a fall in 1-second forced expiratory volume (FEV_1), which can be rapidly and reproducibly measured by spirometry. Increasing doses of aerosolized methacholine or histamine are delivered by nebulizer, and the provocative dose causing a 20% fall in FEV_1 is designated PD_{20}.

Physical challenges with exercise, cold dry isocapnic hyperventilation, or ultrasonically nebulized distilled water have also been standardized for detecting nonspecific bronchial hyperirritability. The mechanisms involved are not understood precisely, although these physical stimuli possibly stimulate bronchial mast cells to release mediators nonimmunologically, whereas histamine and methacholine act directly on bronchial smooth muscle. In all cases of nonspecific testing, maximal bronchoconstriction is achieved in about 5 minutes, with reversion to baseline in 15–20 minutes without a late-phase response (Fig 29–3). Rarely, methacholine may produce a prolonged, severe episode of asthma that requires treatment. The procedures can be performed in an outpatient setting, but emergency equipment should be available in the event of a severe induced asthma attack.

Any one of these tests can be used to assist in diagnosis of asthma in patients with a history of symptoms but negative tests for reversible airway obstruction. Under these conditions a negative methacholine challenge test rules out asthma. However, a positive test indicating airway hyperirritability may be obtained in other conditions such as (1) allergic rhinitis, especially during the pollen season; (2) following a viral respiratory infection or recent immunization with influenza or live measles vaccine; (3) in some relatives of asthmatics; and (4) in a small portion of the normal population. The test has been especially helpful in diagnosis and screening for potential occupational asthma. Recent clinical studies suggest that it might be used in monitoring allergen immunotherapy for asthma.

2. ANATOMIC TESTS

Visualization of paranasal sinuses, lungs, and the gastrointestinal tract may require x-ray, computed tomography, or endoscopy.

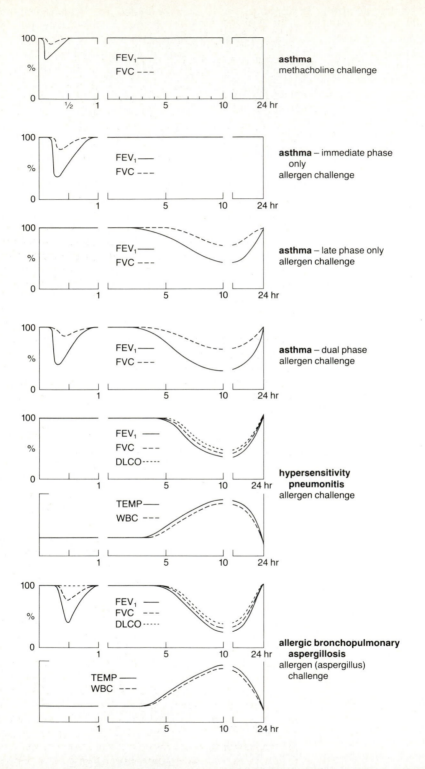

Figure 29–3. Bronchial provocation tests for detection of nonspecific bronchial hyperirritability (methacholine challenge) or immunologic reactivity (allergen challenge). Shown are the responses in patients with asthma (IgE antibody sensitivity), hypersensitivity pneumonitis (principally T cell-mediated sensitivity), and allergic bronchopulmonary aspergillosis (combined IgE and IgG antibody sensitivities). FEV$_1$, forced expiratory volume in 1 second; FVC, forced vital capacity; DLCO, diffusing capacity for carbon monoxide; TEMP, temperature; WBC, leukocyte count.

3. TISSUE DIAGNOSIS

When appropriate, samples of nasal or sinus secretions, sputum, bronchoalveolar fluid, gastrointestinal secretions, stool, or blood can be examined for inflammatory cell content. These studies, as well as histopathology of biopsy specimens from tissues of patients with suspected allergic disease, may confirm the type of inflammation associated with a particular type of allergic response, but they do not identify the causative allergen.

4. ALLERGY SKIN TESTING

A variety of skin test methods are used in the clinical diagnosis of each type of allergic disease. The skin test is a bioassay for the presence or absence of an immune response to a specific allergen that sets off a particular effector mechanism of inflammation. The skin is a convenient organ to test, since it is equipped with all of the elements necessary for eliciting a localized controlled allergic reaction, even though the disease is targeted to another organ.

For diagnosis, skin testing occupies an intermediate position between in vitro tests, which demonstrate specific immune response only, and in vivo provocation tests, which demonstrate the ability of the diseased target organ to respond immunologically to the allergen. Skin tests require some skill in performance and interpretation, but they have many advantages. The tests are convenient, inexpensive, and safe if done properly. Results are available with no delay beyond the time required for the allergic response. There is no possibility of sample (ie, patient) error. Many suspected allergens can be tested simultaneously. Discomfort is usually minimal.

The principal disadvantage of skin testing is the need to discontinue certain inhibitory drugs. Occasionally, skin testing is prohibited for lack of available skin because of generalized dermatitis. The procedure may be unacceptable to some small children and adults. The potential for a systemic reaction or flare of the disease exists, but these are exceedingly unlikely with proper precautions.

Patch Tests

The patch test simulates allergic contact dermatitis on a small patch of skin to which a known concentration of allergen is applied. It is therefore a true provocative test of the disease. In most cases of allergic contact dermatitis, the allergen is a chemical that couples to skin protein, yielding a hapten-protein conjugate. This conjugate then reacts with sensitized cutaneous T lymphocytes to liberate lymphokines, which produce localized cell-mediated inflammation at the site of contact with the test allergen.

A. Method: The concentration of allergen, usually a chemical, is determined by prior testing of several allergic and nonallergic subjects. It must be high enough to elicit a positive reaction in the former but not high enough to cause skin irritation in the latter. Two test methods are available. In the open patch method a drop of acetone extract is applied to the skin. The acetone quickly dries, depositing the test chemical on the skin site, which is left uncovered and inspected after 48 hours. In the closed patch method the allergen in petrolatum is applied to a pad taped to the skin. After 48 hours the pad is removed and the site is inspected. A positive test consists of erythema, papules, or vesicles. If the test is negative, the site should be examined again at 72 and 96 hours, because weak reactions may appear later. Multiple tests can be performed simultaneously. Preferred areas for testing are the back, forearms, or upper arms.

Twenty chemicals cause most cases of allergic contact dermatitis (see Chapter 33). This set of patch test reagents is available from the American Academy of Dermatology. Textbooks on contact dermatitis should be consulted for proper concentrations of many other known contact sensitizers.

Systemic corticosteroid drugs inhibit cell-mediated hypersensitivity and should be discontinued prior to testing. Antihistamines and other antiallergy drugs need not be discontinued.

B. Indications: The patch test is indicated for diagnosis of allergic contact dermatitis if the cause is not apparent by history and distribution of the lesions. When the disease is caused by a topical medication, cosmetic, or other product containing a number of chemical components, each component should be tested separately so that allergen elimination can be specific.

C. Adverse Effects: A strongly positive test in a patient with severe allergy may cause considerable itching and discomfort, in which case the patch should be removed in less than 48 hours. Patch testing during the active phase of contact dermatitis may exacerbate the disease. Whenever possible, the dermatitis should be cleared by treatment before the test is begun. Occasionally the test itself can induce sensitivity, so the selection of test allergens should be limited to those suspected clinically.

D. Photopatch Test: This is a test for photoallergic contact dermatitis. The procedure is identical to the patch test, except that the test site is exposed to ultraviolet light or sunlight after the patch is removed, and the reaction is read after 24 hours and again after 48 hours. A control site is a patch test to the allergen without light exposure.

Cutaneous Tests

The cutaneous test (prick test, puncture test, epicutaneous test) introduces into the dermis, at a single point, a minute quantity of allergen sufficient to react with IgE antibodies fixed to cutaneous mast cells for release of mediators to produce a visible wheal and erythema (Fig 29–4A). It is the procedure least likely to produce systemic anaphylaxis, because of the small amount of allergen introduced into the skin. For the same reason it is also unlikely to elicit an Arthus or cell-mediated skin reaction.

For routine diagnosis in atopic and anaphylactic diseases, a single drop of concentrated aqueous allergen extract in buffered saline diluent at pH 6.0 is placed on the skin, which is then pricked lightly with a needle point at the center of the drop. After 20 minutes the reaction is graded and recorded as indicated in Table 29–4. A negative diluent control must be included. Positive controls of histamine or a nonspecific mast cell mediator-releasing agent such as codeine, or both, may be included. The skin of the back, volar aspect of the forearms, or upper arms can be used. Fifty or more allergens can be tested at one time on the back, but test sites should be at least 3.5 cm apart. A result of 2 + or greater is positive. A result of 0 or 1 + should be repeated by using the intracutaneous method. A late phase reaction is not usually elicited by prick testing.

Another cutaneous testing method is the scratch test, in which a short linear scratch is made in the skin, to which the allergen is then applied. It is not recommended because it frequently causes nonspecific irritation, it is painful, and occasionally it causes scarring.

Any drug with antihistaminic (H_1-receptor blocking) activity must be discontinued for an appropriate period (24 hours or longer, depending upon the drug) prior to testing. Some drugs prescribed for other diseases, notably the tricyclic antidepressants, are potent antihistaminics. Corticosteroids, theophylline, sympathomimetic drugs, and cromolyn do not inhibit immediate skin test reactions and need not be withdrawn prior to testing.

Intradermal Tests

In the intradermal skin test (intracutaneous test), a measured quantity of allergen is introduced into the skin for detection of IgE-mediated (atopic or anaphylactic), IgG-mediated (immune complex), or effector T lymphocyte-mediated (cellular or delayed hypersensitivity) responses (Fig 29–4B). It is therefore used in diagnosis of several different types of allergic diseases.

Intradermal tests should be applied to the arm only, so that a tourniquet can be used in the event of an unexpected systemic reaction. The allergen extract must be nontoxic and free of microbial contaminants. A tuberculin syringe with 27-gauge needle is

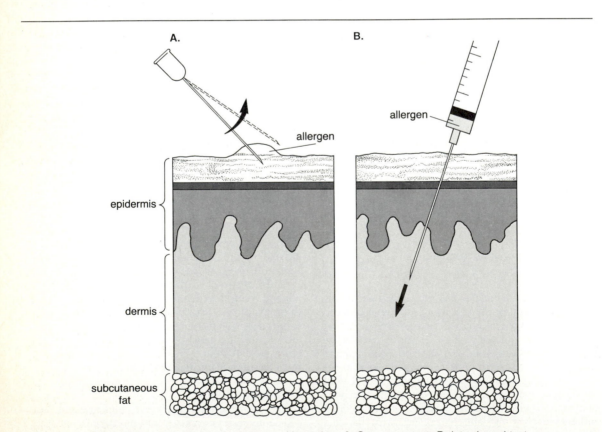

Figure 29–4. The technique of allergy skin testing. **A:** Cutaneous test. **B:** Intradermal test.

Table 29–4. Wheal-and-erythema skin tests.

Test	Reaction	Appearances
Prick	Neg	No wheal or erythema.
	1+	No wheal; erythema < 20 mm in diameter.
	2+	No wheal; erythema > 20 mm in diameter.
	3+	Wheal and erythema.
	4+	Wheal with pseudopods; erythema.
Intracutan-eous	Neg	Same as control.
	1+	Wheal twice as large as control; erythema < 20 mm in diameter.
	2+	Wheal twice as large as control; erythema > 20 mm in diameter.
	3+	Wheal 3 times as large as control; erythema.
	4+	Wheal with pseudopods; erythema.

used, and the volume to be injected depends upon the immunologic effector mechanism under study.

For IgE-mediated sensitivities, the recommended volume ranges from 0.005 to 0.02 mL, but is usually 0.01 mL. Larger volumes are unnecessary and cause confusing results. In most cases, intradermal testing in suspected IgE-mediated diseases is performed only for allergens giving 0 to 1+ responses to prior prick testing (see above), since the intradermal test is approximately 1000 times more sensitive. The reaction is read in 20 minutes (Table 29–4). A 1:500 (wt/vol) dilution of most common inhalant allergens is satisfactory for diagnosis of atopic allergy. A negative diluent control is necessary. A positive histamine or histamine-release control, or both, is optional.

After the immediate wheal and erythema subside, a late-phase 6–12-hour reaction appears in some cases. The diagnostic significance of the late-phase skin reaction is currently uncertain.

Serial dilution (skin endpoint) titration is a semiquantitative form of intradermal testing in which 5- or 10-fold increasing concentrations of allergen extract are tested for each allergen until a positive result occurs. Skin test sensitivity correlates roughly with clinical target organ sensitivity, but the main purpose of serial titration is to determine a starting dose for immunotherapy that will avoid the risk of systemic reaction. It is routinely used in testing for Hymenoptera insect venom anaphylaxis, but some allergists routinely titrate atopic allergens in testing. The method requires many more injections than the standard 2-stage prick and single-dose intradermal test, which can be quantitated by the size of the reaction.

Antihistamine drugs inhibit the intradermal wheal-and-erythema skin test reactions, as discussed above.

Intradermal testing can be used to detect circulating IgG antibodies in a suspected Arthus reaction. The cutaneous Arthus reaction is grossly similar to the late-phase IgE antibody reaction in appearance and timing, except that there is no preceding immediate-phase wheal and erythema and a high concentration of injected allergen is required to elicit a positive test. Immune-complex allergic reactions are infrequent in clinical practice (see Chapter 32), and IgG antibodies can be easily detected in vitro, so the Arthus skin test has not been standardized and is rarely used. A preliminary prick test should be done so that the procedure can be withheld if the patient has a significant (coincidental) IgE sensitivity to the allergen.

The tuberculin test is an intradermal test for cell-mediated hypersensitivity or immunity. It is performed by injecting 0.10 mL of the test allergen intradermally. There is a delayed (onset after 12 hours or more) response of erythema, induration, and tenderness. A positive test consists of induration 10 mm or greater in diameter at 48 hours. The test is not used in clinical diagnosis of cell-mediated allergies (see Chapter 19), but it is used extensively for detecting immunity in certain infections and in assessing cellular immunodeficiency (see Chapter 22).

Passive Transfer Testing

The immediate wheal-and-erythema skin test reaction in atopy or anaphylaxis can be transferred from the allergic patient to a nonallergic subject by injecting serum containing the IgE antibody from the former into the skin of the latter, proving an antibody causation for the disease. This is known as the Prausnitz-Küstner reaction. Cell-mediated skin test reactions, on the other hand, can be transferred by specifically sensitized effector T lymphocytes and not by serum antibodies. These serum or cell passive transfer procedures have been invaluable in research and have been used to a limited extent in the past for diagnosis. Their use in clinical practice is no longer justified, because of the risk of transmitting blood-borne microorganisms and the availability of the other testing methods discussed below.

5. IN VITRO TESTS

The need for in vitro diagnostic tests for allergies that use blood (or occasionally other body fluids) stems from the potential danger, the perceived discomfort, and the subjectivity of in vivo tests. In vitro tests can provide precision, reproducibility, and efficiency. Blood samples can be stored so that serial testing of samples drawn at different times can be performed simultaneously under identical conditions. In vitro tests are especially well suited for large-scale population screening and for testing allergens that are potentially toxic or irritating. They are useful in situations in which in vivo testing is thwarted by other factors, eg, the inability to do skin tests in a patient with extensive dermatitis or in an uncooperative child.

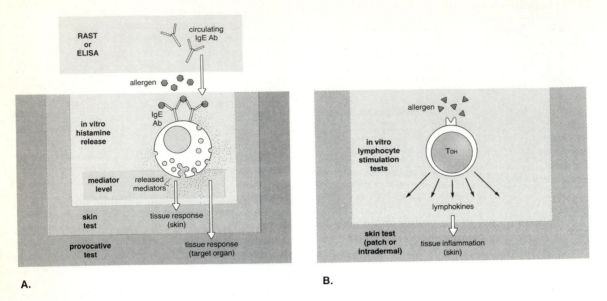

Figure 29–5. Schematic diagram showing the components of IgE-mediated (**A**) and T cell-mediated (**B**) allergic reactions that are detected by various diagnostic procedures.

In vitro tests, however, frequently measure only isolated components of the complex events in an allergic reaction (Fig 29–5). The clinical expression of allergy requires not only an immune response (the sensitized state), but also a properly reactive target tissue or organ, and exposure to a sufficient amount of allergen by an appropriate route of exposure to the allergen. The reaction can be further modified by extraneous factors such as age, endogenous endocrine hormone output, psychologic factors, and medications. All in vitro tests have limitations in sensitivity and are dependent upon the quality of the allergen and reagents and upon other technical factors. Results of any test must always be interpreted in the context of the history, physical examination, and other diagnostic tests.

Tests for IgE Antibodies

Quantitative measurement of allergen-specific IgE antibodies in serum requires special methods to detect the extremely minute quantities (picograms per milliliter) found in allergic patients. The standard technique is the radioallergosorbent test (RAST). This is a 2-phase (solid/liquid) system using an insolubilized allergen that is incubated first in the test serum to react with allergen-specific antibodies and then in radiolabeled heterologous anti-human IgE to detect the allergen-specific antibodies of the IgE isotype. The method is diagrammed and described in Fig 29–6. The test requires purified preparations of allergens and anti-human IgE. The RAST uses a cellulose disk as the insoluble immunosorbent to which protein allergens are coupled covalently with cyanogen bromide. There are a number of modifications of this method using other immunosorbents and other detection labeling systems (various chemicals detected by fluorescence or colorimetry).

Disadvantages of these in vitro methods are both biologic and technical. The quantity of serum IgE antibody is not necessarily a direct reflection of biologically relevant mast cell-fixed antibody. The test result is falsely positive in patients with a high total IgE level because of nonspecific binding of allergen to some immunosorbents, and it is falsely low in desensitized patients with high levels of IgG antibody. Like all other allergy tests, results must be interpreted in the context of the clinical history and examination.

Tests for IgG Antibodies

These are discussed in Chapter 18.

Tests of Immune Complexes

These are discussed in Chapter 18.

Lymphocyte Stimulation

This is discussed in Chapter 19.

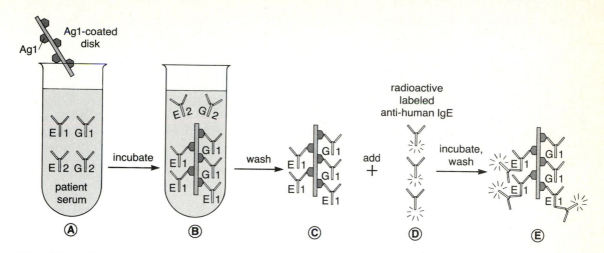

Figure 29–6. Diagram of radioallergosorbent test (RAST). **A:** A disk coated with the test allergen (Ag1) is incubated with serum of a patient with allergy to Ag1, as well as to other allergens (Ag2). **B:** IgE antibodies to Ag1 (E1) and IgG antibodies to the same allergen (G1) react with the Ag1-coated disk, whereas IgE and IgG antibodies (E2, G2) do not, and they remain in the serum. **C,D:** After being washed, the disk is incubated with a radiolabeled heterologous antibody to human IgE. **E:** After the disk is washed to remove unreacted labeled anti-IgE, the amount of radioactivity measured in a gamma counter is proportionate to the quantity of specific IgE antibody (E1) in the patient's serum. IgG antibodies to the same allergen (G1) on the disk do not react with the anti-human IgE antibody.

6. PROVOCATIVE TESTS

Occasionally it is desirable to test the target (respiratory, gastrointestinal, or cutaneous) tissue responsiveness to the allergen under controlled conditions. The patch test for immediate contact urticaria or delayed contact dermatitis is such a procedure. In the nasal provocation test, changes in nasal airway resistance and visible signs of congestion and rhinorrhea are observed after exposure to quantitative allergen challenge. Timed changes in bronchial airway flow rate or resistance are measured by bronchial provocation. Oral challenge with food or drug may be done to observe subjective gastrointestinal symptoms, appearance of skin eruptions, or objective changes in airway resistance.

A positive provocation test does not prove an immunologic basis for the disease, and except for patch testing, they are not used for routine diagnosis. Provocation testing is, however, an invaluable research tool for studying pathogenetic mechanisms and drug efficacy in allergic disease.

Allergen Bronchoprovocation Testing

Inhalational challenge with aerosolized allergen extracts to provoke a bronchial or pulmonary reaction under controlled conditions in the laboratory is of limited use in clinical practice. It is applicable in testing for allergic asthma and hypersensitivity pneumonitis (Fig 29–3).

The method of nebulizing and delivering known quantities of allergen extract is the same as for the methacholine challenge test (see above). Aqueous allergen extracts in several dilutions are prepared in buffered saline. An initial titration skin testing is necessary to determine a safe starting dose for bronchial challenge.

For testing in patients with allergic asthma, a measurement sensitive to acute airway obstruction is used, as in the methacholine challenge, and the dose-response result is presented in the same fashion. Usually the change in FEV_1 is expressed by determination of PD_{20}. Provocation tests have been done with the common inhalant atopic allergens, occupational allergens, and various chemicals. A fall in FEV_1 begins in 10 minutes or less, peaks at 20–30 minutes, and then returns to baseline. This immediate-phase asthmatic response occurs slightly later after allergen challenge than is the case for methacholine, histamine, or physical challenge. It is likely to be more severe and unpredictable, and it may require treatment with an inhaled bronchodilator drug. There may be a late-phase asthmatic response beginning at 4–6 hours, peaking at 8–12 hours, and clearing by 24 hours. Allergen challenges may cause isolated early or late responses, or both. Therefore, pulmonary function monitoring should be continued at hourly intervals after the immediate phase has subsided. Because of the possibility of late-phase responses, allergen bronchoprovocation should be performed in a hospital with appropriate facilities for detecting and treating these reactions. A positive late-phase response may increase the patient's nonspecific bronchial hyperirritability for several days, so if a second allergen is to be tested, this should be done at least 1 week later.

The indications for provocation testing in clinical practice are limited. For routine diagnosis of atopic asthma, bronchoprovocation with allergen gives results that correlate well with skin tests, but patients with only allergic rhinitis may also have specific bronchial response to inhaled allergen extract. A positive test to a suspected causative agent of occupational asthma does not necessarily mean that the asthma is immunologic. For example, bronchoprovocation with isocyanates produces specific immediate and late asthmatic responses in workers with clinical isocyanate asthma, even though the illness does not correlate well with an IgE (or other) immune response to this chemical. Allergen bronchoprovocation may be useful to monitor desensitization therapy.

Allergen bronchoprovocation is especially helpful in cases of suspected hypersensitivity pneumonitis. The method of delivery of allergen is the same as in tests for asthma, but pulmonary function measurements should be sensitive to measures of restrictive lung disease. The fall in forced vital capacity (FVC) and diffusing capacity for CO, as well as fever and leukocytosis, begin 4–6 hours after challenge, reach maximum effect at 8 hours, and return to normal values by 24 hours in patients with acute hypersensitivity pneumonitis.

To quantitate and standardize allergen challenges, it is necessary to use aerosolized aqueous extracts. The procedure therefore does not simulate natural allergic asthma or hypersensitivity pneumonitis caused by particulate allergens, as in the case of pollen and mold asthma, in which the inhaled material is in the form of particles up to 60 μm in diameter. Particles of this size, when inhaled naturally, do not reach the tracheobronchial tree, in contrast to liquid aerosols 1–5 μm in diameter, which do so readily.

Nasal Provocation Testing

An objective quantitative test of nasal mucosal reactivity to allergen or nonimmunologic stimulus is not available for routine diagnosis because of technical difficulties in assessing nasal reactivity. Present methods of rhinomanometry for measuring nasal airway resistance are limited by artifacts and poor patient acceptance. Nasal airflow is subject to anatomic factors, atmospheric conditions, psychologic stimuli, and physiologic fluctuations. Quantitation of rhinorrhea, sneezing, or itching is crude and subjective. Nasal provocation testing has been useful in research but not in clinical practice.

Elimination Diet Testing

Dietary elimination and challenge with foods suspected of causing urticaria or exacerbating atopic dermatitis, asthma, and gastrointestinal or other symptoms are commonly used by allergists. The procedure is not standardized but, rather, is tailored to each individual diagnostic situation. Elimination diets aim to alleviate ongoing symptoms. One or more foods, depending upon history, are eliminated until symptoms disappear. If symptoms are intermittent, a preliminary diet-symptom record may reveal the food(s) to be eliminated. If necessary, all natural foods are eliminated and nutrition is maintained by artificial diet, but restrictive diets should not be continued for more than 2 weeks. If symptoms clear, the eliminated foods are reintroduced one at a time to determine which food or foods provoke the allergic reaction or symptoms. A positive food challenge is repeated several more times for verification, but a single negative result generally rules out allergy to that food. There are no standard time limits for elimination or challenge, but, traditionally, most allergists accept a positive challenge within 2 hours to the same food on 3 successive trials as valid proof of a cause-and-effect relationship, although other information would be necessary to determine the mechanism. The clinical features of the induced reaction and evidence by skin or in vitro test of the relevant immune response will distinguish allergic reactions from toxic, digestive, metabolic, or psychologic responses to the food.

These elimination challenge maneuvers are subjective and greatly prone to erroneous diagnosis of food allergy because of physician and patient bias. A history of an acute allergic reaction to a single food allergen, supplemented if necessary by elimination and challenge testing and accompanied by IgE antibody detected by skin or in vitro test, is sufficient for diagnosis and therapeutic elimination of that food. In other situations in which delayed reactions, atypical or elusive symptoms and signs, and multiple suspect foods might lead to a nutritionally inadequate therapeutic elimination diet, the method of double-blind oral provocation testing should be employed.

Oral Provocation Testing

Double-blind food challenges are critical in defining the role of foods in allergic diseases. The procedure is simple and inexpensive enough to be used in clinical practice, although it is time-consuming. Patients with a history of anaphylaxis to a food should not be deliberately challenged.

Freeze-dried foods are packed into large opaque gelatin capsules. Each capsule can contain up to 600 mg of dry food. Lactose or a food to which the patient is not allergic can be used as a placebo control. The patient swallows a specified dose determined by the number of capsules and is observed for symptoms, signs, and an appropriate objective measure such as a pulmonary function test. The observation time and measurements are based on the history.

The order and frequency of active and placebo challenges are determined by a double-blind protocol. If a severe reaction is anticipated, increasing doses are given, starting as low as 10 mg of dried food and increasing to an amount corresponding to the amount suspected to cause a reaction by history. As much as 8 g can be consumed in capsule form by most patients. Some foods can be disguised in flavored milk shakes. A negative double-blind food challenge should be confirmed by an open dietary trial of the same food, since freeze-drying and encapsulating the food could conceivably change its allergenicity. When properly performed, this procedure is a powerful tool for avoiding an unsubstantiated diagnosis of food allergy when the test is negative. It is important to remember that a positive response shows only an intolerance to the food and does not prove an allergic pathogenesis.

REFERENCES

General

Kaplan AR: *Allergy.* Churchill Livingtone, 1985.

Lockey RF, Bukantz SC (editors): Primer on allergic and immunologic diseases, second edition. *JAMA* 1987; **258**:2829. (Entire issue.)

Middleton E, Reed C, Ellis E (editors): *Allergy: Principles and Practice,* 3rd ed. Mosby, 1988.

Patterson R (editor): *Allergic Diseases: Diagnosis and Management,* 3rd ed. Lippincott, 1985.

Samter M (editor): *Immunologic Diseases,* 4th ed. Little, Brown, 1988.

Sheldon JM, Mathews KP, Lowell RG: *Manual of Clinical Allergy,* 2nd ed. Saunders, 1967.

Diagnosis

Adkinson NF: The radioallergosorbent test in 1981: Limitations and refinement. *J Allergy Clin Immunol* 1981; **67**:87.

AMA Council on Scientific Affairs: In vivo diagnostic testing and immunotherapy for allergy. Part I. *JAMA* 1987;**258**:1363.

AMA Council on Scientific Affairs: In vivo diagnostic testing and immunotherapy for allergy. Part II. *JAMA* 1987; **258**:1505.

AMA Council on Scientific Affairs: In vivo testing for allergy. Report II. *JAMA* 1987;**258**:1639.

Berstein M et al: Double-blind food challenge in the diagnosis of food sensitivity in the adult. *J Allergy Clin Immunol* 1982;**70**:205.

Bock SA et al: Appraisal of skin tests with food extracts for diagnosis of food hypersensitivity. *Clin Allergy* 1978;**8**:559.

Bruce CA et al: Diagnostic tests in ragweed-allergic asthma: A comparison of direct skin tests, leukocyte histamine release and quantitative bronchial challenge. *J Allergy Clin Immunol* 1974;**53**:230.

Cockcroft DW: Bronchial inhalation tests. I. Measurement of nonallergic bronchial responsiveness. *Ann Allergy* 1985;**55**:527.

Cockcroft DW: Bronchial inhalation tests. II. Measurement of allergic and occupational bronchial responsiveness. *Ann Allergy* 1987;**59**:89.

Terr AI: In vivo tests for immediate hypersensitivity. *Annu Rev Med* 1988;**39**:135.

Townley RJ, Hopp RJ: Inhalation methods for the study of airway responsiveness. *J Allergy Clin Immunol* 1987; **80**:111.

30

The Atopic Diseases

Abba I. Terr, MD

GENERAL CONSIDERATIONS

Definition

Atopy refers to an inherited propensity to respond immunologically to many common naturally occurring inhaled and ingested allergens with the continual production of IgE antibodies. Allergic rhinitis and allergic asthma are the most common manifestations of clinical disease following exposure to these environmental allergens. Atopic dermatitis is less common. Allergic gastroenteropathy is still rarer and may be transient. Two or more of these clinical diseases can coexist in the same patient at the same time or at different times during the course of the illness. Atopy can also be asymptomatic (Fig 30–1).

Nonallergic rhinitis, asthma, and eczematous dermatitis occur in a significant number of patients without atopy, ie, in the absence of IgE-mediated allergy. There is a statistical association of elevated total serum IgE and blood and tissue eosinophilia with atopy, but these features are not always present in atopy, and they frequently occur in a variety of nonatopic conditions.

IgE antibodies also cause nonatopic allergic diseases—anaphylaxis and urticaria-angioedema (see Chapter 31)—and they are important in acquired immunity to parasites. A low level of IgE production is present in the normal population.

Thus, the definition of atopy is restricted to a condition with certain specific immunologic and clinical features. Nevertheless, it is a condition that affects a significant portion of the general population, usually estimated at 10–30% in developed countries. The etiology of atopy involves complex genetic factors. Clinical disease requires both genetic predisposition and environmental allergen exposure.

Immunology

A detailed description of the immunopathogenesis of IgE-mediated diseases is given in Chapter 11. Both mast cells and basophils have high-affinity IgE cell membrane receptors for IgE (FcεRI). Mast cells are abundant in the mucosa of the respiratory and gastrointestinal tracts and in the skin, where atopic reactions localize. The physiologic effects of the mediators released or activated immunologically by these cells are responsible for the functional and pathologic features of the immediate and late phases of atopic diseases. The important mediators of IgE allergy are histamine, chemotactic factors, prostaglandins, leukotrienes, and platelet-activating factor.

In allergic rhinoconjunctivitis the reaction occurs entirely at the local tissue level. Contact with allergenic particles such as pollen grains, fungus spores, dust, or skin scales from a pet is followed promptly by absorption of soluble allergenic protein at the mucosal surface. There, the relevant IgE antibody on the mucosal mast cell reacts with allergen, causing prompt mediator release and clinical symptoms. It is not clear whether the bronchial reaction in asthma requires inhalation of smaller particles, such as pollen fragments, capable of reaching the lower respiratory airways or whether allergic asthma is initiated by soluble allergen reaching the bronchial mucosa through the circulation. In atopic dermatitis, ingestion of allergenic food can flare the skin lesions, in which case exposure to the allergen must be via the circulation. The dermatitis can also be activated by direct topical exposure in instances of house dust mite allergy.

Atopic patients typically have multiple allergies; ie, they have IgE antibodies to and symptoms from

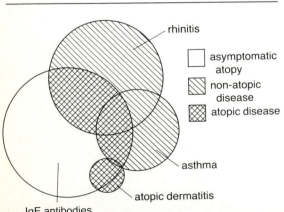

Figure 30–1. Interrelationships of atopy, atopic diseases, and IgE antibodies to environmental allergens.

many environmental allergens. As expected, the total serum IgE level is higher on average in the atopic population than in a comparable nonatopic population, although there is sufficient overlap that a normal serum IgE concentration does not rule out atopy. In general, total IgE in serum is higher in patients with allergic asthma than in those with allergic rhinitis and higher still in those with atopic dermatitis. Some nonatopic diseases are associated with a high serum total IgE (Table 30–1). Although measurement of total serum IgE is not a useful diagnostic indicator of atopy and does not measure specific IgE antibody, several studies show that the presence of IgE in cord serum is a predictor of subsequent atopy.

Since mast cell-bound and not circulating IgE antibodies are functionally important in initiating atopic reactions upon exposure to allergen, measurement of the total quantity of IgE fixed to high-affinity mast cell and basophil receptors (FcϵRI) might be more relevant to atopy. There is no technique for making such a measurement currently, but estimates of skin mast cell-bound IgE by threshold-dilution skin testing with heterologous anti-IgE show that the tissue IgE level is much higher in atopic individuals than in the normal population.

It has been suggested that antibodies of the IgG4 subclass may also fix to mast cells and basophils. The mast cell affinity for IgG4 appears to be low, and evidence that IgG4 antibodies can trigger mediator release in the presence of allergens is controversial. There is no indication that human atopic disease pathogenesis involves IgG4 antibodies.

Etiology

The etiology of atopy is unknown. Epidemiologic, family, and twin studies, as well as animal experiments, provide substantial evidence that genetic factors are involved in the propensity for atopy, in the regulation of total IgE production, and in the production of IgE antibodies to specific epitopes. However, a genetic basis for the various disease manifestations is not established. Several family studies have shown associations of human leukocyte antigen (HLA) types with enhanced production of antibody of IgE (and other) isotypes to a particular allergen. Genetic control of the total level of serum IgE is independent of genes in the major histocompatibility complex (MHC).

One theory based on the study of in vitro IgE antibody production by blood lymphocytes suggests that atopic allergy may arise through abnormal regulation by helper and suppressor T lymphocytes of the differentiation of B cells committed to IgE production into IgE antibody-secreting plasma cells. These regulatory T cells exert their effect through the secretion of protein IgE-binding factors that either enhance or suppress the differentiation of B cells.

A second theory suggests that the defect in atopy resides at the level of absorption of environmental allergens at respiratory and gastrointestinal surfaces prior to processing of the allergen for the immune response. The theory proposes that there is a normal protective mucosal barrier to exogenous antigens which is defective in atopy. Some support for this theory comes from the observation that levels of IgG antibodies to inhalant and food allergens are higher in atopic than nonatopic individuals, although these IgG antibodies are not believed to cause disease.

A third theory of atopy proposes a single defect for both the enhanced production of allergen-specific IgE antibodies and the hyperreactivity of target tissues to the mediators released from mast cells by IgE antibody. Immune cells and bronchial smooth muscle cells are both under autonomic control. Thus, an inherited (or perhaps acquired) autonomic imbalance such as β-adrenergic blockade or cholinergic overactivity could account for both enhanced IgE antibody production and target organ hyperreactivity. There is no direct evidence for defective autonomic control of IgE antibody production in atopy, although there is some indirect evidence for functional β-adrenergic blockade in the asthmatic airway and in atopic eczematous skin.

Environmental factors play a role in etiology. An accumulation of clinical experience suggests that the initial age of exposure to a particular food or pollen may determine the intensity of the subsequent IgE antibody response. A concurrent viral respiratory infection during environmental allergen exposure may have an adjuvant effect on both specific and total IgE production. Tobacco smoking may exert a similar effect. However, if the total level of serum IgE at the time of birth predicts future development of atopy, acquired factors would probably have only a secondary or permissive role.

Table 30–1. Diseases associated with elevated total serum IgE.

Disease	Possible Explanation of Elevated IgE
Allergic rhinitis	Multiple atopic allergies.
Allergic asthma	Multiple atopic allergies.
Atopic dermatitis	Multiple allergies and linkage to a non-MHC gene.
Allergic bronchopulmonary aspergillosus	Unknown; varies with disease activity.
Parasitic diseases	IgE antibodies associated with protective immunity.
Hyper-IgE syndrome	Unknown.
Ataxia-telangiectasia	T-suppressor cell defect?
Wiskott-Aldrich syndrome	Unknown.
Thymic alymphoplasia	Unknown.
IgE myeloma	Neoplasm of IgE-producing plasma cells; IgE is monoclonal.
Graft-versus-host reaction	Transient T suppressor cell defect?

Finally, the relationship between IgE-mediated atopic allergy and IgE-mediated immunity in helminthiasis offers an interesting opportunity to speculate about etiology. Atopic allergy is a prominent clinical problem in developed countries which are largely free of helminthic infestation. In populations in which these infections are endemic, serum IgE levels are typically high because of ongoing IgE stimulation, and it can be assumed that tissue mast cells are chronically saturated with parasite-specific IgE antibodies. The IgE mast cell-mediated immune mechanism has a selective advantage for the host under these circumstances. In a population free of parasitic infections, however, the IgE immune system may be vestigial for immunity but still available to react adversely to innocuous environmental allergens.

ATOPIC ALLERGENS

The allergens responsible for atopic disease are derived principally from natural airborne organic particles, especially plant pollens, fungal spores, and animal and insect debris, and from ingested foods. The ability of different pollens, molds, or foods to sensitize for IgE allergy varies, so that some of these environmental allergens are intrinsically more sensitizing than others, irrespective of the amount of exposure.

Pollen Allergens

The allergenic pollens are from wind-pollinated (anemophilous) flowering plants. There are far fewer of these plants than insect-pollinated (entomophilous) plants, but they discharge large numbers of lightweight, buoyant pollens that are dispersed over a wide area by wind currents. Within each local geographic area the common allergenic trees, grasses, and weeds pollinate during specific and predictable seasons, producing the corresponding seasonal respiratory symptoms in allergic patients.

The number of pollen-producing plants potentially capable of causing allergy is enormous, but those of proven allergenicity are limited. The major taxa and representative examples are listed in Table 30–2. Within each botanic subclass there are many species that cause allergy. Natural, cultivated, and ornamental plants all may produce allergenic pollen. Plants with attractive flowers are generally insect-pollinated, producing small amounts of heavy pollen that does not become airborne, and thus they are usually not the cause of inhalant allergy.

Allergenic pollen grains are mostly spherical, 15–50 μm in diameter, and they can usually be identified morphologically by light microscopy (Fig 30–2). Air sampling for identifying and quantitating pollens is done by volumetric impaction devices such as the rotorod or rotoslide sampler (Fig 30–3).

Table 30–2. Botanic classifications of pollinating plants frequently associated with atopic respiratory allergy.[1]

Botanic Classification[2]	Common Names of Typical Plants
Division Microphyllophyta	Club mosses
Division Pteridophyta	Ferns
Division Pinophyta	
Subdivision Pinicae	Conifers
Division Magnoliophyta	Flowering plants
Class Liliopsida	
Subclass Commelinidae	Grasses, sedges
Subclass Arecidae	Palms, cattails
Class Magnoliopsida	
Subclass Hamamelididae	Nettles, beeches
Subclass Caryophyllidae	Chenopods, sorrels
Subclass Dilleniidae	Willows, poplars
Subclass Rosidae	Maples, ashes
Subclass Asteridae	Ragweeds, sages

[1] Adapted and reproduced, with permission, from Weber RW, Nelson HS: Pollen allergens and their interrelationships. *Clin Rev Allergy* 1985;**3**:291.
[2] Classification system of Takhtajan.

Several representative examples of pollen seasons are shown in Fig 30–4.

Mold Allergens

Fungi are multicellular eukaryotic organisms that are abundant and ubiquitous. They are saprophytic, growing on a variety of dead or decaying organic material, where they flourish in direct relation to temperature and humidity. They reproduce sexually or asexually, producing airborne spores, some of which are allergenic.

Allergy to fungal spores is an important cause of disease in many atopic patients. However, specific diagnosis is hampered by the confusing taxonomic classification and nomenclature because of the enormous biologic complexity of fungi in their morphologic, reproductive, and ecologic behavior. It is difficult to obtain pure spores of many species for immunologic testing. Seasonal patterns of spores in air samples are poorly defined, making clinical correlation especially problematic. Mold spores range in size from 1 to 100 μm in diameter (Fig 30–2). Volumetric impaction samplers that are used for pollen counting are inefficient in trapping spores, so sampling by these devices does not yield quantitative data for spores. Table 30–3 lists some of the fungi most frequently associated with atopic allergy.

Arthropod Allergens

There are more than 50,000 species of mites. The house dust mites, *Dermatophagoides pteronyssinus* and *D farinae*, are the most common of all of the known atopic allergens. These tiny arachnids, barely visible to the naked eye, are found in house dust samples throughout the world but are most prevalent in warm, humid climates. They are especially abundant in bedding, upholstery, and blankets, where their natural substrate, desquamated human skin

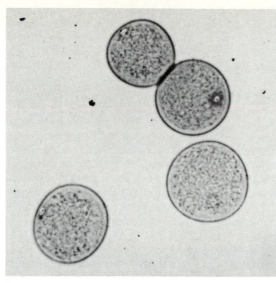

A.

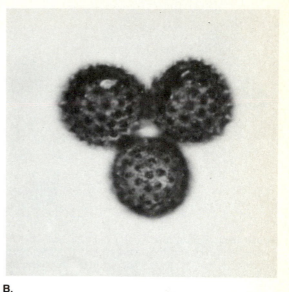

B.

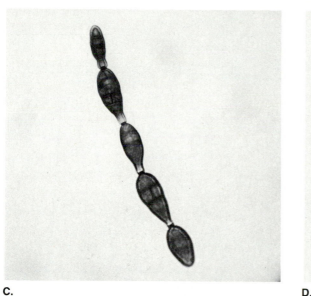

C.

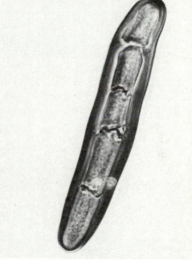

D.

Figure 30–2. Photomicrographs of several common pollens (**A:** grass [30 μm in diameter]; **B:** ragweed [20 μm in diameter]), and mold spores (**C:** *Alternaria* [70 μm in length]; **D:** *Helminthosporium* [80 μm in length]. Courtesy of William R. Solomon, MD)

scales, are likely to be found. The two species cross-react extensively but not completely. House dust contains other uncharacterized allergens, but they are of minor importance compared with *Dermatophagoides* spp. IgE antibodies and environmental exposure to these mite allergens correlate especially well with atopic asthma and atopic dermatitis, because exposure is by inhalation and dermal contact, respectively.

Other allergenic mites such as *Euroglyphus maynei, Lepidoglyphus destructor,* and *Acarus siro*—

storage mites that infest grains—may cause occupational allergy in grain handlers.

Various species of cockroaches are insect pests in homes and restaurants, especially in large cities where there is overcrowding and poor hygiene. Several studies have now documented high rates of sensitivity to cockroach allergen among allergic patients in inner-city populations; this often occurs as an isolated allergy. Other "endemic" causes of respiratory allergy are the emanations and debris of certain insects that swarm in huge numbers seasonally in spe-

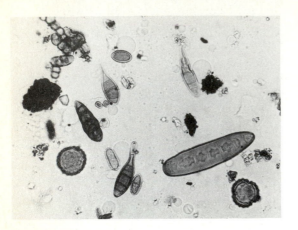

Figure 30–3. Typical "catch" of a volumetric air sampler showing pollen grains, mold spores, insect debris, plant particles, dust, and unidentified particles. (Courtesy of William R. Solomon, MD.)

cific locales. Examples of such insects include caddis fly and mayfly at the eastern and western ends, respectively, of Lake Erie; the green nimitti midge, *Cladotanytarsus lewisi,* in the Sudan; and Lepidoptera in Japan.

Animal Allergens

Atopic allergy to household pets, especially cats and dogs, has always been easily recognized because patients sensitive to these animals experience immediate intense attacks of asthma when in the same house with an animal to which they are allergic. Other animals encountered in domestic, occupational, and recreational settings also cause allergy. The source of the allergen may be in the dander (horse, dog), saliva (cat), or urine (rodents).

Food Allergens

Allergenic components of foods can induce IgE antibodies that may be responsible for either atopic

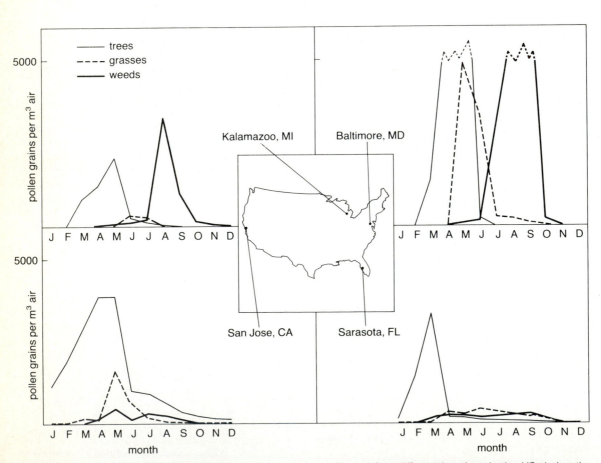

Figure 30–4. Representative examples of quantitative pollen counts at four different locations in the US during the same year (1984). Data from the American Academy of Allergy and Immunology Pollen and Mold Committee.

Table 30–3. Common fungal aeroallergens

Basidiomycetes	Phycomycetes	Ascomycetes
Ustilago	Mucor	Eurotium
Ganoderma	Rhizopus	Chaetomium
Alternaria		
Cladosporium		
Aspergillus		
Sporobolomyces		
Penicillium		
Epicoccum		
Fusarium		
Phoma		
Botrytis		
Helminthosporium		
Stemphylium		
Cephalosporium		

Table 30–4. List of highly purified allergens isolated by mid-1986.[1]

Grass pollens
  Lolium perenne (perennial rye) [5][2]
  Phleum pratense (timothy) [4]
  Dactylis glomerata (orchard or cocksfoot)
  Poa pratensis (Kentucky blue; June)
Weed pollens
  Ambrosia artemisiifolia or elatior (short ragweed) [6]
  Ambrosia trifida (giant ragweed)
  Salsola pestifer (Russian thistle)
Tree pollens
  Alnus incana (alder)
  Betula verrucosa (silver birch)
  Corylus avellana (hazel)
  Cryptomeria japonica (Japanese cedar)
House dust mites (Dermatophagoides spp)
  D pteronyssinus [2]
  D farinae
  D microceras
Nonbiting midges (Chironomus spp)
  C thummi thummi
Animals
  Felis domesticus (cat)
  Equus caballus (horse) [3]
  Bos domesticus (domestic cattle) [3]
  Rattus norvegicus (rat) [2]
Fungal spores
  Alternaria alternata
  Cladosporium herbarum [2]
Ingestants
  Gallus callarias (cod)
  Gallus domesticus (chicken; egg white) [3]
  Ascaris suum

[1]Modified and reproduced, with permission, from Marsh DG et al: Allergen nomenclature. *J Allergy Clin Immunol* 1987; **80**:639.
[2]In some cases multiple allergens have been purified. The number is indicated in brackets.

or nonatopic (anaphylactic) reactions. IgE antibodies to foods frequently exist in atopic patients without causing any reaction when the food is eaten. The factors that operate to convert asymptomatic sensitivity to symptomatic disease are currently unknown. IgG antibodies to many food antigens occur in most people, but they have no known pathogenic significance.

Virtually any food is capable of causing allergy on ingestion and many have been shown to do so in isolated cases, but certain foods are more likely to be allergenic than others. Seafoods are a particularly prominent cause of allergy in areas where fish is a staple in the diet. Crustaceans and mollusks are an important cause of anaphylaxis and anaphylactoid reactions. Legume, cow's milk, and egg white allergies are also common. Wheat, corn, chocolate, and citrus fruits, on the other hand, are often implicated in causing a variety of symptoms that are not characteristic of allergy in patients lacking IgE antibodies to these foods.

The allergenicity of a particular food protein can be changed by heating or cooking. A reaction can occur to the raw food only or to the cooked form only, or to both.

Occupational allergy, especially asthma from the inhalation of airborne food allergens, is a significant problem for many food handlers.

Allergen Extracts

Pollens, molds, foods, and animal and insect emanations are biologically complex materials made up of a mixture of numerous chemicals, many of which have allergenic potential. Aqueous extracts used in testing for IgE antibodies in allergic patients may contain a number of different allergens in addition to nonallergenic soluble compounds. There is an ongoing effort to isolate, purify, analyze, characterize, name, and standardize every important atopic allergen, and much progress has been made to date (Table 30–4). Availability of these purified materials will help to resolve clinical problems such as cross-reactivity among plants or foods. Purified allergens

are essential reagents for research studies on structure-function relationships and for genetic studies.

Crude aqueous extracts are useful for clinical testing and immunotherapy. For many years, standardization of extracts has been based on weight/volume or total protein content, neither of which reflects the allergen content accurately. Recently, standardization of allergen content either by endpoint skin test titration or by radioallergosorbent test (RAST) inhibition has been introduced, and the term Allergen Unit (AU) is now used to denote bioequivalence. A comparison of these methods is shown in Table 30–5.

ALLERGIC RHINITIS

Major Immunologic Features

- Allergic rhinitis is the most common clinical expression of atopic hypersensitivity.
- IgE-mediated allergy is localized in the nasal mucosa and conjunctiva.
- Pollens, fungal spores, dust, and animal danders are the usual atmospheric allergens.

General Considerations

Allergic rhinitis (also known as allergic rhinocon-

Table 30–5. Approximate equivalence of different methods for expressing allergen content in extracts used for testing and immunotherapy.

Method	Units
Weight/volume (W/V)	1:20
Protein nitrogen units/mL (PNU/mL)	10,000
Allergy units/mL (AU/mL)	100,000
Noon units/mL	100
Micrograms of protein/mL	100

junctivitis or hay fever) is the most common manifestation of an atopic reaction to inhaled allergens. More than 20 million persons in the US suffer from this disease. It is a chronic disease, which may first appear at any age, but the onset is usually during childhood or adolescence.

Epidemiology

Allergic rhinitis occurs in 10–12% of the US population. The prevalence and morbidity rate are influenced by the geographic distribution of the common allergenic plants and dust mite. The disease affects both sexes equally. It persists for many years if untreated. It is never fatal, but it does cause considerable morbidity and time lost from school or work.

Clinical Features

A. Symptoms: A typical attack consists of profuse watery rhinorrhea, paroxysmal sneezing, nasal obstruction, and itching of the nose and palate. Postnasal mucus drainage causes sore throat, clearing of the throat, and cough. There is usually an accompanying allergic blepharoconjunctivitis, with intense itching of the conjunctiva and eyelids, redness, tearing, and photophobia. In some patients, conjunctivitis may occur in the absence of nasal symptoms. The disease occurs seasonally in patients with pollen allergy. It may be present year-round if the sensitivity is to a perennial allergen such as house dust, or there may be perennial symptoms with seasonal exacerbations in patients with multiple allergies. Diurnal variation may suggest a household allergen, and symptoms that disappear on weekends suggest an occupational allergy. Severe attacks are often accompanied by systemic malaise, weakness, fatigue, and, sometimes, muscle soreness after intense periods of sneezing. Fever is absent. Swelling of the nasal mucosa may lead to headache because of obstruction of the ostia of the paranasal sinuses.

B. Signs: Rhinoscopy shows a pale, swollen nasal mucosa with watery secretions. The conjunctivae are hyperemic and edematous. There may be eyelid swelling from edema. Lower-eyelid ecchymoses—probably from eye-rubbing—are called "allergic shiners." These changes revert to normal when there is no allergen exposure and the patient is asymptomatic.

C. Laboratory Findings: Eosinophils are numerous in the nasal secretions, but this is not diagnostic, since nasal eosinophilia is found in some patients with nonallergic rhinitis and in those with asthma. Blood eosinophilia is present during symptomatic periods. The presence of any eosinophils in conjunctival scrapings, however, is probably diagnostic. Sinus x-rays, tympanometry, and audiometry may be indicated if an associated sinusitis or otitis media is suspected.

Immunologic Diagnosis

The diagnosis of allergic rhinitis is established by the history and physical findings during the symptomatic phase. Diagnosis of the specific allergic sensitivities in each case is then determined by skin testing for a wheal-and-flare response or by in vitro testing. Selection of allergens for detection of specific IgE antibodies by skin or in vitro test is based on the patient's history and on the known local environmental allergens.

Differential Diagnosis

Chronic nonallergic (vasomotor) rhinitis is a common disorder of unknown cause in which the primary complaint is nasal congestion, usually associated with postnasal drainage. It differs from allergic rhinitis by the absence of sneezing paroxysms or eye symptoms, and rhinorrhea is minimal. Congestion may be unilateral or bilateral, and it often shifts with position. Symptoms occur year-round and are generally worse in cold weather or in dry climates. The nasal mucosa is unusually sensitive to irritants such as tobacco smoke, fumes, and smog. Symptoms usually begin in adult life. The disease is more common among women, and it may begin during pregnancy. Examination shows swollen, erythematous nasal mucosa and strands of thick, mucoid postnasal discharge in the pharynx. Allergy skin tests are negative or unrelated to the symptoms. In nonallergic vasomotor rhinitis, the nasal secretions may or may not contain eosinophils, so nasal eosinophilia is not a reliable sign of allergy but may indicate a preasthmatic state. There is a good therapeutic response to decongestants and humidification, but antihistamines are usually not effective.

Rhinitis medicamentosa denotes the severe congestion that occurs from the rebound effect of excessive use of sympathomimetic nasal sprays or nose drops. In this disease, the mucosa is often bright red and swollen, but these changes are reversible with complete avoidance of nose drops or sprays, even if they have been used excessively for many years.

Infectious rhinitis is almost always due to a virus, and most patients with allergic rhinitis can distinguish their allergic symptoms from those of the common cold, which usually produces fever, an erythematous nasal mucosa, and an exudate in the nasal secretions that is polymorphonuclear rather than eosinophilic. Primary bacterial or fungal infections of the nasal passages are rare.

Some hormones may produce nasal congestion. This is common in pregnancy or with the use of oral contraceptive drugs. Nasal congestion occurs frequently in myxedema. Certain drugs produce nasal congestion (Table 30–6).

Anatomic obstructions may occur from foreign bodies in the nose, tumors, nasal septal deviation or spurs, and nasal polyps. Nasal polyposis is a constitutional condition independent of atopy and allergic rhinitis, but it is associated with asthma, aspirin sensitivity, sinusitis, and eosinophilia. Nasal polyps also occur in children with cystic fibrosis. Anatomic lesions are best detected by fiberoptic rhinoscopy after the application of a topical decongestant.

Vernal keratoconjunctivitis is a disease of unknown cause that usually affects children, producing giant papillary excrescences of the palpebral conjunctivae with symptoms of intense itching and a stringy exudate. The exudate contains eosinophils, mast cells, basophils, and plasma cells, suggesting an immunologic basis, but search for an allergic cause is usually unrewarding. Reversible giant papillary conjunctivitis is caused in some patients by the use of soft contact lenses.

Immunologic Pathogenesis

Soluble allergens from inhaled pollens, spores, and other aeroallergenic particles are rapidly eluted on contact with the moist mucous membranes of nasal mucosa and conjunctivae. Contact with the corresponding IgE antibody on local mast cells and basophils releases the various mast cell-associated mediators described in Chapter 13. Symptoms of sneezing, rhinorrhea, congestion, and pruritis appearing within minutes are caused by the effects of endogenously liberated histamine, leukotrienes, and prostaglandin D_2 in the early-phase allergic response. Chemotactic factors produce an inflammatory exudate that produces the more persistent congestion and nonspecific tissue hyperirritability of the late-phase response. The hyperirritability lowers the nasal threshold to both allergic and irritant stimuli such as temperature changes, irritant particles and gases, sunlight, and ingested alcohol, thereby accentuating the effect of other allergens and prolonging symptoms after cessation of the allergen exposure.

A significant number of patients with allergic rhinitis have a coexisting bronchial hyperreactivity in the absence of clinical signs of asthma. It is not known whether this is an intrinsic abnormality related to atopy or an acquired defect from allergen exposure, possibly a component of the late allergic response. The absence of symptomatic asthma may be explained by effective compensating homeostatic mechanisms that are defective or inoperative in asthmatic patients.

Treatment

Treatment consists of environmental measures to avoid allergen exposure, drugs, and desensitization. For any atopic disease, prophylactic treatment by avoidance of allergens is usually the most effective means of treatment. However, avoidance is not always possible or practical, and so medications are needed to control symptoms. In some cases, the immune response itself can be altered by desensitization therapy.

A. Environmental Measures: Avoidance of an allergen is recommended on the basis of a clinical history of symptomatic allergy and not because of a positive skin test alone. Appropriate measures in individual cases may be the removal of household pets, control of house dust exposure by frequent cleaning, and avoidance of dust-collecting toys or other objects in the patient's bedroom. Air-cleaning devices with high-efficiency particle filters may be helpful. Dehumidification and repair of leaking pipes or roofs may be necessary to prevent mold growth. Avoidance of pollen and outdoor molds is not possible unless the patient is able to stay in an air-conditioned home or office. In some cases, the patient might arrange a vacation trip to a pollen-free area during the peak pollen season.

In cases of occupational allergy, every effort should be made to modify the patient's work routine and to employ industrial hygiene measures to avoid allergen exposure, but if these measures fail, a change in the patient's job may be necessary.

B. Drug Treatment: Antihistamines are the most commonly used drugs in allergic rhinitis, although their use is restricted by side effects. New nonsedating antihistamines avoid the most troublesome side effects. Orally administered nasal decongestants may be helpful, either alone or in combination with antihistamines. Sympathomimetic and antihistaminic eye drops are useful for allergic conjunctivitis. Administration of cromolyn by nasal sprays or conjunctival drops 4 times daily is beneficial and is virtually free of any immediate or long-term toxicity.

Systemic corticosteroids can be extremely effec-

Table 30–6. Drugs that may cause nasal congestion.

Drug	Presumed Mechanism
Oral contraceptives	Unknown
Reserpine	Norepinephrine depletion
Guanethidine	Norepinephrine release blockade
Propranolol	Adrenergic blockade
Thioridazine	α-Adrenergic blockade
Tricyclic antidepressants	Norepinephrine uptake blockade
Aspirin (rarely)	Idiosyncratic generation of vasodilating arachidonate metabolite?

tive in relieving symptoms of allergic rhinitis, but since the disease is a chronic, recurrent, benign condition, these drugs should be used with extreme care. The patient with very severe symptoms lasting for only a few days or several weeks each year who does not respond to antihistamines can be given oral prednisone for 1 or 2 weeks in a dosage just high enough to suppress symptoms. Flunisolide or beclomethasone by nasal spray may be equally effective without causing significant systemic corticosteroid effects. Side effects of nasal burning and epistaxis from nasal corticosteroid sprays are more annoying than dangerous, but the potential for mucosal atrophy and septal perforation with prolonged use requires periodic monitoring. Corticosteroid eye drops should be used very sparingly for brief periods only to control acute severe allergic conjunctivitis, with careful monitoring by an ophthalmologist.

C. Desensitization: Allergen injection therapy has been shown in many prospective double-blind controlled trials to be effective in treating allergic rhinitis. Because of the length of treatment required and the potential danger of serious systemic reactions, injection treatment is used in patients whose symptoms are uncontrolled despite appropriate environmental measures and symptomatic medications. The procedure, which is discussed more fully in Chapter 59, must be individualized and coordinated with environmental and drug treatment to be most effective; therefore, it should be initiated and monitored by a trained allergist.

Complications

Sinusitis as a concomitant or complication of allergic rhinitis is a controversial issue. The diagnosis of sinusitis is difficult because of frequent discrepancies between paranasal sinus symptoms and radiographic evidence of pathology. Mild sinus membrane thickening (less than 6 mm) is frequent in allergic rhinitis and could represent noninfectious allergic inflammation. Significant thickening, opacification, and air-fluid levels usually indicate an infectious sinusitis. Obstruction of the sinus ostia by swollen nasal membranes, whether caused by allergy, a common cold, or nonallergic vasomotor rhinitis, can cause secondary sinus infection, but to date there is no direct evidence that the sinus mucosa per se is a target organ in atopy.

Otitis media with or without effusion is common in children, and its causes are multifactorial, usually involving eustachian tube dysfunction and anatomic factors. The disease does not appear more frequently in atopic than in nonatopic children or adults. It is unlikely that inhaled allergen reaches the middle ear or eustachian tube, although tubal obstruction by swollen nasopharyngeal allergic mucosa or dysfunction caused by the allergic mediators could prolong or exacerbate the disease.

Nasal polyps are likewise observed with similar frequency in atopic and normal individuals. Although polyposis is not a complication of allergic rhinitis, management can be hampered by untreated nasal allergy, and vice versa.

Prognosis

Although no definitive studies have been done on the course of untreated allergic rhinitis, symptoms can be expected to recur or persist for many years if not for life. The severity of the symptoms is dependent upon the degree of exposure to the allergen. A patient with a pollen allergy who moves to an area where that pollen-producing plant does not grow will no longer be symptomatic.

ASTHMA

Major Immunologic Features

- Allergic asthma is a manifestation of IgE-mediated allergy localized in the bronchus.
- Important immunologically released or activated mediators are histamine, leukotrienes, and eosinophil chemotactic factor.
- Hyperirritability of bronchial mucosa amplifies the bronchoconstricting effects of mediators.

Definition

Asthma (also known as reversible obstructive airway disease) is a disease characterized by hyperresponsiveness of the tracheobronchial tree to respiratory irritants and bronchoconstrictor chemicals, producing attacks of wheezing, dyspnea, chest tightness, and cough that are reversible spontaneously or with treatment. The disease is chronic and involves the entire airway, but it varies in severity from occasional mild transient episodes to severe, chronic, life-threatening bronchial obstruction. There is an associated eosinophilia in the blood and in respiratory secretions. Episodes of asthma are triggered immunologically by allergen inhalation in patients with atopic allergy.

General Considerations

It is important to understand the role of allergy in asthma. Asthma and atopy may coexist, but only about half of the asthmatic population has atopy and a smaller percentage of atopic patients have asthma. All asthmatic patients—regarders of atopy—have the cardinal features that define asthma: airway hyperreactivity, reversible airway obstruction, and eosinophilia. In those with allergic asthma, attacks are triggered by allergen exposure as well as by other nonallergic factors.

Asthma and atopy are not wholly independent, however, because asthma occurs more frequently among atopic than nonatopic individuals, especially during childhood. It is not known whether predisposition to the 2 conditions is genetically linked or whether atopy enhances the clinical expression of an undefined asthmatic predisposition. A recent large-scale epidemiologic study showed that, contrary to abundant previous evidence, there is a positive statistical correlation of asthma and IgE antibodies in all age groups. Nonetheless, by tradition and clinical usefulness, asthma is often classified into extrinsic and intrinsic subgroups.

A. Extrinsic Asthma: This is also known as allergic, atopic, or immunologic asthma. As a group, patients with extrinsic asthma generally develop the disease early in life, usually in infancy or childhood. Other manifestations of atopy—eczema or allergic rhinitis—often coexist. A family history of atopic disease is common. Attacks of asthma occur during pollen seasons, in the presence of animals, or on exposure to house dust, feather pillows, or other allergens, depending upon the patient's particular allergic sensitivities. Skin tests show positive wheal-and-flare reactions to the causative allergens. Total serum IgE concentration is frequently elevated but is sometimes normal.

B. Intrinsic Asthma: This is also known as nonallergic or idiopathic asthma. It characteristically appears first during adult life, usually after an apparent respiratory infection, so that the term "adult-onset asthma" is sometimes applied. This term is misleading, because some nonallergic asthmatics first develop the disease during childhood and some allergic asthmatics become symptomatic for the first time as adults when they are exposed to the relevant allergen. Intrinsic asthma pursues a course of chronic or recurrent bronchial obstruction unrelated to pollen seasons or exposure to other allergens. Skin tests are negative to the usual atopic allergens. The serum IgE concentration is normal. Blood and sputum eosinophilia is present. Personal and family histories are usually negative for other atopic diseases. Other schemes for classifying asthma into subgroups, eg, aspirin-sensitive, exercise-induced, infectious, and psychologic, merely define external triggering factors that affect certain patients more so than others.

Epidemiology

Asthma is a worldwide disease that has been recognized for centuries, but prevalence figures vary, in part because of differences in definition and methods of case-finding. It is a common disease, which affects approximately 5% of the population of Western countries. There is no reason to suspect that the rate in Asia and Africa is substantially different. Onset during childhood is predominantly before the age of 5 years, and it affects boys more than girls (by about 3:2). The childhood-onset form is usually of the allergic variety. Adult onset may be at any age, but typically it occurs in the fifth decade. Ordinarily it is of the intrinsic type, and it affects women more than men (by about 3:2).

Some recent studies suggest that prevalence is increasing, but this may reflect better diagnosis and not a true change in incidence. Death caused by asthma—about 2000–3000 cases per year in the US—is relatively infrequent, but there are reports recently from several countries, including the US, of increasing asthma mortality rates and some evidence of increasing morbidity rates, despite substantial advances in symptomatic therapy.

Although not a major cause of mortality, asthma remains a leading cause for time lost from work and school.

Clinical Features

A. Symptoms: Asthma may begin at any age. It is characterized by attacks of wheezing and dyspnea that can range in severity from mild discomfort to life-threatening respiratory failure. Some patients are symptom-free between attacks, whereas others are never entirely free of airway obstruction. The asthmatic attack causes shortness of breath, wheezing, and tightness in the chest, with difficulty in moving air during inspiration but more so during expiration. Coughing is usually present, and with prolonged asthma the cough may produce thick, tenacious sputum that can be either clear or yellow. In children, coughing, especially at night, may be the only symptom to suggest the diagnosis. Fever is absent, but fatigue, malaise, irritability, palpitations, and sweating are occasional systemic complaints.

B. Signs: Physical examination during the attack shows tachypnea, audible wheezing, and use of the accessory muscles of respiration. The pulse is usually rapid, and blood pressure may be elevated. Pulsus paradoxus indicates severe asthma. The lung fields are hyperresonant, and auscultation reveals diminished breath sounds, wheezes, and rhonchi but no rales. The expiratory phase is prolonged. In a severe attack with high-grade obstruction, breath sounds and wheezing may both be absent. These are ominous signs, especially if accompanied by pallor and peripheral cyanosis, excitement or anxiety, and inability to speak. Chronic severe asthma in young children may lead to a structural barrel chest deformity.

C. Laboratory Findings: An increased total eosinophil count in the peripheral blood is almost invariably present unless suppressed by corticosteroids or sympathomimetic drugs. There is eosinophilia in nasal secretions. Sputum examination reveals eosinophils, Charcot-Leyden crystals, and Curschmann's spirals.

The chest x-ray may be normal during the attack or may show signs of hyperinflation, and there may be transient scattered parenchymal densities indicating focal atelectasis caused by mucus plugs in scattered portions of the airway. Total serum IgE is usually elevated in childhood allergic asthma and normal in adult intrinsic asthma, but this test lacks specificity in individual cases as a diagnostic screen for either asthma or atopy (Fig 30–5).

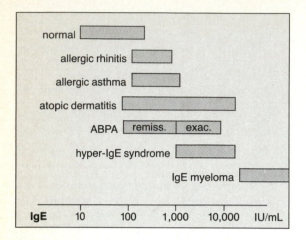

Figure 30–5. Total serum IgE levels in normal individuals and patients with various allergies and IgE disorders. ABPA, Allergic bronchopulmonary aspergillosis.

Pulmonary function tests show the abnormalities of airway obstructive disease. Flow rates and 1-second forced expiratory volume (FEV_1) are decreased, vital capacity is normal or decreased, and total lung capacity and functional residual capacity are usually normal or slightly increased but may be decreased with extreme bronchospasm. Following administration of an aerosolized sympathomimetic bronchodilator, ventilation improves with significant increase in flow rates and FEV_1, indicating the reversible nature of the bronchial obstruction. The lack of response in a patient already receiving large doses of sympathomimetic drugs does not rule out reversibility, and the test should be repeated at a later date after improvement from additional treatment such as hydration, corticosteroids, and chest physical therapy.

Repeated tests of ventilatory function are helpful in the long-term management of the asthmatic patient. Serial determinations of FEV_1, maximal expiratory flow rate, or peak flow rate are easily done in the office or clinic, and they will often detect airway obstruction that may not be apparent to the patient or to the physician on auscultation of the chest.

Inexpensive peak flow rate measurement devices are valuable for daily monitoring at home and work. Information can be used to uncover possible allergens and irritants in the patient's environment and as early warning of a worsening condition requiring more intensive treatment.

Bronchial provocation testing has made a significant contribution to pathophysiologic and pharmacologic research in recent years. These procedures are not necessary for routine diagnosis but are helpful in special circumstances (see Chapter 29). Nonspecific bronchial hyperirritability can be demonstrated by using quantitative challenges with methacholine, his-

tamine, cold air, or exercise. These tests of bronchial hypersensitivity are almost always positive in asthma, but they are not by themselves diagnostic of the disease, since bronchial hyperirritability occurs in a significant number of patients with allergic rhinitis, in normal subjects following viral respiratory infections, and in a small percentage of normal individuals. Since the procedure provokes an asthma attack, it should not be used in the presence of significant bronchial obstruction or if asthma can be diagnosed by other criteria.

Bronchial provocation by inhaling allergens to diagnose specific atopic sensitivities is sometimes useful in suspected occupational asthma, for which measurement of a dose-response effect under controlled conditions is desirable. This may be the case when the patient encounters several potential allergens at work. The patient should be monitored in a hospital for this procedure because of possible severe late-phase reactions.

Pathology

Autopsy on fatal asthma shows hyperinflation of the lungs, hypertrophy and hyperplasia of bronchial smooth muscle, and excessive mucus secretion. Death is usually caused by asphyxiation from mucus plugging of the airways. Microscopic examination shows hypertrophy and hyperplasia of submucosal glands and bronchial smooth muscle, mucosal infiltration with an edematous and mixed cellular inflammatory response especially rich in eosinophils, and epithelial desquamation within mucus plugs. Similar but less intense pathology exists during asymptomatic periods. The pathology therefore reflects both the early phase (smooth muscle contraction, edema, hypersecretion) and late phase (cellular inflammation) of the IgE-mediated allergic response. The gross and microscopic pathology of allergic asthma is indistinguishable from that of nonallergic asthma.

Immunologic Pathogenesis

The cause of asthma is not known. Pathogenesis of the asthmatic attack involves both allergic and nonallergic mechanisms. There is evidence that bronchoconstriction is mediated by an autonomic (vagal) reflex mechanism involving afferent receptors in the bronchial mucosa or submucosa which respond to irritants or chemical mediators and efferent cholinergic impulses, causing bronchial muscle contraction and hypersecretion of mucus. The mast cell-associated mediators (histamine, leukotrienes, prostaglandins, kinins, platelet-activating factor, and chemotactic factors) have properties that can explain the pathologic and functional abnormalities of the asthmatic attack. In the asthmatic patient, the afferent receptors appear to be sensitized to respond to a low threshold of stimulation. It has been proposed that the hyperirritable state of the bronchial mucosa results from defective functioning or blockade of its β-adrenergic receptor, preventing a homeostatic bronchodilating response from endogenous catecholamines. Bronchial hyperirritability is enhanced further during the late phase of the asthmatic reaction.

The linkage between allergen-IgE antibody interaction and release, activation, and secretion of mediators from the mast cell is now firmly established. The means by which nonallergic stimuli such as irritants and viral infections stimulate mast cells is unknown at present, and it is possible that other cells and mediators are involved in nonallergic asthma.

The variety of nonspecific agents that initiate an asthma attack is extensive. Some of these factors are listed in Table 30–7. Some of these items have been shown to increase the underlying bronchial hyperirritability as well, making the patient more sensitive to the effects of other triggers.

Approximately 10% of asthmatic patients have aspirin sensitivity. In these patients, ingestion of aspirin is followed in 20 minutes to 3 hours by an asthmatic attack, which is caused by an idiosyncratic pharmacologic response to the drug. Other nonsteroidal anti-inflammatory drugs cause a similar reaction. These anti-inflammatory drugs inhibit cyclo-oxygenase, the initial enzyme in the synthesis of prostaglandins from cell membrane arachidonic acid, and the quantitative ability of these drugs to provoke asthma is directly related to the ability to inhibit cyclo-oxygenase, indomethacin being the most potent and acetaminophen the least. Nasal polyposis is common in aspirin-sensitive patients.

The mechanism of aspirin-sensitive asthma is idiosyncratic and not immunologic. Since aspirin and related compounds normally inhibit the cyclo-oxygenase pathway of biosynthesis of prostaglandin E_2 (a bronchodilator) from arachidonic acid, it is suspected that in this disease an idiosyncratic response to these drugs favors the local synthesis of either prostaglandin F_{2a} (a bronchoconstrictor) or leukotrienes via the lipoxygenase pathway.

The clinical significance of immediate and late phases of the IgE response is especially clear in asthma. Bronchospastic episodes that occur within minutes upon allergen exposure and are promptly relieved by bronchodilators correspond to the immediate-phase response. Chronic asthma that is poorly responsive to β-adrenergic agonists and theophylline, associated with enhanced nonspecific airway hyperirritability, and dependent upon corticosteroids for reversal, is characteristic of the late-phase allergic response. Bronchial provocation challenge with many of the usual inhaled aeroallergens, ie, pollens, fungi, and dust mite, produce dual early and late asthmatic reaction in untreated allergic asthma.

Exercise-induced and hyperventilation-induced bronchocontriction in asthmatic patients is a consequence of water loss from the airway, which increases the osmolarity of fluid overlying the mucosal epithelial cells. This stimulates mast cells to release mediators, which, in turn, contract bronchial smooth muscle either directly or indirectly through vagal afferent receptor stimulation. Airway cooling, which occurs from inhaling cold air, exaggerates the effect of water loss.

The conceptual model of allergen-IgE antibody-induced allergic disease as discussed in Chapters 11 and 29 is well established. It requires direct contact of allergen with antibodies fixed to tissue mast cells, which then release mediators locally in the target tissues, where the inflammatory pathology and clinical symptoms and signs localize. In atopy the allergen molecule is often encountered as a component of an airborne particle such as a pollen grain or mold spore. In allergic rhonconjunctivitis these particles easily impact on the target conjunctiva and nasal mucosa, completing the direct contact model. In allergic asthma, however, particles at the upper end of this size range would not ordinarily be expected to penetrate as far as the tracheobronchial tree. However, recent immunochemical air-sampling methods have shown that pollen and spore fragments and even droplets containing allergen are inhaled as a significant portion of the ambient allergen load inhaled by the allergic patient.

The allergens commonly associated with allergic asthma and allergic rhinitis are generally similar. However, individual patients may tend to react with rhinitis to pollens and with asthma to molds and animal dander. Very young asthmatic children frequently have food-induced asthma without rhinitis.

Allergic asthma is the usual manifestation of IgE-mediated occupational disease. New occupational in-

Table 30–7. Nonspecific triggers of asthma.

Infections
  Viral respiratory infections
Physiologic factors
  Exercise
  Hyperventilation
  Deep breathing
  Psychologic factors
Atmospheric factors
  SO_2
  NH_3
  Cold air
  O_3
  Distilled water vapor
Ingestants
  Propranolol
  Aspirin
  Nonsteroidal anti-inflammatory drugs
  Sulfites
Experimental inhalants
  Hypertonic solutions
  Citric acid
  Histamine
  Methacholine
  Prostaglandin $F_{2\alpha}$
Occupational inhalant
  Isocyanates

halant allergens are continually being discovered. A partial list is shown in Table 30–8. Occupational asthma may also arise from nonimmunologic sensitivity or irritation to many other substances that fail to induce IgE antibody or other immune responses. In these cases, the cause and pathogenesis are unknown, but possible mechanisms that have been suggested include toxic chemical injury to the bronchial mucosa, irritant stimulation of mast cells or vagal irritant receptors, and β-adrenergic blockade. Patients with atopic allergy to specific allergens, eg, animals, are obviously precluded from working in a job in which they are exposed to these allergens. However, most cases of occupational asthma—both

IgE-mediated and nonimmunologic—occur in nonatopic workers, showing that an unusual high-dose exposure to a potential allergen in an occupational setting can override the requirement for genetic predisposition of atopy.

Immunologic Diagnosis

The diagnosis of asthma is made by history, physical examination, and pulmonary function tests to show reversible bronchial obstruction. Blood and sputum examination for eosinophilia is confirmatory. Chest x-rays are useful primarily to exclude other cardiopulmonary diseases. The methacholine challenge test is reserved for instances in which the

Table 30–8. Occupational allergens causing IgE-mediated allergic asthma.[1]

Allergen	Occupational Exposure
Animal products	
Cows, pigs, poultry, mice, hamsters, rabbits, rats, guinea pigs, bats, dogs, cats, horses	Animal/insect breeders, laboratory workers, veterinarians, breeders
Insect dusts	
Mealworms, storage mites, silk filatures, locusts, bees, cockroaches, flies	Grain handlers, sewerage workers, beekeepers
Sea creatures	
Crabs, shrimp, seasquirt body fluid, fish feed, *Echinodorus plamosus* larvae	Processors, breeders
Plant products	
Dusts, flours, cotton dust, grain dusts, grain flours	Cotton mill and textile workers, grain elevator and bakery workers
Fruits, seeds, leaves, pollens	
Castor beans, green coffee beans	Coffee processors, seamen, laboratory workers
Weeping fig, sunflower pollen, tobacco	Producers, agricultural workers
Organic dyes and inks	
Vegetable, dusts, gums, extracts	
Western red and eastern white cedar (plicatic acid), California redwood, exotic woods	Carpenters, sawmill workers
Colophony (abietic acid)	Electronics workers
Microbial agents	
Alginates, fungal allergens, humidifier contaminants, protozoa, fungi, bacteria	Biotechnology industry, laboratory, office workers
Enzymes	
Subtilisin, papain, pineapple bromelain, pepsin, hog trypsin, pancreatic extracts	Detergent manufacturers, pharmaceutical workers, food processors
Therapeutic agents	
Antibiotics and related compounds, penicillins, cephalosporins, tetracycline, phenylglycine acid chloride, sulfonamides, spiramycin	Pharmaceutical workers, poultry chick breeders
Pharmaceuticals and related compounds	
α-Methyldopa, amprolium hydrochloride, cimetidine, furan-based binder, glycyl compound (salbutamol intermediate), psyllium (bulk laxative)	Pharmaceutical workers, nurses
Piperazine	Medical and veterinary workers
Sterilizing agents	
Chloramine, sulfone chloramides, hexachlorophene	Abattoir, kitchen, hospital workers
Inorganic chemicals	
Metal fumes and salts	Metalworkers
Aluminum, chromium, cobalt, fluoride, nickel, platinum, stainless steel, welding fumes, vanadium, zinc	Chemical industry workers, metal refiners, platers, grinders, welders
Ammonium persulfate	Beauticians
Organic chemicals	
Amines (diamines, ethanolamines, tetramines)	Chemical, electronic, plastic, rubber industry workers, photographers, beauticians, fur handlers
Anhydrides (phthalic, tetrachlorophthalic, trimellitic), azobisformamide, azodicarbonamide	Plastics industry workers, food wrappers

[1]Modified and reproduced, with permission, from Butcher BT, Salvaggio JE: *J Allergy Clin Immunol* 1986;**78**:547.

history is equivocal and pulmonary function is normal.

The history is the primary diagnostic tool for evaluating the presence of allergy and identifying the relevant allergens. In general, inhalant allergens that are important in allergic rhinitis are also implicated in allergic asthma. These include pollens, fungi, animal danders, house dust, and other household and occupational airborne allergens. In young children and infants, allergy to foods may also cause asthma. History and physical findings of other atopic diseases—atopic dermatitis or allergic rhinitis—as well as a family history of atopy increase suspicion that asthma may involve atopic allergy. Skin testing for wheal-and-flare reactions will verify the specific sensitivities. RAST or other in vitro tests may be used in unusual situations when skin testing is contraindicated. Bronchoprovocation allergen testing is used primarily in difficult diagnostic cases of suspected occupational lung disease.

Differential Diagnosis

Chronic bronchitis and emphysema (chronic obstructive lung disease) produce airway obstruction that does not respond to sympathomimetic bronchodilators or corticosteroids, and there is no associated eosinophilia in the blood or sputum. In children acute bronchiolitis, cystic fibrosis, aspiration of a foreign body, and airway obstruction caused by a congenital vascular anomaly must be considered. Benign or malignant bronchial tumors or external compression from an enlarged substernal thyroid, thymus enlargement, aneurysm, or mediastinal tumor may cause wheezing. Acute viral bronchitis may produce enough bronchial inflammation with symptoms of obstruction and wheezing that it may be termed asthmatic bronchitis. Cardiac asthma is a term used for intermittent dyspnea (resembling allergic asthma) caused by left ventricular failure. Carcinoid tumors may occasionally cause attacks of wheezing because of release of serotonin or activation of kinins produced by the neoplasm.

Treatment

Since the cause of asthma is unknown, cure of the basic defect, the hyperirritable bronchial mucosa, is not possible. The aim of treatment is symptomatic control. Environmental measures, drugs, and allergen desensitization may be required.

A. Environmental Control: Irritants such as smoke, fumes, dust, and aerosols should be avoided. If the diagnostic evaluation indicates allergy to animal danders, feathers, molds, or house dust, these should be eliminated from the house.

B. Drug Treatment:

1. Sympathomimetics—β-Adrenergic bronchodilator drugs are effective and are used in the acute attack or for long-term management. Epinephrine has both α- and β-adrenergic effects, but it has a long history of efficacy in acute asthma attacks. It acts rapidly and is given subcutaneously in a dose of 0.2–0.5 mL of 1:1000 aqueous solution. Its duration of action is short, so that if repeated injections are required, long-acting epinephrine (1:200 in suspension) or terbutaline can be used. Albuterol, pirbuterol, metaproterenol, and isoetharine are selective β-adrenergic bronchodilators that are given by inhalation of aerosol. They are available as solutions to be administered by a hand-held nebulizer, in an intermittent positive-pressure breathing device, or in metered-dose pressurized inhalers, but patients must be cautioned that overuse can lead to paradoxic bronchial constriction and worsening of asthma. The β-adrenergic drugs terbutaline, metaproterenol, and albuterol are available as oral sympathomimetic drugs for achieving sustained bronchodilation in chronic asthma. Side effects of nervousness, muscle-twitching, palpitations, tachycardia, and insomnia can occur with all of them.

2. Xanthines—Theophylline and related compounds are especially effective as bronchodilators when used in combination with sympathomimetic drugs. Intravenous aminophylline, 250–500 mg, can be administered fairly rapidly in an acute asthmatic attack, and various oral forms of theophylline are available for long-term use. Absorption of theophylline varies with the drug preparation, the age of the patient, and other factors such as smoking and heart failure. Serum theophylline determination should be utilized to obtain a therapeutic level of 10–20 μg/mL.

3. Corticosteroids—Glucocorticoids are remarkably effective in the treatment of asthma. Even when all other forms of treatment have failed, the response to adequate steroid treatment is so dependable that failure of response might be considered grounds for questioning the diagnosis of asthma. The mechanism of action is unknown, and these drugs are just as effective in reversing asthma in nonallergic patients as in patients suffering allergen-induced attacks. Despite their effectiveness, however, systemic corticosteroids should not be considered primary drugs in the treatment of asthma, and in practice they should be given only when other forms of treatment prove inadequate. The dangers of long-term steroid therapy must be kept in mind by any physician prescribing the drugs.

Treatment is started at high dosage and continued until the obstruction is alleviated, with return of physical findings and flow rates to normal. The dose necessary to achieve this varies with the individual patient, but 30–60 mg of prednisone daily is usually sufficient. An occasional steroid-resistant patient may require a much higher dose because of an abnormally accelerated rate of drug catabolism. After complete clearing of the attack, the daily dose is reduced by slow tapering over many days or weeks to avoid a recurrence of asthma. Long-term alternate-day maintenance therapy minimizes adrenocortical suppression, but not all steroid-dependent asthmatic patients can be controlled in this fashion.

Beclomethasone dipropionate, triamcinolone acetonide, and flunisolide, highly potent corticosteroid drugs, are available in aerosolized form for inhalation. They are effective as long-term maintenance therapy for many steroid-dependent asthmatic patients. Adrenocortical suppression and systemic side effects are virtually absent. When they are used to replace a systemic steroid drug, the dosage of systemic drug must be tapered very slowly to avoid adrenal insufficiency. Inhaled corticosteroids are not useful for treatment of an acute asthma attack.

4. Cromolyn sodium–This drug is available as a powder administered in 20-mg doses by inhalation in a specially designed inhaler or micronized in a metered-dose inhaler. It is not a bronchodilator but is believed to inhibit the release of mediators of immediate hypersensitivity in the lung. It is administered as a long-term prophylactic treatment. It is more effective in younger patients with allergic asthma than in adults, and it frequently prevents exercise-induced bronchospasm. Cromolyn will not reverse an acute attack.

5. Other drugs–Antibiotics are used if secondary bacterial bronchitis or pneumonia occurs. Expectorants and hydration are helpful for thick, tenacious sputum. Inhaled ipratropium bromide, an anticholinergic drug with minimal side effects because of poor absorption, may help to eliminate the asthmatic cough.

C. Desensitization: The effectiveness of injection treatment in pollen hay fever has been shown in several controlled studies, and most allergists believe that allergic asthma responds just as well (see Chapter 59).

D. Treatment of Status Asthmaticus and Respiratory Failure: A severe attack of asthma unresponsive to repeated injections of epinephrine or other sympathomimetic drugs, termed status asthmaticus, is a medical emergency requiring immediate hospitalization and prompt treatment. Factors leading to this condition include respiratory infection, excessive use of respiratory-depressant drugs such as sedatives or opiates, overuse of aerosolized bronchodilators, rapid withdrawal of corticosteroids, and ingestion of aspirin in aspirin-sensitive asthmatic patients.

Immediate determination of arterial blood gases and pH with repeated measurements until the patient responds satisfactorily is necessary for optimal treatment. Injections of terbutaline or epinephrine are continued. If the patient has not been receiving oral theophylline, 250–500 mg of aminophylline may be given intravenously for 10–30 minutes initially, followed by slow intravenous drip with careful attention to toxic symptoms. Serum theophylline determi-

nations are used to maintain the optimal therapeutic level of 10–20 μg/mL of serum. Intravenous corticosteroids are indicated if the patient has previously received steroids, if the attack was caused by aspirin, if excessive aerosolized bronchodilator was a factor in the attack, or if significant CO_2 retention exists. Intravenous hydrocortisone at 4 mg/kg or methylprednisolone at 1 mg/kg, repeated every 2–4 hours, should be given until the patient can be maintained on oral prednisone at 60–80 mg daily in divided doses.

Dehydration usually accompanies status asthmaticus and may give rise to inspissated mucus plugs that further impair ventilation. During the first 24 hours, up to 3–4 L of intravenous fluid may be necessary for rehydration. Oxygen should be supplied by tent, face mask, or nasal catheter to maintain arterial P_{O_2} at about 80–100 mm Hg. Expectorants and chest physical therapy are helpful adjuncts to eliminate mucus plugs. Sedatives should be avoided even in the anxious patient because of the danger of respiratory depression. Antibiotics are used only for concomitant bacterial infection.

Respiratory failure, indicated by an arterial P_{O_2} level above 65 mm Hg and arterial blood pH below 7.25, may require mechanical assistance of ventilation in addition to all the measures listed above. This should be performed by a team of physicians, nurses, and technicians experienced in this form of respiratory therapy.

Complications & Prognosis

The disease is chronic, and its severity may change in an unpredictable fashion. Some children apparently ''outgrow'' asthma in the sense of becoming asymptomatic, but they may continue to show evidence of bronchial lability, and symptoms can reappear later in life. The acute attack can be complicated by pneumothorax, subcutaneous emphysema, rib fractures, atelectasis, or pneumonitis. There is no evidence that emphysema, bronchiectasis, pulmonary hypertension, and cor pulmonale result from long-standing uncomplicated asthma.

Allergic Bronchopulmonary Aspergillosis

This disease occurs almost exclusively in patients with a history of asthma who harbor *Aspergillus* endobronchially and who develop a heterogeneous form of hypersensitivity with both IgE and IgG antibodies to *Aspergillus* antigens (see Chapter 32).

ATOPIC DERMATITIS

Major Immunologic Features

■ It often accompanies atopic respiratory allergy.
■ The clinical course is usually independent of allergen exposure.
■ Very high serum levels of IgE may occur.

Definition

Atopic dermatitis (also known as eczema, neurodermatitis, atopic eczema, or Besnier's prurigo) is a common chronic skin disorder specific to a subset of patients with the familial and immunologic features of atopy. The essential feature is a pruritic dermal inflammatory response, which induces a characteristic symmetrically distributed skin eruption with predilection for certain sites. There is frequent overproduction of IgE by B lymphocytes, possibly caused by abnormal T lymphocyte regulation. Patients often have multiple IgE antibodies to environmental inhalant and food allergens, but the role of these allergens in the dermatitis is uncertain.

General Considerations

Atopic dermatitis is classified as a cutaneous form of atopy because it is associated with allergic rhinitis and asthma in families (and frequently in the same patient) and the serum IgE concentration is often high. However, it is usually difficult to prove that allergy plays a role, because the severity of the dermatitis often does not correlate with exposure to allergens to which the patient reacts positively on skin testing, and allergy desensitization is not effective in this disease. There is evidence for an underlying target organ (ie, skin) abnormality that might be a metabolic or biochemical defect, possibly linked genetically to the high level of serum IgE. Some studies also suggest a partial deficiency in T cell immunity. Atopic dermatitis may begin at any age. Onset in infancy at 3–6 months of age is typical, but it may first appear during childhood or adolescence and occasionally during adult life.

Clinical Features

A. Symptoms: The disease almost always begins in infancy or early childhood. Many cases clear by 2 years of age. Persistence into later childhood and adult life is marked by frequent cycles of remission and exacerbation. Itching is the cardinal symptom. It often worsens at night and is provoked by temperature changes, sweating, exertion, emotional stress, and embarrassment. There is a strong family history of atopy. Scratching and rubbing cause the typical eczematous skin eruption to flare. Itching is also exacerbated by irritants such as wool and by drying agents such as soap and defatting solvents. Ingestion of allergenic foods may cause acute exacerbations. The disease may improve spontaneously during the summer.

B. Signs: The skin is typically dry and scaly. Active skin lesions are characterized by intensely pruritic inflamed papules (prurigo), erythema, and scaling. Scratching produces weeping and excoriations. Chronic lesions are thickened and lichenified. Distribution of the lesions is dependent upon age. In infancy, the forehead, cheeks, and extensor surfaces of the extremities are usually involved. Later, the lesions show a flexural pattern of distribution, with predilection for the antecubital and popliteal areas and the neck. The face, especially around the eyes and ears, is often affected when distribution is more widespread. Staphylococcal pustules are common. Stroking of the skin produces white dermographism, in contrast to the normal erythema and whealing of the triple response of Lewis.

C. Laboratory Findings: Elevated total serum IgE, sometimes extremely high, occurs in 60–80% of cases. A normal level does not rule out the diagnosis.

Epidemiology

Approximately 0.7% of the US population has or has had the disease, but prevalence in children is 4–5%, equally distributed between the sexes. Racial predilection and geographic distribution have not been studied.

Pathology

Grossly, the lesion begins acutely with an erythematous edematous papule or plaque with scaling. Itching leads to weeping and crusting, then to chronic lichenification. Microscopically, the acute lesion is characterized by intercellular edema, and the dermis is infiltrated with mononuclear cells and CD4 lymphocytes. Neutrophils, eosinophils, plasma cells, and basophils are rare, and vasculitis is absent, but degranulated mast cells can be seen. The chronic lesion features epidermal hyperplasia, hyperkeratosis, and parakeratosis. The dermis is infiltrated with mononuclear cells, Langerhans cells, and mast cells. There may be focal areas of fibrosis, including involvement of perineurium of small nerves.

Immunologic Diagnosis

The history and physical examination are almost always diagnostic. Marked elevation of serum IgE is confirmatory, but a normal IgE level does not rule out atopic dermatitis. Biopsy is usually not required.

Because of the uncertainty about specific allergic sensitivities in pathogenesis, skin or in vitro allergy tests will usually produce positive results that may reflect concomitant respiratory allergies or asymptomatic sensitivities rather than causes of the skin disease. In some children with atopic dermatitis there may be positive skin tests to foods that cause acute exacerbation of eczema when those foods are given in a double-blind placebo-controlled oral challenge test. Blood T lymphocyte subset counts are not useful in diagnosis.

Differential Diagnosis

Localized neurodermatitis (lichen simplex chronicus) and allergic or irritant contact dermatitis produce similar eczematous changes of the skin. Seborrhea and dermatophytoses are occasionally confused with atopic dermatitis. Pompholyx (dyshidrosis) with secondary eczema may simulate atopic dermatitis of the hands.

Immunologic Pathogenesis

There is an intrinsic skin abnormality in atopic dermatitis, perhaps analogous to the hyperirritable airway in asthma. Some evidence suggests hyperreactivity to cholinergic stimuli, which might relate to the reduced threshold of the itch response. Increased numbers of mast cells and increased histamine content in the skin have been reported, but the other mast cell-associated chemical mediators have not been thoroughly examined for a role in this disease. Blood basophil counts are normal. Injection of methacholine intradermally initially produces a normal wheal and erythema; this is followed in 2–5 minutes by blanching because of edema. The delayed-blanch response is typical but not diagnostic of atopic dermatitis.

A. Defective Lymphocyte Regulation: Much indirect information suggests a defect in cell-mediated immunity. Delayed hypersensitivity skin test responses to recall antigens, in vitro lymphocyte responses to mitogen and allergen, and the autologous mixed lymphocyte reaction have all been reported to be deficient. Decreased prevalence of naturally acquired and experimentally induced allergic contact dermatitis and increased susceptibility to herpes simplex virus, vaccinia virus, warts, molluscum contagiosum, and dermatophyte skin infections are consistent with a defect in the T cell effector mechanism. Furthermore, many investigations have shown that excessive production of IgE by peripheral blood B lymphocytes in this disease can be accounted for by deficiency in CD8 T lymphocytes. It has been suggested that a defective CD4 helper T lymphocyte population could explain the failure of CD8 T lymphocytes to function as suppressors of IgE production and to achieve sufficient cytotoxicity for effective immunity against secondary skin infections.

B. The Role of Allergy: Atopic respiratory diseases with hypersensitivity to environmental allergens, eosinophilia, elevated serum IgE levels, and a family history of allergy are frequently associated with atopic dermatitis. Nevertheless, it is often difficult to attribute the dermatitis to allergy. The skin lesions rarely flare during pollen seasons, although in some patients there is an association with exposure to house dust, animals, or other environmental allergens. More commonly, food allergy is implicated in children. Milk, corn, soybeans, fish, nuts, and cereal grains are frequently implicated, but other foods may occasionally be important allergens also. Recent controlled food challenges have shown clear-cut exacerbations of the early inflammatory pruritic lesions in selected cases, although the responsible food cannot always be detected by skin testing.

C. Association with Systemic Disorders:

Eczema indistinguishable from atopic dermatitis is found in children with phenylketonuria. The skin lesions of Letterer-Siwe disease are also very similar. Atopic dermatitis without allergy is a feature of several immunologic deficiency disorders, especially Wiskott-Aldrich syndrome, ataxia-telangiectasia, and X-linked hypogammaglobulinemia (see Chapters 23–25).

Treatment

Atopic dermatitis is a chronic disease requiring constant attention to proper skin care, environmental control, drugs, and avoidance of allergens when indicated. Because dry skin enhances the tendency to itch, frequent application of nonirritating topical lubricants is the most important preventive measure. Areas involved with active eczema respond well to topical corticosteroids, but acute involvement of large areas of skin may warrant a brief course of systemic corticosteroids beginning with a high dose and tapering slowly after the acute eruption clears. Oral antihistamines help to control itching. If their sedative effect precludes use during the daytime, a bedtime dose will help to control involuntary scratching during sleep. Frequent bathing or washing, irritating fabrics such as wool, and harsh detergents should be avoided. The hands and fingernails must be kept clean to prevent secondary infection, and if infection does occur, an appropriate antibiotic should be prescribed.

Complications & Prognosis

Atopic dermatitis that persists beyond childhood has an unpredictable tendency to remit spontaneously, even after years of involvement. This is not related to the severity of involvement, the presence or absence of allergy, or treatment. Allergic rhinitis and asthma are not complications but, rather, additional manifestations of the underlying atopic disease.

The most frequent complication is secondary infection, almost always by *Staphylococcus,* as a result of scratching. In the past, the most serious complication was eczema vaccinatum from exposure to vaccinia virus by inadvertent vaccination or contact with a recently vaccinated person in the family or classroom. Eczema herpeticum is a similar condition caused by herpes simplex virus. Topical antibiotics or antihistamines may cause secondary contact dermatitis. Hand dermatitis occurs from excessive contact with water, soap, and solvents in the home and the workplace.

Ophthalmic complications include atopic keratoconjunctivitis, keratoconus, and atopic cataracts.

ALLERGIC GASTROENTEROPATHY

Major Immunologic Features

- Some atopic patients have localized IgE reactions in the gut to an ingested food.

- Gastrointestinal loss of serum proteins and blood may lead to edema and anemia.
- The condition is rare in adults; it is more common but transient in infants.

Definition

Allergic gastroenteropathy (also known as eosinophilic gastroenteropathy) is an unusual atopic manifestation in which multiple IgE food sensitivities are associated with a local gastrointestinal tract mucosal reaction. This produces acute gastrointestinal symptoms, eosinophilia, and gastroenteric loss of fluid, protein, and blood. Extraintestinal allergic symptoms, such as asthma and urticaria, may also be provoked by foods. Other atopic manifestations in the patient and family usually are present.

General Considerations

Allergic gastroenteropathy is the least common expression of atopy. Ingested food allergen reacting with local IgE antibodies in the jejunal mucosa liberates mast cell mediators, causing gastrointestinal symptoms shortly after the meal. Continued exposure to the food produces chronic inflammation, resulting in gastrointestinal protein loss and hypoproteinemic edema. Blood loss through the inflamed intestinal mucosa may be significant enough to cause iron deficiency anemia. In some patients, extraenteric manifestations of atopy may be produced by the same food allergen.

Epidemiology

Very few cases have been reported, but the disease has been described in infants, children, and adults. It is a very rare cause of gastrointestinal symptoms.

Immunologic Pathogenesis

The pathogenesis is that of atopy, as discussed above. The condition may occur more commonly in infants than in adults because of the much greater permeability of the infantile gastrointestinal mucosa to intact proteins. This may account for the transient nature of allergic gastroenteropathy in infants and young children.

The allergic reaction occurs locally in the upper gastrointestinal mucosa. Ingested food allergens react with IgE antibodies fixed to mucosal mast cells, thereby liberating the mediators of hyperemia, increased vascular permeability, and smooth muscle contraction. This results in acute symptoms, chronic loss of blood and plasma protein, and intestinal malabsorption.

Clinical Features

A. Symptoms and Signs: Nausea, vomiting, diarrhea, and abdominal pain occur within 2 hours after ingestion of the allergenic food, and these symptoms resolve on avoidance of the food. Rhinitis, asthma, or urticaria may accompany the intestinal symptoms. Chronic or repeated exposures to allergenic foods in undiagnosed disease may lead to blood loss anemia, abdominal distension, and voluminous foul stools from steatorrhea, edema from hypoalbuminemia, and systemic symptoms of anorexia, weight loss, and weakness. Children may experience growth retardation. Most patients have other manifestations of atopy, including atopic dermatitis, asthma, and allergic rhinitis, and there is usually a family history of atopy.

B. Laboratory Findings: Blood counts show hypochromic microcytic iron deficiency anemia and eosinophilia. Stool examination will reveal gross or occult blood and Charcot-Leyden crystals. Serum albumin is low, and total serum IgE may be elevated. Gastrointestinal x-rays may show mucosal thickening and edema of the small bowel.

Immunologic Diagnosis

A history of chronic or recurrent gastrointestinal symptoms associated with specific foods in an atopic patient should raise a suspicion of this diagnosis, especially if there is accompanying evidence of gastrointestinal blood loss, iron deficiency anemia, intestinal malabsorption, protein-losing enteropathy, other manifestations of atopy, or high serum total IgE.

In reported cases the causative food allergens have been single or multiple. Milk is the usual cause in children. Nursing infants may react to food allergens in breast milk from the maternal diet. The suspected food allergens identified by history can be tested for IgE antibodies by a skin test or RAST. Tests for antibodies to other foods may uncover other allergies, but these should be confirmed by elimination and challenge, preferably performed double-blind. Peroral jejunal biopsy may be necessary in difficult cases.

Pathology

An eosinophilic inflammatory infiltrate in the lamina propria of the upper gastrointestinal tract mucosa is present following allergen exposure and resolves with allergen avoidance.

Differential Diagnosis

Gastrointestinal allergy is overdiagnosed. Patients with food-related gastrointestinal symptoms—even atopic patients—are much more likely to have nonallergic food intolerance. Primary gastrointestinal diseases, reactions to food contaminants, and psychologic food aversion must be considered. Inflammatory bowel diseases, intestinal lymphangiectasia, and primary immunoglobulin deficiencies may produce similar symptoms. In children, lactase and other carbohydrate enzyme deficiencies, phenylketonuria, pancreatic deficiency from cystic fibrosis, and maple syrup urine disease should be ruled out by appropriate tests.

Treatment

Elimination of the allergenic food from the diet is curative. In some cases of milk allergy, boiled milk may be tolerated if the protein allergen is heat-labile. Corticosteroid treatment usually inhibits the reaction, but long-term steroid therapy should be necessary only for patients who do not respond to the elimination diet. There are reports that oral cromolyn in a dose of 200–400 mg given before the allergenic food is eaten inhibits the gastrointestinal allergic reaction, but there are no long-term studies on this form of treatment.

Complications

The major complications of this disease are edema and anemia. Unlike intestinal lymphangiectasia, significant gastroenteric loss of plasma immunoglobulins and lymphocytes does not occur, so susceptibility to infection is usually not a problem. Persistent disease activity may lead to secondary reversible lactose intolerance. Malnutrition can result from undiagnosed disease.

Prognosis

The infantile form of allergic gastroenteropathy is usually transient, but the duration of the disease is unpredictable and is not related to severity of the reaction. No long-term follow-up studies on adults are available.

REFERENCES

General

Ishizaka K: IgE-binding factors and regulation of the IgE antibody response. *Annu Rev Immunol* 1988;**6**:513.

Leskowitz S, Salvaggio J, Schwartz H: A hypothesis for the development of atopic allergy in man. *Clin Allergy* 1972;**2**:237.

Marsh DG, Meyers DA, Bias WB: The epidemiology and genetics of atopic allergy. *N Engl J Med* 1981;**305**:1551.

Terr AI: The atopic worker. *Clin Rev Allergy* 1986;**4**:267.

Allergens

Anderson JA, Sogn DD (editors): *Adverse Reactions to Foods.* NIH Publication no. 84-2442. US Department of Health and Human Services, 1984.

Anderson MC, Baer H, Ohman JL: A comparative study of the allergens of cat urine, serum, saliva, and pelt. *J Allergy Clin Immunol* 1985;**76**:563.

Burge HA: Fungus allergens. *Clin Rev Allergy* 1985;**3**:319.

Platts-Mills TAE, Rawk F, Chapman MD: Problems in allergen standardization. *Clin Rev Allergy* 1985;**3**:271.

Roth A: *Allergy in the World: A Guide for Physicians and Travellers.* University Press of Hawaii, 1978.

Solomon WR: Aerobiology of pollinosis. *J Allergy Clin Immunol* 1984;**74**:449.

Weber RW, Nelson HS: Pollen allergens and their interrelationships. *Clin Rev Allergy* 1985;**3**:291.

Yuninger JW: Allergenic extracts: Characterization, standardization, and prospects for the future. *Pediatr Clin N Am* 1983;**30**:795.

Allergic Rhinitis

Allansmith MR, Ross RN: Ocular allergy. *Clin Allergy* 1988;**18**:1.

Busse W (editor): New directions and dimensions in the treatment of allergic rhinitis. *J Allergy Clin Immunol* 1988;**82**:889.

Connell JT: Quantitative intranasal pollen challenges. 3. The priming effect in allergic rhinitis. *J Allergy Clin Immunol* 1969;**43**:33.

Druce HM, Kaliner MA: Allergic rhinitis. *JAMA* 1988;**259**:260.

Fireman P: Newer concepts in otitis media. *Hosp Pract* 1987;**22**:85.

Friedlaender MH: Ocular allergy. *J Allergy Clin Immunol* 1985;**76**:645.

Mullarkey MF, Gill JS, Webb DR: Allergic and nonallergic rhinitis: Their characterization with attention to the meaning of nasal eosinophilia. *J Allergy Clin Immunol* 1980;**65**:122.

Mygind N, Anggard A: Anatomy and physiology of the nose—pathophysiologic alterations in allergic rhinitis. *Clin Rev Allergy* 1984;**2**:173.

Norman PS: Allergic rhinitis. *J Allergy Clin Immunol* 1985;**75**:531.

Todd NW: Allergy as a cause of otitis media. *Immunol Allergy Clin N AM* 1987;**7**:371.

Asthma

Barnes PJ: New concepts in the pathogenesis of bronchial hyperresponsiveness and asthma. *J Allergy Clin Immunol* 1989;**83**:1013.

Chan-Yeung M, Lam S: Occupational asthma. *Am Rev Respir Dis* 1986;**133**:686.

Cherniak RM: Continuity of care in asthma management. *Hosp Pract* 1987;**22**:119.

Cohen SH: Advances in the diagnosis and treatment of asthma. Clinical evaluation—allergy and immunology. *Chest* 1985;**87(Suppl)**:S26.

Hargreave FE et al: The origin of airway hyperresponsiveness. *J Allergy Clin Immunol* 1986;**78**:825.

König P: Inhaled corticosteroids—their present and future role in the management of asthma. *J Allergy Clin Immunol* 1988;**82**:297.

Li JTI, O'Connell EJ: Viral infections and asthma. *Ann Allergy* 1987;**59**:321.

Mathison DA, Stevenson DD, Simon RA: Precipitating factors in asthma: Aspirin, sulfites, and other drugs and chemicals. *Chest* 1985;**87(Suppl):**S50.

McFadden ER Jr: Clinical physiologic correlates in asthma. *J Allergy Clin Immunol* 1986;**77**:1.

McFadden ER: Therapy of acute asthma. *J Allergy Clin Immunol* 1989;**84**:151.

Ohman JL: Allergen immunotherapy in asthma: Evidence for efficacy. *J Allergy Clin Immunol* 1989;**84**:133.

Rachelefsky GS, Siegel SC: Asthma in infants and children—treatment of childhood asthma. Part II. *J Allergy Clin Immunol* 1985;**76**:409.

Reed CW: Abnormal autonomic mechanisms in asthma. *J Allergy Clin Immunol* 1974;**53**:34.

Scoggin C: Exercise-induced asthma. *Chest* 1985;**87 (Suppl):**S48.

Siegel SC, Rachelefsky GS: Asthma in infants and children. Part I. *J Allergy Clin Immunol* 1985;**76**:1.

Summer WR: Status asthmaticus. *Chest* 1985;**87 (Suppl):**S87.

Atopic Dermatitis

Businco L, Sampson HA (editors): International symposium on atopic dermatitis: An update. *Allergy* 1989; **44(Suppl 9):**1.

Hanifin JM: Atopic dermatitis. *J Allergy Clin Immunol* 1984;**73**:211.

Oakes RC, Cox AD, Burgdorf WH: Atopic dermatitis: a review of diagnosis, pathogenesis, and management. *Clin Pediatr* 1983;**7**:467.

Sampson HA: The role of food allergy and mediator release in atopic dermatitis. *J Allergy Clin Immunol* 1988;**81**:635.

Sampson HA, McCaskill CC: Food hypersensitivity and atopic dermatitis: Evaluation of 113 patients. *J Pediatr* 1985;**107**:669.

Stone SP, Muller SA, Gleich GJ: IgE levels in atopic dermatitis. *Arch Dermatol* 1973;**108**:806.

Allergic Gastroenteropathy

Hutchins P, Waler-Smith JA: The gastrointestinal system. *Clin Immunol Allergy* 1982;**2**:43.

Scudamore HH et al: Food allergy manifested by eosinophilia, elevated immunoglobulin E level, and protein-losing enteropathy: The syndrome of allergic gastroenteropathy. *J Allergy Clin Immunol* 1982;**70**:129.

Waldmann TA, et al: Allergic gastroenteropathy: A cause of excessive gastrointestinal protein loss. *N Engl J Med* 1967;**276**:761.

Walker WA, Hong R: Immunology of the gastrointestinal tract. (2 parts.) *J Pediatr* 1973;**83**:517, 711.

31

Anaphylaxis & Urticaria

Abba I. Terr, MD

The allergic diseases caused by IgE antibodies are separated into 2 chapters in this book. In the previous chapter the atopic diseases were discussed. Atopy is a genetic predisposition to the production of IgE antibodies to common environmental antigens. In this chapter, 2 diseases—anaphylaxis and urticaria—are discussed. These also are caused by IgE antibodies, but they lack the genetically determined propensity and the target organ hyperresponsiveness of atopy, and they have no special predilection for the atopic individual. The immunologic pathogenesis for all IgE-mediated diseases is the same, but separate consideration of atopic and nonatopic diseases is important clinically. There are differences in the mode of exposure to the allergen, genetic factors that influence etiology, diagnostic methods, prognosis, and treatment.

Allergic gastroenteropathy, described in Chapter 30, has features of anaphylaxis, but it is included in the chapter on atopic diseases because it occurs almost exclusively in patients with other atopic manifestations.

ANAPHYLAXIS

Major Immunologic Features
- Systemic anaphylaxis is the occurrence of an IgE-mediated reaction simultaneously in multiple organs.
- The usual causative allergen is a drug, insect venom, or food.
- The reaction can be evoked by a minute quantity of allergen and is potentially fatal.

General Considerations
A. Definitions: **Anaphylaxis** is an acute, generalized allergic reaction with simultaneous involvement of several organ systems, usually cardiovascular, respiratory, cutaneous, and gastrointestinal. The reaction is immunologically mediated, and it occurs upon exposure to an allergen to which the subject had previously been sensitized. **Anaphylactic shock** refers to anaphylaxis in which hypotension, with or without loss of consciousness, occurs. **Anaphylactoid reaction** is one in which the symptoms and signs of anaphylaxis occur in the absence of an allergen-antibody mechanism. In this case, the endogenous mediators of anaphylaxis are released in vivo through a nonimmunologic mechanism.

B. Epidemiology: Anaphylaxis has no known geographic, racial, or sex predilection. It is not common, but prevalence is difficult to determine. It occurs at the rate of 0.4 cases per million per year in the general population, although in hospitals the prevalence is reported to be 0.6 per 1000 patients. The latter figure shows that medications and biologic products are a major cause.

C. Pathology: Grossly there is urticaria and angioedema. The lungs are diffusely hyperinflated, with mucus plugging of airways and focal atelectasis. The microscopic appearance of the lungs is similar to that in acute asthma, with hypersecretion of bronchial submucosal glands, mucosal and submucosal edema, peribronchial vascular congestion, and eosinophilia in the bronchial walls. Pulmonary edema and hemorrhage may be present. Bronchial muscle spasm, hyperinflation, and even rupture of alveoli may be seen microscopically. An important feature of human anaphylaxis is edema, vascular congestion, and eosinophilia in the lamina propria of the larynx, trachea, epiglottis, and hypopharynx. Myocardial ischemia has been found in a high proportion of cases, probably secondary to shock. Occasionally, myocardial infarction may occur. A direct effect of anaphylaxis on the myocardium or coronary arteries has not been shown. The liver, spleen, and other visceral organs are often grossly congested and microscopically hyperemic and edematous. Eosinophils are found in the splenic sinusoids, liver, lamina propria of the upper respiratory tract, and pulmonary blood vessels. Pulmonary edema and intra-alveolar hemorrhage may occur.

Death is usually attributable to asphyxiation from upper airway edema and congestion, irreversible shock, or a combination of these factors. Death occurring after many hours of shock may be from the effects of the late phase of the IgE allergic reaction or secondary to the failure of other organs.

D. Immunologic Pathogenesis: Anaphylaxis requires the presence of IgE antibodies and exposure to the allergen, but it is clear that it occurs in only a very small proportion of patients satisfying these requirements. In some cases the mode and quantity of allergen exposure are important. One example is the inadvertent injection of atopic allergens to atopic persons—a well-recognized risk of diagnostic skin testing and allergen immunotherapy. However, in most instances in which drugs, foods, or insect venoms are the cause, nonimmunologic potentiating factors such as an increased reactivity of mast cells, basophils, or target organs can only be surmised.

Anaphylaxis is the sudden systemic result of the allergen-IgE antibody mast cell-mediator release sequence detailed in Chapters 11 and 29. The result is a sudden profound and life-threatening alteration in functioning of the various vital organs. Vascular collapse, acute airway obstruction, cutaneous vasodilation and edema, and gastrointestinal and genitourinary muscle spasm occur almost simultaneously, although not always to the same degree.

E. Anaphylactic Shock: Hypotension and shock in anaphylaxis reflect generalized vasodilatation of arterioles and increased vascular permeability with rapid transudation of plasma through postcapillary venules. This shift of fluid from intravascular to extravascular spaces produces hypovolemic shock with edema (angioedema) in skin and various visceral organs, pooling of venous blood (especially in the splanchnic bed), hemoconcentration, and increased blood viscosity. Low cardiac output diminishes cardiac return and produces inadequate coronary artery perfusion. Low peripheral vascular resistance can lead to myocardial hypoxia, dysrhythmias, and secondary cardiogenic shock. Stimulation of histamine H_1 receptors in coronary arteries may cause coronary artery spasm. Some patients experience anginal chest pains and, occasionally, myocardial infarction during anaphylaxis. After a prolonged period of shock, organ failure elsewhere may ensue, particularly the kidneys and central nervous system. In some cases shock occurs rapidly before extensive fluid shifts would be expected to occur, suggesting that neurogenic reflex mechanisms might be involved.

F. Urticaria and Angioedema: Histamine and other mediators stimulate receptors in superficial cutaneous blood vessels, causing the swelling, erythema, and itching that characterize urticaria, a hallmark cutaneous feature of systemic anaphylaxis. Increased permeability of subcutaneous blood vessels causes the more diffuse swelling of angioedema, which may account for a substantial volume of fluid loss from the intravascular compartment.

G. Lower Respiratory Obstruction: Bronchial muscle spasm, edema and eosinophilic inflammation of the bronchial mucosa, and hypersecretion of mucus into the airway lumen occur in some patients with anaphylaxis and are indistinguishable from an acute asthmatic attack. Both histamine and leukotrienes have bronchoconstrictor activity, but the former affects the larger proximal airways preferentially, and the latter affects peripheral airways. Airway obstruction leads to impairment of gas exchange with hypoxia, further compounding the vascular effects of anaphylaxis. If this is left untreated, acute cor pulmonale and respiratory failure may occur.

H. Other Effects: Histamine acts on gastrointestinal and uterine smooth muscle, causing painful spasm. Hageman factor-dependent pathways may be activated by basophil and mast cell enzymes during anaphylaxis. One such enzyme has kallikrein activity and has been called basophil kallikrein of anaphylaxis, cleaving bradykinin from high-molecular-weight kininogen. Bradykinin has potent vascular permeability as well as vasodilating, smooth muscle-contracting, and pain-inducing properties, and it is occasionally found in anaphylactic states. Hageman factor activation of the intrinsic clotting mechanism may also explain some of the coagulation abnormalities found in systemic anaphylaxis.

Clinical Features

A. Symptoms and Signs: The reaction begins within seconds or minutes after exposure to the allergen. There may be an initial fright or sense of impending doom, followed rapidly by symptoms in one or more target organ systems: cardiovascular, respiratory, cutaneous, and gastrointestinal.

The cardiovascular response may be peripheral or central. Hypotension and shock are symptoms of generalized arteriolar vasodilatation and increased vascular permeability producing decreased peripheral resistance and leakage of plasma from the circulation to extravascular tissues, thereby lowering blood volume. In some patients without previous heart disease, cardiac arrhythmias may occur. Without prompt treatment by intravascular fluid replacement, prolonged shock may lead to the secondary effects of hypoxia in all vital organs. Death can result from blood volume depletion and irreversible shock or from a cardiac arrhythmia.

The respiratory tract from the nasal mucosa to the bronchioles may be involved. Nasal congestion from swelling and hyperemia of the nasal mucosa and profuse watery rhinorrhea with itching of the nose and palate simulate an acute hay fever reaction. The hypopharynx and larynx are especially susceptible, and obstruction of this critical portion of the airway by edema is responsible for some of the respiratory deaths. Bronchial obstruction from bronchospasm, mucosal edema, and hypersecretion of mucus results in an asthmalike paroxysm of wheezing dyspnea. Obstruction of the smaller airways by mucus may lead to respiratory failure.

The skin is a frequent target organ, with generalized pruritus, erythema, urticaria, and angioedema. Angioedema often involves the eyelids, lips, tongue, pharynx, and larynx. The conjunctival and oropharyngeal mucosa are erythematous and edematous. Occasionally, urticaria may persist for many weeks or months after all other symptoms have subsided.

Gastrointestinal involvement occurs because of contraction of intestinal smooth muscle and mucosal edema, resulting in crampy abdominal pain and sometimes nausea or diarrhea. Similarly, uterine muscle contraction may cause pelvic pain. Abortion can result if the patient is pregnant.

Hemostatic changes can occur but are not often investigated. The intrinsic coagulation pathway is activated, resulting in the possibility of disseminated intravascular coagulation and depletion of clotting factors. Thrombocytopenia may occur, possibly because platelets aggregated by platelet-activating factor (PAF) are sequestered from the circulation. In some cases, circulating heparin or other anticoagulants have been demonstrated.

Convulsions, with or without shock, have been reported rarely. In cases of fatal anaphylaxis, death usually occurs within 1 hour of onset.

B. Laboratory Findings: Laboratory tests are seldom necessary or helpful initially, although certain tests may be used later to assess and monitor treatment and to detect complications. Immediate emergency treatment should never be delayed pending results of laboratory studies. The blood cell counts may be elevated because of hemoconcentration. Eosinophilia may be present. Eosinophil counts may be elevated but are usually normal or low because of the compensatory effect of endogenous or exogenous catecholamines and glucocorticoids. Chest x-ray will show hyperinflation, with or without areas of atelectasis caused by airway mucus plugging. The electrocardiogram may show a variety of abnormalities, including conduction abnormalities, atrial or ventricular dysrhythmias, ST-T wave changes of myocardial ischemia or injury, and acute cor pulmonale. Myocardial infarction may be evidenced by electrocardiographic and serum enzyme changes. Plasma histamine may be elevated.

Clinical Diagnosis

The diagnosis of systemic anaphylaxis in a patient observed during an acute attack should be established or suspected as rapidly as possible by the symptoms and physical findings of hypotension, urticaria, angioedema, and laryngeal or bronchial obstruction, or any combination of these. Appropriate treatment should be instituted as soon as the condition is suspected. After the reaction is successfully treated, diagnostic efforts are directed to the cause.

Immunologic Diagnosis

The history is essential in determining the allergen responsible for an anaphylactic reaction. Skin testing or in vitro tests merely establish the presence of an IgE immune response to an allergen. This information is not in itself diagnostic, but must be consistent with the history. Ingestion of a food or drug; parenteral administration of a drug, vaccine, blood product, or other biologic material; or an insect sting occurring shortly (usually 1 hour or less) before the onset of symptoms raises suspicion that this is the cause. If the patient has experienced more than one episode, evidence of exposure to a common allergen should be sought.

Identification of the specific allergen may require persistent detective work. A reaction to milk may be caused by penicillin contamination. A reaction to a viral vaccine may be caused by egg white from the egg embryo in which the virus was cultured. Occasionally, a reaction occurs after injection of 2 agents with high anaphylactic potential (eg, penicillin and horse serum) or after a meal including several different "allergenic" foods such as fish, legumes, nuts, or berries.

The diagnosis is confirmed by detecting the presence of IgE antibody to the suspected allergen. In most cases, the immediate wheal-and-flare skin test is the most reliable procedure, especially if the allergen is a protein. Systemic reactions to skin tests have occurred in highly sensitive individuals, so testing should be done initially by the cutaneous-prick method. If the test is negative, intradermal testing to diluted sterile extracts of known potency can then be done.

To minimize the risk of anaphylaxis to the skin test itself, serial-titration testing with 10-fold-increasing concentrations of allergen is recommended when testing with protein allergens. Table 31-1 lists several recommended starting concentrations.

Skin testing in cases of suspected Hymenoptera venom anaphylaxis has been shown to be reliable if freshly reconstituted lyophilized venom extracts are used for testing. Testing with standard food extracts may yield false-negative reactions if the allergen is labile. Prick testing with direct application of the native food itself to the skin may yield a positive test, but some foods contain vasoactive chemicals producing false-positive reactions.

Skin testing with haptenic drugs is generally not reliable. Certain drugs cause nonspecific histamine release, producing a wheal-and-flare reaction in normal individuals (Table 31-2). Immunologic activation of mast cells requires a polyvalent allergen, so a negative skin test to a univalent haptenic drug does not rule out anaphylactic sensitivity to that drug.

IgE antibodies to major and minor penicillin allergy determinants are detected by wheal-and-flare skin tests. Penicilloyl-polylysine (6×10^{-5} mol/L solution) elicits a positive skin test in most patients with "major determinant sensitivity," ie, a history of late urticaria or drug rash, but not anaphylaxis.

Table 31-1. Starting intracutaneous skin test concentrations.

Allergen	Starting Concentration
Hymenoptera venoms	0.001 µg/mL
Insulin	0.001 U/mL
Horse serum	1:1000 dilution

Table 31–2. Drugs that cause nonspecific wheal-and-flare skin reactions.

Aspirin
Codeine
Curare
Histamine
Hydralazine
Meperidine
Morphine
Polymyxin B
Stilbamidine

Table 31–3. Some foods that cause anaphylaxis.

Crustaceans	Seeds
Lobster	Sesame
Shrimp	Cottonseed
Crab	Caraway
Mollusks	Mustard
Clams	Flaxseed
Fish	Sunflower
	Nuts
Legumes	**Berries**
Peanut	**Egg white**
Pea	**Buckwheat**
Beans	**Milk**
Licorice	

"Minor determinant sensitivity" indicates anaphylaxis to penicillin, but the test mixture of minor penicillin allergy determinants is not presently marketed, although a skin test using penicillin G (1000 units/mL) is usually positive in persons with documented anaphylaxis. The test is not recommended if there is an unequivocal history of penicillin anaphylaxis, because of risk of anaphylaxis to the test.

In vitro tests to detect the presence of circulating IgE antibody may be helpful if the test is positive, but a negative result does not rule out anaphylactic sensitivity, because the high affinity of IgE antibodies for mast cell receptors may result in a level of circulating IgE antibodies too low for detection by in vitro methods. The radioallergosorbent test (RAST) is the most frequently used in vitro test for IgE antibody, but it can be used only for protein allergens. Technical factors account for a significant number of false-positive and false-negative results.

Oral provocation challenge testing in cases of anaphylaxis to ingested allergens, such as foods, is not recommended because of the danger of a systemic response.

The presence of IgE antibodies, whether detected by a skin test or an in vitro test, does not diagnose the cause of anaphylaxis without correlation with the patient's history.

Allergens

The allergens responsible for anaphylaxis are different from those commonly associated with atopy. They are usually encountered in a food, a drug, or an insect sting. Foods and insect venoms are complex mixtures of many potential allergens. In only a few cases have the allergens been identified chemically. The same allergen or allergenic epitope may exist naturally in more than one food, drug, or venom, resulting in cross-reactivity.

A. Foods: Any food can contain an allergen for anaphylaxis. Table 31–3 lists some of the more common ones. Peanuts, nuts, fish, and egg white lead the list in frequency.

B. Drugs: Any drug is capable of causing anaphylaxis, although the risk is minimal for most people. Table 31–4 lists drugs and diagnostic agents reported to cause anaphylaxis in patients with drug-specific IgE antibody. Heterologous proteins and

polypeptides are the most likely to induce this type of sensitivity. However, most drugs used today are organic chemicals, which function immunologically as haptens. Anaphylaxis can occur from parenteral, oral, or topical drug administration. In some cases the amount needed to cause a systemic reaction can be extremely small; eg, a reaction in penicillin-allergic patients has been produced by minute amounts of penicillin in the milk obtained from penicillin-treated cows.

Anaphylaxis to blood and blood components may be caused by food allergens in donor blood or, rarely, by passive transfer of IgE antibodies to a food or drug when the transfusion recipient ingests that allergen shortly before or after the transfusion.

C. Insect Venoms: Anaphylaxis occurs from stings of Hymenoptera insects (Table 31–5), occasionally from biting insects such as deer flies, kissing bugs, and bedbugs, and rarely from snake venom. The venom of Hymenoptera insects is a complex biologic fluid containing several enzymes and other active constituents. There are multiple al-

Table 31–4. Some drugs and diagnostic agents that cause anaphylaxis.

Heterologous proteins and polypeptides	Haptenic drugs
Hormones	Antibiotics
Insulin	Penicillin
Parathormone	Streptomycin
Adrenocorticotropic	Cephalosporin
hormone	Tetracycline
Vasopressin	Amphotericin B
Relaxin	Nitrofurantoin
Enzymes	Diagnostic agents
Trypsin	Sulfobromophthalein
Chymotrypsin	Sodium dehydrocholate
Chymopapain	Vitamins
Penicillinase	Thiamine
Asparaginase	Folic acid
Vaccines	Others
Toxoids	Barbiturates
Allergy extracts	Diazepam
Polysaccharides	Phenytoin
Dextran	Protamine
Iron-dextran	Aminopyrine
Acacia	Acetylcysteine

Table 31–5. Hymenoptera insects.

Honeybee (*Apis mellifera*)
Yellow jacket (*Vespula* spp)
Hornet (*Dolichovespula* spp)
Wasp (*Polistes* spp)
Fire ant (*Solenopsis* spp)

lergens for human anaphylaxis, some specific to a particular species and others cross-reactive among species and genera. Allergens in honeybee venom include phospholipase A, hyaluronidase, phosphatase, and melittin.

The sting of a single insect is sufficient to produce a severe, even fatal anaphylactic reaction in sensitive patients. Sensitization occurs from prior stings, and if patients are allergic to a common or cross-reacting antigen they may have an anaphylactic reaction after being stung by any species of Hymenoptera insect. There is no evidence that other allergic diseases, including atopy and drug anaphylaxis, predispose to Hymenoptera anaphylaxis.

D. Other Allergens: There have been several cases of anaphylaxis occurring in women during intercourse because of allergy to a glycoprotein allergen in seminal fluid. There is one report of a woman sensitized to exogenous progesterone administered as a drug. She subsequently had anaphylaxis to endogenous progesterone and was cured by oophorectomy.

Anaphylactoid Reactions

A reaction clinically and pathologically identical to anaphylaxis can occur without the participation of an IgE antibody and corresponding allergen. This phenomenon is called an anaphylactoid reaction. (The term "anaphylactoid" is sometimes used inappropriately to refer to mild IgE-mediated anaphylactic reaction.)

A. Exercise-Induced "Anaphylaxis": A number of cases have been described. In some the reaction occurs only in association with eating, sometimes related to a specific food. During exercise the plasma histamine level rises, suggesting that nonimmunologic mast cell stimulation might be triggered by an endogenous factor, possibly endorphin. The reason for individual susceptibility is unknown, although a familial tendency has been reported, possibly because of a genetic defect. Many cases, however, are transient, suggesting a role for acquired factors.

B. Cholinergic Anaphylactoid Reaction. Exercise, emotions, and overheating provoke reactions in this rare condition. The plasma histamine level rises when there is an increase in core body temperature. Patients may have a positive methacholine urticarial skin test. A proposed mechanism is an abnormal reactivity of mast cells to the compensatory cholinergic response in thermoregulation when the core body temperature is elevated. This disease is an exaggerated form of cholinergic urticaria, described later in this chapter.

C. "Aggregate Anaphylaxis": Administration of gamma globulin for prophylaxis in patients with common variable immunodeficiency or other immunodeficiency diseases can cause anaphylactoid reactions. High-molecular-weight aggregated gamma globulin is probably responsible, since immunoglobulin aggregates can activate complement through the classic pathway and ultracentrifugation of the preparation to eliminate aggregates prevents such reactions. Aggregated immunoglobulins simulate the effect of antigen and corresponding specific IgG or IgM complement-activating antibodies, generating anaphylatoxins C3a, C4a, and C5a from the parent complement components C3, C4, and C5, respectively. Anaphylatoxins are capable of activating mast cells for mediator release, thereby producing the anaphylactoid reaction.

D. Non-IgE Anaphylaxis: Some patients with selective absence of IgA produce IgG anti-IgA antibodies following transfusion of IgA-containing plasma in whole blood or blood products. In such patients, subsequent administration of transfused IgA may cause anaphylaxis, presumably from complement activation and anaphylatoxin generation by circulating complexes of IgA and anti-IgA. An alternative explanation would involve antibodies of the IgG4 subclass. Several laboratories have reported that IgG4 antibodies can activate mast cells for mediator release in the presence of antigen. There is no direct proof yet that IgG4 "short-term sensitizing" antibodies are involved in systemic anaphylaxis.

E. Anaphylactoid Reactions From Ionic Compounds: Radiographic iodinated contrast media, especially when used for intravenous pyelography or cholangiography, produce anaphylactoid reactions that are frequently mild, causing only hives or itching. However, they may be severe, causing shock. In one case in 100,000, these reactions are fatal. The reaction can occur on first exposure and does not necessarily recur on subsequent exposure. Attempts to demonstrate specific antibodies to the compounds have been unrewarding. The reaction may be related to the ionic nature of these compounds, since newer nonionic contrast media appear less likely to cause such reactions.

The antibiotic polymyxin B is also a highly charged ionic compound that causes anaphylactoid reactions in some patients.

F. Other Causes: Polysaccharides such as dextran, gums, and resins produce anaphylactoid reactions by unknown mechanisms, probably direct mast cell activation. Certain drugs, especially the opiates, curare, and *d*-tubocurarine, behave similarly (Table 31–6).

G. Idiopathic Anaphylaxis. A few patients ex-

Table 31–6. Drugs and additives that cause anaphylactoid reactions.

Nonsteroidal anti-inflammatory drugs
  Aspirin
  Aminopyrine
  Fenoprofen
  Flufenamic acid
  Ibuprofen
  Indomethacin
  Mefenamic acid
  Naproxen
  Tolmetin
  Zomepirac

Opiate narcotics
  Morphine
  Codeine
  Meperidine

Mannitol
Radiographic iodinated contrast media
Curare and _d_-tubocurarine
Dextran

perience recurrent attacks of anaphylaxis without knowledge of exposure to an antecedent allergen. Exhaustive exploration of the history and careful observation of subsequent attacks will sometimes reveal an unsuspected allergen, but most of these cases appear to be truly idiopathic. Recurrent idiopathic anaphylaxis, like idiopathic chronic urticaria-angioedema, occurs predominantly in women between 20 and 60 years of age.

Differential Diagnosis

Anaphylactic and anaphylactoid reactions are identical in presentation. The former is produced by an antigen-antibody reaction, whereas the latter is caused by nonimmunologic release of mediators, so that the distinction must be determined by demonstrating whether the causative substance is an allergen.

Anaphylactic shock must be differentiated from other causes of circulatory failure, including primary cardiac failure, endotoxin shock, and reflex mechanisms. The most common form of shock that simulates anaphylactic shock is vasovagal collapse, which may occur from the injection of local anesthetics, particularly during dental procedures. In this case, there is pallor without cyanosis, nausea, bradycardia, and an absence of respiratory obstruction and cutaneous symptoms.

The Jarisch-Herxheimer reaction occurs several hours after antimicrobial treatment of syphilis or onchocerciasis. It is characterized by fever, shaking chills, myalgias, headaches, and hypotension. Unlike anaphylaxis, it can be prevented by pretreatment with corticosteroids.

Aspirin and nonsteroidal anti-inflammatory drugs affect a certain subset of asthmatic patients, producing an acute asthmatic reaction that may include nasal congestion, erythema, facial swelling, and shock.

Sulfite additives in certain foods and drugs may affect some asthmatics with a similar anaphylactic-like reaction. These nonimmunologic phenomena are discussed in Chapter 30.

Treatment

Treatment of anaphylaxis and anaphylactoid reactions is the same. It must be started promptly, so a high index of suspicion is necessary, and the diagnosis must be made rapidly. Once anaphylaxis is suspected, aqueous epinephrine, 1:1000 solution, is injected intramuscularly or subcutaneously in a dose of 0.2–0.5 mL for adults or 0.01 mL/kg of body weight for children. The dose is repeated in 15–30 minutes, if necessary. If the reaction was caused by an insect sting or injected drug, 0.1–0.2 mL of epinephrine, 1:1000 solution, can be infiltrated locally to retard absorption of the residual allergen. When anaphylaxis occurs in a patient receiving a β-adrenergic blocking drug, the reaction may be especially resistant to epinephrine, so that higher doses may be required. A tourniquet should be applied proximally if the injection or sting is on an extremity. The patient should then be examined quickly but thoroughly to assess the involved target organs, so that subsequent treatment is appropriate to the physiopathologic abnormalities.

A. Shock: The patient should be recumbent with the legs elevated in Trendelenberg's position. An intravenous line, preferably by catheter, facilitates drug administration. Intravenous epinephrine can be given in a dose of 1–5 mL, 1:10,000 solution, for adults and 0.01–0.05 mL/kg for children if systolic blood pressure is below 60. Other vasopressor drugs, such as dopamine, can be administered while blood pressure and pulse rate are being monitored. The specific treatment for shock, however, is fluid infused rapidly. Normal saline may be satisfactory, although as much as 6 L or more in 12 hours may be necessary. Initially, 1 L should be given every 15–30 minutes while vital signs and urine output are monitored. Plasma or other colloid solutions might be required. It may be necessary to monitor fluid replacement by measuring central venous pressure.

B. Laryngeal Edema: Examination of the airway for the presence of laryngeal obstruction should be done early. Establishing an effective airway is lifesaving. Passage of an endotracheal tube may be difficult because of the swelling. Puncture of the cricothyroid membrane with a 14- or 16-gauge short needle will provide an airway, but it is too dangerous to attempt in a child. Cricothyrotomy is the preferred method if treatment must be done outside a hospital. In the hospital, surgical tracheostomy is preferred.

C. Bronchial Obstruction: The treatment is the same as for acute asthma. Intravenously, aminophyllin at 6 mg/kg in 20 mL of dextrose in water given over 10–15 minutes serves as a loading dose, to be followed by 0.9 mg/kg/h. If the patient is an asthmatic and is receiving theophylline currently, a lower dose is necessary, and theophyllin blood level determinations should be utilized. If bronchospasm persists, nebulized β-adrenergic bronchodilators can be given by intermittent positive-pressure breathing. Hydrocortisone or methylprednisolone injections intramuscularly are used if the patient has recently received steroid therapy for asthma or for another condition. Oxygen by nasal catheter at 4–6 L/min is necessary if Pa_{CO_2} is less than 55 mm Hg. In the event of respiratory failure with Pa_{CO_2} above 65 mm Hg, intubation and mechanical assistance of ventilation are necessary.

D. Urticaria, Angioedema, and Gastrointestinal Reactions. These manifestations are not life-threatening and respond well to antihistamines. If they are mild, an oral antihistamine tablet is adequate. If they are severe, diphenhydramine, 50 mg (1–2 mg/kg for children), can be given intramuscularly or intravenously.

Monitoring treatment is vital in severe cases of anaphylaxis. Measurement of vital signs, examination of upper and lower airway potency, measurement of arterial blood gases, and electrocardiography are best accomplished in the emergency room or intensive care unit. All patients should be observed for 24 hours after satisfactory treatment, except in very mild cases.

Histamine H_2 receptor-blocking drugs, such as cimetidine or ranitidine, have been advocated as an adjunct to H_1 receptor antagonists, but their effectiveness has yet to be evaluated. Corticosteroid drugs have no antianaphylactic actions and should not be expected to alleviate the immediate acute life-threatening manifestations, although there may be special indications, as noted above. Complications such as cardiac arrythmias, hypoxic seizures, and metabolic acidosis are treated in the usual way.

The management of anaphylaxis from a Hymenoptera insect sting is the same as for any anaphylactic reaction. In honeybee stings, the venom sac and stinger usually remain in the skin and should be removed promptly by scraping with a knife or fingernail. Local reactions usually require only cold compresses to ease pain and reduce swelling, but extensive local inflammation may require brief corticosteroid therapy.

Prevention

A. Avoidance: Once the diagnosis of anaphylaxis has been established and the cause has been determined, prevention of future episodes is essential. In the case of food or drug allergy, the allergen and potential cross-reacting allergens must be thoroughly avoided. Insect-sensitive patients should avoid outdoor food and garbage, flowers, perfumes, mowing the lawn, and walking barefoot outdoors. Pretreatment with antihistamines and corticosteroids prior to radiography requiring administration of a contrast medium reduces the risk of a reaction in patients who have experienced a prior radiographic anaphylactoid reaction. Patients with IgA deficiency who require blood products should be transfused from donors with absent IgA (see Chapter 24).

Any physician or nurse who administers drugs by injection should be prepared to treat a possible anaphylactic reaction by having appropriate drugs available, and patients should remain under observation for 15–20 minutes after any injection.

B. Anaphylaxis kit: Patients with anaphylactic sensitivity to Hymenoptera insects or food should carry at all times a small kit containing a preloaded syringe of epinephrine and an antihistamine tablet. Epinephrine or a β-adrenergic drug in a metered-dose inhaler is not a reliable means of protection for anaphylactic shock.

C. Desensitization: Hymenoptera venom desensitization has been shown to be highly effective, as judged by responses to subsequent natural stings. Treatment is recommended for patients who have experienced systemic anaphylaxis after a sting and who have a significant positive skin test to one or more venoms. The maintenance dose for venom desensitization, 100 μg of each venom, is usually achieved in 12 weeks or less on weekly increasing doses. It should be continued at intervals of 4–6 weeks indefinitely.

Insulin-allergic diabetic patients and an occasional penicillin-sensitive patient may require desensitization.

Complications

Death from laryngeal edema, respiratory failure, shock, or cardiac arrhythmia usually occurs within minutes after onset of the reaction, but in occasional cases irreversible shock persists for hours. Permanent brain damage may result from the hypoxia of respiratory or cardiovascular failure. Urticaria or angioedema may recur for months after penicillin anaphylaxis. Myocardial infarction, abortion, and renal failure are other potential complications.

Prognosis

It is usually assumed that in anaphylaxis each succeeding exposure results in a more severe reaction. However, experience with cases of anaphylaxis to penicillin, Hymenoptera venom, and food indicates that this is not necessarily the case. If sufficient time elapses without contact with the allergen, there may be a decrease or loss of sensitivity in some patients. There is no method to predict changes in sensitivity, but it can sometimes be documented by periodic testing. Immunotherapy for stinging-insect sensitivity is strikingly effective in favorably altering the prognosis, and desensitization can occasionally abrogate penicillin anaphylaxis for a short time to permit the drug to be used safely. The prognosis must always be guarded by the knowledge that IgE immunologic memory may be lifelong. Anaphylactoid drug reactions follow various courses. Patients who react adversely to radiographic iodinated contrast media will usually tolerate subsequent exposure to the same contrast medium without reaction, but statistically a reaction is more likely to occur in a patient who had experienced a prior reaction.

URTICARIA & ANGIOEDEMA

Major Immunologic Features
- Acute urticaria-angioedema is a cutaneous form of anaphylaxis.
- IgE-mediated allergies to foods or drugs are common causes.
- Chronic or recurrent disease is usually nonimmunologic and of unknown cause.

General Considerations

Urticaria (also known as hives) and angioedema (also known as angioneurotic edema) can be considered a single illness characterized by vasodilatation and increased vascular permeability of the skin (urticaria) or subcutaneous tissues (angioedema). It is a localized cutaneous form of anaphylaxis and is one of the manifestations of systemic anaphylaxis. The same IgE antibody mechanism is responsible for the pathogenesis of allergic urticaria-angioedema and for that of systemic anaphylaxis, and the lists of the usual allergens are identical. Idiopathic (nonallergic) urticaria-angioedema is analogous to the anaphylactoid reaction. In contrast to anaphylaxis, urticaria is a benign condition and is much more common.

A. Epidemiology. Urticaria affects about 20% of the population, usually as a single or occasional acute attack.

B. Pathology. A variety of histopathologic lesions have been described, but these correlate poorly with the clinical presentation. They include edema, nonnecrotizing vasculitis, necrotizing vasculitis, perivasculitis, and a variety of different inflammatory reactions in the skin.

C. Pathogenesis: Urticaria and angioedema are the visible manifestations of localized cutaneous or subcutaneous edema from the increased permeability of blood vessels, probably postcapillary venules. Since injection of histamine into the skin simulates the spontaneous wheals, erythema, and pruritis of a typical urticarial lesion, it is generally accepted that endogenous histamine liberation is the mechanism responsible for the disease. The fact that subcutaneous tissue is looser and contains fewer nerve endings explains the more diffuse swelling and less severe itching in angioedema. Elevated levels of histamine in venous blood draining areas of induced urticaria have been repeatedly demonstrated. Other mediators from mast cells, particularly leukotrienes, are also believed to contribute to the pathophysiology.

D. Immunologic Pathogenesis: Many cases of acute urticaria and angioedema have been shown to have an allergic cause. In these cases, IgE antibody fixed to cutaneous or subcutaneous mast cells triggers mediator release or activation, as in anaphylaxis or atopy. Other potential immunologic pathways for mast cell mediator liberation, eg, the complement-derived anaphylatoxin pathway, have not been shown to operate in this disease. Idiopathic urticaria-angioedema and the various physical urticarias described below lack an allergen-antibody etiology. The precise means by which cutaneous mast cells are stimulated under these circumstances is unknown.

Clinical Features

A. Symptoms and Signs: Urticaria appears as multiple areas of well-demarcated edematous plaques that are intensely pruritic. They are either white with surrounding erythema or red with blanching when stretched. Individual lesions vary in diameter from a few millimeters to many centimeters. They are circular or serpiginous. Regardless of the duration of the illness, individual lesions are evanescent, lasting from 1 to 48 hours. They may appear anywhere on the skin surface, but often have a predilection for areas of pressure. Angioedema appears as diffuse areas of nondependent, nonpitting swelling without pruritis, with predilection for the face, especially periorbital and perioral areas. Swelling can occur in the mouth and pharynx as well.

Acute urticaria lasts for a few hours or a few days and is most likely to be associated with an identifiable cause, including allergy, nonspecific drug effect, infection, or physical factors. Chronic or recurrent urticaria persists with variable causes over a period of many weeks to years. Urticaria and angioedema may appear together in the same patient.

B. Laboratory Findings: There are no abnormal laboratory tests, except for the specific procedures described below.

Clinical Diagnosis

The diagnosis is immediately apparent on inspection of the skin.

Immunologic Diagnosis

A complete medical and environmental history and physical examination are usually necessary to determine the cause. Allergic urticaria may arise from exposure to allergens by ingestion or injection (most commonly), direct skin contact (less frequently), and inhalation (rarely). The discussion on common allergies in anaphylaxis earlier in this chapter applies to acute allergic urticaria.

Food allergy is diagnosed by careful dietary history, use of elimination diets, and appropriate food challenges. Drug allergy requires close scrutiny of the patient's recent drug history, elimination of suspected drugs, and occasionally deliberate challenge, although skin testing is helpful for certain drugs such as penicillin. The diagnosis of cold urticaria is made by applying an ice cube to the forearm for 5 minutes and observing localized urticaria after the skin has been rewarmed. Similar tests with application of heat, ultraviolet light, vibration, pressure, or water to a test area of the skin are appropriate if the history suggests these causes.

Cholinergic urticaria is suggested by the typical appearance of the lesions and exercise provocation. The methacholine skin test is positive in only one-third of patients.

Diagnostic tests for parasitic or other infections, lymphomas or other neoplasms, or connective tissue diseases are generally indicated only if the history and physical examination would have suggested such diseases in the absence of urticaria. It should be emphasized that in most cases of chronic recurrent urticaria, no cause is found even with the most diligent search.

Causes

A. Allergy: Ingestant allergens are much more frequent causes of urticaria than are inhalants. Any food or drug can cause hives. Occult sources of drugs such as penicillin in milk and the use of proprietary medications such as laxatives, headache remedies, and vitamin preparations must be considered. Food and drug additives are occasionally responsible. Insect sting allergy may cause urticaria without any other signs of systemic anaphylaxis.

B. Physical Causes: Dermographism, the whealing reaction that is an exaggerated form of the triple response of Lewis, occurs following scratching or stroking of the skin in 5% of the population. Another common phenomenon, unrelated to dermographism, is the appearance of hives after showering.

Cold urticaria may be induced locally by cooling of the skin on contact with cold. The hives often appear only upon rewarming. Occasionally generalized hives are provoked by cooling a portion of the body. Patients are in danger of shock when swimming in cold water. The diagnostic ice cube test is performed by applying an ice cube to the forearm for 5 minutes and then allowing the cooled area to rewarm. Hives appear at the site during the test or shortly afterwards. Occasionally the reaction can be passively transferred by serum to the skin of an unaffected individual.

Familial cold urticaria is a rare autosomal dominant disorder in which cold produces fever, chills, joint pains, and hives.

Urticaria and angioedema induced by heat, sunlight, water, or vibration are different syndromes and are rare. Pressure urticaria is a common feature of all forms of urticaria. However, delayed-pressure urticaria resulting from prolonged sustained pressure producing painful swelling is a distinct entity.

Cholinergic urticaria is a disease of unknown cause in which small (1–3-mm) wheals with prominent surrounding flare appear after exercise, heat, or emotional stress. Elevated body temperature is necessary for the reaction, which is believed to be initiated by a cholinergic response that triggers mast cell release. Other symptoms including hypotension and gastrointestinal cramping may accompany the urticaria and angioedema.

C. Vasculitis: Urticaria is reported as a symptom in some patients with systemic lupus erythematosus (SLE), systemic sclerosis, polymyositis, leukocytoclastic vasculitis, palpable purpura, hypocomplementemia, and cryoglobulinemia, but there is no convincing explanation for the association.

D. Neoplasms: Urticaria or angioedema is occasionally reported in a patient with neoplasm, especially Hodgkin's disease and lymphomas, but a cause-and-effect relationship is difficult to document. Rarely, angioedema from C1 esterase deficiency is caused by a lymphoma. This is discussed in Chapter 28.

E. Cyclo-Oxygenase Inhibitors: Aspirin and nonsteroidal anti-inflammatory drugs frequently precipitate acute or chronic urticaria. They also potentiate idiopathic urticaria or urticaria from other causes. The mechanism is unknown. There are many reports that food and drug additives, most notably tartrazine yellow dye and the preservative sodium benzoate, also cause or exacerbate hives, but the evidence is unimpressive.

F. Emotions: Precipitation of hives by emotional stress or other psychologic factors is a frequent clinical observation, but explanation of this phenomenon requires further study.

G. Idiopathic Urticaria-Angioedema: This category encompasses most cases of chronic urticaria-angioedema, because exhaustive diagnostic studies are unrevealing in the large majority of patients with recurrent urticaria lasting for more than 6 weeks.

Differential Diagnosis

The characteristic appearance of urticaria and angioedema, coupled with a history of rapid disappearance of the individual lesions, leaves little chance of incorrect diagnosis.

Multiple insect bites may evoke wheals, but careful inspection will show the bite punctum at the center of the lesion. Angioedema can be distinguished from ordinary edema or myxedema by its absence from dependent areas of localization and by its evanescent appearance.

Hereditary angioedema is a rare condition that produces periodic swelling and may be accompanied by abnormal pain and laryngeal edema. Urticaria does not occur in this disease. The disease is suspected when there is a similar family history of recurrent episodes unrelated to exposure to allergens. The diagnosis is made by finding decreased serum C4 and is confirmed by the absence of C1 esterase inhibitor activity in the serum. It is described in greater detail in Chapter 28.

Urticaria pigmentosa is an infiltration of the skin with multiple mast cell tumors that appear as tan macules which urticate when rubbed or stroked. It may be accompanied by visceral mast cell tumors (systemic mastocytosis).

Treatment

Urticaria caused by foods or drugs is treated by avoidance of the offending agents, although hyposensitization to a drug might be attempted in the rare instances in which no alternative drug is available. Urticaria associated with infection is self-limited if the infection is adequately treated. In cases of physical allergy, protective measures to avoid heat, sunlight, or cold must be advised.

Drug treatment is a useful adjunct in the management of all patients, whether or not the cause has been found, but a good response to symptomatic treatment should not deter the physician from efforts to find an underlying cause. Antihistamine drugs are the principal method of treatment, but they must be given in adequate dosage. H_1 receptor antagonists have a proven but inconsistent effectiveness in treating urticaria. The combined use of H_1 and H_2 receptor blockers is frequently recommended but of unproven value for this disease. Epinephrine injections may relieve hives transiently and should be used in treating angioedema involving the pharynx or larynx. Corticosteroids are usually ineffective and should not be used to treat urticaria of unknown cause.

Complications & Prognosis

Urticaria is a benign disease. Since it is a cutaneous form of anaphylaxis, an excessive dose of allergen or physical triggering agent could result in life-threatening systemic anaphylaxis. Angioedema can obstruct the airway if localized in the larynx or adjacent structures.

REFERENCES

Anaphylaxis

Casale TB, Keahery TM, Kaliner M: Exercise-induced anaphylactic syndromes: Insights into diagnostic and pathophysiologic features. *JAMA* 1986;**255**:2049.

James LP, Austen KF: Fatal systemic anaphylaxis in man. *N Engl J Med* 1964;**270**:597.

Sheffer AL: Anaphylaxis. *J Allergy Clin Immunol* 1985; **75**:227.

Smith PL et al: Physiologic manifestations of human anaphylaxis. *J Clin Invest* 1980;**66**:1072.

Valentine MD: Insect venom allergy: Diagnosis and treatment. *J Allergy Clin Immunol* 1984;**73**:299.

Wiggins CA, Dykewicz MS, Patterson R: Idiopathic anaphylaxis: Classification, evaluation and treatment of 123 patients. *J Allergy Clin Immunol* 1988; **82**:849.

Urticaria & Angioedema

Hirschmann JV et al: Cholinergic urticaria. *Arch Dermatol* 1987;**123**:462.

Kauppinen I, Juntunen K, Lanki H: Year book: Urticaria in children: Retrospective evaluation and follow-up. *Allergy* 1984;**39**:469.

Matthews KP: Urticaria and angioedema. *J Allergy Clin Immunol* 1983;**72**:1.

Soter NA, Wasserman SI: Physical urticaria/angioedema: An experimental model of mast cell activation in humans. *J Allergy Clin Immunol* 1980; **66**:358.

Tas J: Chronic urticaria: A survey of one hundred hospitalized cases. *Dermatologica* 1967;**135**:90.

Wanderer AA et al: Clinical characteristics of cold-induced systemic reactions acquired in cold urticaria syndromes: Recommendations for prevention of this complication and a proposal for a diagnostic classification of cold urticaria. *J Allergy Clin Immunol* 1986;**78**:417.

32 Immune-Complex Allergic Disease

Abba I. Terr, MD

This chapter will discuss allergic diseases mediated by immune complexes of allergen with IgG or IgM antibodies. Activation of complement by immune complexes generates chemotactic and vasoactive mediators that cause tissue damage by a combination of immune-complex deposition, alterations in vascular permeability and blood flow, and the action of toxic products from inflammatory cells. The pathology of immune complexes has been extensively studied in animals, and the process is detailed in Chapter 11. The mechanisms of tissue injury caused by immune complexes in these allergic diseases are believed to occur also in a variety of nonallergic diseases discussed elsewhere in this book. These include systemic lupus erythematosus (Chapter 36), vasculitis (Chapter 39), glomerulonephritis (Chapter 41), rheumatoid arthritis (Chapter 36), and acute allograft rejection (Chapter 60).

In addition to the classic immune-complex allergic diseases, this chapter will include a discussion of allergic bronchopulmonary aspergillosis. In this disease a 2-phase immunologic mechanism is involved, in which immune complexes of *Aspergillus* antigens and IgG antibodies produce bronchial inflammation and bronchopulmonary tissue destruction only in the presence of a concomitant IgE response to the allergen.

THE ARTHUS REACTION

In 1903 Arthus showed that the intradermal injection of a protein antigen into a hyperimmunized rabbit produced local inflammation which progressed to a hemorrhagic necrotic lesion that ulcerated. Later investigations established that the Arthus phenomenon is a localized cutaneous inflammatory response to the deposition of immune complexes in dermal blood vessels. It therefore serves as a model system for all immune complex-mediated diseases.

Arthus reactions are rare in humans. Hemorrhagic necrosis at the site of injection of a drug or an insect bite or sting could suggest an Arthus reaction, but the distinction from a toxic reaction or secondary infection requires laboratory or immunohistochemical evidence of the relevant immune complexes. A mild Arthus reaction occurs commonly at the site of allergy desensitization injections after sufficient

doses of injected allergens have been given to generate IgG "blocking" antibodies (see Chapter 30). Because the level of IgG antibodies achieved in allergy therapy is relatively low, the cutaneous and subcutaneous tissue inflammation produces only mild erythema and induration, which begins several hours after the injection and usually subsides in less than 24 hours.

The immunologic pathogenesis is dependent upon antigen and antibody concentrations necessary to form immune complexes capable of initiating complement activation. Intermediate-sized complexes are the most damaging to tissues. Large insoluble complexes are rapidly cleared by the mononuclear phagocyte system, and small complexes fail to activate complement receptors. Immune complexes activate complement through reaction of the Fc portion of antibody with the Fc receptor on C1q. Liberation of C3a and C5a anaphylatoxins activates mast cells to release permeability factors, permitting localization of the immune complexes along the endothelial cell basement membrane. A coincidental IgE antibody response could theoretically achieve the same effect as complement-generated anaphylatoxins. Chemotactic factors from various complement components attract neutrophils. Neutrophils, macrophages, lymphocytes, and other cells with membrane Fc receptors are activated. Activated neutrophils release toxic chemicals such as oxygen-containing free radicals, generate proteolytic enzymes from cytoplasmic granules, and phagocytose the immune complexes.

SERUM SICKNESS

Major Immunologic Features
- Serum sickness is a systemic immune-complex complement-dependent reaction to an extrinsic antigen.
- The severity of the disease is antigen dose-dependent.
- The typical reaction produced by heterologous serum can occur in milder forms from other drugs.

General Considerations
Serum sickness (also known as serum disease)

was a common disease when heterologous antiserum was used as passive immunization in the treatment of a number of infectious and toxic illnesses in the pre-antibiotic era. Today, "serum therapy" with foreign (usually equine) serum or gamma globulin is restricted to a very few toxic diseases and the use of antilymphocyte or antithymocyte globulin for immunosuppressive therapy. A mild serum sickness reaction may occasionally be caused by other drugs, especially sulfonamides, penicillin, and cephalosporins.

A. Definition. Serum sickness is an acute, self-limited allergic disease caused by immune complex-activated complement-generated inflammation after injection of a protein or haptenic drug. The cardinal features are fever, dermatitis, lymphadenopathy, and joint symptoms.

B. Epidemiology. Serum sickness is caused by therapeutic injection of foreign material that is potentially antigenic as well as therapeutic. Therefore, its prevalence depends on the prevalence of certain forms of medical treatment. Therapeutic injections of large quantities of heterologous serum produce serum sickness in proportion to the dose. The attack rate was approximately 90% when a 200-mL dose of horse serum was given. Fractionated gamma globulin preparations are less likely to cause the disease than is whole serum. There are no prevalence statistics available today, but reports of serum sickness are now uncommon.

C. Immunologic Pathogenesis: The pathogenesis of human serum sickness is believed to be similar to the mechanism of "one-shot" serum sickness produced experimentally in immunized rabbits (Fig 32–1). Following a single large dose of injected antigen there is a brief period of equilibration followed by slow degradation of antigen over several days while the primary antibody response is initiated. Antibody synthesis leads to antibody release into the circulation, where antigen-antibody complexes gradually form under conditions of moderate antigen excess. Intermediate-sized complexes deposit in small blood vessels in various organs, triggering the events that are described above in the Arthus reaction. This gives rise to the clinical and pathologic manifestations of disease, and at the same time free antigen is removed more rapidly from the circulation as antibody production and immune-complex formation increases. The circulating complexes then shift to antibody excess, thereby decreasing in size and clearing more rapidly. Finally, free antibody circulates, no further lesions appear, and healing occurs.

The optimal conditions for serum sickness obtain during the primary antibody response of the previously immunized host. With subsequent exposures to the same antigen, the anamnestic antibody response facilitates rapid antigen clearance and greatly reduces the amount and persistence of immune complexes in the circulation.

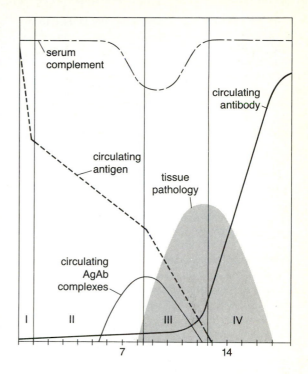

Figure 32–1. Immunologic events in experimental "one-shot" serum sickness in rabbits. The pathogenesis of human serum sickness is similar. A single high dose of antigen is given intravenously on day 0. ***Phase I:*** Equilibration of antigen between blood and tissues. ***Phase II:*** Primary antibody response. Near the end of this phase, antibody combines with antigen to form circulating immune complexes. ***Phase III:*** Tissue pathology and progression of clinical disease. Circulating complexes activate complement and deposit in tissues. The serum complement level falls transiently, and residual antigen is rapidly cleared from the blood. ***Phase IV:*** Remission. Antigen is no longer available, and the level of circulating antibody rises. No further immune complexes form, complement levels return to normal, pathologic lesions repair, and symptoms subside.

Clinical Features

A. Symptoms and Signs: The disease begins 4–21 days (usually 7–10 days) after exposure. The first sign is often a pruritic rash, which may be urticarial, maculopapular, or erythematous. There may be angioedema, and the injection site usually becomes inflamed. Fever, lymphadenopathy, arthralgias, and myalgias complete the clinical presentation. Joint swelling and redness may occur, and occasionally there are headache, nausea, and vomiting. Recovery takes 7–30 days. Clinically significant cardiac or renal involvement is unusual. There may be neurologic involvement, usually in the form of mononeuritis involving especially the brachial plexus. Rarely there may be polyneuritis, Guillain-Barré syndrome, or even meningoencephalitis.

Serum sickness reactions to most drugs used today are much milder than was the disease caused by horse serum injections.

B. Laboratory Findings: There is slight leukocytosis. Plasma cells in the bone marrow are increased in number and may appear in the blood. There may be eosinophilia, but this is not characteristic. The erythrocyte sedimentation rate is increased. Circulating immune complexes and reduced levels of serum complement components are often detected in disease caused by heterologous serum, but they are not usually detected in drug-induced serum sickness (for detection methods, see Chapter 18). Mild proteinuria, hematuria, and casts, transient electrocardiographic abnormalities, and pleocytosis are not unusual.

Immunologic Diagnosis

There is no specific diagnostic test. The diagnosis is made on the basis of a compatible history of typical symptoms at an appropriate interval after drug administration, along with the physical and laboratory evidence. The disease is almost always benign and self-limited, with good prospects for complete recovery, so invasive tests such as tissue biopsy are not indicated.

Treatment

Treatment should be conservative and symptomatic. Aspirin and antihistamines are effective. A short high-dose course of oral corticosteroids is warranted if symptoms are severe.

Complications & Prognosis

Complications are rare. Occasionally laryngeal edema may cause respiratory obstruction. The neuritis rarely is permanent.

ALLERGIC BRONCHOPULMONARY ASPERGILLOSIS (ABPA)

Major Immunologic Features

- Both IgE and IgG antibodies to *Aspergillus* are involved in the pathogenesis of pulmonary disease.
- IgE antibodies are directed to spore allergens.
- IgG antibodies are directed to mycelial allergens.
- There is nonspecific elevation of serum IgE level during acute exacerbations of disease.

General Considerations

Allergic bronchopulmonary aspergillosis (ABPA) is an unusual but not rare illness of young atopic adults with allergic asthma caused by a concomitant IgE and IgG antibody response to the ubiquitous fungus *Aspergillus fumigatus*. The disease may occur in infants and children. It causes bronchiectasis and other destructive lung changes, but tissue damage can be prevented if the condition is diagnosed and treated properly.

A. Epidemiology: Most cases have been reported in the US and United Kingdom, but the disease probably occurs throughout the world. Prevalence rates are not available. With rare exceptions, it is a disease of persons with atopic asthma, but it is also associated with cystic fibrosis (see below). It has not been reported as an occupational disease. There is no known genetic predilection other than that related to atopy, and no human leukocyte antigen (HLA) association has been found.

B. Immunologic Pathogenesis: *A fumigatus* is ubiquitous in the air and soil, and it may be found indoors where moisture and organic matter favor mold growth. Occasional cases are caused by *A ochraceous* or *A terreus*. Exposure to *Aspergillus* is universal, but there is no evidence that excessive environmental exposure causes the disease. However, high-dose exposure may trigger acute attacks in the sensitized subject.

The pathogenesis of the disease is not entirely clear. There is general consensus that ABPA is an allergic disease that requires both IgE and IgG antibodies to *Aspergillus* and that their corresponding immunologic effector mechanisms cause the tissue damage (see Chapter 11). Inhalation of *Aspergillus* spores causes an immediate IgE-mediated bronchospastic reaction to an allergen in the spore, thereby trapping the organisms in the intraluminal mucus of the larger proximal bronchi. When the spores germinate and produce mycelia, the reaction of IgG antibodies to a different mycelial antigen produces tissue damage and inflammation, probably from immune complex-activated complement-derived products. Repeated episodes weaken the bronchial wall, leading to focal bronchiectasis. The significance of pathologic evidence of T cell-mediated inflammation in disease pathogenesis is unknown. The inflammatory process extends to peribronchial lung parenchyma, causing acute inflammatory infiltrates and ultimately chronic parenchymal destruction and fibrosis.

C. Pathology: The disease is confined to the lungs, where pathologic effects are 2-fold: those of the underlying asthma, and those associated with the acute inflammatory episodes and its sequelae. *Aspergillus* hyphae and inflammatory cells can be found in mucus plugs. The adjacent bronchial wall is infiltrated with mononuclear cells and eosinophils. A similar infiltrate affects peribronchial tissues, producing areas of interstitial pneumonia. There is a notable absence of granulocytic inflammation and vasculitis. Immunofluorescence studies have generally not shown immune-complex deposits, although these have been demonstrated in the late-onset skin test site in this disease (see below). The reason for this discrepancy, which weakens the argument for immune-complex pathogenesis, is not clear, but it may reflect the timing of the biopsy studies. Areas of chronic inflammation show noncaseating granulomas. Bronchiectasis and pulmonary fibrosis are late effects in the disease. The pathology, like the clinical manifestations, is variable.

Clinical Features

A. Symptoms and Signs: The clinical picture of ABPA is that of asthma with superimposed acute episodes of fever, cough productive of mucus plugs, chest pains, and malaise. There may be hemoptysis. Other nonspecific symptoms include headache, arthralgias, and myalgias. Some patients present with chronic lung damage, which suggests that the acute inflammatory episodes may be asymptomatic. Physical findings are those of asthma, as well as rales over areas of pulmonary infiltration.

B. Laboratory Findings: The diagnosis of ABPA is readily confirmed by objective evidence for the appropriate immune responses. Intradermal skin testing elicits a dual IgE antibody-mediated wheal-and-flare reaction to *A fumigatus* extract, followed by an Arthus reaction. Immunofluorescence at the height of the late response 6–12 hours after the intradermal injection shows deposition of immunoglobulins and C3, distinguishing this response from a late-phase IgE reaction. Prick testing may not be sensitive enough to elicit the IgG antibody Arthus response, but it is usually sufficient for the immediate IgE wheal and flare.

Serum precipitins to *Aspergillus* are found in about 70% of cases, and most of the remainder will be positive if the serum is concentrated 5-fold. IgG and IgE antibodies in serum can also be detected by radioallergosorbent test (RAST) or enzyme-linked immunosorbent assay (ELISA).

The total serum IgE level is characteristically high in this disease, and the level varies directly with disease activity. The mechanism for this is not known, but IgE levels have important diagnostic and prognostic significance. The majority of the excess IgE cannot be accounted for by *Aspergillus*-specific antibody, suggesting that some aspect of the active phase of ABPA inhibits T lymphocytes with suppressor activity for IgE-bearing B lymphocytes. Eosinophilia is present in blood and sputum, as in any case of asthma. Smear and culture of mucus plugs or sputum may yield the *Aspergillus* organism.

Pulmonary-function testing reveals reversible airway obstruction, but the acute inflammatory episodes can be distinguished from simple asthma by reduction in diffusing capacity. In chronic disease, obstruction may be only partially reversible and a restrictive component may be prominent. Bronchial provocation testing with *Aspergillus* extract produces a dual immediate bronchospastic component followed by a late-phase obstructive-restrictive compo-

nent accompanied by fever and leukocytosis (see Fig 29–3).

The chest x-ray may reveal a variety of findings, but it may also be normal. There is no pathognomonic radiologic finding in this disease. Abnormalities that do occur may be found in many other lung diseases. During the acute phase, mucus plugs may produce focal areas of atelectasis or even segmental or lobar collapse. The peribronchial inflammation appears as migratory infiltrates especially in the upper lobes and hilar areas. Chronic disease from repeated acute insults may cause volume loss, particularly in the upper lobes. Bronchiectasis revealed by bronchography or tomography is saccular and proximal, less commonly cylindrical.

Clinical Diagnosis

The diagnosis of ABPA is made on the basis of certain clinical and laboratory findings. There is no single diagnostic test. Table 32–1 lists diagnostic criteria. The diagnosis is definite when all 7 major criteria are met and probable when 6 are met. All major and minor criteria can be found in other illnesses, but the critical importance of a definitive diagnosis is the ability to use corticosteroids to prevent irreversible pulmonary damage. Any patient with a history of asthma and recurrent pulmonary infiltrates not otherwise explained should be given a diagnostic skin test with *Aspergillus*. Absence of the immediate reaction virtually rules out ABPA, but if the test is positive, a search for serum precipitins and radiographic evidence of bronchiectasis is indicated.

Differential Diagnosis

A fumigatus can cause other respiratory diseases. Invasive aspergillosis is an opportunistic infection that may complicate immunosuppression caused by drugs or disease, as discussed in Chapter 56. Aspergilloma is a localized growth of the organism invading a lung cavity or cyst. It typically induces a very marked precipitating antibody response, with a negative Arthus skin test, probably because of antibody excess at the skin site. *Aspergillus* hypersensi-

Table 32–1. Diagnostic criteria for ABPA.[1]

Major criteria
1. Episodic bronchial obstruction
2. Peripheral blood eosinophilia
3. Positive immediate skin reactivity
4. Serum precipitating antibodies
5. Elevated serum IgE
6. History of pulmonary infiltrates
7. Central bronchiectasis

Minor criteria
1. *A fumigatus*-positive sputum culture
2. History of expectorating brown plugs or flecks
3. Arthus (late) skin reactivity

[1]Reproduced, with permission, from Slavin RG: Allergic bronchopulmonary aspergillosis. *Clin Rev Allergy* 1985;**3**:167.

tivity pneumonitis is a rare cause of farmer's lung. Finally, the organism is an atopic allergen in some cases of allergic asthma.

The variable clinical and radiologic features of the disease mimic other pulmonary diseases, including asthma with periodic mucus plugging or intercurrent viral infections, tuberculosis, hypersensitivity pneumonitis, pulmonary infiltration with eosinophilia (PIE syndrome), mucoid impaction, and bronchocentric granulomatosis.

ABPA in Cystic Fibrosis

By using the criteria of Table 32–1, the diagnosis of ABPA is made more frequently in children with cystic fibrosis than in the atopic asthmatic population. It is difficult to be sure whether this reflects a fundamental predisposition or a secondary opportunistic effect. Both atopy and *Aspergillus* infections are prevalent in children with cystic fibrosis, setting the stage for the necessary immune response involved in the pathogenesis of ABPA. Markedly elevated and fluctuating serum IgE levels, eosinophilia, and dramatic x-ray resolution of infiltrates with corticosteroid treatment are important diagnostic clues that ABPA is present in this disease.

Treatment

The diagnosis is important, because prompt high-dose systemic corticosteroid therapy causes prompt resolution of the acute allergic inflammatory episode and prevents the occurrence of long-term irreversible bronchial and parenchymal lung tissue damage. The mechanism of the therapeutic effect can only be surmised, but it is probably anti-inflammatory rather the immunosuppressive. An initial dose of 60 mg of prednisone daily in divided doses should be maintained until there is clinical and radiologic cure of the episode, after which a slowly tapering dose with maintenance at 20–30 mg once on alternate days should prevent relapses. It is useful to monitor total serum IgE levels, which fall during remissions and rise again with recurrences. There is some evidence that the serum IgE rise might precede the clinical exacerbation. Serial chest x-rays should also be part of the monitoring process.

The concurrent asthma is treated in the standard fashion, including desensitization if indicated, except for injections of *Aspergillus* extract, which might theoretically enhance the IgG antibody response and hence worsen the disease. Inhaled corticosteroids are not indicated for acute attacks, but they can be used to control the asthma between attacks. Chest physiotherapy and inhaled bronchodilators are helpful adjuncts to improve expectoration of mucus plugs, but antifungal drugs are of unproven benefit.

Complications & Prognosis

Table 32–2 is a scheme for staging untreated disease. The course is variable and unpredictable and may depend upon factors of environmental exposure, so that not all patients proceed through all stages. Nevertheless, early recognition and adequate treatment prevent deterioration in pulmonary function and subsequent development of chronic airway obstruction and restrictive disease with pulmonary fibrosis. Occasionally, aspergilloma may develop in a bronchiectatic or emphysematous cyst in ABPA. Cor pulmonale is likely to occur in stage V disease.

Table 32–2. Proposed stages of increasing severity and chronicity in ABPA.[1]

Stage	Description
I	Acute episode responsive to systemic corticosteroids
II	Remission
III	Recurrent exacerbations
IV	Recurrent exacerbations with steroid-dependent severe asthma
V	Pulmonary fibrosis, irreversible obstruction, advanced x-ray changes, cavitation and upper lobe contraction, severe bronchiectasis, emphysema

[1]Reproduced, with permission, from Patterson, R et al: Allergic bronchopulmonary aspergillosis: Staging as an aid to management. *Ann Intern Med* 1982;**96**:286.

REFERENCES

Serum Sickness

Bielory L et al: Human serum sickness: A prospective analysis of 35 patients treated with equine antithymocyte globulin for bone marrow failure. *Medicine* 1988;**67**:40.

Erffmeyer JE: Serum sickness. *Ann Allergy* 1986;**56**:105.

Naguwa SM, Nelson BL: Human serum sickness. *Clin Rev Allergy* 1985;**3**:117.

Allergic Bronchopulmonary Aspergillosis

Greenberger PA, Patterson R: Allergic bronchopulmonary aspergillosis and the evaluation of the patient with asthma. *J Allergy Clin Immunol* 1988;**81**:646.

Laufer P et al: Allergic bronchopulmonary aspergillosis in cystic fibrosis. *J Allergy Clin Immunol* 1984;**73**:44.

Patterson R et al: Allergic bronchopulmonary aspergillosis: Staging as an aid to management. *Ann Intern Med* 1982;**96**:286.

Slavin RG: Allergic bronchopulmonary aspergillosis. *Clin Rev Allergy* 1985;**3**:167.

Cell-Mediated Hypersensitivity Diseases

33

Abba I. Terr, MD

Acquired immunity to many infectious diseases is mediated by specifically sensitized effector T lymphocytes (TDH cells). This is dramatically evident in the marked susceptibility to many bacterial, fungal, viral, and other infections that characterizes patients with congenital (Chapters 26 and 27) and acquired (Chapter 55) T cell deficiency. The effector T lymphocyte also is responsible for certain forms of allergy, frequently referred to as delayed hypersensitivity.

This chapter will discuss a very common form of T cell-mediated allergy, allergic contact dermatitis, and a much less common disease, hypersensitivity pneumonitis. Allergic contact dermatitis is a pure form of T cell hypersensitivity, whereas hypersensitivity pneumonitis is a complex disease that may assume several forms clinically with a corresponding immunologic complexity involving antibodies and T cells, and a combination of both, depending upon factors of allergen dose and the form and the duration of allergen exposure. Hypersensitivity pneumonitis is included in this chapter because T cell mechanisms rather than antibody-mediated mechanisms are predominant in most clinically recognized cases.

ALLERGIC CONTACT DERMATITIS

Major Immunologic Features
- It is mediated by specifically sensitized T cells.
- It is most often caused by contact with haptenic chemicals.
- Patch testing is efficient and accurate in diagnosis.

General Considerations
A. Definition: Allergic contact dermatitis (also known as eczematous contact allergy) is an eczematous skin disease caused by cell-mediated hypersensitivity to an environmental allergen. Both sensitization and elicitation of the reaction involve contact of the allergen with the skin. Allergens causing the disease are numerous and common and include both natural and synthetic chemicals.

B. Epidemiology: The disease occurs world-wide and affects both sexes and all age groups. The most common allergen, pentadecylcatechol, found in poison ivy and poison oak, affects 50% of the US population clinically and another 35% subclinically.

C. Immunologic Pathogenesis: Allergic contact dermatitis is mediated by cutaneous T cell hypersensitivity. In this process, the Langerhans cell, a skin macrophage, functions as the antigen-processing cell at the local site of allergen penetration. It is uncertain whether the site of origin of the sensitized T lymphocyte is the skin, the regional lymph nodes, or elsewhere. Sensitization on primary contact takes several days. Once sensitization occurs, it lasts for years, if not for life, and is generalized. Reactions can be elicited anywhere on the skin. In some instances systemic reactions have been provoked when the allergen enters the body by ingestion or injection.

Many important sensitizing allergens are organic chemicals, and some are metals. It is assumed that they function as haptens, but the source and nature of the host carrier protein in the skin are unknown.

D. Pathology: The inflammatory response in allergic contact dermatitis is characterized by perivenular cuffing with lymphocytes, epidermal-cell vesiculation and necrosis, appearance of basophils and eosinophils, interstitial fibrin deposition, and dermal and epidermal edema.

Clinical Features
A. Symptoms and Signs. The skin eruption appears acutely as erythema, swelling, and vesiculation. In severe cases there may be extensive blistering, scaling, and weeping. In chronic milder disease, papules and scaling are more prominent. The lesion is pruritic or frankly painful if severe. The rapidity of onset after contact is directly proportionate to the degree of sensitivity and may range from 6 hours to several days.

The location of the eruption on the skin is helpful in diagnosing the cause. Certain areas of skin, such as the eyelids, react more easily than others, such as the palms. Metal dermatitis, usually caused by sensitivity to nickel, appears in discrete patches corresponding to the area of contact with jewelry, watches, or metal objects on clothing. A variety of allergens, such as dyes and fabric finishes, are found in clothing, causing a skin eruption on areas of skin covered by the apparel. Volatile allergens affect exposed areas, usually the face and arms. Rhus dermatitis from poison oak or poison ivy produces an especially severe disease with prominent vesicles and bullae, and there are characteristic streaks of vesicles corresponding to brushing of the skin by the plant leaves.

B. Laboratory Findings. There are none.

Allergens

The list of known allergens is enormous and theoretically unlimited. All types of chemicals can produce this disease, but metallic inorganic compounds and organic chemicals are the most likely, in contrast to the protein allergens that dominate in the other types of allergic conditions. The reason for this is unknown but is probably associated with the unique handling of foreign materials by the skin. The most common contact allergens are listed in Table 33–1.

Clinical Diagnosis

Diagnosis is suggested by the physical appearance of the eruption and distribution of lesions. By history, reactions may appear suddenly or present as a chronic, low-grade, smoldering dermatitis. The history must then be directed to monitoring exposures in the home, work, and recreational environment for possible allergens.

Immunologic Diagnosis

The diagnosis is confirmed by patch testing, a time-honored, well-standardized procedure which is both an immunologic skin test and a provocation test that reproduces the disease "in miniature." Standard patch test allergens in concentrations that elicit aller-

gic but not irritant reactions are available commercially for a number of the common contact sensitizers (Table 33–1). Reactions are read in 48 hours for localized eczema at the patch test site (Table 33–2).

Differential Diagnosis

Eczema refers to a general pattern of response of the skin to a variety of injurious stimuli. Scratching of the skin from any pruritic dermatosis can cause eczematization. The most common causes are atopic dermatitis; localized or generalized neurodermatitis; skin infection by bacteria or fungi; primary contact irritation by chemicals, foods, saliva, sweat, or urine; and dyshidrosis.

Treatment

The disease responds to systemic corticosteroids, which should be given as early as possible. Small localized areas of involvement can be treated with a topical steroid cream. Applications of cool, wet dressings containing Burow's solution (aluminum acetate) are helpful for acute lesions. Chronic lichenified dermatitis requires a potent fluorinated steroid ointment with an occlusive dressing. Extensive areas of involvement or severe bullous lesions should be treated with a brief oral burst of high-dose prednisone or with intramuscular triamcinolone or methylprednisone. An antibiotic may be indicated for secondary infection. Antihistamines are generally not effective for controlling the pruritis.

Prognosis

A cure is to be expected if the correct allergen is identified and avoided. However, exposure to a cross-reacting allergenic chemical may cause a recurrence. Chromate allergy tends to be chronic, despite avoidance.

Prevention

The only means of prevention of the dermatitis in a sensitized patient is avoidance. The Landsteiner-Chase phenomenon of tolerance to contact sensitivity in guinea pigs by prior oral ingestion of allergen has no practical application in humans. Some patients with mild nickel sensitivity can tolerate jewelry that is treated with a protective coating. Rhus dermatitis can probably be lessened, if not prevented, if the skin is thoroughly washed with water immediately after contact.

Desensitization with oral or injected Rhus extract

Table 33–1. Common contact allergens and concentrations used in patch testing.

Benzocaine 5%
Mercaptobenzothiazole 1%
Colophony 20%
p-Phenylenediamine 1%
Imidazolidinyl urea 2%
Cinnamic aldehyde 1%
Lanolin alcohol 30%
Carba mix 3%
Neomycin sulfate 20%
Thiuram mix 1%
Formaldehyde 1%
Ehtylenediamine dihydrochloride 1%
Epoxy resin 1%
Quaternium 15 2%
p-tert-Butylphenol formaldehyde resin 1%
Mercapto mix 1%
Black rubber mix 0.6%
Potassium dichromate 0.25%
Balsam of Peru 25%
Nickel sulfate 2.5%

Table 33–2. Patch test interpretation.

Result	Interpretation
−	No reaction
±	Mild erythema
+	Definite erythema
+ +	Erythema and papules
+ + +	Erythema, papules, and vesicles

or pentadecylcatechol has advocates in clinical practice, but there is, as yet, no sound evidence of effectiveness. Some patients appear to lose sensitivity after repeated natural exposure, a phenomenon known as "hardening," but this also remains to be documented.

PHOTOALLERGIC CONTACT DERMATITIS

Major Immunologic Features
■ Allergen requires activation by ultraviolet light.
■ Immunologic mechanism is identical to that of allergic contact dermatitis.

General Considerations
A. Definition: Photoallergic contact dermatitis is an uncommon eczematous skin disease caused by cell-mediated hypersensitivity to certain environmental chemicals that require sunlight activation to render them allergenic. The skin eruption appears on sun-exposed areas of skin only.

B. Epidemiology: The disease has been associated primarily with drugs or chemical constituents of topical products such as soaps, cosmetics, and topical drugs. It therefore appears from time to time in epidemic form when a new product is introduced. The epidemic subsides when the product is withdrawn from the market once the photosensitivity potential is discovered.

C. Immunologic Pathogenesis: The mechanism is identical to ordinary allergic contact dermatitis, except that the causative chemical agent must be activated by the ultraviolet component of sunlight to become allergenic. The mechanism of allergen activation is unknown. Two theories have been proposed. Ultraviolet radiation may cause an alteration in tertiary structure to generate the necessary allergen epitope, or, alternatively, free radicals generated by ultraviolet light may be necessary for binding of the hapten chemical to skin carrier protein.

D. Pathology: The pathology is indistinguishable from that of allergic contact dermatitis.

Clinical Features
The dermatitis varies in its clinical appearance from an exaggerated sunburn to typical eczema to a severe vesiculobullous dermatosis. The distribution corresponds to sunlight exposure, but severe reactions may involve partially covered areas of skin as well. The eruption caused by a topically applied sensitizer is limited to the area of application.

Clinical Diagnosis
The disease is diagnosed by the combination of dermatitis in a sun-exposed distribution and a history of concurrent exposure to a known or suspected photoallergic sensitizer. A high index of suspicion facilitates diagnosis.

Immunologic Diagnosis
Photopatch testing is a modification of the standard patch test. The suspected agent is applied in the standard fashion for patch testing, and then the site is exposed to artificial ultraviolet light or sunlight. A test site not exposed to light is used as a control. The appearance of an eczematous eruption at the light-exposed site is a positive test.

Differential Diagnosis
Certain chemicals and drugs produce dermatitis in sun-exposed areas of skin in all individuals, provided that sufficient amounts of the compound accumulate in the skin and that there is exposure to a particular wavelength of ultraviolet light. These are called phototoxic reactions and are not mediated immunologically. Differential diagnosis also includes ordinary contact dermatitis, sunburn, and other causes of photosensitivity.

Allergens
Some of the important drugs and chemicals that cause photoallergic and phototoxic contact dermatitis are listed in Table 33–3. Some drugs taken systemically produce photodermatitis.

Treatment
Avoidance of the sensitizing agent and sunlight and treatment with topical corticosteroids are usually sufficient. Systemic corticosteroids may be required in severe cases.

Prognosis
Occasionally the dermatitis will persist despite avoidance measures. The reason for this is unknown.

HYPERSENSITIVITY PNEUMONITIS

Major Immunologic Features
■ Primary pathogenetic mechanism involves the effector T cell.

Table 33–3. Some topical causes of photoallergic and phototoxic reactions.

Photoallergic	Phototoxic
Drugs	Drugs
Sulfonamides	Sulfonamides
Phenothiazines	Phenothiazines
Soaps containing halogenated salicylanilides	Plant oils
	Psoralens
Sunscreen agents	Coal tar and its derivatives
p-Aminobenzoate esters	in dyes, perfumes, and
	other synthetics
Benzophenones	Acridine
Fragrances	Anthracene
	Phenanthrene

- Antibody precipitins are useful to establish exposure to the allergen.
- Allergens are frequently biologic organisms or their products.

General Considerations

Hypersensitivity pneumonitis (also known as extrinsic allergic alveolitis) has been known as an occupational disease for well over 200 years, but it was first recognized as an allergic disease just 30 years ago. The concept that it is a pulmonary Arthus reaction caused by immune complexes of inhaled allergen and precipitating IgG antibodies was then widely held. Recently, persuasive evidence from clinical, pathologic, epidemiologic, and experimental studies has shown that the disease is mediated predominantly by T lymphocyte (cellular) effector mechanisms. It shares some pathologic features with sarcoidosis and the pneumoconioses, but it differs from the former disease by having a recognized environmental cause, and from the latter group of diseases by its immune responses to inhaled material. Hypersensitivity pneumonitis, like allergic asthma, is produced by inhaled allergens, and in fact there are allergens that can cause either disease. However, IgE antibodies play no known role in the pathogenesis of hypersensitivity pneumonitis.

A. Definition: Hypersensitivity pneumonitis is an allergic disease of the lung parenchyma with inflammation in the alveoli and interstitial spaces induced immunologically by acute or chronic inhalation of a wide variety of inhaled materials. The disease may present in an acute, subacute, or chronic form. It is not currently possible to ascribe all features of the illness to a single immunologic mechanism. There is evidence for several different immune pathways that operate separately or concurrently, but the most compelling mechanism of pathogenesis is allergen-specific cell-mediated hypersensitivity. Intersitial pneumonitis is the primary clinical manifestation for all forms of the disease.

B. Epidemiology: Cases have been reported worldwide. The disease is most frequently associated with occupational allergens, which determine its prevalence and geographic, age, and sex distribution. Males aged 30–50 years are therefore usually affected. Farmer's lung, the prototype and most widely reported form of hypersensitivity pneumonitis, is caused by thermophilic actinomycetes, usually from warm, moist, moldy hay, and therefore the disease predominates in wet regions and especially among dairy farmers. Several surveys suggest that 2–4% of farmers have been affected. Bird handler's disease (also known as bird fancier's lung, pigeon breeder's disease, and bird breeder's disease) has been diagnosed in 15–21% of exposed individuals. Humidifier lung disease occurs in 23–71% of those exposed to contaminated humidifiers. Many published reports identify a single case or a small epidemic in a workplace. Once recognized, elimination of the environmental source of the allergen eliminates the disease.

C. Allergens: Hundreds of sources of allergens have been reported to cause hypersensitivity pneumonitis, usually in single cases. Some of the more common ones are shown in Table 33–4. The exact allergenic chemical has been isolated infrequently, but they include a variety of heterologous proteins and organic or inorganic compounds. In many cases the chemical identification has been made by serologic or skin testing in the affected patient. As explained below, precipitins and skin tests may be epiphenomena, so definitive identification of the allergen requires bronchial provocation testing.

The allergens have a variety of environmental sources. The most common ones are microorganisms, especially bacteria and fungal spores, and animal products such as feathers and particles of dried excreta. The few industrial chemicals so far identified with this disease have been highly reactive ones, such as isocyanates and anhydrides. Many cases have been clearly associated with a product such as inhaled dust from a food or contaminated water without identification of the source, although microbial contamination is usually suspected.

To date most reported cases have been occupational, because these are more likely to be acute illnesses from high-dose exposure easily traced to the workplace by a history of an epidemic in a particular occupational site. The relatively few instances of disease caused by domestic exposure have been traced to thermophilic actinomycetes, fungi, mites, amebae, pet birds, and unknown organisms in contaminated water of home or automobile air conditioners, heaters, vaporizers, and evaporative air coolers. These tend to cause chronic and insidious pulmonary impairment. Physicians should be aware of this potential cause of "idiopathic" pulmonary fibrosis.

The allergen must be inhaled in a form, such as an aerosol or particle, that is capable of reaching the alveoli during normal respiration. Particulates, whether in the form of an organic dust or microorganism, must be less than 3 μm in diameter.

Many of the allergens associated with hypersensitivity pneumonitis have biologic properties, in addition to allergenicity, which may be important in causing disease. The thermophilic actinomycetes, which are classified in the same botanical order as *Mycobacterium tuberculosis,* are immunologic adjuvants for both antibody synthesis and cell-mediated immunity. Many of the allergens can activate alveolar macrophages and the alternative complement pathway nonimmunologically. The role of these properties in disease pathogenesis is being actively investigated.

D. Pathology: The histopathology of hypersensitivity pneumonitis depends upon the stage of dis-

Table 33–4. Allergens causing hypersensitivity pneumonitis.

Allergen	Source	Disease
Bacteria		
Thermophilic actinomycetes	Contaminated hay or grains	Farmer's lung
	Contaminated bagasse	Bagassosis
	Mushroom compost	Mushroom worker's lung
Bacillus subtilis	Contaminated walls	Domestic hypersensitivity pneumonitis
Streptomyces albus	Contaminated fertilizer	*Streptomyces* hypersensitivity pneumonitis
Fungi		
Aspergillus spp	Moldy barley	Malt worker's lung
	Moldy tobacco	Tobacco worker's lung
	Compost	Compost lung
Aureobasidium, Graphium spp	Redwood bark, sawdust	Sequoiosis
	Contaminated sauna water	Sauna worker's lung
	Contaminated humidifier	Humidifier lung
Cryptostroma corticale	Maple bark	Maple bark disease
Penicillium casei	Moldy cheese	Cheese worker's lung
Sacchoromonospora viridis	Dried grass	Thatched roof disease
Various undetermined puffball spores	Moldy dwellings	Domestic hypersensitivity pneumonitis
	Mold in cork dust	Suberosis
	Lycoperdon puffballs	Lycoperdonosis
Alternaria, Penicillium spp.	Wood pulp, dust	Woodworker's lung
Insects		
Sitophilus granarius (wheat weevil)	Infested flour	Wheat miller's lung
Organic chemicals		
Isocyanates	Various industries	Chemical worker's lung
Miscellaneous		
Pituitary snuff	Medication	Pituitary snuff taker's lung
Coffee bean protein	Coffee bean dust	Coffee worker's lung
Rat urine protein	Laboratory rats	Laboratory worker's lung
Animal fur protein	Animal pelts	Furrier's lung
Unknown	Contaminated tap water	Tap water hypersensitivity pneumonitis

ease. Very few patients have been examined in the acute phase immediately after exposure. Such patients show involvement of centrilobular respiratory bronchioles, alveoli, and blood vessels with intense infiltration by granulocytes, monocytes, and plasma cells. There is Arthus-like vasculitis of alveolar capillaries. Some studies show bronchiolar destruction. There is alveolar-wall thickening, but without necrosis. Immunofluorescence studies show deposition of immunoglobulins, C3, and fibrin in and around affected blood vessels. Thus, any role of precipitating antibodies causing immune-complex deposition and complement-mediated Arthus-like vasculitis, alveolitis, and terminal bronchiolitis would be restricted to the early acute illness after allergen exposure.

The subacute phase, beginning within 3 weeks of exposure, is characterized by noncaseating granulomas in the interstitial spaces accompanied by lymphocytes and plasma cells with only occasional eosinophils and no vasculitis. Mild bronchiolitis obliterans is seen in 50% of cases.

Chronic disease is characterized by persistence of the subacute pathology. There are lymphocytes in alveolar walls, and interstitial fibrosis accompanies the granulomatous and mononuclear interstitial and alveolar inflammation. There is no eosinophilia, and immunofluorescence shows no immunoglobulin or complement deposits. Monoclonal antibody reagents reveal the presence of activated macrophages and T lymphocytes, predominantly CD8 cells.

The histopathology of hypersensitivity pneumonitis is not pathognomonic, with the possible exception of histiocytes with foamy cytoplasm surrounded by lymphocytes, which are seen in the chronic phase.

E. Pathogenesis: The allergic pathogenesis of hypersensitivity pneumonitis was first suspected in farmer's lung because of the granulomatous interstitial inflammation, a hallmark of T cell-mediated immunity. However, the discovery of precipitating antibodies to extracts of thermophilic actinomycetes in patient sera led to a persisting concept that this is an immune-complex disease, even after many studies showed that precipitins correlated with exposure to allergens and not necessarily to the presence of pulmonary disease. As explained above, an Arthus mechanism could be operative in the acute pneumonitis that occurs 4 hours after exposure and clears in 24 hours. However, the clinical manifestations, pathology, disease induced in animal models, epidemiologic data, and recent investigations of bronchoalveolar lavage samples all point to a complicated mechanism of disease involving specific cell-mediated immunity, immunoregulatory and immunogenetic factors, and nonspecific biologic effects of the inhaled material, but only a minor role, if any, for circulating antibodies. The disease is primarily a function of the local pulmonary mucosal cellular immune system, which is poorly reflected in peripheral-blood samples. The role of mucosal IgA has not been fully explored. Both IgA and IgG antibodies are present in bronchoalveolar lavage fluid in proportion to allergen exposure, but IgA and not IgG antibody titers are higher in patients than in exposed persons without disease.

Unlike IgE-mediated diseases, allergen exposure by inhalation must be either intensive and massive or prolonged. It has been calculated that a farmer working with moldy hay may inhale 750,000 fungal spores per minute.

In experimental disease in animals, inhalation of soluble antigens produces a very mild disease or an acute hemorrhagic Arthus alveolitis analogous to human illness in workers exposed occupationally to high doses of trimellitic anhydride or isocyanate who develop high-titer circulating and alveolar-fluid antibodies and a restrictive infiltrative pulmonary disease with hemoptysis and anemia. On the other hand, the typical human hypersensitivity pneumonitis is best reproduced in animals by inhalation of particulate antigens that elicit alveolitis and interstitial granulomas, specific local and systemic cell-mediated hypersensitivity, activation of alveolar macrophages, local lymphokine production in alveolar fluid, and precipitins. Allergen inhalation challenge responses can be passively transferred by sensitized lymphocytes, and the disease can be inhibited with corticosteroids, with antimacrophage serum, and by neonatal thymectomy, all of which are consistent with cellular hypersensitivity.

Animal experiments in mice shed some light on the development and variability of the human disease. By using high- and low-responder strains, it has been shown that the disease is associated with a deficiency in allergen-specific suppressor T lymphocytes in the lung. The deficiency is determined by a dominant gene or genes linked to the immunoglobulin V_H haplotype, but not to H-2 (analogous to human HLA) genes. Repeated exposure to the allergen causes a phenomenon of desensitization, with disappearance of infiltrates, refractoriness to disease by other, unrelated allergens, and cell-mediated anergy in some animals but not others. The anergic state is caused by an allergen-nonspecific suppressor macrophage, whose presence is controlled by a single recessive gene. Animals lacking this gene have sustained granulomatous disease and have failed to develop anergy. These intriguing experiments stress the role of genetic factors of immunoregulation that probably also control susceptibility to and expressions of the disease in humans.

Many of the allergens identified with this disease have intrinsic biologic effects that may be important in pathogenesis. These include adjuvant properties causing nonspecific stimulation of the immune system, activation of macrophages, and nonimmunologic activation of the alternative complement pathway.

Clinical Features

A. Symptoms: Clinical patterns are wide-ranging, but they may be classified into acute, subacute, and chronic forms. Acute reactions are single or multiple episodes of dyspnea, cough, malaise, fever, chills, and chest pain. Each episode begins 4–8 hours after a high-dose allergen exposure and clears within 24 hours. Weight loss and hemoptysis are rare. Subacute disease begins insidiously over a period of weeks, resulting in cough, dyspnea, and weight loss. The cough is initially dry and later productive. Dyspnea may become progressively profound, and there may be cyanosis. Chronic disease occurs from low-dose continuous exposure, as in the case of hypersensitivity to a single bird in the home. Fatigue and weight loss may be the first indication of illness. Gradual progressive dyspnea may be overlooked or denied until it is noticed at rest.

B. Signs: During acute reactions, the temperature is elevated to 39.5 °C. The patient appears acutely ill, with tachypnea and tachycardia. There are bilateral crackling rales, especially at the lung bases, and occasional rhonchi and wheezes, but the lungs may be clear. In chronic disease, breath sounds are diminished and there may be a prolonged expiratory phase if an obstructive component is present.

C. Laboratory Findings: In acute disease there is usually slight leukocytosis without eosinophilia. The erythrocyte sedimentation rate is normal or mildly elevated. In chronic disease, serum immunoglobulin levels may be slightly increased and low-titer rheumatoid factor and antinuclear antibody may be present.

Pulmonary-function tests performed during the acute phase of the disease reveal a reversible restrictive pattern with reduced lung compliance and reduced diffusing capacity. Arterial blood gases show hypoxemia. The spirometric findings in chronic disease are those of irreversible restriction with or without an accompanying obstructive component due to bronchiolitis obliterans. In some patients there may be an additional element of bronchial hyperirritability.

Chest x-ray findings are highly variable. During an acute episode the typical pattern of the interstitial and alveolar filling infiltrate is one of multiple bilateral small nodules sparing the apices and bases. Less common findings are patchy pneumonia or a normal x-ray. In chronic disease a fibrotic linear pattern with or without nodules increases in intensity toward the periphery. There may be loss of volume that is most marked in upper lobes, honeycombing, and cor pulmonale-induced cardiac enlargement. The disease does not cause pleural effusion or thickening, hilar adenopathy, calcification, cavitation, atelectasis, or coin lesions.

The classification described above should not obscure the fact that hypersensitivity pneumonitis is highly variable, and individual cases are frequently "atypical." Clinical manifestations depend upon the frequency, intensity, and chemical and physical properties of the allergen exposure, as well as on host factors. Clinical descriptions have been dominated by occupational syndromes such as farmer's lung, bagassosis, and bird handler's disease. Many unique case reports have been published because of quaint names and unusual allergen sources, such as New Guinea thatched roof lung (contaminated thatch), paprika slicer's lung (*Mucor stalonifer*), Bible printer's lung (contaminated ink), and coptic lung (mummy cloth wrappings).

Clinical Diagnosis

The history is important, as in any allergic disease. Because of the variable nature of hypersensitivity pneumonitis and wide range of environmental sources for the allergens, the diagnosis requires a high degree of suspicion. Any patient with a history of recurrent pneumonia of uncertain etiology, "idiopathic" restrictive or fibrotic lung disease, or unexplained pulmonary abnormality on chest x-ray is a prime suspect. The environmental, especially occupational, history is essential for providing clues for possible causative allergens.

There are no pathognomonic signs from physical examination, routine laboratory tests, or chest x-rays. Even pulmonary-function testing may not show evidence of the restrictive abnormality between acute attacks of early disease. Lung biopsy is likewise not pathognomonic, since histopathology is similar to that of other interstitial diseases, but it is useful mainly to rule out other diagnoses.

Immunologic Diagnosis

Serum antibodies are not usually involved in disease pathogenesis, but their presence nevertheless will at least establish the fact of exposure. There are usually large quantities of precipitating antibodies, especially in early or acute disease, but they may disappear after a prolonged period of allergen avoidance. Ouchterlony analysis is usually adequate to detect precipitins (see Chapter 19), but occasionally the more sensitive radioimmunoassay, radioallergosorbent test (RAST), enzyme-linked immunosorbent assay (ELISA), and complement fixation test are necessary. Serum complement component levels are normal or occasionally increased with acute allergen exposure.

When precipitating antibodies are present in serum, an intradermal skin test will elicit a cutaneous Arthus reaction, characterized by localized diffuse edema and mild inflammation and erythema appearing at 4–6 hours and subsiding completely by 24 hours. Commercial test antigens are available for extracts of fungi and diluted avian serum. Many crude extracts of allergens known to cause this disease, eg, thermophilic actinomycetes, are too irritating for skin testing. The Arthus skin test, like the precipitin test, is an indication of exposure and is not diagnostic of the disease.

Bronchial provocation testing with allergen extract currently has the highest sensitivity and specificity for diagnosis, but it is an experimental procedure because of technical limitations and danger. It must be done in a hospital with 24-hour monitoring. A reversible restrictive lung defect begins at 4–6 hours, peaks at 8 hours, and resolves by 24 hours. Although the timing of response is similar to a late-phase asthmatic response, the abnormality in pulmonary function is different (see Fig 29–3).

Examination of bronchoalveolar lavage fluid for humoral and cellular components has been reported to date for only a few cases of subacute disease. The procedure is still experimental, and the diagnostic usefulness unknown.

A simple no-cost alternative to bronchial provocation is "on-site" challenge to observe changes in symptoms, lung auscultation, pulmonary functions, and chest x-ray by trial exposure of the patient to the suspected environment (eg, home or work) after an adequate period of avoidance. If an acute reaction is provoked, the site must be investigated to uncover the causative allergen. Environmental assessment might require the specialized services of engineers, microbiologists, or others.

Differential Diagnosis

Pulmonary mycotoxicosis (atypical farmer's lung) is a recently described disorder caused by acute massive exposure to moldy silage. The disease is characterized by fever, chills, and coughing that last for several days to a week. There are diffuse infiltrations on chest x-ray and fungal organisms in alveoli and bronchioles, but no serum precipitins. The cause is unknown, but the illness is probably a toxic pneumonitis from a fungal product. Recurrent infectious pneumonias, other causes of interstitial lung disease, asthma, allergic bronchopulmonary aspergillosis, and pneumoconioses must also be differentiated from hypersensitivity pneumonitis.

Treatment

Systemic corticosteroid therapy is indicated for resolution of acute reactions and for terminating and reversing severe or progressive disease. The drug should not be used as an alternative to avoidance of the allergen, but it may be necessary to protect the patient by suppressing inflammation if the allergen source has not been identified. Inhaled corticosteroids are not indicated.

Complications

Respiratory failure and cor pulmonale may result from chronic disease. Bronchiolitis obliterans may lead to irreversible obstructive pulmonary disease. Death from respiratory failure is possible during any phase of the disease.

Prognosis

Prognosis for recovery is good in the acute or subacute stages once the cause has been identified and avoided. However, some patients with bird handler's disease have progressive pulmonary insufficiency even with complete avoidance of birds. On the other hand, farmers can continue to have some exposure to thermophilic actinomycetes without progressive illness as long as the acute febrile symptomatic attacks are avoided.

Prevention

Avoidance is the only means of preventing this disease. Effective treatment therefore requires a specific immunologic diagnosis whenever possible, since the same allergen may be found in different environments (Table 33–4). The purpose of avoidance is prevention of irreversible lung disease.

Occupational preventive measures are obvious for the currently recognized causes. Proper workplace hygiene, filters and masks where appropriate, and other measures should be employed. Diseases caused by allergens in homes, automobiles, and offices are best prevented by physician awareness of the disease.

REFERENCES

Allergic Contact Dermatitis

Adams RM: *Occupational Skin Diseases,* 2nd ed. Grune & Stratton, 1989.

Fisher AA: *Contact Dermatitis,* 3rd ed. Lea & Febiger, 1986.

Mallory SB: Allergic contact dermatitis. *Immunol Allergy Clin North Am* 1987; **7**:407.

Hypersensitivity Pneumonitis

Fink NJ: Hypersensitivity pneumonitis. *J Allergy Clin Immunol* 1984;**74**:1.

Novey HS (editor): Hypersensitivity pneumonitis. *Clin Rev Allergy* 1983;**1**:449. (Entire issue.)

Salvaggio JE: Hypersensitivity pneumonitis. *J Allergy Clin Immunol* 1987;**79**:558.

Drug Allergy

34

H. James Wedner, MD

Adverse reactions to therapeutic agents are a significant problem in the practice of medicine. The spectrum of adverse reactions to drugs comprises (1) side effects, toxic reactions, and drug interactions that are the result of unwanted pharmacologic properties of the therapeutic agent(s) in question; (2) idiosyncratic reactions, which occur in a variable proportion of the population and whose cause is unknown; and (3) immunologic reactions, which depend on the ability of the drug or its hydrolysis or biotransformation products to interact with the immune system and to invoke humoral or cellular immune mechanisms. Adverse reactions resulting from an immunologic mechanism make up a substantial portion of the spectrum. Although this chapter is concerned with reactions based upon immunologic mechanisms, the entire spectrum of reactions must be kept in mind when approaching the problem of adverse reactions to drugs, because the clinical presentations of the reactions may be similar although the mechanisms differ. It is imperative that the underlying mechanism be established since the therapeutic approach will differ depending upon the type of reaction that has occurred.

Some texts define drug allergy as any reaction that results from an immune mechanism, whereas others limit the term to reactions mediated by IgE antibody directed against the drug or one of its metabolic products. This chapter discusses all immunologically mediated drug reactions and then concentrates on those resulting from IgE antibody-dependent release of mediators of anaphylaxis from sensitized mast cells and basophils and those caused by the nonimmunologic release of mediators from mast cells and basophils. The latter have been called "anaphylactoid" or "pseudoallergic" reactions. They are important since the symptoms of allergic and pseudoallergic reactions are identical.

IMMUNOLOGIC BASIS OF DRUG ALLERGY

General Considerations

Although the frequency of reactions to various drugs varies widely, it is probable that any drug is capable of inducing the production of humoral or cellular immune responses. In many cases, the resulting immune reaction is not detrimental. For example, a large proportion of individuals treated with intravenous penicillin develop IgG antibodies to penicillin or penicillin biotransformation products. In the vast majority of instances these antibodies do not result in either the appearance of a drug reaction or a decrease in the effectiveness of the drug. This is also true for patients treated with bovine or porcine insulin. Thus, the demonstration of antibodies or sensitized T cells directed against a drug does not indicate that this immune response will necessarily result in a drug reaction.

Drugs are capable of inducing allergic reactions by any of the hypersensitivity mechanisms that are discussed in Chapter 29, ie, IgE-mediated, cytotoxic-antibody-mediated, immune-complex-mediated, and T effector cell-mediated mechanisms. However, to induce these reactions, a drug must be immunogenic. Since most drugs are of low molecular weight, they are in and of themselves nonimmunogenic. Only when the drug is capable of interacting with tissue proteins and serving as a hapten will it induce an immune response. Some drugs, such as insulin or pituitary snuff (used as a source of antidiuretic hormone), are large polypeptides or proteins and therefore are capable of interacting with immunoreactive cells in their native state. A few relatively low-molecular-weight drugs such as polymyxin appear to be immunogenic without tissue conjugation. Although the exact mechanism is currently unknown, immunogenicity is probably related to the ability of these drugs to form long-chain polymers.

Metabolic Biotransformation & Haptenation

Most haptenic drugs conjugate to tissue protein via a covalent bond. In rare cases the bond may be noncovalent but of sufficient affinity for the drug-protein complex to remain intact during antigen processing and presentation. For this reason the ability of any drug to induce an immune response depends upon the tissue reactivity of that drug. Thus, drugs that easily form covalent bonds will be more immunogenic than those which are relatively unreactive. It is not necessary, however, that the native drug be highly reactive, since its hydrolysis or biotransformation products may serve as the haptens. For this reason, a thorough knowledge of the biotransformation products of a drug is critical in the evaluation of drug allergies, but, unfortunately, these products are not known for most drugs. This limits the ability to predict the immunogenicity of a given drug and, as discussed below, the ability to test for the presence of a drug allergy.

Early studies of patients with known allergy to penicillin demonstrated that only a small percentage of these patients reacted to penicillin G; the majority reacted to the penicilloyl moiety, which is generated by the cleavage of the β-lactam ring, and others reacted to the penilloate group generated by the cleavage of the 5-membered thiazolidine ring (Fig 34–1). This led to the development of accurate methods for detecting allergy to penicillin and other β-lactam drugs, as discussed below. Similarly, only a small percentage of patients allergic to sulfonamides react by skin tests to the native drug, so skin testing is not an accurate predictor of allergic reactivity for this class of drugs. On the other hand, Prausnitz-Küstner passive transfer of serum from sulfonamide-allergic patients to nonallergic individuals results in a wheal and flare at the site of the injection when the recipient ingests the drug. This suggests that metabolism of the drug results in a reactive molecule which, on conjugation to circulating proteins, is capable of interacting with and activating the locally sensitized mast cells.

The immune response generated by certain drugs that are highly tissue reactive may be directed neither to the drug or its metabolic by-products nor to the host tissue but rather to a new antigenic determinant, which is the result of the combination of the drug with a specific tissue protein. This is the mechanism of thrombocytopenia following the ingestion of quinine, an antimalarial drug. In this case, the patient produces an IgG antibody with specificity for quinine, which is bound to the surface of the platelet. The quinine-platelet interaction has generated a new antigenic determinant that does not cross-react with other blood cells or tissues. The exact immunologic mechanisms of most other tissue-specific drug reactions are currently unknown.

Finally, the interaction between a drug and a tissue protein or other tissue component may alter the tissue protein at a site distant from the actual binding of the drug to the protein. This now altered tissue protein can then be recognized as foreign by the immune system and can serve as an immunogen for either humoral or cell-mediated immune responses. This mechanism is of some importance, since the antibodies or cytotoxic T cells generated may be capable of recognizing not only the altered protein but also the protein in its native state. This is the mechanism of some types of drug-induced autoimmunity. A good example of this phenomenon is the systemic lupus erythematosus syndrome associated with the drug hydralazine. Some of these reactions may then persist long after the drug has been withdrawn. The various modes of hapten-carrier interaction in drug allergy are illustrated in Fig 34–2.

Other Factors in Drug Allergenicity

The type of immune response that will be generated by a given drug depends upon (1) the chemical nature of the drug, (2) the route of presentation (ingestion, injection, or application to the skin), and (3) the genetic makeup of the individual. Certain drugs produce a humoral immune response, whereas others more commonly induce T cell immunity. This difference most probably results from differences in tissue reactivity of the drug.

The site of presentation of the drug markedly in-

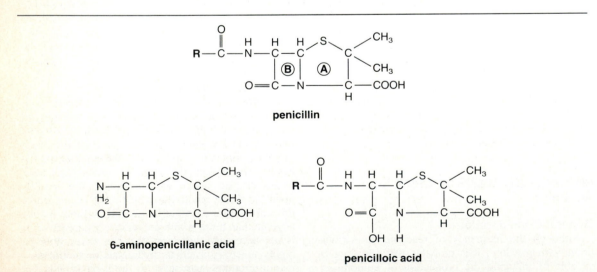

Figure 34–1. Penicillin and 2 allergenic biotransformation products. **A:** Thiazolidine ring; **B:** β-lactam ring.

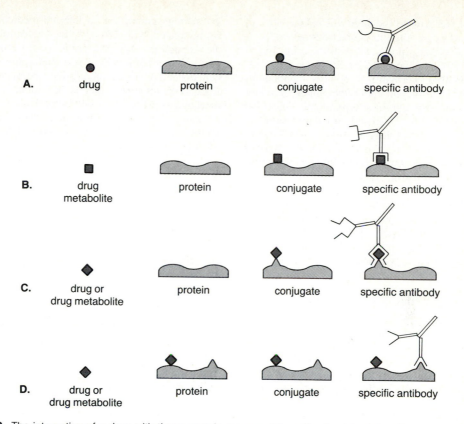

Figure 34–2. The interaction of a drug with tissue protein may result in antibodies (shown) or T cells directed against various determinants. **A:** The specific antibodies are directed against the native molecule. **B:** The antibodies are directed against a hydrolysis or biotransformation product of the drug. **C:** The antibodies are directed against a new determinant formed by the interaction of the drug or drug metabolite and the protein. **D:** Conjugation of the drug or its metabolites results in a conformational change in the tissue protein, which is then recognized as foreign by the immune system.

fluences both the ability of the drug to induce an adverse immunologic reaction and the type of reaction. In general, drugs are far more likely to induce an immune reaction when they are given parenterally (subcutaneously, intramuscularly, or intravenously) than when given orally or applied to the skin. For example, IgE and IgG antibodies to penicillin or its derivatives are produced in a greater proportion of individuals treated intravenously than in those treated orally with comparable doses of the drug.

The route of presentation may also determine the type of immune response (antibody or T cell) associated with a given drug. For example, antihistaminic drugs are rarely allergenic when given by the oral or parenteral route but frequently induce T cell sensitization when applied topically to the skin, causing allergic contact dermatitis.

Clinical Manifestations

An adverse reaction to a drug can be considered to be allergic if (1) the patient has antibodies or sensitized T cells with specificity for the drug, a drug metabolite, or a drug-tissue conjugate, and (2) the chemical features of the reaction are consistent with recognized immunologically induced inflammation (see Chapter 29). In some instances the adverse reaction closely follows the introduction of a drug and the reaction appears to be immunologic, but extensive immunologic studies fail to demonstrate drug-specific antibodies or T cells. This might be explained by failure to identify the appropriate antigen. Drug fever may be an example of this phenomenon. A number of drugs are commonly associated with episodic or persistent fever, which remits upon withdrawal of the drug and recurs promptly when the drug is readministered. Although it has long been suspected that drug fever is an immunologic phenomenon, studies to date have failed to provide a convincing immunologic mechanism.

As noted above, any type of hypersensitivity reaction may cause drug allergy. In some cases, the type of immune response determines the location of reaction. For example, the vast majority of reactions that are T cell-mediated produce dermatitis. Repeated application of the drug to the skin will induce a T cell response and cause allergic contact dermatitis localized to areas of skin in contact with the drug. Ingestion or injection of the drug generally causes a diffuse eczematoid dermatitis or, less commonly, erythema multiforme of either the minor or major (Stevens-Johnson syndrome) type, toxic epidermal necrolysis, or, in rare cases, erythema nodosum.

The manifestation of drug allergy mediated by antibody depends to a great extent upon the type of antibody. Reactions attributed to IgE antibodies include pruritus, urticaria, angioedema, and systemic anaphylaxis. IgG antibodies to drugs result in cytotoxicity or immune-complex deposition with complement-mediated inflammation. These may be tissue specific, as discussed above, or they may be generalized, with multiple organ involvement, eg, in patients with serum sickness.

DIAGNOSIS OF DRUG ALLERGY

Ideally, the diagnosis of drug allergy is made by in vivo or in vitro testing with the drug or its reactive metabolites. For this reason, the most important aspect of the diagnostic evaluation is an accurate and comprehensive history, with special attention to 3 areas.

Nature of Symptoms

First, the nature of the symptoms helps to differentiate immunologic reactions from toxic or idiosyncratic reactions. Isolated gastrointestinal complaints following the institution of antibiotic therapy, pain at the site of drug injection, headache associated with nitroglycerine therapy, or fever and malaise following an influenza inoculation are all predictable side effects that do not have an immunologic basis. The nature of the reaction must be placed in the context of other diseases that might have similar symptoms. For example, patients with systemic lupus erythematosus often present with symptoms resembling those of an allergic drug reaction. On the other hand, allergic drug reactions may stimulate other illnesses.

Previous Drug History

Second, knowledge of the drugs that the patient has taken in the past and whether any of these drugs has been associated with an adverse reaction may reveal that a current allergic response is caused by the same or similar class of drug that caused a previous allergic reaction. On the other hand, the fact that a patient has taken a drug in the past without difficulty suggests that other causes for the patient's illness should be explored, but it does not rule out a newly developed drug sensitivity.

The history may be all the more difficult when patients are taking multiple medications; more often than not, this is the case. It has been estimated that the average patient on an internal-medicine ward is being treated with 10 separate medications, and in the outpatient setting it is not unusual to find patients on 5 or more medications. It is therefore very important that all of these medications be accurately defined. For inpatients this is best done by using a thorough chart review. For outpatients it is best to recommend that they bring all of their medications with them or, if this is not possible, that they bring a list of all their medications.

As noted above, certain drugs are frequently associated with allergic reactions, whereas reactions to others are very uncommon. For example, allergic reactions to digitalis glycosides are extremely rare, whereas reactions to some antibiotics are very common. Thus, in a patient taking both of these classes of drugs, it is far more likely that the antibiotic, rather than the cardiac glycoside, is the cause of the problem.

Temporal Relationship

Third, the temporal relationship between the institution of drug therapy and the onset of the reaction is important. Immunologic reactions may occur at different times following drug therapy. IgE antibody reactions to drugs generally start within 30–60 min following administration of the drug. Allergic contact dermatitis is expected to have a latency period averaging 48–72 hours following application of the drug. The latency period in serum sickness is usually 7 days. In contrast to a reaction in a patient sensitized during a prior course of the drug, sensitization and reaction to a current drug course will cause a longer latency period for appearance of an adverse reaction. Thus, one might see the onset of symptoms of an IgE reaction 7–14 days following the introduction of the drug. It is unlikely but not impossible for a patient who has been on a drug for a long period to develop a de novo sensitization to that drug. It is also unlikely for a patient to develop a reaction to a drug after therapy with that agent has been discontinued, but this might occur with the use of depot medications, which are released into the body over a long period.

In Vivo Tests

It is sometimes possible to confirm a suspected allergic drug reaction by using in vivo testing.

A. Patch or Skin Tests: In vivo testing includes prick or intradermal skin testing for IgE sensitivity, patch testing for delayed-type hypersensitivity, and provocative-dose challenges. The wheal-and-erythema skin test cannot be used to diagnose IgE-mediated allergy to drugs that nonspecifically release the mediators of anaphylaxis from mast cells. A list of such drugs is found in Chapter 31.

When performing skin tests for IgE-mediated drug allergy or patch tests for allergic contact dermatitis, the immunogenic form of the drug (native drug or metabolite) must be used. In addition, for patch testing, the drug in question must not be irritating, as sufficient irritation can produce a false-positive result.

B. Provocative Tests: The provocative-dose challenge is a method whereby the patient is given increasing doses of the drug, beginning with small doses and increasing to the full therapeutic dose, and is observed for signs of an allergic response, at which point the drug is withdrawn. It must be remembered that the use of challenge testing is not without danger. It is reserved for instances when no alternative therapy is available (see p. 428) and when the benefit of the drug far outweighs the potential harm. These tests must be performed only where adequate facilities and personnel are available to treat acute medical emergencies.

In Vitro Tests

These are designed to identify either the antibody that is reacting with a drug hapten or the drug determinant that can stimulate sensitized T cells. For IgE antibody-mediated reaction, the radioallergosorbent test (RAST) or enzyme-linked immunosorbent assay (ELISA) is applicable when the antigenic determinant is known and available. As noted above, the lack of knowledge of the true immunogen for most drugs has limited this type of testing. A RAST is available for detecting IgE antibodies to the penicilloyl determinant, and recently an ELISA for identifying allergy to the sulfonamide group has been developed. Tests of IgG or IgM antibodies are available for only a limited number of allergenic drugs.

For suspected cell-mediated reaction to drugs, lymphocyte activation assays have been used (see Chapter 19). These test the ability of the drug or a drug-protein conjugate to induce the proliferation of T lymphocytes. Lymphocyte activation analysis is relatively simple to perform; however, the 3–5 days necessary to complete the test and the need for appropriate culture facilities have limited its use in practice.

TREATMENT OF DRUG ALLERGY

Since there are only a few drugs for which accurate in vivo or in vitro testing is available, a suspected drug reaction must be treated without such confirmation. There are 3 steps that can be taken. First, any drug not necessary for the care of the patient is discontinued. Second, for drugs that cannot be eliminated, an alternative drug with similar pharmacologic properties but a different chemical structure should be substituted. Finally, in cases when no alternative drug is available and the allergic reaction is mild and not life-threatening, it may be possible to continue the drug and treat the patient symptomatically. If possible, the drug should be discontinued

temporarily for a short time to confirm that it was the cause of the reaction.

PENICILLIN ALLERGY

Penicillin and the other β-lactam antibiotics are a frequent cause of all types of immunologic drug reactions including IgE-mediated anaphylaxis and urticaria, serum sickness, T cell-mediated contact dermatitis, and antibody-mediated cytolysis. However, by far the most common and potentially dangerous penicillin reactions are those resulting from the production of specific IgE. As a group, the β-lactam antibiotics are the most common cause of IgE-mediated allergic reactions to drugs. This class of drugs includes the penicillins, the cephalosporins, the cephamycins, the penems, and the monobactams (Fig 34–3). The penicillins have a β-lactam ring conjugated to a 5-membered thiazolidine ring. They differ from the cephalosporins in that the latter class has a 6-membered rather than a 5-membered sulfur-containing ring. The cephamycins are similar to the cephalosporins but have a methoxy group attached to the β-lactam ring. Penems are a large class that resemble the penicillins, with the exception that the 5-membered ring contains a carbon or oxygen in place of the sulfur. Finally, the monobactams are the only class of drug that do not have a second ring conjugated to the β-lactam ring.

Skin Testing

Specific skin test reagents are available to evaluate patients with suspected penicillin allergy. Skin testing with penicillin G is effective in demonstrating allergic reactivity in only a small percentage of patients. However, conjugation of penicillin to protein following cleavage of the β-lactam ring has provided a skin test reagent that shows a positive correlation with clinical allergic sensitivity in more than 75% of all penicillin-allergic individuals, and so the penicilloyl group has been termed the "major determinant." Fewer patients react with penicilloic acid (7%) and with penicillin G (6%). These 2 molecules are presumed to conjugate to tissue proteins in the skin, thereby providing determinants other than the penicilloyl group. They are called the "minor determinants." In practice, penicilloyl-polylysine is used to test for the major determinant since polylysine is a relatively nonimmunogenic molecule. This reagent is available commercially. The minor determinants, however, are not yet available commercially, although methods for their production and use have been published.

There are a number of protocols for skin testing in cases of suspected penicillin allergy. In one protocol, penicillin G and penicilloic acid are prepared at a concentration of 3.3 mg/mL and diluted 1:100 and 1:10,000. Penicilloyl-polylysine is used at a concentration of 6×10^{-5} mol/L. Skin prick or scratch

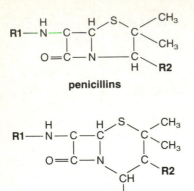

penicillins

cephalosporins

cephamycins

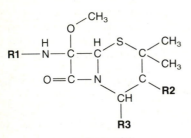

penems (X = O or C)

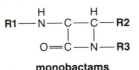

monobactams

Figure 34–3. Core structures of the 5 groups of β-lactam antibiotics. R1, R2, R3,; side chains; X, oxygen atom or CH₂ in penems.

testing is performed first with the most dilute concentration and then with the more concentrated solution if there is no reaction to the first test. If the scratch test is negative, intradermal testing is performed in a similar fashion. A positive skin test is defined as one in which the wheal and flare is greater than in a saline control performed at the same time. The patient is considered to be allergic to penicillin if there is a positive skin test to any of the reagents at any dilution.

The penicillin skin test has proven to be highly predictive. In one study with more than 1500 skin tests, only a single patient with negative skin tests had an acute anaphylactic reaction when given penicillin in full therapeutic doses. Patients who have a positive skin test are at risk for a systemic allergic reaction; in several studies the reaction rate was more than 25%. Thus, patients who are skin test positive will need to be desensitized before full therapeutic doses of this drug can be used.

A number of factors have been shown to correlate with skin test positivity to penicillin. For example, 100% of patients who reported a previous anaphylactic reaction to penicillin were skin test positive and 75% of patients with serum sickness had positive tests. In our studies, more than 40% of patients with other symptoms of an immunologic response to penicillin were skin test positive, although other studies have reported a significantly lower percentage. Skin test positivity correlates with the time course of the reaction during penicillin therapy. Immediate reactions in previously sensitized patients and reactions appearing 7–10 days after the institution of drug therapy in previously unsensitized patients are associated with the highest percentage of positive skin tests.

The time elapsed since the reported allergic reaction is also critical. Skin tests may be negative for several days or weeks after a systemic reaction before becoming positive. The tests remain positive over the next several years and then gradually decline, so that by 10 years following a reaction, fewer than 10% of history-positive patients are still skin test positive. This demonstrates that although drug-induced IgE may persist over a relatively long period, the IgE levels will eventually decline in the absence of further antigenic stimulation.

Patients who present a history of penicillin allergy but are skin test negative can be given penicillin in full therapeutic doses with no greater risk of reaction than those without a history of penicillin allergy. Several studies have demonstrated that patients with a positive history and negative skin tests who are treated with oral penicillin or its analogs are rarely resensitized, and therefore skin testing following therapy is not necessary. In contrast, patients who receive high-dose intravenous penicillin are frequently (70%) resensitized and therefore should be retested at 6–8 weeks following the cessation of therapy.

It has been estimated that at least 250 patients in the USA die each year from anaphylactic reactions to parenteral penicillin. By contrast, there are only 6 reported cases of anaphylactic deaths from oral penicillin, and the number of reported nonfatal anaphylactic reactions from oral penicillin is less than 100. For this reason, we have chosen to use the oral route for penicillin desensitization.

Desensitization to Penicillin

The desensitization procedure is reserved for patients with a history of penicillin allergy and in whom the skin test is positive or cannot be performed. There should be no alternative antibiotic available, and the infection should be serious enough to risk the dangers of anaphylaxis from the treatment. If the patient meets these criteria, one of several protocols can be used. In one protocol, the patient is given increasing doses of oral phenoxymethyl penicillin beginning at 100 units and progressing until 400,000–800,000 U (250 to 500 mg) has been given. The drug is then given intravenously. This procedure has been performed in more than 100 patients, and in only 2 instances has it failed because of unacceptable reactions. In about one-third of patients there is minor skin reaction, but these reactions have not precluded achieving desensitization.

Others have preferred to use an intravenous desensitization. This method, in general, has a higher reaction rate but is effective, particularly when no oral form of the drug is available. Until recently this has been the case for patients sensitive to the third-generation cephalosporins (see below). Oral preparations of the third-generation cephalosporins should be used for desensitization when available.

Cross-Reactions with Other β-Lactams

The chemistry of penicillin metabolites has been studied, and the chemical structure of the allergenic epitopes is now established. Similar studies have not been carried out for the related antibiotics. Therefore, cross-reactivity of anti-penicillin IgE antibodies with the other β-lactam antibiotics has been evaluated only by in vitro tests such as RAST or ELISA inhibition or by clinical studies. Although many of the data are speculative, some generalizations can be made. Natural or semisynthetic penicillins tend to cross-react with one another. In addition, the cross-reactivity between penicillin and the first-generation cephalosporins appears to be relatively high (greater than 50%), particularly in patients with extreme sensitivity. The cross-reactivity between penicillin and the second- and third-generation cephalosporins is significantly lower than for the first-generation drugs. However, there is some cross-reactivity, and there are reports of at least 3 anaphylactic deaths resulting from the use of every second- and third-generation cephalosporin available in the USA. Only the monobactams appear to lack cross-reactivity with penicillin.

The problem of cross-reactivity is further complicated by the fact that some patients have IgE antibodies not to the β-lactam ring but rather to side-chain determinants. For these individuals, who may also have anti-β-lactam IgE as well, the cross-reactivity will depend on the similarity of the side chain. For example, aztreonam and ceftazidime contain the same side chain. Similarly, piperacillin and cephapyrizone contain identical side chains.

SULFONAMIDE ALLERGY

The sulfonamide drugs cause acute allergic reactions in a significant percentage of patients. The class of drugs is used for a variety of therapeutic uses; it includes the sulfonamide antibiotics such as sulfisoxazole and sulfamethoxazole, the diuretics furosemide and hydrochlorothiazide, and the angiotensin-converting enzyme (ACE) inhibitor captopril. The frequency of cross-reactivity among members of this class of drugs is not known. Patients sensitized to one sulfonamide may or may not react when treated with other sulfonamides. Skin testing is unreliable in confirming or rejecting the clinical history of an allergic reaction. Therefore, patients with a history of sensitivity to one member of this class should avoid all sulfonamide drugs. Alternative antibiotics are readily available: ethacrinic acid can be substituted for furosemide, and enalapril and alternative ACE inhibitors or another class of antihypertensive drug can be used to replace captopril.

Recently, an ELISA has been developed that uses sulfonamide conjugated with human serum albumin as antigen, but the test has yet to be studied in a sufficient number of patients to be used with confidence for diagnosis of sulfonamide allergy.

Experience with desensitization is very limited, and severe immediate reactions have been reported, so its use should be considered only in the very rare situations where a sulfonamide antibiotic is the only effective treatment for a life-threatening disease. Sulfonamides can cause severe skin reactions such as Stevens-Johnson syndrome. These are not amenable to desensitization. Thus, the potential danger from the administration of sulfonamides to sensitive individuals is significantly greater than for penicillin.

INSULIN ALLERGY

Insulin is a frequent cause of allergic reactions. Both IgG and IgE antibodies may be induced by therapeutic insulin, but these antibodies may or may not cause allergic reactions. However, several syndromes are related to anti-insulin antibodies. Insulin allergic reactions may be local or systemic, and their onset can be either immediate or delayed. The immediate local reaction is mediated by IgE antibodies. It generally consists of local swelling and erythema, and, in contrast to other IgE-mediated reactions, it is often painful rather than pruritic. However, the delayed local reaction that occurs 4–12 hours following injection is an Arthus reaction resulting from IgG anti-insulin antibodies. Immediate and delayed systemic reaction are both IgE mediated.

The relationship of clinical cross-reactivity and the amino acid sequences of insulins from different animal species is not clear. Patients may be sensitized to either bovine insulin, which differs from human insulin by 3 amino acids in the α chain, or to porcine insulin, which differs from human insulin by a single amino acid in the β chain (Fig 34–4). Some patients are sensitized to proinsulin, which contaminates many insulin preparations. However, many patients sensitive to insulin will react not only to the bovine and porcine varieties but also to human insulin. This is a true cross-reactivity, because insulin-sensitive patients who are treated with recombinant human insulin will also react. Patients treated exclusively with recombinant human insulin, however, do not develop either IgE or IgG antibodies.

Treatment of patients with local reactions to insulin is largely symptomatic. The use of oral antihistamines or concomitant injection of the antihistamine with the insulin is effective in most cases. For very severe local reactions, insulin can be injected with corticosteroids (dexamethasone is preferred because it is compatible with most insulin preparations); however, the dose of corticosteroid must be relatively low (0.75 mg of dexamethasone or equivalent) to avoid steroid-induced gluconeogenesis.

For immediate systemic reactions, single-component (beef, pork, or human) insulin should be tried first. If the patient reacts to all of these, skin testing with beef, pork, and human insulin, followed by rapid desensitization, generally to human insulin, will usually be effective. It is preferable to have the patient discontinue insulin for several days prior to the desensitization if possible.

Most studies have demonstrated that there is a rapid decline in the anti-insulin IgE levels in desensitized patients. The mechanism for this decline is not known. However, patients who undergo desensitization to insulin must be cautioned that there should not be lapses in therapy, because this may lead to reappearance of IgE antibodies and allergic reaction when insulin therapy is resumed.

Patients with high levels of anti-insulin IgG antibodies are usually insulin resistant. The treatment of insulin resistance is beyond the scope of this chapter, and the reader is referred to standard texts.

PSEUDOALLERGIC REACTIONS

Many drugs can induce the release of mediators of anaphylaxis from mast cells or circulating basophils by nonimmunologic means. Although IgE production is not involved, the symptoms of anaphylactic and anaphylactoid reactions are identical (see Chapter 31). Many of these drugs are capable of causing significant reactions in a certain portion of the treated population.

Radiocontrast media, particularly the ionic forms, are perhaps the best examples of drugs that cause pseudoallergic reactions. Other common drugs include aspirin and other nonsteroidal anti-inflammatory drugs (NSAID), curare and its derivatives, the opiate analgesics, and some local anesthetics. The reason for the susceptibility of only a portion of the treated population to nonimmunologic urticaria and anaphylactoid reactions to these drugs is not known. Several strategies have been developed for safe administration of drugs that cause pseudoallergic reactions. For patients who have previously reacted to radiocontrast media, pretreatment with H_1 and H_2 receptor-blocking antihistamines and corticosteroids has proven highly effective. Patients with sensitivity to aspirin or other NSAID are best treated by avoiding these drugs; however, oral "desensitization" to aspirin successfully prevents reactions to aspirin and other NSAID.

species	amino acid sequence variations			
	A-chain position			B-chain position
	8	9	10	30
human	Thr-Ser-Ile			Thr
pig, dog, sperm whale	Thr-Ser-Ile			Ala
cattle, goat	Ala-Ser-Val			Ala

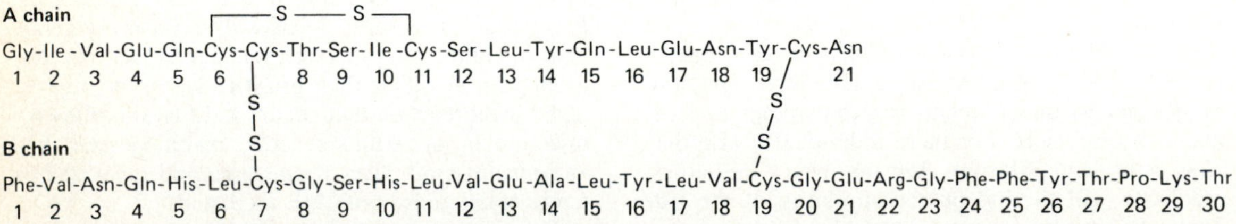

A chain

Gly-Ile-Val-Glu-Gln-Cys-Cys-Thr-Ser-Ile-Cys-Ser-Leu-Tyr-Gln-Leu-Glu-Asn-Tyr-Cys-Asn
1 2 3 4 5 6 8 9 10 11 12 13 14 15 16 17 18 19 21

B chain

Phe-Val-Asn-Gln-His-Leu-Cys-Gly-Ser-His-Leu-Val-Glu-Ala-Leu-Tyr-Leu-Val-Cys-Gly-Glu-Arg-Gly-Phe-Phe-Tyr-Thr-Pro-Lys-Thr
1 2 3 4 5 6 7 8 9 10 11 12 13 14 15 16 17 18 19 20 21 22 23 24 25 26 27 28 29 30

Figure 34–4. Covalent structure and variations of human and animal insulins. (Reproduced, with permission, from Ganong WF: *Review of Medical Physiology*, 14th ed. Appleton & Lange, 1989.)

CONCLUSIONS

Immunologically mediated drug hypersensitivity makes up a significant portion of the overall spectrum of adverse reactions to drugs. The variety of immune responses to drugs accounts for the spectrum of drug allergy. Although the proportion of treated patients who will react to a given drug or class of drugs varies widely, it is most likely that any drug is capable of inducing an adverse immunologic reaction, and so any drug must be considered a possible cause of an individual patient's reaction.

The majority of drugs are considered to be haptens and therefore must conjugate to tissue protein in vivo to be immunogenic. Unfortunately, the actual immunogen is not known for most drugs. This has made the development of accurate in vivo or in vitro tests difficult. Thus, for most drug classes, an accurate clinical history is the only diagnostic test for suspecting a particular drug as the cause of a patient's reaction. When the history suggests a candidate, its effect can then be confirmed by testing. When testing is not possible, drug withdrawal and, if necessary, rechallenge will confirm the patient's sensitivity.

It is only in a minority of situations that continuation of or reintroduction of the drug will be necessary. In this case, pretreatment protocols, provocative challenge, and drug desensitization procedures are available. However, the best treatment for drug allergy is the use of a different drug with similar pharmacologic properties but different chemical (ie, antigenic) structure.

REFERENCES

Adverse reactions to radiocontrast media. *Invest Radiol* 1980;**15(Suppl 6):**S1. (Entire issue.)

Carrington DM, Earl HS, Sullivan TJ: Studies of human IgE to a sulfonamide determinant. *J Allergy Clin Immunol* 1987;**79:**442.

Hansbrough JR, Wedner HJ, Chaplin DD: Anaphylaxis to intravenous furosemide. *J Allergy Clin Immunol* 1987;**80:**538.

Levine BB, Zolov DM: Prediction of penicillin allergy by immunological tests. *J Allergy* 1969;**43:**231.

Parker CW et al: Hypersensitivity to penicillenic acid derivatives in human beings with penicillin allergy. *J Exp Med* 1982;**115:**821.

Ring J: Pseudoallergic reactions. In: *Allergy: Theory and Practice,* 2nd ed. Korenblat PE, Wedner HJ (editors). Grune & Stratton, 1989 (in press).

Sullivan TJ et al: Desensitization of patients allergic to penicillin by orally administered beta-lactam antibiotics. *J Allergy Clin Immunol* 1982;**69:**275.

Sullivan TJ et al: Skin testing to detect penicillin allergy. *J Allergy Clin Immunol* 1981;**68:**171.

Wedner HJ: Adverse reactions to drugs. Pages 640–646 in: *Current Pediatric Therapy,* 12th ed. Gellis SS, Kagan BM (editors). WB Saunders, 1986.

Wedner HJ: Protocols for penicillin desensitization. Appendix A, p 423 in: *Allergy: Theory and Practice.* Korenblat PE, Wedner HJ (editors). Grune & Stratton, 1984.

Mechanisms of Disordered Immune Regulation

Alfred D. Steinberg, MD

Are there autoimmune diseases? Yes. There are numerous diseases that have characteristic autoimmune concomitants. Are these diseases initiated by an immune reaction against a self antigen? Although the answer to this question is unknown, it may ultimately be "no" or "very few." That is, most of the autoimmune disorders ultimately may be found to be induced by one or more foreign agents. Nevertheless, grouping these diseases serves the purpose of considering the common aspects of autoimmunity. Moreover, our conceptual framework of autoimmunity tends to direct both our investigations and our therapy. This framework has changed over the years (Table 35-1). We now recognize that self-reactivity is critical to normal immune responsiveness and immune regulation. Therefore, it is now conceptually more difficult to understand why some anti-self-immune responses are useful whereas others induce immune-mediated pathology. Moreover, when immunology was an adjunct to microbiology, it was expected that Koch's postulates would be applicable to autoimmune diseases. This view was reinforced by early studies of induction of organ-specific autoimmune diseases in animals by injection of lymphocytes from animals with disease that had been induced by immunization with target organ extracts in adjuvants. More recently it has become apparent that Koch's postulates are very difficult—both in principle and in practice—to apply in spontaneously occurring disorders that are multifactorial in etiology, such as the autoimmune diseases.

DISEASE MECHANISMS

A limited number of effector mechanisms characterize immune responsiveness. These include anaphylactic, cytotoxic, antigen-antibody-complex-mediated, and cell-mediated processes, which ultimately contribute to disease manifestations. Although the effector mechanisms may be understood, at least in general terms, for many diseases, the factors that initiate and regulate such processes often are uncertain. This chapter will therefore emphasize approaches to understanding initiation and perpetuation factors in the genesis of autoimmune diseases.

Cross-Reactivity & Molecular Mimicry

It has long been held that one possible mechanism of induction of autoimmunity might be immunization with an antigen that cross-reacts with a self antigen. That is, one or more antigenic determinants on the foreign antigen would induce an immune response that would simultaneously be directed against a self antigen by virtue of the similar structures of the foreign antigen and self antigen. Such an immune response could be humoral or cell-mediated. For example, the human immune response to group A β-hemolytic streptococci includes a component that is directed at self antigens in the heart and, if sufficiently vigorous, can lead to acute rheumatic fever.

In addition to cross-reactivity, in which the antigenic determinants are similar but not identical, recent studies have demonstrated areas of identity between viruses and self antigens. This has been called **molecular mimicry.** For example, there are many instances in which a sequence of 5 amino acids has been found in common between a given foreign antigen and a self antigen. Even longer homologous stretches have been found between self antigens and retroviral proteins, bacterial proteins, herpesvirus glycoprotein, and others. The molecular mimicry observed has been proposed as the cause of the autoimmune disease characterized by an immune response

Table 35–1. Autoimmune diseases: a conceptual framework.

Some degree of self-reactivity is normal
  A. Mechanism of development of self reactivity
    1. CD 4 T cell interaction with class II MHC plus antigen
    2. CD 8 T cell interaction with class I MHC plus antigen
    3. Anti-idiotype antibodies
    4. Anti-idiotypic T cells
  B. Quantitative aspects of disease may be critical: how much of a given antibody or T cell specificity; how many immune complexes; how much of a given cytokine; etc
  C. Diseases are multifactorial
    1. Genetic basis (multiple genes may be important)
    2. Environmental agents

against the relevant self antigen. Such a construction would be plausible if molecular mimicry were an extremely improbable event.

What is the probability of molecular mimicry? One can provide a gross estimate of the chance that a sequence of 5 amino acids on a human protein and a foreign protein might be identical on a random basis. For the estimate we will assume that (1) the average protein has 300 amino acids, (2) the 20 amino acids are distributed randomly and independently, and (3) the primary structure is critical to cross-reactivity. A 5-amino-acid sequence has a probability of $1/20^5$, or 3×10^{-7}. If there are 300 amino acids per protein, there are more than 200 possible pentapeptides in each of the human and foreign proteins. Therefore, we have to multiply 3×10^{-7} by 200 for the foreign protein and again by 200 for the self protein, which gives 10^{-2}. Thus, such calculations give approximately a 1% chance that a foreign and a human protein, each 300 amino acids long, will have a pentapeptide in common.

Many pentapeptides may not be readily accessible to the immune system in the 3-dimensional configuration of the native protein or the intracellular location of the protein. Moreover, many pentapeptides of self antigens may not be immunogenic because the relevant T cell specificities have not developed, possibly because of deletion in the thymus. Even if immunogenic, the pentapeptides might induce low-affinity antibody, which is not pathogenic. On the other hand, an immunogenic carrier, to which T cell clones have not been deleted in the thymus, which induces a vigorous immune response to a self pentapeptide adjacent to the carrier might be particularly pathogenic.

Since there are approximately 20,000 human genes capable of producing a protein, many potential 5-amino-acid sequences might share identical sequences with foreign proteins. In fact, a priori, it is highly probable that for any foreign protein there is a 5-amino-acid sequence of identity in some human (self) protein. Similarly, for every self protein, there is a strong probability that some foreign protein will have a 5-amino-acid sequence in common with it. Therefore, molecular mimicry should be the rule rather than the exception. However, demonstrating that a 5-amino-acid sequence is important in autoimmunity is another more difficult issue.

In addition to cross-reactivity and molecular mimicry as pathogenetic factors in the induction of disease, immunogenic foreign antigens could combine with self antigens and thereby induce an immune response to the self antigen. For example, virus-encoded antigens expressed on mammalian cell surfaces could act as carriers for self antigens adjacent to them on the cell membrane. In such a concept, the self antigen would appear as a hapten to which an immune response could not be induced without an immunogenic carrier.

Idiotypy & Autoimmunity

Idiotypy constitutes a normal self-self interaction (Table 35–1). Idiotypy in B cells consists of a set of B cells with receptors that recognize unique epitopes on antibodies produced by other B cells. Similarly, T cells have receptors able to recognize epitopes on other T cells or on antibody molecules. As a result, such idiotypic B cells or T cells can be activated by self antigens. It has been postulated that some degree of idiotypic response plays a role in normal immune regulatory processes. It is also possible that perturbation of the idiotype networks gives rise to pathogenic immune responses. Moreover, idiotypic interactions could serve as amplification systems for autoimmunity rather than as down-regulatory forces, in a manner similar to the induction of immunity by anti-idiotypic antibody simulating the role of antigen.

It is possible that the molecular mimicry described above acts in concert with idiotypy as a possible mechanism of autoimmunity. Many viruses utilize normal host receptors for their attachment to and entry into host cells. Therefore, the invading virus must contain a structure homologous with and presumably antigenically cross-reactive with a normal ligand for that receptor. If the host makes an immune response to that part of the foreign agent, it will be making an immune response resembling an autoimmune response to the normal ligand. In addition, the production of antibody to the normal ligand can trigger an anti-idiotype response to that antibody; such an anti-idiotype might represent an antibody reactive with the receptor itself. In such a manner, a virus or other microorganism that utilizes a receptor might be able to induce an autoimmune response to that receptor. This mechanism may be important in the induction of such antireceptor disorders as myasthenia gravis, anti-insulin receptor antibody syndrome, and Graves' disease. More generally, anti-idiotype autoantibodies could easily be the natural consequence of a normal immune response. If the external agent that induced such a response persisted, the stimulus to autoantibody production also would be maintained. If the stimulus were intermittent, the resulting autoimmune response also might be stimulated intermittently. The same reasoning would hold for T cell idiotypy.

A. Loss of Normal Tolerance; Central Versus Peripheral Effects: In order for many of these previously described mechanisms to operate, self tolerance must be broken. Normal self-tolerance mechanisms include (1) deletion of certain self-reactive cells during development and (2) peripheral suppression of unwanted responses later in life. Deletion of self-reactive cells would probably be limited to cells capable of high-affinity interactions with self determinants. If low-affinity anti-self cells were also deleted, there would probably be deletion of critical cells with the potential for high-affinity interactions with foreign pathogens. However, it is possible that the deletion process is imperfect, allowing a fraction of high-affinity anti-self cells to emerge. Therefore, functional loss of tolerance to important self antigens and resultant development of autoimmune disease could occur by the following mechanisms: (1) a defect in the deletion process, either a global defect or a specific one, allowing the emergence of an increased percentage of high-affinity anti-self cells; (2) excessive peripheral expansion of the few randomly nondeleted high-affinity cells that ''normally'' escape deletion; (3) excessive peripheral expansion of normally nondeleted low-affinity cells, which might increase the probability of emergence of pathogenic anti-self responses; (4) because of molecular mimicry, deletion, by normal deletion processes, of cells potentially reactive with specific microorganisms sharing epitopes with self antigens in that genetic type (in other individuals such cells are not deleted and are used to prevent chronic infection by certain foreign pathogens); (5) excessive deletion of self-reactive cells, which allows, by molecular mimicry, persistent infections that induce ''autoimmune'' diseases.

B. Central Mechanisms: It is now known that processes within the thymus delete a substantial proportion of certain potentially self-reactive clones. A defect in these central deletion processes could underlie the generation of autoimmunity. Studies of possible lack of intrathymic deletion, especially in organ-specific diseases involving immune responses to specific antigenic determinants, are needed to clarify this issue.

C. Peripheral Mechanisms: Peripheral mechanisms for controlling self-reactive cells include tolerance and suppression. Mechanisms that suppress and mechanisms that interfere with suppression (contrasuppression), are being reevaluated. It is likely that some mechanisms of suppression of humoral immunity simultaneously increase cellular immunity and vice versa. Differential stimulation of helper T cell subtypes may be critical for these effects. Nevertheless, impaired suppression or excessive contrasuppression may be important contributors to autoimmunity.

In some instances, these phenomena may be the result of excess cytokine production or even bystander stimulation. For example, a vigorous immune response to a foreign pathogen could lead to sufficient polyclonal immune stimulation that autoimmune phenomena are allowed to occur. Such a process might contribute to the autoimmune manifestations of such diseases as tuberculosis, leprosy, malaria, and trypanosomiasis. Similar excess production of stimulatory cytokines may contribute to idiopathic autoimmune diseases.

Experimental tolerance is a well-established mechanism for preventing immunity to specific foreign antigens. For example, immunity to heterolo-gous gamma globulins administered in an immunogenic form can be prevented by treatment with deaggregated gamma globulin before the immunogenic form is administered. This form of tolerance can be prevented by providing a B cell stimulus (eg, bacterial lipopolysaccharide) at the time of the deaggregated gamma globulin injection.

Interleukin-1 (IL-1), which is induced by agents that interfere with tolerance, probably plays a critical role in preventing tolerance. Impaired experimental tolerance and loss of self tolerance are features of mouse strains predisposed to systemic autoimmunity. Increased production of stimulatory cytokines most probably leads to both the defective tolerance and the heightened immunity that characterize murine systemic lupus erythematosus.

In multifactorial organ-specific as well as generalized autoimmune diseases, increased immunity and decreased suppression, which is often antigen nonspecific, are among the predisposing factors. These nonspecific factors, however, do not negate a role for specifically sensitized T cells that recognize a critical self epitope, or the important role of cognate cellular interactions in tolerance induction and immunity. Antigen-specific defects in either tolerance or immunity also play critical roles in such disorders.

D. Animal Models of Rheumatoid Arthritis: The multifactorial pathogenesis of autoimmune disease (Table 35–1) is illustrated by the example of experimental rheumatoid arthritis in swine (Table 35–2). If the cause of arthritis in group 5 was unknown, identification of single causes, such as *Erysipelothrix, Mycoplasma,* trauma to the joints as a result of walking on cement floors, or a genetic basis of disease would be correct but only partially so, since the disease in full expression is multifactorial. The data suggest that genetic factors, at least 2 infectious agents, and other environmental factors (cement floors) all contribute to the disease experienced by group 5.

E. Other Organ-Specific Diseases and a Possible Role for Class II MHC Expression: Most autoimmune diseases preferentially affect a single tissue or organ system. As a result, the details of pathogenesis depend upon the particular immune responses involved in the individual disorder. Organ-specific autoimmune diseases may be primarily cell-

Table 35–2. Multifactorial etiology of rheumatoid arthritis-like disease in swine.

Factor	Arthritis
1. Swine of the wrong type (wrong genes) regardless of other manipulations	Trivial
2. *Erysipelothrix insidiosa*	Mild
3. *Mycoplasma hyorhinis*	Mild
4. 2 + 3 (housed on dirt)	Moderate
5. 2 + 3 (housed on cement)	Severe

mediated or antibody-mediated; however, several different mechanisms may contribute to glandular destruction. In many cases, immunity to specific receptors probably is induced by anti-idiotypic effects (see above) or molecular mimicry (see above). For other diseases, a genetic predisposition to specific immunity may be critical. Table 35–3 summarizes the etiologic factors gleaned from many studies of animal models of autoimmune diseases as they may apply to human disease.

It is established that antigen presentation to T cells occurs in the context of self major histocompatibility complex (MHC) molecules. As a result, aberrant expression of MHC molecules on tissues normally expressing very little MHC could lead to the "presentation" of self determinants in association with the aberrantly expressed MHC. Such a process might, for example, be induced by an infection that induces the MHC or by interferon production as a result of either viral or immune effects. It is likely that such MHC expression represents a mechanism producing secondary inflammation of certain endocrine organs in an autoimmune process.

It has become apparent that the central nervous system bears important analogies to the rest of the body in terms of MHC expression and interferon effects. For example, astroytes can be induced by interferon to express MHC molecules and present antigens to T cells. As a result, viral infections of the central nervous system can induce immune and potentially autoimmune central nervous system effects. Consistent with such a view, interferon exacerbates multiple sclerosis and increases the immune response to myelin basic protein.

One aspect that has not yet been stressed is the possibility that an immune deficiency, either global or restricted, predisposes to autoimmune disease. Individuals who fail to clear infections of specific or varied types may develop chronic inflammatory diseases. For example, many individuals with hypogammaglobulinemia or with complement deficiencies develop rheumatic diseases. Patients with ankylosing spondylitis may be predisposed to disease because the HLA-B27 gene they carry allows an immune response to a common antigenic determinant shared by the HLA-B27 antigen and certain bacteria. Alterna-

tively, this molecular mimicry could allow persistence of certain bacteria by virtue of self tolerance to HLA-B27 and a failure of cross-reactive immune responses against the bacteria.

F. Commentary on the Pathogenesis of SLE:

Systemic lupus erythematosus (SLE) differs from many other autoimmune diseases in the relative organ nonspecificity of the disorder. Patients with SLE produce large amounts of antibodies reactive with epitopes on a variety of nuclear, cytoplasmic, and cell surface antigens. Although it is a complex disease, SLE provides a number of insights into autoimmune pathogenesis. Several different factors appear capable of predisposing to disease: genetic factors that increase humoral immunity, impaired clearance of immune complexes, defective immune regulation, and exogenous agents that stimulate humoral immunity. Thus, a decreased number of receptors for immune complexes on erythrocytes predisposes to impaired clearance of immune complexes and their increased deposition in tissues. Relatively unusual antibodies may underlie specific pathologic events. For example, antibodies reactive with platelet phospholipids may predispose to in situ thromboses and hence induce pulmonary infarcts or strokes.

In SLE, autoantibody production may be antigen-driven and T cell-dependent. On the other hand, SLE often is characterized by polyclonal B cell activation. Patients have marked increases in numbers of activated and immunoglobulin-producing circulating B cells and increased numbers of B cells producing anti-hapten antibodies.

Studies on murine lupus show that a substantial portion of the immune systems of both normal strains and strains predisposed to autoimmunity are devoted to autoantibody production: approximately 1% to anti-DNA and another 1% to anti-T cell antibodies. The increase in numbers of autoantibody-producing cells early in the life of mice with lupus results not from a skewing of the B cell repertoire toward autoantibody production but from an increase in total numbers of immunoglobulin-secreting cells, of which autoantibody-producing cells are a relatively constant fraction. This polyclonal B cell activation is fertile soil for autoimmune disease to arise. Later in life, T cell-dependent responses become progressively more important in the induction of autoantibody synthesis. The polyclonal expansion precedes antigen-specific responses. The same sequence probably holds for some humans with SLE. Polyclonal activation may interfere with development or maintenance of self tolerance and hence may predispose to production of pathogenic autoantibodies. Moreover, a switch to active SLE is associated with a switch from IgM to IgG autoantibody production, substituting a long-lived isotype for a much shorter-lived one. Therefore, even without any change in total numbers of immunoglobulin-secreting cells,

---

Table 35–3. Etiologic factors from animal models of autoimmune disease.

1. Genetic susceptibility
   a. Initial infection
   b. Perpetuation
   c. Severity of reaction
2. Initial insult(s): virus, bacterium, mycoplasma, etc (more than one may contribute to disease)
3. Factors allowing perpetuation
   a. Impaired immune regulation
   b. Excessive inflammatory response
   c. Impaired degradation or clearance of foreign antigens
   d. Trauma

there would be a substantial increase in serum autoantibody.

Conclusions

From the foregoing it might seem surprising that everyone does not have autoimmune diseases. In fact, we all have many autoantibodies. The difference between health and disease may be only a 10–20-fold difference in the quantity of certain immune responses. There are many mechanisms by which normal immune regulatory processes can go awry. Autoimmune diseases result when there is a disruption of such normal processes to a sufficient extent to bring about pathogenic autoimmunity.

Diseases that we recognize as single entities may, in fact, be syndromes with different underlying mechanisms by which the common disorder arises. Appropriate therapy for such individuals probably requires an understanding of the specific underlying mechanisms.

REFERENCES

General

Smith HR, Steinberg AD: Autoimmunity—A perspective. *Ann Rev Immunol* 1983;**1**:175.

Molecular Mimicry

Beck S, Barrell BG: Human cytomegalovirus encodes a glycoprotein homologous to MHC class-I antigens. *Nature* 1988;**331**:269.

Dale JB, Beachey EH: Protective antigenic determinant of streptococcal M protein shared with sarcolemmal membrane protein of human heart. *J Exp Med* 1982;**156**:1165.

Jahnke U, Fischer EH, Alvord EC Jr: Sequence homology between certain viral proteins and proteins related to encephalomyelitis and neuritis. *Science* 1985;**229**:282.

Krisher K, Cunningham MW: Myosin: A link between streptococci and heart. *Science* 1985;**227**:413.

Oldstone MBA: Molecular mimicry and autoimmune disease. *Cell* 1987;**50**:819.

Oppliger IR et al: Human rheumatoid factors bear the internal image of the Fc binding region of staphylococcal protein A. *J Exp Med* 1987;**166**:702.

Query CC, Keene JD: A human autoimmune protein associated with U1 RNA contains a region of homology that is cross-reactive with retroviral p30-gag antigen. *Cell* 1987;**51**:211.

Idiotypy & Autoimmunity

Gaulton EN, Greene MI: Idiotypic mimicry of biological receptors. *Annu Rev Immunol* 1986;**4**:253.

Helenius A et al: Human and murine histocompatibility antigens are cell surface receptors for Semliki Forest virus. *Proc Natl Acad Sci USA* 1978;**75**:3846.

Klinman DM, Steinberg AD: Idiotypy and autoimmunity. *Arthritis Rheum* 1986;**29**:697.

Plotz PH: Autoantibodies are anti-idiotypic antibodies to antiviral antibodies. *Lancet* 1983;**2**:824.

Powell TJ et al: Induction of effective immunity to Moloney murine sarcoma virus using monoclonal anti-idiotypic antibody as immunogen. *J Immunol* 1989;**142**:1318.

Steinberg AD: Idiotype regulation of autoantibody production. Pages 21–44 in: *Recent Advances in Autoimmunity and Tumor Immunology.* Dammacco F (editor). Edi-Ermes Publisher, 1988.

Loss of Immunologic Tolerance

Ben-Nun A, Wekerle H, Cohen IR: The rapid isolation of clonable antigen-specific T lymphocyte lines capable of mediating autoimmune encephalomyelitis. *Eur J Immunol* 1981;**11**:195.

Kappler JW, Roehm N, Marrack P: T cell tolerance by clonal elimination in the thymus. *Cell* 1987;**49**:273.

Kappler JW et al: Self-tolerance eliminates T cells specific for Mls-modified products of the major histocompatibility complex. *Nature* 1988;**332**:35.

Kappler JW et al: A T cell receptor Vbeta8 segments that imparts reactivity to a class II MHC product. *Cell* 1987;**49**:263.

Kisielow P et al: Tolerance in T-cell receptor transgenic mice involves deletion of nonmature CD4$^+$8$^+$ thymocytes. *Nature* 1988;**333**:742.

Kotzin BL, Babcock SK, Herron LR: Deletion of potentially self-reactive T cell receptor specificities in L3T4$^-$, Lyt-2$^-$ T cells of *lpr* mice. *J Exp Med* 1988;**168**:2221.

Laskin CA et al: NZB T cells actively interfere with the establishment of tolerance to BGG in radiation chimeras. *J Immunol* 1983;**131**:1121.

MacDonald H et al: T-cell receptor Vbeta8 use predicts reactivity and tolerance to Mls^a-encoded antigens. *Nature* 1988;**332**:40.

Matzinger P, Zamoyska R, Waldmann H: Self tolerance is H-2 restricted. *Nature* 1984;**308**:738.

Smith HR et al: Induction of autoimmunity in normal mice by thymectomy and administration of polyclonal B cell activators: Association with contrasuppressor function. *Clin Exp Immunol* 1983;**51**:579.

Steinberg AD: Tolerance and autoimmunity. In: *Internal Medicine*, 3rd ed. Stein JH (editor). Little, Brown, 1990.

Steinberg AD et al: Approach to the use of antigen nonspecific immunosuppression in systemic lupus erythematosus and other rheumatic autoimmune diseases. *J Autoimmun* 1988;**1**:575.

Weigle WO et al: The effect of lipopolysaccharide desensitization on the regulation of in vivo induction of immunologic tolerance and antibody production and in vitro release of IL-1. *J Immunol* 1989;**142**:1107.

Weigle WO et al: Modulation of the induction and circumvention of immunological tolerance to human gammaglobulin by interleukin-1. *J Immunol* 1987;**138**:2069.

Role of MHC-II (Ia) Expression

Fontana A et al: Astrocytes as antigen presenting cells. *J Neuroimmunol* 1986;**12**:15.

Panitch HS et al: Treatment of multiple sclerosis with gamma interferon: Exacerbations associated with activation of the immune system. *Neurology* 1987;**37**:1097.

Steinberg AD: Diseases of Ia, real and theoretical: A proposal for a new classification of a subset of immune mediated diseases. Pages 926–933 in: *Regulation of the Immune System (UCLA Symposium)* Cantor H, Chess L, Sercarz E (editors). Alan R. Liss, 1984.

Traugott U, Lebon P: Interferon-gamma and Ia antigens are present on astrocytes in active chronic multiple sclerosis lesions. *J Neuroimmunol* 1988;**84**:257.

Wong GHW et al: Inducible expression of H-2 and Ia antigens on brain cells. *Nature* 1984;**310**:688.

Systemic Lupus Erythematosus

Bernard NF, Eisenberg RA, Cohen PL: H-2 linked Ir gene control of T cell recognition of the Sm nuclear autoantigen and the aberrant response of autoimmune MRL/Mp− +/+ mice. *J Immunol* 1985;**134**:3812.

Blaese RM, Grayson J, Steinberg AD: Elevated immunoglobulin secreting cells in the blood of patients with active systemic lupus erythematosus: Correlation of laboratory and clinical assessment of disease activity. *Am J Med* 1980;**69**:345.

Budman DR et al: Increased spontaneous activity of antibody-forming cells in the peripheral blood of patients with active systemic lupus erythematosus. *Arthritis Rheum* 1977;**20**:829.

Klinman DM, Steinberg AD: Systemic autoimmune disease arises from polyclonal B cell activation. *J Exp Med* 1987;**165**:1755.

Klinman DM, Eisenberg RA, Steinberg AD: Development of the autoimmune B cell repertoire in MRL-*lpr/lpr* mice. *J Immunol* 1990;**144**:506.

36

Rheumatic Diseases

Kenneth H. Fye, MD, & Kenneth E. Sack, MD

Many of the major rheumatologic disorders are autoimmune in nature. Therefore, a thorough understanding of the mechanisms of the immune response is essential to an understanding of these diseases. Of particular importance is information in Chapter 35 which describes mechanisms of disordered immune regulation. This chapter will discuss the rheumatologic diseases with proved or hypothesized immunologic pathogenesis.

SYSTEMIC LUPUS ERYTHEMATOSUS (SLE)

Major Immunologic Features
- High-titer antinuclear antibodies (diffuse or outline pattern on immunofluorescence) are present.
- Anti-double-stranded DNA and anti-Sm antibodies are present.
- Serum complement levels are depressed.
- Immunoglobulin and complement are deposited along glomerular basement membrane and at the dermal-epidermal junction.
- Numerous other autoantibodies are present.

General Considerations

Osler described the systemic manifestations of systemic lupus erythematosus (SLE) in 1895. Prior to that time, lupus was considered to be a disfiguring but nonfatal skin disease. It is now known to be a chronic systemic inflammatory disease that follows a course of alternating exacerbations and remissions. Multiple organ system involvement characteristically occurs during periods of disease activity. The cause is not known. The disease affects predominantly females (4:1 over males) of childbearing age; however, the age at onset ranges from 2 to 90 years. It is more prevalent among nonwhites (particularly blacks) than whites. The disease also occurs in certain strains of mice (MRL/1, NZB).

Immunologic Pathogenesis

The discovery of the lupus erythematosus (LE) cell phenomenon (see Immunologic Diagnosis, below) marked the start of the modern era of research into the pathogenesis of SLE. This initial clinical observation led to the finding of multiple antinuclear factors, including antibodies to DNA, in the sera of patients with SLE. Further studies of renal eluates from patients with SLE established the importance of DNA-containing immune complexes in the causation of lupus glomerulonephritis. Reduced serum complement and the presence of antibodies to double-stranded (ds) DNA are hallmarks of active SLE, distinguishing this entity from other lupus variants. It is not known whether viral or host DNA is the immunogen for anti-DNA antibody formation.

Additional autoantibody activity is also associated with SLE. Lymphocytotoxic antibodies (with predominant specificity for T lymphocytes) occur in many patients with SLE. Cold-reactive IgM and warm-reactive IgG anti-T cell antibodies can interfere with T cell function. Such antibodies are capable of killing T lymphocytes in the presence of complement and of coating peripheral blood T cells so as to interfere with HLA typing. These antibodies have specificity for T cell surface antigens and can be released from the lymphocyte cell surface in the form of specific antigen-antibody complexes. Such complexes may themselves attach to and block the function of other lymphocytes or may contribute to immune complex deposition, leading to vasculitis and nephritis. Family studies have demonstrated a genetic susceptibility to the development of SLE. Autoantibody formation in SLE is in part genetically determined; eg, patients with HLA-DR2 are more likely to produce anti-ds-DNA antibodies, those with HLA-DR3 produce anti-SS-A and anti-SS-B antibodies (Table 36-1), and those with HLA-DR4 and HLA-DR5 produce anti-Sm and anti-RMP antibodies.

Autoantibody formation is partially prevented through the action of T regulatory lymphocytes called suppressor T cells. Although the mechanism of suppression is unknown, such suppressor T cells probably play an important role in immunologic tolerance and self-nonself discrimination. A defect in suppressor T cell activity has also been observed in human beings with SLE; however, this defect may be due to anti-T cell antibody activity and may not represent a primary suppressor T cell deficiency.

SLE, like many rheumatic disorders, occurs predominantly in women. Studies have demonstrated that estrogens enhance anti-DNA antibody formation

Table 36–1. Antinuclear antibodies.

Pattern	Antigen	Associated Diseases
Peripheral	Double-stranded DNA	SLE
Homogeneous	DNA-histone complex	SLE, occasionally other connective tissue disease
Speckled	Sm (Smith antigen)	SLE
	RNP (ribonucleoprotein)	Mixed connective tissue disease, SLE, Sjögren's syndrome, scleroderma, polymyositis
	SS-A (Ro)	Sjögren's syndrome, SLE
	SS-B (La)	Sjögren's syndrome, SLE
	Jo-1	Polydermatomyositis
	Scl-70	Scleroderma
	Centromere	CREST syndrome
	RANA (rheumatoid-associated nuclear antigen) (nuclear antigen induced by EBV)	Rheumatoid arthritis
Nucleolar	Nucleolus-specific RNA	Scleroderma
	PM-Sc1	Polymyositis

and increase the severity of renal disease in animal models. Androgens have an opposite effect on both anti-DNA antibody production and renal disease.

Pathology

There are numerous characteristic pathologic changes in SLE:

(1) The verrucous endocarditis of Libman-Sacks consists of ovoid vegetations, 1–4 mm in diameter, which form along the base of the valve and, rarely, on the chordae tendineae and papillary muscles.

(2) A peculiar periarterial concentric fibrosis results in the so-called "onion skin" lesion seen in the spleen.

(3) The pathognomonic finding in SLE, the "hematoxylin body," consists of a homogeneous globular mass of nuclear material that stains bluish purple with hematoxylin. Hematoxylin bodies have been found in the heart, kidneys, lungs, spleen, lymph nodes, and serous and synovial membranes. It should be emphasized that patients with fulminant SLE involving the central nervous system, skin, muscles, joints, and kidneys may not have any distinctive pathologic abnormalities at autopsy.

Clinical Features

A. Symptoms and Signs: SLE presents no single characteristic clinical pattern. The onset can be acute or insidious. Constitutional symptoms include fever, weight loss, malaise, and lethargy. Every organ system may become involved.

1. Joints and muscles—Polyarthralgia or arthritis is the most common manifestation of SLE (90%). The arthritis is symmetric and can involve almost any joint. It may resemble rheumatoid arthritis, but bony erosions and severe deformity are unusual.

Avascular necrosis of bone is common in SLE. The femoral head is most frequently affected, but other bones may also be involved. Corticosteroids, which are major therapeutic agents in SLE, may play a role in the pathogenesis of this complication. Myalgias, with or without frank myositis, are common.

2. Skin—The most common skin lesion is an erythematous rash involving areas of the body chronically exposed to ultraviolet light. Relatively few patients with SLE develop the classic "butterfly" rash or the characteristic erythematous rash over the fingertips and palms. In some cases, the rash is similar in appearance to that of discoid lupus erythematosus. The rash may resolve without sequelae or may result in scar formation, atrophy, and hypo- or hyperpigmentation. A non-scarring skin lesion termed subacute cutaneous lupus erythematosus occurs predominantly in patients with anti-SS-A antibodies. In addition, bullae, patches of purpura, urticaria, angioneurotic edema, patches of vitiligo, subcutaneous nodules, and thickening of the skin may be seen. Vasculitic lesions, ranging from palpable purpura to digital infarction, are common. Alopecia, which may be diffuse, patchy, or circumscribed, is also common. Mucosal ulcerations, involving both oral and genital mucosa, are present in about 15% of cases.

3. Polyserositis—Pleurisy is frequently present. Although one-third of cases have pleural fluid, massive effusion is rare. Involvement of the pleura produces pleuritic chest pain and shortness of breath. Pericarditis is the commonest form of cardiac involvement and can be the first manifestation of SLE. The pericarditis is usually benign, with only mild chest discomfort and a pericardial friction rub, but severe pericarditis leading to tamponade can occur. Peritonitis alone is extremely rare, although 5–10% of patients with pleuritis and pericarditis have concomitant peritonitis. Manifestations of peritonitis include abdominal pain, anorexia, nausea and vomiting, and, rarely, ascites.

4. Kidneys—Renal involvement is a frequent and serious feature of SLE. Seventy-five percent of patients have nephritis at autopsy. The study of renal tissue by light microscopy, immunofluorescence, and electron microscopy has revealed 5 histologic lesions associated with rather distinctive clinical features. (1) Mesangial glomerulonephritis is characterized by hypercellularity and the deposition of immune complexes in the mesangium. This is a benign form of lupus nephritis. (2) In focal glomerulonephritis, segmental proliferation occurs in less than 50% of glomeruli. Immune complexes are deposited in the mesangium and in the subendothelium of the glomerular capillary. Focal glomerulonephritis is often a benign process, but may progress to a diffuse proliferative lesion. (3) Diffuse proliferative glomerulonephritis is characterized by extensive cellular proliferation in more than 50% of glomeruli. Immune complexes are deposited largely in subendothelial distribution. This process frequently leads to renal failure. (4) In membranous glomerulonephritis, glomerular cellularity is normal, but the capillary basement membrane is thickened. Immune complexes are deposited mainly in subepithelial and intramembranous areas. This lesion may be associated with the development of renal failure. (5) Sclerosing glomerulonephritis is defined by an increase in mesangial matrix glomerulosclerosis, capsular adhesions, fibrous crescents, interstitial fibrosis with tubular atrophy, and vascular sclerosis. This lesion portends a poor prognosis and is not responsive to drugs.

It must be emphasized that a benign renal lesion may evolve into a more serious one.

Systemic hypertension is a common finding in acute or chronic lupus nephritis and may contribute to renal dysfunction.

5. Lungs—Clinically apparent lupus pneumonitis is unusual. When a pulmonary infiltrate develops in a patient with SLE, particularly one being treated with corticosteroids or immunosuppressive drugs, infection must be the first diagnostic consideration. The commonest form of lupus pulmonary involvement is restrictive interstitial lung disease, which may be asymptomatic and detectable only by pulmonary function tests. The chest x-ray is usually normal but may show "platelike" atelectasis or interstitial fibrosis with "honeycombing." Other pulmonary manifestations include pulmonary hypertension, alveolar hemorrhage, pneumothorax, hemothorax, and vasculitis.

6. Heart—Clinically apparent myocarditis occurs rarely in SLE but when present may result in congestive heart failure with tachycardia, gallop rhythm, and cardiomegaly. Arrhythmias are unusual and are considered a preterminal event. The verrucous endocarditis of SLE, with the characteristic Libman-Sacks vegetations, is usually diagnosed only at autopsy. Thickening of the aortic valve cusps with resultant aortic insufficiency can occur. Coronary artery disease, possibly related to corticosteroid therapy, is being detected with increasing frequency.

7. Nervous system—Cerebral involvement is a life-threatening complication of SLE. Disturbances of mentation and aberrant behavior, such as psychosis or depression, are the commonest manifestations of central nervous system involvement. Convulsions, cranial nerve palsies, aseptic meningitis, migraine headache, peripheral neuritis, and cerebrovascular accidents may also occur.

8. Eyes—Ocular involvement is present in 20–25% of patients. The characteristic retinal finding (the cytoid body) is a fluffy white exudative lesion caused by focal degeneration of the nerve fiber layer of the retina secondary to retinal vasculitis. Scleritis is also a manifestation of ocular vasculitis. Corneal ulceration occurs in conjunction with Sjögren's syndrome (see below).

9. Gastrointestinal system—Gastrointestinal ulceration due to vasculitis can occur in SLE but is uncommon. Pancreatitis is not unusual, and acute and chronic hepatitis may occur.

10. Hematopoietic system—See Laboratory Findings, below.

11. Vascular system—Small-vessel vasculitis commonly occurs in active SLE. Cutaneous manifestations of small-vessel disease include splinter hemorrhages, periungual occlusions, finger pulp infarctions, and atrophic ulcers. Gastrointestinal manifestations include abdominal pain, diarrhea, hemorrhage, pancreatitis, and cholecystitis. The "stocking-glove" peripheral neuropathy commonly encountered in SLE is due to small-vessel vasculitis. Medium-vessel arteritis, involving arteries 0.5–1 mm in diameter, also occurs in SLE. Manifestations range from bowel infarction to mononeuritis multiplex to cerebrovascular accidents. Hypercoagulation leading to arterial and venous occlusive disease is seen in patients with antiphospholipid antibodies called lupus anticoagulants (see below). Reynaud's phenomenon occurs in 15% of patients with SLE.

12. Sjögren's syndrome—Five to 10% of patients with SLE develop the sicca complex (keratoconjunctivitis sicca, xerostomia).

13. Drug-induced lupuslike syndrome—Certain drugs may provoke a lupuslike picture in susceptible individuals. The most commonly implicated drugs, hydralazine and procainamide, can induce arthralgias, arthritis, skin rash, and, less commonly, fever and pleurisy. Nephritis and central nervous system involvement are thought not to occur. The antinuclear antibodies typical of drug induced lupus are anti-single stranded DNA (ss) and antihistone antibodies. The disease usually remits when the drug is discontinued. The list of agents that produce a lupuslike syndrome includes phenytoin, trimethadione, isoniazid, penicillamine, methyl- and propylthiouracil quinidine, ethoxysuximide, and chlorpromazine.

B. Laboratory Findings: Anemia is the most common hematologic finding in SLE. Eighty percent of patients present with a normochromic, normocytic anemia due to marrow suppression. A few develop Coombs-positive hemolytic anemia. Leukopenia and thrombocytopenia are common. Urinalysis may show hematuria, proteinuria, and erythrocyte and leukocyte casts. The sedimentation rate is high in almost all cases but frequently does not correlate with disease activity. Serologic abnormalities are described in the section on immunologic diagnosis (below). The synovial fluid in SLE is yellow and clear, with a low viscosity. The leukocyte count does not exceed 4000/μL, most of which are lymphocytes. Complement levels are low. The pleural effusion of SLE is a transudate with a predominance of lymphocytes and a total leukocyte count of no more than 3000/μL. A hemorrhagic pleural effusion is very rare. In central nervous system lupus, the cerebrospinal fluid protein concentration is sometimes elevated, and there is occasionally a mild lymphocytosis. Patients with nonfocal central nervous system disease may have antineuronal antibodies in cerebrospinal fluid.

C. X-Ray and Other Findings: Chest x-ray may reveal cardiomegaly (due either to pericarditis or myocarditis), pleural effusion, platelike atelectasis, or interstitial fibrosis with a "honeycomb" appearance. Joint x-rays may show soft tissue swelling and mild osteopenia but rarely show erosions. The lumbar puncture, cerebrospinal fluid, EEG, and radionuclide brain scan are abnormal in many cases of central nervous system involvement.

Immunologic Diagnosis

A. Proteins and Complement: Most patients with SLE (80%) present with elevated α_2- and γ-globulins. Hypoalbuminemia is occasionally present. The serum complement is frequently reduced in the presence of active disease because of increased utilization due to immune complex formation, reduced synthesis, or a combination of both factors. Several complement components, including C3 and C4, and total hemolytic complement activity are decreased while the activity of the attack complex of complement, C5–9, is increased during disease activity. The serum of patients with active SLE occasionally contains circulating cryoglobulin consisting of IgM/IgG aggregates and complement.

B. Autoantibodies:

1. LE cell phenomenon—This phenomenon was first described in the bone marrow of patients with SLE. It reflects the presence of IgG antibody to deoxyribonucleoprotein. However, this relatively cumbersome and insensitive technique is only of historic interest.

2. Antinuclear antibodies (ANA)—Immunoglobulins of all classes may form antinuclear antibodies. The indirect immunofluorescence technique was introduced in 1957. Six different morphologic patterns of immunofluorescent staining have been described, 4 of which have clinical significance (Fig 36-1 and Table 36-1).

a. The "homogeneous" ("diffuse" or "solid") pattern is the morphologic expression of antihistone antibodies and occurs in patients with systemic or

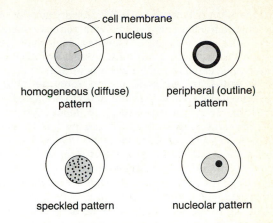

Figure 36–1. Patterns of immunofluorescent staining for antinuclear antibodies.

drug-induced lupus erythmatosus. In this pattern, the nucleus shows diffuse and uniform staining.

b. The "peripheral" ("shaggy" or "outline") pattern is the morphologic expression of anti-ds-DNA antibodies. The outline pattern is best seen when human leukocytes are used as substrate. It is characteristic of active SLE.

c. The "speckled" pattern reflects the presence of antibodies directed against non-DNA nuclear constituents. The anti-ENA (extractable nuclear antigen) assay detects antibodies against 2 saline-extractable nuclear antigens, the Sm (Smith) antigen and RNP (ribonucleoprotein) antigen. Antibodies against the Sm antigen are characteristic of SLE. High titers of anti-RNP antibodies are the hallmark of mixed connective tissue disease, but low-titer anti-RNP antibodies may occur in SLE. Other antinuclear antibodies have been described in Sjögren's syndrome, rheumatoid arthritis, scleroderma, CREST syndrome (see p. 453), and polymyositis-dermatomyositis.

d. The "nucleolar" pattern is caused by the homogeneous staining of the nucleolus. It has been suggested that this antigen may be the ribosomal precursor of ribonucleoprotein. This pattern is most often associated with scleroderma or polymyositis-dermatomyositis.

A positive ANA test must be interpreted with caution because (1) the serum of a patient with any rheumatic disease may contain many autoantibodies to different nuclear constituents, so that a "homogeneous" pattern may obscure a "speckled" or "nucleolar" pattern; (2) different antibodies in the serum can be present in different titers, so that by diluting the serum one can change the pattern observed; (3) the stability of the different antigens is different and can be changed by fixation or denaturation; and (4) the pattern observed appears to be influenced by the types of tissues or cells used as substrate for the test.

The ANA determination is occasionally positive in normal individuals, in patients with various chronic diseases, and in the aged. However, high titers are most often associated with SLE. Absence of ANA is strong evidence against a diagnosis of SLE.

3. Anti-DNA antibodies and immune complexes—Three major types of anti-DNA antibodies can be found in the sera of lupus patients: (1) anti-single-stranded or "denatured" DNA (ss-DNA); (2) anti-double-stranded or "native" DNA (ds-DNA); and (3) antibodies that react to both ss-DNA and ds-DNA. These antibodies may be either IgG or IgM immunoglobulins. High titers of anti-ds-DNA antibodies are essentially seen only in SLE. In contrast, anti-ss-DNA antibodies are not specific and can be found in other autoimmune diseases, eg, rheumatoid arthritis, chronic active hepatitis, and primary biliary cirrhosis. Antibodies to ss-DNA occur in drug-induced lupuslike syndrome. Antibodies to DNA can be quantitatively measured by RIA or ELISA techniques (see Chapter 18). Complement-fixing and high-avidity anti-ds-DNA antibodies may be associated with the development of renal disease. The amount of antibody correlates well with disease activity, and the antibody titer frequently decreases when patients enter remission.

Circulating immune complexes are present in the sera of patients with active disease. However, different assay techniques are required to detect complexes of different sizes, and there is controversy about how closely the level of soluble circulating immune complexes correlates with disease activity.

4. Antierythrocyte antibodies—These antibodies belong to the IgG, IgA, and IgM classes and can be detected by the direct Coombs test. The prevalence of these antibodies among SLE patients ranges from 10% to 65%. Hemolytic anemia does occasionally occur and, when present, is associated with a complement-fixing warm antierythrocyte antibody.

5. Circulating anticoagulants and antiplatelet antibodies—Antiphospholipid antibodies, called lupus anticoagulants, develop in 10–15% of patients with SLE. These antibodies are often associated with a false-positive VDRL and possess activity against cardiolipin. Although these anticoagulants prolong the partial thromboplastin and prothrombin times, hemorrhagic complications are rare. Paradoxic thrombotic states may develop owing to actions of antiphospholipid antibodies on platelets, vascular endothelial cells, or erythrocytes. Patients with antiphospholipid antibodies are at increased risk for thrombotic events, and women with these antibodies are subject to recurrent spontaneous abortions. Specific anti-factor VIII antibodies have also been described. These antibodies are potent anticoagulants and may be associated with bleeding. Antiplatelet antibodies are found in 75–80% of patients with SLE. These antibodies inhibit neither clot retraction nor thromboplastin generation in normal blood. They probably induce thrombocytopenia by direct effects on platelet surface membrane.

6. False-positive serologic test for syphilis—A false-positive VDRL test is seen in 10–20% of patients with SLE. The serologic test for syphilis can be considered an autoimmune reaction, because the antigen is a phospholipid present in many human organs (see above).

7. Rheumatoid factors—Almost 30% of patients with SLE have a positive latex fixation test for rheumatoid factors.

8. Anticytoplasmic antibodies—Numerous anticytoplasmic antibodies (antimitochondrial, antiribosomal, antilysosomal) have been found in patients with SLE. These antibodies are not organ- or species-specific. Antiribosomal antibodies are found in the sera of 25–50% of patients. The major antigenic determinant is ribosomal RNA. Antimitochondrial antibodies are more common in other diseases (eg, primary biliary cirrhosis) than in SLE.

C. Tissue immunofluorescence

1. Kidneys—Irregular or granular accumulation of immunoglobulin and complement occurs along the glomerular basement membrane and in the mesangium in patients with lupus nephritis. On electron microscopy, these deposits are seen in subepithelial, subendothelial, and mesangial sites.

2. Skin—Almost 90% of patients with SLE have immunoglobulin and complement deposition in the dermal-epidermal junction of skin that is *not* involved with an active lupus rash. The immunoglobulins are IgG or IgM and appear as a brightly staining homogeneous or granular band. Patients with discoid lupus erythematosus show deposition of immunoglobulin and complement only in involved skin.

Differential Diagnosis

The diagnosis of SLE in patients with classic multisystem involvement and a positive ANA test is not difficult. However, the onset of the disease can be vague and insidious and can therefore present a perplexing diagnostic problem. The polyarthritis of SLE is often similar to that seen in viral infections, infective endocarditis, mixed connective tissue disease, rheumatoid arthritis, and rheumatic fever. When Raynaud's phenomenon is the predominant complaint, progressive systemic sclerosis should be considered. SLE can present with a myositis similar to that of polymyositis-dermatomyositis. The clinical constellation of arthritis, alopecia, and a positive VDRL suggests secondary syphilis. Felty's syndrome (thrombocytopenia, leukopenia, splenomegaly in patients with rheumatoid arthritis) can simulate SLE. Takayasu's disease should be considered in a young woman who presents with arthralgias, fever, and asymmetric pulses. The diagnosis of SLE can be facilitated by finding anti-ds-DNA or a high titer of ANA (outline pattern) in serum.

Some patients with discoid lupus erythematosus may develop leukopenia, thrombocytopenia, hypergammaglobulinemia, a positive ANA, and an elevated sedimentation rate. Ten percent of patients with discoid lupus erythematosus have mild systemic symptoms. The frequent presence of anti-ds-RNA in discoid lupus erythematosus suggests that SLE and discoid lupus erythematosus are part of a single disease spectrum.

Treatment

The efficacy of the drugs used in the treatment of SLE is difficult to evaluate, since spontaneous remissions do occur. There are few controlled studies, because it is difficult to withhold therapy in the face of the life-threatening disease that can develop in fulminant SLE. Depending on the severity of the disease, no treatment, minimal treatment (aspirin, antimalarials), or intensive treatment (corticosteroids, cytotoxic drugs) may be required.

When arthritis is the predominant symptom and other organ systems are not significantly involved, high-dose aspirin or another fast-acting nonsteroidal anti-inflammatory drug may suffice to relieve symptoms. When the skin or mucosa is predominantly involved, antimalarials (hydroxychloroquine or chloroquine) and topical corticosteroids are very beneficial. Because high-dosage antimalarial therapy may be associated with irreversible retinal toxicity, these drugs should be used judiciously and in low doses.

Systemic corticosteroids in severe SLE can suppress disease activity and prolong life. The mode of action is unknown, but the immunosuppressive and anti-inflammatory properties of these agents presumably play a significant role in their therapeutic efficacy. High-dosage corticosteroid treatment (eg, prednisone, 1 mg/kg/d orally) decreases immunoglobulin levels and autoantibody titers and suppresses immune responses. High-dosage corticosteroid therapy is recommended in acute fulminant lupus, acute lupus nephritis, acute central nervous system lupus, acute autoimmune hemolytic anemia, and thrombocytopenic purpura. One or more courses of ''pulse'' therapy (ie, 15 mg/kg/d intravenously for 3 days) may be effective in patients with recalcitrant disease. The course of corticosteroid therapy should be monitored by the clinical response and meticulous follow-up of laboratory and immunologic parameters—complete blood count with reticulocyte and platelet counts, urinalysis, anti-ds-DNA titer, and complement levels.

If the clinical and immunologic status of the patient fails to improve or if serious side effects of corticosteroid therapy develop, immunosuppressive therapy with cytotoxic agents such as cyclophosphamide, chlorambucil, or azathioprine is indicated. Recent work suggests that intravenous ''pulse'' therapy with cyclophosphamide is a practical and effective means of treating lupus nephritis. Because of serious complications (cancer, marrow suppression, infection, and liver and gastrointestinal toxicity), immunosuppressive agents should be used with discretion.

Complications & Prognosis

SLE may run a very mild course confined to one or a few organs, or it may be a fulminant fatal disease. Renal failure and central nervous system lupus were the leading causes of death until the corticosteroids and cytotoxic agents came into widespread use. Since then, the complications of therapy, including atherosclerosis, infection, and cancer, have become common causes of death. The 5-year survival rate of patients with SLE has markedly improved over the past decade and now approaches 80–90%.

RHEUMATOID ARTHRITIS

Major Immunologic Features

- Monomeric and pentameric IgM and IgG rheumatoid factors exist in serum and synovial fluid.
- There is decreased complement in synovial fluid.
- Vasculitis and synovites are present.

General Considerations

Rheumatoid arthritis is a chronic, recurrent, systemic inflammatory disease primarily involving the joints. It affects 1–3% of people in the USA, with a female to male ratio of 3:1. Constitutional symptoms include malaise, fever, and weight loss. The disease characteristically begins in the small joints of the hands and feet and progresses in a centripetal and symmetric fashion. Elderly patients may present with more proximal large-joint involvement. Deformities are common. Extra-articular manifestations are characteristic of the rheumatoid process and often cause significant morbidity. Extra-articular manifestations include vasculitis, atrophy of the skin and muscle, subcutaneous nodules, lymphadenopathy, splenomegaly, and leukopenia.

Immunologic Pathogenesis

The cause of the unusual immune responses and subsequent inflammation in rheumatoid arthritis is unknown. HLA-D4 and HLA-DR4 occur in approximately 70% of patients with rheumatoid arthritis. Some patients who are negative for HLA-D4 and HLA-DR4 carry the HLA-DR1 gene. It is possible that these and perhaps other genetic determinants impart susceptibility to an unidentified environmental factor, such as a virus, that initiates the disease process. Although no virus particles have ever been identified, theoretically an antigenic stimulus leads to the appearance of an abnormal IgG that results in the production of rheumatoid factor and the eventual development of rheumatoid disease (Fig 36–2).

There is a possible relationship between Epstein-

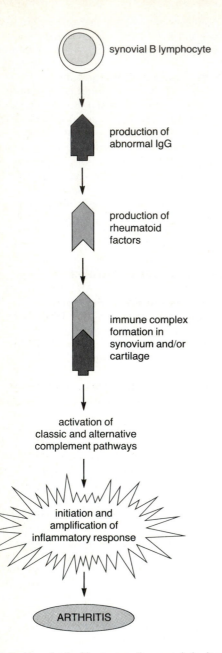

synovial B lymphocyte

production of
abnormal IgG

production of
rheumatoid
factors

immune complex
formation in
synovium and/or
cartilage

activation of
classic and alternative
complement pathways

initiation and
amplification of
inflammatory response

ARTHRITIS

Figure 36–2. Hypothetical immunopathogenesis in rheumatoid arthritis.

tionship of EBV with rheumatoid arthritis remains speculative.

Whatever the primary stimulus, synovial lymphocytes produce IgG that is recognized as foreign and stimulates an immune response within the joint, with production of IgG, monomeric IgM, and pentameric IgM anti-immunoglobulins, ie, rheumatoid factors. The presence of IgG aggregates or IgG-rheumatoid factor complexes results in activation of the complement system via the classic pathway. Breakdown products of complement accumulate within the joint and amplify the activation of complement by stimulation of the alternative (properdin) system. Activation of the complement system results in a number of inflammatory phenomena, including histamine release, the production of factors chemotactic for PMN and mononuclear cells, and membrane damage with cell lysis (see Chapter 11). There is a marked influx of leukocytes into the synovial space. Prostaglandins and leukotrienes produced by inflammatory cells are thought to play a major role in mediation of the inflammatory process. In addition, activated lysosomes and enzymes released into the synovial space by leukocytes further amplify the inflammatory and proliferative response of the synovium. The mononuclear infiltrate characteristically seen within the synovium includes perivascular collections of helper T cells and interstitial collections of suppressor T cells, B lymphocytes, lymphoblasts, plasma cells, and macrophages. The immunologic interaction of these cells leads to the liberation of lymphokines responsible for the accumulation of macrophages within the inflammatory synovium and to continued immunoglobulin and rheumatoid factor synthesis. Immune complexes in articular cartilage attract PMN, which damage cartilage by releasing proteases and collagenase.

Rheumatoid factor may play a role in the causation of extra-articular disease. Patients with rheumatoid vasculitis have high titers of monomeric and pentameric IgM and IgG rheumatoid factors. Antigen-antibody complexes infused into experimental animals in the presence of IgM rheumatoid factor induce necrotizing vasculitis. Theoretically, immune complexes initiate vascular inflammation by the activation of complement. Pulmonary involvement is associated with the deposition of 11S and 15S protein complexes containing aggregates of IgG in the walls of pulmonary vessels and alveoli. 19S IgM rheumatoid factor has also been detected in arterioles and alveolar walls adjacent to cavitary nodules. Rheumatoid factors do not initiate the inflammatory process that causes rheumatoid disease, but they probably perpetuate and amplify that process.

Clinical Features
A. Symptoms and Signs:
1. Onset—The usual age at onset is 20–40 years. In most cases the disease presents with joint mani-

Barr virus (EBV), a known polyclonal B cell stimulator, and rheumatoid arthritis. Rheumatoid arthritis patients have a high frequency of precipitating serum antibody (RA precipitin [RAP]) that reacts specifically with a nuclear antigen from a human lymphoblastoid cell line containing EBV. This antigen (RA nuclear antigen [RANA]) is expressed only in EBV-infected cells. However, because of the high frequency of RAP in normal controls, any causal rela-

festations; however, some patients first develop extra-articular manifestations, including fatigue, weakness, weight loss, mild fever, and anorexia.

2. Articular manifestations—Patients experience stiffness and joint pain, which are generally worse in the morning and improve throughout the day. These symptoms are accompanied by signs of articular inflammation, including swelling, warmth, erythema, and tenderness on palpation. The arthritis is symmetric, involving the small joints of the hands and feet, ie, the proximal interphalangeals, metacarpophalangeals, the wrists, and the subtalars. Large joints (knees, hips, elbows, ankles, shoulders) commonly become involved later in the course of the disease, although in some patients large joint involvement predominates. The cervical spine may be involved; the thoracic and lumbosacral spine is usually spared.

Periarticular inflammation is common, with tendonitis and tenosynovitis resulting in weakening of tendons, ligaments, and supporting structures. Joint pain leads to muscle spasm, limitation of motion, and, in advanced cases, muscle contractions and ankylosis with permanent joint deformity. The most characteristic deformities in the hand are ulnar deviation of the fingers, the "boutonnière" deformity (flexion of the proximal interphalangeal joints and hyperextension of the distal interphalangeal joints resulting from volar slippage of the lateral bands of the superficial extensor tendons), and the "swan neck" deformity (hyperextension of the proximal interphalangeal joints and flexion of the distal interphalangeal joints resulting from contractures of intrinsic hand muscles).

3. Extra-articular manifestations—Twenty to 25% of patients (particularly those with severe disease) have subcutaneous or subperiosteal nodules, so-called rheumatoid nodules. Rheumatoid nodules consist of an irregularly shaped central zone of fibrinoid necrosis surrounded by a margin of large mononuclear cells with an outer zone of granulation tissue containing plasma cells and lymphocytes. They are thought to be a late stage in the evolution of a vasculitic process, probably induced by the deposition of circulating immune complexes. These are usually present over bony eminences, with the most common sites of nodule formation being the olecranon bursa and the extensor surface of the forearm. Nodules are firm, nontender, round or oval masses that can be movable or fixed. They may be found in the myocardium, pericardium, heart valves, pleura, lungs, sclera, dura mater, spleen, larynx, and synovial tissues.

Lung involvement includes pleurisy, interstitial lymphocytic pneumonitis or fibrosis, and Caplan's syndrome (development of large nodules in the lung parenchyma of patients with rheumatoid arthritis who also have pneumoconiosis). The manifestations of rheumatoid cardiac disease include pericarditis, myocarditis, valvular insufficiency, and conduction disturbances.

Several types of vasculitis occur in rheumatoid arthritis. The most common type is a small-vessel obliterative vasculitis that leads to peripheral neuropathy. Less common is a subacute vasculitis associated with ischemic ulceration of the skin. The rarest form of rheumatoid vasculitis is a necrotizing vasculitis of medium and large vessels indistinguishable from polyarteritis nodosa. The major neurologic abnormalities in rheumatoid arthritis involve peripheral nerves. In addition to the peripheral neuropathy associated with vasculitis, there are a number of entrapment syndromes due to impingement by periarticular inflammatory tissue or amyloid on nerves passing through tight fascial planes. The carpal tunnel syndrome is a well-known complication of wrist disease; however, entrapment can also occur at the elbow, knee, and ankle. Destruction of the transverse ligament of the odontoid results in atlantoaxial subluxation. This generally causes no symptoms but may be associated with cord or nerve root impingement.

Sjögren's syndrome (keratoconjunctivitis sicca and xerostomia) occurs in up to 30% of patients. Myositis with lymphocytic infiltration of involved muscle is rare. Ocular involvement ranges from benign inflammation of the surface of the sclera (episcleritis) to severe inflammation of the sclera, with nodule formation. Scleronodular disease can lead to weakening and thinning of the sclera (scleromalacia). A catastrophic but rare complication of scleromalacia is perforation of the eye with extrusion of vitreous (scleromalacia perforans).

4. Felty's syndrome—Felty's syndrome is the association of rheumatoid arthritis, splenomegaly, and neutropenia. Possible mechanisms of the hematologic abnormalities seen in these patients include anti-stem cell antibodies, antigranulocyte antibodies, and splenic sequestration of immune complex-coated polymorphonuclear leukocytes. The syndrome almost always develops in patients with high rheumatoid factor titers and rheumatoid nodules, although the arthritis itself is frequently inactive. Other features of hypersplenism and lymphadenopathy may also be present. These patients are at increased risk of developing bacterial infections.

B. Laboratory Findings: A normochromic, normocytic anemia and thrombocytosis are common among patients with active disease. The sedimentation rate is elevated, and the degree of elevation correlates roughly with disease activity.

The synovial fluid is more inflammatory than that seen in degenerative osteoarthritis or SLE. The synovial fluid protein concentration ranges from 2.5 g/dL to more than 3.5 g/dL. The leukocyte count is usually 5000–20,000/μL (rarely higher than 50,000/μL). Two-thirds of the cells are PMN that discharge lysosomal enzymes into the synovial fluid, presumably leading to depolymerization of synovial hyaluronate, decreased viscosity, and a poor mucin clot. The glucose level may be low or normal. Rheumatoid factor can be found in synovial fluid, and complement is often depressed.

The rheumatoid pleural effusion is an exudate containing less than 5000 mononuclear or polymorphonuclear leukocytes per microliter. Protein exceeds 3g/dL, and glucose is often reduced below 20 mg/dL. Rheumatoid factors can be detected, and complement levels are usually low.

C. X-Ray Findings: The first detectable x-ray abnormalities are soft tissue swelling and juxta-articular demineralization. The destruction of articular cartilage leads to joint space narrowing. Bony erosions develop at the junction of the synovial membrane and the bone just adjacent to articular cartilage. Destruction of the cartilage and laxity of ligaments lead to maladjustment and subluxation of articular surfaces. Spondylitis is usually limited to the cervical spine, with osteoporosis, joint space narrowing, erosions, and finally subluxation of the involved articulations.

Immunologic Diagnosis

The most important serologic finding is the elevated rheumatoid factor titer, present in over 75% of patients. Rheumatoid factors are immunoglobulins with specificity for the Fc fragment of IgG. Most laboratory techniques detect pentameric IgM rheumatoid factor, but rheumatoid factor properties are also seen in monomeric IgM, IgG, and IgA. Pentameric IgM rheumatoid factor may combine with IgG molecules to form a soluble circulating high-molecular-weight immunoglobulin complex in the serum.

In rheumatoid arthritis, serum protein electrophoresis may show increased α_2-globulin, polyclonal hypergammaglobulinemia, and hypoalbuminemia. Cryoprecipitates composed of immunoglobulins are often seen in rheumatoid vasculitis. Serum complement levels are usually normal but may be low in the presence of active vasculitis. Many patients have antinuclear antibodies.

Several tests are available in the laboratory to detect rheumatoid factor. The earliest test, now rarely used, was the streptococcal agglutination reaction. The latex fixation test is now the most commonly used method for detection of rheumatoid factor. Aggregated γ-globulin (Cohn fraction II) is adsorbed onto latex particles, which then agglutinate in the presence of rheumatoid factor. The latex fixation test is not specific but is very sensitive, resulting in a high incidence of false-positive results. The sensitized sheep erythrocyte test (Rose-Waaler test) depends on specific antibody binding and is the most specific test in common use. Sheep erythrocytes are coated with rabbit antibody against sheep erythrocytes. The sensitized sheep erythrocytes then agglutinate in the presence of rheumatoid factor.

It is important to emphasize that a negative rheumatoid factor by routine laboratory procedures does not exclude the diagnosis of rheumatoid arthritis. The so-called seronegative patient may have IgG or IgM rheumatoid factor or circulating IgG-anti-IgG complexes. Conversely, rheumatoid factors are not unique to rheumatoid arthritis. Rheumatoid factor is also present in patients with SLE (30%), in a high percentage (90%) of patients with Sjögren's syndrome, and less often in patients with scleroderma or polymyositis. Positive agglutination reactions with the latex test also occur in patients with a number of chronic inflammatory conditions including chronic active hepatitis, kala-azar, sarcoidosis, neoplasia, and syphilis. The sensitized sheep erythrocyte test is usually negative in these conditions. In some chronic infectious diseases such as leprosy and tuberculosis, both the latex and the sensitized sheep erythrocyte tests may be positive. In subacute bacterial endocarditis, both tests may be positive during active disease and revert to negative as patients improve. The transient appearance of rheumatoid factor has been noted following vaccinations in military recruits. Epidemiologic studies have shown that a small number of normal people also have rheumatoid factors. A large proportion of the elderly have a positive latex test, though the sensitized sheep erythrocyte test is generally negative.

Differential Diagnosis

In the patient with classic articular changes, bony erosions of the small joints of the hands and feet, and a positive rheumatoid factor, the diagnosis of rheumatoid arthritis is not difficult. Early in the disease, or when extra-articular manifestations dominate the clinical picture, other rheumatic diseases (including SLE, Reiter's syndrome, gout, psoriatic arthritis, degenerative osteoarthritis, and the peripheral arthritis of chronic inflammatory bowel disease) or infectious processes may mimic rheumatoid arthritis. Patients with SLE can be distinguished by their characteristic skin lesions, renal disease, and diagnostic serologic abnormalities. Reiter's syndrome occurs predominantly in young men, generally affects joints of the lower extremity in an asymmetric fashion, and is often associated with urethritis and conjunctivitis. Gouty arthritis is usually an acute monoarthritis with negatively birefringent sodium urate crystals present within the white cells of inflammatory synovial fluid. Psoriatic arthritis is usually asymmetric and often involves distal interphalangeal joints and produces nail changes. Degenerative arthritis is characterized by Heberden's nodes, lack of symmetric joint involvement, and involvement of the distal interphalangeal joints. The peripheral arthritis of bowel disease usually occurs in large weight-bearing joints and is often associated with bowel symptoms. The polyarthritis associated with rubella vaccination, parvovirus infection, HBsAg antigenemia, sarcoidosis, and infectious mononucleosis can mimic early rheumatoid arthritis.

Treatment

A. Physical Therapy: A rational program of physical therapy is vital in the management of patients with rheumatoid arthritis. Such a program should consist of an appropriate balance of rest and exercise and the judicious use of heat or cold therapy. The patient may require complete or intermittent bed rest on a regular basis to combat inflammation or fatigue. In addition, specific joints may have to be put at rest through the use of braces, splints, or crutches. An exercise program emphasizing active range-of-motion movements helps to maintain strength and mobility. Heat or cold is valuable in alleviating muscle spasm, stiffness, and pain. Many patients need a hot shower or bath to loosen up in the morning, and others cannot perform their exercises adequately without prior heat treatment. Heating pads or paraffin baths are often used to apply heat to specific joints. In some patients ice massage is more effective than heat. Physical and occupational therapists provide valuable help in devising an appropriate physical therapy program.

B. Drug Treatment:

1. Salicylates—Salicylates are the mainstay of medical therapy of rheumatoid arthritis. Although its exact mechanism of action is uncertain, it effectively inhibits the production of prostaglandins thereby reducing inflammation. The doses used to attain therapeutic levels (ie, 20–30 mg/dL) range from 3.6 to 6.5 g per day in divided doses. High-dosage aspirin therapy is associated with numerous side effects. Tinnitus—with or without hearing loss—is reversible with a decrease in dosage. Gastric distress is common but can be partly alleviated by liberally using antacids, histamine H_2 receptor blockers, or sucralfate and by encouraging patients to take their aspirin with meals. Some patients can avoid gastric irritation by using enteric-coated aspirin. Microscopic blood loss from the gastrointestinal tract is common and is not an indication for stopping aspirin therapy. Since aspirin does decrease platelet adhesiveness, its use should be avoided in patients with a bleeding diathesis or those receiving coumarin anticoagulants.

2. Other nonsteroidal drugs—Several other nonsteroidal anti-inflammatory agents such as fenoprofen, ibuprofen, naproxen, sulindac, tolmetin, mefenamic acid, ketoprofen, diclofenac, carprofen, indomethacin, and piroxicam are useful in patients with rheumatoid arthritis. Combining 2 or more nonsteroidal anti-inflammatory agents provides little or no additional benefit over maximum doses of single agents and may increase gastrointestinal toxicity.

3. Antimalarial drugs—Many rheumatologists advocate the use of antimalarial drugs for prolonged periods in patients with severe disease. Their mechanism of action is unclear, but they appear to affect monocyte function. The antimalarial drugs act slowly, often requiring 1–6 months of treatment for maximum therapeutic benefit. The preparations and dosages most often used are chloroquine, 250 mg orally daily, and hydroxychloroquine, 200–400 mg orally daily. The toxic side effects of these agents include skin rashes, nausea and vomiting, myopathy, and both corneal and retinal damage. Eye toxicity is rare at the low doses used in rheumatoid arthritis, but patients should have ophthalmologic examinations every 4–6 months while on antimalarial therapy.

4. Gold salt therapy—Although associated with a high incidence of toxic side effects, parenteral gold salt therapy is of significant benefit to many patients. Gold acts as a lysosomal membrane stabilizer and may chiefly affect macrophage function. It is administered intramuscularly, with an initial test dose of 10 mg of gold salt. If no toxic reactions occur after the test dose, the patient receives 50 mg of gold salt intramuscularly every week until clinical benefit ensues, at which time the interval between injections is gradually increased to every 3–4 weeks. If no benefit occurs after a total of 1500 mg has been administered, gold should be considered ineffective. Toxic side effects occur in 40% of patients and include dermatitis, photosensitivity, stomatitis, thrombocytopenia, agranulocytosis, hepatitis, aplastic anemia, peripheral neuropathy, nephritis with nephrotic syndrome, ulcerative enterocolitis, pneumonitis, and keratitis. Before each dose, the patient should be evaluated for possible toxic side effects. A urine protein measurement, hematocrit, leukocyte count, and platelet count should be obtained. Liver function tests should be performed periodically. Toxic side effects may necessitate temporary or permanent withdrawal of the drug. Corticosteroids and dimercaprol may be of benefit if life-threatening toxicity occurs.

An oral gold salt preparation, auranofin, is now available. Its main effect may be on macrophage-T cell interactions.

Side effects, although similar to those of parenteral gold salt preparations, may occur less frequently. Diarrhea, however, is more common. The usual dose is 3 mg twice daily. As with parenteral gold preparations, it may take 3–6 months to achieve therapeutic benefit.

5. Penicillamine—Penicillamine is also useful in the treatment of rheumatoid arthritis. It may work through its inhibitory effect on helper T cell activity. Like gold, penicillamine is a slow-acting nonsteroidal anti-inflammatory agent, and it may take up to 6 months for a therapeutic response to become apparent. The incidence of drug toxicity is similar to that of parenteral gold, so during the initiation of therapy patients should be seen every other week for evaluation. Routine laboratory monitoring studies should include a complete blood count, platelet count, and urinalysis. The initial dose of 250 mg orally daily is increased by 125–250 mg every 4–12 weeks until improvement occurs or until the patient is receiving a maximum dose of 750 mg daily. Most patients require no more than 500 mg/d. Toxic side effects include rash, loss of sense of taste, nausea and vomiting, anorexia, proteinuria, agranulocytosis, aplastic anemia, and thrombocytopenia. Less commonly, myasthenia, myositis, Goodpasture's syndrome, pemphigus, bronchiolitis, and a lupuslike syndrome may be seen. Prior gold toxicity does not preclude the use of penicillamine.

6. Corticosteroids—Intermittent intra-articular injection of corticosteroids is useful for the patient with only a few symptomatic joints. Relief may last for months. However, multiple intra-articular corticosteroid injections in weight-bearing joints should be avoided, since they may lead to degenerative arthritis. Low-dose systemic corticosteroids may be indicated in patients who do not respond to NSAIDs or other remittive therapy. The usual dose is 5–10 mg of prednisone daily. Withdrawal from corticosteroids should be gradual, since clinical exacerbation of arthritis or steroid withdrawal syndrome may occur. Long-term systemic corticosteroid treatment results in hyperadrenocorticism and disruption of the pituitary-adrenal axis. Manifestations of corticosteroid toxicity include weight gain, moon facies, ecchymoses, hirsutism, diabetes mellitus, hypertension, osteoporosis, avascular necrosis of bone, cataracts, myopathy, mental disturbances, activation of tuberculosis, and infections.

7. Immunosuppressive agents—The antimetabolite methotrexate has been shown to induce dramatic improvement in patients with severe disease. Side effects include marrow suppression, liver toxicity, oral ulcers, and teratogenesis. Alkylating agents (eg, chlorambucil, cyclophosphamide) and purine analogs (eg, mercaptopurine, azathioprine) have also been used in the treatment of rheumatoid arthritis. However, these drugs are associated with major toxic side effects including an increased incidence of neoplasm and infection. They should, therefore, be used with great caution.

C. Orthopedic Surgery: Surgery is often an essential part of the general management of the patient with rheumatoid arthritis to correct or compensate for joint damage. Arthroplasty is employed to maintain or improve joint motion. Arthrodesis can be used to correct deformity and alleviate pain, but it results in loss of motion. Early synovectomy might prevent joint damage or tendon rupture and will decrease pain and inflammation in a given joint, but the synovium often grows back and symptoms return.

Complications & Prognosis

Several clinical patterns of rheumatoid arthritis are apparent. Spontaneous remission may occur, usually within 2 years after the onset of the disease. Some patients have brief episodes of acute arthritis with longer periods of low-grade activity or remission. Rare patients will have sustained progression of active disease resulting in deformity and death. The development of classic disease within 1 year of the onset of symptoms, an age of less than 30 years at onset of disease, and the presence of rheumatoid nodules and high titers of rheumatoid factor are unfavorable prognostic factors.

Follow-up of patients after 10–15 years shows that 50% are stationary or improved, 70% are capable of full-time employment, and 10% are completely incapacitated. Death from vasculitis or atlantoaxial subluxation is rare. Fatalities are more often associated with sepsis or the complications of therapy.

JUVENILE ARTHRITIS

Major Immunologic Features
- Overt or "hidden" rheumatoid factors exist.
- There are antinuclear antibodies.

General Considerations

Juvenile arthritis is not a single disease but a group of disorders that cause arthritis in individuals under 16 years of age. It may present as a systemic illness (Still's disease) or as a seronegative polyarthritis. The prognosis in these instances is good. The incidence of the disease peaks in boys at age 2 and again at age 9, while in girls it peaks between 1 and 3 years of age. Less commonly, juvenile arthritis presents as a pauciarticular process involving 4 or fewer joints. The outlook for girls with pauciarticular disease is excellent, whereas boys with pauciarticular disease may eventually develop ankylosing spondylitis. In older children, juvenile arthritis occasionally presents as a seropositive polyarticular disease that follows a course identical to that of adult rheumatoid arthritis. Although upper respiratory infections and trauma have both been implicated as precipitating factors, the roles of infection, trauma, and heredity in the pathogenesis of the disease are unclear. The onset of the disease may be as early as 6 weeks of life, but most children are between 2 and 5 or between 9 and 12 years of age at onset. Juvenile arthritis is a major cause of fever of undetermined origin in children.

Immunologic Pathogenesis

The basic immunopathogenic mechanisms in juvenile arthritis are unknown. However, both humoral and cellular defects occur in these patients. Diffuse hypergammaglobulinemia, involving IgG, IgA, and IgM, is present. Rheumatoid factors of all immunoglobulin classes have been detected. Approximately 10% of children with juvenile arthritis have a positive latex fixation test for IgM rheumatoid factor. The sera from some patients with negative latex fixation tests may actually contain IgM rheumatoid factors. Two major theories have been offered in an attempt to explain the presence of these "hidden" rheumatoid factors in juvenile arthritis. First, IgM rheumatoid factor may bind avidly to native IgG in the patient's serum and therefore may not be able to bind IgG coating the latex particles. Second, an abnormal IgG may be present that preferentially binds IgM, thereby blocking latex fixation. Cold-reacting (4 °C) pentameric IgM rheumatoid factors (cryoglobulins) are associated with severe disease.

Serum components of both the classic and alternative (properdin) complement systems are elevated, although this elevation is less in patients who have rheumatoid factors or severe disease. Elevation of serum complement may reflect a secondary overcompensation in response to increased consumption, or possibly a general increase in protein synthesis. Studies of the metabolism of complement actually demonstrate hypercatabolism. The depression of complement in synovial fluid is probably secondary to complement activation by immune complexes, similar to that seen in rheumatoid arthritis.

Preliminary studies suggest that patients with juvenile arthritis possess certain HLA tissue types with greater than expected frequencies. Thus, patients with early-onset pauciarticular disease tend to be HLA-DR5- or HLA-DR8-positive, while those with late-onset pauciarticular disease tend to be HLA-B27-positive. Patients with rheumatoid factor-positive polyarticular disease tend to be HLA-D4-positive, and those with systemic disease tend to be HLA-DR5-positive.

Clinical Features
A. Symptoms and Signs:
1. Onset—
a. Twenty percent of children, usually under age 4, present with high, spiking fever, an evanescent rash, polyserositis, hepatosplenomegaly, and lymphadenopathy (Still's disease).

b. Forty percent of patients present with polyarthritis (more than 4 joints involved during the first 6 months of illness), sometimes accompanied by low-grade fever and malaise. In 25% of this group, the onset is in late childhood and is associated with rheumatoid factor.

c. Forty percent of patients present with few systemic manifestations and asymmetric involvement of only one or 2 joints. Slightly more than 50% of these patients are young girls with antinuclear antibodies who are particularly likely to develop iridocyclitis.

2. Joint manifestations—Even in the presence of severe arthritis, young children may not complain of pain but may instead limit the use of an extremity. The knees, wrists, ankles, and neck are common sites of initial involvement. Early involvement of the hip is extremely rare in young children with pauciarticular disease. Older children occasionally develop symmetric involvement in the small joints of the hands (metacarpophalangeal, proximal interphalangeal, and distal interphalangeal) similar to that seen in adults. In seronegative patients, the metacarpophalangeal joints may be spared. With severe hand involvement, children are more likely to develop radial rather than ulnar deviation. Involvement of the feet may lead to hallux valgus or hammer toe deformity. Achillobursitis and achillotendinitis may cause tender, swollen heels. Older boys with pauciarticular disease commonly develop ankylosing spondylitis.

3. Systemic manifestations—Fever, often with a high evening spike, is characteristic of Still's disease. Anorexia, weight loss, and malaise are common. Most children with Still's disease develop an evanescent, salmon-colored maculopapular rash that coincides with periods of high fever. Occasional patients manifest cardiac involvement. Pericarditis occurs commonly but rarely leads to dysfunction or constriction. Myocarditis is an unusual manifestation of the cardiac disease, but, when present, can lead to heart failure.

Cases of acute pneumonitis or pleuritis have been described, but chronic rheumatoid lung disease is rarely seen in patients with juvenile arthritis.

Iridocyclitis occurs most commonly in young girls with pauciarticular disease and can precede articular involvement. It often persists even when joint disease becomes quiescent. Iridocyclitis often runs an insidious course and is best monitored by frequent slit lamp examinations, at least through puberty.

Lymphadenopathy and hepatosplenomegaly are associated with severe systemic disease and are uncommon in patients with chiefly articular manifestations.

Subcutaneous nodules occur in children with polyarticular disease, usually in association with a positive test for rheumatoid factor.

Rarely, Still's disease occurs in adults. Characteristic manifestations include high spiking fevers, evanescent rash, arthritis, and elevated leukocyte count and hepatic enzyme levels.

4. Complications—The major complication of juvenile arthritis is impairment of growth and development secondary to early epiphyseal closure. This is particularly common in the mandible, causing micrognathia, and in the metacarpals and metatarsals, leading to abnormally small fingers and toes. The extent of growth impairment usually correlates positively with the severity and duration of disease but may also reflect the growth-inhibiting effects of steroids. Children in whom arthritis begins before age 9 occasionally undergo increased growth of an affected extremity. Vasculitis and encephalitis are occasionally observed in patients with juvenile arthritis. Secondary amyloidosis occurs rarely.

B. Laboratory Findings: Mild leukocytosis (15,000–20,000/μL) is the rule, but some patients develop leukopenia. A normochromic microcytic anemia, an elevated erythrocyte sedimentation rate, and an abnormal C-reactive protein occur commonly. Because an elevated ASO titer is so frequently encountered, this test cannot be used to differentiate juvenile arthritis from rheumatic fever. Positive tests for rheumatoid factor occur in older children with polyarticular disease, while antinuclear antibodies are found both in patients with polyarticular disease and in young patients with pauciarticular disease. ANA almost never occur in Still's disease. Serum protein electrophoresis shows an increase in acute-phase reactants (α-globulins) and a polyclonal increase of γ-globulin. The synovial fluid in active juvenile rheumatoid arthritis is exudative, with a leukocyte count of 5000–20,000/μL (mostly neutrophils), a poor mucin clot, and decreased glucose compared to serum glucose. Mononuclear cells may predominate in the synovial fluid of patients with pauciarticular disease.

C. X-Ray Findings: Radiographic changes early in the disease include juxta-articular demineralization, periosteal bone accretion, premature closure of the epiphyses, cervical zygapophyseal fusion (particularly at C2-3), osseous overgrowth of the interphalangeal joints, and erosion and narrowing of the joint space. Carpal arthritis with ankylosis is seen as a late manifestation of Still's disease.

Immunologic Diagnosis

Currently, the diagnosis of juvenile arthritis is based on clinical criteria. Although certain abnormalities of immunoglobulins, complement, and cellular immunity are compatible with the diagnosis of juvenile arthritis, no specific immunologic test is diagnostic.

Differential Diagnosis

The diagnosis of juvenile arthritis is extremely difficult, since the disease can present with non-specific constitutional signs and symptoms in the absence of arthritis. Other causes of fever, particularly infections and cancer, must be considered. Leukemia can present in childhood with fever, lymphadenopathy, and joint pains. Rheumatic fever closely resembles juvenile arthritis, particularly early in the disease, but the patient with juvenile arthritis tends to have higher spiking fevers, lymphadenopathy and hepatosplenomegaly in the absence of carditis, and a more refractory, long-lasting arthritis. Rheumatic fever patients are more likely to have evidence of recent streptococcal infection, including elevated titers of antihyaluronidase, antistreptokinase, and antistreptodornase antibodies. In addition, patients with rheumatic fever tend to have a less intense leukocytosis and respond more dramatically to low doses of salicylates. An expanding skin lesion followed in weeks or months by arthritis suggests the diagnosis of Lyme disease, an inflammatory arthropathy caused by the spirochete *Borrelia burgdorferi*. Rheumatic diseases that may begin in childhood, such as SLE or dermatomyositis, can be differentiated by their different clinical course, different organ system involvement, and characteristic serologic abnormalities.

When juvenile arthritis presents primarily with arthritis, examination of synovial fluid is of paramount importance in excluding infection.

Treatment

The major goals of therapy are to relieve pain, prevent contractures and deformities, and promote normal physical and emotional development. These goals are best achieved by a comprehensive program of physical, medical, and, when necessary, surgical therapy.

A. Physical Therapy: As in the treatment of adult rheumatoid arthritis, rest is an important part of physical therapy. Complete rest is indicated during exacerbations and may be necessary for short afternoon periods on a routine basis. Specific joints can be put at rest by the use of splints, collars, and braces that support the joint and help prevent deformity. Judicious use of heat will decrease pain and muscle spasm and is particularly useful before exercising. Exercise promotes muscle strength, encourages growth, and prevents deformity.

B. Drug Treatment:

1. Salicylates—The disease responds to aspirin at a dosage level of 90–130 mg/kg/d given in 4–6 divided doses. Tinnitus and decreased hearing are poor indicators of aspirin toxicity in children. Irritability, drowsiness, or intermittent periods of hyperpnea are early signs of salicylate intoxication. Therefore, it is essential to monitor blood salicylate levels during aspirin therapy. Acidosis and ketosis may develop in infants. Respiratory alkalosis, due to primary stimulation of the respiratory center, occurs in older children.

2. Remittive agents—Children with refractory arthritis may benefit from injectable or oral gold, antimalarials, penicillamine, or methotrexate.

3. Corticosteroids—Intra-articular corticosteroid injections are useful in pauciarticular disease. Systemic corticosteroids are reserved for patients with myocarditis, vasculitis, refractory iridocyclitis, or Still's disease that is unresponsive to aspirin therapy. Patients with iridocyclitis may require prolonged corticosteroid therapy. In children, the major toxic effects of corticosteroid therapy include subcapsular cataract formation, vertebral osteoporosis and collapse, infection, premature skeletal maturation with diminished growth, and pseudotumor cerebri with intracranial hypertension.

C. Surgical Treatment: The aims of surgery in juvenile arthritis are to relieve pain and maintain or improve joint function. Synovectomy may diminish pain due to chronic synovitis, but long-term effectiveness is questionable. Synovectomy for severe extensor tenosynovitis of the hand may prevent tendon rupture. Tendon release procedures help relieve joint contractures. Hip replacement is of benefit in selected cases but should be delayed as long as possible, since in some children hip cartilage may regenerate with continued weight bearing.

Complications & Prognosis

Seventy percent of patients experience a spontaneous and permanent remission by adulthood. Patients with Still's disease tend to have several recurrences per year. Patients presenting with oligoarthritic disease, particularly if they are female, tend to remain oligoarthritic, while those presenting with polyarthritis remain polyarthritic. Rarely, the disease persists into adulthood. This usually occurs in children with symmetric polyarthritis similar to that seen in adults. Sometimes a patient with juvenile arthritis in apparent remission develops rheumatoid arthritis as an adult. In an occasional unfortunate case, the disease is relentless and crippling. Small-joint involvement, positive serum rheumatoid factor, and onset in later childhood all portend a poor prognosis.

SJÖGREN'S SYNDROME

Major Immunologic Features

- Lymphocytes and plasma cells infiltrate involved tissues.
- There is hypergammaglobulinemia, rheumatoid factor, and antinuclear antibodies, including specific acid-extractable nuclear antigens.
- There are autoantibodies against salivary duct antigens.

General Considerations

Sjögren's syndrome is a chronic inflammatory disease of unknown cause characterized by diminished lacrimal and salivary gland secretion resulting in keratoconjunctivitis sicca and xerostomia. There is dryness of the eyes, mouth, nose, trachea, bronchi, vagina, and skin. In half of patients, the disease occurs as a primary pathologic entity (primary Sjögren's syndrome). In the other half, it occurs in association with rheumatoid arthritis or other connective tissue disorders. Ninety percent of patients with Sjögren's syndrome are female. Although the mean age at onset is 50 years, the disease does occur in children.

Immunologic Pathogenesis

It has been hypothesized that patients with Sjögren's syndrome have an abnormal immunologic response to one or more unidentified antigens, perhaps viral antigens or virus-altered autoantigens. This ab-

normal response is characterized by excessive B cell and plasma cell activity, manifested by polyclonal hypergammaglobulinemia and the production of rheumatoid factor, antinuclear factors, cryoglobulins, and anti-salivary duct antibodies. Immunofluorescence studies have shown both B and T helper lymphocytes and plasma cells infiltrating involved tissues. Large quantities of IgM and IgG are synthesized by these infiltrating lymphocytes. In patients with coexisting macroglobulinemia, monoclonal IgM may be synthesized in the salivary glands. Excessive B cell activity could be due either to a primary B cell defect or to defective T lymphocyte regulation, since there is evidence of decreased suppressor T cell function in patients with Sjögren's syndrome.

Pathology

Histologically, there is lymphocytic infiltrate in exocrine glands of the respiratory, gastrointestinal, and vaginal tracts as well as glands of the ocular and oral mucosa. Histologic demonstration of lymphocytic infiltration in a biopsy specimen taken from the minor labial salivary glands is the most specific and sensitive single diagnostic test for Sjögren's syndrome.

Clinical Features

A. Symptoms and Signs:

1. Oral—Dryness of the mouth is usually the most distressing symptom and is often associated with burning discomfort and difficulty in chewing and swallowing dry foods. Polyuria and nocturia develop as the patient drinks increasing amounts of water in an effort to relieve these symptoms. The oral mucous membranes are dry and erythematous, and the tongue becomes fissured and ulcerated. Severe dental caries is often present. Half of patients have intermittent parotid gland enlargement with rapid fluctuations in the size of the gland. The parotid gland in Sjögren's syndrome is firm in contrast to the soft parotid enlargement characteristic of diabetes mellitus or alcohol abuse. Oral candidiasis can be a complication of Sjögren's syndrome.

2. Ocular—The major ocular finding is keratoconjunctivitis sicca. Symptoms include burning, itching, decreased tearing, ocular accumulation of thick mucoid material during the night, photophobia, pain, and a "gritty" or "sandy" sensation in the eyes. Decreased tearing is demonstrated by an abnormal Schirmer test. Slit lamp examination reveals punctate rose bengal or fluorescein staining of the conjunctiva and cornea, strands of corneal debris, and a shortened tear film break-up time. Severe ocular involvement may lead to corneal ulceration, vascularization with opacification, or perforation.

3. Miscellaneous—Dryness of the nose, posterior oropharynx, larynx, and respiratory tract may lead to epistaxis, dysphonia, recurrent otitis media, tracheobronchitis, or pneumonia. The vaginal mucosa is also dry, and women with the disease commonly complain of dyspareunia. Active synovitis is a common finding, particularly in patients who also have rheumatoid arthritis. Twenty percent of patients with primary Sjögren's syndrome complain of Raynaud's phenomenon. Ten percent of patients have extraglandular lymphocytic infiltrates, particularly in the kidneys, lungs, lymph nodes, and muscles. A few such patients develop lymphoma.

B. Laboratory Findings: Anemia, leukopenia, and an elevated erythrocyte sedimentation rate are common features. Parotid salivary flow is less than the normal 5 mL/10 min/gland. Secretory sialography with radiopaque dye demonstrates glandular disorganization. Salivary scintigraphy with Tc99m pertechnetate reveals decreased parotid secretory function.

Immunologic Diagnosis

No immunologic test is diagnostic for Sjögren's syndrome. However, a myriad of nonspecific immunologic abnormalities occur in these patients.

A. Humoral Abnormalities: Hypergammaglobulinemia is seen in half of patients. Although serum protein electrophoresis usually shows a polyclonal hypergammaglobulinemia, occasional patients develop a monoclonal IgM paraproteinemia, usually of the kappa type. Patients who develop lymphoma sometimes become severely hypogammaglobulinemic and show disappearance of autoantibodies. Rheumatoid factors can be detected by the latex fixation test in 90% of patients with Sjögren's syndrome. ANA in a speckled or homogeneous pattern is present in 70% of patients. Many of these antinuclear antibodies are directed against acid-extractable nuclear antigens. Antibodies against one such antigen, termed SS-B, are relatively specific for patients with primary Sjögren's syndrome. Antibodies against a second acid-extractable nuclear antigen, SS-A, may be found in Sjögren's syndrome alone or in Sjögren's syndrome associated with SLE. Patients with Sjögren's syndrome and rheumatoid arthritis have neither anti-SS-A nor anti-SS-B antibodies. Autoantibodies against salivary duct antigens have been detected in 50% of patients with Sjögren's syndrome associated with rheumatoid arthritis.

B. Cellular Abnormalities: Thirty percent of patients with Sjögren's syndrome have decreased lymphocyte responses to mitogenic stimulation. A few patients also have decreased numbers of circulating T lymphocytes in the peripheral blood (see Immunologic Pathogenesis, above).

C. HLA Associations: HLA typing studies suggest a genetic predisposition to the development of Sjögren's syndrome. The prevalence of both HLA-DR3 and HLA-B8 is increased in patients with primary Sjögren's syndrome and Sjögren's syndrome with SLE.

Differential Diagnosis

The diagnosis of Sjögren's syndrome can be made on the basis of 2 of the 3 classic manifestations of xerostomia, keratoconjunctivitis sicca, and rheumatoid arthritis. However, the varied and multisystemic nature of the disease may obscure the diagnosis. Any patient with a rheumatic disease—eg, SLE, rheumatoid arthritis, or scleroderma—should be observed for Sjögren's syndrome; likewise, any patient with Sjögren's syndrome should be examined for the purpose of ruling out other rheumatic diseases. Other causes of bilateral parotid swelling include nutritional deficiencies, endocrine disorders, sarcoidosis, drug reactions, infections, amyloid and obesity. Parotid gland cancer must always be considered in a patient with unilateral parotid swelling.

Treatment

A. Symptomatic Measures:

1. Oral—Patients must be urged to maintain fastidious oral hygiene, with regular use of fluoride toothpaste, mouthwashes, and regular dental examinations. Frequent sips of water and the use of sugarless gum or candy to stimulate salivary secretion are sometimes helpful in relieving xerostomia. Many patients find aerosolized preparations of artificial saliva helpful. A bedroom humidifier will help decrease nocturnal xerostomia and nasal dryness.

2. Ocular—Artificial tears alleviate ocular symptoms and protect against ocular complications. Shielded glasses offer protection against the drying effects of wind. Therapy for refractory ocular complications includes mucolytic agents, punctal occlusion, soft contact lenses, and partial tarsorrhaphy.

B. Systemic Measures: Sjögren's syndrome can usually be controlled with symptomatic therapy. Nonsteroidal anti-inflammatory drugs are useful in the treatment of the nonerosive arthritis of Sjögren's syndrome. Corticosteroids or immunosuppressive agents may be useful in treating patients with severe or life-threatening disease, such as lymphoma, Waldenström's macroglobulinemia, or massive lymphocytic infiltration of vital organs.

Complications & Prognosis

In the vast majority of patients, significant lymphoproliferation is confined to salivary, lacrimal, and other mucosal glandular tissue, resulting in a benign chronic course of xerostomia and xerophthalmia. Rarely, patients develop significant extraglandular lymphoid infiltration or neoplasia.

Splenomegaly, leukopenia, and vasculitis with leg ulcers may occur. Hypergammaglobulinemic purpura, often associated with renal tubular acidosis, has been described and may be a presenting complaint. Five percent of patients with Sjögren's syndrome develop chronic autoimmune thyroiditis. Other associations include primary biliary cirrhosis, chronic active hepatitis, gastric achlorhydria, pancreatitis, renal and pulmonary lymphocytic infiltration, cryoglobulinemia with glomerulonephritis, hyperviscosity syndrome, and adult celiac disease. Neuromuscular complications include polymyositis, peripheral or cranial (particularly trigeminal) neuropathy, and cerebral vasculitis. Rarely, patients with Sjögren's syndrome develop lymphoid cancer, immunoblastic sarcoma, or Waldenström's macroglobulinemia. The lymphoma is often a monoclonal B cell neoplasm containing intracellular IgM-κ immunoglobulin.

PROGRESSIVE SYSTEMIC SCLEROSIS

Major Immunologic Features

- Antinuclear antibodies with a speckled or nucleolar pattern occur.
- Anticentromere antibodies occur in patients with CREST syndrome.
- Antibodies against an acid-extractable nuclear antigen occur.

General Considerations

Progressive systemic sclerosis is a disease of unknown cause characterized by abnormally increased collagen deposition in the skin. The course is usually slowly progressive and chronically disabling, but it can be rapidly progressive and fatal because of involvement of internal organs. It commonly begins in the third or fourth decade of life. Children are occasionally affected. The prevalence of the disease is 4–12.5 cases per million population. Women are affected twice as often as men, and there is no racial predisposition.

Immunologic Pathogenesis

The association of progressive systemic sclerosis with Sjögren's syndrome and, less often, with thyroiditis or primary biliary cirrhosis—and the serologic abnormalities seen in the majority of cases (presence of ANA, rheumatoid factor, polyclonal hypergammaglobulinemia)—are suggestive of an immunologic aberration in these patients. At present, there is scanty evidence for a humoral mechanism in the pathogenesis of the disease, although a serum factor toxic to vascular endothelium has been identified. Humoral factors may stimulate increased collagen production by fibroblasts. Immunoglobulins have not been found at the dermal-epidermal junction in scleroderma, although examination of the fibrinoid lesions seen in the walls of renal arterioles has revealed the presence of immunoglobulins and complement. The ability of lymphocytes to destroy embryonic fibroblasts in tissue cultures may indicate an alteration in cellular immunity in these patients. However, in contrast to other autoimmune diseases,

cellular infiltration in scleroderma is minimal or absent in all organs except the synovium, where impressive collections of lymphocytes and plasma cells can be seen. Unfortunately, research on the pathogenesis of progressive systemic sclerosis is severely hampered by the absence of an animal model.

Pathology

Biopsy of clinically involved skin reveals thinning of the epidermis with loss of the rete pegs, atrophy of the dermal appendages, hyalinization and fibrosis of arterioles, and a striking increase of compact collagen fibers in the reticular dermis.

Synovial findings range from an acute inflammatory lymphocytic infiltration to diffuse fibrosis with relatively little inflammation.

The histologic changes seen in muscles include interstitial and perivascular inflammatory infiltration followed by fibrosis and myofibrillar necrosis, atrophy, and degeneration.

In patients with renal involvement, the histologic appearance of the kidney is similar to that of malignant hypertensive nephropathy, with intimal proliferation of the interlobular arteries and fibrinoid changes in the intima and media of more distal interlobular arteries and of afferent arterioles.

There is increased collagen deposition in the lamina propria, submucosa, and muscularis of the gastrointestinal tract. Small-vessel changes similar to those that occur in the skin may also result. With loss of normal smooth muscle, the large bowel is subject to development of the characteristic widemouthed diverticula and to infiltration of air into the wall of the intestine (pneumatosis cystoides intestinalis).

Clinical Features

A. Symptoms and Signs:

1. Onset—Frequently Raynaud's phenomenon heralds the onset of the disease; it occurs in at least 90% of patients. Progressive systemic sclerosis frequently begins with skin changes, but in one-third of patients polyarthralgias and polyarthritis are the first manifestations. Skin involvement may be limited to the hands, forearms, feet, or face or may be more diffuse with extensive truncal involvement. Initial visceral involvement without skin manifestations is very unusual. In the so-called CREST syndrome—*c*alcinosis, *R*aynaud's phenomenon, *e*sophagal dysmotility, *s*clerodactyly, and *t*elangiectases—the disease may remain stable for many years.

2. Skin abnormalities—There are 3 stages in the clinical evolution of scleroderma. In the edematous phase, symmetric nonpitting edema is present in the hands and, rarely, in the feet. The edema can progress to the forearms, arms, upper anterior chest, abdomen, back, and face. In the sclerotic phase, the skin is tight, smooth, and waxy and seems bound down to underlying structures. Skin folds and wrinkles disappear. The hands are involved in most patients, with painful, slowly healing ulcerations of the fingertips in half of those cases. The face appears stretched and masklike, with thin lips and a "pinched" nose. Pigmentary changes and telangiectases are frequent at this stage. The skin changes may stabilize for prolonged periods and then either progress to the third (atrophic) stage or soften and return to normal. It should be emphasized that not all patients pass through all the stages. Subcutaneous calcifications, usually in the fingertips (calcinosis circumscripta), occur more often in women than in men. The calcifications vary in size from tiny deposits to large masses and may develop over bony prominences throughout the body.

3. Joints and muscles—Articular complaints are very common and may begin at any time during the course of the disease. The arthralgias, stiffness, and frank arthritis seen in progressive systemic sclerosis may be difficult to distinguish from those of rheumatoid arthritis, particularly in the early stages of the disease. Involved joints include the metacarpophalangeals, proximal interphalangeals, wrists, elbows, knees, ankles, and small joints of the feet. Flexion contractures caused by changes in the skin or joints are common. Muscle involvement is usually mild but may be clinically indistinguishable from that of polymyositis, with muscle weakness, tenderness, and pain of proximal muscles of the upper and lower extremities.

4. Lungs—The lungs are frequently involved in progressive systemic sclerosis, either clinically or at autopsy. A low diffusion capacity is the earliest detectable abnormality, preceding alterations in ventilation or clinical and radiologic evidence of disease. Dyspnea on exertion is the most frequently reported symptom. Orthopnea, paroxysmal nocturnal dyspnea, chronic cough, hemoptysis, chest pain, and hoarseness are also manifestations of pulmonary involvement. Pleurisy (with associated pleural friction rub) can also occur. Pulmonary fibrosis may occur early in the disease in patients with diffuse truncal involvement but occurs later in disease, often in association with pulmonary hypertension, in patients with CREST syndrome. Patients with diffuse pulmonary involvement have intimal proliferation of small and medium-sized pulmonary arteries and arterioles and may have an intense bronchiolar epithelial proliferation.

5. Heart—Because of the frequency of pulmonary fibrosis, cor pulmonale is the commonest cardiac finding. Myocardial fibrosis, leading to digitalis-resistant left-sided heart failure, carries a poor prognosis. Cardiac arrhythmias and conduction disturbances are common manifestations of myocardial fibrosis. Pericarditis is usually asymptomatic and is found incidentally at autopsy. Although 40% of patients have pericardial effusion by electrocardiography, tamponade is extremely rare.

6. Kidneys—Renal involvement is an uncommon but life-threatening development in patients with diffuse disease. Although renal insufficiency may follow an indolent course, it frequently presents as rapidly progressive oliguric renal failure with or without malignant hypertension.

7. Gastrointestinal tract—The gastrointestinal tract is commonly affected. The esophagus is the most frequent site of involvement, with dysphagia or symptoms of reflux esophagitis occurring in 80% of patients. Gastric and small bowel involvement presents with cramping, bloating, and diarrhea alternating with constipation. Hypomotility of the gastrointestinal tract with bacterial overgrowth may result in malabsorption. Colonic scleroderma is associated with chronic constipation.

8. Sjögren's syndrome—Sicca syndrome is seen in 5–7% of patients.

9. Uncommon clinical manifestations—Biliary cirrhosis or mononeuropathy, either cranial or peripheral, may rarely be associated with progressive systemic sclerosis.

10. Mixed connective tissue disease—Mixed connective tissue disease is a syndrome with features of scleroderma, rheumatoid arthritis, SLE, and polymyositis-dermatomyositis. The manifestations of the disease include arthritis, Raynaud's phenomenon, scleroderma of the fingers, muscle weakness and tenderness, interstitial lung disease, and a skin rash resembling either dermatomyositis or SLE. These patients have a high-titer speckled pattern of ANA and antibody to the ribonuclease-sensitive component of extractable nuclear antigen (eg, RNP). Renal disease is unusual in these patients. The disease appears to respond to moderate doses of corticosteroids.

B. Laboratory Findings: The normochromic normocytic anemia of chronic inflammatory disease is occasionally seen in progressive systemic sclerosis. Microangiopathic anemia can also occur. An elevated erythrocyte sedimentation rate and polyclonal hypergammaglobulinemia are common. A positive speckled or nucleolar pattern ANA is frequently encountered.

C. X-Ray Findings:

1. Bones—Thickening of the periarticular soft tissues and juxta-articular osteoporosis are seen in involved joints. Absorption of the terminal phalanges is often associated with soft tissue atrophy and subcutaneous calcinosis.

2. Chest—Characteristically, a diffuse increase in interstitial markings is seen in the lower lung fields of patients with moderate to severe pulmonary involvement. "Honeycombing," nodular densities, and disseminated pulmonary calcifications may also be seen.

3. Gastrointestinal tract—Upper gastrointestinal series often reveal decreased or absent esophageal peristaltic activity, even in patients without symptoms of dysphagia. Long-standing disease leads to marked dilation of the lower two-thirds of the esophagus. Gastrointestinal reflux is present in the majority of cases, and ulcers or strictures of the lower esophagus due to peptic esophagitis are commonplace. With gastrointestinal involvement, barium is often retained in the second and third portions of the duodenum. Intestinal loops become dilated and atonic, with irregular flocculation and hypersegmentation.

The barium enema may reveal large, wide-mouthed diverticula along the antimesenteric border of the colon.

4. Renal arteriography—Marked changes are seen on renal arteriography in patients with scleroderma kidney. Irregular arterial narrowing, tortuosity of the interlobular arterioles, persistence of the arterial phase, and absence of a nephrogram phase are typical findings.

Immunologic Diagnosis

Polyclonal hypergammaglobulinemia is a frequent serologic abnormality in progressive systemic sclerosis. The fluorescent ANA test shows a speckled or nucleolar pattern in 70% of cases. Thirty percent of patients with diffuse truncal involvement have antibodies against topoisomerase (anti-Scl-70 antibodies). Seventy-five percent of patients, particularly those with CREST syndrome, have anti-centromere antibodies.

Differential Diagnosis

When classic skin changes and Raynaud's phenomenon are associated with characteristic visceral complaints, the diagnosis is obvious. In patients presenting with visceral or arthritic complaints and no skin changes, the diagnosis is difficult. In many cases, only the presence or absence of antibodies to ribonuclease-sensitive extractable nuclear antigen (RNP) makes it possible to differentiate scleroderma from mixed connective tissue disease. Patients with eosinophilic fascitis present with marked thickening of the skin similar to that seen in the edematous phase of scleroderma. However, Raynaud's phenomenon and visceral involvement are rare in eosinophilic fascitis, and fibrosis and inflammatory cell infiltration are seen in the deep facial layers, whereas in scleroderma the fibrosis occurs predominantly in the dermis. The differential diagnosis also includes scleromyxedema, polyvinyl chloride toxicity, carcinoid syndrome, phenylketonuria, porphyria cutanea tarda, amyloidosis, Werner's syndrome, and progeria.

Treatment

There is at present no cure for progressive systemic sclerosis. Sympathectomy has resulted in only transient relief of vascular symptoms, but vasodilating agents, particularly calcium channel-blockers, have provided relief for patients with severe Raynaud's phenomenon. Corticosteroids have no effect on the visceral progression of the disease, though they are beneficial in scleroderma with myositis and in mixed connective tissue disease. Colchicine has limited efficacy in treatment of the cutaneous manifestations of the disease. Penicillamine is often effective in the treatment of cutaneous scleroderma, and evidence suggests that it may be of benefit in slowing the progression of visceral disease.

Patients should avoid exposure to cold and should wear gloves to protect their hands. Tobacco should be avoided. Skin ulcers require careful antiseptic care. Cor pulmonale and left-sided heart failure may be treated with diuretics and digitalization, although the response is often poor. Antibiotics may be beneficial in decreasing intestinal bacterial overgrowth that leads to malabsorption.

Hypertensive crisis in renal disease associated with progressive systemic sclerosis is very difficult to control even with potent hypotensive agents. Angiotensin-converting enzyme inhibitors may be of benefit in treating the renal disease associated with scleroderma. The arthritis can usually be controlled with aspirin and other fast-acting nonsteroidal anti-inflammatory drugs. Skin lubricants can alleviate dryness and cracking.

Complications & Prognosis

Spontaneous remissions occur, but the usual course of the disease is one of relentless progression from dermal to visceral involvement. Involvement of the heart, lungs, or kidneys is associated with a high mortality rate. Aspiration pneumonia resulting from esophageal dysfunction is a complication in advanced disease.

Although the prognosis for any given patient is extremely variable, the overall 5-year survival rate for progressive systemic sclerosis is approximately 40%.

POLYMYOSITIS-DERMATOMYOSITIS

Major Immunologic Features

- Cytotoxin is produced by lymphocytes incubated with autologous muscle.
- There is lymphocytic and plasma cell infiltration of involved muscle.
- Antibodies to the nuclear antigens Jo-1, PM-Scl, and RNP are present.

General Considerations

Polymyositis-dermatomyositis is an acute or chronic inflammatory disease of muscle and skin that may occur at any age. Women are affected twice as commonly as men. There is no racial preponderance. The incidence of the disease is one per 200,000 population.

Polymyositis-dermatomyositis can be subclassified into 5 categories: (1) idiopathic polymyositis, (2) idiopathic dermatomyositis, (3) polymyositis-dermatomyositis associated with cancer, (4) childhood polymyositis-dermatomyositis, and (5) polymyositis-dermatomyositis associated with other rheumatic diseases (Sjögren's syndrome, SLE, progressive systemic sclerosis, mixed connective tissue disease).

Immunologic Pathogenesis

Although the precise pathogenetic mechanisms are unknown, there is a great deal of evidence that autoimmunity may play a role in disease causation. Experimental polymyositis has been induced in rats and guinea pigs by the injection of allogeneic muscle tissue in Freund's complete adjuvant. Polymyositis-dermatomyositis may coexist with other autoimmune diseases.

A. Humoral Factors: Polyclonal hypergammaglogulinemia is common in patients with polymyositis-dermatomyositis, and rheumatoid factors and antinuclear antibodies occur in 20% of cases. In children, focal deposits of complement, IgG, and IgM have been seen in vessel walls of involved skin and muscle. Some patients with polymyositis-dermatomyositis have been shown to produce antibodies both against a component of the extractable nuclear antigen and against purified human skeletal muscle myoglobin.

B. Cellular Factors: There is evidence that cellular immunity plays a role in the pathogenesis of polymyositis-dermatomyositis. Lymphocytes from patients with polymyositis-dermatomyositis, after incubation with normal autologous muscle, produce a lymphokine that is toxic to monolayers of human fetal muscle cells. The lymphocytes in the muscle infiltrate of patients with polymyositis-dermatomyositis produce this lymphotoxin upon simple incubation of involved muscle. Thus, the lymphocytes of patients with polymyositis-dermatomyositis may respond to their own muscle antigens as if they were foreign (Fig 36–3). It is not known whether this is a primary defect in antigen recognition by the lymphocytes or whether these muscle antigens are cross-reactive with an unidentified foreign antigen. Polymyositis has been induced in rats and guinea pigs by the transfer of sensitized lymphoid cells.

Pathology

Biopsy of involved muscles is diagnostic in only 50–80% of cases. Therefore, a normal muscle biopsy does not rule out the diagnosis of polymyositis-dermatomyositis in a patient with a characteristic clinical picture, muscle enzyme elevations, and an abnormal electromyogram. The histologic findings in acute and subacute polymyositis-dermatomyositis include (1) focal or extensive primary degeneration of muscle fibers, (2) signs of muscle regeneration (fiber basophilia, central nuclei), (3) necrosis of muscle fibers, and (4) a focal or diffuse lymphocytic infiltration. Chronic myositis leads to a marked variation in the cross-sectional diameter of muscle fibers and a variable degree of interstitial fibrosis.

Clinical Features

A. Symptoms and Signs:

1. Onset—Although the symptoms may begin abruptly, the onset of the disease is usually insidious.

2. Muscle involvement—The commonest manifestation is weakness of involved striated muscle. The proximal muscles of the extremities are most often affected, usually progressing from the lower to the upper limbs. The distal musculature is involved in only 25% of patients. Weakness of the cervical muscles with inability to raise the head and weakness of the posterior pharyngeal muscles with dysphagia and dysphonia are also seen. Facial and extraocular muscle involvement is unusual. Muscle pain, tenderness, and edema also occur.

3. Skin involvement—The characteristic rash of dermatomyositis, present in approximately 40% of patients, consists of raised, smooth or scaling, dusky red plaques over bony prominences of the hands, elbows, knees, and ankles. An erythematous telangiectatic rash may appear over the face and sun-exposed areas. Less commonly seen is the pathognomonic "heliotrope" rash of the face (a dusky, lilac suffusion of the upper eyelids). One-fourth of pa-

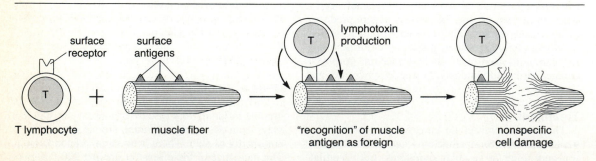

Figure 36–3. Defective "recognition" in polymyositis.

tients have various dermatologic manifestations ranging from skin thickening to scaling eruptions to erythroderma.

4. Cancer—Some patients with polymyositis-dermatomyositis are found to have a concomitant malignant tumor. In patients older than 40 years of age, the association between polymyositis-dermatomyositis and cancer appears to be more common. Removal of the tumor may result in a dramatic improvement in the polymyositis-dermatomyositis.

5. Miscellaneous features—A mild transitory arthritis is not unusual. Sjögren's syndrome occurs in 5–7% of cases. In children, vasculitis may result in gastrointestinal ulceration with abdominal pain, hematemesis, and melena. Patients with severe muscle disease are particularly susceptible to the development of interstitial pneumonia and pulmonary fibrosis. Raynaud's phenomenon occurs occasionally.

B. Laboratory Findings: An elevated erythrocyte sedimentation rate and a mild anemia are very common. Half of patients have elevated α_2- and γ-globulins on serum protein electrophoresis. Myoglobinemia and myoglobinuria are often seen. Up to 20% of patients with acute polymyositis have nonspecific T wave abnormalities on the ECG.

1. Muscle enzymes—When muscle cells are injured, a number of muscle enzymes, including glutamic-oxaloacetic transaminase, creatine phosphokinase, and aldolase, are released into the blood. The serum enzyme elevation reflects the severity of muscle damage as well as the amount of muscle mass involved.

2. Urinary creatine—Creatine is normally produced in the liver and transported via the circulatory system to the musculature. After attaching to receptor sites on the muscle cell surface, it is carried into the cell, where it is converted to creatinine. Polymyositis-dermatomyositis and other myopathies lead to a decrease in the number of cell surface receptors, causing an increase in circulating creatine that is quickly cleared by the kidneys. An increase in the urine creatine concentration is the most sensitive laboratory test for muscle damage and is a valuable indicator of disease activity. It is the first detectable laboratory abnormality in relapse of disease.

3. Electromyography—When involved muscles are examined, 70–80% of patients will demonstrate myopathic changes on electromyography. These changes are nonspecific but can point to the diagnosis of myositis. They include (1) spontaneous "sawtooth" fibrillatory potentials and irritability on insertion of the test needle; (2) complex polyphasic potentials, often of short duration and low amplitude; and (3) salvos of repetitive high-frequency action potentials (pseudomyotonia).

Immunologic Diagnosis

The diagnosis must be based on the nonimmunologic clinical and laboratory data discussed above.

However, antibodies to the nuclear antigen Jo-1 occur in a substantial number of patients with polymyositis, particularly those with pulmonary involvement. Antibodies to PM-Scl (a nucleolar antigen) are more common in patients with polymyositis and scleroderma. Anti-RNP antibodies occur most frequently in patients with myositis as a component of mixed connective tissue disease.

Differential Diagnosis

At least 3 of the following criteria must be present for a definite diagnosis of polymyositis: (1) weakness of the shoulder or pelvic girdle, (2) biopsy evidence of myositis, (3) elevation of muscle enzymes, and (4) electromyographic findings of myopathy. Typical skin changes must also be present for a definite diagnosis of dermatomyositis. A number of diseases can affect muscles and lead to clinical and laboratory abnormalities that are identical to those seen in polymyositis-dermatomyositis. The diagnostic criteria outlined above cannot be strictly applied in patients with infection, sarcoidosis, muscular dystrophy, SLE, progressive systemic sclerosis, mixed connective tissue disease, drug-induced myopathy (alcohol, clofibrate), rhabdomyolysis, and various metabolic and endocrine disorders (McArdle's syndrome, hyperthyroidism, myxedema, acid maltase deficiency, carnitine palmityl transferase deficiency, and AMP deaminase deficiency). A diligent search for occult cancers should be made in any patient who develops polymyositis-dermatomyositis as an adult.

Treatment

A. Corticosteroids: Prednisone, 60–80 mg orally daily, will usually decrease muscle inflammation and improve strength. The dose is tapered slowly, with clinical and laboratory monitoring. Creatinuria is the most sensitive index of disease activity and is often the first indication of relapse as corticosteroid dosage is reduced. However, assessment of muscle strength and determination of serum enzyme levels are usually sufficient indicators of disease activity. Some patients require chronic prednisone therapy (5–20 mg daily) to control the disease.

B. Cytotoxic Agents: Methotrexate and azathioprine have each been used with success in patients who do not respond to corticosteroids or who develop severe complications of corticosteroid therapy.

Complications & Prognosis

Polymyositis-dermatomyositis is a chronic disease characterized by spontaneous remissions and exacerbations. Most patients respond to corticosteroid therapy. Patients with severe muscle atrophy show little response to either corticosteroid or other immunosuppressive therapy. When the disease is associated with cancer, the prognosis depends on the response to tumor therapy.

BEHÇET'S DISEASE

Behçet's disease is a chronic recurrent inflammatory disease affecting adults of both sexes. The major manifestations of the disease are aphthous stomatitis, iritis, and genital ulcers. Other findings include vasculitis (particularly of the skin), arthritis, meningomyelitis, enterocolitis, erythema nodosum, thrombophlebitis, and epididymitis. The differential diagnosis includes viral (herpes simplex) or chlamydial (inclusion conjunctivitis, lymphogranuloma venereum) infections, Reiter's syndrome, inflammatory bowel disease, Stevens-Johnson syndrome, oral pemphigus, and SLE. A pustular lesion appearing after needle puncture of the skin is highly suggestive of Behçet's disease.

Genetic and environmental factors probably play a role in pathogenesis. Some studies show an increased prevalence of HLA-B5 and HLA-B51 in Behçet's disease. There is also evidence suggesting that a virus may play a role in disease causation. Antibodies against various human mucosal antigens have been detected, and indirect immunofluorescence has demonstrated vascular deposition of immunoglobulins as well as circulating anticytoplasmic antibodies. Recent studies have demonstrated a decrease in circulating helper T lymphocytes. Furthermore, lymphocytes and plasma cells are prominent in the perivascular infiltrate of Behçet's vasculitis. Amyloidosis may develop in these patients.

Local corticosteroids are useful in the treatment of mild ocular and oral disease. Systemic corticosteroids are helpful in the treatment of systemic manifestations, but chlorambucil is thought to be the most useful agent for treating ocular disease. Unproved remedies include whole-blood transfusions, transfer factor, levamisole, colchicine, cyclosporine, and thalidomide.

ANKYLOSING SPONDYLITIS

Ankylosing spondylitis is a chronic progressive inflammatory disorder involving the sacroiliac joints, spine, and large peripheral joints. Ninety percent of cases occur in males, with the usual age at onset being the second or third decade of life.

The disease begins with the insidious onset of low back pain and stiffness, usually worse in the morning. Symptoms of the acute disease include pain and tenderness in the sacroiliac joints and spasm of the paravertebral muscles. Findings in advanced disease include ankylosis of the sacroiliac joints and spine, with loss of lumbar lordosis, marked dorsocervical kyphosis, and decreased chest expansion. Peripheral arthritis, when present, usually involves the shoulder or hips. Twenty-five percent of patients also have iritis or iridocyclitis. Carditis with or without aortitis is seen in 10% of patients, with 1–4% progressing to insufficiency of the aortic valves. Rare complications include pericarditis and pulmonary fibrosis.

Patients with ankylosing spondylitis are seronegative for rheumatoid factor. Hypergammaglobulinemia and ANA are not seen in ankylosing spondylitis, but an elevated erythrocyte sedimentation rate and a mild anemia are common during active disease. Electrocardiographic abnormalities, such as atrioventricular block, left or right bundle branch block, and left ventricular hypertrophy reflect cardiac involvement. X-rays of the sacroiliac joints reveal osteoporosis and erosions early in the disease and sclerosis with fusion in advanced disease. Calcification of the anterior longitudinal ligament of the spine and squaring of the vertebrae are seen on lateral x-rays of the spine. Ossification of the outer margins of the intervertebral disk (syndesmophyte formation) may lead to fusion of the spine.

On pathologic examination, these patients have a chronic proliferative synovitis very similar to that of rheumatoid arthritis. The characteristic skeletal change in advanced disease is ossification of the sacroiliac joints and interspinous and capsular ligaments. Pathologic cardiac findings include focal inflammation and fibrous thickening of the aortic wall and the base of the valve cusps.

The physical findings in patients with severe osteoarthritis of the spine may resemble those of patients with end-stage ankylosing spondylitis. However, degenerative osteoarthritis begins much later in life, does not extensively involve the sacroiliac joints, and is characterized radiographically by osteophytes rather than syndesmophytes. The differentiation of ankylosing spondylitis from other diseases associated with sacroiliitis and spondylitis, such as psoriatic arthritis, Reiter's syndrome, regional enteritis, and ulcerative colitis, depends upon the presence or absence of the clinical and radiologic characteristics of those diseases.

The basic pathogenesis of ankylosing spondylitis is unknown. Although the presence of mononuclear cells in acutely involved tissue and the histologic similarity of the synovitis to rheumatoid arthritis suggest a possible immunologic mechanism, there are no data to support autoimmune pathogenesis. There is a strong genetic predisposition to ankylosing spondylitis. Several members of the same family are often involved, and twin concordance for ankylosing spondylitis has been described. Furthermore, 90% of patients with ankylosing spondylitis have HLA-B27, compared with about 8% in the white US population. The gene that determines this specific cell surface antigen may be linked to other genes that determine pathologic autoimmune phenomena or that lead to an increased susceptibility to infectious or environmental agents. Alternatively, there may be molecular mimicry between the HLA-B27 epitope and an infectious agent, resulting in the production of a cross-reacting autoantibody. The recently described homology between an epitope of HLA-B27 and *Klebsiella pneumoniae* lends credence to this concept.

The treatment of ankylosing spondylitis consists of giving anti-inflammatory agents to decrease acute inflammation and relieve pain and of instituting physical therapy to maintain muscle strength and flexibility. Therapy is designed to maintain a position of function even if ossification and ankylosis progress. Posturing exercises (lying flat for periods during the day, sleeping without a pillow, breathing exercises), the judicious use of local heat, and job modification are all part of a rational physical therapy program. Total hip replacement may offer considerable relief to patients with ankylosis of the hips, although recurrent ankylosis is sometimes a problem.

REITER'S SYNDROME

Reiter's syndrome is clinically defined as a triad consisting of arthritis, urethritis, and conjunctivitis. However, the arthritis is frequently accompanied by only one of the other characteristic manifestations. Although Reiter's syndrome usually affects men, it may also occur in women and children. The arthritis is recurrent or chronic, migratory, asymmetric, and polyarticular, involving primarily joints of the lower extremity. Fever, malaise, and weight loss occur commonly with episodes of acute arthritis. The urethritis is of unknown cause and often asymptomatic. The conjunctivitis is mild, but 20–50% of patients develop iritis. Balanitis circinata, painless oral ulcerations, and keratoderma blennorrhagicum (thick keratotic lesions of the palms and soles) are mucocutaneous manifestations. Complications include spondylitis and carditis.

Most patients have a mild leukocytosis. The urethral discharge is purulent, and smear and culture are usually negative for *Neisseria gonorrhoeae*. Synovial fluid is sterile, with a leukocyte count of 2000–50,000/μL, mostly PMN. The classic radiographic finding is fluffy periosteal proliferation of the heels, ankles, metatarsals, phalanges, knees, and elbows. Bony erosions may be seen in severe cases but rarely, if ever, occur in upper extremities.

Major diseases in the differential diagnosis include gonococcal arthritis, psoriatic arthritis, ankylosing spondylitis, Lyme arthritis, and the arthritis of inflammatory bowel disease. Patients with psoriatic arthritis occasionally develop urethritis or conjunctivitis. The differentiation of psoriatic arthritis and Reiter's syndrome is difficult to make on the basis of the skin lesion, since keratoderma blennorrhagicum is histologically indistinguishable from pustular psoriasis. Reiter's syndrome can be differentiated from ankylosing spondylitis by the presence of the urethritis and conjunctivitis, the prominent involvement of distal joints, and the presence of asymmetric radiologic changes in the sacroiliac joints and spine.

In Reiter's syndrome, the arthritis is thought to be an immunologic response to infection elsewhere in the body. Predisposing infectious agents include shigellae, salmonellae, gonococci, mycoplasmas, chlamydiae, yersiniae, and *Campylobacter*. The manifestations of Reiter's syndrome appear to be more severe in AIDS. Eighty percent of patients with Reiter's syndrome have HLA-B27. It is not known whether this antigenic marker imparts an increased susceptibility to environmental or infectious agents or is associated with an unusual immune response gene.

Salicylates, indomethacin, or one of the newer nonsteroidal agents may be used to control acute inflammation. Immunosuppressive drugs, such as methotrexate or azathioprine, may be necessary in treatment of patients with recalcitrant disease. Although the acute attack usually subsides in a few months, recurrences are common and some patients develop a chronic deforming arthritis.

PSORIATIC ARTHRITIS

Psoriatic arthritis is a chronic, recurrent, asymmetric, erosive polyarthritis that occurs in 5–7% of patients with psoriasis. The onset of the arthritis may be acute or insidious and is usually preceded by skin disease. It characteristically involves the distal interphalangeal joints of the fingers and toes and may involve the hips, sacroiliac joints, and spine. Distal interphalangeal joint disease is frequently accompanied by nail pitting or onycholysis secondary to psoriasis of the nail matrix or nail bed. Constitutional signs and symptoms, such as fever and fatigue, may occur. Severe erosive disease may lead to marked deformity of the hands and feet (arthritis mutilans), and marked vertebral involvement can result in ankylosis of the spine.

An elevated erythrocyte sedimentation rate and a mild anemia are common. Hyperuricemia is occasionally seen in patients with severe skin disease. Serum immunoglobulin levels are normal, and rheumatoid factor is absent. Synovial fluid examination reveals a leukocyte count of 5000–40,000/μL, mostly PMN. Characteristic x-ray findings include "pencil cup" erosions, fluffy periosteal proliferation, and bony ankylosis of peripheral joints. Sacroiliac changes, including erosions, sclerosis, and ankylosis similar to that in Reiter's syndrome, occur in 10–30% of patients.

The major diseases that must be differentiated from psoriatic arthritis include rheumatoid arthritis, ankylosing spondylitis, and Reiter's syndrome. Psoriatic arthritis is differentiated from rheumatoid arthritis by the absence of rheumatoid factor and subcutaneous nodules, the involvement of distal interphalangeals, the characteristic x-ray findings of psoriatic arthritis, and the presence of psoriasis. The presence of the skin lesion, the involvement of distal interphalangeals, and differences in the radiologic appearance of the spine help differentiate psoriatic arthritis from ankylosing spondylitis. The differentiation of psoriatic arthritis from Reiter's syndrome is particularly difficult, since both diseases are associated with HLA-B27 and involve the sacroiliac joints and spine and since keratoderma blennorrhagicum is histologically indistinguishable from pustular psoriasis. A helpful clinical distinction is the greater likelihood of upper extremity involvement in psoriatic arthritis.

The cause of psoriasis and psoriatic arthritis is unknown. Genetic factors appear to play a role in disease causation. Psoriasis and rheumatic diseases are found in family members of approximately 15% of patients. Patients with psoriasis and peripheral arthritis have an increased prevalence of haplotypes HLA-DR4, A26, and Bw38. Forty-five percent of patients with spondylitis have HLA-B27. Other HLA antigens may be associated with peripheral psoriatic arthritis. The high prevalence of genetic markers might be associated with an increased susceptibility to unknown infectious or environmental agents or to primary abnormal autoimmune phenomena. However, no immunologic pathogenetic mechanism has yet been demonstrated.

Skin and arthritic manifestations require therapy. Topical corticosteroids, coal tar and ultraviolet light, or immunosuppressive drugs can be used to treat the skin disease. Treatment of arthritis is similar to that of rheumatoid arthritis.

RELAPSING POLYCHONDRITIS

Relapsing polychondritis is a rare disease characterized by recurrent episodes of inflammatory necrosis involving cartilaginous tissues of the ears, nose, upper respiratory tract, and peripheral joints. It often begins abruptly with swollen, painful, erythematous lesions of the nose or ears, usually associated with fever. Destruction of supporting cartilaginous tissues leaves patients with characteristic "floppy ear" and "saddle nose" deformities and can lead to collapse of the trachea. The commonest cause of death in these patients is airway obstruction. Recurrent episcleritis, anterior inflammatory ocular disease, auditory and vestibular defects, systemic vasculitis, necrotizing glomerulitis, vasculitis, and arthritis are other manifestations of relapsing polychondritis. Aortic insufficiency due to destruction and dilatation of the aortic valve ring occurs rarely.

Laboratory abnormalities include an elevated erythrocyte sedimentation rate, increased serum immunoglobulins, a false-positive VDRL, and mild anemia. Pathologic examination reveals infiltration of the cartilage-connective tissue interface with lymphocytes, plasma cells, and PMN. As the lesion evolves, the cartilage loses its basophilic stippling and stains more acidophilic. Eventually, the cartilage becomes completely replaced by fibrous tissue.

The pathogenesis of this disease is unknown. However, there is some evidence that autoimmune phenomena play a role. Immunofluorescence has revealed the presence of immune complexes at the fibrocartilaginous junction. Antibodies to human cartilage and to type II collagen are frequently present but also occur in other rheumatic diseases. Electron microscopy reveals electron-dense deposits of lysosomal origin in involved cartilage. In some patients with relapsing polychondritis, cartilage antigen will induce lymphocyte activation and lymphocyte production of migration inhibitory factor (MIF).

Corticosteroids, dapsone, colchicine, and nonsteroidal anti-inflammatory agents have been used with success in the treatment of relapsing polychondritis.

RELAPSING PANNICULITIS
(Weber-Christian Disease)

Relapsing panniculitis is a rare syndrome characterized by recurrent episodes of discrete nodular inflammation and nonsuppurative necrosis of subcutaneous fat. Most patients are women. Painful, erythematous nodules usually appear over the lower extremities but may involve the face, trunk, and upper limbs and progress to local atrophy and fibrosis. Occasionally, they may undergo necrosis, with the discharge of a fatty fluid. Constitutional signs, including fever, usually accompany an acute episode. Histologically, one sees edema, mononuclear cell infiltration, fat necrosis, perivascular inflammatory cuffing, and endothelial proliferation. The differential diagnosis includes superficial thrombophlebitis, polyarteritis nodosa, necrotizing vasculitis, erythema induratum, erythema nodosum, and factitious disease.

The cause of relapsing panniculitis is not known, and in fact the syndrome may be simply a nonspecific response to any one of a number of inciting factors, including trauma, cold, exposure to toxic chemicals, and infection. It has been seen in patients with SLE, rheumatoid arthritis, diabetes mellitus, sarcoidosis, tuberculosis, withdrawal from corticosteroid therapy, acute and chronic pancreatitis, and pancreatic carcinoma. An autoimmune mechanism is suggested by the presence of hypocomplementemia, circulating immune complexes, and the association of relapsing panniculitis with several autoimmune diseases. The only autoantibodies demonstrated to date are circulating leukoagglutinins.

Acute episodes respond to corticosteroid therapy. Prostaglandin inhibitors, antimalarial drugs, and immunosuppressive drugs have been used to treat severe disease.

HEREDITARY COMPLEMENT DEFICIENCIES & COLLAGEN VASCULAR DISEASES

Complement deficiency is seen in one in a million normal adults and is associated with various rheumatoid diseases. C2 deficiency is the most common hereditary complement deficiency (see Chapters 14 and 28).

Deficiencies of C1r, C1s, C2, C4, C5, C6, C7, C8, and C1 esterase have all been associated with lupuslike syndromes. Hereditary complement deficiency could lead to an increased susceptibility to infectious agents, which may then stimulate the autoimmunity. Lack of complement could impair clearance of immune complexes. Alternatively, a neighboring gene predisposing to autoimmune phenomena could be inherited along with the defective gene for complement production.

HYPOGAMMAGLOBULINEMIA & ARTHRITIS

Hypogammaglobulinemia is an acquired or congenital disorder that may involve all or any one of the specific classes of immunoglobulin (see Chapter 24). Hypogammaglobulinemia is associated with infections, chronic inflammatory bowel disease, sarcoidosis, SLE, scleroderma, Sjögren's syndrome, polymyositis-dermatomyositis, and cancer. Patients with classic adult and juvenile rheumatoid arthritis may develop hypogammaglobulinemia.

Hypogammaglobulinemia patients may develop a seronegative, symmetric arthritis, with morning stiffness, occasional nodule formation, and radiographic evidence of demineralization and joint space narrowing. Bony erosions are rarely seen. Biopsy of the synovium reveals chronic inflammatory changes without plasma cells. Despite the reduction of serum immunoglobulins, immunoglobulin may be detected in the inflammatory synovial fluid. Total hemolytic complement is commonly depressed in the synovial fluid, suggesting immune complex formation.

Hypogammaglobulinemia may increase susceptibility to infection by unidentified viruses that may induce the autoimmune phenomena (including arthritis) in these patients.

Hypogammaglobulinemic arthritis may improve after the administration of gamma globulin.

REFERENCES

Systemic Lupus Erythematosus

Arnett F et al: Systemic lupus erythematosus: Current state of the genetic hypothesis. *Semin Arthritis Rheum* 1984;**14**:24.

Balow JE et al: Lupus nephritis. *Ann Intern Med* 1987;**106**:79.

Budman D, Steinberg A: Hematologic aspects of systemic lupus erythematosus: Current comments. *Ann Intern Med* 1977;**86**:220.

Dubois EL: Antimalarials in the management of discoid and systemic lupus erythematosus. *Semin Arthritis Rheum* 1978;**8**:35.

Fritzler MJ: Antinuclear antibodies in the investigation of rheumatic diseases. *Bull Rheum Dis* 1985;**35(6)**:1.

Haupt H et al: The lung in systemic lupus erythematosus: Analysis of the pathologic changes in 120 patients. *Am J Med* 1981;**71**:791.

Hughes GRV, Harris NN, Gharavi AE: The anticardiolipin syndrome. *J Rheumatol* 1986;**13**:486.

Levin RE et al: A comparison of the sensitivity of the 1971 and 1982 American Rheumatism Association criteria for the classification of systemic lupus erythematosus. *Arthritis Rheum* 1984;**27**:530.

Mandell BF: Cardiovascular involvement in systemic lupus erythematosus. *Semin Arthritis Rheum* 1987;**17**:126.

McCluskey R: The value of renal biopsy in lupus nephritis. *Arthritis Rheum* 1982;**25**:867.

McCune WJ, Golbus J: Neuropsychiatric lupus. *Rheum Dis N Am* 1988;**14**:149.

Steinberg A et al: Systemic lupus erythematosus: Insights from animal models. *Ann Intern Med* 1984;**100**:714.

Tan EM et al: 1982 Revised criteria for the classification of systemic lupus erythematosus. *Arthritis Rheum* 1982;**25**:1271.

Urman JD, Rothfield NF: Corticosteroid treatment in systemic lupus erythematosus: Survival studies. *JAMA* 1977;**238**:2272.

Wilson J et al: Mode of inheritance of essential C3b receptors on erythrocytes of patients with systemic lupus erythematosus. *N Engl J Med* 1982;**307**:981.

Zwaifler N, Bluestein H: The pathogenesis of central nervous system manifestations of systemic lupus erythematosus. *Arthritis Rheum* 1982;**25**:862.

Rheumatoid Arthritis

Arnett FC et al: The American Rheumatism Association 1987 revised criteria for the classification of rheumatoid arthritis. *Arthritis Rheum* 1988;**31**:315.

Feigenbaum SL, Masi AT, Kaplan SB: Prognosis in rheumatoid arthritis: A longitudinal study of newly diagnosed younger adult patients. *Am J Med* 1979;**66**:377.

Hunder A, Bunch T: Treatment of rheumatoid arthritis. *Bull Rheum Dis* 1982;**32**:1.

Hurd ER: Extra-articular manifestations of rheumatoid arthritis. *Semin Arthritis Rheum* 1979;**8**:151.

Krane SM: Aspects of the cell biology of the rheumatoid synovial lesion. *Ann Rheum Dis* 1981;**40**:433.

Kremer JM, Lee JK: A long-term prospective study of the use of methotrexate in rheumatoid arthritis. *Arthritis Rheum* 1988;**31**:577.

Scott D et al: Systemic rheumatoid vasculitis: A clinical and laboratory study of 50 cases. *Medicine* 1981;**60**:288.

Stastny P: Association of the B-cell alloantigen DRw4 with rheumatoid arthritis. *N Engl J Med* 1978;**298**:869.

Zvaifler N: New perspectives on the pathogenesis of rheumatoid arthritis. *Am J Med* 1988;**85(Suppl 4A):**12.

Juvenile Arthritis

Cassidy J et al: A study of classification criteria for a diagnosis of juvenile rheumatoid arthritis. *Arthritis Rheum* 1986;**29**:274.

Fink C: Treatment of juvenile arthritis. *Bull Rheum Dis* 1982;**32**:21.

Howard JF, Sigsbee A, Glass DN: HLA genetics and inherited predisposition to JRA. *J Rheumatol* 1985;**12**:7.

Moore T, Weiss T: Immunologic studies in juvenile arthritis. *Bull Rheum Dis* 1982;**32**:25.

Schaller JG, Wedgwood RJ: Juvenile rheumatoid arthritis: A review. *Pediatrics* 1972;**50**:940.

Sjögren's Syndrome

Alexander E et al: Sjögren's syndrome: Association of anti-Ro (SSA) antibodies with vasculitis, hematologic abnormalities, and serologic hyperactivity. *Ann Intern Med* 1983;**98**:155.

Daniels T: Labial salivary gland biopsy in Sjögren's syndrome: Assessment as a diagnostic criterion in 362 suspected cases. *Arthritis Rheum* 1984;**27**:147.

Fox R et al: Primary Sjögren's syndrome: Clinical and immunopathologic features. *Semin Arthritis Rheum* 1984;**14**:77.

Fox R et al: Sjögren's syndrome. Proposed criteria for classification. *Arthritis Rheum* 1986;**29**:577.

Fye KH et al: Relationship of HLA-Dw3 and HLA-B8 to Sjögren's syndrome. *Arthritis Rheum* 1978;**21**:337.

Zulman J, Jaffe R, Talal N: Evidence that the malignant lymphoma of Sjögren's syndrome is a monoclonal B-cell neoplasm. *N Engl J Med* 1978;**299**:1215.

Progressive Systemic Sclerosis

Barnett A et al: A survival study of patients with scleroderma over 30 years (1953–1983): The value of a simple cutaneous classification in the early stages of disease. *J Rheumatol* 1988;**15**:276.

Nimelstein S et al: Mixed connective tissue disease: A subsequent evaluation of the original 25 patients. *Medicine* 1980;**59**:239.

Rocco V, Hurd E: Scleroderma and sclerodermalike disorders. *Semin Arthritis Rheum* 1986;**16**:22.

Rodnan GP: Progressive systemic sclerosis and penicillamine. *J Rheumatol* 1981;**8(Suppl 7):**116.

Rodnan GP: When is scleroderma not scleroderma? *Bull Rheum Dis* 1981;**31**:7.

Subcommittee for Scleroderma Criteria of the American Rheumatism Association Diagnostic and Therapeutic Criteria Committee: Preliminary criteria for the classification of systemic sclerosis (scleroderma). *Arthritis Rheum* 1980;**23**:581.

Polymyositis-Dermatomyositis

Benbasset J et al: Prognostic factors in polymyositis/dermatomyositis: A computer-assisted analysis of ninety-two cases. *Arthritis Rheum* 1985;**28**:249.

Bohan A, Peter JB: Polymyositis-dermatomyositis. (2 parts.) *N Engl J Med* 1975;**292**:344, 403.

Bunch TW: Prednisone and azathioprine for polymyositis: Long-term follow-up. *Arthritis Rheum* 1981;**24**:45.

Hochberg M et al: Adult onset polymyositis/dermatomyositis: An analysis of clinical and laboratory features and survival in 76 patients with a review of the literature. *Semin Arthritis Rheum* 1986;**15**:168.

Behçet's Disease

James D: "Silk route disease" (Behçet's disease). *West J Med* 1988;**148**:433.

O'Duffy J et al: Summary of the Third International Conference on Behçet's Disease. *J Rheum* 1983;**10**:154.

Shimizu T et al: Behçet's disease (Behçet syndrome). *Semin Arthritis Rheum* 1979;**8**:223.

Ankylosing Spondylitis

Ahearn J, Hochberg M: Epidemiology and genetics of ankylosing spondylitis. *J Rheumatol* 1988;**15**:22.

Calin A et al: Ankylosing spondylitis—an analytical review of 1500 patients: The changing pattern of disease. *J Rheumatol* 1988;**15**:1234.

Moll JMH et al: Associations between ankylosing spondylitis, psoriatic arthritis, Reiter's disease, the intestinal arthropathies, and Behçet's syndrome. *Medicine* 1974;**53**:343.

Reiter's Syndrome

Aho K et al: Reactive arthritis. *Clin Rheum Dis* 1985;**11**:25.

Calin A, Fries J: An "experimental" epidemic of Reiter's syndrome revisited: Follow-up evidence on genetic and environmental factors. *Ann Intern Med* 1976;**84**:564.

Fox R et al: The chronicity of symptoms and disability in Reiter's syndrome: An analysis of 131 consecutive patients. *Ann Intern Med* 1979;**9**:190.

Neuwelt C et al: Reiter's syndrome: A male and female disease. *J Rheum* 1982;**9**:268.

Wilkens RF et al: Reiter's syndrome: Evaluation of preliminary criteria for definite disease. *Arthritis Rheum* 1981;**24**:844.

Psoriatic Arthritis

Laurent M: Psoriatic arthritis. *Clin Rheum Dis* 1985;**11**:61.

Polychondritis

Ebringer R et al: Autoantibodies to cartilage and type II collagen in relapsing polychrondritis and other rheumatic diseases. *Ann Rheum Dis* 1981;**40**:473.

McAdam LP et al: Relapsing polychondritis: Prospective study of 23 patients and a review of the literature. *Medicine* 1976;**55**:193.

Panniculitis

Förström L, Winkelmann RK: Acute panniculitis as a clinical and histopathological study of 34 cases. *Arch Dermatol* 1977;**113**:909.

Panush R et al: Weber-Christian disease: Analysis of 15 cases and review of the literature. *Medicine* 1985; **64**:181.

Hereditary Complement Deficiency

Agnello V: Complement deficiency states. *Medicine* 1978;**57**:1.

Frank M: Complement in the pathophysiology of humm disease. *N Engl J Med* 1987;**316**:1525.

Moore T, Weiss T: Mediators of inflammation. *Semin Arthritis Rheum* 1985;**14**:247.

Hypogammaglobulinemia & Arthritis

Ammann AJ, Hong R: Selective IgA deficiency: Presentation of 30 cases and a review of the literature. *Medicine* 1971;**50**:223.

Grayzel AI et al: Chronic polyarthritis associated with hypogammaglobulinemia: A study of two patients. *Arthritis Rheum* 1977;**20**:887.

Webster ADB et al: Polyarthritis in adults with hypogammaglobulinemia and its rapid response to immunoglobulin treatment. *Br Med J* 1976;**1**:1314.

37

Endocrine Diseases

James R. Baker, Jr, MD

In the 30 years since the first demonstration of the immune basis for thyroiditis, autoimmune disease has been identified as a major cause of dysfunction of all endocrine organs. It is now apparent that such diverse disorders as idiopathic Addison's disease, type I diabetes mellitus, and the polyglandular endocrinopathy syndromes all have an autoimmune basis in common. Although primary therapy for these disorders remains the replacement of hormones depleted as a result of autoimmune destruction of endocrine organs, research is now being conducted into the genesis of the autoimmune process itself. It is hoped that through this research some treatment could be developed to abort the autoimmune process before the gland is destroyed, thereby allowing normal endocrine function to continue.

MECHANISM OF DEVELOPMENT OF AUTOIMMUNE ENDOCRINE DISEASE

Endocrine disease has become a favored model for the study of autoimmune pathogenesis. Two major factors in the development of human autoimmunity have been identified specifically through the study of endocrine disorders. The first is the discovery of aberrant expression of class II human leukocyte antigens (HLA) (see Chapter 4) on the surface of target cells in autoimmune disease (Fig 37–1). It is postu-

lated that autoimmunity begins with an inflammatory process, possibly of infectious origin, in an endocrine organ. The inflammatory cells in the gland produce gamma interferon and other cytokines, which induce the aberrant de novo expression of class II HLA molecules on endocrine cell membranes. After expression of class II major histocompatibility complex (MHC) molecules, endocrine cells may function as antigen-presenting cells for their own cellular proteins, which are recognized by autoreactive T and B cells. This leads to enzymatic and oxidative destruction of endocrine cells, which further releases cellular proteins for processing by antigen-presenting cells, propagating the autoimmune response. Either abnormalities in the presentation of antigen owing to allogenic specificities in class II MHC or inappropriate recognition of the class II HLA-antigen complex as a result of their inherited differences in the T cell antigen receptor structure can cause these autoantigens to be recognized as foreign.

Another possible mechanism of autoimmune endocrine disease involves anti-idiotypic antibodies (Fig 37–2). This is best illustrated by examining the potential relationship between these antibodies, hormones, and receptors. An antibody against a binding site on a hormone will have a conformational similarity to the receptor for the hormone. If an antibody is then generated against the binding site, or idiotype, of the first antibody, the second antibody will have a conformation structure similar to the hor-

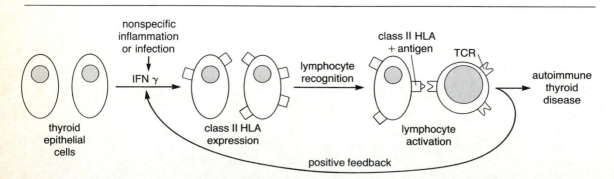

Figure 37–1. Initiation of autoimmunity through class II HLA expression. The expression of class II HLA results in lymphocyte activation, which causes the production of more lymphokines. These cause feedback stimulation of HLA expression and produce cytotoxic cells, which can destroy epithelial cells.

464

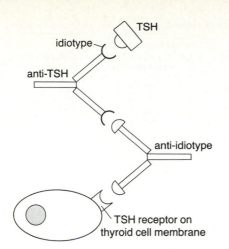

Figure 37–2. Anti-idiotype production of antireceptor antibodies. The antihormone antibody results in a second, anti-idiotypic antibody, which then recognizes the hormone receptor on the cell.

mone, thereby binding to the receptor. The finding of antibodies directed against insulin, thyroid-stimulating hormone (TSH), and other hormones in patients with autoimmune endocrine diseases suggests that anti-idiotype antibodies may play a role in the production of antibodies against the endocrine tissues.

ORGAN-SPECIFIC AUTOANTIBODIES

The presence of organ-specific autoantibodies is often utilized as an adjunct to the diagnosis and occasionally the management of some autoimmune disorders. Table 37–1, showing the relative sensitivity and specificity of autoantibodies in different diseases, should be referred to during study of this chapter.

One of the other hallmarks of autoimmune endocrine diseases is the presence of organ-specific autoantibodies in the sera of affected patients.

Organ-specific antibodies are defined by several methods, including their binding to tissue as determined by immunohistologic staining and the binding of specific proteins, lipids, carbohydrates, and hormones in immunoassays. In addition, autoantibody activity is defined by the inhibition of hormone binding to receptor or through physiologic alterations of organ and cells physiology in vitro. However, there are difficulties in the use of these autoantibodies in diagnosis and evaluation of autoimmune diseases. There are often inconsistencies in the way many of the bioassays are conducted, leading to variability in sensitivity of autoantibody results. Also, in immunoassays for antibodies to ill-defined antigens, differences in the antigen preparation can cause variable results.

Often, even well-characterized autoantibodies are not specific for an associated autoimmune disorder. This raises concern about the pathogenic role of the autoantibody in the autoimmune disorder. A good example of this is the presence of antithyroglobulin antibodies in healthy relatives of patients with autoimmune thyroid disease and in some healthy elderly individuals. In contrast, some antibodies found in only a small proportion of patients with autoimmune disease, such as insulin receptor antibodies, correlate well with disease activity in those patients (Table 37–1). Thus, it is always important to evaluate autoantibody findings in the context of the patient's clinical situation.

THYROID AUTOIMMUNE DISEASES

CHRONIC THYROIDITIS (Hashimoto's Disease)

Major Immunologic Features
- There is lymphocytic infiltration of the thyroid gland.
- Antibodies to thyroid antigens are present.
- There is cellular sensitization to thyroid antigens.

General Considerations
Hashimoto's thyroiditis is an inflammatory disorder of unknown etiology, which results in progressive destruction of the thyroid gland. It is found most commonly in middle-aged and elderly females, but it also occurs in other age groups, including children, in whom it may cause goiter. Although it is distributed throughout the world without racial or ethnic restriction, it occurs more commonly in families where another member has an autoimmune thyroid disease. It is observed in conjunction with Graves' disease in a form of autoimmune-overlap syndrome. In addition, it is associated with other autoimmune disorders such as systemic lupus erythematosus (SLE), chronic active hepatitis, dermatitis herpetiformis, and scleroderma. Although no formal mode of inheritance is recognized, there have been reported associations with several class II HLA antigens, including DR4 and DR5. However, these associations are not consistent among different ethnic populations.

Pathology
The hallmark of Hashimoto's thyroiditis is lymphocytic infiltration that almost completely replaces the normal glandular architecture of the thyroid (Fig 37–3). Plasma cells and macrophages abound, whereas scattered through this infiltrate are dying

Table 37–1. Specificity and sensitivity of autoantibodies.

Autoantigen/Autoantibody	Associated Autoimmune Disease	Percentage of Patients Having Autoantibody (Sensitivity)	Specificity for Disorder
Thyroid peroxidase (microsomal antigen)	Hashimoto's thyroiditis	80–95	High
	Graves' disease	50–80	Low
	Subacute thyroiditis	30–50	Moderate
	Idiopathic hypothyroidism	50–80	Moderate
Thyroglobulin	Hashimoto's thyroiditis	40–70	Moderate
	Graves' disease	20–40	Low
	Subacute thyroiditis	10–30	Moderate
	Idiopathic hypothyroidism	10–30	Low
Thyroid-stimulating immunoglobulin (TSI)	Graves' disease	50–90	High
	Hashimoto's thyroiditis	10–20	Low
	Idiopathic hypothyroidism	0–5	ND[1]
Thyroid growth-stimulating immunoglobulin (TGSI)	Graves' disease	20–50	Moderate
	Hashimoto's thyroiditis	0–5	ND
	Idiopathic hypothyroidism	0–5	ND
Thyrotropin binding-inhibitory immunoglobulin (TBII)	Graves' disease	50–80	High
	Hashimoto's thyroiditis	5–10	Low
	Idiopathic hypothyroidism	10–20	Moderate
Anti-islet cell antibodies	Type I diabetes mellitus	35–80	High
Anti-insulin antibodies	Type I diabetes mellitus	20–60	Low
	insulin resistance	0–2	High
Antibodies to insulin receptors	Type I diabetes mellitus	5–10	Low
	Type B insulin resistance	90–100	High
Antibodies to adrenal cortex	Addison's disease	30–60	High

[1]ND, not determined.

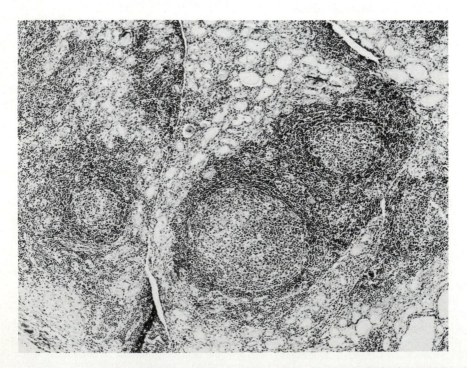

Figure 37–3. Pathology of Hashimoto's thyroiditis. Note the germinal centers and the lack of normal thyroid architecture. (Original magnification ×100.)

thyroid cells with acidophilic granules called Aske-nasze cells. Formations of germinal centers often give the impression that the thyroid gland is being converted into a lymph node. Lymphocytes infiltrating the thyroid are mainly B cells and CD4 T cells, although CD8 cytotoxic T cells have been cloned from Hashimoto's glands.

Clinical Features

Hashimoto's thyroiditis is primarily associated with symptoms of altered thyroid function. Early in the course of the disease the patient is usually euthyroid but may experience clinical hyperthyroidism due to the inflammatory breakdown of thyroid follicles with release of thyroid hormones. In contrast, late in the disease the patient is often hypothyroid because of progressive destruction of the thyroid gland. The most common eventual outcome of Hashimoto's disease is hypothyroidism.

A consistent physical sign seen in Hashimoto's disease is an enlarged thyroid gland. The goiter is often large and "rubbery" and may feel nodular, similar to its condition in other goitrous diseases. Often, lymph nodes surrounding the gland become enlarged. Rarely, patients will show symptoms of generalized vasculitis with urticaria and nephritis, and this has been associated with the presence of circulating immune complexes.

General laboratory findings are not helpful in making the diagnosis and relate primarily to the thyroid status of the patient. Patients with hyperthyroidism are differentiated from those with Graves' disease by the demonstration of patchy or decreased uptake on a radioiodine scan of the thyroid.

Immunologic Diagnosis

The hallmark of the diagnosis of Hashimoto's disease is the presence of circulating autoantibodies to thyroglobulin and thyroid microsomal antigen (now known to be the enzyme thyroid peroxidase). These antibodies were first detected by immunofluoresence (Fig 37–4), but they are now measured by tanned-

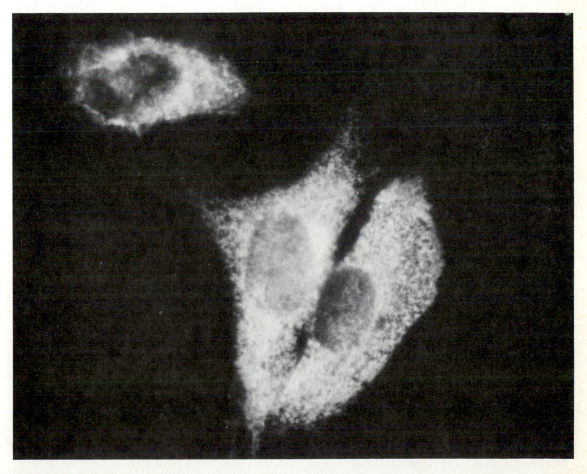

Figure 37–4. Immunofluorescent staining of a cultured human thyroid cell by antithyroglobulin antibodies showing the distribution of the antigen. (Original magnification × 400.) (Courtesy of Donald Sellitti.)

cell hemagglutination or ELISA (see Chapter 18). They are present in the serum of more than 90% of Hashimoto's disease patients, with antimicrosomal antibodies being more common and of higher titer than antithyroglobulin antibodies. In patients without serum antibodies, autoantibody production may be localized to the intrathyroidal lymphocytes and plasma cells.

Other thyroid antibodies are often present in Hashimoto's disease patients, including antibodies that displace TSH from its receptor or thyroid cells and others that stimulate thyroid cells to produce hormones. Other important thyroid antigens stimulate the production of autoantibodies, since multiple unidentified protein bands are recognized by Hashimoto's sera in Western blots of thyroid membranes. In addition, lymphocytes of these patients proliferate in response to thyroid antigens.

Differential Diagnosis

One must differentiate Hashimoto's disease from other forms of goiter. This is usually done by using clinical criteria with the help of antithyroid antibody titers. On occasion, the rapid enlargement of one lobe of the thyroid gland will be confused with thyroid cancer or thyroid lymphoma, which are observed with an increased incidence in Hashimoto's glands. In these cases, needle biopsy of the nodule may be helpful, whereas computed tomograms or magnetic resonance images of the neck can be used to evaluate cervical adenopathy.

Treatment

Treatment of Hashimoto's disease usually consists of thyroid hormone replacement for hypothyroidism. If the patient has a symptomatic goiter, doses of thyroid hormone that suppress TSH secretion can often decrease the size of the gland. Rarely, thyroidectomy will be necessary for an unusually large or painful gland.

Prognosis

While the prognosis of Hashimoto's disease is excellent, serial thyroid function tests, especially TSH levels, are necessary to monitor the requirement for thyroid hormone replacement.

TRANSIENT THYROIDITIS SYNDROMES

Major Immunologic Features

■ There is "giant cell" infiltration of the thyroid.
■ There is transient production of antithyroid antibodies.

General Considerations

Several heterogeneous, self-limited thyroiditis syndromes have been described that have in common a transient immune activity against the thyroid. The 2 most common are subacute (de Quervain's) thyroiditis and postpartum thyroiditis. Subacute thyroiditis is possibly caused by a viral infection of the thyroid gland. It has a seasonal and geographic distribution common to infections with mumps virus, coxsackie virus, and echo virus. Patients with this disorder usually have an acute phase of thyroiditis in which the gland may be painful and antithyroid antibodies may be present. At this time, patients are thyrotoxic, with an elevated serum T4 and decreased radioiodine uptake. Progressive euthyroid and hypothyroid periods of 4–8 weeks may follow before thyroid functions finally normalize.

Similar in clinical course, postpartum thyroiditis is a common disorder which usually presents within 3 months of delivery. Patients may be either hypo- or hyperthyroid, and a significant percentage of affected individuals develop chronic thyroid dysfunction. Of interest, patients who have this disorder often have recurrent courses with subsequent pregnancies.

Postpartum thyroiditis occurs in about 5–8% of pregnant women and, unlike subacute thyroiditis, is not thought to be related to a viral infection of the thyroid. Supporting this are the presence of antithyroid antibodies preceding the onset of clinical disease and an association with HLA-DR3 and -DR5 haplotypes.

Pathology

Although the lymphocytic infiltrate seen in subacute thyroiditis is similar to that in Hashimoto's disease, 2 findings in subacute thyroiditis are distinctive. First, giant cells with a small center of thyroid colloid can be seen (this is known as colloidophagy) and the follicular infiltration tends to progress to form granulomas. These findings are not seen in postpartum thyroiditis, however.

Clinical Features

Subacute thyroiditis and postpartum disease have in common the clinical presentation of rapidly enlarging thyroid gland with signs of thyroid dysfunction. Subacute thyroiditis has a much more acute course than postpartum disease and is more commonly associated with pain and tenderness in the area of the gland. Postpartum thyroiditis and other types of transient thyroiditis without pain or other symptoms are sometimes termed "silent" thyroiditis.

Subacute thyroiditis is also accompanied by an elevated erythrocyte sedimentation rate. Both syndromes can cause "low-uptake" toxicosis, in that they can produce elevated serum levels of thyroid hormones in the face of low to normal levels of radioactive iodine uptake.

Immunologic Diagnosis

Antibodies to thyroglobulin and thyroid microsomes (peroxidase enzyme) are present acutely in both syndromes; however, they tend to be transient and of low titer in subacute thyroiditis. Thyroid-stimulating antibodies have also been demonstrated in postpartum disease.

Treatment & Prognosis

In most cases thyroid function returns to normal within several months in both disorders. Patients with subacute thyroiditis who have especially painful glands may be treated with anti-inflammatory drugs. Postpartum patients who are clinically hypothyroid can benefit from thyroid hormone replacement. There is some evidence that the persistence of antithyroid antibodies identifies patients who will have protracted hypo- or hyperthyroidism. This finding offers a means for monitoring patients for eventual therapy with thyroid hormone or antithyroid drugs.

GRAVES' DISEASE

Major Immunologic Features

- Antibodies against thyroid antigens are present that stimulate thyroid cell function and displace TSH binding.
- There is class II HLA expression on the surface of thyroid cells.
- There is associated autoimmune ophthalmopathy and dermopathy.

General Considerations

Graves' disease is an autoimmune disorder of unknown etiology, which presents as thyrotoxicosis with a diffuse goiter. It is unique among autoimmune disorders since it is probably caused by autoantibodies that actually stimulate thyroid cellular activity. In addition, patients with Graves' disease often have associated phenomena of ophthalmopathy and a proliferative dermopathy, which appear to be autoimmune in nature. The endocrine, skin, and eye disorders are most commonly seen in combination. However, they can exist separately and often have different clinical courses even when they coexist in the same patient.

Graves' disease is most common in the third and fourth decades of life and has a marked female predominance of 7:1. Unlike Hashimoto's disease, it rarely occurs in children but often occurs in individuals past the fifth decade of life. It is a relatively common disorder, occurring in 0.1–0.5% of the general population.

Graves' disease was among the first autoimmune disorders noted to have an association with HLA haplotypes. There is a strong association with DR3 in whites and with Bw35 and Bw46 in Asians. Also, the disease tends to occur in families and is associated with the same HLA and Gm haplotypes in affected kindred. The disease seems to be associated with a type of "autoimmune susceptibility" in some families, since other family members often have autoimmune disorders such as Hashimoto's disease and antibodies to gastric parietal cells and intrinsic factor.

Pathology

Thyroid glands from patients with Graves' disease present a uniformly enlarged and diffuse goiter. Microscopic analysis reveals small thyroid follicles with hyperplastic epithelium, but little colloid. Although there is often a lymphocytic and plasma cell infiltrate, it is much less intense and does not have the associated destruction of normal tissue seen in Hashimoto's disease. These findings resolve in patients treated with antithyroid drugs.

Immunofluoresence analysis indicates that a high proportion of thyroid cells express HLA-DR antigens on their surface. In addition, analysis of the lymphocyte subsets in the gland reveals both CD4 and CD8 T cells and B cells.

Clinical Features

Graves' disease typically present with diffuse goiter and thyrotoxicosis. The signs of hyperthyroidism are heat intolerance, hand tremor, nervousness, irritability, warm moist skin, weight loss, muscle reflex changes, hyperdynamic cardiovascular status with tachycardia, hyperdefecation, and changes in mental status. The exception to this is in the elderly, in whom apathetic hyperthyroidism may present with tachycardia as the sole clinical manifestation. Patients with accompanying ophthalmopathy may have proptosis, lid lag, and a characteristic "stare." Dermopathy usually presents as a swelling in the pretibial area (myxedema), and in the feet, face, or hands.

Laboratory findings are those of hyperthyroidism, with elevated levels of total and free T3 and T4. TSH levels in this disease are low or undetectable because the stimulation of the thyroid gland is exogenous rather than from the pituitary axis and the elevated levels of the thyroid hormones cause a feedback inhibition of pituitary TSH secretion.

The thyroid gland in patients with Graves' disease always shows an increased uptake of radioactive iodine. A diffuse homogeneous uptake on a radio isotopic scan of the thyroid is almost pathognomonic of Graves' disease.

Immunologic Diagnosis

The immunologic diagnosis of Graves' disease rests on the identification of antithyroid antibodies with the ability to alter thyroid cell function. These antibodies tend to fall into 3 catagories (Fig 37–5): (1) antibodies that stimulate the production of cAMP (thyroid-stimulating immunoglobulins, or TSI); (2) antibodies causing proliferation of thyroid cells as measured by the incorporation of [^{3}H] thymidine into their DNA (thyroid growth-stimulating immunoglobulins [TGSI]); (3) antibodies that displace the

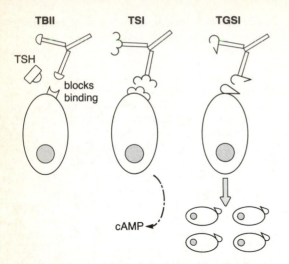

Figure 37–5. The 3 classes of antithyroid antibodies associated with Graves' disease. TBII antibodies block binding of TSH to its receptor, whereas TSI antibodies stimulate the production of cAMP, and TGSI antibodies cause proliferation of thyroid cells. Whether these three antibodies bind to a single antigen, separate antigens, or separate epitopes on a single antigen is still unknown.

binding of TSH from its receptor (thyroid binding-inhibitory immunoglobulins [TBII]). Although these antibodies have been found in several other disorders, especially Hashimoto's thyroiditis, their presence in the appropriate clinical setting is virtually pathognomonic of Graves' disease. In addition, monitoring the function of these antibodies may, in some cases, correlate with the clinical course of the disease and its response to antithyroid drugs.

Initial efforts to measure the activity of TSI involved injecting IgG fractions from patients with Graves' disease into animals and measuring thyroid activity. This test has been replaced by the Fisher rat thyroid line 5 (FRTL-5). These cells are grown in culture with IgG from patients with Graves' disease, and the effect on cell function (either the production of cAMP or the incorporation of [^{3}H] thymidine) is measured. The ability of the IgG to displace TSH from its receptor is still measured as described more than 15 years ago. The test involves the incubation of IgG with porcine thyroid membranes and radiolabeled TSH. The amount of TSH bound to the membrane is then calculated and compared with the amount bound in the presence of control IgG or unlabeled TSH. This results in a "percent displacement" of radiolabeled TSH, which gives a relative activity of the IgG. The recent identification and sequencing of the TSH receptor should allow classification of the specific function of these autoantibodies.

Differential Diagnosis

The differential diagnosis of Graves' disease includes exclusion of other thyroid disorders with hyperthyroidism such as Hashimoto's disease, pituitary tumors, or thyroid adenomas. Most of these can be ruled out by determining that the thyroid gland has a diffuse increase in iodine uptake. The presence of ophthalmopathy and dermopathy also supports the diagnosis of Graves' disease.

Treatment

The initial treatment of Graves' disease involves the inhibition of symptomatic β-adrenergic hyperstimulation with β-adrenergic blocking agents. Therapy with drugs to inhibit thyroid cell function is also given soon after diagnosis. These drugs, propylthiouracil and methimazole, offer several advantages in the treatment of Graves' disease. They not only inhibit the production of thyroid hormones, relieving hyperthyroidism, but also decrease the size and vascularity of the goiter, making it more amenable to definitive therapy with surgery or radioactive iodine. Of interest, these drugs may also interrupt the perpetuation of the underlying autoimmune process, possibly through the resolution of the hyperthyroidism, as thyroid hormones appear to have nonspecific immunostimulatory activities in vitro.

Definitive therapy for Graves' disease involves the destruction of the thyroid gland, either by ^{131}I or by complete surgical removal of the gland. Although personal preference and experience often dictate which therapy is used, surgery has been the therapy of choice in women of childbearing age because of the potential risks of radiation to the gonads and fetus. Recent studies do not show risk to the ovaries, however, and radioiodine is becoming increasingly popular in premenopausal women once pregnancy is ruled out.

Prognosis & Complications

The prognosis for most patients is very good once their thyroid function is controlled. The most serious problems in Graves' disease often come from the associated ophthalmopathy and dermopathy, which in some cases do not respond to treatments that normalize thyroid function. Treatment with corticosteroids will provide relief in some cases, but occasionally the ophthalmopathy progresses to a point that vision is threatened. At that point, radiotherapy or surgical decompression of the orbit is often required. More aggressive treatment protocols with immunosuppressive drugs such as cyclosporine have shown some success in reversing the autoimmune process in these patients.

PRIMARY HYPOTHYROIDISM

Major Immunologic Features
- There is lymphocytic infiltration of the thyroid gland.
- Antithyroid antibodies can be present.

General Considerations

Primary hypothyroidism, or thyroid atrophy, is the most common cause of hypothyroidism (other than iatrogenic ablation) in adults. Much like the other autoimmune thyroid diseases, it is more common in women than men and occurs most often from age 40 to 60 years. The atrophy probably results from asymptomatic or unrecognized thyroiditis with resulting progressive destruction of the gland. However, some data suggest that some of these cases are related to antibodies which block TSH binding to its receptor, thereby inhibiting the trophic effect of the hormone. Thyroid atrophy also occurs as part of the polyglandular syndromes (see below).

Pathology

The thyroid is markedly atrophic and often fibrotic. In some cases there is residual lymphocytic infiltration.

Clinical Features

Although most patients demonstrate the usual findings of hypothyroidism and a small, impalpable thyroid gland, some present with palpable fibrosis in the area of the thyroid gland. Laboratory findings include elevated TSH levels with low (or low normal) levels of circulating thyroid hormones. TSH response to thyrotropin-releasing hormone (TRH) administration is often exaggerated, indicating an increased state of activation of the pituitary axis.

Immunologic Diagnosis

Antithyroid antibodies are found in a high proportion of patients (> 80%), but they are not necessary for the diagnosis. No other specific immunologic tests are available.

Treatment & Prognosis

Treatment consists of thyroid hormone replacement. Most patients do well with this therapy. However, replacement is required throughout the rest of the patient's life.

DISORDERS OF THE ENDOCRINE PANCREAS

TYPE I DIABETES MELLITUS

Major Immunologic Features

- There is lymphocytic infiltration of the islets of Langerhans.
- There are antibodies against multiple components of islet beta cells.
- There is HLA-DR expression on the beta cells.
- There is some evidence for partial responses to immunosuppressive therapy.

General Considerations

Type I diabetes mellitus is a disorder in which the destruction of the insulin-producing beta cells of the pancreatic islets of Langerhans results in a deficiency of insulin. This is in contrast to the defect in type II diabetes mellitus, in which resistance of target organs to the effects of insulin is present. Although type I diabetes mellitus has only recently been associated with an immune pathogenesis, it is now clear that there is an autoimmune cause in the great majority of patients with this disorder. The postulated sequence of events leading to islet cell destruction is similar to the scheme outlined in Fig 37–1. After an initiating event such as a viral infection, an inflammatory response to beta cells of the islets results. This inflammation is characterized by HLA-DR expression on the beta cells and lymphocytic infiltration of the islets. Subsequently, either a persistent stimulation of the immune system or a defect in immune regulation allows the propagation of the autoimmune response in a genetically predisposed individual. This causes destruction of the beta cells and leads to insulin deficiency.

The hypothesis that a viral infection is the initial insult leading to the development of type I diabetes mellitus in humans is unproven. There is, however, much evidence in favor of this hypothesis including reports of the development of type I diabetes mellitus following infections with viruses such as mumps virus, cytomegalovirus, influenza virus, and rubella virus, as well as a direct relationship between viral infection and diabetes in experimental animals. Mumps virus, coxsackie virus types B3 and B4, and reovirus type 3 can infect and destroy human islet cells in vitro. As yet, however, there is no direct causal link between the common occurrence of infections with these viruses and the rare event of developing autoimmune diabetes mellitus. It seems that the heterogeneous genetic susceptibility to development of autoimmunity is what has made identification of a specific environmental cause difficult.

Epidemiologic studies support the concept of a genetic susceptibility to develop type I diabetes mellitus. Seen almost entirely in individuals under the age of 30 years, it has a peak age of onset between 10 and 14 years. It occurs predominantly in whites and has a prevalence of approximately 0.25% in both the USA and Europe. Unlike most other autoimmune disorders, males are more commonly affected than females, by a small margin. The incidence of this disorder has increased slightly over the past 50 years. There are also seasonal fluctuations.

The genetics of type I diabetes mellitus have come under intense study recently. It is well documented that more than 90% of patients have HLA-DR3, -DR4, or both and that there is a negative association with HLA-DR2. An additive risk occurs when both HLA-DR3 and -DR4 are present. However, few individuals who have the HLA-DR3 and -DR4 haplotypes develop type I diabetes mellitus. A closely linked genetic abnormality to these HLA haplotypes may explain this paradox. Restriction analysis of the HLA-DQ β-chain genes indicates a unique nucleotide in position 56 in patients susceptible to type I diabetes mellitus who also have the HLA-DR3/4 haplotype. This DQ region gene may thus be the true "disease susceptibility" gene.

Pathology

Patients show evidence of lymphocytic infiltration in the pancreatic islets even before evidence of glucose intolerance is noted. This inflammatory lesion progresses to cause specific destruction of the beta cells with atrophy and scarring of the islets. The other endocrine cells in the islets usually remain functional.

Immunofluorescence staining of the islet inflammation reveals several interesting findings. First, there is HLA-DR expression on the beta cells, as well as on the infiltrating lymphocytes. The majority of these lymphocytes stain positively with monoclonal antibodies for CD8, indicating a cytotoxic/suppressor phenotype. Antibody-producing cells are also seen, and antibody and complement components are present on the surface of the beta cells.

Clinical Features

The signs and symptoms are well known and are beyond the scope of this chapter. Unlike type II disease, there is a true insulin deficiency in type I diabetes mellitus, which leaves the patient prone to greater fluctuations in blood glucose concentration and to subsequent ketosis.

The laboratory diagnosis still rests on the documentation of elevated blood glucose concentrations. A fasting blood glucose level greater than 140 mg/dL in the appropriate clinical setting is diagnostic for diabetes. If the fasting glucose concentration is normal, the use of a glucose tolerance test may be helpful, but this is controversial. The level of hemoglobin A1c is helpful primarily in monitoring the ongoing control of blood glucose concentrations in patients on therapy.

Immunologic Diagnosis

Presently, no immunologic test is useful clinically. Antibodies to both islet cell cytoplasm and membranes can be identified by using immunofluo-

rescence; however, these antibodies are not helpful in determining whether a susceptible individual will develop the disease. In the future, genetic analysis of HLA polymorphisim or antibodies against a specific pancreatic antigen may serve this purpose. In this regard, the recent description of antibodies to a 64-kilodalton antigen that precede the development of clinical glucose intolerance may be a useful marker to follow.

Treatment

Treatment of diabetes requires normalization of blood glucose concentrations by using oral hypoglycemic drugs or insulin injections. Most type I diabetes mellitus patients require insulin, and the availability of human insulin may allow better therapy for some patients with insulin antibodies. Segmental pancreas or islet cell transplantation may offer a more physiologic form of insulin replacement in the future.

There have now been many trials of immunosuppressive therapy to attempt to reverse the inflammatory process that causes islet cell destruction (Fig 37–5). Although most of these trials were started a short time after the development of glucose intolerance, there have been some (Table 37–2) successful increases in C peptide levels and clinical improvement in blood glucose control, obviating a need for insulin injections. All of these drugs have potentially severe toxicity and require larger-scale clinical trials before they go into general use.

ADRENAL INSUFFICIENCY (Addison's Disease)

Major Immunologic Features

■ Circulating antibodies against adrenal cells are present.
■ Complement is fixed on the surface of adrenal cells.
■ It is associated with other autoimmune diseases.

General Considerations

Since the decline of tuberculosis, idiopathic Addison's disease is the most common form of adrenal insufficiency, accounting for 70–80% of all cases. The prevalence is relatively low, only 40–50 cases per million, and it tends to affect young individuals

Table 37–2. Immunotherapy trials in type I diabetes mellitus.

Drug	C Peptide Increase Period	Insulin Therapy-Free Period
Prednisone	24 mo	Transient
Alpha interferon	None	None
Prednisone, antithymocyte globulin, and azathioprine	12 mo	3–26 mo
Cyclosporine	> 12 mo	12 mo (25% of subjects)

in their third or fourth decade. The female-to-male ratio is lower than that seen in other autoimmune disorders, only 1.8:1. It can present as an isolated disorder or in combination with other autoimmune diseases. It is most commonly seen as part of a polyglandular syndrome (see below), which accounts for up to 40% of the cases of this disease. The disease is associated with HLA-DR3/4 in a manner similar to type I diabetes mellitus, except when part of a polyglandular syndrome.

Pathology

Grossly, adrenal glands from patients with idiopathic Addison's disease show progressive scarring and atrophy. Microscopic examination often reveals a lymphocytic infiltrate early in the course of the disease, and immunofluoresence shows antibody and complement fixed to cortical cells.

Clinical Features

Idiopathic Addison's disease is usually slowly progressive, with the development of clinical manifestations such as salt wasting, hypotension, anorexia, malaise, and hyperpigmentation occurring so gradually that they can easily be undetected. Serum levels of adrenocorticotropic hormone (ACTH) are often elevated long before clinical disease develops. The finding of small, noncalcified adrenal glands on x-ray or computed tomography of the abdomen helps to differentiate this disorder from adrenal insufficiency secondary to carcinoma (primary or metastatic) and tuberculosis. The laboratory diagnosis rests on the lack of a cortisol (and possibly aldosterone) response to ACTH administration.

Immunologic Diagnosis

Serum antibodies against adrenal cortical cells are demonstrable by immunofluorescence in up to 80% of cases.

Treatment

Treatment consists of corticosteroid hormone replacement and, when needed, replacement of mineralocorticoid hormones. No trials of immunosuppressive therapy have been published.

LYMPHOCYTIC ADENOHYPOPHYSITIS

Lymphocytic adenohypophysitis is a rare disorder characterized by the rapid development of hypopituitarism without evidence of pituitary adenoma. It occurs most often in women during or after pregnancy. Although the incidence of this disorder is unknown, the finding of antibodies against pituitary cells in 18% of patients with Sheehan's syndrome suggests that at least some of these patients may have had an autoimmune basis for their hypopituitarism. It also

occurs as part of a polyglandular syndrome (as discussed below), in which it has been associated with isolated deficiencies of gonadotropic hormones.

PREMATURE OVARIAN FAILURE

Evidence is accumulating that some individuals may have an autoimmune basis for premature gonadal failure. There have been several cases in which autoimmune oophoritis is associated with other autoimmune endocrine diseases, especially adrenal insufficiency. This is especially true in polyglandular syndromes.

IDIOPATHIC HYPOPARATHYROIDISM

This is another uncommon disorder seen primarily in polyglandular autoimmune syndromes. Although antibodies against parathyroid tissue commonly occur in the polyglandular syndromes, their presence does not correlate with overt hypoparathyroidism. It has been reported that antibodies from patients with this disorder cause complement-mediated cytolysis of parathyroid cells, suggesting that a subset of antibodies may have pathogenic significance.

AUTOIMMUNE POLYGLANDULAR SYNDROMES

Major Immunologic Features

- There are circulating antibodies against multiple endocrine organs.
- There is evidence of HLA-DR expression on affected cells.
- There is genetic susceptibility to autoimmunity.

General Considerations

Polyglandular syndromes are groupings of multiple endocrine dysfunctions of autoimmune origin in a genetically susceptible individual. There were initially many versions of these syndromes identified by multiple eponyms; however, recently a classification scheme for these disorders has been developed (Table 37–3).

A. Type I Syndrome: The type I syndrome is a disorder that occurs in childhood, usually before the age of 10 years, with a slight female predominance. It was previously known as mucocutaneous candidiasis endocrinopathy. The most common association is between candidiasis and hypoparathyroidism (> 70% of cases), but 40–70% of patients also go on to develop adrenal insufficiency. With the exception of gonadal failure, which occurs in approximately 40% of patients, the other autoimmune endocrine disorders are less common in the type I

Table 37–3. Classification of polyglandular syndromes.

Syndrome	Major Criteria	Minor Criteria
Type I	Candidiasis Adrenal failure Hypoparathyroidism	Gonadal failure Alopecia Malabsorption Chronic hepatitis
Type II	Adrenal failure Thyroid disease Type I diabetes mellitus	Gonadal failure Vitiligo Nonendocrine autoimmune disease
Type III[1]	Thyroid disease	a. Type I diabetes b. Gastric disease c. Nonendocrine autoimmune disease

[1]Type III is composed of thyroid disease plus only one of a, b, or c.

syndrome. There is, however, an association with chronic active hepatitis (10–15% of cases), alopecia areata, malabsorption, and pernicious anemia.

The pathogenesis of this disorder is unknown, but the problems with chronic fungal infection suggest a defect in cell-mediated immunity. Autoantibodies against cells from most affected organs are also seen in a large percentage of patients.

Although type I polyglandular syndrome occurs sporadically, it is more commonly seen as a familial disorder with inheritance suggestive of an autosomal recessive trait. It has not, however, been associated with a particular HLA haplotype.

B. Type II Syndrome: Type II polyglandular syndrome was originally known as Schmidt's syndrome. It tends to occur most often between the ages of 20 and 30 years and has a 2:1 female predominance. It is a rare disorder, with a prevalence of 20 per million. It is characterized by the presence of a second, autoimmune disorder (usually diabetes or thyroid disease or both) with idiopathic Addison's disease. Gonadal failure occurs in a smaller percentage of cases, and nonendocrine autoimmune disorders have been occasionally noted.

Although at least half the cases of type II polyglandular are familial, the mode of inheritance is unknown. Both autosomal dominant and recessive patterns have been suggested, and there is also a high frequency of HLA-DR3 in these patients. Autoantibodies against cells of the affected organs are present in the majority of patients, and there have also been reports of alterations in cell-mediated immunity.

C. Type III Syndrome: Type III polyglandular syndrome is the least well characterized but probably the most common of the disorders. It is defined by the presence of autoimmune thyroid disease with another autoimmune disorder. This syndrome is composed of at least 3 clinical entities. The first is the association of diabetes mellitus with autoimmune thyroid disease. The second is the association of autoimmunity against gastric components such as parietal cells or intrinsic factor in association with au-

toimmune thyroid disease. The association of any other organ-specific autoimmune disorder, such as myasthenia gravis, with autoimmune thyroid disease comprises the third component. Patients with type III polyglandular syndrome, by definition, do not have Addison's disease.

The cause of type III polyglandular syndrome is unclear, but it tends to primarily involve female patients (7:1 female predominance) who have HLA-DR3-associated autoimmune disease. Again, organ-specific autoantibodies are present in the sera of patients with this disorder.

D. Other Considerations: The pathology, symptoms, and treatment of patients with the polyglandular syndromes are the same as for the individual autoimmune disorders, with a few important exceptions. Patients with type I polyglandular syndrome should have their candidiasis treated with ketoconazole. This not only provides symptomatic relief, but also may help resolve some of the defects in cell-mediated immunity. In addition, all patients with the polyglandular syndromes should be monitored for the development of other autoimmune disorders associated with their syndrome. This will prevent missing disorders such as Addison's disease, which may develop later in the course of the syndrome.

REFERENCES

General

Bach JF: Antireceptor or antihormone autoimmunity and its relationship with the idiotype network. *Adv Nephrol* 1987;**16**:25.

Belcher M: Receptors, antibodies and disease. *Clin Chem* 1984;**30(7)**:1137.

Bottazzo GF et al: Organ-specific autoimmunity: A 1986 overview. *Immunol Rev* 1986;**94**:137.

Buse JB, Eisenbarth GS: Autoimmune endocrine disease. *Vitam Horm* 1985;**42**:253.

Chaplin DD, Kemp ME: The major histocompatibility complex and autoimmunity. *Year Immunol* 1986–87; **3**:179.

De Baets MH: Autoimmune endocrine diseases. *Year Immunol* 1986;**2**:289.

Monroe JG, Greene MI: Anti-idiotypic antibodies and disease. *Immunol Invest* 1986;**15**:263.

Pujol-Borrell R et al: Inappropriate major histocompatibility complex class II expression by thyroid follicular cells in thyroid autoimmune disease and by pancreatic beta cells in type I diabetes. *Mol Biol Med* 1986;**3**:159.

Thyroid Diseases

Baker JR Jr et al: Seronegative Hashimoto thyroiditis with thyroid autoantibody production localized to the thyroid. *Ann Intern Med* 1988;**108**:26.

Bottazzo GF, Doniach D: Autoimmune thyroid disease. *Annu Rev Med* 1986;**37**:353.

Burman KD, Baker JR Jr: Immune mechanisms in Graves' disease. *Endocr Rev* 1985;**6**:183.

Jacobson DH, Gorman CA: Endocrine opthlmopathy: Current ideas concerning etiology, pathogenesis and treatment. *Endocr Rev* 1984;**5**:200.

Weetmen AP, McGregor AM: Autoimmune thyroid disease: Developments in our understanding. *Endocr Rev* 1984;**5**:309.

Type I Diabetes Mellitus

Dobersen MJ, Chase HP: Immunologic aspects of type I diabetes. *Pediatrician* 1983–85;**12**:173.

Henson V et al: Molecular genetics of insulin-dependent diabetes mellitus. *Mol Biol Med* 1986;**3**:129.

Lernmark A et al: Islet-specific immune mechanisms. *Diabetes Metab Rev* 1987;**3**:959.

Neumer C, Brandt R, Zuhlke H: The major histocompatibility complex and diabetes mellitus. *Exp Clin Endocrinol* 1987;**89**:112.

Skyler JS: Immune intervention studies in insulin-dependent diabetes mellitus. *Diabetes Metab Rev* 1987; **3**:1017.

Addison's Disease

Betterle C et al: Complement-fixing adrenal autoantibodies as a marker for predicting onset of idiopathic Addison's disease. *Lancet* 1983;**1**:1238.

Burke CW: Adrenocortical insufficiency. *Clin Endocrinol Metab* 1985;**14**:947.

Latinne D et al: Addison's disease: Immunological aspects. *Tissue Antigens* 1987;**30**:23.

Scheithauer BW, Kovacs K, Randall RV: The pituitary gland in untreated Addison's disease. A histologic and immunocytologic study of 18 adenohypophyses. *Arch Pathol Lab Med* 1983;**107**:484.

Vita JA et al: Clinical clues to the cause of Addison's disease. *Am J Med* 1985;**78**:461.

Lymphocytic Adenohypophysitis & Hypoparathyroidism

Brandi ML et al: Antibodies cytotoxic to bovine parathyroid cells in autoimmune hypoparathyroidism. *Proc Natl Acad Sci USA* 1986;**83**:8366.

Guay AT et al: Lymphocytic hypophysitis in a man. *J Clin Endocrinol Metab* 1987;**64**:631.

Homberg JC: Hypoparathyroidism, ovarian insufficiency and adrenal insufficiency of autoimmune origin. *Rev Prat* 1986;**36**:3505.

McDermott MW et al: Lymphocytic adenohypophysitis. *Can J Neurol Sci* 1988;**15**:38.

Polyglandular Syndromes

Ahonen P: Autoimmune polyendocrinopathy candidosis ectodermal dystrophy (APECED): Autosomal recessive inheritance. *Clin Genet* 1985;**27**:535.

Appleboom TM, Flowers FP: Ketoconazole in the treatment of chronic mucocutaneous candidiasis secondary to autoimmune polyendocrinopathy candidiasis syndrome. *Cutis* 1982;**30**:71.

Brun JM: Juvenile autoimmune polyendocrinopathy. *Horm Res* 1982;**16**:308.

Leshin M: Polyglandular autoimmune syndromes. *Am J Med Sci* 1985;**290**:77.

Neufeld M, MacLaren NK, Blizzard RM: Autoimmune polyglandular syndromes. *Pediatr Ann* 1980;**9**:154.

38 Hematologic Diseases

J. Vivian Wells, MD, FRACP, FRCPA, & James P. Isbister, FRACP, FRCPA

There are many areas in hematology that are significantly affected by immunologic processes. An important group of disorders—the autoimmune hemolytic anemias, autoimmune neutropenias, and immune thrombocytopenias—are characterized by immunologic destruction of circulating blood cells. Even hematopoietic precursor cells in the bone marrow may be destroyed or suppressed by immunologic mechanisms, as seen in pure erythrocyte aplasia and some cases of aplastic anemia. Another large group of hematologic disorders—the plasma cell dyscrasias, lymphotic leukemias, and lymphomas—represent abnormal proliferations of primary cells of the immune system (see Chapter 48).

This chapter will be devoted primarily to hematologic disorders in which immunologic cells or mechanisms play a major role. The chapter discusses immunologic disorders of leukocytes, erythrocytes, and coagulation.

disease. These patients may be asymptomatic or may have recurrent infections. Antigranulocyte antibodies have been detected by a variety of procedures, including the utilization of anti-immunoglobulin antisera with fluorescence or antiglobulin consumption techniques, functional assays, and cytotoxicity assays. The presence of leukoagglutinins does not correlate well with leukopenia. Bone marrow function is relatively normal in autoimmune neutropenia, with myeloid hyperplasia and a shift to the left in maturation often observed, presumably in response to increased peripheral granulocyte destruction. The autoantibody may also suppress bone marrow myeloid cell growth in vitro and in vivo. Autoimmune neutropenia often responds to splenectomy and treatment with corticosteroids or immunosuppressive drugs.

Autoimmune neutropenia may also be seen in systemic lupus erythematosus (SLE), Felty's syndrome (rheumatoid arthritis, splenomegaly, and severe neu-

WHITE LEUKOCYTE DISORDERS

LEUKOPENIA

Leukopenia is defined as a reduction in the number of circulating leukocytes below 4000/μL. Granulocytopenia may be caused either by decreased granulocyte production by the bone marrow or by increased granulocyte utilization or destruction. Decreased granulocyte production occurs in aplastic anemia, leukemia, and other diseases marked by bone marrow infiltration; many drugs also cause leukopenia by this mechanism. Increased granulocyte utilization or destruction occurs in hypersplenism, autoimmune neutropenia, and some forms of drug-induced leukopenia. The major causes of leukopenia are listed in Table 38–1.

1. AUTOIMMUNE NEUTROPENIA

Autoimmune neutropenia may occur as an isolated disorder or secondary to an underlying autoimmune

Table 38–1. The major causes of leukopenia.

Infections
  Viral—rubella
  Bacterial—typhoid fever, miliary tuberculosis brucellosis
  Rickettsial
Therapy
  Ionizing radiation
  Cytotoxic drugs
  Drugs
    Selective neutropenia
    Agranulocytosis
    Aplastic anemia
Hematologic diseases
  Megaloblastic anemia
  Acute leukemia
  Myelodysplasia
  Aplastic anemia
  Multiple myeloma
  Paroxysmal nocturnal hemoglobinuria
  Leukoerythroblastic anemia
    Metastatic carcinoma
Autoimmune neutropenia
  Hypersplenism
  SLE
  Felty's syndrome
Chronic idiopathic neutropenia
Cyclic neutropenia
Miscellaneous
  Anaphylaxis
  Hypopituitarism

tropenia), and other autoimmune disorders. There is some evidence that immune neutropenia in these disorders may be caused by adsorption of immune complexes onto the neutrophil membrane with premature cell destruction rather than by an antibody directed at specific neutrophil antigens. Some patients with Felty's syndrome also appear to have depressed granulocyte production by the bone marrow, probably also on an immunologic basis.

2. DRUG-INDUCED IMMUNE NEUTROPENIA

Although most drugs produce neutropenia by bone marrow suppression, some may cause neutropenia by the attachment of drug-antibody immune complexes to the surface of the granulocytes, with premature cell destruction. This "innocent bystander" mechanism is known to occur in drug-induced immune hemolytic anemia and thrombocytopenia. Cephalothin causes granulocytopenia in approximately 0.1% of patients given the drug, probably by this mechanism.

3. AGRANULOCYTOSIS

Agranulocytosis is characterized by the total absence of granulocytes and granulocyte precursors from the peripheral blood and bone marrow. This most often results from exposure of the patient to certain drugs, eg, aminopyrine, dipyrone, and phenylbutazone. Patients with agranulocytosis usually present with infections—often serious, life-threatening ones. Prior to the antibiotic era, agranulocytosis was almost invariably fatal. Patients now usually recover with intensive antibiotic treatment and granulocyte transfusions when necessary. Unlike drug-induced aplastic anemia, agranulocytosis usually resolves spontaneously within a few days to a few weeks after discontinuing the offending drug.

Although antigranulocyte antibodies or leukocyte drug-dependent antibodies generally have not been demonstrated in agranulocytosis, there is circumstantial evidence that immunologic damage to peripheral blood and bone marrow granulocytic cells is the mechanism of cell destruction, at least in some cases. Such patients often develop agranulocytosis after taking the responsible drug for weeks or months. If they recover from the agranulocytosis after the drug is discontinued and later are rechallenged with a small test dose of the same drug, acute agranulocytosis occurs immediately, associated with the acute onset of fever, chills, and hypocomplementemia.

ERYTHROCYTE DISORDERS

The erythrocyte disorders in which immune processes play an important role are the immune hemolytic anemias, paroxysmal nocturnal hemoglobinuria, and aplastic anemia and related disorders.

IMMUNE HEMOLYTIC ANEMIAS

The immune hemolytic disorders are classified in Table 38–2. The classification is based on the behavioral characteristics of antibodies involved and whether there is a demonstrable underlying disease or not. The clinical picture may be one of an acute self-limiting hemolytic disorder but is more often chronic. Since correct identification of the type of antibody is essential to correct diagnosis in patients with suspected immune hemolytic anemia, the immunologic laboratory investigation of such patients will be discussed before the individual diseases.

Table 38–2. Classification of immune hemolytic anemias.

Autoimmune hemolytic anemias
A. Warm-antibody types
1. Idiopathic warm autoimmune hemolytic anemia (AIHA)
2. Secondary warm autoimmune hemolytic anemias
   a. SLE and other autoimmune disorders
   b. Chronic lymphocytic leukemia, lymphomas, etc
   c. Hepatitis and other viral infections
B. Cold-antibody types
1. Idiopathic cold agglutinin syndrome
2. Secondary cold agglutinin syndrome
   a. *Mycoplasma pneumoniae* infection; infectious mononucleosis and other viral infections
   b. Chronic lymphocytic leukemia, lymphomas, etc
3. Paroxysmal cold hemoglobinuria
   a. Idiopathic
   b. Syphilis, viral infections

Drug-induced immune hemolytic anemias
1. Drug absorption mechanism
2. Membrane modification mechanism
3. Immune complex mechanism

Partial list of drugs:

Aminosalicylic acid (PAS)	Methyldopa
Antihistamines	Penicillin
Carbromal	Phenacetin
Cephalothin	Pyramidon
Chlorinated hydrocarbons	Quinidine
Chlorpromazine	Quinine
Dipyrone	Rifampin
Insulin	Stibophen
Isoniazid	Sulfonamides
Levodopa	Sulfonylureas
Mefenamic acid	Tetracyclines
Melphalan	

Alloantibody-induced immune hemolytic anemias
A. Hemolytic transfusion reactions
B. Hemolytic disease of the newborn
C. Allograft-associated anemias

Immunologic Laboratory Investigations

There are 2 basic groups of immunologic tests necessary to properly investigate patients with suspected immune hemolytic anemias: (1) tests to detect and characterize antibodies involved in the hemolytic process, and (2) tests to aid in diagnosis of possible underlying disease processes. Tests that define underlying disorders include detection of anti-DNA antibodies and antinuclear antibody (ANA) in SLE, rheumatoid factors in rheumatoid arthritis, and monoclonal B cells in chronic lymphocytic leukemia.

The serologic tests used to characterize antibodies in serum and on erythrocytes are basic blood-banking procedures, with the addition of monospecific antisera to identify specific proteins on erythrocytes and titration techniques to precisely quantitate antibody activity. Laboratory evaluation of such patients can be considered in terms of a series of questions: (1) Are the erythrocytes of the patient coated with immunoglobulin, complement components, or both? (2) How heavily are the erythrocytes sensitized? (3) What antibodies are eluted from the erythrocytes? (4) What antibodies are present in the serum?

Routine screening is performed by means of the direct antiglobulin (Coombs) test by tube or slide agglutination (see Chapter 20) using antisera with broad specificity. Subsequent evaluation requires testing the red cells with dilutions of monospecific antisera, especially antisera to IgG and C3. The activity of the autoantibody is examined at different temperatures to see whether the temperature of maximal activity identifies it as a ''warm'' or ''cold'' antibody.

False-negative and false-positive results can be obtained in direct antiglobulin tests. Approximately 20% of all patients with immune hemolytic anemias will have a negative or only weakly positive direct antiglobulin test unless the antiserum contains adequate titers of antibodies to complement components, especially C3. A positive direct antiglobulin test may be seen in situations other than autoantibodies on erythrocytes and does not necessarily mean autoimmune hemolytic anemia. Causes of such reactions include the following: (1) antibody formation against drugs rather than intrinsic erythrocyte antigens (see below); (2) damage to the erythrocyte membrane due to infection or cephalosporins, leading to nonimmunologic binding of proteins; (3) in vitro complement sensitization of erythrocytes by low-titer cold antibodies (present in many normal individuals) in clotted blood samples stored at 4 °C prior to separation; (4) delayed transfusion reactions; and (5) unknown mechanisms. The above reactions are generally weak and can be differentiated by clinical and detailed serologic studies.

Serologic investigations of the patient's serum and erythrocyte eluates should then answer another series of questions: (1) Are antibodies present? (2) Do they act as agglutinins, hemolysins, or incomplete antibodies? (3) What is their thermal range of activity? (4) What is their specificity?

The patient's serum is tested both undiluted and with fresh added complement against untreated and enzyme-treated pools of erythrocytes. Enzyme treatment enhances the sensitivity of the Ii system or abolishes activity in the case of the Pr system. The tests are run at both 37 °C and 20 °C and examined at 1 hour for agglutination and lysis. Cold agglutinin titration at 4 °C is also performed. Erythrocyte eluate is similarly tested.

Specialized tests may be performed to detect antibodies to drugs (eg, penicillin) in cases of drug-induced immune hemolytic anemia.

The specificity of the antibodies is tested at different temperatures with a panel of erythrocytes of different Rh genotypes and with cells of different types in the Ii blood group system (see below).

The results of the serologic investigations are then correlated with clinical and other laboratory investigations to establish a definitive diagnosis.

1. WARM AUTOIMMUNE HEMOLYTIC ANEMIA

Major Immunologic Features

■ There is a positive direct antiglobulin (Coombs) test.

■ Associated lymphoreticular cancer or autoimmune disease may be present.

■ Splenomegaly is common.

General Considerations

Warm-antibody autoimmune hemolytic anemia is the most common type of immune hemolytic anemia. It may be either idiopathic or secondary to chronic lymphocytic leukemia, lymphomas, SLE, or other autoimmune disorders or infections (Table 38–2). The idiopathic form may follow overt or subclinical viral infection.

Clinical Features

A. Symptoms and Signs: Patients usually present with symptoms of anemia and hemolysis. There may also be manifestations of an underlying disease, eg, lymphadenopathy, hepatosplenomegaly, or manifestations of autoimmune disease.

B. Laboratory Findings: Normochromic normocytic or slightly macrocytic anemia is usually present; spherocytosis is common, and nucleated erythrocytes may occasionally be found in the peripheral blood. Leukocytosis and thrombocytosis are often present, but occasionally (especially in SLE) leukopenia and thrombocytopenia are seen. There is usually a moderate to marked reticulocytosis. The bone marrow shows marked erythroid hyperplasia with plentiful iron stores. There is an increase in the serum level of indirect (unconjugated) bilirubin. Stool and urinary urobilinogen may be greatly increased. Transfused blood has a shortened survival time.

Immunologic Diagnosis

The results of the serologic tests discussed above are summarized in Table 38–3. The most common pattern is IgG and complement on erythrocytes, with IgG in the eluate. The eluate generally has no activity if the erythrocytes are sensitized only with complement.

Warm hemolysins active against enzyme-treated erythrocytes occur in 24% of sera, but warm serum agglutinins or hemolysins against untreated erythrocytes are rare. The indirect antiglobulin test (see Chapter 20) is positive at 37 °C in approximately 50–60% of patients' sera tested with untreated erythrocytes but in 90% of serum samples tested with enzyme-treated erythrocytes. This warm antibody is usually IgG but rarely may be IgM, IgA, or both.

The specificity of antibodies in warm antibody autoimmune hemolytic anemia is very complex, but the main specificity is directed against determinants in the Rh complex (see below). Identification is generally performed by blood banks or hematology laboratories with reference panels of erythrocytes of rare types.

Differential Diagnosis

Congenital nonspherocytic hemolytic anemia, hereditary spherocytosis, and hemoglobinopathies can usually be differentiated by the family history, routine hematologic tests, hemoglobin electrophoresis, and a negative direct antiglobulin test.

Treatment

A. General Measures: Treatment of the primary disease is necessary when autoimmune hemolytic anemia is secondary to an underlying disease process. Blood transfusions may be necessary for life-threatening anemia but should be avoided when possible, since the transfused cells are rapidly destroyed. Careful serologic studies are needed to minimize the risks of serious hemolytic transfusion reactions, and successful cross-matching can be difficult or impossible in this situation. Alloantibodies are more common and are difficult to detect.

B. Specific Measures: Hemolysis can be controlled with relatively high doses of corticosteroids in most patients. The steroids are fairly rapidly tapered and then slowly reduced until the clinical state, hemoglobin level, and reticulocyte count indicate the appropriate maintenance dose. Occasionally it is possible to gradually withdraw steroids completely. Regular monitoring is necessary since relapses often occur in patients in remission.

Monitoring generally includes serologic studies, eg, direct and indirect antiglobulin tests, and these may show improvement with reduced amounts of IgG and complement on erythrocytes and lower antibody titers or a negative antibody test. However, there is no consistent correlation between clinical response and serologic tests; prednisone often induces clinical remissions in patients with warm-antibody

Table 38–3. Summary of serologic findings in patients with autoimmune hemolytic anemia.[1]

Disease Group	Erythrocytes			Serum		
	Direct Antiglobulin Test	**Eluate**	**Immunoglobulin Type**	**Serologic Characteristics**		**Specificity**
Warm antibody type	IgG 30% IgG + complement 50% Complement 20%	IgG IgG No activity	IgG (rarely also IgA or IgM)	Positive indirect antiglobulin test 50% Agglutination of enzyme-treated erythrocytes 90% Hemolysis of enzyme-treated erythrocytes 24% Agglutination of untreated erythrocytes (20 °C) 20% Agglutination or hemolysis of untreated erythrocytes (37 °C) Very rare		Rh system (often with a "nonspecific" component)
Cold agglutinin syndrome	Complement	No activity	IgM (rarely IgA)	High-titer cold agglutinin (usually 1:1000 at 4 °C) up to 32 °C; monoclonal IgM in chronic disease		Anti-I usually (can be anti-i or anti-Pr)
Paroxysmal cold hemoglobinuria (very rare)	Complement	No activity	IgG	Potent hemolysin also agglutinates normal cells. Biphasic (usually sensitizes cells in cold up to 15 °C and hemolyzes them at 37 °C)		Anti-P blood group

[1]Modified from Petz LD, Garratty G: Laboratory correlations in immune hemolytic anemias. Page 139 in: *Laboratory Diagnosis of Immunologic Disorders.* Vyas GN, Stites DP, Brecher G (editors). Grune & Stratton, 1975.

autoimmune hemolytic anemia despite persistently positive direct antiglobulin tests.

If prednisone therapy fails or if unacceptable side effects occur, splenectomy is usually performed. Since splenectomy often produces long-term remissions in patients with idiopathic autoimmune hemolytic anemia, splenectomy is the treatment of choice if hemolysis persists after 2–3 months of corticosteroids. ^{51}Cr-labeled erythrocyte survival studies can be used to identify abnormal splenic erythrocyte sequestration prior to splenectomy; however, clinical remissions may occur after splenectomy even when abnormal splenic sequestration cannot be documented. Continued significant hemolysis or late relapse sometimes occurs after splenectomy and requires therapy with steroids with or without other immunosuppressive agents.

Other immunosuppressive drugs include oral azathioprine (1.0–1.5 mg/kg/d for at least 3 months), cyclophosphamide at low dosage (1.0–1.5 mg/kg/d), or cyclosporine.

Prognosis

The prognosis of idiopathic warm-antibody autoimmune hemolytic anemia is fairly good; however, relapses are not infrequent, and death sometimes occurs. The prognosis of secondary warm autoimmune hemolytic anemia is determined by the underlying disease, eg, SLE or lymphoma.

2. COLD-AGGLUTININ SYNDROMES

These diseases may also be primary or may be secondary to infections or the lymphomas (Table 38–2). The infections include mycoplasmal pneumonia and infectious mononucleosis and other viral infections.

The clinical features are often those of the underlying disease. Cold-reactive symptoms such as Raynaud's phenomenon, livedo reticularis, or vascular purpura are seen in some patients. Hemolysis is generally mild but may occasionally be severe, especially in cases secondary to lymphoreticular cancer. The onset may be acute in cases secondary to infection. The idiopathic form is generally gradual in onset and runs a chronic and usually benign course in older patients.

These diseases usually are characterized by very high serum titers of agglutinating IgM antibodies which react optimally in the cold. These patients have cold-agglutinin titers in the thousands or millions, whereas normal individuals may have low-titer IgM cold agglutinins, and patients with chronic parasitic infections and most patients with *Ancylostoma* infection have titers up to 1:500. The presence of hemolysis is determined by the thermal range of the cold agglutinin. The high-titer, narrow-thermal-range antibodies will cause acral ischemic symp-toms. Some, however, may have a low titer but a thermal range reacting up to 37 °C. The specificity of the IgM is generally anti-I in the Ii system, but occasionally it is anti-i or anti-Pr (Table 38–3). In chronic idiopathic cases or cases associated with lymphoreticular malignancy, the cold agglutinin is generally a monoclonal IgM-κ paraprotein. The direct antiglobulin test is always positive using antiserum to C3.

Treatment consists of keeping the patient warm and waiting for spontaneous resolution in acute cases. Chronic cases sometimes respond to chlorambucil in low doses. Corticosteroids and splenectomy are probably not helpful, unless an underlying lymphoma is present.

The prognosis is generally good except for patients with severe underlying disease such as malignant lymphoma.

3. DRUG-INDUCED IMMUNE HEMOLYTIC ANEMIA

Many cases of immune hemolytic anemia have been reported in association with drug administration; the most common examples are included in Table 38–2. There are 3 stages in the investigation of a patient with suspected drug-induced hemolytic anemia: a history of intake of the drug, confirmation of hemolysis, and serologic tests. Detailed serologic tests are necessary to confirm the diagnosis, since different drugs produce hemolysis by different mechanisms. The immunopathologic mechanisms and clinical and laboratory features are summarized in Table 38–4. The mechanisms are classified as immune complex formation, hapten adsorption, nonspecific adsorption, and other, unknown mechanisms.

(1) Immune-complex formation: Circulating preformed immune complexes between the drug and antibody to the drug sensitize the erythrocyte ("innocent bystander" phenomenon). Quinine in low doses is a typical example. There is great variability in clinical features and serologic findings.

(2) Drug (hapten) adsorption: The drug acts as a hapten in that it is bound to the erythrocyte membrane and stimulates the production of a high titer of antidrug antibodies.

(3) Nonspecific adsorption: The drug affects the erythrocytes so that various nonimmunologic proteins are adsorbed onto erythrocytes and give a positive Coombs test. This does not result generally in marked hemolysis.

(4) Unknown mechanisms: This type is exemplified by the positive Coombs test that develops within 3 months in 20% of patients treated with methyldopa. The IgG that coats erythrocytes in these patients does not have antibody activity against the drug, and the drug is not required in in vitro tests.

Table 38–4. Summary of immunopathologic mechanisms and clinical and laboratory features in drug-induced immune hemolytic disorders.[1]

Mechanism	Drugs	Clinical Findings	Serologic Evaluation	
			Direct Antiglobulin Test	Antibody Characterization
Immune complex formation (drug + antidrug antibody)	Quinine, quinidine, phenacetin	History of small doses of drugs. Acute intravascular hemolysis and renal failure. Thrombocytopenia occasionally found.	Complement (IgG occasionally also present).	Drug + patient's serum + enzyme-treated erythrocytes → Hemolysis, agglutination, or sensitization. Antibody often complement-fixing IgM. Eluate generally nonreactive.
Drug adsorption to erythrocyte membrane (combination with high-titer serum antibodies to drug)	Penicillins, cephalosporins	History of large doses of drugs. Other allergic features may be absent. Usually subacute extravascular hemolysis.	IgG (strongly positive if hemolysis occurs). Rarely, weak complement sensitization also present.	Drug-coated erythrocytes + serum → Agglutination or sensitization (rarely hemolysis). High-titer antibody. Eluate reacts only with antibiotic-coated erythrocytes.
Membrane modification (nonimmunologic adsorption of proteins to erythrocytes)	Cephalosporins	Hemolytic anemia rare.	Positive with reagents with antibodies to a variety of serum proteins.	Drug-coated erythrocytes + serum → Sensitization to antiglobulin antisera in low titer.
Unknown	Methyldopa	Gradual onset of hemolytic anemia. Common.	IgG (strongly positive if hemolysis occurs).	Antibody sensitizes normal erythrocytes without drug. Antibody in serum and eluate identical to warm antibody. No in vitro tests demonstrate relationship to drug.

[1]Adapted from Garratty G, Petz LD: Drug-induced immune hemolytic anemia. *Am J Med* 1975:**58**:398.

The hemolysis may be acute and severe, but only rarely is blood transfusion required. The main treatment is to stop treatment with the offending drug and monitor the patient to be sure the hemolysis disappears. The prognosis is therefore excellent.

4. PAROXYSMAL COLD HEMOGLOBINURIA

This rare disease may be transient or chronic and constitutes 10% of the cold autoimmune hemolytic anemias. It may occur as a primary idiopathic disease or secondary to syphilis or viral infection. It is characterized clinically by signs of hemolysis and hemoglobinuria following local or general exposure to cold. Symptoms may include combinations of fatigue, pallor, aching and pain in the back, legs, or abdomen, chills and fever, and the passing of dark-brown urine. The symptoms may appear from within a few minutes to a few hours after exposure to cold.

The disease is characterized by the presence of the classic biphasic Donath-Landsteiner antibody. This polyclonal IgG antibody sensitizes erythrocytes in the cold (usually below 15 °C), so that complement components are detected on the erythrocytes by the direct antiglobulin test after rewarming. Heavily sensitized cells are hemolyzed when warmed to 37 °C. The antibody has specificity for the P antigen.

Acute attacks are treated symptomatically, and postinfectious cases generally resolve spontaneously, but transfusion is often necessary.

5. HEMOLYTIC DISEASE OF THE NEWBORN

Immunologic Pathogenesis

During pregnancy, very small amounts of fetal blood are leaked into the maternal circulation, especially during the last trimester. However, this is usually not enough to trigger antibody formation in the mother. During delivery, when the placenta is detached, bleeding of cord blood into the mother's circulation can elicit an immune response to fetal erythrocyte alloantigens.

Hemolytic disease of the newborn results from the mother's antibodies crossing the placenta and destroying fetal erythrocytes. This leads to hemolytic anemia and hydrops in the newborn infant. Hyperbilirubinemia occurs as a postnatal complication.

The first child is seldom affected by the hemolytic disease, but the chances for alloimmunization increase with each incompatible pregnancy. The primary stimulus for immunization can also be a previous incompatible blood transfusion or abortion.

Formation of Rh antibodies is the most common form of alloimmunization to give rise to clinically important disease. Antibodies to blood groups A and B (see Chapter 20) may also cause hemolysis of fetal cells if the maternal antibodies are IgG and thus capable of crossing the placenta. In these cases, the mother belongs usually to group O and the baby to group A. In fact, ABO immunization during pregnancy occurs more often than Rh immunization, but it seldom results in serious problems. If the fetus secretes soluble A or B substances, the maternal antibodies become neutralized before they cause damage to erythrocytes. A or B substances are present not only on erythrocytes but also on other tissues, including the placental endothelium. Therefore, many of the antibodies are consumed by these cells.

Clinical Features

The most frequent signs in the newborn are anemia and rapidly developing jaundice, which is usually present within the first 24 hours (in contrast to the physiologic icterus that occurs later). The infant's response to the anemia is marked reticulocytosis and erythroblastosis. As bilirubin accumulates in the plasma, it may cross the blood-brain barrier and cause damage to the nervous system (kernicterus). Severe alloimmunization causes fetal hydrops, and the fetus may die in utero. In these cases, if the father is homozygous for the relevant blood group, the prognosis is very poor for future babies.

Immunologic Diagnosis

Since the cause of the disease is antibody on erythrocyte membrane, the direct Coombs test is usually positive. In ABO incompatibility, it is often negative. The reason for this is somewhat unclear, but the relatively small amount of IgG antibody and the adsorption by other tissues may result in so few antibody molecules on the erythrocyte surface that the conventional Coombs method is not able to detect them. Thus, a negative direct Coombs test does not rule out an immunologic cause for neonatal icterus. If antibodies are not found in the mother's serum, however, immune hemolysis is unlikely.

Alloimmunization should be detected during pregnancy. In many countries, all Rh-negative women are screened for the presence of blood group antibodies during pregnancy. As the number of D immunizations decreases, the relative proportion of immunizations to other blood groups has increased. Consequently, antibody screening should not be restricted to Rh-negative women. No reliable screening test is available for ABO disease, although several assays for detection of clinically important IgG anti-A or anti-B have been used.

When unexpected antibodies are found in the mother's serum, the father's blood groups should be determined. If the father is negative for the relevant blood group, there is no risk; if he is heterozygous, the baby has only a 50% chance of being affected. Increasing antibody titer or a history of previously ill children increases suspicion that the fetus can be affected, and amniocentesis is done to determine the concentration of bile pigments and possibly antibodies in the amniotic fluid. With these procedures and with ultrasound examination, the presence and seriousness of the hemolytic disease can be assessed. Detectable amounts of antibodies sometimes develop in the serum so late in the pregnancy that they remain unnoticed until the time of delivery. Alloimmunization should always be suspected if the bilirubin level starts rising rapidly in an anemic newborn infant.

Treatment & Prevention

Treatment can be started during the last trimester of pregnancy if the results of amniocentesis and antibody determinations indicate that the fetus has serious disease. Compatible blood is injected into the abdominal cavity of the fetus and is rapidly absorbed into the circulation. Direct intravascular transfusion may be achieved by fetoscopy as early as 18 weeks, but only in specialized centers. The blood should be free of viable leukocytes to avoid the risk of subsequent graft-versus-host disease. Intrauterine transfusions may help the fetus to survive until mature enough to live outside the uterus. The last weeks of pregnancy are the most critical time for the fetus. Careful monitoring of clinical data by the obstetrician and neonatologist may prompt a decision to deliver the affected baby prior to term.

Immediately after delivery, the infant's blood group is determined and the cord cells are tested by the direct Coombs technique. If the baby is affected, exchange transfusions are usually needed, although in mild cases phototherapy with ultraviolet light or close supervision of bilirubin levels may be sufficient.

Women who have antibodies to the fetal erythrocytes should deliver in hospitals that have facilities and experience in exchange transfusion. Despite modern advances in the treatment of hemolytic disease of the newborn, the mortality rate in severe intrauterine cases remains high.

Over 90% of Rh-negative women having Rh-positive offspring do not form anti-D antibodies. The immunization of the rest can be prevented by giving the mother $100\mu g$ concentrated anti-D (Rh_o) immunoglobulin within 72 hours of delivery if she does not have any preexisting anti-D antibodies. Since it is not possible to predict who will make antibodies, all Rh-negative women with an Rh-positive baby must be given prophylaxis. Since Rh antigens are detectable in an embryo a few weeks postconception, anti-D immunoglobulin should also be given to Rh-negative women who have aborted.

The mechanism of inhibition of antibody synthesis is unclear, but rapid destruction and clearance of Rh-positive cells from the circulation seem to play a role. In experimental conditions, Rh-positive cells coated with blood group antibodies other than anti-D are quickly destroyed and anti-D antibodies are not formed. Mothers with anti-A or anti-B antibodies reacting with fetal cells produce Rh antibodies less often than in ABO-compatible pregnancies.

Systematically applied anti-D prophylaxis has reduced the number of immunized women from about 7–8% to a little over 1% if measured by the number of Rh-negative women with antibodies after 2 consecutive Rh-positive babies. Several reasons have been suggested for the few failures: immunization early during the pregnancy (not starting at the time of delivery); abnormally large volume of fetal blood leaking into the maternal circulation with insufficient anti-D immunoglobulin; and unusual sensitivity of the maternal immune system to the antigen D.

PAROXYSMAL NOCTURNAL HEMOGLOBINURIA

This rare disease is now known to cover a wide spectrum of clinical presentations. It can occur in adults as a chronic hemolytic anemia with acute exacerbations. It may follow other hematologic disorders such as idiopathic or drug-induced bone marrow aplasia and may terminate in acute myelogenous leukemia. The intravascular hemolysis causes intermittent hemoglobinemia and hemoglobinuria. This activity fluctuates throughout the day; the classic nocturnal timing of hemoglobinuria is seen in only 25% of cases. Venous thrombosis is a recognized complication.

The diagnosis is suggested by the findings of intermittent or chronic intravascular hemolysis, iron deficiency, hemosiderinuria, a low leukocyte alkaline phosphatase value, and frequently pancytopenia. The diagnosis of paroxysmal nocturnal hemoglobinuria is confirmed by any of the following tests: the acid hemolysis (Ham) test, the sugar water test, and the inulin test. These tests are presumably expressions of the 2 presently known abnormalities in paroxysmal nocturnal hemoglobinuria, ie, the exquisite sensitivity of paroxysmal nocturnal hemoglobinuria erythrocytes to complement lysis and the abnormally low acetylcholinesterase activity in the erythrocyte membrane. Patients' cells are lysed by approximately 4% of the amount of complement required to lyse normal erythrocytes. These tests demonstrate the sensitivity to complement lysis of paroxysmal nocturnal hemoglobinuria erythrocytes but do not elucidate the fundamental underlying cause of paroxysmal nocturnal hemoglobinuria. The alternative complement pathway may well be involved in this disease, as suggested by the inulin test, since inulin activates this pathway. However, serum complement studies are normal, no antibody has been identified either in the serum or on erythrocytes, and no abnormalities have been defined in membrane lipids and phospholipids. Electron microscopy shows a pitted surface on erythrocytes, but this has not been correlated with the functional complement abnormalities.

Treatment is mainly symptomatic but otherwise unsatisfactory. Transfusions are often required, and reactions are not infrequent. Androgens may be useful if there is underlying bone marrow hypoplasia. Corticosteroids and splenectomy are probably not useful. Rarely, bone marrow transplantation may be possible.

APLASTIC ANEMIA & RELATED DISORDERS

Some cases of aplastic anemia and related disorders may be immunologic in origin.

Pure Erythrocyte Aplasia

This rare form of anemia is characterized by a marked reduction or absence of bone marrow erythroblasts and blood reticulocytes, with normal granulopoiesis and thrombopoiesis. It occurs as an acquired disorder in adults, either in an idiopathic form or associated with thymoma (in 30–50% of cases), lymphoma, other tumors, or certain drugs. Patients usually present with progressive anemia requiring transfusion support. Bone marrow examination confirms the diagnosis. Thymoma is present in a small number of patients. Other immunologic abnormalities, such as hypogammaglobulinemia, monoclonal gammopathy, autoimmune hemolytic anemia, myasthenia gravis, and features of SLE may be seen in patients with pure erythrocyte aplasia.

Many patients with pure erythrocyte aplasia, with or without thymoma, have serum antibodies that react with bone marrow erythroblasts. These IgG antibodies have been demonstrated by immunofluorescence microscopy, with staining of nuclei of bone marrow erythroblasts. These antibodies fix complement and are specifically cytotoxic for erythroblasts. It has also been demonstrated that plasma from patients with pure erythrocyte aplasia suppresses erythropoiesis by normal bone marrow when cultured in vitro, while bone marrow from patients with pure erythrocyte aplasia shows normal erythropoiesis when cultured in vitro in normal plasma. This plasma factor suppressing erythropoiesis in pure erythrocyte aplasia is an IgG antibody.

Patients with pure erythrocyte aplasia usually require total erythrocyte transfusion support. Patients with thymomas should have these tumors removed; this will produce a remission in about 30% of these patients. Patients with idiopathic pure erythrocyte aplasia and those who do not respond to thymectomy should be treated with immunosuppressive drugs. Corticosteroids are usually used first, but few patients respond, and most are subsequently treated with cyclophosphamide plus prednisone. This combination produces remissions in 30–50% of patients, but relapses may occur when drugs are discontinued. Splenectomy has also been advocated for refractory patients with pure erythrocyte aplasia, as has plasma exchange.

Diamond-Blackfan Syndrome

This disorder, also known as congenital hypoplastic anemia, represents the congenital form of pure erythrocyte aplasia seen in infants. Anemia is usually noted in the first year of life but may occur later. These patients must be distinguished from patients with transient erythroblastopenia of infancy and childhood, which is a less serious, self-limited disorder.

Aplastic Anemia

Aplastic anemia is defined as pancytopenia due to bone marrow aplasia. Patients with severe aplastic anemia have no hematopoietic precursor cells present in their bone marrow and must be supported with erythrocyte and platelet transfusions and antibiotics. Problems exist with continuing transfusion support; even with optimal supportive care, severe aplastic anemia rarely undergoes spontaneous remission, and there is a 75–90% mortality rate. Treatment with high doses of androgens may benefit some patients, but few patients with severe aplasia respond. Bone marrow transplantation produces long-term remissions in over 50% of patients with severe aplastic anemia, and early bone marrow transplantation is currently considered the treatment of choice for younger patients with a histocompatible matched sibling.

In the past, aplastic anemia was usually associated with exposure to toxic drugs or chemicals (benzene, chloramphenicol, arsenicals, gold, anticonvulsants, etc). Recent series, however, indicate that most patients have no such exposure and no other associated illness, so that they are classified as having idiopathic aplastic anemia. Although it is possible that these patients have been exposed to unknown or inapparent environmental toxins, recent studies indicate that at least some of these cases are due to immunologic causes. Lymphocytes from the bone marrow of about one-third of patients with aplastic anemia have been shown to suppress the growth of or kill granulocyte colonies from normal bone marrow in vitro. When these abnormal suppressor lymphocytes are separated from the marrow granulocytic stem cells or killed with a specific cytotoxic antilymphocyte serum, increased granulocyte colony formation occurs. Other investigators found that peripheral blood lymphocytes from patients with aplastic anemia may suppress erythropoiesis of normal bone marrow when cultured in vitro.

Trials have confirmed the efficacy of antilymphocyte globulin (ALG) in selected patients, with response in approximately 50% of patients. Other proven approaches may be effective in small numbers of patients, eg, high-dose methyl prednisolone, splenectomy, or cyclosporin.

Major research activities have been directed to cloning the genes for various growth factors (GM-CSF, G-CSF, M-CSF, IL-3, etc [see Chapter 7]). Recombinant engineering methods are being used to produce these compounds, and numerous trials are in progress to assess their role in stimulating hematopoietic activity in clinical settings.

The major therapeutic approach in severe aplastic anemia is bone marrow transplantation (see Chapter 60).

Aplastic anemia, therefore, may result from at least 3 different defects involving the stem cells, the hematopoietic environment, or suppressor cells. A review of 14 patients with aplastic anemia studied by in vitro bone marrow cultures found evidence that 8 patients had defects in their stem cells. One patient had a defective hematopoietic environment, and 5 patients had increased suppressor cell activity. Characterization of the nature of the defects would permit more rational management of patients with aplastic anemia, since those patients with evidence of increased suppressor cell activity would be considered for treatment with immunosuppressive drugs or antithymocyte globulin (ATG) and those with obvious stem cell defects would be considered for early bone marrow transplantation.

PLATELET DISORDERS

Thrombocytopenia may be caused by decreased platelet production, increased platelet destruction, or abnormal platelet pooling. Immunologic thrombocytopenias, the subject of this section, are caused by increased platelet destruction, usually following platelet sensitization with antibody. Thrombocytopenias from decreased platelet production (aplastic anemia, leukemias, etc) have already been discussed with regard to immunologic features. Thrombocytopenia due to abnormal platelet pooling in an enlarged spleen (hypersplenism) is generally not associated with immunologic abnormalities.

Immunologic Mechanisms of Platelet Destruction

Several immunologic mechanisms of platelet damage leading to thrombocytopenia have been described. Platelet autoantibodies sensitize circulating platelets in idiopathic thrombocytopenic purpura and related disorders, leading to premature destruction of these cells in the spleen and other parts of the monocyte-macrophage system (see following section). Platelet alloantibodies may develop after multiple transfusions with blood products, or maternal sensitization can occur during pregnancies. Such platelet alloantibodies are becoming a major problem in long-term platelet support for patients with bone marrow failure. Alloantibodies may cause shortened platelet survival after transfusion or produce immediate platelet lysis with severe fever and chill reactions. Shortened platelet survival appears to be mediated by non-complement-dependent IgG or IgM antibodies similar to autoantibodies seen in idiopathic thrombocytopenic purpura. Platelet lysis, on the other hand, appears to be mediated by complement-dependent cytotoxic antibodies. These alloantibodies are directed primarily at HLA antigens, but non-HLA platelet antigens may also be involved. Alloantibody-dependent lymphocyte-mediated cytotoxicity has also been described in some patients. Neonatal thrombocytopenia due to passive transfer of maternal alloantibody or autoantibody is fortunately rare but may be life-threatening when it occurs.

Other immunologic mechanisms of platelet destruction include development of antibodies to drugs or other antigenic substances (haptens) adsorbed to the platelet membrane and adsorption of preformed antigen-antibody complexes onto the platelet membrane, with rapid removal of these sensitized cells from the circulation ("innocent bystander" phenomenon). The reactions are often complement-dependent. These mechanisms occur in drug-induced immune thrombocytopenia, in some infections, and in autoimmune disorders such as SLE. It has been suggested that cell-mediated immunity, ie, lymphocyte activation, may alone be able to cause platelet damage and thrombocytopenia. Lymphocyte activation has been observed in response to autologous platelets in some patients with idiopathic thrombocytopenic purpura. Whether this represents a true cellular immune response or whether the lymphocytes are reacting to immune complexes or otherwise altered platelets remains uncertain. Finally, it is known that bacterial endotoxin can cause thrombocytopenia directly, usually involving activation of the complement system. Antibodies are not required for this reaction.

Table 38–5 shows a classification of immunologic thrombocytopenias that are discussed in more detail in the following section.

IDIOPATHIC THROMBOCYTOPENIC PURPURA

Major Immunologic Features

- Antiplatelet antibodies are demonstrable on platelets and in serum.
- Platelet survival is shortened.
- There is a therapeutic response to prednisone and splenectomy.

Table 38–5. Classification of immune thrombocytopenias.

Idiopathic (autoimmune) thrombocytopenic purpura (ITP)
Secondary autoimmune thrombocytopenias
  SLE and other autoimmune disorders
  Chronic lymphocytic leukemia, lymphomas, some
    nonlymphoid malignancies
  HIV infection
  Infectious mononucleosis and some other infections
Drug-induced immune thrombocytopenias (partial list of drugs)

Acetazolamide	Imipramine
Allymid	Meprobamate
Aminosalicylic acid (PAS)	Methyldopa
Antazoline	Novobiocin
Apronalide	Phenolphthalein
Aspirin	Phenytoin
Carbamazepine	Quinidine
Cephalothin	Quinine
Chlorothiazide	Rifampin
Digitoxin	Spironolactone
Factor VIII concentrate	Stibophen
Heparin	Sulfamethazine
Hydrochlorothiazide	Thioguanine

Posttransfusion purpura
Thrombotic thrombocytopenic purpura (TTP)
Neonatal immune thrombocytopenias
  Due to autoantibodies (ITP)
  Due to alloantibodies (maternal sensitization)
Due to alloantibodies (destruction of transfused platelets)
  Sensitization from previous transfusions
  Maternal sensitization during pregnancies

General Considerations

Idiopathic thrombocytopenic purpura is an autoimmune disorder characterized by increased platelet destruction by antiplatelet autoantibody. IgG autoantibodies sensitize the circulating platelets, leading to accelerated removal of these cells by the macrophages of the spleen and at times the liver and other components of the monocyte-macrophage system. Although there is a compensatory increase in platelet production by the bone marrow (total platelet turnover may be 10–20 times the normal rate), thrombocytopenia occurs, and, depending on the severity, gives rise to the 2 typical clinical features of the disease: purpura and bleeding.

Idiopathic thrombocytopenic purpura most often occurs in otherwise healthy children and young adults. Childhood idiopathic thrombocytopenic purpura often occurs within a few weeks following a viral infection, suggesting possible cross-immunization between viral and platelet antigens, or adsorption of immune complexes, or a hapten mechanism. Adult idiopathic thrombocytopenic purpura is less often associated with a preceding infection. An identical form of autoimmune thrombocytopenia can also be associated with SLE, chronic lymphocytic leukemia, lymphomas, nonlymphoid cancers, infectious mononucleosis, and other viral and bacterial infections. Certain drugs can also cause immune thrombocytopenia, and these can produce a clinical picture that is indistinguishable from idiopathic thrombocytopenic purpura.

Although adult and childhood idiopathic thrombocytopenic purpura appear to have similar basic pathophysiologic features, there are significant differences in their course and therefore their treatment. The features of idiopathic thrombocytopenic purpura in children and adults are compared in Table 38–6. Most children have spontaneous remissions within a few weeks to a few months, and splenectomy is rarely necessary. Adult patients, on the other hand, rarely have spontaneous remissions and usually require splenectomy within the first few months after diagnosis. Idiopathic thrombocytopenic purpura has been described in many AIDS patients. It is now recognized more frequently in patients infected with HIV who have not yet had an AIDS-associated disease. This is now referred to as HIV-associated immune thrombocytopenic purpura.

Immunologic Diagnosis

Harrington and coworkers first showed in 1951 that the plasma from patients with idiopathic thrombocytopenic purpura caused thrombocytopenia when transfused into normal human recipients. Techniques to detect antiplatelet antibodies are shown in Table 38-7. The so-called immuno-injury techniques (platelet factor 3 release, ^{14}C-serotonin release) detect antiplatelet antibodies in the serum of 60–70% of adult patients with idiopathic thrombocytopenic purpura. Recent methods for detecting platelet-autoantibody complexes by lymphocyte activation or ingestion by granulocytes, or competitive binding assays or antiglobulin tests for the measurement of antiplatelet antibodies on the platelet surface have shown positive results in almost all patients with idiopathic thrombocytopenic purpura.

Platelet Kinetics

^{51}Cr-platelet kinetic studies show that all patients with idiopathic thrombocytopenic purpura and other types of autoimmune thrombocytopenia have markedly shortened platelet survival times ($t_{1/2}$ 0.1–30

Table 38–7. Tests for platelet autoantibodies in idiopathic thrombocytopenic purpura (ITP).

Method	Percent Positive
Standard immunologic tests (agglutination, complement fixation, etc)	0
Transfusion of plasma from patients with ITP into normal donors	63–75
Platelet factor 3 release	65–70
^{14}C-serotonin release	60
Lymphocyte activation by autologous platelets	70
Lymphocyte activation by platelet-antibody immune complexes	90 +
Phagocytosis of platelet-antibody immune complexes by granulocytes	90 +
Measurement of platelet-associated IgG by competitive binding assays	90 +
Radiolabeled Coombs antiglobulin test	90 +
Fluorescein-labeled Coombs antiglobulin	90 +
Enzyme-linked immunosorbent assay (ELISA)	90 +

hours; normal $t_{1/2}$ 100–120 hours) and have normal or only slightly subnormal platelet recoveries at t_0 (40–80%; normal 60–80%). About 75% of patients have splenic platelet sequestration, and 25% have both splenic and hepatic sequestration. Patients with thrombocytopenia due to an enlarged splenic platelet pool can be easily distinguished from patients with autoimmune thrombocytopenia by these kinetic methods. Although it was believed initially that determination of the sites of platelet sequestration might be useful in predicting the response to splenectomy, a recent report shows no significant difference in response rates based on presplenectomy platelet sequestration patterns. Both groups in this report had an 85–90% complete remission rate at 2 years' follow-up postsplenectomy.

Clinical Features

A. Symptoms and Signs: The onset may be acute, with sudden development of petechiae, ecchymoses, epistaxis, and gingival, gastrointestinal, or genitourinary tract bleeding. Alternatively, the disease may be gradual in onset and chronic in course. Often, however, chronic idiopathic thrombocytopenic purpura is slowly progressive or suddenly becomes acute.

B. Laboratory Findings: The platelet count is usually less than 20,000–30,000/μL in acute cases, and 30,000–100,000/μL in chronic cases. There may be moderate anemia due to blood loss and iron deficiency. The leukocyte count is normal or slightly increased but may be low in SLE. Platelets are often larger than normal on peripheral blood smear, and no immature leukocytes are present. The bone marrow shows normal or increased numbers of megakaryocytes and is otherwise normal. The megakaryocytes may be normal or immature in appearance but at times are larger than normal with increased numbers of nuclei.

Table 38–6. Idiopathic thrombocytopenic purpura in children and adults

Parameter	Children	Adults
Peak age incidence (yr)	2–6	20–30
Sex incidence (M:F)	1:1	1:3
Clinical onset	Acute	Gradual
Antecedent infection	Common	Uncommon
Average duration of disease	1 month	Months to years
Spontaneous remission	90%	10–20%
Presenting platelet count	< 20 × 10⁹/L	(30–50) × 10⁹/L

Differential Diagnosis

All causes of thrombocytopenia must be considered when evaluating a patient with suspected idiopathic thrombocytopenic purpura (Table 38–8). Patients with idiopathic thrombocytopenic purpura characteristically feel and look well, and all physical and laboratory findings are normal except for thrombocytopenia and the associated purpura and possible bleeding. Patients with "consumptive" thrombocytopenias, on the other hand, tend to be acutely ill, often with fever and evidence of multisystem disease, especially renal disease. These patients generally have microangiopathic hemolytic anemia, the fragmented erythrocytes being a critical diagnostic finding on the peripheral blood smear. Abnormalities of clotting function are also often present. Patients with acute leukemia, aplastic anemia, and other serious bone marrow disorders are also often acutely ill, and bone marrow examination is diagnostic. Patients with hypersplenism sufficient to cause thrombocytopenia usually have an easily palpable spleen; hypersplenism alone rarely causes a platelet count of less than 50,000/μL.

Secondary causes of autoimmune thrombocytopenia, such as SLE, must be ruled out by appropriate laboratory tests. If a patient with apparent idiopathic thrombocytopenic purpura has been taking any suspicious drugs, the possibility of drug-induced thrombocytopenia must be considered. In some areas, HIV-associated disease is now the most common cause of thrombocytopenic purpura, especially in males between 20 and 50 years of age. Testing for antibodies to HIV is an essential part of the assessment of idiopathic thrombocytopenic purpura.

Table 38–8. Differential diagnosis of thrombocytopenic purpuras.

Thrombocytopenias due to increased platelet destruction
  Immune thrombocytopenias
    Idiopathic thrombocytopenic purpura
    Secondary autoimmune thrombocytopenias
    Drug-induced immune thrombocytopenias
    Posttransfusion purpura
    Neonatal immune thrombocytopenias
    Thrombocytopenia due to use of factor VIII concentrate
    HIV infection
  Consumptive thrombocytopenias
    Thrombotic thrombocytopenic purpura
    Hemolytic-uremic syndrome
    Disseminated intravascular coagulation
    Vasculitis
    Sepsis
  Hypersplenism
Thrombocytopenias due to decreased platelet production
  Bone marrow suppression by drugs, alcohol, toxins, infections
  Aplastic anemia
  Leukemias and other bone marrow cancers
  Megaloblastic anemia
  Refractory anemias, preleukemia, hematopoietic dysplasia

Treatment

Splenectomy is the treatment of choice for adult patients with idiopathic thrombocytopenic purpura who have persistent symptomatic thrombocytopenia. Corticosteroids are usually able to increase the platelet count temporarily but probably do not alter the course of the underlying disease, and most patients relapse when steroid use is tapered or discontinued. Adults rarely have spontaneous remissions. Splenectomy is therefore usually necessary in adults with idiopathic thrombocytopenic purpura within the first few months after diagnosis. Large doses of steroids over long periods should be avoided in these patients, as 75–90% will have prolonged complete remissions following splenectomy. Immunosuppressive therapy with cytotoxic drugs should generally not be used until the patient has had the benefit of splenectomy; this is particularly true for younger patients, since these drugs may cause serious late adverse effects.

Vincristine seems to be a valuable agent in patients with autoimmune thrombocytopenia who do not respond to splenectomy, who relapse after an initial response to splenectomy, or in whom the risk of splenectomy is unacceptable. A significant increase in platelet count occurs in 70–80% of patients with refractory autoimmune thrombocytopenia treated with vincristine. Vincristine appears to be more effective, less toxic, and better tolerated than cyclophosphamide or other standard immunosuppressive drugs. Its mechanism of action in increasing the platelet count in autoimmune thrombocytopenia remains uncertain; it appears to work by a different mechanism from other immunosuppressive drugs. Other therapeutic modalities include intravenous immunoglobulin. Intravenous gamma globulin (IVGG) may be used as a short-term measure in adults prior to splenectomy, if corticosteroid has failed to maintain a satisfactory platelet count at an acceptable dose. IVGG is also used in patients with HIV-associated immune thrombocytopenic purpura, prior to splenectomy, where one would prefer not to use long-term immunosuppressive and cytotoxic therapy. More recently, the antiviral agent zidovudine (AZT) has been reported as effective in raising platelet counts in patients with HIV-associated immune thrombocytopenic purpura.

Children with mild or moderately severe idiopathic thrombocytopenic purpura should be observed without therapy. In children who require active treatment, IVGG is the treatment of choice. A 5-day course of 400 mg/kg/d is given. Many patients respond for only a short time, and repeat courses may be necessary. Corticosteroids may be given when severe thrombocytopenia and bleeding occur, although the platelet count does not respond as consistently to steroids in children as in adults. Splenectomy should be considered in children only when severe thrombocytopenia persists for 3–6 months, since most children will have had a spontaneous remission by that time. The postsplenectomy state is much more likely to predispose to serious or overwhelming infection in young children than in adults. Immunosuppressive drugs should generally not be used in children.

DRUG-INDUCED IMMUNE THROMBOCYTOPENIAS

The principal drugs that may cause immune thrombocytopenic purpura are listed in Table 38–5. The best-studied example was the sedative apronalide (Sedormid) (no longer in use); the drugs most commonly used in clinical practice that can produce immune thrombocytopenic purpura are sulfonamides, thiazide diuretics, chlorpropamide, quinidine, heparin, and gold. A syndrome resembling acute drug-induced immune thrombocytopenia has also been observed in heroin addicts, although the mechanism of this kind of thrombocytopenia has not been proved. Further reports have confirmed the increasing frequency of the heparin-induced thrombosis thrombocytopenia syndrome. This unusual combination includes clinical features of hemorrhagic tendencies due to development of thrombocytopenia in patients treated with heparin for thrombosis. It appears that the heparin-dependent IgG-class antibody induces thromboxane synthesis and aggregation of the platelets.

There is a variable period of sensitization after initial exposure to the drug, but subsequent drug reexposure is rapidly followed by thrombocytopenia. Patients therefore usually give a history of having taken the drug in the past for at least several weeks if this is their first exposure. A very small plasma concentration of the drug and very small amounts of antibody may induce severe thrombocytopenia. The drug itself generally shows only weak and reversible binding to the platelet; the thrombocytopenia in most cases appears to be caused by adsorption of the drug-antibody complexes to the platelet membrane with complement activation.

Treatment consists mainly of withdrawal of the offending drug (or all drugs) and monitoring for return of normal platelet counts, generally within 7–10 days. Thrombocytopenia may persist if the drug is excreted slowly. When a patient who is taking a number of suspicious drugs is first seen, it is often impossible to tell whether the patient has drug-induced immune thrombocytopenia or idiopathic thrombocytopenic purpura. In vitro tests can now be used in some centers to confirm drug-antibody reactions involving platelets. In vivo drug challenges of sensitized patients for confirmation of drug-induced immune thrombocytopenia should be avoided, since they are too hazardous.

POSTTRANSFUSION PURPURA

There are 2 types of posttransfusion purpura. The first is due to dilution and occurs during massive blood replacement, as in the treatment of hemorrhage and shock. Further bleeding from the dilutional thrombocytopenia may complicate clinical management. The second type, which is due to alloantibodies, is an acute severe thrombocytopenic state appearing about 1 week after transfusion of a blood product. It occurs almost exclusively in women. It is mediated by an alloantibody, usually directed against the platelet PL_A^1 antigen. Platelets both with and without the PL_A^1 antigen are destroyed.

The diagnosis is suspected when acute thrombocytopenia occurs 7–10 days after blood transfusion. Coagulation studies are normal, and the bone marrow shows abundant megakaryocytes. The anti-PL_A^1 antibody is detected in the plasma.

Gradual recovery from posttransfusion purpura usually occurs in 1–6 weeks. Corticosteroids do not appear to alter the course of the disease. Massive exchange transfusions have been associated with more rapid recovery, but severe transfusion reactions often occur. Aggressive plasma exchange has also been shown to be effective without the risks of severe transfusion reactions.

COAGULATION DISORDERS

HEMOPHILIA & VON WILLEBRAND'S DISEASE

Classic hemophilia and von Willebrand's disease are both congenital bleeding disorders caused by abnormalities of the factor VIII molecule complex. Hemophilia is an X-linked disorder characterized by severe deficiency of factor VIII procoagulant activity (VIII:C), which is measured in clotting assays. Von Willebrand's disease is an autosomally inherited disorder also characterized by a deficiency of VIII:C, but it is also associated with defective platelet function, resulting in a prolonged bleeding time. The abnormal platelet function in von Willebrand's disease is due to a deficiency of factor VIII-related protein (VIIIR), which is also known as von Willebrand factor (vWF). vWF activity is measured by testing the ability of plasma to support platelet agglutination by the antibiotic ristocetin or ristocetin cofactor (VIIIR:RC) activity. The gene for factor VIII is located near the tip of the long arm of the X chromosome (Xq 2.8/Ter).

Heterogeneous antibodies made to purified factor VIII detect antigenic determinants on VIIIR (VIIIR:Ag). VIIIR:Ag has been found to be normal in patients with classic hemophilia, indicating that these patients have a normal amount of the basic factor VIII molecule but that they lack the portion of the molecule necessary for normal procoagulant activity. The heterologous antibodies therefore appear to recognize antigenic determinants distinct from the functional site responsible for procoagulant activity. Patients with von Willebrand's disease, on the other hand, have reduced levels of both VIII:C and VIIIR:Ag, indicating a true deficiency of factor VIII complex molecules. Measurement of VIII:C and VIIIR:Ag can therefore be used to differentiate between classic hemophilia and von Willebrand's disease and in most cases can differentiate between female carriers of hemophilia (heterozygotes) and normal individuals. Measurement of ristocetin cofactor (VIIIR:RC) can also be used to identify patients with von Willebrand's disease. Studies with antibodies have helped to clarify the relationships of the factor VIII complex. More recently, studies with molecular genetics have clarified carrier detection and inheritance patterns.

Human antibodies to factor VIII, unlike heterologous antibodies, are usually directed at antigenic determinants at the functional procoagulant site of factor VIII (VIII:CAg), and these antibodies are capable of blocking factor VIII clotting activity. These antibodies sometimes develop in patients with severe hemophilia after they have been transfused with factor VIII-containing blood products and sometimes develop spontaneously in otherwise healthy individuals. When present in high titer, they cause a severe hemorrhagic disorder that is difficult to correct with factor VIII transfusions, since the transfused factor VIII is simply inactivated by the factor VIII antibodies (see next section).

Many hemophiliacs treated in the early 1980s with factor VIII concentrate have developed AIDS, and approximately 1% of confirmed AIDS patients are hemophiliacs. AIDS is now the most common cause of death in hemophiliacs. Centers have switched from treating the hemophiliac with factor VIII concentrate derived from large donor pools back to using cryoprecipitate derived from a single donor. Infectivity can be abolished by heating the preparation.

It is hoped that in the future, recombinant engineered factor VIII will be available to overcome problems with supply, purity, and cross-infection.

CIRCULATING INHIBITORS OF COAGULATION

Abnormal bleeding is occasionally due to circulating inhibitors that block one or more plasma coagu-

lation factors. These inhibitors, also called endogenous circulating anticoagulants, have in most cases been shown to be IgG antibodies. Inhibitors against factor VIII and against the prothrombin activator complex (''lupus inhibitor'') occur most often, but inhibitors directed against factors V, IX, XIII, and vWF have also been reported. There are rare reports of human monoclonal proteins (especially IgM) with antibody activity directed against clotting components, eg, factor VIII, phospholipid. Inhibitors may appear abruptly and be associated with life-threatening hemorrhage or may be chronic and associated with little or no bleeding.

Factor VIII inhibitors develop in 5–20% of patients with classic hemophilia after they have been transfused with factor VIII-containing blood products; genetic factors appear to determine which patients develop inhibitors. Factor VIII inhibitors also occasionally occur spontaneously in women postpartum, in patients with autoimmune disorders such as SLE, and in older patients without demonstrable underlying disease. Rarely, the paraprotein in a monoclonal gammopathy has specific inhibitor activity against factor VIII or other clotting factors.

High-titer factor VIII inhibitors (antibodies) often cause serious bleeding and require aggressive treatment. Patients with serious bleeding can be given several times the calculated amount of factor VIII to saturate the inhibitor, provided the inhibitor titer is not too high. When bleeding cannot be stopped, even after giving large amounts of factor VIII, activated prothrombin complex concentrates should be given, as these will often stop the bleeding by providing activated clotting factors which bypass the factor VIII step. If this is unsuccessful, aggressive large-volume plasma exchange can be used to remove the inhibitor.

A recent study found that combination therapy with factor VIII, cyclophosphamide, vincristine, and prednisone (CVP) was highly effective in the eradication of factor VIII inhibitors in nonhemophiliacs, but not in hemophiliacs.

Anticardiolipin Antibody (Lupus Anticoagulant)

The lupus anticoagulant was so named because of its initial identification in association with SLE, but the term has turned out to be a slight misnomer. The lupus anticoagulant appears to be an IgG anticardiolipin antibody, explaining false-positive syphilis screening serologic tests. Anticardiolipin antibody should be suspected in patients with a prolongation of the partial thromboplastin time, but it is associated only with classic SLE in a minority of patients and is not associated with an in vivo hemostatic defect. Paradoxically, the lupus anticoagulant is associated with a venous and arterial thrombotic tendency. A distinct syndrome has been identified in recent years, with recurrent arterial and venous thrombosis, recurrent abortion due to placental infarction, and thrombocytopenia. Venous thrombosis may occur in unusual sites, such as hepatic, renal, retinal, and mesenteric veins. Classic SLE serologic tests in this group of patients are often negative. Specialized tests are necessary to further categorize this unusual hemostatic defect.

Recently, circulating coagulation inhibitors similar to lupus anticoagulant were reported in AIDS patients with active opportunistic infections. The inhibitors tended to disappear with successful resolution of the infection.

REFERENCES

Leukopenias

Blumfelder TM, Logue GL, Shimm DS: Felty's syndrome: Effects of splenectomy upon granulocyte count and granulocyte-associated IgG. *Ann Intern Med* 1981; **94:**623.

Cines DB et al: Granulocyte-associated IgG in neutropenic disorders. *Blood* 1982;**59:**124.

Goldman JM: Granulocytes, monocytes, and their benign disorders. Chapter 11 in: *Postgraduate Haematology.* Hoffbrand AV, Lewis SM (editors). Heinemann, 1989.

Levitt LJ, Ries CA, Greenberg PL: Pure white-cell aplasia: Antibody-mediated autoimmune inhibition of granulopoiesis. *N Engl J Med* 1983;**308:**1141.

Lieschke GJ et al: Effects of bacterially synthesized recombinant human granulocyte-macrophage colony-stimulating factor in patients with advanced malignancy. *Ann Intern Med* 1989;**110:**357.

Minchinton RM, Waters AH: The occurrence and significance of neutrophil antibodies. *Br J Haematol* 1984; **56:**521.

Negrin RS: Treatment of myelodysplastic syndromes with recombinant human granulocyte colony-stimulating factor. *Ann Intern Med* 1989;**110:**976.

Sieff CA: Hemopoietic growth factors. *J Clin Invest* 1987;**79:**1549.

Erythrocyte Disorders

Beal RW, Isbister JP: *Blood Component Therapy in Clinical Practice.* Blackwell, 1985.

Camitta BM, Storb R, Thomas ED: Aplastic anemia. (2 parts.) *N Engl J Med* 1982;**306:**645, 712.

Dessypris EN et al: Mode of action of the IgG inhibitor of erythropoiesis in transient erythroblastopenia of childhood. *Blood* 1982;**59:**114.

Engelfriet CP, Van Loghem JJ, Von Dem Borne AEGK: *Immunohaematology.* Elsevier, 1984.

Gale RP et al: Aplastic anemia: Biology and treatment. *Ann Intern Med* 1981;**95:**477.

Gordon-Smith EC, Hows J: Acquired haemolytic anaemias. Chapter 7 in: *Postgraduate Haematology.* Hoffbrand AV, Lewis SM (editors). Heinemann, 1989.

Marsh JCW et al: Survival after antilymphocyte globulin therapy for aplastic anemia depends on disease severity. *Blood* 1987;**70:**1046.

Petz LD, Garratty G: *Acquired Immune Hemolytic Anemias.* Churchill Livingstone, 1980.

Queenan JT: Current management of the Rh-sensitized patient. *Clin Obstet Gynecol* 1982;**25:**293.

Rosse WF, Parker CJ: Paroxysmal nocturnal hemoglobinuria. *Clin Hematol* 1985;**14:**105.

Rote NS: Pathophysiology of Rh isoimmunization. *Clin Obstet Gynecol* 1982;**25:**243.

Vincent PC: Haemopoietic inhibitors in aplastic anemia: A review. *Pathology* 1982;**14:**25.

Platelet Disorders

Abrams DI et al: Antibodies to human T-lymphotropic virus type III and development of acquired immunodeficiency syndrome in homosexual men presenting with immune thrombocytopenia. *Ann Intern Med* 1986;**104:**47.

Bussel JB, Hilgartner MW: The use and mechanism of action of intravenous immunoglobulin in the treatment of immune haematologic disease. *Br J Haematol* 1984;**56:**1.

Chong BH et al: Heparin-induced thrombocytopenia: Association of thrombotic complications with heparin-dependent IgG antibody that induces thromboxane synthesis and platelet aggregation. *Lancet* 1982;**2:**1246.

Firkin BG: *The Platelet and Its Disorders.* MTP Press, 1984.

Hardisty RM: Platelet disorders. Chapter 22 in: *Postgraduate Haematology.* Hoffbrand AV, Lewis SM (editors). Heinemann, 1989.

Karpatkin S: Autoimmune thrombocytopenic purpura. *Semin Hematol* 1985;**22:**260.

Karpatkin S, Nardi MA, Hymes KB: Immunologic thrombocytopenic purpura after heterosexual transmission of human immunodeficiency virus (HIV). *Ann Intern Med* 1988;**109:**190.

Kelton JG: The measurement of platelet-bound immunoglobulins: An overview of the methods and the biological relevance of platelet-associated IgG. *Prog Hematol* 1983;**13:**163.

Leaf AN et al: Thrombotic thrombocytopenic purpura associated with human immunodeficiency virus type 1 (HIV-1) infection. *Ann Intern Med* 1988;**109:**194.

Oksenhendler E et al: Zidovudine for thrombocytopenic purpura related to human immunodeficiency virus (HIV) infection. *Ann Intern Med* 1989;**110:**365.

Ratnoff OD: Coincident classic hemophilia and "idiopathic" thrombocytopenic purpura in patients under treatment with concentrates of antihemophilic factor (factor VIII). *N Engl J Med* 1983;**308:**439.

Coagulation Disorders

Cohen AJ, Philips TM, Kessler CM: Circulating coagulation inhibitions in the acquired immunodeficiency syndrome. *Ann Intern Med* 1986;**104:**175.

DeShazo RD et al: An immunologic evaluation of hemophiliac patients and their wives: Relationships to the acquired immunodeficiency syndrome. *Ann Intern Med* 1983;**99**:159.

Eyster ME et al: Long term follow-up of hemophiliacs with lymphocytopenia or thrombocytopenia. *Blood* 1985; **66**:1317.

Gastineau DA et al: Lupus anticoagulant: An analysis of the clinical and laboratory features of 219 cases. *Am J Hematol* 1985;**19**:265.

Lederman MM et al: Impaired cell-mediated immunity in patients with classic hemophilia. *N Engl J Med* 1983;**308**:79.

Lian ECY, Larcada AF, Chiu AYZ: Combination immunosuppressive therapy after factor VIII infusion for acquired factor VIII inhibitor. *Ann Intern Med* 1989; **110**:774.

Lottenberg R, Kentro TB, Kitchens CS: Acquired hemophilia. A natural history study of 16 patients with factor VIII inhibitors receiving little or no therapy. *Arch Intern Med* 1987;**147**:1077.

Slocombe GW et al: The role of intensive plasma exchange in the prevention and management of haemorrhage in patients with inhibitors to factor VIII. *Br J Haematol* 1981;**47**:577.

39

Cardiac & Vascular Diseases

Thomas R. Cupps, MD

CARDIAC DISEASES

A variety of immunologic diseases probably involve cardiac tissues without causing any clinically relevant effects; nevertheless, there are several recognized syndromes characterized by clinically significant immune-mediated damage of the pericardium, myocardium, and endocardium.

PERICARDIAL DISEASES

Relapsing Pericarditis

This is a disease of unknown cause, characterized by chronic recurrent episodes of pericardial inflammation. Other disease processes associated with pericarditis, including infection, neoplasm, and collagen vascular disease, should be actively excluded. Chest pain and shortness of breath with or without pericardial effusion make up the characteristic pattern during an episode of pericarditis. Complications including pericardial tamponade, hemopericardium, and constrictive pericarditis have been reported. Nonsteroidal anti-inflammatory drugs, such as indomethacin and ibuprofen, constitute the initial form of treatment. Some patients with relapsing pericarditis develop a chronic pattern, which requires treatment with corticosteroids. A subset of these patients may become corticosteroid-dependent, requiring prolonged suppressive treatment. Pericardiectomy may be considered in patients who cannot be successfully treated medically.

An immunologic pathogenesis for this disease is presumed, largely on the basis of histopathology, which includes infiltration by acute and chronic inflammatory cells and fibrin deposition.

Postinfarction Syndrome & Postpericardiotomy Syndrome

Pericardial inflammation also occurs following damage to cardiac tissue after myocardial infarction, cardiac surgery, or trauma. Postinfarction (Dressler's) syndrome is characterized by chest pain, profound malaise, fever, pericardial inflammation and effusion, leukocytosis with or without pleural effusion, pulmonary infiltrates, arthralgia, or transient arthritis that develops 2–3 weeks following surgical or traumatic opening of the pericardium. The presence of myocyte antibodies detected by immunofluorescence and rising titers of antiviral antibodies suggests that these syndromes may be associated with a concurrent or reactivated viral illness triggering the immunologic response that produces the characteristic clinical syndrome. Increasing titers of antibodies to coxsackie-virus type B, cytomegalovirus, and adenovirus occur frequently. The response is therefore not limited to a particular type of virus. The postinfarction syndrome occurs in 3% or fewer of patients with myocardial infarction. The presence of a pericardial friction rub during the first several days postinfarction increases the likelihood of developing the syndrome. The postpericardiotomy syndrome occurs in approximately 25% of patients following surgical intervention or blunt trauma to the heart. Rare complications include pericardial tamponade and restrictive pericarditis. Nonsteroidal anti-inflammatory agents will suppress the clinical symptoms in most cases. A brief course of corticosteroid therapy may be required in the more severe cases. These syndromes generally run a self-limited course lasting several weeks to several months.

MYOCARDIAL DISEASES

Autoimmune Myocarditis

This is a rare disease characterized by an aberrant immune response that damages myocardial tissue and is generally seen as part of a systemic autoimmune syndrome. Autoimmune myocarditis is associated most commonly with polymyositis-dermatomyositis and systemic lupus erythematosus (SLE) and less commonly with rheumatoid arthritis, scleroderma, mixed connective tissue disease, and sarcoidosis. Little is known about the etiology of autoimmune myocarditis. The presence of mononuclear cell infiltrates in the myocardium and the association with immunologically mediated diseases suggest an autoimmune pathogenesis. Autoimmune myocarditis may present with signs and symptoms of congestive heart failure, arrhythmias, or conduction abnormalities. Chest pain from an associated pericarditis may also be present. Findings on chest radiograph, echocardiogram, and electrocardiogram may reflect diffuse myocardial dysfunction and rhythm or conduction abnormalities. Other laboratory studies may suggest the diagnosis of an associated autoimmune disease. There is an increased occurrence of the anti-ribonucleoprotein (RNP) autoantibody in patients with SLE who develop autoimmune myocarditis. Autoimmune myocarditis generally responds rapidly and dramatically to corticosteroid therapy. The outlook is generally favorable, with the patient's prognosis being determined by the underlying disease.

Autoimmune myocarditis is differentiated clinically from viral myocarditis by its association with SLE, rheumatoid arthritis, myositis, and, less commonly, scleroderma. Favorable response to immunosuppressive and anti-inflammatory treatment is also a distinguishing feature. However, the histopathology of mononuclear cell infiltration in autoimmune and viral pericarditis is identical.

Dilated Cardiomyopathy

A subset of patients with dilated cardiomyopathy may have a component of myocarditis. This disease is associated with low cardiac output and ejection fraction, in contrast to the hypertrophic and restrictive forms of cardiomyopathy. Transvenous endomyocardial biopsy studies in patients with nonischemic dilated cardiomyopathy demonstrate a 15–25% prevalence of myocarditis. The clinical presentation, including signs and symptoms associated with congestive heart failure, rhythm, and conduction disturbances, is similar whether or not myocarditis is present. Treatment with immunosuppressive drugs including corticosteroids may result in a short-term improvement in myocardial function but does not appear to alter the long-term prognosis. The role of chronic immunosuppressive therapy in dilated cardiomyopathy remains to be defined. Treatment is directed at the underlying congestive heart failure. The prognosis is guarded and is associated with the cardiac functional status. Selected patients may be considered for cardiac transplantation.

ENDOMYOCARDIAL DISEASES

The association of eosinophilia with endomyocardial fibrosis is recognized in a number of clinical syndromes including **tropical endomyocardial fibrosis, Löffler's endomyocardial disease, eosinophilic leukemia,** and the **hypereosinophilic syndrome.** It has been suggested that these clinical entities may represent a spectrum of a single disease process. Morphologic abnormalities of eosinophils include decreased numbers of crystalloid granules, vacuolation, and hypersegmentation. Presumably,

aberrant tissue invasion and inappropriate degranulation of the eosinophils result in the endomyocardial pathology, which involves both ventricles. Three stages of the disease are recognized: (1) an acute stage with infiltration of eosinophils and myocytolysis; (2) an intermediate thrombotic stage, in which a thickened endocardium is covered by thrombus; and (3) a fibrotic stage, in which dense fibrosis occurs in the endocardium and myocardium. An immunologic pathogenesis is presumed because of the eosinophilia. In these conditions there is a marked tendency for clot formation with fibrosis on resolution of the clots, and it is possible that the eosinophilia is secondary to this process.

The clinical presentation is that of a restrictive cardiomyopathy with a pattern of biventricular involvement. Emboli from intraventricular thrombi may be a prominent clinical component of the disease. Therapy is directed at the management of the cardiac dysfunction and thromboembolic complications. Treatment with prednisone and hydroxyurea may benefit patients with hypereosinophilic syndrome. Surgical intervention (endomyocardiectomy, thrombectomy, or valve replacement) may benefit carefully selected patients. Despite therapeutic intervention, the prognosis remains guarded.

VASCULAR DISEASES: THE VASCULITIDES

Vasculitis is defined as a clinicopathologic process characterized by inflammation and necrosis of blood vessels. The clinical spectrum ranges from a primary disease involving exclusively blood vessels to an involvement of vessels as a relatively insignificant component of another systemic disease. Because vasculitis can potentially involve any blood vessel, a complex and often confusing array of clinical syndromes results (Table 39–1). The vasculitides are a heterogeneous group of clinical syndromes, and therefore no single cause explains the pathophysiology of all of the inflammatory vessel diseases. The best-characterized mechanism is immune complex-mediated vasculitis. The elements necessary for the expression of this process include (1) soluble immune complexes larger than 19S formed in slight antigen excess, (2) increased vascular permeability with passive deposition of complexes in the vessel wall, (3) activation of complement with subsequent attraction of polymorphonuclear neutrophils (PMN) to the site of immune-complex deposition, and (4) release of inflammatory mediators and disruption of vascular integrity. Other potential mechanisms are less well established. Aberrant regulation of T cell,

Table 39–1. Classification of the vasculitides.

Systemic necrotizing vasculitis
Polyarteritis nodosa
Allergic angiitis and granulomatosis
"Polyangiitis overlap syndrome"
Associated diseases (connective-tissue diseases, hepatitis B, cytomegalovirus infection, hairy cell leukemia)

Small-vessel (hypersensitivity) vasculitis
Henoch-Schönlein purpura
Serum sickness
Other drug-related vasculitides
Vasculitis associated with food, foreign protein, or other exogenous antigens
Vasculitis associated with a systemic disease (Table 39–2)
Hypocomplementemic urticarial vasculitis
Congenital deficiencies of the complement system
Erythema elevatum diutinum

Behçet's disease

Wegener's granulomatosis

Arteritis of larger arteries
Temporal (cranial) arteritis
Takayasu's arteritis
Large-artery arteritis-complicating diseases such as ankylosing spondylitis, Reiter's syndrome, relapsing polychondritis, and Cogan's syndrome
Aortitis-associated syphilis

Thromboangiitis obliterans (Buerger's disease)

Isolated angiitis of the central nervous system

Mucocutaneous lymph node syndrome (Kawasaki's disease)

Miscellaneous vasculitis syndromes

B cell, monocyte-macrophage and endothelial cell function may be important in some of the vasculitides. Other factors that determine disease activity include the class of blood vessel affected, the pattern of organ system involvement, and the relative sensitivity of involved tissue to the effects of ischemia. These are important in defining the clinical manifestations of the different vasculitic syndromes. With the exception of the small vessel (hypersensitivity) vasculitis, the vasculitides are relatively rare syndromes.

SMALL-VESSEL (HYPERSENSITIVITY) VASCULITIS

Major Immunologic Features
- Small vessels undergo inflammation.
- It is an immune complex-mediated process.

General Considerations
Small-vessel vasculitis, which includes a heterogeneous group of clinical syndromes, is characterized by inflammation of arterioles, capillaries, and venules. The most commonly involved vessel is the venule, producing a venulitis. Skin involvement is characteristic of small-vessel vasculitis, although any organ system can be affected. Immune-complex deposition is an important mechanism in at least a subset of cases of small-vessel vasculitis. A variety of agents have been suggested as causal factors in hypersensitivity vasculitis; these include (1) microorganisms (bacteria, mycobacteria, viruses, and parasites), (2) foreign proteins (animal serum and monoclonal antibodies), (3) chemicals (insecticides, herbicides, and petroleum products), and (4) drugs (antibiotics, antihypertensives, antiarrhythmics, nonsteroidal anti-inflammatory drugs, antirheumatic drugs, and others). The chemicals and drugs are presumed to function as haptens, binding covalently to unknown host carrier molecules and thereby eliciting an immune response. Small-vessel vasculitis can also occur in association with a wide variety of systemic diseases. It most commonly occurs in the fifth decade of life, with a slight female predominance.

Pathology
The most common histologic pattern is a neutrophilic leukocyte infiltrate of the postcapillary venules with leukocytoclasis (presence of nuclear debris), fibrinoid necrosis, endothelial swelling, and disruption of vascular integrity (Fig 39–1). Patterns of mixed acute and chronic inflammatory infiltrates, as well as a chronic infiltrate composed predominantly of lymphocytes, are also recognized.

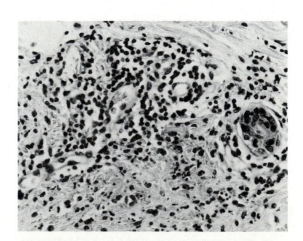

Figure 39–1. Skin biopsy from a patient with hypersensitivity vasculitis. A venulitis with a mixed cellular infiltrate is seen. A mononuclear-cell infiltrate around a venule is present in one area of the biopsy, while a neutrophil infiltrate with early leukocytoclasis (presence of nuclear debris) is seen in an adjacent area. Hematoxylin and eosin stain. (Original magnification × 330.) (Reproduced, with permission, from Cupps TR, Fauci AS: The vasculitides. In: *Major Problems in Internal Medicine.* Vol 21. Smith LH [editor]. Saunders, 1981.)

Clinical Features

A nonblanching palpable purpuric lesion (palpable purpura) is characteristic. Other associated skin findings include papular, petechial, and ulcerative lesions. The lesions tend to recur in crops varying in number from a few to more than a 100. Each crop resolves over 2–4 weeks. The lesions have a symmetric distribution and are most often found in dependent areas, particularly the distal lower extremities. Vasculitis produces pain, a burning sensation, or dependent edema in up to 40% of patients. Evidence of joint, kidney, lung, gastrointestinal, or peripheral nervous system involvement is present in the minority of cases.

Immunologic Diagnosis

No specific laboratory test is diagnostic for small-vessel vasculitis. The following tests may or may not be abnormal: sedimentation rate, cryoglobulins, immune complexes, rheumatoid factor, and serum complement levels. A biopsy of a newly developing skin lesion should establish the diagnosis.

Differential Diagnosis

Once the diagnosis of small-vessel vasculitis is established, the patient should be evaluated for evidence of visceral involvement or an associated underlying disease process.

Treatment

Treatment should be directed at eliminating any inciting agent or treating any underlying systemic disease. A brief course of corticosteroid therapy or period of bed rest may expedite the resolution of an acute flare. Lengthy regimens of high-dose or split-dose daily corticosteroid treatment should be avoided. Analgesics may be required for symptomatic relief.

Complications & Prognosis

With rare exceptions, small-vessel vasculitis does not progress to life-threatening complications. The disease may be self-limited or, less commonly, develop a chronic recurrent pattern.

SYNDROMES ASSOCIATED WITH SMALL-VESSEL VASCULITIS

Several subgroups of hypersensitivity vasculitis have distinctive clinicopathologic patterns and are considered separate syndromes. In clinical practice these subsets may overlap. In this section the unique features of Henoch-Schönlein purpura, Behçet's disease, urticarial vasculitis, and small-vessel vasculitis associated with systemic disease processes are reviewed.

1. HENOCH-SCHÖNLEIN PURPURA

This syndrome, a distinctive subset of the small-vessel vasculitides, is characterized by the nonthrombocytopenia purpuric skin lesions, arthralgias, colicky abdominal pain with bleeding, and renal disease. It is the systemic form of small-vessel vasculitis. Deposition of IgA containing immune complexes with activation of the alternative complement pathway may be an important pathophysiologic mechanism. The majority of patients have symptoms of an upper respiratory tract infection prior to the onset of their disease. Other suspected causes including drugs (antibiotics and thiazides), foods (milk, fish, eggs, rice, nuts, beans, and others), and immunizations may appear to precipitate the disease clinically. There is a slight male predominance. The peak age of onset is between the ages of 4 and 7 years, although the disease does occur in adults. The disease has a seasonal variation, with the peak incidence reported in spring. The histopathology is a diffuse leukocytoclastic vasculitis involving small vessels of any involved organ system. In the bowel, hemorrhage may occur in the submucosal surface or subserosal areas. The kidneys show focal or diffuse glomerulonephritis. The clinical manifestation varies with age. In children, symptoms localized to skin, gut, and joints predominate. In adults, the disease presents predominantly with skin findings, whereas initial complaints related to the gastrointestinal tract or joints are present in fewer than one-quarter of patients. The cutaneous lesion of Henoch-Schönlein purpura evolves through the following phases: (1) an initial small urticarial lesion that may be pruritic; (2) a pink maculopapular spot that develops over several hours; (3) maturation of this spot to a raised, darkened lesion; (4) progression the following day to a 0.5–2-cm maculopapular lesion which, in some cases, may become a confluent patch; and (5) final resolution in 2 weeks without scarring. Arthralgias without synovitis tend to follow a migratory pattern involving most commonly the large joints of the lower extremities. Abdominal symptoms including colicky pain, nausea, vomiting, and blood loss are present in the majority of patients. Life-threatening gastrointestinal tract problems such as major bleeding, bowel perforation, or intussusception are present in fewer than 5% of patients. The most common form of intussusception is ileoileal. The mean age of patients with this complication is 6 years, although intussusception has been reported in young adults. Clinically, the diagnosis of intussusception is suggested in a patient with a worsening clinical course, an unchanging abdominal mass, bright-red rectal bleeding, and the clinical pattern of complete bowel obstruction. Kidney involvement is characteristically very mild, although a few patients may develop progressive renal failure. Radiographic studies of the bowel may be useful in diagnosing an intussusception. IgA containing immune complexes may be present. These complexes, however, are not pathognomonic and are not detected by C1q assay, although the Raji cell assay may be positive. A skin biopsy will establish the vasculitic nature of the process, and immunofluorescence showing IgA deposition in vessel walls will further support the diagnosis of Henoch-Schönlein purpura.

The differential diagnosis for a patient presenting with rash, abdominal pain, and joint symptoms includes, in part, inflammatory bowel disease, *Yersinia* enterocolitis, meningococcemia, Rocky Mountain spotted fever, rheumatic fever, and viral infections. The disease usually resolves spontaneously after one or more recurrent episodes; consequently, the prognosis of even untreated patients is excellent. Therapy consists of supportive care and symptomatic relief. Timely surgical intervention may be required for the rare patients with life-threatening bowel complications. In the small number of patients with renal involvement with progressive functional impairment, corticosteroid therapy may be required.

2. BEHÇET'S DISEASE

Behçet's disease is characterized by recurrent episodes of oral ulcers, eye lesions, genital ulcers, thrombophlebitis, and other cutaneous lesions. The characteristic pathologic lesion is a venulitis, although vessels of any size in any organ system can be affected.

The primary lesion is a small-vessel vasculitis, presumably reflecting an antibody- or T cell-mediated response, although no antigenic epitope has yet been identified as a cause. Serum complement levels are normal, but circulating immune complexes may be present. There are studies showing complement deposition in lesions, but it is not known whether this is a primary or secondary event.

The oral lesions begin as raised erythematous areas with progression to shallow, punched-out lesions with yellow necrotic bases. These are discussed further in Chapter 40. The genital ulcers have similar appearance and follow a similar time course. Ocular involvement is most frequently observed in the anterior chamber, with iridocyclitis and hypopyon, which generally resolve without long-term complications. Involvement of the posterior structures is less frequent, but recurrent episodes over several years may lead to impaired vision. Renal, cardiovascular, and gastrointestinal tract involvement occurs in a minority of patients. In the absence of central nervous system or bowel involvement, the prognosis is good. No drug is uniformly successful in the treatment of Behçet's disease, but favorable results have been reported with indomethacin, colchicine, levamisole, corticosteroids, and cytotoxic agents. The need for early aggressive therapy of central nervous system disease has been emphasized.

3. HYPOCOMPLEMENTEMIC URTICARIAL VASCULITIS

This disease is a clinicopathologic entity characterized by a reduction of the early complement components in serum, persistent urticaria, and a pattern of leukocytoclastic vasculitis. Characteristically, there is a selective depression of the C1q component of complement because of the binding of C1q by IgG molecules through the $F(ab)'_2$—not Fc—portion of the molecule. The clearance of C1q is increased. The primary clinical feature of this disease is a persistent urticarial eruption, with lesions lasting a day or longer. Additional findings may include angioedema with occasional laryngeal involvement, joint symptoms, abdominal distress, neurologic abnormalities, and glomerulonephritis. The characteristic complement profile is a depressed C1q level with near-normal C1r and C1s levels. Other complement components including C2, C3, and C4 may be depressed. The alternative pathway complement components are normal. Diseases such as SLE, urticaria-angioedema, and inherited partial C3 deficiency may present with a similar clinical pattern. Antihistamines, anti-inflammatory drugs (indomethacin), and immunosuppressive agents have been tried, but their therapeutic efficacy has not been established.

4. SMALL-VESSEL VASCULITIS ASSOCIATED WITH SYSTEMIC DISEASES

Small-vessel vasculitis occurs in association with a wide variety of systemic diseases (Table 39–2). It

Table 39–2. Systemic diseases associated with small-vessel vasculitis.

Systemic vasculitides
Systemic necrotizing vasculitis of the polyarteritis nodosa group (particularly the Churg-Strauss syndrome and the polyangiitis overlap group), Wegener's granulomatosis, Behçet's disease, Henoch-Schönlein purpura

Collagen vascular diseases
SLE, rheumatoid arthritis, Sjögren's syndrome, dermatomyositis, scleroderma, rheumatic fever, sarcoidosis, C2 deficiency, mixed cryoglobulinemia

Neoplasms
Lymphoproliferative neoplasms, carcinoma

Infections
Bacterial (endocarditis), viral, mycobacterial, rickettsial

Miscellaneous syndromes
Chronic active hepatitis, inflammatory bowel disease, primary biliary cirrhosis, retroperitoneal fibrosis, Goodpasture's syndrome, relapsing polychondritis, α-antitrypsin deficiency, celiac disease, and others

generally resolves when the underlying disease process is adequately treated.

SYSTEMIC NECROTIZING VASCULITIS

Systemic necrotizing vasculitis is a category that includes polyarteritis nodosa, allergic angiitis and granulomatosis (Churg-Strauss syndrome), and the "polyangiitis overlap syndrome." These diseases have in common a multisystem necrotizing vasculitis of small and medium-sized muscular arteries.

1. POLYARTERITIS NODOSA

Major Immunologic Features
- There is necrotizing vasculitis of small- and medium-sized muscular arteries.
- It is an immune complex deposition disease.

General Considerations
Classic polyarteritis nodosa is a necrotizing vasculitis of small and medium-sized muscular arteries. Involvement of renal and visceral arteries with sparing of the pulmonary circulation is characteristic. Immune-complex deposition in involved arteries is considered to be the relevant pathophysiologic mechanism. In patients with polyarteritis nodosa in association with chronic hepatitis B virus infection, hepatitis B surface antigen, IgM, and complement components can be demonstrated in early vasculitic lesions. With more than 1000 cases reported, polyarteritis nodosa is considered an uncommon but not rare disease. The male-to-female ratio is 2.5:1. The mean age at onset is 45 years, although the disease occurs at both extremes of age.

Pathology
Involvement of the kidneys, heart, abdominal organs, and nervous system (both central and peripheral nervous systems) is characteristic. With the exception of the bronchial arteries, the pulmonary vessels are uninvolved. The vasculitic lesions are segmental and have a predilection for branching and bifurcating points of small- and medium-sized muscular arteries (Fig 39–2). Arterioles, venules, and veins are characteristically spared, and granuloma formation is rare. Destruction of the media and internal elastic lamina with aneurysm formation is characteristic. Endothelial proliferation, vessel wall degeneration with fibrinoid necrosis, thrombosis, ischemia, and infarction are present to various degrees. Lesions at all stages of evolution, including (1) the degenerative stage, (2) the acute inflammatory stage, (3) the chronic inflammatory stage, and (4) healing with scarring, may be present at any

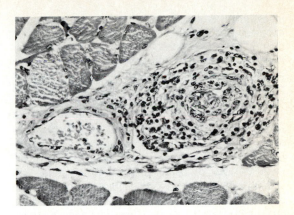

Figure 39–2. Muscle biopsy from a patient with classic polyarteritis nodosa. A necrotizing vasculitis of a small, muscular artery with a predominantly mononuclear-cell infiltrate is seen. The adjacent vein is not involved. Hematoxylin and eosin stain. (Original magnification × 330.) (Reproduced, with permission, from Cupps TR, Fauci AS: The vasculitides. In: *Major Problems in Internal Medicine.* Vol 21. Smith LH [editor]. Saunders, 1981.)

given time. Renal pathology includes the presence of vasculitis, hypertensive changes, and glomerulonephritis.

Immunologic Pathogenesis
Polyarteritis nodosa is associated with various infections, especially hepatitis B but also tuberculosis, streptococcal infections, and otitis media. Evidence for an exogenous antigen causing the vasculitis is strongest when hepatitis B virus is present. The surface antigen of the virus is present at higher concentrations in plasma than are other viral antigens. It is found in immune complexes, and it can also be detected in tissues. Immune complexes containing IgM antibody could bind to the surface antigen nonspecifically, so definite proof that the vasculitis is caused by a viral antigen-antibody immune complex is lacking.

Host factors predisposing to development of polyarteritis nodosa could include failure of the mononuclear phagocyte system to clear circulating complexes and defective immune regulation. To date, no human leukocyte antigen (HLA) association has been reported.

Clinical Features
Nonspecific signs and symptoms are common at the presentation of polyarteritis nodosa; these include weakness, abdominal pain, leg pain, neurologic symptoms, fever, and cough. The nonspecific nature of the presentation and the relatively uncommon occurrence of polyarteritis nodosa may contribute to the difficulty in establishing the diagnosis. Kidney

involvement is common but tends to be asymptomatic. Arthritis, arthralgia, or myalgia occurs in more than half of the patients, as does hypertension. Diffuse renal vasculitis with secondary hyperreninemia appears to be an important cause of hypertension in patients with polyarteritis nodosa. The peripheral nervous system is involved in half of the cases. Several patterns of involvement are recognized. Mixed motor-sensory involvement with a pattern of mononeuritis multiplex suggests the diagnosis of vasculitis. There is clinical evidence for abdominal involvement in 45% of patients. Nausea, vomiting, and abdominal pain, which may suggest pancreatitis, are present. Less common manifestations of gastrointestinal tract disease include "intestinal angina" (postprandial abdominal pain, anorexia, and weight loss), malabsorption, and steatorrhea. Although rare, bowel infarction is a life-threatening complication, which requires rapid diagnosis and prompt surgical intervention.

Skin involvement is present in 40% of patients. The most common pattern is a maculopapular rash. In addition, subcutaneous painful nodules or livedo reticularis (a red to blue netlike mottling of the skin) can be seen. Clinical involvement of the heart is present in one-third of patients. Cardiac disease may be secondary to the hypertension, coronary vasculitis, or pericarditis. Central nervous system involvement including stroke, altered mental status, and seizures can be seen in one-quarter of patients. At autopsy there are changes secondary to hypertension as well as active vasculitis. Similarly, retinal vessel involvement from hypertension and vasculitis is recognized in patients with polyarteritis nodosa.

Abnormal laboratory studies include elevated erythrocyte sedimentation rate, leukocytosis, anemia, thrombocytosis, and cellular casts in the urinary sediment, indicating glomerular disease. Angiographic evaluation is important in establishing the diagnosis (Fig 39–3). Two abnormalities suggest the diagnosis of polyarteritis nodosa: (1) aneurysms (vascular dilatation with a circular appearance), and (2) changes in vessel caliber (these tend to have an asymmetric pattern). The aneurysms in a given individual tend to be similar in size, ranging most commonly between 1 and 5 mm. Angiography will establish the diagnosis of polyarteritis nodosa in approximately 80% of cases; consequently, a negative study does not totally exclude the diagnosis.

Immunologic Diagnosis

There may be immune complexes, cryoglobulins, rheumatoid factor, and reduced level of complement components, but no specific immunologic test is diagnostic. The histologic diagnosis of systemic necrotizing vasculitis can be established from a variety of tissue sites. Biopsies taken from symptomatic sites such as skeletal muscle or nerves have a higher diagnostic yield than those from asymptomatic sites.

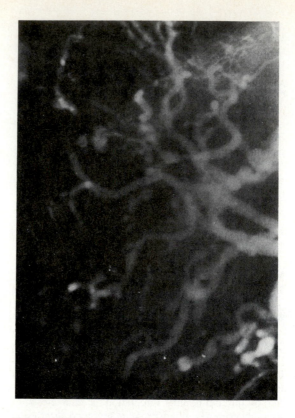

Figure 39–3. Hepatic angiogram from a patient with classic polyarteritis nodosa. Multiple saccular aneurysms and areas of symmetric narrowing are seen.

Differential Diagnosis

Because the initial signs and symptoms of polyarteritis nodosa are nonspecific, vasculitis should be considered in all patients with an undiagnosed systemic illness. At initial presentation many patients with polyarteritis nodosa are believed to have a neoplasm, infection, or other collagen vascular disease. The presence of an abnormal urinary sediment, recent onset of hypertension, or mononeuritis multiplex suggests the diagnostic possibility of vasculitis. A number of diseases occur in association with polyarteritis nodosa, including infections (hepatitis B virus infection, acute otitis media, endocarditis, and streptococcal infection), collagen vascular diseases (SLE, rheumatoid arthritis, Sjögren's syndrome, and others), and neoplasms (hairy cell leukemia).

Treatment

Although corticosteroids alone are generally recommended in the less fulminant cases of polyarteritis nodosa, cyclophosphamide is the treatment of choice in severe progressive polyarteritis nodosa. The drug is started at 2 mg/kg as a single daily oral dose, with monitoring of the leukocyte count to avoid a total leukocyte count of less than 3000 cells/mm^3. Prednisone (60 mg orally per day) is also started during the induction period of 10–14 days. After this induction period, a taper to an alternate-day schedule is initiated. The taper to alternate-day prednisone administration is generally completed in 2–3 months.

Complications & Prognosis

Cyclophosphamide will induce long-term clinical remissions in patients with systemic necrotizing vasculitis, including those who have been refractory to other treatment modalities. Meticulous control of hypertension is needed for several reasons. One reason is the potential for accelerated atherosclerosis in arteries damaged by the necrotizing vasculitis. Another major reason is that kidneys initially damaged by vasculitis or glomerulonephritis should be protected from the additional insult of poorly controlled blood pressure. Angiotensin-converting enzyme inhibitors may be particularly effective in this clinical setting.

2. ALLERGIC ANGIITIS & GRANULOMATOSIS (Churg-Strauss Syndrome)

Major Immunologic Features

- There is vasculitis of blood vessels of various type and sizes (including small- and medium-sized muscular involvement).
- Pulmonary involvement is common.

General Considerations

Allergic angiitis and granulomatosis is a rare disease characterized by a granulomatous vasculitis of multiple organ systems. Although vascular lesions identical to the pattern seen in polyarteritis nodosa may be present, this disease is unique for the following findings: (1) frequency of involvement of pulmonary vessels, (2) vasculitis of blood vessels of various types and sizes (small- and medium-sized muscular arteries, veins, and small vessels), (3) intra- and extravascular granuloma formation, (4) eosinophilic tissue infiltrates, and (5) association with severe asthma and peripheral eosinophilia. The pathophysiology of this syndrome appears to be similar to the pattern described for polyarteritis nodosa. There is a slight male predominance, and the mean age at the onset of disease is 44 years. In one series of patients with systemic necrotizing vasculitis, approximately 30% of patients had a clinical pattern of allergic angiitis and granulomatosis.

Pathology

In autopsy studies, the frequent involvement of the spleen and pulmonary vessels with sparing of central nervous system contrasts with the pattern seen in polyarteritis nodosa. In addition to the pattern of arteritis seen in polyarteritis nodosa, involvement of smaller vessels is commonly seen. Eosinophils and granulomata are seen in and around the vascular infiltrates. The veins are involved in approximately half of the patients, and small-vessel vasculitis is seen in the purpuric skin lesions.

Clinical Features

The clinical manifestation of allergic angiitis and granulomatosis is similar to the pattern seen in polyarteritis nodosa, except for the high frequency of pulmonary signs and symptoms. Asthma and transient pulmonary infiltrates are frequently noted. Symptoms related to the lungs generally precede the diagnosis of systemic vasculitis by 2 years, although the range is from 0 to 30 years. A short duration of pulmonary symptoms has been associated with a poorer prognosis. Peripheral-blood eosinophilia is seen in 85% of cases at some point in the course of the disease.

Immunologic Diagnosis

Elevation of IgE has been reported in allergic angiitis and granulomatosis. In addition to the peripheral biopsy sites described for polyarteritis nodosa, an open-lung biopsy may be useful to establish the diagnosis of necrotizing vasculitis.

Differential Diagnosis

In addition to the differential diagnosis discussed for polyarteritis nodosa, the diagnosis of allergic angiitis and granulomatosis should be considered in patients with bronchospasm and pulmonary infiltrates.

Treatment, Complications, & Prognosis

Treatment and prognosis are similar to those of polyarteritis nodosa. The bronchospasm may persist after successful treatment for the systemic vasculitis, and specific treatment of asthma may be required.

3. POLYANGIITIS OVERLAP SYNDROME

There are patients who share clinical and pathologic features characteristic of both polyarteritis nodosa and allergic angiitis and granulomatosis, as well as other vasculitic syndromes, but do not fit precisely into these strictly defined diagnostic categories. The presence of an overlap syndrome emphasizes that there is a continuum of disease manifestations in patients with systemic necrotizing vasculitis. The approach to the patients in the polyangiitis overlap syndrome group is similar to the one described for other systemic necrotizing vasculitides.

WEGENER'S GRANULOMATOSIS

Major Immunologic Features
- This is a necrotizing granulomatous vasculitis.
- There is focal segmental glomerulonephritis.
- There are antineutrophil cytoplasmic autoantibodies.

General Considerations

Wegener's granulomatosis is a clinicopathologic complex of a necrotizing, granulomatous vasculitis of the upper and lower respiratory tracts, glomerulonephritis, and variable degrees of small-vessel vasculitis. The cause is unknown. Because of the predominant involvement of the upper and lower respiratory tracts in this disease, it has been suggested that an infectious agent or an inhaled antigen may trigger an aberrant immune response. However, no such antigen or infectious agent has been identified as yet. There is a slight male predominance. The majority of cases begin in the fourth or fifth decade of life, although the disease has been described at both extremes of age.

Pathology

Wegener's granulomatosis is characterized by fibrinoid necrosis of predominantly small arteries and veins, with early infiltration of neutrophils followed by mononuclear cells. This is followed by healing with fibrosis. The vasculitis lesions occur at all stages of evolution. Granulomata are well-formed with plentiful multinucleated giant cells. Renal involvement is characterized by a focal segmental glomerulonephritis. Crescent formation can be seen in the more severe cases. Renal vasculitis or granuloma formation is less frequent.

Clinical Features

The most common presenting complaints (present in 85% of patients) involve the upper respiratory tract and include sinusitis, nasal obstruction, otitis, hearing loss, and oropharyngeal symptoms. Lower respiratory tract symptoms occur in 35% of patients; these include cough, sputum production, dyspnea, pleuritic chest pain, and, less commonly, hemoptysis. Other presenting complaints include arthralgias, weight loss, and weakness. Wegener's granulomatosis can involve any organ system, but the lungs are involved in virtually all patients. Lung disease may be asymptomatic, but it can be seen radiographically. In addition to the presenting symptoms of cough and dyspnea, massive pulmonary hemorrhage can be seen, but it is rare. There is evidence of sinus involvement in 95% of patients; this can be complicated by a superimposed bacterial infection. Inflammatory lesions may involve any site in the upper airways. Destruction of the nasal septum results in the saddle nose deformity. A persistent sore throat is a frequent complaint. Shallow oral ulcerations with sharp margins occur. Renal involvement is generally asymptomatic but can be documented in 80% of cases. Functional impairment may progress very rapidly in the absence of appropriate treatment. In contrast to patients with systemic necrotizing vasculitis, renal-vascular hypertension is not a significant clinical problem. Joint symptoms are present in more than half of the patients, but a deforming arthritis is not characteristically seen. Skin involvement including ulceration, vesicles, petechiae, and subcutaneous nodules occurs in almost half of the patients. The eyes are involved in 40% of patients. The most common abnormalities are proptosis secondary to a retro-orbital inflammatory mass and inflammation of the anterior ocular structures (ie, conjunctivitis, episcleritis, scleritis, and corneoscleral ulceration). Vasculitis of the vessels in the optic nerve or retina occurs in 10% of cases. Cardiac involvement is reported in one-quarter of patients. The most common abnormality is pericarditis, but inflammation of other structures including the endocardium, the myocardium, and the coronary vessels has been reported. The nervous system is involved in one-quarter of patients. Different patterns of peripheral nerve involvement, including mononeuritis multiplex, are noted. Involvement of the central nervous system is less common but is a well-recognized complication.

Laboratory studies show leukocytosis, thrombocytosis, elevated sedimentation rate, and presence of C-reactive protein. An abnormal urinary sediment is present in 80% of patients. Hematuria, with or without cellular casts, and proteinuria make up the most common pattern. The most common pattern seen on a chest radiograph is multiple, nodular, bilateral cavitary infiltrates, although virtually any pattern has been described. Computed tomography of the orbits may be useful in diagnosing and monitoring retro-orbital eye involvement.

Immunologic Diagnosis

Polyclonal elevations of IgG and IgA with normal levels of IgM is the characteristic pattern seen in active Wegener's granulomatosis. Elevation is variable. Circulating immune complexes can be detected in some patients. Antineutrophil cytoplasmic autoantibodies can be detected in the majority of patients. These autoantibodies can also occur in patients with SLE and other forms of renal disease. A definitive diagnosis of Wegener's granulomatosis is made by seeing the histologic pattern of granulomatous necrotizing vasculitis on a biopsy. Open-lung biopsy has the highest diagnostic yield. Tissue taken from other sites has an approximately 10% yield in demonstrating the diagnostic pattern. Renal tissue will provide a histologic pattern that is consistent with the diagnosis of Wegener's granulomatosis.

Differential Diagnosis

Wegener's granulomatosis is included in the differential diagnosis of patients with chronic sinusitis or otitis media. Diseases that are associated with a pulmonary-renal syndrome (SLE, Goodpasture's syndrome, thrombotic thrombocytopenia purpura, etc) may be confused with Wegener's granulomatosis during the initial phases.

Treatment

Cyclophosphamide at 2 mg/kg orally as a single daily dose is the preferred treatment. After the initial induction period the total leukocyte count is monitored to adjust the dose of cyclophosphamide. Care should be taken to avoid lowering the leukocyte count below 3000 cells/mm^3. In addition, oral prednisone at 1 mg/kg/d is used. After 2 weeks of daily prednisone, a taper to an alternate-day regimen of prednisone is initiated; the taper is completed after 2–3 months. Treatment should continue until the patient is free of disease for 1 year before the drugs are discontinued; withdrawal should be gradual. The significance of recent observations that trimethoprim-sulfamethoxazole may help in the treatment of Wegener's granulomatosis requires further investigation.

Complications & Prognosis

Treatment with cyclophosphamide and prednisone will put 90% of patients into a sustained remission. Sinus damage by the disease may predispose to recurrent episodes of bacterial sinusitis. Obstruction from scarring of large airways can be seen in patients with severe endobronchial disease. The most common obstructed site is the subglottic region. Potential complications of cyclophosphamide therapy include hemorrhagic cystitis, bladder fibrosis, and, possibly, neoplasia.

TEMPORAL ARTERITIS

Major Immunologic Features

- This is a granulomatous panarteritis.
- It affects the elderly.
- Headache is common, but presenting symptoms are nonspecific.
- It is associated with polymyalgia rheumatica.

General Considerations

Temporal arteritis is a systemic panarteritis affecting any medium-sized or large artery. The disease predominantly affects the elderly, with clinical signs and symptoms resulting from vasculitis in branches of the carotid artery. Although studies suggest immune complex-mediated, antibody-mediated, and cell-mediated immune mechanisms, the precise cause is unknown. There is a slight female predominance, and the average age at onset of the disease is 70 years. More than 95% of cases occur in patients older than 50 years. The age-specific incidence per 100,000 population per year increases with age, rising from 1.7 in the sixth decade to 55.5 for patients older than 80 years.

Pathology

The disease is characterized by a panarteritis consisting of mononuclear cells, multinucleated giant cells, PMN, and eosinophils. The major site of involvement is the media, with smooth muscle necrosis and interruption of internal elastic membrane. The inflammatory lesions have a segmental pattern.

Clinical Features

The presenting signs and symptoms of temporal arteritis have a nonspecific pattern. The most frequent presenting complaints of headache, malaise, and fatigue are common symptoms in an older population. Less-common presenting problems include jaw or extremity claudication, fever, arthralgias, chronic sore throat, and tender scalp nodules. Headache is the most common manifestation. The pain has a continuous, boring quality with intermittent exacerbations. Although the pain is most commonly located over the distribution of the temporal artery, radiation to the neck, face, jaw, or tongue occurs. Although abnormalities along the course of the temporal artery, including tenderness, absent pulse, and nodules, are seen in half of the patients, these findings appear later in the course of disease. Other findings include hair loss, erythema, and necrosis along the course of the temporal artery. Eye problems including visual impairment, blindness, amaurosis fugax, and diplopia, occur in more than one-third of patients. Although temporal arteritis may present with sudden blindness, the majority of patients will have other symptoms for an average of 3.5 months prior to developing visual impairment. Because the loss of vision is the result of ischemic optic neuritis in the majority of cases, the funduscopic examination may be normal for several days after the onset of blindness.

Jaw claudication (pain brought on by chewing or talking and relieved by rest) occurs in one-third of patients and suggests the diagnosis of temporal arteritis. Polymyalgia rheumatica, a syndrome characterized by proximal muscle pain, periarticular pain, and morning stiffness, occurs in approximately half of the patients with temporal arteritis. Conversely, up to 50% of patients presenting with symptoms of polymyalgia rheumatica may have a positive temporal artery biopsy.

Laboratory abnormalities include a normochromic, normocytic anemia, elevated alkaline phosphatase, and mild elevation of hepatic transaminases.

Immunologic Diagnosis

The sedimentation rate, total IgG, and acute-phase reactants are characteristically elevated. The diagnosis is established by finding the characteristic panarteritis on a temporal artery biopsy. Because of the segmental nature of the inflammation, the need for generous biopsy specimens and serial sectioning has been emphasized.

Differential Diagnosis

Because of the nonspecific nature of the majority of presenting symptoms, temporal arteritis can be confused with a wide variety of disease processes including neoplasia, chronic infection, abnormal thyroid function, and other connective-tissue diseases.

Treatment

Prednisone at 40–60 mg/d orally is the initial treatment. As manifestations of the disease are suppressed, an attempt should be made to taper the dose of the drug. Although some patients may be adequately treated with 6 months of therapy, most will require a more prolonged course, for 1–2 years. Prednisone should be tapered to the minimum effective dose, generally in the range of 7.5–10 mg/d.

Complications & Prognosis

Corticosteroids are effective in suppressing the symptoms of temporal arteritis and preventing visual impairment. In general, visual impairment is not reversible once present. Other than loss of vision, the major complication of this disease is the morbidity associated with prolonged corticosteroid use in an elderly population.

TAKAYASU'S ARTERITIS

Major Immunologic Features

- There is inflammation and stenosis of large and intermediate-sized arteries.
- There is frequent involvement of the aortic arch.

General Considerations

Takayasu's arteritis is characterized by inflammation and stenosis of large and intermediate-sized arteries with frequent involvement of the aortic arch and its branches. There is a marked female predominance (about 9:1). The disease generally presents between the ages of 15 and 20 years. Although originally recognized in Asian women, Takayasu's arteritis has a worldwide distribution.

Pathology

Takayasu's arteritis is characterized by a panarteritis of large elastic arteries, with infiltration of all layers of the artery wall by mononuclear cells and giant cells. Other findings include intimal prolifera-

tion fibrosis, disruption of elastic lamina, and vascularization of the media. Aneurysms, dissection, and hemorrhage are less common. In descending order of frequency, the following arteries are involved: subclavian artery (85%), descending aorta (58%), renal artery (56%), carotid artery (43%), ascending aorta (30%), abdominal aorta (20%), vertebral artery (17%), iliac artery (16%), innominate artery (15%), and pulmonary artery (15%).

Clinical Features

Two clinical stages, an initial inflammatory phase and a chronic occlusive phase, are recognized in Takayasu's arteritis. The initial inflammatory phase occurs in 70% of patients and is characterized by a pattern of systemic inflammation including fever, night sweats, malaise, weakness, myalgias, and arthralgias. A migratory arthritis, episcleritis, iritis, and painful skin nodules are less common. A mean of 8 years (range, several months to several decades) may separate the initial inflammatory phase from clinical expression of the occlusive phase. Symptoms during the chronic phase reflect ischemia of the involved organ systems. Signs of vascular insufficiency are present in almost all patients. The pulse of the radial, ulnar, and carotid arteries is decreased or absent in 98% of patients. Bruits can be detected in 86% of patients. Symptoms of claudication or pain over the distribution of an artery occur in approximately one-third of patients. Central hypertension is present in half of the cases. Blood pressure determinations of the lower extremities more reliably reflect the true central blood pressure in the presence of severe aortic arch involvement. Sixty percent of patients experience difficulty in looking up, resulting in the characteristic "face-down" position. Patients assume this position to avoid transient decreases in visual acuity and narrowing of visual fields caused by a further decrement of compromised blood flow to the central nervous system. Ischemic changes to the retina and anterior structures of the eye are seen in a minority of patients. Cardiac symptoms are present in one-third of patients. Palpitations and congestive heart failure (right- and left-sided failure) secondary to hypertension are the most common manifestations. Less commonly, cardiac ischemia (secondary to coronary arteritis), aortic insufficiency, myocarditis, and pericarditis have been reported. Routine blood tests may show a mild anemia and leukocytosis.

Immunologic Diagnosis

The erythrocyte sedimentation rate is generally elevated. IgG, IgA, and IgM may be elevated, while the rheumatoid factor and antinuclear antibodies are generally negative. Arteriography is important in the diagnosis and management of Takayasu's arteritis. Arteriographic abnormalities include symmetric narrowing to complete occlusion of large arteries with collateralization of flow. Aneurysms, including both saccular and fusiform patterns, can be seen. Other noninvasive tests to measure blood flow may be useful for serial follow-up evaluations.

Differential Diagnosis

Other causes of aortitis including syphilis, mycotic aneurysm, rheumatic fever, Reiter's syndrome, and ankylosing spondylitis should be excluded. Vascular occlusion secondary to emboli can also mimic Takayasu's arteritis.

Treatment

Corticosteroids are usually effective in suppressing the inflammatory symptoms. The use of 30 mg of prednisone followed by a taper to a chronic maintenance therapy in the range of 5–10 mg per day has been suggested. The use of a chronic maintenance regimen may prevent the long-term vascular complications and improve survival. Cyclophosphamide may be useful in treating patients who develop progressive occlusive disease despite corticosteroid therapy. Vascular surgery may prove useful in selected cases.

Complications & Prognosis

In 2 large series a 10% mortality rate was noted. The most common cause of death was congestive heart failure, and the second most common was myocardial infarction. Less common causes of death were renal failure and central nervous system hemorrhage.

THROMBOANGIITIS OBLITERANS (Buerger's Disease)

This syndrome is characterized by inflammatory occlusive vascular disease of the intermediate to small arteries and veins of the extremities. Three histopathologic phases of the disease are recognized: (1) neutrophil infiltrate of the vessel wall associated with microabscesses and thrombosis, (2) a subacute phase with mononuclear cell and giant cell infiltrates, and (3) a chronic phase with fibrosis and recanalization of the thrombus. The disease predominantly affects males younger than 40 years of age with a significant smoking history. The most common presenting symptoms are lower-extremity claudication or migratory thrombophlebitis. Less than 5% of patients present with upper-extremity problems. During the course of the disease the majority of patients will develop Raynaud's syndrome, and upper-extremity involvement will be seen in 90% of cases. Systemic symptoms are characteristically absent. Protection of ischemic tissue and cessation of tobacco use are imperative. Carefully selected patients may benefit from surgical intervention. Morbidity from tissue loss may be great, but survival is not affected.

Circulating immune complexes have been reported by some investigators but not others. There are no diagnostic immunologic tests. It is not known whether tobacco has a toxic or immunologic effect in this disease. However, the possibility of an immune pathogenesis is raised by the close resemblance of the histopathology in the early phase of the disease with that of a hyperacute graft rejection.

OTHER VASCULITIC SYNDROMES

1. ISOLATED ANGIITIS OF THE CENTRAL NERVOUS SYSTEM

This is a distinct clinicopathologic entity characterized by vasculitis restricted to the vessels of the central nervous system. The arteriole is the most commonly affected vessel, although any size of vessel can be affected. The disease generally presents with a pattern of higher-cortical dysfunction or severe headache and progresses to a pattern of multifocal neurologic deficits. Immunosuppressive therapy is successful in inducing long-term clinical remissions.

2. ERYTHEMA NODOSUM

This is a clinical syndrome characterized by recurrent crops of painful nodular lesions and is generally associated with infection (mycobacterial, fungal, or bacterial) or with sarcoidosis. The histopathology is characterized by acute and chronic inflammation of the dermis and subcutaneous tissue including a vasculitic component.

3. COGAN'S SYNDROME

This disease is seen in young adults and is characterized by episodes of acute interstitial keratitis and vestibuloauditory dysfunction. An aortitis may be seen in a subset of these patients. Other rare vasculitic syndromes are recognized and are reviewed in the general references.

REFERENCES

General

Cupps TR, Fauci AS: The vasculitides. Vol 21 in: *Major Problems in Internal Medicine.* Smith LH (editor). Saunders, 1981.

Fan PT et al: A clinical approach to systemic vasculitis. *Semin Arthritis Rheum* 1980;**9**:4.

Fauci AS, Haynes BF, Katz P: The spectrum of vasculitis: Clinical, pathologic, immunologic, and therapeutic considerations. *Ann Intern Med* 1978;**89**:660.

Hurst JW et al (editors): *The Heart: Arteries and Veins.* McGraw-Hill, 1986.

Pericardial Disease

Burch GE, Colcolough HL: Postcardiotomy and postinfarction syndromes: A theory. *Am Heart J* 1970;**80**:290.

Connolly DC, Burchell HB: Pericarditis: A ten year survey. *Am J Cardiol* 1961;**7**:7.

Engle, MA et al: Viral illness and the postpericardiotomy syndrome: A prospective study in children. *Circulation* 1980;**60**:1151.

Kossowsky WA, Alan FL, Spain DM: Reappraisal of the postmyocardial infarction Dressler's syndrome. *Am Heart J* 1981;**102**:954.

Lichstein E et al: Current incidence of postmyocardial infarction (Dressler's) syndrome. *Am J Cardiol* 1982; **50**:1269.

Myocardial Disease

Borenstein DG et al: The myocarditis of systemic lupus erythematosus: Association with myositis. *Ann Intern Med* 1978;**89**:619.

Kereiakes DJ, Parmley WW: Myocarditis and cardiomyopathy. *Am Heart J* 1984;**108**:1318.

Mason JW, Billingham ME, Ricci DR: Treatment of acute inflammatory myocarditis assisted by endomyocardial biopsy. *Am J Cardiol* 1980;**45**:1037.

Endomyocardial Disease

Chusid MJ et al: The hypereosinophilic syndrome: Analysis of fourteen cases with review of the literature. *Medicine* 1975;**54**:1.

Olsen EGJ, Spry CJF: The pathogenesis of Löffler's endomyocardial disease, and its relationship to endomyocardial fibrosis. Chap 12, pp 281–303, in: *Progress in Cardiology,* 8th ed. Yu PN, Goodwin JF (editors). Lea & Febiger, 1979.

Roberts WC, Liegler DG, Carbone PP: Endomyocardial disease and eosinophilia: A clinical and pathologic spectrum. *Am J Med* 1969;**46**:28.

Spry CJF, Tai PC: Studies on blood eosinophils: II. Patients with Löffler's cardiomyopathy. *Clin Exp Immunol* 1976;**24**:423.

Small-Vessel Vasculitis

Ballard HS, Eisinger RP, Gallo G: Renal manifestations of the Henoch-Schönlein syndrome in adults. *Am J Med* 1970;**49**:328.

Chajek T, Fainaru M: Behçet's disease: Report of 41 cases and a review of the literature. *Medicine* 1975;**54**:179.

Cream JJ, Gumpel JM, Peachy RDG: Schönlein-Henoch purpura in the adult: A study of 77 adults

with anaphylactoid or Schönlein-Henoch purpura. *Q J Med* 1970;**39**:461.

Cupps TR, Fauci AS: Cutaneous vasculitis. Pages 136–140 in: *Current Therapy in Allergy and Immunology 1983–1984.* Lichtenstein LM, Fauci AS (editors). BC Decker, 1983.

Winkelman RK, Ditto WB: Cutaneous and visceral syndromes of necrotizing or "allergic" angiitis: A study of 38 cases. *Medicine* 1964;**43**:59.

Wisnieski JJ, Naff GB: Serum IgG antibodies to C1q in hypocomplementemic urticarial vasculitis syndrome. *Arthritis Rheum* 1989;**32**:1119.

Systemic Necrotizing Vasculitis

Chumbley LC, Harrison EG, DeRemee RA: Allergic granulomatosis and angiitis (Churg-Strauss syndrome): Report and analysis of 30 cases. *Mayo Clin Proc* 1977;**54**:477.

Fauci AS et al: Cyclophophamide therapy of severe systemic necrotizing vasculitis. *N Engl J Med* 1979; **301**:235.

Leib ES, Restivo C, Paulus HE: Immunosuppressive and corticosteroid therapy of polyarteritis nodosa. *Am J Med* 1979;**67**:41.

Levitt RY, Fauci AS: Polyangiitis overlap syndrome: Classification and prospective clinical experience. *Am J Med* 1986;**81**:79.

Travers RL et al: Polyarteritis nodosa: A clinical and angiographic analysis of 17 cases. *Semin Arthritis Rheum* 1979;**8**:184.

Wegener's Granulomatosis

Burton CW, Todd JR, King JW: Wegenergranulomatosis and trimethoprim-sulfamethoxazole: Complete remission after a twenty-year course. *Ann Intern Med* 1987;**106**:840.

Falk RJ, Jennette JC: Anti-neutrophil cytoplasmic autoantibodies with specificity for myeloperoxidase in patients with systemic vasculitis and idiopathic necrotizing and crescentic glomerulonephritis. *N Engl J Med* 1988; **318**:1651.

Fauci AS, Wolff SM: Wegener's granulomatosis: Studies in eighteen patients and a review of the literature. *Medicine* 1973;**52**:535.

Fauci AS et al: Wegener's granulomatosis: Prospective clinical and therapeutic experience with 85 patients for 21 years. *Ann Intern Med* 1983;**98**:76.

Haynes BF et al: The ocular manifestations of Wegener's granulomatosis: Fifteen years experience and review of the literature. *Am J Med* 1977;**63**:131.

Temporal Arteritis

Goodman BW Jr: Temporal arteritis. *Am J Med* 1979; **67**:839.

Hamilton CR Jr, Shelley WM, Tumulty PA: Giant cell arteritis: Including temporal arteritis and polymyalgia rheumatica. *Medicine* 1971;**50**:1.

Huston KA et al: Temporal arteritis: A 25-year epidemiologic, clinical, and pathologic study. *Ann Intern Med* 1978;**88**:162.

Takayasu's Arteritis

Fraga A et al: Takayasu's arteritis: Frequency of systemic manifestations (study of 22 patients) and favorable response to maintenance steroid therapy with adrenocorticosteroids (12 patients). *Arthritis Rheum* 1972;**15**:617.

Hall, S et al: Takayasu arteritis: A study of 32 North American patients. *Medicine* 1985;**64**:89.

Ishikawa K: Natural history and classification of occlusive thromboaortopathy (Takayasu's disease). *Circulation* 1978;**57**:27.

Lupi-Herrara E et al: Takayasu's arteritis: Clinical study of 107 cases. *Am Heart J* 1977;**93**:94.

Shelhamer JH et al: Takayasu's arteritis and its therapy. *Ann Intern Med* 1985;**103**:121.

Thromboangiitis Obliterans

Goodman RM et al: Buerger's disease in Israel. *Am J Med* 1965;**39**:601.

Lie JT: Thromboangiitis obliterans (Buerger's disease) in women. *Medicine* 1986;**65**:65.

McKusick VA et al: Buerger's disease: A distinct clinical and pathologic entity. *JAMA* 1962;**181**:93.

Shionoya S et al: Diagnosis, pathology, and treatment of Buerger's disease. *Surgery* 1974;**75**:695.

Other Syndromes

Cupps TR, Moore PM, Fauci AS: Isolated angiitis of the central nervous system: Prospective diagnostic and therapeutic experience. *Am J Med* 1983;**74**:97.

Haynes BF et al: Cogan syndrome: Studies in thirteen patients, long-term follow-up and a review of the literature. *Medicine* 1980;**59**:426.

40

Gastrointestinal, Hepatobiliary, Oral, & Dental Diseases

Stephen P. James, MD, Warren Strober, MD, & John S. Greenspan, BDS, PhD, FRCPath

As reviewed in Chapter 15, the gastrointestinal tract is normally a site of intense immunologic activity. The gastrointestinal lumen contains a complex mixture of harmless (and necessary) bacterial flora, potential pathogens, and large quantities of complex macromolecules capable of eliciting immune responses. The mucosal immune system has evolved mechanisms to down regulate immune responses to harmless flora and food antigens, while eliciting protective responses to pathogens. The diseases reviewed in this chapter are thought to be the result of aberrations of the mucosal immune response to harmless exogenous antigens or autoantigens, resulting in inappropriate injury to the host, or diseases such as hepatitis in which the immunologic host response to a pathologic agent is an important component of the disease process.

GASTROINTESTINAL DISEASES

Stephen P. James, MD, & Warren Strober, MD

GLUTEN-SENSITIVE ENTEROPATHY

Major Immunologic Features
- There is hypersensitivity to cereal grain proteins (gliadins).
- Antigliadin antibodies are present.
- The lamina propria is infiltrated with lymphocytes and plasma cells, associated with villous atrophy.
- It is associated with HLA-DR3 and -DR7.
- It may be associated with dermatitis herpetiformis.

General Considerations
Gluten-sensitive enteropathy (celiac sprue, nontropical sprue) is a disease of the small intestine that is characterized by villous atrophy and malabsorption. It is caused by hypersensitivity to cereal grain storage proteins (gluten or gliadin, a substance derived from gluten) found in wheat, barley, and oats.

The disease is most common in whites and occurs only occasionally in African blacks and not in Asians. It is either limited to the intestine or associated with a vesicular skin disease, dermatitis herpetiformis.

Pathology
The inflammatory lesions are restricted to the small-intestinal mucosa, with the most severe changes being in the area most often in contact with ingested gluten, the proximal small intestine. Gliadin challenge studies show that the disease begins with subepithelial edema and thickening of the basement membrane followed by an influx of inflammatory cells. The latter initially consists of polymorphonuclear leukocytes, but these are soon replaced by lymphocytes and plasma cells. Although IgA plasma cells increase in number and continue to predominate, there is a disproportionate increase in IgG plasma cells; in contrast, few if any IgE plasma cells appear. These inflammatory changes are accompanied by shortening and eventual flattening of the villi and lengthening of the crypts; the latter is indicative of a marked increase in epithelial cell turnover (Fig 40–1). When dermatitis herpetiformis is present, the intestinal lesions are similar to (but usually milder

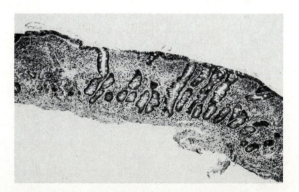

Figure 40–1. Gluten-sensitive enteropathy. Jejunal biopsy shows complete loss of villi, elongation of crypts, and lymphocytic infiltrate in a severe case.

than) those when it is absent, while the skin lesions consist of subepidermal collections of inflammatory cells near areas of fluid accumulation. A characteristic feature of the skin lesions is the presence of granular deposits of IgA and complement in both lesional and normal skin.

Immunologic Pathogenesis

Gluten-sensitive enteropathy is most probably due to a specific immunologic hyperreactivity to gliadin, which leads to the induction of gliadin-specific lymphocytes in the mucosa. Consistent with this hypothesis, patients have antibody responses to gliadin that are quantitatively and qualitatively distinct from those found in the other gastrointestinal tract diseases. They also have gliadin-specific T cell-mediated responses that are not seen in controls. Further evidence of an immunologic origin comes from organ culture studies that show that gliadin is not toxic by itself, but instead requires the participation of an endogenous effector mechanism. In addition, 80–90% of patients both with and without dermatitis herpetiformis bear a particular complex of HLA antigens including HLA-B8, HLA-DR3, HLA-DR7, and certain DP and DQ locus antigens. This finding suggests that particular immune response genes are the basis of the inappropriate antigliadin immune responses that are presumably causing the disease.

Clinical Features

In gluten-sensitive enteropathy alone, the clinical course is dominated by gastrointestinal tract symptoms and malabsorption, whereas when dermatitis herpetiformis is present the course is dominated by a vesicular skin eruption and the intestinal disease is usually absent. The intestinal symptoms of gluten-sensitive enteropathy are highly variable and consist of weight loss, diarrhea, symptoms due to nutritional deficiencies, and growth failure in children. When dermatitis herpetiformis is present, the skin disease consists of a vesicular, intensely pruritic skin eruption on extensor and exposed surfaces. Typical laboratory findings in gluten-sensitive enteropathy include evidence of malabsorption: increased fecal fat, abnormal D-xylose absorption, vitamin deficiencies, anemia, and, in severe cases, biochemical evidence of osteomalacia and abnormal coagulation due to vitamin K deficiency. Intestinal contrast studies during active disease show dilatation and thickening of the proximal small bowel. The intestinal biopsy is the most important specific diagnostic test, particularly in association with gluten challenge studies.

Immunologic Diagnosis

The diagnosis of gluten-sensitive enteropathy is established by demonstrating villous atrophy in the small-bowel biopsy, which resolves with removal of gluten from the diet and which reappears with gluten challenge. Antigliadin antibodies are present in active disease, but their presence is not entirely specific, unless they are present in high titers and are of the IgA class. The presence of HLA-B8, -DR3, or -DR7 is supportive of the diagnosis but not pathognomonic.

Differential Diagnosis

The differential diagnosis includes all intestinal diseases causing malabsorption. However, small-bowel biopsy showing villous atropy and inflammation considerably narrows the diagnostic possibilities to gluten-sensitive enteropathy, tropical sprue, hypogammaglobulinemia, and some forms of intestinal lymphoma.

Treatment

Treatment consists of lifelong elimination of gluten-containing foods from the diet. It is recommended that such treatment be instituted even in patients with mild disease because a major complication of gluten-sensitive enteropathy is an increased prevalence of small-bowel carcinoma and lymphoma, and it is thought that reduction of chronic inflammation by gluten restriction may diminish the risk of this complication. Nutritional supplements should be instituted as needed in patients with active disease. Very severe disease, particularly associated with severe villous atrophy and small-bowel ulceration, may respond to corticosteroids. When dermatitis herpetiformis is present, both the intestinal and skin lesions can also be treated with a gluten-free diet. However, more usually, diaminodiphenylsulfone (dapsone), an anti-inflammatory agent that provides good control of the skin lesions, is used.

Complications & Prognosis

Unrecognized and untreated gluten-sensitive enteropathy may lead to severe debility and death, but following treatment, patients usually return to normal health and have a normal life expectancy. As noted above, the incidence of intestinal carcinoma and lymphoma is increased. Recently it has been shown that intestinal lymphoma is most often a CD8 T cell lymphoma. Patients with long-standing intestinal changes may be relatively unresponsive to a gluten-free diet and may require corticosteroid therapy. Rarely, patients develop villous atrophy associated with severe intestinal ulceration (ulcerative iliojejunitis), a syndrome that in some instances becomes life-threatening.

NON-GLUTEN (NON-GLIADIN) HYPERSENSITIVITY

Major Immunologic Features

- There is IgE-mediated hypersensitivity or gluten-sensitive enteropathy-like hypersensitivities.

■ There are ill-defined mucosal abnormalities marked by eosinophilic infiltration or villous atrophy of the mucosa.

General Considerations

Several conditions marked by hypersensitivity to food substances other than gluten (gliadin) also occur. These include IgE-mediated food allergy localized to the gastrointestinal tract, usually associated with nongastrointestinal allergic symptoms. The causative food substance in this case can induce an increase in mucosal IgE plasma cells and mast cell degranulation, which may lead to a severe protein-losing enteropathy. Treatment consists of eliminating the offending food from the diet (see Chapter 30).

A second type of hypersensitivity is due to food substances that induce a clinical picture nearly identical to that in gluten-sensitive enteropathy: villous atrophy and malabsorption developing days to weeks after exposure to the causative substance. This condition is more or less limited to young children and is most frequently caused by cow's milk protein; however, soy, egg, and wheat proteins have also been implicated. It frequently occurs after a gastrointestinal infection and resolves spontaneously after the age of 3 years. It may be due to immaturity of the mucosal immune system and hence an inability to develop immunologic tolerance to food antigens.

Finally, there is an ill-defined group of gastrointestinal tract hypersensitivity states marked by either eosinophilic infiltration of the bowel or villous atrophy and not definitely associated with a causative food or other agent. In some cases these conditions may be due to a self-perpetuating inflammation that was initiated by an inappropriate immune response, whereas in other cases it may be due to an autoimmune process.

CROHN'S DISEASE

Major Immunologic Feature

■ There is transmural granulomatous inflammation of the bowel wall.

General Considerations

Crohn's disease (regional ileitis, granulomatous ileitis, or colitis) is a syndrome of unknown origin characterized by transmural inflammation of the bowel wall. It occurs worldwide, but is most common in persons of European origin. The prevalence ranges from 10 to 70 per 100,000, and it is much more common in industrialized countries. There is a slight female predominance. The disorder can begin at any age, but most typically begins between 15 and 30 years of age. There is a familial aggregation of cases but no clear mode of inheritance.

Pathology

Crohn's disease may involve any part of the alimentary tract from the mouth to the anus, although most patients fall into one of the typical patterns of the disease, having predominant involvement of the ileocolic, small-intestinal, or colonic/anorectal regions. The gross pathology of Crohn's disease is characterized by transmural inflammation of the bowel wall, often in a discontinuous fashion, with ulceration, strictures, and fistulae being typical findings. The histopathologic findings are those of a discontinuous granulomatous inflammatory process (true granulomas are found in about 60% of surgically resected specimens) (Fig 40–2), crypt abscesses, fissures, and aphthous ulcers. The inflammatory infiltrate is mixed, consisting of lymphocytes (both T and B cells), plasma cells, macrophages, and neutrophils. There is a disproportionate increase in IgM- and IgG-secreting plasma cells compared with IgA-secreting cells, but the latter are also increased. The number of T cells is increased, but a normal proportion of CD4 and CD8 cells is maintained.

Crohn's disease (like ulcerative colitis, below) is found primarily in industrialized countries, suggesting that one or more environmental factors are important in pathogenesis; however, no such factors have yet been identified. Infection with *Mycobacterium paratuberculosis* species has been suggested as a cause, but recent evidence makes it more likely that this organism is a commensal that does not have an etiologic role. Because of the failure to identify a specific causative infectious microorganism, it has been suggested that the disease has a primary immunologic basis. One leading possibility in this regard is that the mucosal inflammation in Crohn's disease is the result of abnormality of mucosal T cell regulation, which leads to an inappropriate mucosal im-

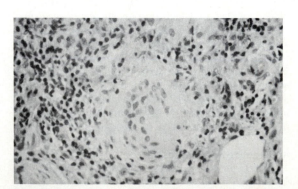

Figure 40–2. Crohn's disease. Rectal biopsy shows mucosal granuloma.

mune response to ubiquitous intestinal antigens (see Chapter 15). In support of this concept are the facts that (1) the inflammatory lesion in Crohn's disease begins as a follicular collection of lymphocytes which resembles a normal (if inappropriate) immune response; (2) patients manifest excessive responses to oral antigen challenge; and (3) several immuno-regulatory defects have been identified, including the presence of circulating suppressor T cells and abnormal lymphokine secretory patterns in the mucosa. However, these data are not conclusive, and additional work is needed to establish an immunologic origin.

Clinical Features

Typical symptoms include abdominal pain, anorexia, weight loss, fever, diarrhea, perianal discomfort and discharge, and extraintestinal symptoms involving the skin, eyes, and joints. The manifestations vary somewhat according to the predominant pattern of intestinal involvement. Extraintestinal manifestations are not unusual and include arthritis, erythema nodosum, pyoderma gangrenosum, aphthous mouth ulcers, uveitis, anemia, urinary calculi, and sclerosing cholangitis. Typical laboratory abnormalities include anemia (chronic disease, iron deficiency, vitamin B_{12} deficiency, folate deficiency), leukocytosis, thrombocytosis, elevation of the erythrocyte sedimentation rate, hypoalbuminemia, electrolyte abnormalities (in severe diarrhea), and presence of occult blood in the stool. Many radiographic abnormalities may be present in small-bowel and colon contrast studies. These include aphthous ulceration, linear ulceration, edema, and thickening of the bowel wall (Fig 40–3), as well as strictures, fissures, fistulae, and mass lesions (inflammatory mass or abscess); the chronic inflammation also may lead to a characteristic "cobblestone" pattern. When the areas involved are accessible, endoscopy provides a direct method of evaluating disease activity and permits collection of biopsy material for pathologic confirmation as well as screening for colon carcinoma.

Immunologic Diagnosis

Multiple abnormalities of immune function have been described, but none has diagnostic specificity.

Differential Diagnosis

Diseases sometimes having an appearance similar to Crohn's disease are appendicitis, diverticulitis, intestinal neoplasia, and intestinal infections (*M tuberculosis, Chlamydia, Yersinia entercolitica, Campylobacter jejuni, Entamoeba histolytica, Cryptosporidium,* herpes simplex virus, cytomegalovirus, *Salmonella,* and *Shigella*). A combination of stool cultures, intestinal biopsies, and clinical follow-up are usually sufficient to exclude these possibilities.

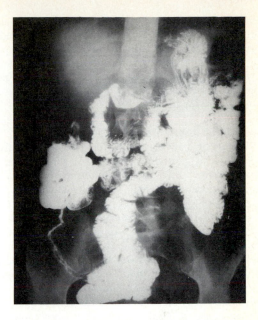

Figure 40–3. Crohn's disease. Small-bowel barium contrast x-ray shows marked narrowing of the terminal ileum due to transmural inflammation.

Treatment

The anti-inflammatory drug sulfasalazine is useful in treating mildly active colonic Crohn's disease and is commonly used in an attempt to maintain remission of disease, although a National Cooperative Crohn's Disease trial did not prove that such prophylaxis is effective. Metronidazole is similar in efficacy to sulfasalazine and appears to be particularly useful for perianal disease, although its side effects (seizures, peripheral neuropathy, disulfuram-like reaction to alcohol) may be significant. In more severe active disease, corticosteroids are effective in treating acute exacerbations and possibly in maintaining remission in some patients. There is no evidence, however, that corticosteroids prevent the progression of subclinical disease. Azathioprine and 6-mercaptopurine are used as steroid-sparing drugs in patients who require chronic corticosteroids and are not amenable to surgical therapy; in addition, it has been suggested but not proved that these drugs may have a role in long-term prophylaxis. There may be a long delay in the onset of action of these drugs (6 months). Antidiarrheal drugs provide symptomatic relief in some patients. Dietary management with elemental diets or total parenteral nutrition are useful for improving the nutritional status of patients and in inducing symptomatic improvement of acute disease, but diet alone does not induce sustained clinical remissions. Antibiotics are used in treating secondary small-bowel bacterial overgrowth and in treatment of pyogenic complications. Cyclosporine is currently under investigation in controlled trials; early, uncontrolled experience with this drug indicates that it produces improvement in some but not all patients with severe Crohn's disease. Finally, surgical treatment is necessary when the disease is not controlled medically and when various complications occur (see below).

Complications & Prognosis

Patients typically have recurrent episodes of active disease with periods of intervening quiescence. However, they often have low-grade symptoms even during periods of apparent disease inactivity, and the disease has high social and economic costs. Approximately two-thirds of patients require surgery at some time during their life for diseases not treatable with tolerable doses of steroids or for complications such as obstruction, abscess, fistula, hemorrhage, or megacolon. However, the disease is clearly not curable by surgical resection and recurs at a rate approaching 90% in very long-term follow-up. The mortality rate of Crohn's disease is approximately twice that in the general age-matched population, although most mortality occurs early in the course of the disease and there is only a small increase in mortality in patients with long-standing disease. The incidence of intestinal carcinoma is increased, but the frequency is much lower than that associated with ulcerative colitis.

ULCERATIVE COLITIS

Major Immunologic Features
- Colonic mucosa is chronically inflamed, with ulceration of the epithelial layer.
- Anticolon antibodies are present.

General Considerations

Idiopathic ulcerative colitis is a disease of unknown origin characterized by chronic inflammation of the colonic mucosa. As with Crohn's disease, ulcerative colitis is found primarily in industrialized nations, although it does occur worldwide. The prevalence ranges from 37 to 80 per 100,000 with a slight female predominance. Although it was previously reported to be much more common in Jews, this finding was probably due to selection bias. There are two peaks of incidence: one in the third decade and one in the fifth decade. There is a significant familial association but no clear pattern of inheritance.

Pathology

Ulcerative colitis, in contrast to Crohn's disease, is limited to the colon and involves mainly the superficial layers of the bowel. In addition, the inflammation is continuous and is not associated with granulomas. Typically, the disease is found in the distal colon and rectosigmoid area, but it extends proximally to involve the entire colon in more severe cases. Gross pathologic findings include edema, increased mucosal friability, and frank ulceration. Histologic features are crypt abscesses consisting of accumulations of polymorphonuclear cells adjacent to crypts, necrosis of the epithelium, and surrounding accumulations of chronic inflammatory cells (Fig 40–4). Over time, there is distortion of the crypt architecture. Finally, in long-standing disease, epithelial-cell dysplasia and colonic carcinoma may be found.

As in Crohn's disease, the immunopathogenesis is uncertain. Autoantibodies reactive with mucin-associated antigens or with colonic epithelial-cell antigens have been identified in patients. These antibodies have in some cases been demonstrated to cross-react with bacterial cell wall antigens and have been identified in relatives of patients. Other studies have shown that lymphocytes from patients with ulcerative colitis can be cytotoxic for colonic epithelial cells; although not completely proven, this is probably due to arming of Fc receptor-bearing cytotoxic cells with anti-epithelial cell antibodies. These findings suggest that primary immunologic mechanisms, possibly involving an autoimmune component, are the basis of the disease. Overall, the disease mechanism appears to be similar but not identical to that underlying Crohn's disease.

Clinical Features

The clinical features are highly variable. The onset may be insidious or abrupt. Symptoms include diarrhea, tenesmus, and relapsing rectal bleeding. With fulminant involvement of the entire colon, toxic megacolon, a life-threatening emergency, may occur. Extraintestinal manifestations include arthritis, pyoderma gangrenosum, uveitis, and erythema nodosum. As mentioned above, colonic dysplasia

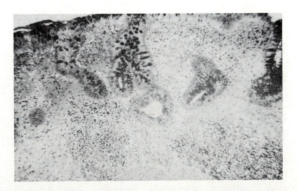

Figure 40–4. Ulcerative colitis. Rectal biopsy shows distortion of crypts and lymphoid aggregates.

and carcinoma may ensue in long-standing disease. Typical laboratory abnormalities include anemia (chronic disease, iron deficiency), leukocytosis, thrombocytosis, elevation of the erythrocyte sedimentation rate, electrolyte abnormalities (in severe diarrhea), and the presence of occult blood in stool. A barium enema study may demonstrate ulcerations and, in more severe disease, pseudopolyps. In chronic disease the colon may be shortened, narrowed, and tubular. Colonoscopy is useful for direct assessment of the degree and extent of inflammation, for biopsy confirmation of the diagnosis, and for screening for dysplasia and carcinoma.

Immunologic Diagnosis

No immunologic test is specific for the disease. Anti-colon epithelial-cell antibodies have been identified in research laboratories, but they have not been shown to be of diagnostic utility.

Differential Diagnosis

The differential diagnosis is similar to that listed above for Crohn's disease, with the addition of ischemic colitis, radiation-induced enteritis, and pseudomembranous colitis. It is occasionally difficult to distinguish between Crohn's disease of the colon and ulcerative colitis. Such differentiation is usually based on the fact that Crohn's disease, but not ulcerative colitis, is a discontinuous lesion and is associated with granulomatous inflammation.

Treatment

As in the case of Crohn's disease, sulfasalazine and related salicylate-containing drugs are effective in mild cases, and corticosteroid drugs are effective in severe cases. Sulfasalazine is used to maintain remission, although with variable results. Topical administration of either salicylates or corticosteroids is effective in some patients, particularly those with disease limited to distal bowel, and is associated with decreased side effects compared with systemic use. Supportive measures such as administration of iron and antidiarrheal agents are sometimes indicated. Azathioprine and 6-mercaptopurine are sometimes used in refractory corticosteroid-dependent cases.

Complications & Prognosis

Ulcerative colitis patients usually respond to medical therapy and enjoy a reasonable quality of life without surgical intervention. However, patients with severe intractable disease or with megacolon may require colectomy. In contrast to Crohn's disease, surgery completely eliminates the disease. In patients who have the disease for longer than 2 decades, the incidence of colon carcinoma increases significantly, and so patients should be subjected to periodic screening examinations. Whether the presence of colonic dysplasia is an indication for prophylactic colectomy is controversial.

ALPHA HEAVY-CHAIN DISEASE

Major Immunologic Features

- The small intestine is infiltrated with malignant, α-chain-producing B cells.
- α-Heavy chain protein is present in serum.

General Considerations

The immunoproliferative intestinal diseases consist of a rare group of premalignant or malignant lymphomas that are limited mostly to the small bowel. The pathognomonic feature is infiltration of the bowel by aberrant B cells, which produce α heavy chains. The diseases are usually found in underdeveloped countries, especially in the Middle East, and generally in young patients of low socioeconomic status. It has been suggested that the disease begins as a response to excessive antigenic stimulation as a result of infectious agents in the setting of malnutrition, since it may respond initially to antibiotic administration. The diffuse infiltration of the intestine is associated with villous flattening and malabsorption. Mucosal ulceration and small-bowel obstruction may occur with progression. The diagnosis is established by intestinal biopsy and the presence of α heavy chain in the serum.

PERNICIOUS ANEMIA

Major Immunologic Features

- Anti-parietal cell antibodies are present.
- Anti-intrinsic factor antibodies are present.

General Considerations

Pernicious anemia is an autoimmune disease in which there is progressive destruction of the gastric fundic glands, leading to atrophic gastritis, achlorhydria, loss of production of intrinsic factor, and vitamin B_{12} malabsorption. The disease presents insidiously with megaloblastic anemia and rarely with neurologic complications due to vitamin B_{12} deficiency. Recognition and treatment of the disease prior to onset of neurologic symptoms is important to prevent irreversible neurologic damage. There is an increased familial incidence and an association with other autoimmune diseases, particularly those involving the thyroid and adrenal glands. Other associations include vitiligo, hypoparathyroidism, and common variable hypogammaglobulinemia. Most patients with pernicious anemia have anti-parietal cell antibodies, and the majority have anti-intrinsic factor antibodies. The fact that such antibodies are found with increased frequency in unaffected family members as well as in patients with other autoimmune diseases suggests that (1) the disease has a genetic component and (2) these antibodies do not cause disease by themselves. This fact, as well as other data, suggests that the disease is caused primarily by T cell-mediated immune damage to the stomach. Routine laboratory abnormalities in pernicious anemia include the presence of megaloblastic anemia, vitamin B_{12} deficiency, and increased serum gastrin. The diagnosis is confirmed by the demonstration of achlorhydria and an abnormal Shilling test, which corrects with addition of intrinsic factor. Treatment consists of vitamin B_{12} replacement. Patients with pernicious anemia have an increased incidence of gastric polyps and gastric carcinoma, and therefore attention to gastric symptoms and screening for occult blood in the stool are indicated.

WHIPPLE'S DISEASE

Major Immunologic Features
■ There is massive infiltration of the lamina propria with periodic acid-Schiff-positive macrophages.
■ There are secondary T cell abnormalities.

General Considerations
Whipple's disease is a rare infectious disease caused by one or more bacteria, which as yet are not well defined. Characteristic features include abdominal pain, diarrhea, weight loss, and a variety of central nervous system manifestations. The diagnosis is established by intestinal biopsy, which discloses free-lying bacteria and the characteristic presence of large numbers of macrophages containing bacterial cell wall debris (periodic acid-Schiff-positive material) in the lamina propria. The infection is not limited to the gastrointestinal tract and can involve the heart, lungs, serosal surfaces, joints, and central nervous system. In the gastrointestinal tract, the cell infiltration leads to "clubbed" villi, lymphatic obstruction, malabsorption, and protein-losing enteropathy. These patients suffer progressive inanition. In addition, when lymphatic obstruction is severe, they may lose lymphocytes into the gastrointestinal tract, become lymphopenic, and develop a secondary T cell immunodeficiency. The cause of the disease is unclear, but it may be due to an inability to respond immunologically to particular bacterial antigens. In any case, the disease frequently responds to antibiotic therapy.

HEPATOBILIARY DISEASES

Stephen P. James, MD, & Warren Strober, MD

Several diseases of the liver and biliary tract have important immunologic features in pathogenesis. These include acute viral hepatitis (Table 40–1), chronic hepatitis, and primary sclerosing cholangitis.

HEPATITIS A

Major Immunologic Feature
■ There are antibodies to HAV (IgG antibodies are long-lived).

General Considerations
Hepatitis A is an acute liver infection caused by a

Table 40–1. Viral and serological characteristics of hepatitis.

| Type | Viral Markers | | Serological Markers | |
	Antigen	Characteristics	Antibody	Characteristics
Hepatitis A	HAAg (hepatitis A antigen)	Found in stool during incubation and transiently during acute symptomatic phase.	IgM anti-HAV IgG anti-HAV	Acute hepatitis Long-lived antibody found during convalescence
Hepatitis B	HBsAg B surface antigen	Viral coat; present in acute and chronic phase.	Anti-HBe	Found during convalescence
	HBcAg	Core antigen found in nuclei of infected hepatocytes.	IgM anti-HBc IgG anti-HBc	Acute hepatitis High titer in chronic hepatitis
	HBeAg	Virus-encoded protein of unknown function; marker of active viral replication.	Anti-HBe	Found after resolution of active replication
	DNA polymerase (HBV DNA)	Found in serum during active replication.		
Hepatitis D	Delta antigen	Found primarily in hepatocyte nuclei and occasionally in serum during active infection.	Anti-delta	High titer in chronic infection
	HBV markers	Requires coinfection with HBV.		
Non-A, non-B, hepatitis	None currently available		None currently available	

small RNA picornavirus (hepatitis A virus, HAV). The virus may cause dramatic epidemics or appear sporadically. Transmission is virtually always by the fecal-oral route. During acute viral hepatitis, there is ballooning and acidophilic degeneration of hepatocytes and portal and periportal infiltration with mononuclear cells. In severe disease, there may be massive necrosis of the liver. HAV particles may be identified in the cytoplasm of infected hepatocytes. Young children with hepatitis A may be asymptomatic, whereas adults usually have nausea, vomiting, dark urine, abdominal pain, and fatigue. Hepatomegaly, abdominal tenderness, and jaundice are typical findings in symptomatic patients. HAV is one of the causes of fulminant hepatitis, which is associated with hepatic encephalopathy and a high mortality rate. Although a relapsing course may rarely occur, the disease usually resolves completely. Typical laboratory features include striking elevations of the serum aminotransferases.

It is thought that the mechanism of liver injury in hepatitis A is not due to the virus itself but rather to the immune response to viral antigens present on the surface of the hepatocytes. In this regard, cytolytic CD8 T cells, which specifically kill hepatitis A–infected target cells, have been shown to be present in the liver in hepatitis A patients. It is thought that variability in the outcome of acute hepatitis A infection, ie, mild versus fulminant disease, might be due in part to genetically controlled differences in the magnitude of the immune response to the virus.

Immunologic Diagnosis

The diagnosis is confirmed by the presence of IgM anti-HAV antibodies. IgG antibodies are long-lived and may persist for the life of the host, and their presence signifies immunity to infection.

Differential Diagnosis

The differential diagnosis of acute hepatocellular necrosis includes acute viral hepatitis from other viruses; toxic hepatitis due to drugs, chemicals, or physical agents; acute fatty liver associated with pregnancy; acute reactivation of chronic hepatitis; fulminant Wilson's disease; and Reye's syndrome.

Treatment

Hepatitis A usually resolves quickly, and there is no evidence of a long-lasting carrier state. Treatment is supportive. No vaccine currently exists, but prophylaxis for close contacts with immune serum globulin is indicated.

HEPATITIS B

Major Immunologic Features

- In acute hepatitis there are HBsAg, HBeAg, and IgM anti-HBc in serum.

- In acute hepatitis (convalescent phase) there is IgG anti-HBs in serum.
- In chronic hepatitis (active viral replication phase) there are HBV DNA, DNA polymerase, HBsAg, HBeAg, and high-titer IgG anti-HBc in serum.
- In chronic hepatitis (viral integration phase) there are HBsAg, anti-HBc, and anti-HBe in serum.
- HBV is not cytopathic; immune mechanisms are thought to cause hepatocyte necrosis.

General Considerations

Hepatitis B virus (HBV) infection is a double-stranded DNA virus of worldwide distribution. The mode of transmission is parenteral or maternal-infant. Individuals at risk for infection include recipients of blood or blood products, drug addicts, dialysis patients, male homosexuals, some health care workers, and infants born to HBV-infected mothers. The risk of chronic infection is higher in infants, immunosuppressed patients, patients with lymphoid cancer, and children with Down's syndrome. Infection has many possible outcomes, including an acute asymptomatic infection or symptomatic hepatitis, a chronic carrier state with or without development of chronic or progressive liver disease, fulminant hepatitis, and hepatocellular carcinoma. Other syndromes associated with HBV include polyarteritis nodosa, aplastic anemia, glomerulonephritis, and essential mixed cryoglobulinemia.

Pathology

The histologic features of acute HBV infection include ballooning and eosinophilic degeneration of hepatocytes, the presence of focal areas of necrosis of hepatocytes, and lymphocytic infiltration of the parenchyma and portal areas. In more severe cases, extensive areas of necrosis of hepatocytes may be present in central and mid zones, which may lead to collapse of the reticulin framework, giving the pattern of "bridging necrosis." In chronic HBV infection, the pathologic findings are variable. In chronic carriers who are clinically well, there may be no histopathologic abnormalities. Alternatively, there may be variable degrees of hepatic inflammation ranging from scattered focal areas of hepatocyte necrosis and lymphocyte infiltration of portal tracts to more severe inflammation, resulting in disruption of the limiting plate between the portal tract and the parenchyma. The latter features are known as piecemeal necrosis. In addition, "ground-glass" hepatocytes, which contain large amounts of hepatitis B surface antigen (HBsAg), may be visible in hematoxylin-and-eosin-stained sections. Chronic type B hepatitis may progress to cirrhosis and hepatocellular carcinoma. Specific antibody staining for HBsAg or hepatitis B core antigen (HBcAg) in acute hepatitis B shows little detectable viral antigen in the liver. In chronic hepatitis, large amounts of HBsAg and (if viral replication is active) HBcAg may be found in hepatocytes.

There is no evidence that HBV is cytopathic, and thus it is thought that hepatocyte injury is mediated by the immune response against the virus. In this regard, evidence has been presented that lymphocytes derived from the liver or circulation of patients with hepatitis B infection are cytotoxic for autologous hepatocytes, but the specificity and mechanism of this cytotoxicity have not yet been completely defined.

Clinical Features

The symptoms of hepatitis B infection are highly variable. As many as half the cases of acute infection are anicteric, and patients have no symptoms or mild nonspecific symptoms of a viral illness. Symptoms described above for acute hepatitis A may occur in typical symptomatic cases. Acute hepatitis B is occasionally preceded by a serum sickness-like syndrome. Approximately 5–10% of patients develop chronic infection (lasting more than 6 months). They often have had a mild or asymptomatic acute infection. During the phase of active viral replication, nonspecific symptoms or symptoms of acute viral hepatitis may be present. With progressive chronic hepatitis, symptoms attributable to cirrhosis or hepatic decompensation may supervene.

Physical findings in acute hepatitis B infection are few. Icterus may be present, the liver may be enlarged and mildly tender, and splenomegaly is sometimes present. In chronic hepatitis B infection, there are often no physical abnormalities until chronic liver damage occurs; at that point, findings common to other chronic liver diseases are seen.

Laboratory findings of acute hepatitis B are similar to those of hepatitis A. In chronic hepatitis B, the serum aminotransferase levels are highly variable and may be normal. However, if significant liver damage is present, hypoalbuminemia and prolongation of the prothrombin time may occur.

Immunologic Diagnosis

Serum immunologic findings in hepatitis B infection are variable, depending on the length and clinical outcome of the infection (Fig 40–5). During acute infection, both HBsAg and IgM anti-HBc are present; in addition, HBV, DNA, and a viral protein antigen known as HBeAg make a transient appearance. With resolution of the acute infection, HBsAg disappears (usually after 1–6 months) and anti-HBsAg appears and persists for years. In chronic infection, the serum findings are variable and depend on the stage of the natural history of the infection. HBsAg is often present in very high titers, as is anti-HBc, but anti-HBs is absent. During the period of active viral replication, HBeAg, DNA polymerase, and HBV DNA are also present. Patients with asymptomatic chronic infection may have episodes of acute reactivation that correlate with the appearance of markers of active viral replication. Eventually, evidence of viral replication may disappear, and there is seroconversion to anti-HBe positivity.

Differential Diagnosis

The serologic diagnosis of acute and chronic hep-

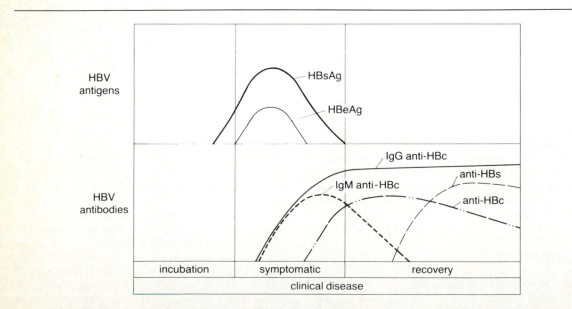

Figure 40–5. Hepatitis B antigens and antibody titers during the course of an acute hepatitis B infection.

atitis B infection is usually definitive. In the setting of chronic hepatitis B infection, an apparent relapse should prompt a search for other possible cases of liver disease including superimposed delta hepatitis (see below) or drug-induced hepatotoxicity.

Treatment

Acute hepatitis B usually resolves completely, and supportive care is needed only for severe hepatitis. In chronic hepatitis, use of specific antiviral agents is considered experimental at present. Although the liver injury in chronic hepatitis B is thought to be immunologically mediated, immunosuppressive drugs alone do not favorably alter the outcome, and their withdrawal may be associated with an acute exacerbation. Since acute exacerbations are occasionally associated with resolution of chronic hepatitis, experimental trials of combinations of corticosteroids followed by antiviral agents are currently being conducted.

Prevention

Screening of blood products for hepatitis B virus has nearly eliminated blood products as a mode of transmission. Individuals at high risk of acquiring hepatitis B should be immunized with HBsAg vaccine, which is safe and confers long-lasting immunity in most individuals.

HEPATITIS D
(Delta Hepatitis)

Major Immunologic Features
- It is caused by a defective virus requiring the presence of HBV infection (hepatitis B markers present in serum).
- Anti-delta antibody is present in serum.

General Considerations

Hepatitis D is caused by a small defective (ie, unable to replicate in the absence of another virus) RNA virus (delta agent), which requires the presence of hepatitis B virus for replication and production of infectious particles. The virus may be associated with acute or fulminant hepatitis due to coinfection with HBV, or it may cause a superimposed acute or chronic hepatitis in patients with chronic hepatitis B infection. The virus is found worldwide and has caused epidemics with high mortality rates. Transmission is primarily parenteral. Since inflammation is not a prominent feature, it is thought that the virus is directly cytopathic. Diagnosis is established by the presence of serum anti-delta antibody and consistent clinical features. There is no effective specific treatment; however, it may be prevented by immunization for hepatitis B, since this prevents the hepatitis B infection necessary for hepatitis D virus replication.

HEPATITIS C
(Non-A, Non-B Hepatitis)

Major Immunologic Features
- It presents as acute and chronic hepatitis similar to hepatitis B.
- There is a specific immunoassay for antibody to viral protein.

General Considerations

Epidemiologic evidence has indicated for many years that hepatitis is caused by more than one virus; hepatitis which is due neither to HAV nor to HBV has been classified as non-A, non-B hepatitis. Non-A, non-B hepatitis is not due to either of these viruses or any other virus known to cause hepatitis, such as cytomegalovirus. Recent research has revealed a protein encoded by what appears to be the major putative viral agent of non-A, non-B hepatitis in the USA, and an immunoassay for antibodies to the peptide has been developed. Approximately 80% of transfusion-associated chronic non-A, non-B hepatitis patients in Japan and Italy had antibodies according to this test; approximately 60% of patients with chronic non-A, non-B hepatitis in the USA without any known source of hepatitis were positive, but only about 15% of patients with acute, resolving transfusion-associated hepatitis in Japan were positive. Thus, it appears that a viral protein has been identified that may be the major cause of chronic transfusion-associated non-A, non-B hepatitis. This agent has been named hepatitis type C virus, although to date it has not been successfully propagated in vitro. Now that a serologic test is available, further epidemiologic study is required to define the prevalence of infection with this agent in the general population and to define its characteristics. There is epidemiologic evidence to suggest that at least one additional viral agent has yet to be identified as a cause of hepatitis. Non-A, non-B hepatitis viruses cause both acute and chronic hepatitis, with the latter more likely to occur than in HBV disease. The pathogenesis of tissue injury in hepatitis C is unknown. At present, treatment of hepatitis C with antiviral agents remains experimental. Avoidance of commercial blood donors has diminished the incidence of posttransfusion non-A, non-B hepatitis, and presumably the development of new assays for hepatitis C virus will further diminish the transmission of this virus by transfusion.

AUTOIMMUNE CHRONIC ACTIVE HEPATITIS

Major Immunologic Features
- There are autoantibodies to smooth-muscle and liver membranes.

- There is polyclonal hypergammaglobulinemia.
- There is HLA-B8/DR3 association.
- There is destruction of hepatocytes associated with portal infiltration of lymphocytes.

General Considerations

Autoimmune hepatitis is a rare form of chronic hepatitis of unknown cause and is associated with various autoimmune phenomena. The disease usually affects women and is more common in individuals of northern European descent. The great majority of cases are sporadic. Of interest, there is a significant association with HLA-B8/DR3 as well as an association with the Gm allotype of IgG, termed "ax." For unknown reasons the incidence of the disease has been declining.

Pathology

The major histologic finding in the liver, one not specific to this disease and mentioned before in relation to hepatitis B infection, is piecemeal necrosis, in which there is necrosis of hepatocytes in the periportal region, disruption of the limiting plate of the portal tract, and local infiltration of lymphoid cells (Fig 40–6). The degree of piecemeal necrosis is variable, but in some patients it may lead to bridging necrosis and cirrhosis. The lymphoid cells infiltrating lesions of autoimmune hepatitis consist of plasma cells and CD4-positive T cells. There are immunoglobulin deposits on hepatocytes.

The mechanism of liver damage in autoimmune hepatitis is unknown. Although autoantibodies against the liver have been shown to be present, it is not clear that they play a role in liver damage. Lymphocyte-mediated killing of autologous hepatocytes has been demonstrated in vitro; however, the specificity and mechanism of this killing are uncertain.

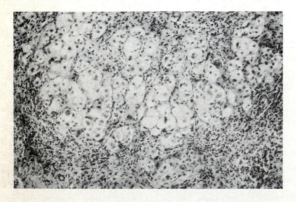

Figure 40–6. Chronic HBV infection. Liver biopsy shows ballooning of hepatocytes and piecemeal necrosis typical of chronic active hepatitis.

Clinical Features

Typical symptoms of autoimmune hepatitis include easy fatigability, jaundice, dark urine, abdominal pain, anorexia, myalgia, delayed menarche, and amenorrhea. Late in the disease, symptoms attributable to progressive chronic liver disease may supervene. Abnormal physical findings include hepatomegaly, jaundice, splenomegaly, spider nevi, and cushingoid features. Common laboratory findings include elevation of serum aminotransferase levels and hypergammaglobulinemia.

Immunologic Diagnosis

There are no serologic features that are diagnostic of the disease. However, polyclonal hypergammaglobulinemia is typically found, and autoantibodies are common, particularly antinuclear antibodies and smooth-muscle antibodies. In addition, antibodies against liver membrane antigens are present. Antimitochondrial antibodies are usually absent and, when present, are found in low titer. Serologic markers of hepatitis viruses are absent. The presence of HLA-B8 supports the diagnosis.

Differential Diagnosis

Since there are no specific diagnostic tests, viral hepatitis and drug- or chemical-induced liver injury must be excluded as well as rare liver diseases such as Wilson's disease and other metabolic liver diseases such as α_1-antitrypsin deficiency. Primary biliary cirrhosis may have features that overlap those of autoimmune hepatitis, but this disease is associated with the presence of antimitochondrial antibodies (see below). Primary sclerosing cholangitis is occasionally misdiagnosed as autoimmune hepatitis, but this disease is associated with characteristic radiographic abnormalities of the biliary system.

Treatment

Unlike those with viral hepatitis, patients with severe autoimmune hepatitis respond favorably to corticosteroid treatment. This therapy may prevent or retard the development of cirrhosis and may improve survival.

PRIMARY BILIARY CIRRHOSIS

Major Immunologic Features

- Associated autoimmune syndromes are frequent.
- There is a high titer of antimitochondrial antibodies in most patients.
- Serum IgM with abnormal properties is elevated.
- There is lymphocytic infiltration and destruction of intrahepatic bile ducts.

General Considerations

Primary biliary cirrhosis is a chronic disease of

unknown cause, primarily affecting middle-aged women. It is characterized by chronic intrahepatic cholestasis due to chronic inflammation and necrosis of intrahepatic bile ducts and progresses insidiously to biliary cirrhosis. Although syndromes resembling primary biliary cirrhosis may follow ingestion of drugs such as chlorpromazine or contraceptive steroids, no toxic or infectious agent has been identified. It has been suggested that primary biliary cirrhosis is an autoimmune disease because of the frequent association of other autoimmune syndromes, the presence of autoantibodies, and histologic features of the disease. Its prevalence has been estimated to be 2.3–14.4 per 100,000. The distribution of the disease is worldwide, without predilection for any racial or ethnic groups. The usual age at diagnosis is in the fifth and sixth decades, but age at onset varies widely from the third to the ninth decade. Ninety percent of patients are female. Familial aggregation has been reported but is rare; however, although there is no known HLA association, the incidence of immunologic abnormalities has been reported to be increased in family members.

Pathology

The histologic abnormalities in the liver have been divided into 4 stages, although they overlap, and more than one stage may be found in biopsies from the same patient. The earliest changes (stage I) are most specific and consist of localized areas of infiltration of intrahepatic bile ducts with lymphocytes and necrosis of biliary epithelial cells; these lesions may have granulomas in close proximity (Fig 40–7). In stage II there is proliferation of bile ductules, prominent infiltration of portal areas with lymphoid cells, and early portal fibrosis. Stage III is character-

ized by reduction of the inflammatory changes, paucity of bile ducts in the portal triads, and increased portal fibrosis. In stage IV, fibrosis is prominent in biliary cirrhosis and a marked increase in hepatic copper is found. Thus, the pathologic process is characterized by slowly progressive, spotty destruction of bile ducts, with associated inflammation and fibrosis and, ultimately, cirrhosis. Hepatocellular necrosis is not a prominent feature, although there are occasional cases of primary biliary cirrhosis-chronic active hepatitis overlap syndromes with piecemeal necrosis. Immunofluorescence shows predominantly IgM plasma cells in portal triads and deposition of IgM. CD4 T cells predominate in portal triads, but CD8 T cells have been observed in close proximity to damaged epithelial cells. HLA-DR antigen expression is increased on biliary epithelial cells, a finding associated with autoimmunity (see Chapter 35).

Although the mechanisms of liver injury in this disease are unknown, the presence of associated autoimmune syndromes and other features suggests that primary biliary cirrhosis is an autoimmune disease. Patients frequently have circulating immune complex-like materials, abnormalities of the complement cascade, and nearly always antimitochondrial antibodies. These antibodies have different specificities, the most prevalent being against the E2 component of pyruvate dehydrogenase, which is present on the inner mitochondrial membrane. In recent years, ample evidence of immunoregulator abnormalities have been found, and it is thought that these underlie the autoimmunity.

Clinical Features

The onset of symptoms is typically insidious, and as many as half of all patients are asymptomatic at diagnosis. Typical symptoms include pruritus, fatigue, increased skin pigmentation, arthralgias, and dryness of the mouth and eyes. Jaundice and gastrointestinal bleeding from varices are uncommon presentations. There may be no abnormalities on physical examination. Typical findings that occur with disease progression include hepatomegaly, splenomegaly, skin hyperpigmentation, excoriations, xanthomata, xanthelasma, spider telangiectasia, and, late in the disease, deep jaundice, petechiae, purpura, and signs of hepatic decompensation. In addition, symptoms or signs of the many associated autoimmune syndromes may be present. The most common include keratoconjunctivitis sicca, arthritis, hypothyroidism, scleroderma (CREST variant), Raynaud's phenomenon, and pulmonary alveolitis.

Common laboratory abnormalities include elevation of serum alkaline phosphatase and γ-glutamyl transpeptidase. Total bilirubin is normal early in the disease but increases progressively as the disease advances. Hypercholesterolemia is also common. Nonspecific laboratory changes of hepatic decompensa-

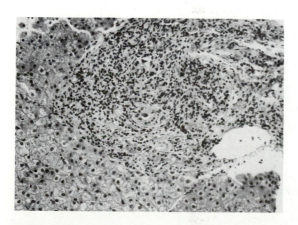

Figure 40–7. Primary biliary cirrhosis. Percutaneous liver biopsy shows bile duct surrounded by dense lymphoid infiltrate typical of stage I disease.

tion are found late in the disease. Cholangiography is normal early in the course of the disease but may reveal distortion of bile ducts due to cirrhosis late in the disease.

Immunologic Diagnosis

The nearly pathognomonic immunologic feature of primary biliary cirrhosis is the presence in high titer of non-species-specific, non-organ-specific antibodies against the inner-membrane components of mitochondria. Antimitochondrial antibodies are found in other autoimmune syndromes, but only in low titer. Less than 10% of primary biliary cirrhosis patients lack these antibodies. Many other autoantibodies are commonly found in patients but are not useful in diagnosis. Other immunologic abnormalities such as circulating immune complex-like materials, complement abnormalities, and abnormalities of lymphocyte function are not useful in diagnosis.

Differential Diagnosis

Chronic cholestasis may follow the administration of drugs such as chlorpromazine, but this does not lead to progressive loss of bile ducts, and it resolves following withdrawal of the drug. Hepatic sarcoidosis may closely mimic primary biliary cirrhosis, but mitochondrial antibodies are absent. Graft-versus-host disease may be found in patients with primary biliary cirrhosis, but in the former disease the basement membrane around bile ducts remain intact. Hepatic allograft rejection may also be associated with nonsuppurative destructive cholangitis.

Treatment

Medical treatment includes supportive treatment such as anion exchange resins to relieve pruritus and administration of lipid-soluble vitamins for nutritional deficiencies. Attempts to suppress the primary inflammatory process have been disappointing. Corticosteroids are considered to be contraindicated because of their tendency in uncontrolled studies to exacerbate metabolic bone disease, complicating the disease. Azathioprine and colchicine may improve survival marginally. D-Penicillamine does not increase survival and is associated with severe side effects. Cyclosporine has been used on an investigational basis but has not yet been proved to be efficacious. The only treatment for end-stage disease is hepatic transplantation.

Complications & Prognosis

Progressive disease is often associated with metabolic bone disease and may lead to chronic hepatic decompensation. Survival from the time of diagnosis is highly variable; asymptomatic patients may have a normal life span. For symptomatic patients, survival from diagnosis is about 12 years. Patients with end-stage disease may be excellent candidates for transplantation, and the long-term prognosis in patients who survive the procedure is good.

PRIMARY SCLEROSING CHOLANGITIS

Major Immunologic Features

- There is chronic inflammation and fibrosis of intrahepatic and extrahepatic bile ducts.
- It is frequently associated with inflammatory bowel disease.

General Considerations

Primary sclerosing cholangitis is a disease of unknown origin characterized by inflammation and fibrosis of both intrahepatic and extrahepatic bile ducts. The disease occurs primarily in young men but may be found in children and older adults. It is often associated with chronic inflammatory bowel disease (usually ulcerative colitis). It is usually progressive and leads to biliary cirrhosis. In addition, it has a significant association with cholangiocarcinoma.

The symptoms are similar to those of other chronic cholestatic diseases and include fatigue, pruritus, hyperpigmentation, xanthelasma, and jaundice. Patients may have fever and abdominal pain associated with superimposed acute bacterial cholangitis. Symptoms of underlying inflammatory bowel disease may be prominent, mild, or absent. Extrahepatic manifestations (other than inflammatory bowel disease) are unusual. Laboratory findings are generally similar to those in primary biliary cirrhosis; however, it is distinct from the latter disease in that antimitochondrial antibodies are absent.

The most important laboratory test is cholangiography, which demonstrates tortuosity and areas of dilatation and stricture of either intrahepatic bile ducts, extrahepatic bile ducts, or both.

The liver biopsy is usually abnormal but is often not diagnostic; the abnormalities may, in fact, occasionally resemble those in primary biliary cirrhosis or autoimmune hepatitis. A characteristic feature that does occur is a fibrous-obliterative process in which segments of bile ducts are replaced by solid cords of connective tissue, leading to an ''onion skin'' appearance. The differential diagnosis includes biliary stricture secondary to stones, surgery, or neoplasia. Like primary biliary cirrhosis, treatment is supportive (eg, antibiotics for cholangitis), and the underlying disease has proved resistant to treatment with anti-inflammatory agents. Patients with localized areas of high-grade obstruction in large bile ducts may benefit from palliative surgical procedures to relieve obstruction. Patients with advanced disease who have not had prior surgery may be excellent candidates for hepatic transplantation.

ORAL & DENTAL DISEASES

John S. Greenspan, BDS, PhD, FRCPath

The mouth is the portal of entry for a variety of antigens, including numerous microorganisms, into the alimentary and respiratory systems. Normally, these antigens do not cause disease and are flushed away with swallowed saliva into the distal parts of the alimentary tract. The mucosal barrier, continual desquamation of oral epithelium, toothbrushing, and other forms of mouth cleaning mechanically protect the mouth. Immunologic defense mechanisms, particularly secretory IgA antibodies, probably prevent adherence of microorganisms to mucosal and tooth surfaces by aggregating them and possibly rendering them more susceptible to phagocytosis.

Several of the most important oral diseases, including caries, the common forms of gingival and periodontal disease, oral herpes simplex virus infections, candidal infections, and the oral manifestations of primary and secondary immunodeficiency, especially AIDS, are due to an imbalance between oral organisms and the host response. This imbalance results from hypersensitivity or immunologic deficiency. Alternatively, particularly in the case of dental caries and chronic inflammatory periodontal disease, specific pathogenic microorganisms may directly damage the tissues regardless of the status of the host response.

Another group of oral diseases in which immunologic factors have been implicated are those in which oral tissues are a target for autoimmune reactions. Manifestations may be confined to the mouth or may involve other systemic organs. Many are mucocutaneous diseases, several are rheumatoid diseases (these are discussed in Chapters 36 and 42), and others involve mainly the gastrointestinal tract. The role of tumor immune mechanisms in oral homeostasis and the part that defects in these mechanisms play in the cause and pathogenesis of oral precancerous lesions and mucosal malignancy constitute a rapidly growing field of interest. Tumor immune mechanisms are probably important but must be considered in the context of other factors including oncogenic viruses and chemical carcinogens.

LOCAL ORAL DISEASES INVOLVING IMMUNOLOGIC MECHANISMS

1. INFLAMMATORY PERIODONTAL DISEASES: GINGIVITIS & PERIODONTITIS

Major Immunologic Features

- Bacterial dental plaque induces inflammation of tissues immediately surrounding the teeth.
- The local responses of the host are not effective in eliminating the bacteria, which continue to adhere to the tooth surfaces. Humoral and cellular immunity are both involved in these responses.
- Local responses include complement activation, infiltration of leukocytes, release of lysosomal enzymes and cytokines, and production of a serous gingival crevicular exudate.
- Inflammatory agents from the bacteria and immunopathologic reactions of the host result in gingivitis and periodontitis.

General Considerations

Inflammation of the supporting tissues of the teeth produces one of the most common forms of human diseases. Depending on its severity, the destructive process may involve both the gingiva (gingivitis) and the periodontal ligament and alveolar bone surrounding and supporting the teeth (periodontitis). Periodontitis may involve both the direct cytotoxic and proteolytic effects of dental plaque and the indirect pathologic consequences of the host immune response to the continued presence of bacterial plaque microorganisms (Fig 40–8).

Dental plaque consists of a mass of bacteria that adheres tenaciously to the tooth surfaces. In gingivitis, the plaque generates inflammation of the gingival tissue without affecting the underlying periodontal ligament and bone. In periodontitis, attachment between the gingiva and the involved teeth is lost, subgingival bacterial plaque forms on the root surfaces, and bone loss is clinically apparent (Figs 40–9 and 40–10). Elimination of the plaque usually stops the inflammatory process. In children with poor oral hygiene, gingivitis is common but periodontitis is rare.

The microflora of the dental plaque is complex, comprising many different strains of bacteria including gram-positive rods and cocci and gram-negative rods, cocci, and filamentous forms. In general, the healthy gingival crevice contains only a few gram-positive streptococcal and facultative *Actinomyces*

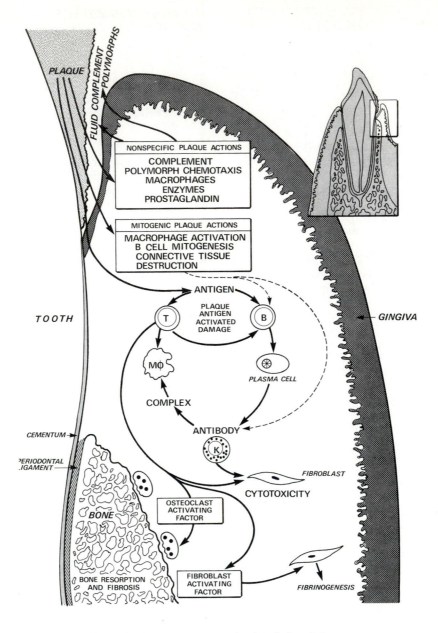

Figure 40–8. The pathogenesis of periodontal disease.

species. As gingivitis develops, many more gram-negative organisms are found, including *Fusobacterium nucleatum, Bacteroides intermedius,* and *Haemophilus* species. Many motile rods and spirochetes are also seen. In advanced adult periodontitis, the organisms usually cultured are predominantly gram-negative anaerobic rods such as *Bacteroides gingivalis, B intermedius,* and *F nucleatum.* Furthermore, phase-contrast examination shows that as many as

50% of organisms from such lesions are motile rods and spirochetes. There is some indirect evidence for a relationship between particular forms of periodontal disease and specific microorganisms. Thus, elevated levels and increased frequency of serum antibodies to *Actinobacillus actinomycetemcomitans, Capnocytophaga* spp, and *Eikenella corrodens* are found in localized juvenile periodontitis (rapidly progressive periodontitis) (see below).

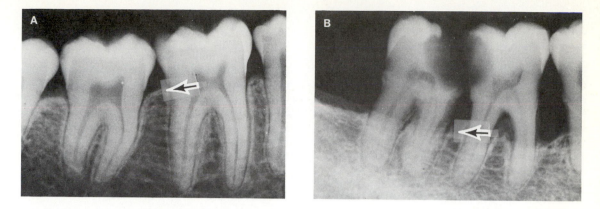

Figure 40–9. Radiographs of the lower molars of a 25-year-old man with a normal periodontium (**A**) and a 45-year-old man with advanced periodontitis and severe dental caries (**B**). In the patient with periodontitis, more than half of the supporting alveolar bone has been destroyed (arrows). (Courtesy of GC Armitage.)

Immunologic Pathogenesis

A delicate balance exists between dental plaque organisms and the host response. In healthy individuals, the immunologic response provides a well-regulated specific defense against infiltration by plaque substances. The tissue-destructive mechanisms thought to be involved in periodontal disease include direct effects of plaque bacteria, polymorphonuclear-induced damage, neutrophil complement-mediated damage initiated by both antibody and the alternative pathway, and cell-mediated damage.

Clinically apparent gingivitis is probably the result of an exaggerated response to bacterial plaque. Individuals with mild gingivitis have, in addition to a continued polymorphonuclear infiltration, a gingival influx of a few T lymphocytes. However, those with prolonged severe gingivitis and severe periodontitis have an influx composed mainly of B lymphocytes and plasma cells, with resulting IgG antibody production. Most noteworthy in severe periodontal disease is the extremely low proportion of gingival plasma cells committed to IgG2 production, while serum levels of the other IgG subclasses are normal. The proportions of antibodies of IgG3, IgG1, or IgG4 subclasses with specific antibody activity for plaque antigens in the gingival tissues are unknown. This unusual local IgG subclass response may indicate a degree of nonspecific activation of B lymphocytes arriving in the inflamed area, possibly caused by a variety of mechanisms involving bacterial mitogens and proteases. The bacteria may also activate the alternative complement pathway. Associated with gingivitis is the generation of a serum exudate known as crevicular fluid, which flows from around the teeth and contacts the dental plaque. This exu-

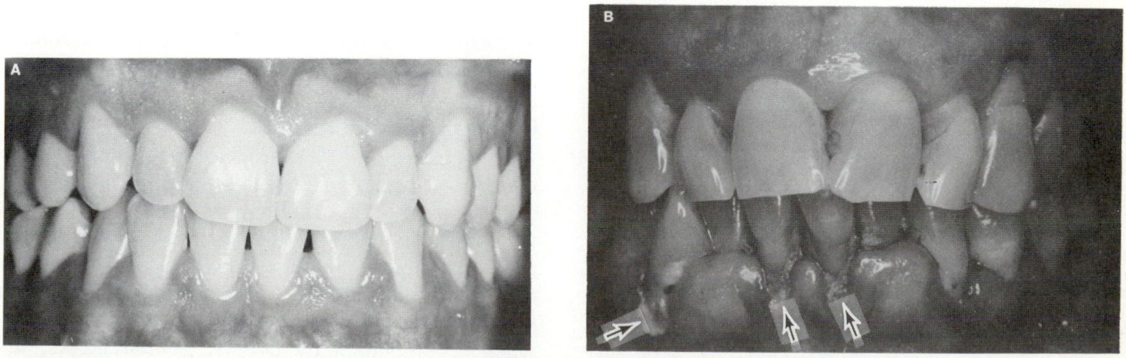

Figure 40–10. Clinical appearance of the anterior teeth and periodontal tissues of a 22-year-old man with healthy gingiva (**A**) and a 48-year-old man with advanced periodontitis (**B**). Note the heavy deposits of plaque and calculus (arrows) in the patient with periodontitis. Marked gingival inflammation is particularly noticeable around the lower anterior teeth. Most teeth have either pocket formation or extensive gingival recession. (Courtesy of GC Armitage.)

date, like serum, contains functional complement components as well as low levels of specific antibodies to the various plaque antigens.

The onset of flow of crevicular fluid is an important stage in the progression of periodontal disease. Crevicular fluid complement is rapidly activated by a combination of effects. These include activation of the classic pathway by IgG and IgM antibodies to subgingival plaque antigens; activation of the alternative complement pathway by endotoxins and peptidoglycan from gram-negative and gram-positive microorganisms, respectively; and activation of complement components by host and bacterial proteolytic enzymes. Complement activation results first in the release of C3a and C5a, which cause additional edema and increase crevicular fluid flow, and subsequently in chemotactic attraction of polymorphonuclear leukocytes. Other chemotactic factors are produced directly by the plaque microorganisms. The release of proteolytic enzymes with collagenase and trypsinlike activities by host cells is believed to damage tissue and activate additional complement components and subsequent release of prostaglandin E. In vitro, prostaglandin E can induce bone resorption through its effect on osteoclasts.

Cell-mediated immunity may also play a role in the progression of periodontal disease. In some studies, individuals with periodontal disease generally exhibit increased peripheral blood T lymphocyte reactivity to plaque antigens. Yet, for reasons unknown, in severe gingivitis and severe periodontitis the local T cell response to the plaque is conspicuously small. Bone destruction in periodontal disease may be mediated by lymphokines including osteoclast-activating factor as well as by parathyroid hormone and prostaglandins. Individuals with reduced immunologic capacity, notably primary immunodeficiency and immunodeficiency secondary to treatment associated with kidney transplantation, do not have more gingival and periodontal disease than do normal controls. However, severe periodontal disease is seen in association with HIV infection.

Immunologic Diagnosis

Lymphocytes from individuals with periodontal disease are more responsive to dental plaque antigens in vitro than are lymphocytes from normal individuals, but no clear relationships have been found between disease severity and serum or salivary antibody levels. At present, immunologic tests are not generally useful in the diagnosis of gingivitis and periodontitis. Most individuals with inflammatory periodontitis have gingivitis, but the clinical symptoms of the latter may be masked by fibrosis.

Treatment

Although gingivitis and periodontitis are apparently caused by dental bacterial plaque, there is a reluctance to treat this disease with antibiotics be-

cause elimination of one group of organisms by antibiotics may lead to the emergence of antibiotic-resistant strains. However, some clinicians use local application of tetracycline depending on the severity of the periodontal disease. Treatment may range from simply good routine oral hygiene to periodontal surgery. Reduction of plaque accumulation to an absolute minimum is essential for the arrest of gingivitis or the reduction of periodontal ligament destruction and bone loss. Topical antibacterial agents, notably chlorhexidine, are valuable for this purpose.

2. JUVENILE PERIODONTITIS

In a small percentage of the population, periodontal bone loss occurs very rapidly, sometimes within 2–5 years. In this condition—juvenile periodontitis, formerly known as periodontosis—conventional periodontal treatment is ineffective. There is a characteristic gram-negative anaerobic flora, different from that in the more slowly progressive form of periodontitis. Short-term antibiotics are probably useful in these cases, but there is no evidence that the results of such treatment are permanent. Several reports suggest that defects in granulocyte or monocyte function may be involved.

RECURRENT ORAL ULCERATION
(Aphthous Stomatitis)

Major Immunologic Features
- Lymphocyte infiltration is present at the earliest stage of the lesion.
- Circulating antibodies to oral mucous membranes are present in some patients and may cross-react with oral organisms.
- Cellular immunity to the same antigens is reported.
- Circulating immune complexes are found in some patients.
- There is association with HLA-B12.
- Response to topical or systemic corticosteroids is favorable.

General Considerations

After caries and chronic periodontal disease, oral ulceration probably represents the most common lesion of the mouth. Although oral ulcers can be due to a large number of diseases, the most common form is recurrent oral ulceration (aphthous stomatitis). Recurrent oral ulcers usually occur alone, but may be a local manifestation of Behçet's disease when accompanied by uveitis, genital ulcers, and perhaps lesions of other systems. Estimates of the prevalence of recurrent oral ulceration vary, but probably 20% of the population experience it. The condition may recur only once or twice a year or may be so frequent that a new set of ulcers overlaps a previous group. There is slight evidence of a familial incidence. Emotional and nutritional factors may play a causative role, and an association has been suggested with changes in the hormone status during the menstrual cycle. Extensive searches for specific bacterial or viral causes have been unsuccessful. A possible role for herpes simplex virus type 1 has again been raised by the observation that part of the herpes simplex virus genome is present and transcribed in peripheral blood mononuclear cells of patients with recurrent aphthae and Behçet's disease. Additional evidence also indicates a possible role for *Streptococcus sanguis,* since this organism has been cultured from the ulcers and patients exhibit delayed hypersensitivity reactions to the organism and significant inhibition of leukocyte migration by antigens of this organism in vitro. However, the organism is a common commensal. One study has shown reduced lymphocyte transformation to *S sanguis* in patients compared with controls. A likely role for bacterial or viral agents in this disease is that of cross-reacting antigens, which elicit host responses to autologous oral mucous-membrane antigens.

Immunologic Pathogenesis

Patients have a raised level of circulating antibody to a saline extract of fetal oral mucous membrane. Slightly raised levels of the same antibody have been found in other ulcerative conditions, but in lower titers. The antibodies are of the agglutinating and complement-fusing types, suggesting that antibody cytotoxicity might be involved in the tissue destruction. However, some studies show poor correlation between the level of anti-mucous membrane antibody and clinical features of the disease. In addition, 2 other mechanisms could explain the presence of circulating autoantibodies of this type. The antibodies may cross-react with antigens of an organism present in the mouth, such as *S sanguis* or a virus, and oral mucous membrane epithelial cells. Alternatively, the antibodies may be a response to exposed tissue antigens from chronic ulcerations that had previously been protected from the immune system. Attempts to show that patient serum containing significant titers of this antibody has a direct cytotoxic effect against oral epithelial cells have been unsuccessful. Thus, it is unlikely that a cytotoxic anti-oral mucosal antibody is directly involved in the pathogenesis.

Interest in the role of cellular immunity in the pathogenesis of recurrent oral ulceration was aroused by the observation that the earliest histologic changes involve the presence of an infiltrate of lymphocytes. Other cells do not appear until a later stage. Furthermore, patients with recurrent oral ulceration have peripheral blood lymphocytes that are sensitized to oral mucous-membrane antigen. These 2 observations support the hypothesis that a cell-mediated hypersensitivity mechanism might be involved in the pathogenesis of the lesion. Lymphocytes from some patients with recurrent oral ulceration are cytotoxic to oral epithelial cells. The antigen eliciting the cytotoxic reaction has not been identified. It might be one or more epithelial cell surface autoantigens, determinants cross-reacting with an infecting organism or organisms, or food or microbial antigens attached to oral epithelial cell surfaces or even by a hapten. Increased antibody-dependent cellular cytotoxicity has been found, but the identity of the population of lymphocytes involved in these reactions is also unknown. There is at present no acceptable hypothesis linking oral mucous membrane autoantigens and effector mechanisms, although transient defects in immunoregulation have been postulated.

Patients with Behçet's disease and recurrent oral ulceration show elevated levels of serum C9 and of circulating soluble immune complexes. IgG and C3 have also been demonstrated in the basement membrane zone of the lesions. It is not clear whether these observations are clues to the immunologic pathogenesis of the disease or represent epiphenomena. There is also some evidence for an increased incidence of HLA-B12 in recurrent oral ulceration.

Treatment & Prognosis

Effective treatment depends on identification of any underlying systemic disease. In such cases, treatment of the systemic condition usually leads to cure of the oral ulceration. For the remaining group, uncomplicated by known systemic disease, several treatment forms are available. They are the use of topical corticosteroids, antibiotics, and immunostimulants. The most effective topical corticosteroids available are 0.1% triamcinolone in Orabase, 2.5-mg tablets of hydrocortisone sodium succinate, and 0.025% fluocinonide in Orabase. Some cases of major aphthous ulceration are sufficiently severe to warrant the use of systemic prednisone. Tetracycline mouth rinses have been used with some success in the herpetriform variety of recurrent oral ulceration. The treatment of Behçet's disease is discussed in Chapter 36.

ACQUIRED IMMUNODEFICIENCY SYNDROME (AIDS)

The oral mucosa is particularly hospitable to opportunistic pathogens. Thus, primary and recurrent herpes simplex virus, varicella-zoster virus, and several fungi, notably *Candida* species, are frequent features of primary immunodeficiency syndromes (see Chapter 23). The same conditions, as well as a number of others, are seen in patients whose immune systems are compromised by chemotherapy, those receiving bone marrow transplants, patients with leukemia or lymphoma, and those with clinical expressions of HIV-induced immunosuppression.

The oral features of AIDS include Kaposi's sarcoma, non-Hodgkin lymphoma, and severe oral candidiasis as well as persistent herpesvirus lesions (herpes simplex virus and varicella-zoster virus). Other conditions seen in AIDS and other HIV disease include severe periodontal disease, oral warts, and the recently described lesion known as oral hairy leukoplakia.

Hairy leukoplakia is seen on the tongue in HIV immunosuppressed patients. Ninety-nine percent of patients are HIV virus antibody-positive, and the majority of those tested carry the virus in blood lymphocytes. This lesion has characteristic histopathologic features suggestive of human papillomavirus, further evidence for the presence of which is provided by antigen staining. However, no human papillomavirus DNA is found by hybridization techniques. Instead, clear evidence for the presence of Epstein-Barr virus (EBV) comes from immunocytochemistry with monoclonal antibodies, from electron-microscopic morphology, and from DNA studies with EBV probes. Southern blot hybridization provides evidence for the presence of EBV DNA in complete linear virion form and in very high copy number. At the time of diagnosis of hairy leukoplakia, about 20% of patients have AIDS, but a very large number of those who are AIDS-free when first seen subsequently develop AIDS, with mean conversion rates at 48% at 16 months and 83% at 30 months, mostly with *Pneumocystis carinii* pneumonia.

Oral hairy leukoplakia is a significant indicator of HIV-induced immunosuppression and is highly predictive of the subsequent development of AIDS. It appears to be one of only 2 oral lesions specifically associated with HIV infection. It is the first form of oral leukoplakia consistently associated with a virus or viruses. The mechanism whereby HIV favors oral opportunistic infection presumably involves viral elimination of helper T cells and thus the loss of cell-mediated immunity to herpesviruses and fungi as well as to other organisms. However, other mechanisms may also mediate the immune defect, including loss of Langerhans cells or their functions as well as polymorphonuclear cell and macrophage aberrations.

ORAL CANDIDIASIS

Major Immunologic Features
- There are many associated immunologic defects.
- It is the most significant oral indication of an underlying immunodeficiency.
- It is a prominent feature of HIV-induced immunodeficiency.

General Considerations
Oral candidiasis is the most common oral fungal disease. It may occur in acute or chronic form at any age. The disease may be a sign of serious life-threatening systemic disease or may be confined to a small part of the oral mucous membrane and have no general significance. *Candida* species are frequent oral commensals, and it has not yet been established whether candidiasis is predominantly of endogenous or exogenous origin.

Immunologic Pathogenesis
The immunologic features of generalized candidiasis are discussed in Chapters 25 and 52. A wide range of immunologic defects have been found, including defects in cytotoxicity to *Candida,* reduced lymphokine production, failure of anticandidal antibody response of one or more classes, generalized cytotoxicity defects, failure of lymphocyte activation to candidal antigen, absence of the delayed hypersensitivity skin test to *Candida* or to many antigens, and presence of an abnormal suppressor T cell population. However, immunologic defects alone do not explain the pathogenesis of candidiasis. High glucose levels in diabetics and low levels of serum iron transferrin and blood folate are also important factors. Granulocyte defects have been shown in some patients, as have defects in leukocyte myeloperoxidase. A few patients have been described in whom antibody production to *Candida* and other antigens was raised while cellular immune function was depressed.

Immunologic Diagnosis
The diagnosis of thrush is based upon the clinical appearance and history. The immunologic approach is directed toward establishing the nature of the immunologic defect, if any. Although immunologic investigation of patients with oral candidiasis is still predominantly a research tool, it is likely that subtypes of patients will be identified and that specific immunologic treatment will be directed toward the correction of localized defects in cell-mediated immunity. The differential diagnosis of candidal leukoplakia from other white oral lesions involves smear, culture, and biopsy.

Treatment & Prognosis
Treatment of localized oral candidiasis consists of elimination of predisposing factors, when known, and administration of topical antifungal therapy. This may be prolonged in the treatment of chronic oral candidiasis. Systemic therapy is used in cases that are resistant to local measures and in generalized mucocutaneous candidiasis.

REFERENCES

General

Brown WR, Strober W: Immunological disease of the gastrointestinal tract. In: *Immunological Diseases.* Samter M et al (editors). Little, Brown, 1988.

James SP: Immunology of hepatobiliary diseases. In: *Immunological Diseases.* Samter M et al (editors). Little, Brown, 1988.

Gluten-Sensitive Enteropathy

Strober, W: Gluten-sensitive enteropathy: An abnormal immunologic response of the gastrointestinal tract to a dietary protein. In: *Gastrointestinal Immunity for the Clinician.* Kirsner JR, Shorter RG (editors). Grune & Stratton, 1985.

Crohn's Disease & Ulcerative Colitis

Strober W, James S: The immunologic basis of inflammatory bowel disease. *J Clin Immunol* 1986;**6:**415.

Primary Biliary Cirrhosis

James SP et al: Primary biliary cirrhosis: A model autoimmune disease. *Ann Intern Med* 1983;**99:**500.

Primary Sclerosing Cholangitis

LaRusso NF et al: Primary sclerosing cholangitis. *N Engl J Med* 1984;**310:**899.

Alpha Chain Disease

Seligman M: Immunochemical, clinical and pathological features of alpha-chain disease. *Arch Intern Med* 1975;**135:**78.

Pernicious Anemia

Kay MD: Immunological aspects of gastritis and pernicious anemia. *Beillieres Clin Gastroenterol* 1987;**1:**487.

Hepatitis

Czaja AJ: Natural history, clinical feature and treatment of autoimmune hepatitis. *Semin Liver Dis* 1984;**4:**1.

Dienstag JL: Non-A, non-B hepatitis: Recognition, epidemiology and clinical features. *Gastroenterology* 1983; **85:**439.

Hoofnagle JH: Chronic type B hepatitis. *Gastroenterology* 1983;**84:**422.

Kuo G et al: An assay for circulating antibodies to a major etiologic virus of human non-A, non-B hepatitis. *Science* 1989;**244:**362.

Rizzetto M et al: Hepatitis delta virus disease. *Prog Liver Dis* 1986;**7:**56.

Periodontal Disease

Engel D et al: Mitogen-induced hyperproliferation response of peripheral blood mononuclear cells from patients with severe generalized periodontitis: Lack of correlation with proportions of T cells and T-cell subsets. *Clin Immunol Immunopathol* 1984;**30:**374.

Genco RB, Mergenhagen SE (editors): *Host-Parasite Interactions in Periodontal Diseases.* American Society for Microbiology, 1982.

Lavine WS et al: Impaired neutrophil chemotaxis in patients with juvenile and rapidly progressing periodontitis. *J Periodontal Res* 1979;**14:**10.

Page RC et al: Rapidly progressive periodontitis: A distinct clinical condition. *J Periodontol* 1983;**54:**197.

Robertson PB et al: Periodontal status of patients with abnormalities of the immune system. *J Periodontol* 1980;**51:**70.

Seymour GJ et al: The identification of lymphoid cell subpopulations in sections human lymphoid tissue and gingivitis in children using monoclonal antibodies. *J Periodontal Res* 1982;**17:**247.

Tew JG et al: Immunological studies of young adults with severe periodontitis. 2. Cellular factors. *J Periodontal Res* 1981;**16:**403.

Recurrent Oral Ulceration

Burnett PR, Wray D: Lytic effects of serum and mononuclear leukocytes on oral epithelial cells in recurrent aphthous stomatitis. *Clin Immunol Immunopathol* 1985; **34:**197.

Eglin RP, Lehner T, Subak-Sharpe JH: Detection of RNA complementary to herpes-simplex virus in mononuclear cells from patients with Behçet's syndrome and recurrent oral ulcers. *Lancet* 1982;**2:**1356.

Gadol N et al: Leukocyte migration inhibition in recurrent aphthous ulceration. *J Oral Pathol* 1985;**14:**121.

Greenspan JS et al: Antibody-dependent cellular cytotoxicity in recurrent aphthous ulceration. *Clin Exp Immunol* 1981;**44:**603.

Greenspan JS et al: Lymphocyte function in recurrent aphthous ulceration. *J Oral Pathol* 1985;**14:**603.

Lindemann RA, Riviere GR, Sapp JP: Oral mucosal antigen reactivity during exacerbation and remission phases of recurrent aphthous ulceration. *Oral Surg* 1985;**60:**281.

Savage NW, Seymour GJ, Kruer BJ: T-lymphocyte subset changes in recurrent aphthous stomatitis. *Oral Surg* 1985;**60:**175.

Acquired Immunodeficiency Syndrome

Greenspan D et al: Oral "hairy" leukoplakia in male homosexuals: Evidence of association with both papillomavirus and a herpes-group virus. *Lancet* 1984;**2:**831.

Greenspan JS et al: Replication of Epstein-Barr virus within the epithelial cells of oral "hairy" leukoplakia, an AIDS-associated lesion. *N Engl J Med* 1985;**313:**1564.

Lozada F et al: Oral manifestations of tumor and opportunistic infection in the acquired immunodeficiency syndrome (AIDS): Findings in 53 homosexual males with Kaposi's sarcoma. *Oral Surg* 1983;**55:**601.

Oral Candidiasis

Aronson IK, Soltani K: Chronic mucocutaneous candidiasis: A review. *Mycopathologia* 1976;**60:**17.

Corbeel L et al: Immunological observations before and after successful treatment of mucocutaneous candidiasis with ketoconazole and transfer factor. *Eur J Pediatr* 1984;**143:**45.

Epstein JB et al: Effects of specific antibodies on the interaction between the fungus Candida albicans and human oral mucosa. *Arch Oral Biol* 1982;**27:**469.

Lehner T: Classification and clinico-pathological features of Candida infections in the mouth. In: *Symposium on Candida Infections.* Winner HI, Hurley RE (editors). Livingstone, 1966.

41

Renal Diseases

Curtis B. Wilson, MD, Alessandro Fornasieri, MD, Phillippe Moullier, MD, PhD,
Winson Tang, MD, & David M. Ward, MB, ChB, MRCP(UK)

Immunologically induced glomerulonephritis and tubulointerstitial nephritis are estimated to be responsible for roughly half of all instances of end-stage renal failure and its consequent mortality, morbidity, and expense. Nephritogenic antibody-antigen reactions most often lead directly or indirectly to glomerular immune deposits. The subsequent activation of humoral and cellular mediator systems produces foci of glomerular inflammation (Table 41–1). Recently, it has been shown experimentally that antibody-induced damage can be restricted to a single glomerular cell type when the surface antigens of that cell are involved.

Immune deposits occur when nephritogenic antibodies react directly with antigens in the kidney. In humans, the major nephritogenic structural antigens are in the glomerular basement membrane (GBM). Antibodies may also react with nonrenal, often exogenous, antigens that have been ''trapped'' in the GBM by physiologic, immunologic, or physicochemical mechanisms such as the reaction of cationic molecules with the polyanionic glomerular capillary wall.

In contrast to the direct reaction of antibody with renal antigens, glomerular injury can occur when antibodies react with soluble antigens in the circulation to form immune complexes, which subsequently ac-

cumulate in the glomerulus. Immune-complex formation is a dynamic process with continual modification of the deposited immune complexes by ongoing interaction with additional antibodies, antigens, or immune complexes from the circulation. The local exchange with tissue-fixed immune complex results in some overlap between the direct and indirect mechanisms of glomerular immune deposit formation. On the basis of identification of nonglomerular exogenous and endogenous antigens and their antibodies in glomeruli, most cases of human glomerulonephritis appear to be caused by the immune-complex mechanism.

In renal biopsy tissue, antibodies reactive with the GBM have a characteristic linear configuration by immunofluorescence microscopy, whereas randomly deposited immune complexes have a granular pattern. However, antibodies directly reactive with fixed glomerular antigens that are distributed irregularly could be confused with immune-complex disease.

In contrast to the humoral mechanisms of glomerulonephritis, there is much less evidence for a contribution by cellular immunity. A cellular immune response has been recognized in some forms of human glomerulonephritis. Sometimes T cells can be identified in nephritic glomeruli, and a role for T

Table 41–1. Immunopathogenesis of humorally mediated renal disease classified by the solubility of the antigen.

Solubility	Mechanism	Antigen	Condition
Insoluble or tissue-fixed antigens	Antibodies react with structural components of the kidney.	GBM	Glomerulonephritis
		TBM	Tubulointerstitial nephritis
		Other glomerular wall antigens	Experimental glomerulonephritis
		Cell surface antigens	Experimental glomerulonephritis, tubulointerstitial nephritis
	Antibodies react with antigens trapped or "planted" in the glomerulus.	Mesangial accumulations, immune-complex components, lectins, cationic materials; possibly bacterial antigens, DNA.	Experimental glomerulonephritis. May contribute to human glomerulonephritis as well.
Soluble antigens	Antibodies react with antigens in the vascular compartment to form circulating immune complexes.	Exogenous antigens: drugs, products of infectious agents, etc.	Glomerulonephritis, tubulointerstitial nephritis, vasculitis
		Endogenous antigens: nuclear antigens, tumor antigens, etc.	
	Antibodies react with antigens in the extravascular fluid near the site of antigen release.	Tubular antigens	Experimental tubulointerstitial nephritis

cells in some forms of experimental glomerulonephritis has been shown by cell transfer studies.

The actual glomerular injury caused by glomerular antibody accumulation results in large part from the action of immunologic mediator systems. The best studied of these are the complement and neutrophil systems. Complement activation generates biologically active fragments that initiate immune adherence, opsonization, histamine release, and leukocyte chemotaxis. Deposition of C5–C9 in human diseases suggests that the membrane attack complex may participate in the glomerular injury. In some situations complement activation can serve to solubilize immune-complex material and may affect immune-complex handling by erythrocyte CR1 receptors. In many forms of glomerulonephritis, neutrophils attracted by products of complement activation accumulate in the glomerular capillary loops, where they can displace the endothelium and release enzymes and other injurious materials, including reactive oxygen species.

In addition to neutrophils and the complement system, macrophages, platelets, and plasma factors including coagulation proteins can contribute to glomerular injury. Glomerular fibrin deposits have been found in patients with glomerulonephritis, usually in association with extracapillary crescent formation. Glomerular cells themselves, particularly mesangial cells, can produce a large variety of mediator molecules including proteases, interleukin-1, tumor necrosis factor, platelet-activating factor, and arachidonic acid metabolites.

ANTI-GLOMERULAR BASEMENT MEMBRANE ANTIBODY-INDUCED GLOMERULONEPHRITIS

Major Immunologic Features
- Linear deposition of immunoglobulin and often of C3 occurs along the GBM.
- Anti-GBM antibodies are usually detectable in serum by radioimmunoassay (RIA), less often by indirect immunofluorescence techniques.

General Considerations

Anti-GBM antibodies can produce glomerulonephritis, Goodpasture's syndrome (glomerulonephritis and pulmonary hemorrhage), and, occasionally, idiopathic pulmonary hemosiderosis. The pathogenicity of these antibodies was demonstrated (1) by transfer to subhuman primates by using anti-GBM antibodies recovered from the serum of or eluted from the kidneys of affected patients and (2) by the observation of recurrence of anti-GBM antibody disease in renal transplants inadvertently placed in patients with residual circulating anti-GBM antibodies.

The nephritogenic GBM antigens appear to be in the noncollagenous carboxyl extension of the type IV procollagen molecule, a region termed NC1. This region of the type IV molecule is involved in intermolecular joining. Of interest, anti-GBM antibodies do not react with the GBM from affected individuals in some kindreds of patients with hereditary nephritis (Alport's syndrome), a condition with GBM abnormalities. Transplantation of a normal kidney to such an individual lacking the reactive antigen may induce nephritogenic anti-GBM antibodies in the recipient.

Little is known about the events responsible for the induction of spontaneous anti-GBM antibodies in humans. There is a suggested genetic association with HLA-DR2. Materials cross-reactive with the GBM have been identified in the urine of animals and humans. Mercuric chloride administered to rats produces a transient anti-GBM antibody response. Both hydrocarbon solvent inhalation and influenza A2 virus infections have been associated with anti-GBM antibody production and Goodpasture's syndrome in a few patients. The duration of the anti-GBM antibody response is self-limited, suggesting that the immunologic stimulus is also transient. Most affected individuals have only a single episode, although 2 or more episodes have been reported.

Less than 5% of human glomerulonephritis is caused by anti-GBM antibodies. There is a bimodal age distribution. Anti-GBM antibody-associated Goodpasture's syndrome is most commonly identified in males in the second to fourth decades of life; however, either sex can be involved, and children under 5 and adults over 70 can be affected. A second grouping of cases occurs in patients older than 50 years. Glomerulonephritis alone is more common in this group, and there is a female predominance.

Pathology

The renal pathology induced by anti-GBM antibodies is related to quantitative and temporal factors of antibody binding. Lesions may vary from mild focal proliferative glomerulonephritis to diffuse proliferative necrotizing glomerulonephritis with crescent formation. The anti-GBM antibody deposits are not visualized by electron microscopy, in contrast to the electron-dense deposits of immune complexes. Tubulointerstitial nephritis in patients with anti-GBM antibody disease is caused by concomitant anti-tubular basement membrane (TBM) antibodies. The pulmonary pathology of Goodpasture's syndrome is intra-alveolar hemorrhage with hemosiderin-laden macrophages in alveoli and sputum.

Clinical Features

Half to two-thirds (depending on age and sex) of patients with anti-GBM antibody glomerulonephritis also have pulmonary hemorrhage and often respiratory impairment. This condition is referred to as

Goodpasture's syndrome. The first symptoms may be either renal or pulmonary, occurring nearly simultaneously or separated by as much as 1 year. Episodes of pulmonary hemorrhage may occur at any time during anti-GBM antibody production. Alteration in the accessibility of the alveolar basement membrane antigen by such factors as fluid overload, toxin exposure (smoking, hydrocarbons), or infection may facilitate the binding of anti-GBM antibodies and precipitate the episodes of lung injury. In many patients, particularly those with Goodpasture's syndrome, influenzalike symptoms precede the onset of renal or pulmonary symptoms. Arthritis is an early complaint in fewer than 10% of patients, and central nervous system involvement may occur infrequently. Overall, about 75% of patients develop renal failure, necessitating dialysis, although the outlook is improving somewhat as a result of early diagnosis and more aggressive treatment. Milder forms of disease account for fewer than 10% of cases. Nephrotic syndrome is unusual in anti-GBM antibody glomerulonephritis.

Immunologic Diagnosis

The diagnosis of anti-GBM antibody disease can be established by finding at least 2 of the following: (1) linear deposits of immunoglobulins along the GBM by immunofluorescence, (2) elution of anti-GBM antibody from renal tissue, and (3) detection of circulating anti-GBM antibody. By immunofluorescence, anti-GBM antibodies appear as linear deposits of IgG and infrequently IgA or IgM along the GBM (Fig 41–1). Linear deposits of IgG are present along the TBM in about 70% of patients and may also be found along the alveolar basement membranes in some patients with pulmonary involvement; however, lung tissue is not as useful for detection of antibody as is kidney. Irregular glomerular IgM deposits may also be present. The linear glomerular deposits of immunoglobulins are accompanied by linear or irregular deposits of C3 in about two-thirds of kidneys from patients with linear IgG deposits. Fibrin may be striking in areas of extracapillary proliferation and crescent formation. When C3 is present, it is usually accompanied by deposits of other components of the classic complement pathway. Nonimmunologic linear accumulations of IgG are sometimes found in kidneys from patients with diabetes mellitus, in kidneys perfused in preparation for transplantation, and in some normal kidneys. These must be distinguished from linear anti-GBM antibody deposits; the latter can be eluted from the renal tissue.

Circulating anti-GBM antibodies are usually detected by indirect immunofluorescence or preferably by the more sensitive RIA. Almost all patients with confirmed anti-GBM antibody deposits have circulating anti-GBM antibodies detected by RIA in serum obtained early in the course of the disease.

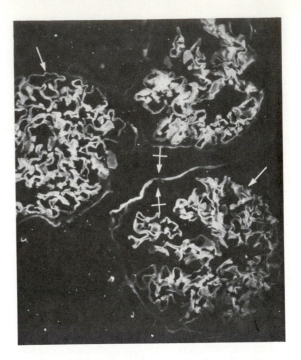

Figure 41–1. Smooth linear deposits of IgG (arrows) representing anti-GBM antibodies are seen outlining the GBM of 3 glomeruli from a young man with Goodpasture's syndrome. The antibody also had reactivity with Bowman's capsule (opposed hatched arrows). (Original magnification × 160.)

Differential Diagnosis

Although anti-GBM antibodies are probably the most frequent cause of Goodpasture's syndrome, immune-complex mechanisms can induce a similar clinical picture; therefore, immunopathologic investigation is essential for correct diagnosis. Some patients with rapidly progressive, crescentic glomerulonephritis (sometimes with pulmonary symptoms) have no detectable anti-GBM antibody or immune-complex deposits.

Treatment

There is no immunologically specific treatment. High-dose corticosteroids are generally helpful in the management of acute pulmonary hemorrhage in patients with anti-GBM antibody-associated Goodpasture's syndrome. To hasten the disappearance of antibodies, repeated and intensive plasmapheresis, in conjunction with immunosuppression, is being tried. Initial results are promising if the combined therapy is instituted before irreversible renal damage has taken place, although confirmatory controlled trials are not yet available.

Complications & Prognosis

The mean duration of the anti-GBM antibody response measured by sensitive RIA is about 15 months; it ranges from a few weeks to 5 years. Immunosuppression and plasmapheresis hasten the disappearance of the anti-GBM antibody. Nephrectomy has no immediate effect on the levels of circulating anti-GBM antibody but may speed its eventual disappearance. The ultimate outcome is influenced by the severity of disease at the initiation of therapy. Initial improvement is not sustained in all patients, so that long-term follow-up is needed. Circulating anti-GBM antibodies can transfer glomerulonephritis to a transplanted kidney, so transplantation should be postponed until circulating anti-GBM antibodies are absent or greatly reduced. Posttransplant immunosuppression may help suppress the recrudescence of the anti-GBM antibody response.

IMMUNE-COMPLEX GLOMERULONEPHRITIS

Major Immunologic Features
- Granular deposits of immunoglobulins and complement occur in glomeruli.
- Circulating immune complexes may be detectable.

General Considerations

The demonstration by immunofluorescence of granular deposits of immunoglobulins in the glomerulus can usually be interpreted as evidence of immune complex-mediated glomerulonephritis. It must be kept in mind that the direct reaction of antibody with irregularly distributed fixed or "planted" antigens, as noted above, could be confused with immune-complex deposits by immunofluorescence; this stresses the need for identification of the antigen-antibody systems involved.

The glomerulus seems to be a uniquely susceptible site for immune-complex accumulation; this is probably related in part to its function as a filter with a fenestrated endothelial lining. Several factors may influence the tissue localization of immune complexes in terms of (1) the characteristics and quantity of immune complexes reaching the glomerulus and (2) local factors within the glomerulus itself. A number of factors influence the delivery of immune complexes to the glomerulus, including the blood flow or its alteration and the systemic clearance of immune complexes by the mononuclear phagocytic system. It has been demonstrated, for example, that patients with autoimmune disease and tissue deposition of immune complexes have defective Fc receptor-mediated phagocytic clearance.

The size of the circulating immune complex, which, in turn, is determined by the relative antigen/antibody ratio, the size, valence, and nature of the antigen, and the antibody class and affinity, also influences the fate of the immune complex. Great antigen excess produces small immune complexes that are not particularly nephritogenic. Great antibody excess produces large, often insoluble immune complexes, which are rapidly removed from the circulation by the mononuclear phagocytic system and are not available for vascular localization. Experimentally, large complexes in antibody excess that are delivered to the circulation leading to the kidney localize in vessels and mesangial areas but are rapidly removed, in contrast to those formed during a period when the antigen/antibody ratio is more closely balanced.

Local factors that affect immune-complex deposition in the glomerulus include permeability and electrical charge of the glomerular capillary wall and the composition of the immune complex. Vasoactive substances released as part of the immune response may enhance vascular permeability and immune-complex localization. The physicochemical properties of the antigen, antibody, and resultant immune complex have a bearing on their affinity for the highly charged glomerular capillary wall. Interchange with circulating antigens and antibodies appears to be particularly important. The size and composition of the immune complex are subject to modification with shifts in the relative concentration of either antigen or antibody. Once localization has begun, antigen, antibody, or immune complexes can interact at the site. The interchange of immune-complex components is influenced by such factors as the location, degree of inflammation, affinity of the antibody reaction, and physicochemical factors. Immune-complex cross-linking via secondary immune reactions with rheumatoid factors or anti-idiotypic antibodies could alter free interchange between the primary immune-complex reactants. Complement activation can solubilize the immune complex and could contribute to immune-complex lability.

Granular immunoglobulin deposits, presumably immune complexes, appear to be responsible for more than 75% of cases of human glomerulonephritis of various histologic types, clinical courses, and demographic presentation (Table 41–2). Immunogenetic factors may influence susceptibility to immune-complex disease with increasing numbers of associations between the HLA-DR system and glomerulonephritis being recognized (Table 41–2). It is not known how the actual gene products are involved in the generation of the disease. The ever-increasing number of antigen-antibody systems identified in immune-complex glomerulonephritis in humans can be divided into exogenous (or foreign) and endogenous (or self) antigens (Table 41–3). However, in most cases of presumed human immune-complex glomerulonephritis, the causative antigen-antibody systems are unknown and screening for antigens is difficult.

Table 41–2. Morphologic, immunopathologic, serologic, and clinical features of the major histologic classifications of immune-complex glomerulonephritis.

Morphology of Glomeruli	Immunofluorescence of Glomeruli (Granular Pattern)	Immunology Laboratory Findings (Serology)	Clinical Presentation and Features
Glomerulonephritis types **Diffuse proliferative glomerulonephritis, including poststreptococcal glomerulonephritis** Diffuse hypercellularity, electron-dense deposits in the mesangia or along GBM. Poststreptococcal form: subepithelial "humps" by electron microscopy.	IgG and C3 scattered along GBM. Variable IgA and IgM. In poststreptococcal form, C3 may be present when immunoglobulin is minimal or absent.	Non-poststreptococcal forms: usually no abnormalities. Decreased C3, C4, and C1q, or presence of immune complex suggests underlying disease (eg, SLE or chronic infection). Poststreptococcal form: increased antistreptolysin O titer, decreased C3 (usually normal C4). Immune complexes and cryoglobulins may be present.	Non-poststreptococcal forms: Microscopic hematuria and/or proteinuria, gross hematuria, hypertension. Onset and course variable. May progress to renal failure. Poststreptococcal form: Acute nephritic syndrome, usually resolves, especially in children. Prevalence variable depending on serotype of streptococcus.
Diffuse proliferative crescent-forming glomerulonephritis Diffuse hypercellularity with extracapillary crescents. Electron microscopy as above.	Heavy fibrinogen-related antigen in areas of crescents. Immunoglobulin and complement as above.	Secondary forms: features of underlying disease as above. Idiopathic form: complement is normal or reduced. Variable immune-complex and cryoglobulin detection.	Rapidly progressive renal failure, even anuric or oliguric from onset. Microscopic or gross hematuria, erythrocyte casts in urine, proteinuria, nephrotic syndrome unusual. Uncommon; more common above age 50.
Focal proliferative glomerulonephritis, including mesangial IgA nephropathy Focal and segmental mesangial hypercellularity, with electron-dense deposits.	IgA often prominent, with or without C3 and IgG, sometimes IgM, in mesangial pattern (often segmental).	Variable increased serum IgA. Often immune complex of IgA class (less reactivity in usual immune-complex assays). Some association with HLA-Bw35 and -DR4.	Microscopic hematuria and/or proteinuria. Recurrent gross hematuria, may accompany intercurrent respiratory infections. Occasionally progresses to renal failure. Prevalent in young adults.
Membranous glomerulonephritis Thickening of GBM, little or no hypercellularity. Subepithelial spikes by silver stains, diffuse subepithelial electron-dense deposits.	IgG and C3 diffusely along the GBM. IgA and IgM unusual in idiopathic form.	Usually no abnormality in idiopathic form. (SLE form described below.)	Proteinuria, often nephrotic syndrome. Slow progression in one-third of cases. In older patients, may rarely be related to neoplasm. Common in adults; unusual before age 15.
Membranoproliferative glomerulonephritis Mesangial proliferation with interposition between endothelium and thickened GBM. At least 2 variants by electron microscopy: type I (subendothelial deposits) and type II (intramembranous dense deposits).	Type I: Heavy C3, some IgG, along GBM; occasional IgA or IgM. Type II: Heavy C3 along GBM. Immunoglobulin deposits uncommon.	Persistent low C3 in most type I and all type II. C4 usually normal. Nephritic factor often present, especially in type II.	Proteinuria, microscopic or gross hematuria, often nephrotic syndrome, often hypertension, usually progresses over several years to renal failure. Type I is somewhat uncommon. Type II is rare. Type II can be associated with partial lipodystrophy.
End-stage (chronic) glomerulonephritis Hyalinized glomeruli, extensive tubulointerstitial destruction. Electron microscopy occasionally detects features of original disease process.	Variable IgG, IgA, IgM, and C3 in least damaged glomeruli. C3 may persist in absence of immunoglobulin deposits.	Abnormalities typical of original disease occasionally persist.	Renal failure, often hypertension, variable degree of proteinuria and/or hematuria. End stage of many morphologic forms of glomerulonephritis.

Table 41–2 (cont'd). Morphologic, immunopathologic, serologic, and clinical features of the major histologic classifications of immune-complex glomerulonephritis.

Morphology of Glomeruli	Immunofluorescence of Glomeruli (Granular Pattern)	Immunology Laboratory Findings (Serology)	Clinical Presentation and Features
Systemic diseases with glomerulonephritis (subclassified according to morphologic type) **Systemic lupus erythematosus** Classified into mesangial only, membranous glomerulonephritis, diffuse proliferative glomerulonephritis, and focal proliferative glomerulonephritis. Resemble lesions listed above. Some transitions from one type to another.	IgG, IgA, IgM (typically all three) and C3 (also C4 and C1q). Patterns of glomerular deposition in accord with morphologic type. Often prominent tubulointerstitial immune deposits.	ANA positive. Decreased C3, C4, and C1q; increased anti-DNA antibody immune complex, with or without cryoglobulins, especially in diffuse proliferative type; often fluctuating with changes in disease activity and can be normalized by immunosuppressive treatment.	Only mild urinary abnormalities with minimal mesangial lesions. Proteinuria and microscopic hematuria, nephrotic syndrome in others; 10–50% progression to end-stage renal failure by 5 years, depending on morphologic type. Rapidly progressive course when crescentic glomerulonephritis. Lupus nephritis affects half or more of all patients with SLE.
Essential mixed Cryoglobulinemia Usually proliferative glomerulonephritis (diffuse, occasionally focal or membranoproliferative).	IgG, IgM, C3 diffusely along the GBM; sometimes massive deposits in capillary lumens. Fibrinogen-related antigen variable.	Decreased C4, cryogloglobulins (especially IgMκ-IgG), rheumatoid factor.	Proteinuria, microscopic hematuria, acute nephritic episodes, hypertension, episodes of purpura. Progresses slowly to renal failure. Rare disease; affects females more than males.
Henoch-Schönlein purpura Focal or diffuse proliferative glomerulonephritis, sometimes crescentic.	IgA prominent, usually with IgG and C3, with or without IgM. Fibrinogen-related antigen frequently prominent.	Variable increased serum IgA. Often immune complex of IgA class (less reactivity in usual immune-complex assays). Some association with HLA-Bw35.	Microscopic hematuria, proteinuria, nephrotic syndrome, acute nephritic syndrome. Generally favorable outcome, but some cases progress to end-stage renal failure. Nephritis occurs in more than half of patients with Henoch-Schönlein purpura.

Pathology

Primary immune-complex glomerulonephritis (ie, glomerulonephritis in patients without identifiable systemic disease) is usually classified histologically into diffuse, focal, and crescent-forming proliferative, membranoproliferative (mesangiocapillary), membranous, and end-stage glomerulonephritis (Table 41–2). The secondary forms of glomerulonephritis (principally those associated with systemic diseases such as systemic lupus erythematosus (SLE), essential mixed cryoglobulinemia, Henoch-Schönlein purpura, and subacute infective endocarditis) are often of a proliferative type, although other histologic variants (noted above) occur. The main histologic patterns are described in Table 41–2 and Fig 41–2. The immune-complex deposits are visualized as electron-dense deposits by electron microscopy and may appear in subepithelial, subendothelial, intramembranous, and mesangial locations (Table 41–2).

Clinical Features

Since immune-complex deposition in glomeruli can induce all histologic forms of glomerulonephritis, the clinical features vary widely depending on the type and severity of glomerulonephritis (Table 41–2). Proteinuria is almost always present and may be mild, moderate, or severe. Nephrotic syndrome occurs when urinary protein loss exceeds the body's capacity to completely replace it, after which serum oncotic pressure decreases and edema develops. Nephrotic syndrome most frequently accompanies membranous glomerulonephritis. Hematuria is more common in patients with proliferative or membranoproliferative histologic findings. The presence of erythrocyte casts in the urinary sediment suggests an acute phase of glomerular inflammation. Acute nephritic syndrome frequently accompanies diffuse proliferative and membranoproliferative glomerulonephritis. It is characterized by hematuria, proteinuria, edema, hypertension, and a reduced glomeru-

Table 41–3. Antigen-antibody systems known to cause or strongly suspected of causing immune-complex glomerulonephritis in humans.

Antigens	Clinical Condition
Exogenous or foreign antigens	
Iatrogenic agents	
Drugs, toxoids, foreign serum	Serum sickness, heroin nephropathy (?), gold nephropathy (?), etc
Infectious agents	
Bacterial: Nephritogenic streptococci, *Staphylococcus albus* and *S aureus*, *Corynebacterium bovis*, enterococci, *Streptococcus pneumoniae*, *Propionibacterium acnes*, *Klebsiella pneumoniae*, *Yersinia enterocolitica*, *Treponema pallidum*, *Salmonella typhi*, *Mycoplasma pneumoniae*	Poststreptococcal glomerulonephritis, infected ventriculoatrial shunts, endocarditis, pneumonia, yersiniasis, syphilis, typhoid fever, pneumonia
Parasitic: *Plasmodium malariae*, *Plasmodium falciparum*, *Schistosoma mansoni*, *Echinococcus granulosus*, *Toxoplasma gondii*	Malaria, schistosomiasis, toxoplasmosis, hydatid disease
Viral: Hepatitis B virus, retrovirus-related antigen, measles virus, Epstein-Barr virus, cytomegalovirus	Hepatitis, leukemia, subacute sclerosing panencephalitis, Burkitt's lymphoma, cytomegalovirus infection
Fungal: *Candida albicans*	Candidiasis
Perhaps others as yet undetermined	Endocarditis, leprosy, kala-azar, dengue, mumps, varicella, infectious mononucleosis, Guillain-Barré syndrome, AIDS (?)
Endogenous or self antigens	
Nuclear antigens	SLE
Immunoglobulin	Cryoglobulinemia
Tumor antigens	Neoplasms
Thyroglobulin	Thyroditis

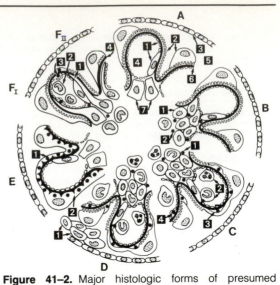

Figure 41–2. Major histologic forms of presumed immune-complex glomerulonephritis. **A:** *Normal glomerular anatomy.* 1, Glomerular endothelial cells, with fenestrated endothelium; 2, glomerular epithelial cells with specialized foot processes; 3, parietal epithelium lining Bowman's capsule; 4, glomerular capillary lumen; 5, urinary space; 6, GBM; 7, the glomerular mesangium, composed predominantly of smooth muscle-like mesangial cells and occasional mononuclear phagocytes. **B:** *Focal proliferative glomerulonephritis.* The lesion is characterized by focal (some glomeruli) and segmental (portions of glomeruli) mesangial hypercellularity (1). Immune deposits of immunoglobulin and C3 (2) are found in the mesangial area. IgA deposits predominate in IgA nephropathy. **C:** *Diffuse proliferative glomerulonephritis.* Extensive and widespread hypercellularity is present with infiltration of polymorphonuclear and mononuclear inflammatory cells (2). Immune deposits of immunoglobulin and C3 may be found in mesangial (1), subepithelial (3), or subendothelial (4) locations. In poststreptococcal proliferative glomerulonephritis, the subepithelial deposits have a characteristic humplike appearance in electron microscopy. **D:** *Diffuse proliferative glomerulonephritis with crescent formation.* In addition to the features of diffuse proliferative glomerulonephritis, macrophages and parietal epithelial cells accumulate in Bowman's space (1) in response to fibrin deposits, which accumulate in this area when severe glomerular capillary wall damage has occurred. The inflammation may be sufficiently intense to cause necrosis in the glomerular tuft. **E:** *Membranous glomerulonephritis.* This is typified by marked thickening of the GBM, the accumulation of immunoglobulin and C3 immune deposits in a subepithelial position (1), and a lack of glomerular hypercellularity. With time, GBM extensions or "spikes" (2) develop between the immune deposits and eventually engulf them. F_I/F_{II}: *Membranoproliferative glomerulonephritis.* Interposition of mesangial cells between the endothelium and the GBM (1) produces a "tram-track" appearance of the glomerular capillary wall. Mesangial hypercellularity and inflammatory cells are present (2). In type I, immune deposits of immunoglobulin and C3 are present predominantly in subendothelial positions (3). In type II, also called densedeposit disease, the GBM is thickened and abnormally electron dense (4). Heavy C3 deposits are seen in the GBM and mesangial areas with little or no immunoglobulin.

lar filtration rate. Hypertension can be present from the outset of any of these diseases or may appear later if the nephritis progresses. The syndrome of rapidly progressive glomerulonephritis resembles that of acute glomerulonephritis except for the rapid progression (within weeks or a few months) toward end-stage renal failure.

Renal failure and chronic glomerulonephritis may follow any form of immune-complex glomerular injury, usually related to the particular histologic type (Table 41–2).

Immunologic Pathogenesis

The presumptive diagnosis of immune-complex glomerulonephritis is based on the finding in renal biopsy of granular deposits of immunoglobulin, usually accompanied by complement, in the glomeruli. IgG is the most common, with IgA or IgM occasionally predominating (Table 41–2). The glomerular immune-complex deposition may diffusely involve all capillary loops in membranous or diffuse proliferative glomerulonephritis (Fig 41–3A). In focal glomerulonephritis the deposits tend to involve only segments of the glomerular capillary wall or mesangium, but may be more widespread than expected from the focal nature of the histologic change, and in some patients the immune-complex deposition is confined to the mesangium (Fig 41–3B).

Predominant IgA deposits are seen in patients with focal glomerulonephritis. The association has been so striking that the term "mesangial IgA nephropathy" has been coined to denote the condition. Circulating IgA-containing immune complexes can be detected in at least 60% of cases of IgA nephropathy, and the rapidity with which hematuria follows an infectious episode suggests that the immune complexes may be formed during antibody excess, possibly with preformed antibody to a common infectious microorganism in the oropharynx. The large, antibody-excess complexes would preferentially accumulate in the mesangium. Alternative explanations for the IgA accumulation have included IgA polymers, fibronectin-immunoglobulin aggregates, and antimesangial antibodies. Fifty percent of patients have raised serum IgA levels and evidence of abnormal regulation of IgA production in vitro, suggesting a primary immune abnormality. Occasionally, patients with similar clinical courses have predominantly IgM mesangial deposits.

In SLE, the immune-complex deposits may be widespread, involving glomeruli and, in 70% of instances, extraglomerular renal tissues as well. Indeed, granular deposits of immunoglobulin and complement in TBM or peritubular capillaries should suggest the diagnosis of SLE. IgA and C1q deposits are prominent in kidneys of patients with SLE.

Immunologic Diagnosis

It is helpful to identify antigen-antibody systems in individuals with immune-complex glomerulonephritis. Serologic evidence of recent streptococcal infections should be excluded. Antibodies for common infections, such as hepatitis B, can be measured. Antinuclear and anti-DNA antibodies should be sought, since SLE glomerulonephritis can occur without other overt organ involvement. The presence of rheumatoid factors or cryoglobulins may provide additional insight into the pathogenic process. However, in most cases, serum antibody testing is unrevealing.

Serum complement levels may be helpful (Table 41–2). C3, C4, and total hemolytic complement (CH_{50}) are normal in the majority of cases of glomerulonephritis, but when abnormalities occur, they are of considerable diagnostic importance. Hypocomplementemia occurs frequently in certain forms of immune-complex glomerulonephritis, especially SLE, essential mixed cryoblobulinemia, and infection-associated glomerulonephritis (poststreptococcal, endocarditis, infected ventriculoatrial shunts, etc). It is also common in membranoproliferative glomerulonephritis, a group of diseases incorporating at least 2 varieties of nephritis with differing pathogenetic mechanisms: type I and type II mem-

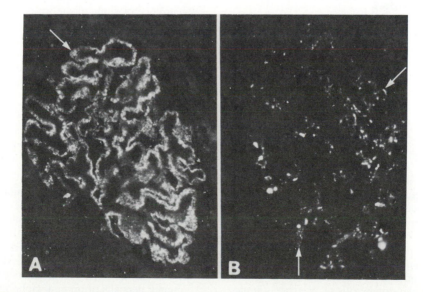

Figure 41–3. Granular deposits of IgG are seen in the glomeruli of patients with immune complex-induced glomerulonephritis. **A:** Heavy diffuse deposits (arrow) are present in a patient with membranous glomerulonephritis and nephrotic syndrome. **B:** Focal granular deposits (arrows), largely confined to the mesangium, are present in a patient with focal proliferative glomerulonephritis and mild proteinuria. (Original magnification × 250.)

branoproliferative glomerulonephritis. Type I is an etiologically heterogeneous group with granular immune-complex deposits. Type II, or "dense-deposit" disease, is identified by electron-dense transformation of the GBM, in which chemical analysis of the GBM suggests an increase in sialic acid-rich GBM glycoproteins, rather than the accumulation of a nonbasement membrane component.

A serum factor, termed nephritic factor, capable of activating the alternative complement pathway, is present in many patients with membranoproliferative glomerulonephritis, particularly type II. Nephritic factor has been shown to be an immunoglobulin with immunoconglutinin properties, capable of reacting with activated components of the alternative complement pathway, specifically the bimolecular complex of C3b and activated factor B, stabilizing its C3 convertase activity.

Several sensitive methods for the detection of circulating immune complexes are available (see Chapter 18). The use of a combination of assays based on different biologic activities of the immune complex enhances the detection of immune complexes in test sera. In general, the immune-complex assays are positive when large amounts of circulating immune complexes are present in patients with SLE and with glomerulonephritis associated with other systemic immune-complex diseases. Immune complexes are found more frequently in acute than in chronic glomerulonephritis and in patients with low levels of complement. The immune-complex assays may be valuable when repeated serially to assess disease activity and response to therapy.

Differential Diagnosis

The simultaneous presence of proteinuria (more than 1 g daily) and urinary casts almost invariably indicates a glomerular disease. The differential diagnosis is extensive and includes familial renal disease, hypertension, SLE, streptococcal infection, viral hepatitis, rheumatoid arthritis, and cryoglobulinemia.

Treatment

The most commonly used drugs are corticosteroids, cyclophosphamide, and azathioprine, and occasionally other "immunosuppressive" therapy used singly or in combination. In general, membranous or membranoproliferative glomerulonephritis does not respond to immunosuppressive treatment, although some investigators believe that corticosteroids may be beneficial. Proliferative forms of immune-complex glomerulonephritis are usually also unresponsive to immunosuppressive therapy, but occasional success continues to encourage its usage. In contrast, the glomerulonephritis of Wegener's granulomatosis seems to respond favorably to cyclophosphamide. Patients with SLE often respond to corticosteroid therapy, and the addition of azathioprine or

cyclophosphamide treatment may sometimes be appropriate.

Ideally, management of immune-complex glomerulonephritis should either eradicate the source of the antigen or inhibit production of the specific antibody. These approaches stress the need for identification of the antigen-antibody systems in each patient. For example, removal of antigen by treating *Treponema pallidum* infection has been beneficial to individuals with syphilitic immune-complex glomerulonephritis, as has removal of malignant tissue in immune-complex glomerulonephritis associated with neoplasia. The use of plasmapheresis and of specific immunoadsorbents to remove circulating antibodies, antigens, or immune complexes is under investigation.

Complications & Prognosis

The prognosis is extremely variable, depending on the histologic form of glomerulonephritis (Table 41–2). Generally, diffuse proliferative forms have worse prognoses than focal proliferative or nonproliferative forms. An exception is diffuse proliferative postinfectious glomerulonephritis, which usually remits in 90% of cases. Complications include progressive loss of glomerular filtration leading to renal failure and the eventual need for dialysis or kidney transplantation. Hypertension may occur with any form of immune-complex glomerulonephritis and is occasionally severe. Proteinuria of the degree found in the nephrotic syndrome may cause hypoalbuminemia (leading to edema or anasarca), depletion of the serum IgG level, and disturbed balance of coagulation factors manifesting as venous thrombosis, pulmonary embolism, or renal vein thrombosis.

Recurrence of some of the forms of glomerulonephritis in kidney transplants has been reported, especially with focal mesangial IgA nephropathy and type II membrano-proliferative glomerulonephritis. However, because recurrence is infrequent in the former and slow in the latter, transplantation is not contraindicated.

TUBULOINTERSTITIAL NEPHRITIS

Major Immunologic Features

- There are extensive interstitial mononuclear cell infiltrates, predominantly T cells.
- In anti-TBM tubulointerstitial nephritis, linear deposits of immunoglobulin usually accompanied by complement are found along the TBM; circulating anti-TBM antibody may be detected.
- In immune-complex tubulointerstitial nephritis, granular deposits of immunoglobulin and complement are found in the TBM, interstitium, or peritubular capillaries; circulating immune complexes may be detected.

■ In presumed cell-mediated tubulointerstitial nephritis, there is no detectable immunoglobulin along the TBM, and no anti-TBM antibody or immune complex is detected in the circulation.

Immune processes that lead to tubulointerstitial nephritis are similar to those described above for the glomerulus. These include anti-TBM antibodies, immune complexes, and cell-mediated immunity. Immune tubulointerstitial nephritis can accompany glomerulonephritis or occur as an independent event. Experimental models of anti-TBM antibody- and immune complex-induced tubulointerstitial nephritis have been developed, and similar processes have been identified in humans. Evidence exists that sensitized cells may transfer or contribute to tubulointerstitial nephritis in experimental models. Despite the conspicuous infiltration of interstitial mononuclear cells, including T cells, the pathogenetic role of cell-mediated immunity, other than in renal allografts, is not well established in humans.

General Considerations

Anti-TBM antibodies occur in about 70% of patients with anti-GBM glomerulonephritis and correlate with greater degrees of interstitial inflammation. Anti-TBM antibodies are occasionally found in drug-induced tubulointerstitial nephritis, in tubulointerstitial nephritis associated with immune complex-induced glomerulonephritis, in renal allografts, and rarely in primary tubulointerstitial nephritis.

In immune-complex tubulointerstitial nephritis, granular deposits of immunoglobulin and complement are found along the TBM, interstitium, or peritubular capillaries. These deposits are present in 50–70% of patients with SLE nephritis and infrequently in those with cryoglobulinemia, Sjögren's syndrome, membranoproliferative and rapidly progressive glomerulonephritis, and primary idiopathic tubulointerstitial nephritis. Tubulointerstitial immunoglobulin deposits may be present in the absence of glomerular immune-complex deposits and have occasionally been found in patients with SLE.

Mononuclear interstitial infiltrates without anti-TBM antibodies or immune complexes are the most common form of tubulointerstitial nephritis in humans. Frequently, the disease appears to be a hypersensitivity reaction to drugs, which may include a wide range of antibiotics, nonsteroidal anti-inflammatory drugs, and diuretics. Other situations in which mononuclear interstitial infiltrates may be prominent include acute allograft rejection, anti-GBM glomerulonephritis, pyelonephritis, sarcoidosis, Sjögren's syndrome, chronic active hepatitis, and idiopathic interstitial nephritis.

Pathology

Depending upon the duration, underlying causes, and severity of disease, renal pathology varies from focal to diffuse mononuclear interstitial infiltrates composed primarily of T lymphocytes and macrophages. Tubular lesions may range from minimal degeneration of the tubular epithelium to necrosis and atrophy. Polymorphonuclear leukocytes may be associated with necrotic tubules. As the inflammation advances, interstitial fibrosis and thickened TBM develop. Eosinophils may be prominent in drug hypersensitivity. The glomerulus is not involved unless there is an associated glomerulonephritis.

Clinical Features

The clinical course is usually that of renal functional impairment without urinary findings suggestive of glomerular disease. When anti-TBM antibody- and immune complex-induced tubulointerstitial nephritis is associated with glomerulonephritis, the features of the glomerulonephritis usually predominate. Evidence of tubular dysfunction manifesting as complete or partial Fanconi's syndrome may occur. When anti-TBM antibodies occur in transplant recipients, their effects may be indistinguishable from those of cell-mediated immune rejection.

Drug-induced tubulointerstitial nephritis usually presents acutely with fever, rash, hematuria, azotemia, and eosinophilia associated with a course of drug therapy. Other features such as pyuria, eosinophiluria, mild proteinuria, flank pain, and arthralgia may also be present, together with an elevated serum IgE level. Progressive renal failure is the general rule unless the offending drug is discontinued.

Immunologic Diagnosis

To distinguish the immune mechanism responsible for the mononuclear infiltrate characteristic of tubulointerstitial nephritis, renal biopsy for immunopathologic studies is needed and should include determination of the phenotypes of the infiltrating cells. Linear deposits of immunoglobulin and complement are found along the TBM (Fig 41–4A) in anti-TBM antibody-associated tubulointerstitial nephritis. As in anti-GBM antibody disease, the specificity should be confirmed by elution studies or detection of circulating anti-TBM antibodies. Rarely, anti-TBM antibodies have been found in drug-induced tubulointerstitial nephritis in which the drug or its metabolites can be detected bound to the TBM.

In immune-complex disease, the tubules, vessels, and interstitium should be carefully examined for immunofluorescent deposits of immunoglobulin (Fig 41–4B) and complement, which are often focal and less intense than are glomerular deposits. Prominent or widespread tubulointerstitial immunoglobulin deposits suggest SLE.

In presumed cell-mediated tubulointerstitial nephritis, no immunoglobulin deposits are found. T lymphocytes are the predominant cells, although a

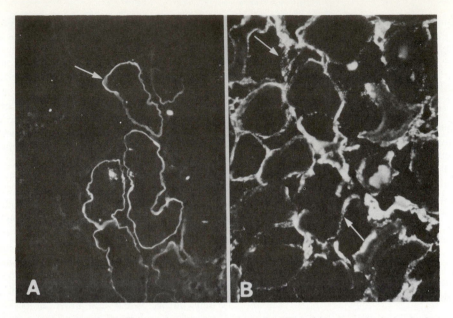

Figure 41–4. **A:** Linear deposits of IgG (arrow) are present along the TBM of focal renal tubules in the renal biopsy of a patient with anti-GBM glomerulonephritis. **B:** Diffuse granular deposits of IgG (arrows) are seen along the TBM of most renal tubules in the renal biopsy of a patient with SLE and immune-complex glomerulonephritis. (Original magnification × 250.)

few B cells are also present. Monoclonal antibodies directed to T cell subsets identify both CD4 (helper/inducer) and CD8 (suppressor/cytotoxic) cells. However, the proportion of CD4 to CD8 cells appears to vary depending upon the underlying cause of disease. CD8 cells are the predominant phenotype found in drug-induced cases, whereas either CD4 or CD8 cells may be the major cells found in renal allograft rejection. The patient's reactivity to the drug can be tested by antibody measurement and lymphocyte proliferation (see Chapter 19).

Treatment

Tubulointerstitial nephritis associated with glomerulonephritis is treated as outlined in the previous sections. In cases of drug-induced tubulointerstitial nephritis, the offending drug should be discontinued immediately and replaced as needed with a structurally unrelated alternative drug. Corticosteroids may aid in quicker resolution of drug-induced tubulointerstitial nephritis.

MINIMAL-CHANGE NEPHROPATHY

General Considerations

Minimal-change nephropathy is the most common cause of nephrotic syndrome in children; however, it causes less than 10% of adult cases. No clear epidemiologic factor has been established. Abnormal T cell function or T cell products have been suggested as possible etiologic factors.

Pathology

Typically, no abnormalities are detected by light microscopy, and no immunoglobulin deposits are found by immunofluorescence. By electron microscopy, there is a diffuse effacement of the epithelial cell foot processes.

Clinical Features

Patients have nephrotic edema and selective proteinuria with no impairment of the renal function, no hypertension, rare microscopic hematuria, and no hypocomplementemia; however, hypoproteinemia may be marked. The disease follows a naturally remitting and relapsing course. Repeated relapses in childhood are often followed by permanent remission in adolescence.

Treatment

Minimal-change nephropathy is particularly corticosteroid-sensitive, so that a rapid remission, in 2–8 weeks, on steroid therapy is considered diagnostic. Relapses may occur, and in these cases steroid treatment may be supplemented with immunosuppressive treatment.

FOCAL GLOMERULOSCLEROSIS

General Considerations

Focal glomerulosclerosis is another common cause of nephrotic syndrome in children and young adults. It is usually an idiopathic disease; however, a similar disease may develop in heroin abusers and in some patients with AIDS. Focal glomerulosclerosis may be difficult to distinguish from minimal-change nephropathy early in the course of the 2 diseases.

Pathology

The glomerular lesion is that of segmental hyalinosis and sclerosis. IgM, C3, and fibrin are present in small quantities in the hyalinized segments of glomeruli, although their immunopathogenic significance is unclear.

Clinical Features

Nephrotic syndrome is common and may be associated with hypertension and microscopic hematuria and then progressive impairment of renal function. A large percentage of cases reach end-stage renal failure within 10 years.

Treatment

Most focal glomerulosclerosis is corticosteroid-resistant, and there is no evidence that any other specific treatment alters the natural history of progression to renal failure. Transplantation is not contraindicated, despite slow and inconsistent recurrence of the same histologic lesion in the transplant.

VASCULITIS

General Considerations

The vasculitides are syndromes with a spectrum of clinicopathologic features with the essential common component of vasculitis, an inflammatory reaction in vessel walls, leading to ischemia of the supplied tissues. Increasing evidence points to an immunologic pathogenesis of the vascular lesions, particularly the deposition of circulating immune complexes triggering the inflammatory process through humoral and cellular mediators. Several vasculitides involve the renal vessels and glomeruli, the major ones being polyarteritis nodosa, Henoch-Schönlein purpura, and Wegener's granulomatosis. These diseases are discussed in Chapter 39.

Pathology

Vasculitis is diagnosed by the presence of segmental vasculitic lesions, with a perivascular inflammatory infiltrate, fibrinoid necrosis, and, in the extreme, aneurysm formation. The lesion may have evidence of coagulation, luminal obliteration, and downstream ischemia.

Polyarteritis nodosa is a necrotizing vasculitis of small and medium-sized muscular arteries with arteriolar and glomerular lesions (often segmental and focal), glomerular necrosis, and proliferative and crescentic glomerulonephritis. Lesions may be present at all stages of development. The lesions in Henoch-Schönlein purpura involve arterioles or venules, usually at similar states of development in the lungs, skin, and kidneys. Proliferative glomerulonephritis occurs in a significant proportion of these patients, with diffuse, granular mesangial deposition of IgA, C3, and fibrin. Wegener's granulomatosis is a necrotizing granulomatous angiitis involving arteries and veins. The renal lesion consists of a proliferative necrotizing glomerulonephritis with crescent formation and granulomatous angiitis.

Clinical Features

Polyarteritis nodosa is a multisystemic disease, and its prognosis is influenced by the degree of kidney involvement. Renovascular hypertension occurs in more than 50% of the cases, and end-stage renal failure is the common cause of death. Henoch-Schönlein purpura occurs more often in boys than in girls and may be triggered by infections and drugs. The role of food allergy is controversial. The diagnosis relies upon the clinical profile, which includes a nonthrombocytopenic purpuric skin rash, arthralgia, abdominal pain, and intestinal hemorrhage. Remissions can occur, with recurrences sometimes years later. The renal lesions can also undergo remissions, and progression of renal disease occurs in a minority of patients. Wegener's granulomatosis occurs equally in both sexes and often involves the upper respiratory tract, the lungs, and the kidneys.

Immunologic Diagnosis

The diagnosis is based on a combination of multisystem vasculitic involvement combined with renal and other biopsy studies. Recently, anti-neutrophil cytoplasmic autoantibodies have been detected by indirect immunofluorescence in patients with Wegener's granulomatosis and microscopic polyarteritis. Although these antibodies are a useful marker of the disease, their etiologic importance has not yet been determined.

Treatment

Besides Henoch-Schönlein purpura, in which remissions can occur when the triggering agent is found and removed, trials of steroids and immunosuppressive therapy have shown beneficial effects on Wegener's granulomatosis and, to a much lesser extent, on polyarteritis nodosa. At the early stage of the latter, plasmapheresis has been recommended. In cases of polyarteritis nodosa associated with hepatitis B virus, trials of antiviral agents associated with plasmapheresis have considerably improved the prognosis.

REFERENCES

Andres G et al: Biology of disease. Formation of immune deposits and disease. *Lab Invest* 1986;**55:**510.

Balow JE, Austin HA III: Clinical aspects of immunologic glomerular diseases. Page 213 in: *Contemporary Issues in Nephrology.* Vol 18. Wilson CB, Brenner BM, Stein JH (editors). Churchill Livingstone, 1988.

Couser WG: Mechanisms of glomerular injury in immune-complex disease. *Kidney Int* 1985;**28:**569.

Couser WG, Baker PJ, Adler S: Complement and the direct mediation of immune glomerular injury: A new prospective. *Kidney Int* 1985;**28:**879.

Glassock RJ et al: Primary glomerular diseases. Page 929 in: *The Kidney,* 3rd ed. Brenner BM, Rector FC Jr (editors). Saunders, 1986.

Glassock RJ et al: Secondary glomerular diseases. Page 1014 in: *The Kidney,* 3rd ed. Brenner BM, Rector FC Jr (editors). Saunders, 1986.

McCluskey RT, Bhan AK: Cell-mediated immunity in renal disease. *Hum Pathol* 1986;**17:**146.

Neilson EG et al: Experimental strategies for the study of cellular immunity in renal disease. *Kidney Int* 1986; **30:**264.

Salant D: Immunopathogenesis of crescentic glomerulonephritis and lung purpura. *Kidney Int* 1987;**32:**408.

Sterzel RB, Lovett DH: Interactions of inflammatory and glomerular cells in the response to glomerular injury. Page 137 in: *Contemporary Issues in Nephrology.* Vol 18. Wilson CB, Brenner BM, Stein JH (editors). Churchill Livingstone, 1988.

Theofilopoulos AN, Dixon FJ: Autoimmune diseases. Immunopathology and etiopathogenesis. *Am J Pathol* 1982;**108:**321.

Vogt A, Batsford S: Local immune complex formation and pathogenesis of glomerulonephritis. *Contrib Nephrol* 1984;**43:**51.

Wilson CB: Antibody reactions with native or planted glomerular antigens producing nephritogenic immune deposits or selective glomerular cell injury. Page 1 in: *Contemporary Issues in Nephrology.* Vol 18. Wilson CB, Brenner BM, Stein JH (editors). Churchill Livingstone, 1988.

Wilson CB: Immune aspects of renal diseases. *JAMA* 1987;**258:**2957.

Wilson CB: Immunologic diseases of the lung and kidney (Goodpasture's syndrome). Page 675 in: *Pulmonary Diseases and Disorders,* 2nd ed. Fishman AP (editor). McGraw-Hill, 1988.

Wilson CB: Study of the immunopathogenesis of tubulointerstitial nephritis using model systems. *Kidney Int* 1989;**35:**938.

Wilson CB, Blantz RC: Nephroimmunopathology and pathophysiology. (Editorial Review.) *Am J Physiol* 1985;**248:**F319.

Wilson CB, Dixon FJ: The renal response to immunological injury. Page 800 in: *The Kidney,* 3rd ed. Brenner BM, Rector FC Jr (editors). Saunders, 1986.

Dermatologic Diseases

42

Sanford M. Goldstein, MD, & Bruce U. Wintroub, MD

Several diseases of the skin have been linked strongly to disordered immune regulation, or, more precisely, to autoimmunity. These diseases are characterized by blistering and by the presence of autoantibodies that bind to various cutaneous structures. The discovery of these autoantibodies has revolutionized the understanding and classification of these diseases. These antibodies also serve as specific and clinically important diagnostic markers. They have been used as reagents to help identify and characterize important proteins in the skin. In the clinical diagnosis and management of blistering disorders, skin biopsy for direct and indirect immunofluorescence is indispensable.

Allergic and infectious diseases of the skin are discussed in other chapters.

BULLOUS PEMPHIGOID

Major Immunologic Features
- There is linear deposition of IgG and C3 at the dermal-epidermal junction.
- Circulating IgG binds to the bullous pemphigoid antigen in the lamina lucida of the dermal-epidermal junction.
- There are immune complexes in blood and in skin lesions.

General Considerations
A. Definition: Bullous pemphigoid is characterized by tense, often pruritic blisters located on the flexor surfaces of the extremities, axilla, groin, and lower abdomen. There is characteristic deposition of IgG or C3 or both at the dermal-epidermal junction, without which the diagnosis is in question.

B. Etiology: In vivo and in vitro models suggest that the binding of IgG to the bullous pemphigoid antigen (named for the disease) at the lamina lucida of the dermal-epidermal junction is an initiating event in the disease. The "major" bullous pemphigoid antigen is a basic glycoprotein (MW 230,000) synthesized by epidermal keratinocytes, although other antigens of lower molecular weight have also been identified by immunoblotting. The primary stimulus for production of the autoantibody is unknown. The disease may be passively transferred to

animals by injection of patient antibody. Bound IgG activates the complement cascade through the classic and alternative complement pathways. Antibody and complement, in addition to mast cell activation in situ, appear to direct the influx of inflammatory cells, including eosinophils, into the area. The release of mediators from inflammatory cells, including proteolytic enzymes, may contribute to the characteristic separation of the epidermis from the dermis. The typical distribution of lesions on the body surface may be correlated with the regional distribution and concentration of the bullous pemphigoid antigen at those sites.

C. Prevalence: The prevalence is unknown. Bullous pemphigoid is an uncommon but not rare disease. There is no sex or race predominance. Although the disease has been identified in children, it is primarily a disease of individuals aged 60 years or older. There are no known patterns of inheritance, and no HLA associations have been found.

Pathology
Biopsies (3–4 mm in diameter) are obtained from the edge of a fresh blister and should also contain perilesional skin. A subepidermal bulla is seen with fibrin, neutrophils, eosinophils, and lymphocytes within the blister cavity (Fig 42–1). The epidermis is

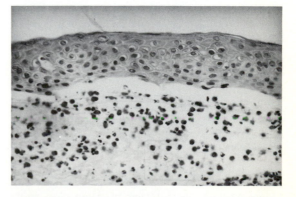

Figure 42–1. Histopathology of bullous pemphigoid. Note the full thickness of epidermis that makes up the blister roof. (Courtesy of Philip LeBoit.)

intact and not necrotic. Biopsy of older lesions may give the false appearance of an intraepidermal blister if the epidermis has begun to regenerate. The dermal infiltrate will vary depending upon whether the base of the clinical lesion is grossly inflamed or normal, the former being characterized by an infiltrate in the papillary dermis similar to that seen in the blister cavity.

Clinical Features

A. Signs and Symptoms: The classic lesion of bullous pemphigoid is a tense blister with a diameter of 1 cm or more, appearing on a normal or erythematous base (Fig 42–2). The tenseness of the blisters in bullous diseases usually correlates with the thickness of the blister roof, which in bullous pemphigoid is full-thickness epidermis (Fig 42–1). The lesions may be very pruritic, but this is variable. Bullae are distributed over the extremities and trunk as noted above and may rupture and then heal. Smaller blisters, called vesicles, are sometimes seen in a clinical

variant called vesicular pemphigoid. Blisters may remain localized to areas such as the lower legs in a variant termed localized pemphigoid. Occasionally, elderly patients present with perplexing and nonspecific papules, urticarial lesions, or widespread red and scaly areas. This presentation is sometimes called "pre-eruptive pemphigoid" and precedes the eruption of blisters. Recognizing these clinical variants will allow one to obtain a skin biopsy for routine stains and direct immunofluorescence. Blisters may be found in the oral cavity in one-third of patients and, rarely, on other mucous membranes, including the esophagus, vagina, and anus.

B. Laboratory Findings: Peripheral eosinophilia and elevated serum IgE were present in 50% and 70% of patients, respectively, in one series. These tests are rarely clinically useful and are not routinely ordered.

Immunologic Diagnosis

Punch biopsies for immunofluorescence studies must be stored in liquid nitrogen or a special holding medium. Linear deposits of IgG are found at the dermal-epidermal junction in 50–90% of patients, and linear deposits of C3 are found at this junction in almost all patients, occasionally in the absence of immunoglobulin deposition (Fig 42–3). Other immunoglobulin classes and complement components are detected less commonly. Indirect immunofluorescence tests, identifying circulating IgG that binds to the dermal-epidermal junction of a target tissue such as monkey esophagus in vitro, are positive in 70% of cases. The direct immunofluorescence patterns of bullous pemphigoid, herpes gestationis, and epidermolysis bullosa acquisita are identical. Epidermolysis bullosa acquisita may be distinguished from the others by electron microscopy. Direct immunofluorescence is positive in only 25% of herpes gestationis cases. Unconfirmed electron microscopy studies suggest that the patterns of binding in bullous pemphigoid and herpes gestationis may be different, but this is not clinically applicable. Immunofluorescence, like all tests, requires clinical and pathologic correlation. An indirect immunofluorescence pattern in bullous pemphigoid may also be seen in epidermolysis bullosa acquisita and herpes gestationis, but they may be separated by using electron microscopy or a substrate split at the dermal-epidermal junction by using NaCl.

Differential Diagnosis

The differential diagnosis includes several diseases characterized by blistering. These may be definitively separated from bullous pemphigoid, most often on the basis of immunofluorescence tests and histopathology and less often by clinical features and natural course. In an elderly patient with tense blisters, the presence of a subepidermal blister on light microscopy and deposition of IgG or C3 or both on

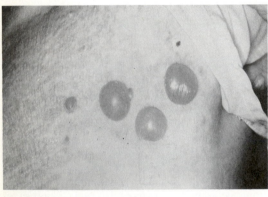

A

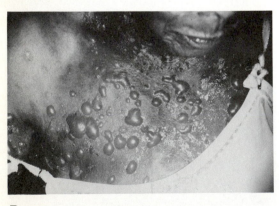

B

Figure 42–2. A: Tense blisters on a red base on the back of a patient with bullous pemphigoid. **B:** Multiple blisters on the chest of a patient. (Courtesy of Richard Odom.)

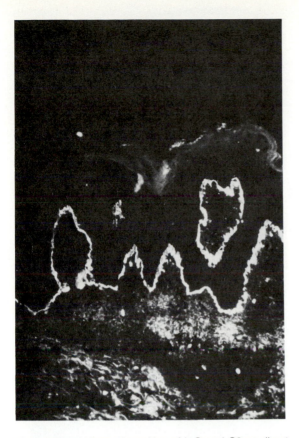

Figure 42–3. Linear deposition of IgG and C3 on direct immunofluorescence of lesional skin. (Courtesy of Richard Odom.)

direct immunofluorescence confirm the diagnosis. However, the same features in a young woman who is pregnant or taking oral contraceptive drugs suggest herpes gestationis. Another diagnostic possibility is a bullous drug eruption, which may be similar histologically, but has negative immunofluorescence studies. Bullous erythema multiforme often shows a few target or bull's-eye lesions with central blisters and will have distinct histologic and immunofluorescence findings. Other blistering diseases, such as cicatricial pemphigoid, dermatitis herpetiformis, pemphigus vulgaris, epidermolysis bullosa acquisita, and porphyria cutanea tarda, are readily distinguished from bullous pemphigoid on clinical grounds and laboratory findings.

Treatment

Treatment in the mildest and most localized cases consists of topical application of potent fluorinated steroids. In more generalized cases, in the absence of contraindications, 60–100 mg of prednisone per day is administered until no new lesions are seen. The steroids may then be slowly tapered. Up to 50%

of patients may experience a remission after total withdrawal of systemic therapy. Recently tetracycline or erythromycin in combination with niacinamide has been used. Although this regimen may be used alone as initial therapy, it appears to be somewhat slower and less effective in clearing the disease. Many clinicians use it concomitantly with corticosteroids or after the disease has been initially controlled with prednisone, to maintain remission during tapering of the prednisone. The use of azathioprine, cyclophosphamide, dapsone, high-dose pulse therapy with steroids, plasma exchange, or cyclosporine has been proposed, but is seldom required.

Prognosis

Bullous pemphigoid is usually a self-limited disease with a benign, if sometimes prolonged, course. Fatal complications may arise in the oldest and most debilitated of patients. The key to successful management is adequate control of the disease while avoiding the complications of systemic corticosteroids. Patients with bullous pemphigoid were thought to have an increased prevalence of internal cancers, but data from several series have refuted this impression. It is possible, but unproven, that patients with negative indirect immunofluorescence tests (''seronegative'') may be at increased risk for neoplasia. Because the disease typically affects older adults, concurrent internal cancers may be expected. Therefore a thorough history and physical examination is indicated in every case.

HERPES GESTATIONIS

Major Immunologic Features

■ IgG and complement are deposited along the dermal-epidermal junction.
■ Circulating IgG antibody to the herpes gestationis antigen is found in the basement membrane zone of skin. The IgG avidly binds complement.
■ It is associated with HLA-DR3 and -DR4.

General Considerations

A. Definition: Herpes gestationis is characterized by extremely pruritic vesicles and bullae appearing during pregnancy. ''Herpes'' refers to the Greek word for ''to creep,'' but this disease has no association with herpes simplex virus or varicella-zoster virus.

B. Etiology: The cause is unknown. The primary stimulus for antibody production is not known, but the antigen appears to be an epidermal protein (MW 180,000) in the basement membrane zone of the skin. It has not been purified to homogeneity. The onset of herpes gestationis appears to require placental tissue, choriocarcinoma, or hydatiform moles; recurrences may be caused by exogenous estrogen alone. Antibodies bound to placental tissue in these patients are not cross-reactive with the skin.

The antibody also reacts with the amnion epithelial basement membrane of second-trimester and full-term placentas, although the significance of this finding is unclear. Fixation of complement and activation of the classic complement pathway may be involved in the blistering seen clinically.

C. Prevalence: Herpes gestationis is rare, ranging from 1:3000–1:10,000 in early studies to 1:50,000 births in recent series. There have been few reports of cases in blacks in the USA, and this may reflect the lower frequency of HLA-DR4 in this population. Between 61 and 83% of patients have the HLA-DR3 haplotype and 45% have both HLA-DR3 and -DR4, compared with 3% of women in the general population. However, the HLA type does not correlate with the duration, severity, or recurrence of disease or with antibody titer. Abnormal regulation of anti-HLA idiotype antibodies during pregnancy was demonstrated in one patient, but the prevalence and significance in this defect in immune regulation are not known.

Pathology

The classic picture on light microscopy of a subepidermal bulla with eosinophils in the blister cavity is seen in only a minority of cases. The papillary dermis shows edema and a mixed perivascular lymphohistiocytic infiltrate with eosinophils. Spongiosis (edema between epidermal cells), with or without eosinophils, liquefactive degeneration, or necrosis in the epidermis, may be present. Eosinophils are an important histologic feature when present (Fig 42–4A).

Clinical Features

A. Signs and Symptoms: The onset is usually in the second or third trimester; in 20% of cases it is in the first few days postpartum. Intense pruritus accompanies and at times precedes the eruption, which often begins around the umbilicus or on the extremities as hivelike plaques, blisters, or rings of vesicles at the edges of hivelike plaques (Figs 42–4B and 42–4C). The disease may worsen at delivery. It tends to recur with subsequent pregnancies and last for weeks to months postpartum, occasionally flaring with ovulation, menstruation, or use of oral contraceptives. Lactation may shorten the natural course of untreated postpartum skin disease. Barring secondary bacterial infection, the blisters heal without scarring.

B. Laboratory Findings: Routine investigations are not clinically useful. Peripheral eosinophilia may occur, with an elevated erythrocyte sedimentation rate. Serum complement concentrations are usually normal.

Immunologic Diagnosis

A skin biopsy at the edge of a fresh blister for direct immunofluorescence testing reveals deposition

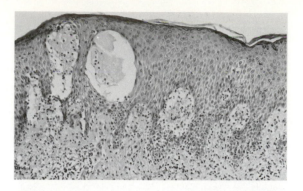

A

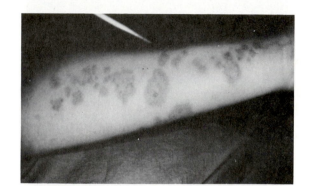

B

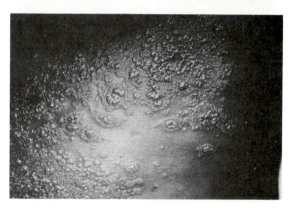

C

Figure 42–4. A: Histopathology of herpes gestationis showing early subepidermal blister formation. The teardrop-shaped vesicle at the left is characteristic of early herpes gestationis. (Courtesy of Philip LeBoit.) **B:** Hivelike and ringed lesions with vesicular edges on the arm of a patient with herpes gestationis. (Courtesy of Richard Odom.) **C:** Rings of vesicles at the edges of plaques in herpes gestationis. (Courtesy of Richard Odom.)

of C3 in virtually all cases. IgG is also found in 25% of biopsy specimens. Indirect immunofluorescence is usually negative. The pattern is identical to that seen in bullous pemphigoid.

Differential Diagnosis

The onset of pruritic, hivelike plaques with tense blisters in a pregnant woman requires punch biopsies for light and immunofluorescence microscopy to confirm the diagnosis. The greatest confusion may exist in cases of herpes gestationis prior to the appearance of blisters, and one must rule out disorders causing pruritus and those causing hivelike rashes. There are reports of a large number of poorly defined pruritic cutaneous syndromes in pregnant women. One should also rule out atopic dermatitis, scabies, and dry skin. Hivelike or edematous plaques may be caused by pruritic urticarial papules and plaques of pregnancy (which, unlike herpes gestationis, typically spares the umbilicus), urticaria, and erythema multiforme, but these may be ruled out by skin biopsy.

Treatment

Treatment should be undertaken in consultation with the patient's obstetrician. Prednisone at 40–60 mg/d controls the disease in most cases within a week, but higher doses should be used in the event of a poor response. The steroid therapy is then slowly tapered over several weeks to a maintenance dose. Some patients improve spontaneously in the third trimester, but the condition flares at delivery. Cytotoxic immunosuppressive agents should be avoided during pregnancy. Antihistamines have little, if any, effectiveness. Dapsone has been used in the past, but its efficacy is questionable and its use in pregnancy is controversial.

Complications & Prognosis

Herpes gestationis tends to recur and appear earlier with subsequent pregnancies. There appears to be no increased risk of fetal or maternal complications, although retrospective data collected in some series suggest an increased number of low-birth-weight and premature infants and, possibly, stillbirths. Ten percent of newborns may exhibit transient mild cutaneous disease. Antibodies may remain detectable in the skin years after the disease has abated.

DERMATITIS HERPETIFORMIS

Major Immunologic Features

■ Granular deposits of IgA and complement components are deposited at the dermal-epidermal junction in dermal papillae in lesional and normal-appearing skin.
■ It is associated with HLA-B8, -DRW3, and -DQw2.
■ There is a critical sensitivity to dietary gluten.

General Considerations

Dermatitis herpetiformis is characterized by pruritic grouped papules, papulovesicles, and vesicles and the granular deposition of IgA in dermal papillae at the dermal-epidermal junction. The cause is unknown. The stimuli for production of IgA antibodies found on the skin, the antigen(s) to which they are bound, and cellular and biochemical causes of the clinical disease remain to be determined. The IgA antibody does not react with gluten or gliadin and may be found in clinically normal-appearing skin. Circulating IgA antibodies are found in only a very few patients. It is presumed that the primary stimulus for the disease occurs in the gastrointestinal tract.

Prevalence estimates range from 10 to 39 persons per 100,000 in Scandinavia, but the rate is much lower in Japan. The rate may relate to the frequency of HLA types. Between 80 and 95% of patients with granular deposits of IgA in normal skin have the HLA-B8 haplotype, and up to 95% have HLA-DRW3. More than 90% of patients may express the HLA antigen DQw2 recognized by monoclonal antibody Te24. HLA-B8 is also associated with "ordinary" gluten-sensitive enteropathy without skin lesions (see Chapter 40).

Pathology

The skin lesions optimal for biopsy are early papules or fresh, unbroken vesicles for light microscopy. Neutrophils are seen at the dermal papillary tips in early lesions that may evolve into subepidermal blisters. Eosinophils and a mild perivascular lymphohistiocytic infiltrate may be seen. Older vesicles and crusted lesions may yield nondiagnostic findings. For direct immunofluorescence tests, biopsy of normal-appearing perilesional skin is recommended.

Clinical Features

Grouped red papules, hivelike plaques, and vesicles are symmetrically distributed on the elbows and knees, upper back, buttocks, and posterior neck and scalp (Fig 42–5). This distribution may be quite helpful to the diagnosis. The lesions are pruritic or may burn or sting. When excoriated, they leave crusted areas.

There are no diagnostic laboratory findings. Endoscopy with biopsy or radiographic studies may detect signs seen in gluten-sensitive enteropathy, but this is neither clinically useful nor necessary for diagnosis or management. More than 70% of patients do not have symptomatic bowel disease.

Immunologic Diagnosis

Biopsy of normal-appearing perilesional skin will reveal granular deposits of IgA along dermal papillae in all patients, and this defines the disease (Fig 42–6). C3 may also be found.

Differential Diagnosis

Vesicles may be seen in a variety of diseases, in-

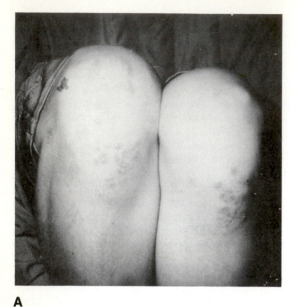

A

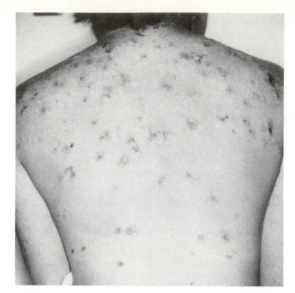

B

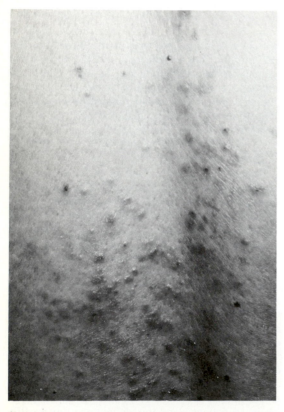

C

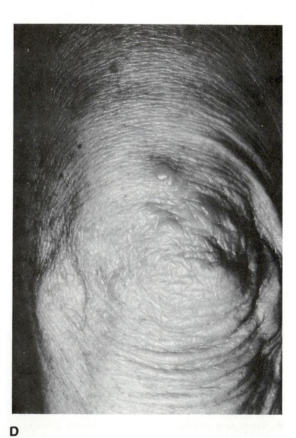

D

Figure 42–5. Dermatitis herpetiformis. **A** and **B:** Typical distribution of lesions on knees and upper back. (Courtesy of Richard Odom.) **C:** Papular lesions on the mid-back. (Courtesy of John Reeves.) **D:** Close-up view of papulovesicular lesions on elbow. (Courtesy of John Reeves.)

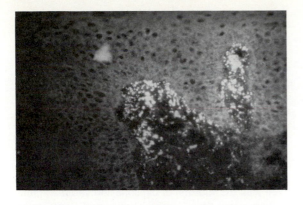

Figure 42–6. Direct immunofluorescence of perilesional skin demonstrates IgA deposition in dermal papillae in dermatitis herpetiformis. (Courtesy of Richard Odom.)

cluding varicella, herpes simplex, and herpes zoster. Cytologic smears and cultures, as well as their nongrouped or asymmetric distribution of lesions, distinguish these diseases from dermatitis herpetiformis. A clinically similar disease with different HLA associations, called linear IgA disease, is characterized by linear deposits of IgA in or below the lamina lucida of the basement membrane zone. Direct immunofluorescence can also rule out diseases such as bullous pemphigoid, herpes gestationis, and chronic bullous disease of childhood, all of which are usually clinically distinguishable as well.

Treatment

Strict avoidance of dietary gluten may control the disease entirely after 1–4 years or may lower the dosage of sulfones required by the vast majority of patients. Moreover, such avoidance in some patients has been shown to lead to a clearing of skin IgA deposits after more than a decade of dietary treatment. It is difficult to follow such a diet, but, in general, it is thought that less than total avoidance will often not be beneficial. A glucose-6-phosphate dehydrogenase (G6PD) level must be determined for all patients prior to therapy with dapsone. Hemolysis may occur at high dapsone doses even in patients with normal G6PD levels. Dapsone at doses of 100–300 mg/d is usually beneficial. Patients on dapsone must be monitored for hemolysis and methemoglobinemia, as well as hepatic, renal, and neurologic complications of therapy.

Prognosis & Associated Diseases

Dermatitis herpetiformis is a chronic disease unless dietary avoidance of gluten is maintained. Even after clearing of lesions, reintroduction of gluten rapidly results in disease exacerbation. Lesions heal without scarring, although pigmentary changes may remain. There are reported associations of dermatitis

herpetiformis with anti-gastric parietal cell antibodies, gastric hypochlorhydria or achlorhydria, antithyroid antibodies, IgA nephropathy, and, possibly, gastrointestinal lymphoma.

EPIDERMOLYSIS BULLOSA ACQUISITA

Major Immunologic Features

- IgG and, less frequently, IgA, IgM, C3, C1q, C4, factor B, and properdin are deposited at the basement membrane zone in the sublamina densa zone.
- Seventy-one percent of blacks and 100% of whites have been reported to have the HLA-DR2 haplotype in one series.

General Considerations

Epidermolysis bullosa acquisita is a blistering disease marked by skin fragility. It occurs on noninflamed skin over the distal extremities and heals with scarring. Immunoelectron microscopy detects linear immunoglobulin deposits in the sublamina dense zone of the dermal-epidermal junction. These may also be seen by immunofluorescence microscopy on the dermal side of skin separated at the dermalepidermal junction after incubation in NaCl.

The cause is unknown. The epidermolysis bullosa acquisita antigen is the globular carboxyterminus of type VII procollagen, which is also synthesized by epidermal cells and fibroblasts in culture. Aggregates of type VII collagen form the anchoring fibrils that bind the epidermis and dermis together. Passive transfer experiments with human epidermolysis bullosa acquisita antibody in animals have not been successful. In vitro organ culture models of the disease indicate that epidermolysis bullosa acquisita antibody fixes complement and directs an influx of leukocytes into the skin, resulting in epidermal-dermal separation.

Pathology

There is a subepidermal blister. Other lesions, especially the dermal infiltrate, are variable and correlate with clinical features. Noninflammatory lesions may resemble porphyria cutanea tarda. Inflammatory lesions resemble bullous pemphigoid, but with a greater predominance of neutrophils.

Clinical Features

A. Signs and Symptoms: Epidermolysis bullosa acquisita is a disease of adult onset with 2 distinct presentations. The "classic presentation" involves acral skin fragility and blisters, which heal with scarring and milia. Alternatively, almost half of all patients have widespread vesicles and bullae on red or noninflamed bases; these are associated with pruritus, erosions, and erythematous plaques. These lesions may be accentuated in skin folds and flexural areas. This second presentation resembles bullous pemphigoid. Patients may also have combinations of both presentations during the evolution of their disease. Some patients also have nail changes, oral lesions, or a scarring process in the scalp, leading to hair loss. Epidermolysis bullosa acquisita may be significantly associated with inflammatory bowel disease, particularly Crohn's disease. Individual patients have been reported to have other systemic diseases including thyroiditis, systemic lupus erythematosus (SLE), diabetes mellitus, or rheumatoid arthritis, but these associations are unclear.

B. Laboratory Findings: Routine tests are generally normal. Twenty-four-hour urine porphyrin levels are normal.

Immunologic Diagnosis

Direct immunofluorescence examination of perilesional skin demonstrates a broad linear band of IgG, C3, and, occasionally, other immune deposits at the dermal-epidermal junction. Immune deposits are not found within dermal blood vessels. This staining pattern is found in other conditions, especially bullous pemphigoid, so it is not pathognomonic for epidermolysis bullosa acquisita. However, 25–50% of patients have positive indirect immunofluorescence of the basement membrane zone below stratified squamous epithelium; the autoantibodies do not cross-react with the lungs and kidneys. When skin that has been split between the epidermis and dermis by incubation in a solution high in salt is used as the substrate for indirect immunofluorescent tests, a characteristic staining of the area on the dermal side helps define epidermolysis bullosa acquisita. In the absence of positive indirect immunofluorescence, immunoelectron microscopy will localize the immune deposits to the sublamina densa fibrillar zone.

Differential Diagnosis

Family history and immunofluorescence tests will help rule out hereditary forms of epidermolysis bullosa. Noninflammatory lesions may clinically and histologically be confused with those of porphyria cutanea tarda, but determination of 24-hour urinary porphyrin excretion and the finding of immune deposits in dermal vessels should be diagnostic of porphyria cutanea tarda. Bullous pemphigoid may be similar clinically and histologically to one presentation of epidermolysis bullosa acquisita. However, immunoelectron microscopy, indirect immunofluorescence on split-skin substrates, the presence or absence of scarring and milia, and the response to treatment will distinguish between the two diseases. Bullous SLE may be indistinguishable from epidermolysis bullosa acquisita clinically, histologically, by immunofluorescence testing, and by Western immunoblot analysis of patient sera against epidermolysis bullosa acquisita antigen. The distinction between patients with both epidermolysis bullosa acquisita and bullous SLE and those with bullous SLE alone is unclear, but patients with bullous SLE are said to respond more readily to dapsone, have less skin fragility, heal without scars and milia, and have a more granular staining pattern at the dermal-epidermal junction on direct immunofluorescence than patients with both epidermolysis bullosa acquisita and bullous SLE.

Treatment

Management is difficult, since patients respond poorly to topical and systemic corticosteroid therapy, even with the addition of dapsone and various immunosuppressive drugs. Initial studies with cyclosporin A have been promising. Currently, an initial trial of prednisone (2 mg/kg) with or without azathioprine has been recommended. Careful and gentle local measures to promote skin cleanliness, control infections, and minimize trauma are important.

Complications & Prognosis

Epidermolysis bullosa acquisita appears to be a chronic, nonremitting disease with great morbidity secondary to pain, scarring, and ultimately disfiguring skin lesions.

PEMPHIGUS VULGARIS & PEMPHIGUS FOLIACEUS

Major Immunologic Features

- IgG is deposited in the intercellular regions in the epidermis.
- Circulating IgG antibody binds to the intercellular regions of stratified squamous epithelium.

General Considerations

Pemphigus vulgaris and pemphigus foliaceus are described together because they are blistering diseases characterized by acantholysis and the deposition of intercellular autoantibodies. They may be distinguished clinically, histologically, and immunologically (Table 42–1). Other pemphigus variants, such as pemphigus erythematosus and pemphigus vegetans, will not be discussed.

Pemphigus vulgaris and pemphigus foliaceus are characterized by widespread blistering and denudation of skin and mucous membranes. They have a distinctive histologic picture demonstrating acantholysis (loss of cohesion) of epidermal cells and a typical pattern on direct immunofluorescence tests. The lesion is superficial in pemphigus foliaceus and deeper in pemphigus vulgaris.

A. Etiology: The cause is unknown. The stimulus for antibody production is unknown, but search for a pemphigus vulgaris "antigen" is under way. Although a rabbit antibody against a glycoprotein (MW 66,000) purified from human foreskin reproduced the disease in newborn mice, other immunoprecipitation and immunoblotting studies have iden-

Table 42–1. Characteristic features of pemphigus vulgaris and pemphigus foliaceus.

Characteristics	Pemphigus Vulgaris	Pemphigus Foliaceus
Frequency	80%	Uncommon
Mucous membranes affected	Almost all	Almost none
Age at onset	Middle age	Varies
Ethnicity	Jewish, Mediterranean	Less clear association
Lesions	Large, flaccid bullae; crusts	Small bullae, mostly crusts, arise on erythematous skin
Course	Severe and fatal if untreated	Causes morbidity, but chronic and less severe
Histopathology	Acantholysis between and above basal cells	Acantholysis superficially and in granular layer
Immunofluorescence, direct and indirect	Identical	Identical except occasionally more superficial in epidermis

tified larger pemphigus vulgaris antigens in the skin. A mechanism of acantholysis in pemphigus has been proposed. Because the addition of pemphigus antibody in high titer to skin in organ culture results in epidermal acantholysis that is blocked by serine protease inhibitors, it is postulated that the cross-linking of pemphigus antigen on epidermal cells by pemphigus antibody induces the secretion of a protease that results in the detachment of epidermal cells from each other. Evidence suggests that plasminogen activator is directly or indirectly involved in acantholysis, but the entire mechanism has not yet been elucidated. Addition of antibody and complement to such systems also results in epidermal separation, but complement is not necessary for acantholysis. The sera of 50–75% of patients with pemphigus foliaceus precipitate desmoglein I, a major component of desmosomes and other desmosome-associated proteins. The epidemiology of pemphigus foliaceus in Brazil suggests an infectious vector in its transmission in that country, but such an agent(s) remains unidentified. Pemphigus has been reported to be associated with the administration of penicillamine and other drugs such as phenylbutazone, although the association with the latter is less clear. Immunoprecipitation and immunoblotting studies suggest that pemphigus vulgaris and pemphigus foliaceus sera do not cross-react with the same antigens.

B. Epidemiology: Pemphigus vulgaris occurs predominantly but not exclusively in persons of Jewish or Mediterranean ancestry. It may occur in all age groups, with an incidence of 0.5–3.2 cases per 100,000 per year, but it is more common in the fourth and fifth decades and is rare after age 60.

Genetics: HLA-A10 was first identified as being more commonly represented among patients with pemphigus vulgaris than in the general population. More recently it has been shown that 95% of pemphigus vulgaris patients are HLA-DR4/DQw3 or HLA-DRw6/DQw1 positive, and it is thought that pemphigus may segregate with the DQ alleles. In a series of 13 DQw1-positive patients with pemphigus vulgaris, all were identified as positive for an allele designated $PV6_\beta$ versus 1 of 13 DR/DQ-matched controls. This allele differs from the normal DQ_β allele in codon 57, where asparagine replaces valine or serine.

Pathology

Skin biopsy shows a suprabasal intraepidermal blister with loss of cohesion of keratinocytes (acantholysis) in pemphigus vulgaris (Fig 42–7). Pemphigus foliaceus demonstrates a superficial subcorneal or subgranular split.

Clinical Features

Pemphigus vulgaris is characterized by blisters that most commonly affect the scalp, chest, umbilicus, and body folds (Fig 42–8). In contrast to the lesions of bullous pemphigoid, these blisters are flaccid and fragile because the epidermal split occurs within the epidermis, resulting in a thinner roof (Fig 42–7). Lesions may easily rupture, and in some cases only crusts and no blisters are seen. Oral lesions may be the initial or, rarely, the only presentation of the disease. Nikolsky's sign (sloughing of the

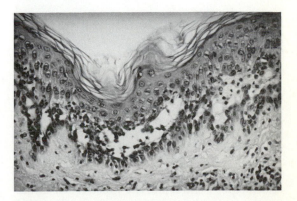

Figure 42–7. Histopathology of pemphigus vulgaris demonstrates intraepidermal blister formation with loss of cohesion of keratinocytes (acantholysis). (Courtesy of Philip LeBoit.)

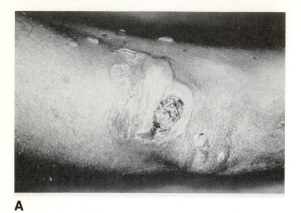

A

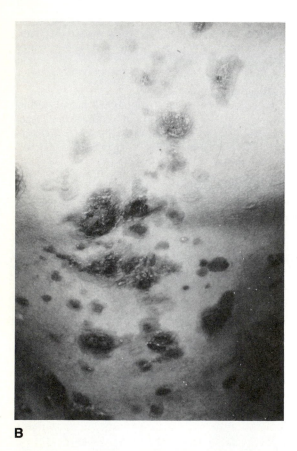

B

Figure 42–8. **A:** Flaccid blister on the elbow of a patient with pemphigus vulgaris (compare with the tense blister in bullous pemphigoid in Fig 42–2). **B:** Crusted and bullous lesions on the chest of a patient with pemphigus vulgaris. (Courtesy of Richard Odom.)

epidermis after lateral pressure with a cotton applicator or tongue blade) is positive in involved skin. Pemphigus foliaceus, with its more superficial histologic process of blistering, may show only scaly, crusted, and superficial erosions without frank blis-

ters. Oral lesions are uncommon in pemphigus foliaceus. Routine laboratory tests are not helpful in diagnosis or management.

Immunologic Diagnosis

Direct immunofluorescence reveals the deposition of IgG in virtually all patients and complement components (mostly C3) in intercellular spaces in the skin, forming a honeycomb pattern (Fig 42–9), in 50% of patients. Complement components are depleted in pemphigus blister fluids. Between 80 and 90% of patients also have circulating IgG that stains the intercellular spaces of stratified squamous epithelium in target substrates such as monkey esophagus or human skin. Although it has been reported that pemphigus foliaceus sera stain the more superficial layers of the epidermis compared with pemphigus vulgaris sera, this seldom is seen in practice. Circulating pemphiguslike antibodies have been found in patients with burns, lepromatous leprosy, morbilliform rashes to penicillin, SLE, myasthenia gravis

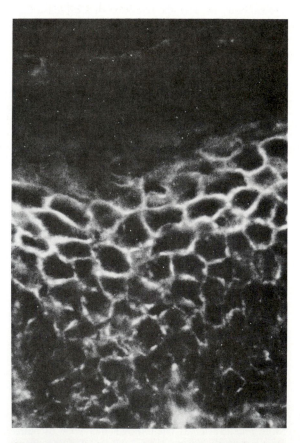

Figure 42–9. Direct immunofluorescence pattern of IgG deposition in pemphigus vulgaris. The immunoglobulins and complement components are deposited in intercellular regions in the epidermis forming a honeycomb pattern. (Courtesy of Denny Tuffanelli.)

with thymoma or thymic hyperplasia, high titers of anti-A or anti-B isohemagglutinins, cutaneous *Trichophyton* infection, erythema multiforme, and cicatricial or bullous pemphigoid. Such antibodies are usually of low titer in the conditions, and the direct immunofluorescence is negative.

Differential Diagnosis

Several diseases may be confused with pemphigus vulgaris. The diagnosis depends upon clinical suspicion when presented with a disease featuring blisters and crusting and biopsy with appropriate immunofluorescence studies. Oral lesions may be confused with aphthous ulcers or oral erythema multiforme. Scalp lesions may appear similar to impetigo. Occasionally pemphigus vulgaris will resemble other pemphigus variants, including pemphigus foliaceus and pemphigus erythematosus, but light microscopy is helpful in this situation. Other blistering eruptions (see above) are readily distinguished by clinical appearance (size, grouping, distribution, and tenseness of blisters), histopathology, and immunofluorescence pattern. Since pemphigus vulgaris and pemphigus foliaceus may be somewhat confused with widespread dermatitis or impetigo, the persistence in empirically treating a patient for these other diseases without a biopsy will often delay the correct diagnosis.

Treatment

Successful treatment of pemphigus vulgaris is a delicate balance of control of this potentially fatal disease and avoidance of fatal complications, especially sepsis, from therapeutic agents. There is much clinical experience, but there are no double-blind controlled studies to guide therapy. It is best to treat pemphigus vulgaris as early in its course as possible. There are several regimens tailored to inducing and then maintaining control of the disease. For treatment of pemphigus vulgaris, systemic corticosteroids beginning with prednisone, 80–120 mg/d in divided doses, alone or in combination with azathioprine, 50 mg 1–3 times daily is one regimen supported by much clinical experience. Lower doses of prednisone may be adequate in some cases of pemphigus foliaceus, but much higher doses of prednisone are sometimes required. Cyclophosphamide, methotrexate, and plasmapheresis have also been used in combination with corticosteroids. The experience with cyclosporin A has been limited and not always successful. The use of gold therapy in pemphigus vulgaris may be considered, but it has not been consistently effective.

Prognosis & Associated Diseases

Pemphigus vulgaris is uniformly fatal if untreated. Many patients may be successfully maintained in remission for years. There are no statistics that permit estimates of average 5- or 10-year survival rates.

The prognosis depends upon adequate therapy to control the disease, with vigilant monitoring and avoidance of adverse side effects. Pemphigus vulgaris has been associated with myasthenia gravis and thymoma. Pemphigus foliaceus tends to be a chronic, relapsing disease, but it is less life-threatening. It, too, may be quite difficult to control.

LINEAR IGA BULLOUS DERMATOSIS

A subset of patients (10%) with vesicles and bullae appear to have a disease that falls between bullous pemphigoid and dermatitis herpetiformis. Like patients with bullous pemphigoid, they have larger bullae than seen in dermatitis herpetiformis, as well as linear deposits of immunoglobulin, usually IgA, but sometimes IgG and C3 as well. Unlike patients with bullous pemphigoid, these patients respond to sulfones but not to corticosteroids, and deposits are at and below the lamina lucida. Other patients have small vesicles like those of dermatitis herpetiformis, but occasionally without the marked symmetry of dermatitis herpetiformis. However, unlike patients with dermatitis herpetiformis, histopathologically they show a linear bandlike infiltrate of polymorphonuclear neutrophils at the dermal-epidermal junction, in addition to papillary neutrophil microabscesses and linear deposits of IgA at the dermal-epidermal junction, in and below the lamina lucida. The disease is now called linear IgA bullous dermatosis. Patients present with vesicles and bullae that may clinically resemble bullous pemphigoid or dermatitis herpetiformis, or both. Direct immunofluorescence is positive for IgA and occasionally other immunoglobulins at and below the lamina lucida. Indirect immunofluorescence may be positive in some cases. Patients have a lower prevalence of HLA-B8 than those with dermatitis herpetiformis (ranging from a normal frequency up to 56% of patients versus 80–95% in dermatitis herpetiformis). They do not have jejunal changes of gluten-sensitive enteropathy, they lack the anti-endomysium antibodies seen in dermatitis herpetiformis and gluten-sensitive enteropathy, they do not benefit from a gluten-free diet, they respond to sulfones, and their disease tends to have a chronic course. The antigen(s) that binds the IgA has not been identified.

DISCOID LUPUS ERYTHEMATOSUS

Major Immunologic Features

- Immunoglobulins and complement components are deposited in lesional skin, particularly older established lesions.
- SLE occurs in some patients with discoid lesions.
- Low or negative antinuclear antibody levels, negative double-stranded and normal CH_{50} and C3 are found in patients without systemic disease.

General Considerations

Discoid lupus erythematosus lesions are round or irregular discrete skin lesions with follicular plugging, which tend to heal with scarring. They are seen in patients without SLE and occasionally in patients with SLE. The major reason for identifying discoid lesions in patients both with and without an established diagnosis of SLE is to treat such lesions aggressively so as to prevent or lessen their progression to disfiguring scarring. In patients presenting with discoid lesions, sufficient history, physical examination, and laboratory tests should be performed to exclude SLE.

Pathology

Biopsy specimens of lesions with erythema, scale, and follicular plugging, stained with hematoxylin and eosin, are usually sufficient to make the diagnosis. In these cases direct immunofluorescence is not necessary. In cases of old, "burned out" discoid lupus erythematosus, or when the light-microscopic picture is nondiagnostic, direct immunofluorescence may be helpful when positive. However, false-positive direct immunofluorescence has occasionally been found in areas of the body that are continually exposed to the sun. Therefore, the diagnosis should not be established by any one particular test or finding, but by the constellation of findings. Specific histologic features include hyperkeratosis and follicular plugging, irregular epidermal atrophy and hyperplasia, and superficial and deep perivascular lymphocytic infiltrate. Immunofluorescence findings include a broad linear band of IgG at the dermal-epidermal junction.

Clinical Features

DLE lesions are round or irregular, sharply bordered lesions characterized by erythema with or without the following: hyperpigmentation, scale, plugging of hair follicles with scaly debris, and telangiectasia. They are most common on the face and less common on the scalp and upper body. Extremity and trunk lesions are often seen with more widespread disease. The inner aspect of the pinna is a characteristic and relatively specific area to see the changes of discoid lupus erythematosus (Fig 42–10). Older lesions become scarred and are characterized by atrophy and decreased to absent pigmentation. Scalp lesions are characterized by follicular plugging, erythema, and loss of hair (Fig 42–11). Loss of hair may be temporary early in the lesion, but will become permanent when the follicle becomes scarred. Lesions may be tender or pruritic.

Differential Diagnosis

The differential diagnosis includes other red and scaly disorders, including psoriasis, seborrheic dermatitis, sarcoid, granuloma annulare, nummular dermatitis, tinea, sclerosing basal-cell carcinoma, and

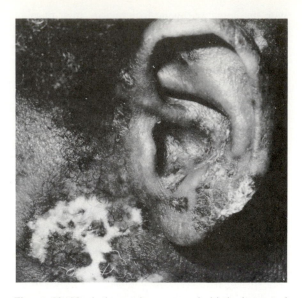

Figure 42–10. Active scaly areas and old depigmented scarred areas on the face and pinna in a patient with discoid lupus erythematosus.

polymorphous light eruption. Scalp lesions may resemble lichen planopilaris, pseudopelade, and tinea infections (*Trichophyton tonsurans*). Examination of the lesion, the rest of the body surface, and a fungal scraping or culture can often differentiate among these conditions.

Laboratory Findings

Since patients and their families will often be concerned or even confused about the possibility of

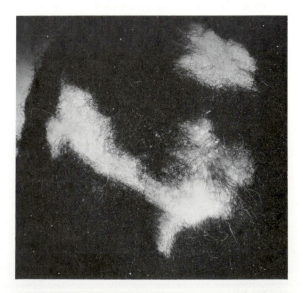

Figure 42–11. Scarring alopecia in patient with discoid lupus erythematosus lesions.

SLE, initial workup should include biopsy, complete blood count, erythrocyte sedimentation rate, antinuclear antibody test, and urinalysis. If the antinuclear antibody test is positive, the physician may order anti-double-stranded DNA, CH_{50}, C3, and other tests appropriate for SLE. Up to two-thirds of discoid lupus erythematosus patients may have at least one mildly abnormal laboratory test.

Treatment

Patients should be instructed to avoid sun exposure and to use sunscreens. Lesions on the face should be initially treated topically with high-potency fluorinated steroids, with close monitoring for steroid-induced skin atrophy. Resistant lesions and all scalp lesions may be treated with intralesional triamcinolone acetonide. Lesions should be treated until no activity (erythema) is present. If these modalities are not effective, an antimalarial drug such as hydroxychloroquine should be given for a 3 month trial after first obtaining an eye examination and G6PD level. Only 60% of patients with discoid lupus erythematosus benefit from antimalarial drugs. Further treatment requires consultation with a dermatologist or physician experienced with this entity. Most patients have a chronic course without developing SLE.

Prognosis

Discoid lupus erythematosus may be especially devastating in black patients, whose lesions may result in scarring with marked depigmentation and peripheral hyperpigmentation. On the scalp permanent hair loss may result. From 5 to 10% of patients presenting only with discoid lupus erythematosus progress to SLE. Laboratory tests and clinical findings that suggest a greater likelihood of progression include a high-titer antinuclear antibody, low leukocyte count, anemia, low platelet count, false-positive VDRL, widespread lesions (generalized discoid lupus erythematosus), and, of course, signs and symptoms of SLE. There is some suggestion that SLE patients with discoid lupus erythematosus lesions may have a better overall prognosis than SLE patients without these lesions.

REFERENCES

Bullous Pemphigoid

Berk MA, Lorincz AL: The treatment of bullous pemphigoid with tetracycline and niacinamide: A preliminary report. *Arch Dermatol* 1986;**122**:670.

Goldstein SM, Wasserman SI, Wintroub BU: Mast cell and eosinophil mediated damage in bullous pemphigoid. In: *Immune Mechanisms in Cutaneous Disease.* Norris D (editor). Dekker, 1989.

Jordan RE, Kawana S, Fritz KA: Immunopathologic mechanisms in pemphigus and bullous pemphigoid. *J Invest Dermatol.* 1985;**85(Suppl)**:72.

Korman N: Bullous pemphigoid. *J Am Acad Dermatol* 1987;**16**:907.

Tivolet J, Barthelemy H: Bullous pemphigoid. *Semin Dermatol* 1988;**7**:91.

Herpes Gestationis

Holmes RC, Black MM: The special dermatoses of pregnancy. *J Am Acad Dermatol* 1983;**8**:405.

Lawley TJ et al: Pruritic urticarial papules and plaques of pregnancy. *JAMA* 1979;**241**:1696.

Shornick JH: Herpes gestationis. *J Am Acad Dermatol* 1987;**17**:539.

Dermatitis Herpetiformis

Fry L: Fine points in the management of dermatitis herpetiformis. *Semin Dermatol* 1988;**7**:206.

Hall RP: The pathogenesis of dermatitis herpetiformis: Recent advances. *J Am Acad Dermatol* 1987;**16**:1129.

Katz SI et al: HLA-B8 and dermatitis herpetiformis in patients with IgA deposits in skin. *Arch Dermatol* 1977;**113**:155.

Epidermolysis Bullosa Acquisita

Crow LL et al: Clearing of epidermolysis bullosa acquista on cyclosporine. *J Am Acad Dermatol* 1988; **19**:937.

Gammon WR et al: Differentiating anti-lamina lucida and anti-sublamina densa anti-BMZ antibodies by direct immunofluorescence on 1.0 M sodium chloride-separated skin. *J Invest Dermatol* 1984;**82**:139.

Roenigk HH Jr, Ryan JG, Bergfeld WF: Epidermolysis bullosa acquista: Report of three cases and review of the literature. *Arch Dermatol* 1971;**103**:1.

Woodley DT et al: Epidermolysis bullosa acquista antigen is the globular carboxyl terminus of type VII procollagen. *J Clin Invest* 1988;**81**:683.

Woodley DT et al: Review and update of epidermolysis bullosa. *Semin Dermatol* 1988;**7**:11.

Pemphigus Vulgaris & Foliaceus

Bystryn JC: Therapy of pemphigus. *Semin Dermatol* 1988;**7**:186.

Korman N: Pemphigus. *J Am Acad Dermatol* 1988; **18**:1219.

Peterson LL, Wuepper KD: Isolation and purification of a pemphigus antigen from human epidermis. *J Clin Invest* 1984;**17**:1113.

Discoid Lupus Erythematosus

Prystowsky SD, Gilliam JN: Antinuclear antibody studies in chronic cutaneous discoid lupus erythematosus. *Arch Dermatol* 1977;**113**:183.

Prystowsky SD, Herndon JH, Gilliam JN: Chronic cutaneous lupus erythematosus (DLE)—a clinical and laboratory investigation of 80 patients. *Medicine* 1975;**55**:183.

Tuffanelli DC: Discoid lupus erythematosus. *Clin Rheum Dis* 1982;**8**:327.

43

Neurologic Diseases

Hillel S. Panitch, MD, Francine J. Vriesendorp, MD, & Paul S. Fishman, MD, PhD

The role of immunologic mechanisms in diseases of the nervous system is the focus of increasing interest and investigation. In acute disseminated encephalomyelitis and acute inflammatory demyelinating polyneuropathy (Guillain-Barré syndrome), the host response to an infectious agent may trigger a direct autoaggressive assault on the nervous system. The pathogenesis of multiple sclerosis is less clear, but evidence from immunogenetic studies, defects of immunoregulation, and responses to immunosuppressive therapy suggests that the immune system is involved in the pathogenesis of the disease. In myasthenia gravis, an antibody response directed against the acetylcholine receptor directly inhibits neuromuscular transmission. In other conditions such as subacute sclerosing panencephalitis, paraneoplastic syndromes, amyotrophic lateral sclerosis, and certain chronic neuropathies, abnormal immune responses are known to occur; however, their significance is uncertain. In Creutzfeldt-Jakob disease and Alzheimer's disease, the role of the immune system in pathogenesis is entirely conjectural.

DEMYELINATING DISEASES

The commonly accepted pathologic criteria for a demyelinating disease are destruction of myelin sheaths of nerve fibers with relative sparing of neurons and axons. Lesions are frequently perivascular in location and are accompanied by mononuclear inflammatory infiltrates, suggesting that immunologic mechanisms participate in their pathogenesis.

ACUTE DISSEMINATED ENCEPHALOMYELITIS

Major Immunologic Features
- It follows infectious diseases or immunizations.
- Inflammatory demyelination occurs in central nervous system white matter.
- There is cellular immunity to myelin basic protein.

General Considerations
Although acute disseminated encephalomyelitis is uncommon, it is important because of the widespread practice of vaccination for prevention of infectious diseases. The onset of clinical illness occurs several days to weeks following vaccination; in the case of natural viral infections, such as measles, rubella, varicella, mumps, and influenza, it can occur concomitantly with the illness (parainfectious) or after the acute phase (postinfectious). Except for measles, in which the incidence of acute disseminated encephalomyelitis is well defined and constant at 1:1000, reliable figures are not available. However, they are all much lower than the incidence following measles. The argument favoring an immunologic pathogenesis of this disorder is based on its similarity to experimental allergic encephalomyelitis, in which animals are immunized with extracts of brain tissue or specific myelin proteins, resulting in an autoimmune response mediated by T lymphocytes.

Pathology
Acute disseminated encephalomyelitis is marked by perivascular mononuclear cell infiltrates in white matter throughout the brain and spinal cord; polymorphonuclear leukocytes and microhemorrhages are seen in the most acute form of the disease. As the lesions age, they become sclerotic, with proliferation of astrocytes and formation of glial scars. The lesions are pathologically all of the same age, reflecting the monophasic nature of the illness.

Clinical Features
Systemic symptoms of fever, malaise, headache, myalgia, nausea, and vomiting generally precede neurologic symptoms by 24–48 hours. Neurologic symptoms and signs develop rapidly thereafter and include pain, paresthesias, motor weakness, spasticity, uncoordination, dysarthria, dysphagia, and respiratory distress. Seizures are common in severe cases and in the acute hemorrhagic form, and widespread brain lesions can lead to stupor and coma. A more restricted form of the same pathologic process may be confined to the spinal cord as acute transverse myelitis.

Immunologic Diagnosis
Cellular immunity to myelin basic protein can sometimes be demonstrated in acute disseminated encephalomyelitis by measuring the activation in

vitro of peripheral blood or spinal fluid lymphocytes during the acute phase of the illness. Antibodies to basic protein appear to play no part in the disease. Cerebrospinal fluid may be abnormal, with mild to moderate pleocytosis and elevated levels of IgG, but there is no evidence that this represents local immunoglobulin synthesis as occurs in multiple sclerosis.

Differential Diagnosis

Acute multiple sclerosis can be difficult to distinguish from acute disseminated encephalomyelitis. Fever and a preceding viral illness or vaccination favor the latter diagnosis. The vasculitis of systemic lupus erythematosus can affect the central nervous system, but neurologic symptoms generally accompany the systemic illness and tend to be more focal than in acute disseminated encephalomyelitis. Primary infections of the nervous system with herpes simplex virus or the arboviruses tend to involve gray as well as white matter, and they produce neuronal dysfunction such as seizures, stupor, and coma early in the illness. Direct isolation of viruses from cerebrospinal fluid and increasing serum antibody titers are helpful in differentiating viral encephalitides from acute disseminated encephalomyelitis. The subacute encephalitis of acquired immunodeficiency syndrome (AIDS) develops more slowly and is not usually associated with focal neurologic deficits. Toxoplasmosis of the central nervous system may be distinguished serologically. Computed tomography and magnetic resonance imaging may be useful in diagnosis; however, a diagnostic brain biopsy is sometimes necessary to exclude a treatable central nervous system infection.

Treatment

Although the course is unpredictable, high doses of corticosteroids may be of value in treatment. The successful prevention of experimental allergic encephalomyelitis with immunosuppressive and immunomodulating agents offers hope that similar treatment may inhibit the attack of sensitized T lymphocytes on the nervous system in acute disseminated encephalomyelitis.

Complications & Prognosis

The mortality rate varies from 1% to 27%, with the highest rates reported in association with measles. Neurologic sequelae persist in 25–40% of survivors. The occasional occurrence of relapses blurs the distinction between this condition and multiple sclerosis in about 5% of cases.

MULTIPLE SCLEROSIS

Major Immunologic Features

■ There is inflammatory demyelination in central nervous system white matter.

■ There are alterations in immunoregulatory T cell function and cytokine production.
■ There are oligoclonal immunoglobulins in cerebrospinal fluid.
■ It responds to immunosuppressive and immunomodulating agents.

General Considerations

Multiple sclerosis is a chronic relapsing disease in which there are signs and symptoms of central nervous system involvement separated both in time and in location in the nervous system. Epidemiologic studies have uncovered important clues about multiple sclerosis, but the cause remains unknown. In high-risk areas the prevalence is 50–100 per 100,000 population, whereas in low-risk areas such as Africa and Japan the rate is less than 5 per 100,000. Individuals who migrate from high-risk to low-risk areas, or vice versa, after age 15 carry with them their native risk of acquiring the disease. In addition, the peak onset is at age 30, with few cases before age 15 or after age 55, suggesting that some critical event in determining the risk of acquiring multiple sclerosis occurs in adolescence. The risk of disease in a first-degree relative is 10–15 times higher than the risk in the general population, and the concordance rate in identical twins is higher than 25%, indicating a strong genetic component. However, localized epidemics of multiple sclerosis have been described, most notably in the Faroe Islands, where the temporal clustering of cases suggests a transmissible cause. Studies of histocompatibility antigens have indicated statistically significant associations with HLA-A3 and HLA-B7 in northern European and North American populations, and higher-level associations with HLA-DR2 and HLA-DQw1 which may be more closely linked to a multiple sclerosis susceptibility gene.

Numerous viruses have been implicated as possible etiologic agents, by the presence of specific antibodies in spinal fluid, identification of viral DNA or RNA in brain tissue or mononuclear cells, and, in some cases, actual viral isolation. However, none of these observations has been consistently confirmed. The pathogenesis is thought to be autoimmune, but current understanding of the disease is continually being modified by new observations. Numerous immunoregulatory defects have been identified, one of the best documented being abnormal suppressor T cell function in acute attacks and in the chronic progressive phase. Although decreases in the CD8 T cell subset are not consistently found, the defect may reside in a loss of CD4 suppressor-inducer cells identified by coexpression of the 2H4 (CD45R) surface antigen with CD4. In addition, there are excessive numbers of activated T cells in the blood and cerebrospinal fluid. These findings may be partially responsible for defective regulation of IgG synthesis within the nervous system. Monocytes and macrophages also appear to play important roles in multiple sclerosis, possibly related to their sensitivity to gamma interferon, which induces class II human leukocyte antigen (HLA) (HLA-DR, -DP, and -DQ) surface antigens and activates macrophages (Fig 43–1). Activated macrophages are prevalent in multiple sclerosis plaques, where they release proteinases and phagocytose myelin. The importance of gamma interferon as an immune activator was recently emphasized by a clinical trial in which patients treated with gamma interferon developed acute exacerbations. Minor viral infections often precipitate attacks; this effect may be mediated by gamma interferon or other cytokines. Within the central nervous system, gamma interferon induces class II antigens on astrocytes, enabling them to present antigens to T cells and to propagate the disease process. Unfortunately, the specific antigen in question is unknown, but it is likely to be a component of myelin such as the basic protein. The autoimmune theory of multiple sclerosis is strengthened by its response to immunosuppressive drugs such as corticosteroids and cyclophosphamide. Alpha and beta interferons, which inhibit the synthesis of gamma interferon and reverse some of its immunostimulatory effects, also may be effective in preventing exacerbations.

Pathology

The lesions of multiple sclerosis are confined to the central nervous system and primarily involve the white matter of the cerebrum, cerebellum, brain stem, and spinal cord. In early active disease they consist of perivascular infiltrates of T lymphocytes and macrophages. In older lesions, macrophage-mediated demyelination is further advanced and large numbers of reactive astrocytes are seen. These lesions or plaques appear to be of different ages and correlate with the appearance of clinical signs and symptoms at different times during the illness. Plasma cells within the plaques secrete oligoclonal IgG into the extracellular and cerebrospinal fluid. The similarities between the lesions of multiple sclerosis and the inflammatory demyelination seen in experimental allergic encephalomyelitis (particularly the relapsing form) suggest that cellular immune mechanisms are involved in the pathogenesis of multiple sclerosis.

Clinical Features

Because multiple sclerosis plaques tend to involve many areas of the central nervous system white matter, the symptoms and signs are extremely varied. The most common manifestations are motor weakness, paresthesias, impairment of visual acuity, and diplopia. Ataxia, urinary bladder dysfunction, impotence, spasticity, and mild to moderate dementia are also common. Symptoms may occur rapidly as acute exacerbations that develop over several days and

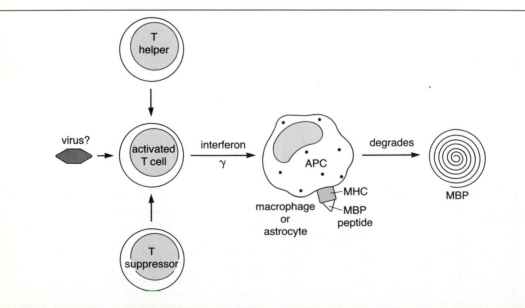

Figure 43–1. Interaction of T cells, cytokines, and antigen-presenting cells in multiple sclerosis. In this simplified representation, activated T cells proliferate, differentiate, enter the central nervous system, and secrete gamma interferon, which induces class II MHC antigens on macrophages and astrocytes. Activated macrophages attack and degrade myelin, take up myelin basic protein (MBP) peptides, and present them to other T cells, amplifying the immune response. Class II MHC containing astrocytes can also present MBP peptides. Suppressor T cells, which are functionally defective in multiple sclerosis patients, fail to regulate the immune response normally.

persist for days to weeks with gradual recovery, or more slowly in the chronic progressive form of the disease. Exacerbations occur at varying intervals and tend to subside with less complete recovery of function and increasing disability as the disease progresses. Visual, auditory, and somatosensory evoked potentials are often abnormal and assist in diagnosis. However, the most important recent diagnostic advance has been the introduction of magnetic resonance imaging, which provides striking visualization of plaques in the cerebral white matter (Fig 43–2).

Immunologic Diagnosis

Despite the many immunologic abnormalities described above, there is no single diagnostic test for multiple sclerosis. Oligoclonal IgG bands are detectable in cerebrospinal fluid by electrophoresis or isoelectric focusing in more than 90% of patients (Fig 43–3). An elevated IgG index (ratio of cerebrospinal fluid to serum IgG corrected for albumin concentration in each compartment) indicates local IgG synthesis, but this can be found in other inflammatory diseases of the nervous system. Myelin basic protein may be detected by radioimmunoassay in the cerebrospinal fluid, but it is largely a reflection of myelin damage and can be seen in other conditions such as head trauma and stroke. Other immunologic findings such as HLA haplotypes, abnormal CD4/CD8 T cell ratios, reduced suppressor cell activity, activated

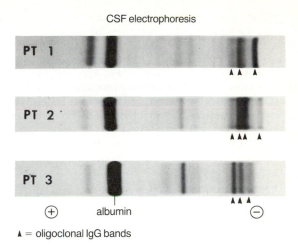

CSF electrophoresis

PT 1

PT 2

PT 3

$\oplus$ albumin $\ominus$

▲ = oligoclonal IgG bands

Figure 43–3. Oligoclonal bands in cerebrospinal fluid (CSF) specimen from a patient with subacute sclerosing parencephalitis. Cerebrospinal fluid electrophoresis pattern in agarose gel demonstrates the phenomenon of oligoclonal banding. In the gamma region (to the right), several dark, distinct bands are noted for all these patients. Similar abnormalities are noted in cerebrospinal fluid specimens from multiple sclerosis patients.

T cells in blood or cerebrospinal fluid, and increased cytokine synthesis are not specific or consistent enough to be useful in diagnosis and, for the present, must be restricted to the research laboratory.

Differential Diagnosis

Acute episodes of multiple sclerosis must be differentiated from structural lesions of the central nervous system such as brain and spinal cord tumors, spondylosis, or vascular malformations. A host of other medical conditions may produce signs, symptoms, spinal fluid findings, and, in some cases, magnetic resonance images that mimic those of multiple sclerosis, and they must be excluded by appropriate testing. These diseases include neurosyphilis, sarcoidosis, systemic lupus erythematosus, Sjögren's syndrome, vitamin B_{12} deficiency, and Lyme disease. Spinal and cerebellar disorders such as Friedreich's ataxia and olivopontocerebellar degeneration can mimic multiple sclerosis, but tend to be familial, chronically progressive, and associated with normal spinal fluid. Finally, tropical spastic paraparesis or HTLV-I-associated myelopathy should be considered. Some cases may be indistinguishable from multiple sclerosis, but the diagnosis of HTLV-I-associated myelopathy may be made if antibody to HTLV-I is present.

Treatment

Corticosteroids or adrenocorticotropic hormone

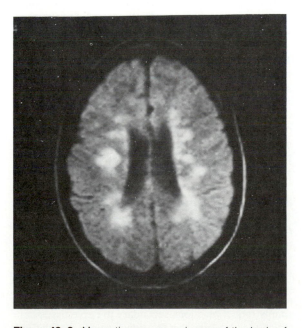

Figure 43–2. Magnetic resonance image of the brain of a multiple sclerosis patient, showing lesions (irregular white areas) in the white matter surrounding the lateral ventricles.

(ACTH) may shorten the duration of acute exacerbations, particularly when optic neuritis is present, but the long-term benefits of such therapy are not striking. Numerous trials of experimental immunotherapy have been undertaken, some with partial success. In one trial intensive immunosuppression with cyclophosphamide combined with ACTH seemed to arrest progression in some patients for periods up to 1 year. Alpha interferon given by subcutaneous injection and beta interferon given either intrathecally or subcutaneously have been reported to prevent exacerbations in patients with relapsing-remitting multiple sclerosis. Copolymer I, a synthetic polypeptide that inhibits experimental allergic encephalomyelitis in animals, was effective in preventing exacerbations in a limited but well-controlled clinical trial. Although there is little evidence for a pathogenic humoral factor in multiple sclerosis, plasmapheresis may result in improvement and should be investigated further. A multicenter study of the effects of cyclosporine in patients with chronic progressive disease showed a statistically significant but biologically minimal effect on the clinical course of the disease. Targeted immunotherapy with monoclonal antibodies directed against subpopulations of activated T cells is in the preliminary stages of investigation. It remains to be seen which, if any, of these therapeutic modalities will survive testing in rigorously controlled double-blind clinical trials.

Complications & Prognosis

The prognosis of multiple sclerosis is difficult to predict because of its extremely variable nature. Benign cases in which patients function normally or with little neurologic deficit are not uncommon, while fulminant cases of acute multiple sclerosis can result in severe disability or death within a few years. Most patients fall between these extremes and continue to have exacerbations and remissions, or chronic progression, for many years. Despite substantial evidence for defective immunoregulation, patients with multiple sclerosis do not have increased susceptibility to other autoimmune disorders, infections, or neoplasms.

ACUTE INFLAMMATORY DEMYELINATING POLYNEUROPATHY (Guillain-Barré Syndrome)

Major Immunologic Features

- It commonly follows acute viral infections.
- There is inflammatory demyelination of peripheral nerves.
- There is cellular and humoral immunity to nerve proteins.

General Considerations

Acute inflammatory demyelinating polyneuropathy, like acute disseminated encephalomyelitis, frequently follows an infectious illness. Upper respiratory infections, exanthems, vaccinations, and viral illnesses such as infectious mononucleosis and hepatitis commonly precede acute inflammatory demyelinating polyneuropathy by 1–3 weeks. Increasing numbers of cases are being reported in patients with AIDS. The disease affects all age groups and is not related to sex, race, or genetic background. The annual incidence is approximately 2 per 100,000.

Pathology

Acute inflammatory demyelinating polyneuropathy is a multifocal demyelinating disease of the peripheral nervous system characterized by perivascular mononuclear-cell infiltrates with segmental demyelination in the areas of inflammation. In areas of most severe involvement, axonal destruction and wallerian degeneration occur. These lesions sometimes show infiltration of polymorphonuclear leukocytes as well as mononuclear cells early in the course of the disease.

Clinical Features

The onset is characterized by rapidly progressive weakness first of the lower extremities, then of the upper extremities, and finally of the respiratory musculature. Weakness and paralysis are frequently preceded by paresthesias and numbness of the limbs, but objective sensory loss is mild and transient. Cranial nerves, most commonly the facial nerve, can be involved. The tendon reflexes are decreased or lost early in the illness, and nerve conduction in affected limbs is moderately to markedly slowed. Cerebrospinal fluid protein is increased in all cases, but frequently not during the first few days of the illness. The cerebrospinal fluid cell count is commonly normal, but elevated when the disease occurs in association with AIDS. The usual clinical course is one of rapid evolution of symptoms over 3 days to 3 weeks with improvement and return to normal function over 6–9 months. However, other patterns such as a more gradual onset, a prolonged period of complete paralysis, recovery with severe residual deficits, and a relapsing course have also been described.

Immunologic Diagnosis

In patients tested early in the course of their illness, high titers of complement-fixing antimyelin antibody of the IgM class have been detected. Clearance of this antibody from the serum often correlates with clinical improvement. Other antinerve and antimyelin antibodies have also been found, but it has not been established whether these are pathogenic or simply reflect reactions secondary to nerve tissue destruction. Spontaneously transformed circulating lymphocytes have been described, as well as lymphocytes that respond to peripheral-nerve myelin proteins by proliferation or lymphokine production.

Both cellular and humoral immune responses are therefore thought to play roles in the pathogenesis of acute inflammatory demyelinating polyneuropathy.

Differential Diagnosis

Neuropathies associated with porphyria or heavy-metal poisoning can be excluded by appropriate blood or urine tests. Acute transverse myelitis or early spinal cord compression may resemble acute inflammatory demyelinating polyneuropathy, but increased reflexes and spasticity occur days to weeks after initial flaccidity, usually with bowel and bladder involvement. Vasculitides such as polyarteritis nodosa can produce peripheral neuropathies, but these tend to present with asymmetric multifocal involvement. Acute myasthenia gravis may resemble acute inflammatory demyelinating polyneuropathy, but is more likely to be associated with oculomotor weakness and generally responds to anticholinesterase drugs. Botulism and tick paralysis, uncommon diseases causing subacute generalized weakness through the effect of their associated toxins on the neuromuscular junction, can usually be distinguished by the clinical history and by neurophysiologic testing.

Treatment

Plasmapheresis, especially if begun as early as possible, is effective in shortening the course of the illness (Fig 43–4). Intensive supportive care, including respiratory assistance, must be given as required. Corticosteroids tend to prolong the duration of illness and are therefore contraindicated, except in some cases of recurrent polyneuropathy.

Complications & Prognosis

Modern methods for assisting and maintaining respiration have resulted in a marked decrease in the mortality rate of acute inflammatory demyelinating polyneuropathy, which currently ranges from 1 to 5%. However, residual neurologic deficits, caused by irreversible axonal disruption and wallerian degeneration, occur in as many as 50% of patients. Respiratory muscle and pharyngeal weakness favor the development of infections, which may be life-threatening, and associated autonomic neuropathy may produce vasomotor instability and cardiac arrhythmias, resulting in sudden death despite adequate respiratory care.

CHRONIC DEMYELINATING POLYNEUROPATHIES

These are uncommon disorders that resemble acute inflammatory demyelinating polyneuropathy pathologically and physiologically but follow a much more indolent and frequently relapsing course. Clinical manifestations include variable degrees of ex-

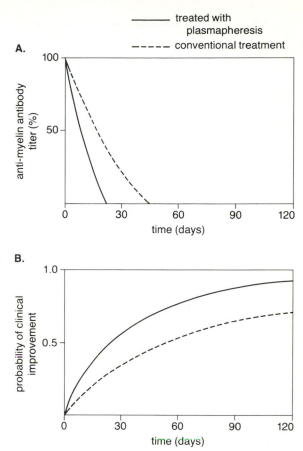

Figure 43–4. Effect of plasmapheresis on antimyelin antibody (**A**) and clinical recovery (**B**) in acute inflammatory demyelinating polyneuropathy (AIDP). Titers decline faster and recovery is more rapid and more nearly complete with plasma exchange, especially when performed during the first week of illness. (Panel A adapted from data provided by CL Koski; panel B adapted from Guillain-Barré Syndrome Study Group Clinical Trial, *Neurology* 1985;**35**:1096.)

tremity weakness and sensory symptoms. Nerve conduction studies show profound slowing with conduction block. Cerebrospinal fluid protein is characteristically increased; deposits of immunoglobulin may be found in peripheral nerves; and complement-fixing antibody to myelin may be detected, suggesting an immune system-mediated process. Patients frequently respond to plasma exchange, long-term corticosteroid treatment (particularly in the relapsing type), or treatment with other immunosuppressive drugs.

Patients with multiple myeloma, Waldenström's macroglobulinemia, and primary systemic amyloidosis sometimes develop peripheral neuropathies in which the pathologic pattern is primarily axonal degeneration with secondary demyelination. The pathogenesis of these conditions has been largely unexplored. However, a group of patients with benign monoclonal gammopathy and peripheral neuropathy have recently aroused interest because of evidence that their circulating paraproteins, usually of the IgM isotype, are monoclonal antibodies directed against the myelin-associated glycoprotein of peripheral-nerve myelin. These autoantibodies react with the carbohydrate portion of the myelin-associated glycoprotein molecule and cross-react with other glycoprotein and glycolipid components of peripheral nerve. Evidence that these antibodies actually initiate demyelination is inconclusive. Nevertheless, plasma exchange and immunosuppression have produced remissions with reversal of conduction block and disappearance of the paraprotein from the serum in some cases. The role of immune cells has not been determined, although mononuclear cell infiltrates are often present in demyelinated areas of peripheral nerve, and secretion of the IgM paraprotein is under T cell control. Not only are these disorders immunologically fascinating in their own right, but they may serve as models for studies of other more common immune system-mediated diseases of the peripheral and central nervous systems.

DISORDERS OF NEUROMUSCULAR TRANSMISSION

Myasthenia gravis and the myasthenic (Eaton-Lambert) syndrome are the neurologic diseases for which an autoimmune pathogenesis is best established.

MYASTHENIA GRAVIS

Major Immunologic Features
- It is commonly associated with thymic hyperplasia or thymoma.
- Pathogenic autoantibodies are directed against the acetylcholine receptor.
- It is often associated with other autoantibodies and autoimmune diseases.

General Considerations
Myasthenia gravis is a disease of unknown cause in which there is muscle weakness due to a disorder of neuromuscular transmission. The frequent occurrence of myasthenia gravis with thymomas, thymic hyperplasia, autoantibodies, and other autoimmune diseases strongly suggests that the immune system is involved in its pathogenesis. Anti-acetylcholine receptor antibody, which binds at the postsynaptic membrane of the neuromuscular junction, interrupts transmission by increasing endocytosis of acetylcholine receptors and forms immune complexes that bind complement, causing further destruction of the postsynaptic membrane (Fig 43–5). The prevalence of myasthenia gravis is 2–10 per 100,000. It occurs at all ages, but different subgroups are recognized. In patients with thymoma, in whom the onset is usually after age 40, there is no sex or HLA antigen association; in patients without thymoma in whom onset is before age 40, there is a female preponderance and association with HLA-A1, -B8, and -DR3; in patients without thymoma in whom the onset is after age 40, there is a male preponderance and association with HLA-A3, -B7, and -DR2.

Pathology
Scattered aggregates of lymphocytes are observed in the muscles. At the neuromuscular junction there is widening of the synaptic cleft and a marked abnor-

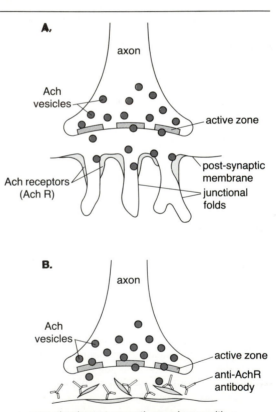

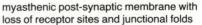

myasthenic post-synaptic membrane with loss of receptor sites and junctional folds

Figure 43–5. Normal (**A**) and myasthenic (**B**) neuromuscular junctions. At the normal junction, acetylcholine (Ach) is released from the nerve terminal and taken up by receptors on the complex folded postsynaptic membrane. In myasthenia gravis, anti-acetylcholine receptor (AchR) antibodies and immune complexes induce complement-mediated destruction of the membrane, with loss of normal folds and receptor sites.

mality of the postsynaptic membrane, with sparse, shallow postsynaptic folds. Eighty percent of patients have hyperplasia of lymphoid follicles with active germinal centers in the medulla of the thymus, whereas 10% have a thymoma (a locally invasive thymic neoplasm), and in the remaining 10% the thymus appears normal.

Clinical Features

Skeletal muscles are normal at rest but become increasingly weak with repetitive use. Weakness is often first noted in the extraocular muscles as diplopia or ptosis, while pharyngeal and facial weakness results in dysphagia and dysarthria. Skeletal-muscle weakness is more often proximal than distal and causes difficulty in climbing stairs, rising from chairs, combing the hair, or even holding up the head. When respiratory muscles are weak, ventilatory assistance is sometimes necessary. Exacerbations can occur spontaneously but are often related to intercurrent infections, surgery, or emotional stress and may result in myasthenic crisis with severe bulbar and respiratory weakness. Except for muscle weakness and depressed reflexes, the neurologic examination is normal. Intravenous injection of edrophonium, a short-acting anticholinesterase, is useful in diagnosis, as it produces dramatic transient improvement of weakness by prolonging the availability of acetylcholine at the postsynaptic receptor.

Immunologic Diagnosis

Anti-acetylcholine receptor antibodies are found in 90% of myasthenia gravis patients and occasionally in thymoma patients without muscle weakness (these patients do not have myasthenia gravis), but they may be absent in patients with purely ocular myasthenia. As they are found in no other neuromuscular disease, their presence in the appropriate clinical setting is diagnostic. Anti-striated-muscle antibodies are often detected in patients with an associated thymoma, but their pathogenic significance is unknown.

Differential Diagnosis

Myasthenia gravis can be differentiated from other myopathies on the basis of its response to anticholinesterase drugs. The various forms of periodic paralysis do not show the oculomotor involvement of myasthenia. The myasthenic (Eaton-Lambert) syndrome usually associated with small-cell carcinoma of the lung can be differentiated by electrodiagnostic studies and by lack of response to anticholinesterase agents. Botulism and tick paralysis can be diagnosed on the basis of the clinical history and electrophysiologic testing.

Treatment

Anticholinesterase drugs such as pyridostigmine and neostigmine are the mainstays of long-term ther-

apy. Thymectomy is beneficial in the majority of cases, and all patients with myasthenia gravis except those with nondisabling ocular myasthenia should be considered for thymectomy. The response to corticosteroids and immunosuppressive agents such as azathioprine has been encouraging. Dramatic improvement also occurs in severely ill patients treated with plasmapheresis, which removes anti-acetylcholine receptor antibodies from the circulation. Plasmapheresis is most effective when combined with immunosuppressive drugs to diminish the rapid increase in anti-receptor antibody that follows plasma exchange.

Complications & Prognosis

The course of myasthenia gravis prior to the widespread use of thymectomy, plasmapheresis, and corticosteroids was one of remission in 25% of cases during the first 2 years and chronic persistent weakness with a 20–30% mortality rate in the remainder. Improvement or complete remission within 5 years can now be expected in up to 90% of patients undergoing thymectomy supplemented by the other treatment modalities. Potential hazards for the myasthenic patient include myasthenic crisis with respiratory impairment, cholinergic crisis with weakness caused by overdosage of anticholinesterase drugs, pulmonary infections resulting from respiratory insufficiency and pharyngeal weakness, and lowered resistance to invading organisms as a result of immunosuppressive therapy.

MYASTHENIC SYNDROME

This condition, also known as Eaton-Lambert syndrome, superficially resembles myasthenia gravis, but commonly spares ocular and bulbar muscles, affects proximal limb muscles, and is characterized by increasing strength with repeated muscle contraction. This phenomenon is reflected electrophysiologically in increased amplitude of motor unit action potentials evoked by rapid repetitive nerve stimulation. Myasthenic syndrome usually occurs as a remote effect of small-cell carcinoma of the lung, or occasionally as an isolated disorder. It is an autoimmune disease mediated by circulating IgG antibodies to components of the presynaptic membrane known as active zones, which function as calcium channels and are important in releasing acetylcholine at the nerve terminal. In cases associated with cancer, the antibodies are presumably directed against tumor cell antigens and cross-react with determinants in the active zones to down-regulate calcium channel activity. The disease can be experimentally transmitted to mice with serum IgG from affected patients and often responds to treatment with plasmapheresis and immunosuppressive drugs.

IMMUNOLOGIC ABNORMALITIES IN OTHER NEUROLOGIC DISEASES

Immunologic findings have been described in several neurodegenerative disorders, but in only one, paraneoplastic cerebellar degeneration, has an autoimmune mechanism clearly been defined. The causes of Alzheimer's disease and amyotrophic lateral sclerosis are unknown, and the significance of immunologic abnormalities is speculative. In subacute sclerosing panencephalitis, progressive multifocal leukoencephalopathy, and Creutzfeldt-Jakob disease, transmissible agents are clearly involved and the role of the immune response is secondary or nonexistent.

PARANEOPLASTIC CEREBELLAR DEGENERATION

This is the best-described syndrome of neural degeneration occurring as an indirect effect of systemic cancer. Patients develop gait instability or ataxia and gross incoordination of their arms and hands. If untreated, the condition can progress to disabling incoordination and unintelligible speech in a few months. Although such degeneration has been described in patients with a variety of cancers, it is strongly associated with carcinomas of the lung and ovary. In patients who present with nervous system disease, an occult tumor may be discovered only after prolonged investigation. Two features dominate the pathology of this condition: extensive loss of Purkinje cells (the major output neuron of the cerebellum) and proliferation of microglial cells. A patchy lymphocytic infiltrate may also be seen. Many patients have serum antibodies that bind to human cerebellum tissue slices. These antibodies are usually polyclonal IgG. An antigenic target has recently been described as a cytoplasmic protein present in both the tumor and Purkinje cells. This condition serves as a model for antibody-mediated paraneoplastic disease, in which antibodies raised as a natural immune defense against tumor cells cross-react with a normal tissue componenet. Purkinje cells in vivo may extract antibody from the cerebrospinal fluid, leading to neuronal degeneration and death (Fig 43–6). Remission of the cerebellar disease may occasionally be seen after successful treatment of the underlying cancer.

AMYOTROPHIC LATERAL SCLEROSIS

Amyotrophic lateral sclerosis causes progressive weakness, atrophy, and fasciculations due to degeneration of motor neurons of the spinal cord. Most patients also show degeneration of corticospinal upper motor neurons, resulting in spasticity, hyperreflexia, and poor control of voluntary movement. The disease progresses inexorably to death, usually within 3–5 years. Survival is poorest in patients who have wasting and weakness of the muscles of the pharynx, chest, and diaphragm, leading to aspiration pneumonia and respiratory failure. Commonly known as Lou Gehrig's disease, amyotrophic lateral sclerosis typically affects males after age 40. Although pathologic examination reveals neuronal loss and glial proliferation without inflammatory cells, an immunologic basis has been proposed for a subgroup of patients with a monoclonal IgM paraproteinemia. Recent work has identified the possible target antigens as glycolipids known as gangliosides, which are normal neural membrane components. Amyotrophic lateral sclerosis patients without paraproteinemia may also have increased antibody titers against gangliosides. Such circulating autoantibodies may either damage motor neurons directly or may be internalized at nerve terminals outside the blood-brain barrier and transported to the cell body, where they interfere with cellular metabolism (Fig 43–6). Several immunosuppressive agents have been tested in patients with amyotrophic lateral sclerosis, but only cyclosporine has shown even a small effect on disease progression. A clinical trial of total lymphoid irradiation is currently in progress, although the significance of immune processes in pathogenesis remains unclear.

ALZHEIMER'S DISEASE

Alzheimer's disease was originally described as a presenile dementia. It is now clear that the same pathology occurs in patients older than 65 years and that it is the commonest cause of senile dementia. Memory and abstract reasoning are affected early in the course of the disease, which can eventually render patients unable to care for themselves. This makes Alzheimer's disease the single largest reason for nursing home care. The disease is defined by its pathologic changes. Large neurons, particularly in the cortex and hippocampus, develop cytoplasmic filamentous abnormalities called ''neurofibrillary tangles.'' Clusters of degenerating nerve terminals mixed with deposits of an amyloid-type protein form senile plaques, the other pathologic hallmark of Alzheimer's disease. Autoantibodies against neuronal antigens have been described, but their role in the pathogenesis of the disease is unclear, and they may represent only a secondary response to neuronal degeneration. Many attempts to transmit Alzheimer's disease by injection of affected brain tissue into primates have failed, but the possibility of a transmissible agent in familial Alzheimer's disease has been raised by recent work showing that hamsters receiving injections of leukocytes from familial

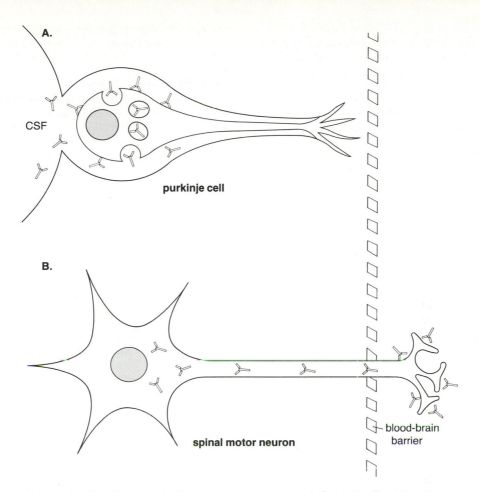

Figure 43–6. Uptake of antibodies by central nervous system neurons. **A:** Cerebellar Purkinje cell, a neuron that does not extend outside the blood-brain barrier. Antibody molecules diffuse from the cerebrospinal fluid (CSF) into the extracellular space, where they may bind to surface antigens and be taken up by endocytosis. **B:** Spinal motor neuron projecting to the neuromuscular junction outside the blood-brain barrier. Antibodies are taken up at the nerve terminal and reach the cell body via retrograde axonal transport.

Alzheimer's disease patients develop spongiform changes in their brains, similar to those found in Creutzfeldt-Jakob disease. At first glance the presence of amyloid plaques in both diseases suggests some similarity between them, but several different proteins can assume an ''amyloid'' configuration, and the amyloid in these two conditions is antigenically distinct. The role of both immunologic and infectious factors in the pathogenesis of Alzheimer's disease is currently in need of further clarification.

SLOW & LATENT VIRUS INFECTIONS OF THE NERVOUS SYSTEM

Subacute Sclerosing Panencephalitis

This is a degenerative and demyelinating central nervous system disease of children that can occur several years after acute infection with measles virus. In countries where an active measles vaccination program has been implemented, the incidence of subacute sclerosing parencephalitis has declined dramatically, but elsewhere it remains a serious pediatric neurologic problem. Manifestations include personality change, dementia, seizures, and myoclonus, which progress rapidly to death in 12–18 months in most cases. Pathologically, there are intranuclear and cytoplasmic inclusion bodies that contain paramyxovirus nucleocapsids. Measles virus antigens can be demonstrated immunohistochemically, and measles virus may be recovered from infected brain tissue by cocultivation techniques. The persistence of the virus in the presence of high titers of antibody suggests an underlying defect in immunity. However, consistent defects in assays of cellular and humoral immunity cannot be identified. Measles virus strains isolated from patients with subacute sclerosing parencephalitis are indistinguishable from wild-type strains, but current evidence suggests that an abortive infection occurs and that mature virions are not produced. Incomplete expression or defective synthesis of particular measles virus proteins may be related to the high antibody titers in serum and cerebrospinal fluid. The accumulation of viral components in brain cells may alter cellular function, but infiltrates of mononuclear cells are also seen in lesions and may contribute to the pathogenic process. Treatment with the antiviral agent inosine pranobex (Isoprinosine), or with alpha interferon by intraventricular injection, has resulted in stabilization and even improvement in some cases.

PROGRESSIVE MULTIFOCAL LEUKOENCEPHALOPATHY

Progressive multifocal leukoencephalopathy is a rare disease of the central nervous system that presents with focal weakness, ataxia, spasticity, visual disturbances, aphasia, dementia, and rapid progression to coma and death within 6 months to 1 year. It occurs most frequently in adult patients with debilitating illnesses associated with some form of immunosuppression. These include lymphomas, leukemias, exogenous immunosuppression given to prevent transplant rejection, and AIDS. A papovavirus known as JC virus has been isolated from brain tissue and may be identified by immunohistochemical or in situ hybridization techniques in oligodendrocytes and astrocytes. Direct infection and destruction of oligodendrocytes causes the characteristic widespread demyelination. Inflammation is minimal or absent, and the cerebrospinal fluid is usually normal. JC virus is a ubiquitous human pathogen, and the majority of normal adults have serum IgG antibodies, indicating prior exposure. The pathogenesis of progressive multifocal leukoencephalopathy is still not completely understood, but it is likely that generalized immunosuppression results in reactivation of a latent papovavirus infection, which selec-

tively attacks oligodendrocytes and astrocytes to produce the typical clinical and pathologic findings of this disease.

Creutzfeldt-Jakob Disease

This progressive degenerative disease is characterized by dementia and myoclonic jerks, with some patients showing ataxia and seizures as well. A vegetative state leading to death usually results within 1 year of diagnosis. Although Creutzfeldt-Jakob disease is a minor cause of dementia in the general population, it has had great impact on our concepts of causes of neurodegenerative disease. It has a distinctive pathology termed spongiform encephalopathy, showing intra- and extraneuronal vacuolization, severe gliosis, and neuronal loss, but no inflammatory changes. This pathology is also seen in kuru, a progressive neurologic disease of the Fore natives of New Guinea, and scrapie, a neurodegenerative disease of sheep. Scrapie was known to be transmissible, and its pathologic similarity to kuru and Creutzfeldt-Jakob disease led to the inoculation of infected brain tissue into primates, which produced a disease similar to Creutzfeldt-Jakob disease, demonstrating that these human diseases were transmissible as well. The infectious agent, called a prion, can have a latency period of several years and is resistant to routine forms of sterilization. The major structural component of the agent is thought to be a protein encoded by a gene found in both infected and normal brain. This protein forms rodlike structures that make up the amyloid plaques in brains of Creutzfeldt-Jakob disease patients. Cannibalism was the probable source of infection for kuru, but the route of transmission of sporadic Creutzfeldt-Jakob disease is less clear. Although inadvertent inoculation with infected tissue can transmit the disease, most affected patients have no history of contact. No agent-specific immune response has been identified in Creutzfeldt-Jakob disease patients, nor does clinical immunosuppression predispose patients to develop the disease, as is the case in progressive multifocal leukoencephalopathy.

REFERENCES

Acute Disseminated Encephalomyelitis

Johnson KP et al: Immune-mediated syndromes of the nervous system related to virus infections. Chap 20, pp 391–434, in: *Handbook of Clinical Neurology.* Vol 34. Vinken PJ, Bruyn GW (editors). North-Holland, 1978.

Johnson RT et al: Measles encephalomyelitis: Clinical and immunologic studies. *N Engl J Med* 1985; **310**:137.

Multiple Sclerosis

Antel JP, Arnason BGW, Medof ME: Suppressor cell

function in multiple sclerosis: Correlation with clinical disease activity. *Ann Neurol* 1979;**5**:338.

Ebers GC et al: A population-based study of multiple sclerosis in twins. *N Engl J Med* 1986;**315**:1638.

Hafler DA et al: In vivo activated T lymphocytes in the peripheral blood and cerebrospinal fluid of patients with multiple sclerosis. *N Engl J Med* 1985; **312**:1405.

Knobler RL et al: Systemic alpha interferon therapy of multiple sclerosis. *Neurology* 1984;**34**:1273.

McFarlin DE, McFarland HF: Multiple sclerosis. *N Engl J Med* 1982;**307**:1183.

Panitch HS et al: Treatment of multiple sclerosis with gamma interferon. *Neurology* 1987;**37**:1097.

Traugott U, Lebon P: Multiple sclerosis: Involvement of interferons in lesion pathogenesis. *Ann Neurol* 1988;**24**:243.

Weiner HL, Hafler DA: Immunotherapy of multiple sclerosis. *Ann Neurol* 1988;**23**:211.

Acute Inflammatory Demyelinating Polyneuropathy

Arnason BGW: Acute inflammatory demyelinating neuropathy. Chap 90, pp 2050–2100, in: *Peripheral Neuropathy*. Vol 1. Dyck PJ et al (editors). Saunders, 1984.

Guillain-Barré Syndrome Study Group: Plasmapheresis and acute Guillain-Barré syndrome. *Neurology* 1985;**35**:1096.

Koski CL et al: Anti-peripheral myelin antibody in patients with demyelinating neuropathy: Quantitative and kinetic determination of serum antibody by complement component 1 fixation. *Proc Natl Acad Sci USA* 1985; **82**:905.

Chronic Demyelinating Polyneuropathies

Dyck PJ, Arnason BGW: Chronic inflammatory demyelinating polyradiculoneuropathy. Chap 91, pp 2101–2114, in: *Peripheral Neuropathy*. Vol 2. Dyck PJ et al (editors). Saunders, 1984.

Latov N et al: Plasma cell dyscrasia and peripheral neuropathy: Identification of myelin antigens that react with human paraproteins. *Proc Natl Acad Sci USA* 1981;**78**:7139.

Mendell JR et al: Polyneuropathy and IgM monoclonal gammopathy: Studies on the pathogenetic role of anti-myelin-associated glycoprotein antibody. *Ann Neurol* 1985;**17**:243.

Myasthenia Gravis & Myasthenic Syndrome

Dau PC et al: Plasmapheresis and immunosuppressive drug therapy in myasthenia gravis. *N Engl J Med* 1977;**297**:1134.

Drachman DB et al: Functional activities of autoantibodies to acetylcholine receptors and the clinical severity of myasthenia gravis. *N Engl J Med* 1982: **307**:769.

Engel AG: Myasthenia gravis and myasthenic syndromes. *Ann Neurol* 1984;**16**:519.

Nagel A et al: Lambert-Eaton myasthenic syndrome IgG depletes presynaptic membrane active zone particles by antigenic modulation. *Ann Neurol* 1988;**24**:552.

Pascuzzi RM, Coslett HB, Johns TR: Long-term corticosteroid treatment of myasthenia gravis: Report of 116 patients. *Ann Neurol* 1984;**15**:291.

Paraneoplastic Cerebellar Degeneration

Anderson NE, Rosenblum MK, Posner JB: Paraneoplastic cerebellar degeneration: Clinical-immunological correlations. *Ann Neurol* 1988;**24**:599.

Henson RA, Urich H: *Cancer and the Nervous System: The Neurological Manifestations of Systemic Malignant Disease*. Blackwell, 1982.

Jaeckle KA et al: Autoimmune response of patients with paraneoplastic cerebellar degeneration to a Purkinje cell cytoplasmic protein antigen. *Ann Neurol* 1985; **18**:592.

Amyotrophic Lateral Sclerosis

Mitsumoto H, Hanson MR, Chad DA: Amyotrophic lateral sclerosis: Recent advances in pathogenesis and therapeutic trials. *Arch Neurol* 1988;**45**:189.

Pestronk A et al: Serum antibodies to Gm1 ganglioside in amyotrophic lateral sclerosis. *Neurology* 1988; **38**:1457.

Alzheimer's Disease

Manuelidis EE et al: Transmission studies from blood of Alzheimer disease patients and healthy relatives. *Proc Natl Acad Sci USA* 1988;**85**:4898.

Selkoe D: Deciphering Alzheimer's disease: The pace quickens. *Trends Neurosci* 1987;**10**:181.

Slow & Latent Virus Infections

Case Records of the Massachusetts General Hospital (case 45-1988): Progressive multifocal leukoencephalopathy. *N Engl J Med* 1988;**319**:1268.

Panitch HS et al: Subacute sclerosing panencephalitis: Remission after treatment with intraventricular interferon. *Neurology* 1986;**36**:562.

Prusiner SB, Gabizon R, McKinley MP: On the biology of prions. *Acta Neuropathol* 1987;**72**:299.

Roberts GW et al: CNS amyloid proteins in neurodegenerative diseases. *Neurology* 1988;**38**:1534.

44

Eye Diseases

Mitchell H. Friedlaender, MD, & G. Richard O'Connor, MD

The eye is frequently considered to be a special target of immunologic disease processes, but proof of the causative role of these processes is lacking in all but a few disorders. In this sense, the immunopathology of the eye is much less clearly delineated than that of the kidney, the testis, or the thyroid gland. Because the eye is a highly vascularized organ and because the rather labile vessels of the conjunctiva are embedded in a nearly transparent medium, inflammatory eye disorders are more obvious (and often more painful) than those of other organs such as the thyroid or the kidney. The iris, ciliary body, and choroid are the most highly vascularized tissues of the eye. The similarity of the vascular supply of the uvea to that of the kidney and the choroid plexus of the brain has given rise to justified speculation concerning the selection of these 3 tissues, among others, as targets of immune complex diseases (eg, serum sickness).

Immunologic diseases of the eye can be grossly divided into 2 major categories: antibody-mediated and cell-mediated diseases. As is the case in other organs, there is ample opportunity for the interaction of these 2 systems in the eye.

ANTIBODY-MEDIATED DISEASES

Before it can be concluded that a disease of the eye is antibody-dependent, the following criteria must be satisfied: (1) There must be evidence of specific antibody in the patient's serum or plasma cells. (2) The antigen must be identified and, if feasible, characterized. (3) The same antigen must be shown to produce an immunologic response in the eye of an experimental animal, and the pathologic changes produced in the experimental animal must be similar to those observed in the human disease. (4) It must be possible to produce similar lesions in animals passively sensitized with serum from an affected animal upon challenge with the specific antigen.

Unless all of the above criteria are satisfied, the disease may be thought of as *possibly* antibody-dependent. In such circumstances, the disease can be regarded as antibody-mediated if only one of the following criteria is met: (1) if antibody to an antigen is present in higher quantities in the ocular fluids than in the serum (after adjustments have been made for the total amounts of immunoglobulins in each fluid); (2) if abnormal accumulations of plasma cells are present in the ocular lesion; (3) if abnormal accumulations of immunoglobulins are present at the site of the disease; (4) if complement is fixed by immunoglobulins at the site of the disease; (5) if an accumulation of eosinophils is present at the site of the disease; or (6) if the ocular disease is associated with an inflammatory disease elsewhere in the body for which antibody dependency has been proved or strongly suggested.

VERNAL CONJUNCTIVITIS & ATOPIC KERATOCONJUNCTIVITIS

These 2 diseases also belong to the group of atopiclike disorders. Both are characterized by itching and lacrimation of the eyes but are more chronic than hay fever conjunctivitis. Furthermore, both ultimately result in structural modifications of the lids and conjunctiva. The immunologic basis for these diseases is not delineated.

Vernal conjunctivitis characteristically affects children and adolescents; the incidence decreases sharply after the second decade of life. Like hay fever conjunctivitis, vernal conjunctivitis occurs only in the warm months of the year. Most of its victims live in hot, dry climates. The disease characteristically produces giant ("cobblestone") papillae of the tarsal conjunctiva (Fig 44–1). The keratinized epithelium from these papillae may abrade the underlying cornea, giving rise to complaints of foreign body sensations.

Atopic keratoconjunctivitis affects individuals of all ages and has no specific seasonal incidence. The skin of the lids has a characteristic dry, scaly appearance. The conjunctiva is pale and boggy. Both the conjunctiva and the cornea may develop scarring in the later stages of the disease. Atopic cataract has also been described. Staphylococcal blepharitis, manifested by scales and crusts on the lids, commonly complicates this disease.

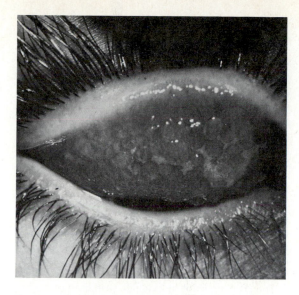

Figure 44–1. Giant papillae ("cobblestones") in the tarsal conjunctiva of a patient with vernal conjunctivitis.

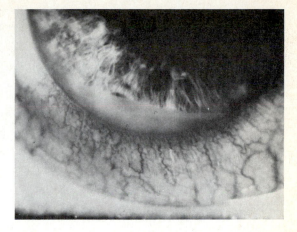

Figure 44–2. Acute iridocyclitis in a patient with ankylosing spondylitis. Note the fibrin clot in the anterior chamber.

RHEUMATOID DISEASES AFFECTING THE EYE

The diseases in this category vary greatly in their clinical manifestations depending upon the specific disease entity and the age of the patient. Uveitis and scleritis are the principal ocular manifestations of the rheumatoid diseases. **Juvenile rheumatoid arthritis** affects females more frequently than males and is commonly accompanied by iridocyclitis of one or both eyes. The onset is often insidious, the patient having few or no complaints and the eye remaining white. Extensive synechia formation, cataract, and secondary glaucoma may be far-advanced before the parents notice that anything is wrong. The arthritis generally affects only one joint (eg, a knee) in cases with ocular involvement.

Ankylosing spondylitis affects males more frequently than females, and the onset is in the second to sixth decades. It may be accompanied by iridocyclitis of acute onset, often with fibrin in the anterior chamber (Fig 44–2). Pain, redness, and photophobia are the initial complaints, and synechia formation is common.

Rheumatoid arthritis of adult onset may be accompanied by acute scleritis or episcleritis (Fig 44–3). The ciliary body and choroid, lying adjacent to the sclera, are often involved secondarily with the inflamation. Rarely, serous detachment of the retina results. The onset is usually in the third to fifth decade, and women are affected more frequently than men.

Reiter's disease affects men more frequently than women. The first attack of ocular inflammation usu-

ally consists of a self-limited papillary conjunctivitis. It follows, at a highly variable interval, the onset of nonspecific urethritis and the appearance of inflamation in one or more of the weight-bearing joints. Subsequent attacks of ocular inflammation may consist of acute iridocyclitis of one or both eyes, occasionally with hypopyon (Fig 44–4).

Immunologic Pathogenesis

Rheumatoid factor, an IgM autoantibody directed against the patient's own IgG, probably plays a major role in the pathogenesis of rheumatoid arthritis. The union of IgM antibody with IgG is followed by fixation of complement at the tissue site and the attraction of leukocytes and platelets to this area. An occlusive vasculitis resulting from this train of events is thought to be the cause of rheumatoid nod-

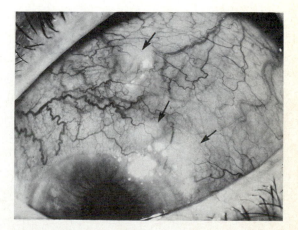

Figure 44–3. Scleral nodules in a patient with rheumatoid arthritis. (Courtesy of S Kimura.)

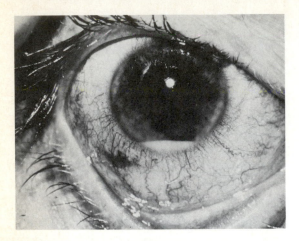

Figure 44–4. Acute iridocyclitis with hypopyon in a patient with Reiter's disease.

ule formation in the sclera as well as elsewhere in the body. The occlusion of vessels supplying nutriments to the sclera is thought to be responsible for the "melting away" of the scleral collagen that is so characteristic of rheumatoid arthritis (Fig 44–5).

Although this explanation may suffice for rheumatoid arthritis, patients with the ocular complications of juvenile rheumatoid arthritis, ankylosing spondylitis, and Reiter's syndrome usually have negative tests for rheumatoid factor, so other explanations must be sought.

Outside the eyeball itself, the lacrimal gland has been shown to be under attack by circulating antibodies. Destruction of acinar cells within the gland and invasion of the lacrimal gland (as well as the salivary glands) by mononuclear cells result in decreased tear secretion. The combination of dry eyes (keratoconjunctivitis sicca), dry mouth (xerostomia), and rheumatoid arthritis (or other collagen-vascular

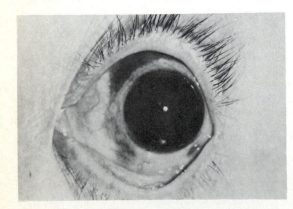

Figure 44–5. Scleral thinning in a patient with rheumatoid arthritis. Note the dark color of the underlying uvea.

disease) is known as Sjögren's syndrome (see Chapter 36).

A growing body of evidence indicates that the immunogenetic background of certain patients accounts for the expression of their ocular inflammatory disease in specific ways. Analysis of the HLA antigen system shows that the incidence of HLA-B27 is significantly greater in patients with ankylosing spondylitis and Reiter's syndrome than could be expected by chance alone. It is not known how this molecule controls specific inflammatory responses.

Immunologic Diagnosis

Rheumatoid factor can be detected in the serum by a number of standard tests involving the agglutination of IgG-coated erythrocytes or latex particles. Unfortunately, the test for rheumatoid factor is not positive in the majority of isolated rheumatoid afflictions of the eye.

The HLA types of individuals suspected of having ankylosing spondylitis and related diseases can be determined by standard cytotoxicity tests with specific antisera. These tests are generally done in tissue typing centers where work on organ transplantation necessitates such studies. X-ray of the sacroiliac area is a valuable screening procedure that may show evidence of spondylitis prior to the onset of low back pain in patients with the characteristic form of iridocyclitis.

Treatment

Patients with uveitis associated with rheumatoid disease respond well to local instillations of corticosteroid drops (eg, dexamethasone 0.1%) or ointments. Orally administered corticosteroids must occasionally be resorted to for brief periods. Salicylates given orally in divided doses with meals are thought to reduce the frequency and blunt the severity of recurrent attacks. Atropine drops 1% are useful for the relief of photophobia during the acute attacks. Shorter-acting mydriatics such as phenylephrine 10% should be used in the subacute stages to prevent synechia formation. Corticosteroid-resistant cases, especially those causing progressive erosion of the sclera, have been treated successfully with immunosuppressive drugs such as chlorambucil. Hydroxychloroquine, an antimalarial drug, has been useful in the treatment of Sjögren's syndrome and other collagen-vascular diseases. Eye examinations at 6 to 12-month intervals are recommended, since deposits in the cornea and retina have been reported with high-dose Plaquenil therapy.

OTHER ANTIBODY-MEDIATED DISEASES

The following antibody-mediated diseases are infrequently seen by the practicing ophthalmologist.

Systemic lupus erythematosus (SLE), associated with the presence of circulating antibodies to DNA, produces an occlusive vasculitis of the nerve fiber layer of the retina. Such infarcts result in cytoid bodies or "cotton-wool" spots in the retina (Fig 44–6).

Pemphigus vulgaris produces painful intraepithelial bullae of the conjunctiva. It is associated with the presence of circulating antibodies to an intercellular antigen located between the deeper cells of the conjunctival epithelium.

Cicatricial pemphigoid is characterized by subepithelial bullae of the conjunctiva. In the chronic stages of this disease, cicatricial contraction of the conjunctiva may result in severe scarring of the cornea, dryness of the eyes, and, ultimately, blindness. Pemphigoid is associated with local deposits of tissue antibodies directed against one or more antigens located in the basement membrane of the epithelium.

Lens-induced uveitis is a rare condition that may be associated with circulating antibodies to lens proteins. It is seen in individuals whose lens capsules have become permeable to these proteins as a result of trauma or other disease. Interest in this field dates back to 1903, when Uhlenhuth first demonstrated the organ-specific nature of antibodies to the lens. Witmer showed in 1962 that antibody to lens tissue may be produced by lymphoid cells of the ciliary body.

CELL-MEDIATED DISEASES

This group of diseases appears to be associated with T-cell-mediated immunity (delayed hypersensi-

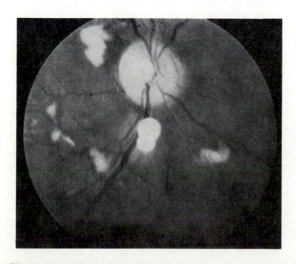

Figure 44–6. Cotton-wool spots in the retina of a patient with SLE.

tivity). Various structures of the eye are invaded by mononuclear cells, principally lymphocytes and macrophages, in response to one or more chronic antigenic stimuli. In chronic infections such as tuberculosis, leprosy, toxoplasmosis, and herpes simplex, the antigenic stimulus has clearly been identified as an infectious agent in the ocular tissue. Such infections are often associated with delayed skin test reactivity following the intradermal injection of an extract of the organism.

More intriguing but less well understood are the granulomatous diseases of the eye for which no infectious cause has been found. Such diseases are thought to represent cell-mediated, possibly autoimmune processes, but their origin remains obscure.

OCULAR SARCOIDOSIS

Ocular sarcoidosis is characterized by a panuveitis with occasional inflammatory involvement of the optic nerve and retinal blood vessels. It often presents as iridocyclitis of insidious onset. Less frequently, it occurs as acute iridocyclitis, with pain, photophobia, and redness of the eye. Large precipitates resembling drops of solidified "mutton fat" are seen on the corneal endothelium. The anterior chamber contains a good deal of protein and numerous cells, mostly lymphocytes. Nodules are often seen on the iris, both at the pupillary margin and in the substance of the iris stroma. The latter are often vascularized. Synechiae are commonly encountered, particularly in patients with dark skin. Severe cases ultimately involve the posterior segment of the eye. Coarse clumps of cells ("snowballs") are seen in the vitreous, and exudates resembling candle drippings may be seen along the course of the retinal vessels. Patchy infiltrations of the choroid or optic nerve may also be seen.

Infiltrations of the lacrimal gland and of the conjunctiva have been noted on occasion. When the latter are present, the diagnosis can easily be confirmed by biopsy of the small opaque nodules.

Immunologic Pathogenesis

Although many infectious or allergic causes of sarcoidosis have been suggested, none has been confirmed. Noncaseating granulomas are seen in the uvea, optic nerve, and adnexal structures of the eye as well as elsewhere in the body. The presence of macrophages and giant cells suggests that particulate matter is being phagocytized, but this material has not been identified.

Patients with sarcoidosis are usually anergic to extracts of the common microbial antigens such as those of mumps, *Trichophyton, Candida,* and *Mycobacterium tuberculosis.* As in other lymphoproliferative disorders such as Hodgkin's disease and chronic lymphocytic leukemia, suppression of T cells immunity impairs normal delayed hypersensitivity responses to common antigens. Meanwhile, circulating immunoglobulins are usually detectable in the serum at higher than normal levels.

Immunologic Diagnosis

The diagnosis is largely inferential. Negative skin tests to a battery of antigens to which the patient is known to have been exposed are highly suggestive, and the same is true of the elevation of serum immunoglobulins. Biopsy of a conjunctival nodule or scalene lymph node may provide positive histologic evidence of the disease. X-rays of the chest reveal hilar adenopathy in many cases. Elevated levels of serum lysozyme or serum angiotensin-converting enzyme may be detected. A gallium scan, utilizing gallium 67, may be useful in detecting clinically unapparent lesions.

Treatment

Sarcoid lesions of the eye respond well to corticosteroid therapy. Frequent instillations of prednisolone acetate 1% eye drops generally bring the anterior uveitis under control. Atropine drops should be prescribed in the acute phase of the disease for the relief of pain and photophobia; short-acting pupillary dilators such as phenylephrine should be given later to prevent synechia formation. Systemic corticosteroids are sometimes necessary to control severe attacks of anterior uveitis and are always necessary for the control of retinal vasculitis and optic neuritis. The latter condition often accompanies cerebral involvement and carries a grave prognosis.

SYMPATHETIC OPHTHALMIA & VOGT-KOYANAGI-HARADA SYNDROME

These 2 disorders are discussed together because they have certain common clinical features. Both are thought to represent autoimmune phenomena affecting pigmented structures of the eye and skin, and both may give rise to meningeal symptoms.

Clinical Features

Sympathetic ophthalmia is an inflammation in the second eye after the other has been damaged by penetrating injury. In most cases, some portion of the uvea of the injured eye has been exposed to the atmosphere for at least 1 hour. The uninjured or "sympathizing" eye develops minor signs of anterior uveitis after a period ranging from 2 weeks to several years. Floating spots and loss of the power of accommodation are among the earliest symptoms. The disease may progress to severe iridocyclitis with pain and photophobia. Usually, however, the eye remains relatively quiet and painless while the inflammatory disease spreads around the entire uvea.

Despite the presence of panuveitis, the retina usually remains uninvolved except for perivascular cuffing of the retinal vessels with inflammatory cells. Papilledema and secondary glaucoma may occur. The disease may be accompanied by vitiligo (patchy depigmentation of the skin) and poliosis (whitening) of the eyelashes.

Vogt-Koyanagi-Harada syndrome consists of inflammation of the uvea of one or both eyes characterized by acute iridocyclitis, patchy choroiditis, and serous detachment of the retina. It usually begins with an acute febrile episode with headache, dysacusis, and occasionally vertigo. Patchy loss or whitening of the scalp hair is described in the first few months of the disease. Vitiligo and poliosis are commonly present but are not essential for the diagnosis. Although the initial iridocyclitis may subside quickly, the course of the posterior disease is often indolent, with longstanding serous detachment of the retina and significant visual impairment.

Immunologic Pathogenesis

In both sympathetic ophthalmia and Vogt-Koyanagi-Harada syndrome, delayed hypersensitivity to melanin-containing structures is thought to occur. Although a viral cause has been suggested for both disorders, there is no convincing evidence of an infectious origin. It is postulated that some insult, infectious or otherwise, alters the pigmented structures of the eye, skin, and hair in such a way as to provoke delayed hypersensitivity responses to them. Soluble materials from the outer segments of the photoreceptor layer of the retina have recently been incriminated as possible autoantigens. Patients with Vogt-Koyanagi-Harada syndrome are usually Asians, which suggests an immunogenetic predisposition to the disease.

Histologic sections of the traumatized eye from a patient with sympathetic ophthalmia may show uniform infiltration of most of the uvea by lymphocytes, epithelioid cells, and giant cells. The overlying retina is characteristically intact, but nests of epithelioid cells may protrude through the pigment epithelium of the retina, giving rise to **Dalen-Fuchs nodules.** The inflammation may destroy the architecture of the entire uvea, leaving an atrophic, shrunken globe.

Immunologic Diagnosis

Skin tests with soluble extracts of human or bovine uveal tissue are said to elicit delayed hypersensitivity responses in these patients. Several investigators have recently shown that cultured lymphocytes from patients with these 2 diseases undergo transformation to lymphoblasts in vitro when extracts of uvea or rod outer segments are added to the culture medium. Circulating antibodies to uveal antigens have been found in patients with these diseases, but such antibodies are to be found in any patient with long-standing uveitis, including those suffering from several infectious entities. The spinal fluid of patients with Vogt-Koyanagi-Harada syndrome may show increased numbers of mononuclear cells and elevated protein in the early stages.

Treatment

Mild cases of sympathetic ophthalmia may be treated satisfactorily with locally applied corticosteroid drops and pupillary dilators. The more severe or progressive cases require systemic corticosteroids, often in high doses, for months or years. An alternate-day regimen of oral corticosteroids is recommended for such patients in order to avoid adrenal suppression. The same applies to the treatment of patients with Vogt-Koyanagi-Harada disease. Occasionally, patients with long-standing progressive disease become resistant to corticosteroids or cannot take additional corticosteroid medication because of pathologic fractures, mental changes, or other reasons. Such patients may become candidates for immunosuppressive therapy. Chlorambucil and cyclophosphamide have been used successfully for both conditions. More recently, cyclosporin A has shown promise in the treatment of corticosteroid-resistant uveitis.

OTHER CELL-MEDIATED DISEASES

Giant cell arteritis (temporal arteritis) (see Chapter 39) may have disastrous effects on the eye, particularly in elderly individuals. The condition is manifested by pain in the temples and orbit, blurred vision, and scotomas. Examination of the fundus may reveal extensive occlusive retinal vasculitis and choroidal infarcts. Atrophy of the optic nerve head is a frequent complication. Such patients have an elevated erythrocyte sedimentation rate. Biopsy of the temporal artery reveals extensive infiltration of the vessel wall with giant cells and mononuclear cells.

Polyarteritis nodosa (see Chapter 39) can affect both the anterior and posterior segments of the eye. The corneas of such patients may show peripheral thinning and cellular infiltration. The retinal vessels reveal extensive necrotizing inflammation characterized by eosinophil, plasma cell, and lymphocyte infiltration.

Behçet's disease (see Chapter 36) has an uncertain place in the classification of immunologic disorders. It is characterized by recurrent iridocyclitis with hypopyon and occlusive vasculitis of the retinal vessels. Although it has many of the features of a delayed hypersensitivity disease, dramatic alterations of serum complement levels at the very beginning of an attack suggest an immune complex disorder. Furthermore, high levels of circulating immune complexes have recently been detected in patients with this disease. Most patients with eye symptoms are positive for HLA-B5 (subtype B51).

Contact dermatitis (see Chapter 33) of the eyelids represents a significant though minor disease caused by delayed hypersensitivity. Atropine, perfumed cosmetics, materials contained in plastic spectacle frames, and other locally applied agents may act as the sensitizing hapten. The lower lid is more extensively involved than the upper lid when the sensitizing agent is applied in drop form. Periorbital involvement with erythematous, vesicular, pruritic lesions of the skin is characteristic.

Phlyctenular keratoconjunctivitis (Fig 44-7) represents a delayed hypersensitivity response to certain microbial antigens, principally those of *Mycobacterium tuberculosis*. It is characterized by acute pain and photophobia in the affected eye, and perforation of the peripheral cornea has been known to result. The disease responds rapidly to locally applied corticosteroids. Since the advent of chemotherapy for pulmonary tuberculosis, phlyctenulosis is much less of a problem than it was 30 years ago. It is still encountered occasionally, however, particularly among Native Americans and Alaskan Eskimos. Rarely, other pathogens such as *Staphylococcus aureus* and *Coccidioides immitis* have been implicated in phlyctenular disease.

Acquired Immunodeficiency Syndrome (AIDS) (see Chapter 55) is commonly associated with ocular disorders, seen mainly in homosexual men, intravenous drug abusers, and hemophiliacs. Cotton-wool exudates are the most common ocular sign. They have the same appearance as those seen in SLE (Fig 44-6), but it is not known whether the cotton-wool spots of AIDS have the same pathogenesis. As is the case with SLE, patients suffering from AIDS may have elevated serum immune complexes.

In addition to cotton-wool spots, AIDS patients may develop Kaposi's sarcoma of the conjunctiva or

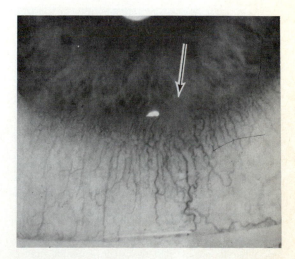

Figure 44-7. Phlyctenule (arrow) at the margin of the cornea. (Courtesy of P Thygeson.)

lids as well as chorioretinitis associated with any one of a number of different opportunistic pathogens such as cytomegalovirus, *Cryptococcus, Toxoplasma,* or *Candida.* These patients have a fundamental disorder of cell-mediated immunity reflected in reduced levels of CD4 cells and chronic infection by HIV. These patients often die of systemic opportunistic infections such as *Pneumocystis carinii* pneumonia or toxoplasmal encephalitis. Since cotton-wool spots are an early sign of AIDS, the ophthalmologist may be the first physician to alert the patient to the existence of this serious disorder.

CORNEAL GRAFT REACTIONS

General Considerations

Blindness due to opacity or distortion of the central portion of the cornea is a remediable disease (Fig 44–8). If all other structures of the eye are intact, a patient whose vision is impaired solely by corneal opacity can expect great improvement from a graft of clear cornea into the stroma, and a single-layered endothelium. Although the surface epithelium may be sloughed and later replaced by the recipient's epithelium, certain elements of the stroma and all of the donor's endothelium remain in place for the rest of the patient's life. This has been firmly established by sex chromosome markers in corneal cells when donor and recipient were of opposite sexes. The endothelium must remain healthy in order for the cornea to remain transparent, and an energy-dependent pump mechanism is required to keep the cornea from

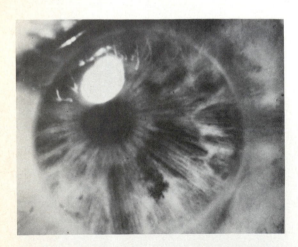

Figure 44–8. A cornea severely scarred by chronic atopic keratoconjunctivitis into which a central graft of clear cornea has been placed. Note how distinctly the iris landmarks are seen through the transparent graft.

swelling with water. Since the recipient's endothelium is in most cases diseased, the central corneal endothelium must be replaced by healthy donor tissue.

A number of foreign elements exist in corneal grafts that might stimulate the immune system of the host to reject this tissue. In addition to those mentioned above, the corneal stroma is regularly perfused with IgG and serum albumin from the donor, although none—or only small amounts—of the other blood proteins are present. While these serum proteins of donor origin rapidly diffuse into the recipient stroma, these substances are theoretically immunogenic.

Although the ABO blood antigens have been shown to have no relationship to corneal graft rejection, the HLA antigen system probably plays a significant role in graft reactions. HLA incompatibility between donor and recipient has been shown by several authors to be significant in determining graft survival, particularly when the corneal bed is vascularized. It is known that most cells of the body possess these HLA antigens, including the endothelial cells of the corneal graft as well as certain stromal cells (keratocytes). The epithelium has been shown by Hall and others to possess a non-HLA antigen that diffuses into the anterior third of the stroma. Thus, while much foreign antigen may be eliminated by purposeful removal of the epithelium at the time of grafting, that amount of antigen which has already diffused into the stroma is automatically carried over into the recipient. Such antigens may be leached out by soaking the donor cornea in tissue culture for several weeks prior to engraftment.

Immunologic Pathogenesis

Both antibody and cellular mechanisms have been implicated in corneal graft reactions. It is likely that early graft rejections (within 2 weeks) are cell-mediated reactions. Cytotoxic lymphocytes have been found in the limbal area and stroma of affected individuals, and phase microscopy in vivo has revealed an actual attack on the grafted endothelial cells by these lymphocytes. Such lymphocytes generally move inward from the periphery of the cornea, making what is known as a "rejection line" as they move centrally. The donor cornea becomes edematous as the endothelium becomes compromised by an accumulation of lymphoid cells.

Late rejection of a corneal graft may occur several weeks to many months after implantation of donor tissue into the recipient eye. Such reactions may be antibody-mediated, since cytotoxic antibodies have been isolated from the serum of patients with a history of diseased area. Trauma, including chemical burns, is one of the most common causes of central corneal opacity. Others include scars from herpetic keratitis, endothelial cell dysfunction with chronic corneal edema (Fuch's dystrophy), keratoconus, and opacities from previous graft failures. All of these conditions represent indications for penetrating corneal grafts, provided the patient's eye is no longer inflamed and the opacity has been allowed maximal time to undergo spontaneous resolution (usually 6-12 months). It is estimated that approximately 10,000 corneal grafts are performed in the USA annually. Of these, about 90% can be expected to produce a beneficial result.

The cornea was one of the first human tissues to be successfully grafted. The fact that recipients of corneal grafts generally tolerate them well can be attributed to (1) the absence of blood vessels or lymphatics in the normal cornea and (2) the lack of presensitization to tissue-specific antigens in most recipients. Reactions to corneal grafts do occur, however, particularly in individuals whose own corneas have been damaged by previous inflammatory disease. Such corneas may have developed both lymphatics and blood vessels, providing afferent and efferent channels for immunologic reactions in the engrafted cornea.

Although attempts have been made to transplant corneas from other species into human eyes (xenografts), particularly in countries where human material is not available for religious reasons, most corneal grafts have been taken from human eyes (allografts). Except in the case of identical twins, such grafts always represent the implantation of foreign tissue into a donor site; thus, the chance for a graft rejection due to an immune response to foreign antigens is virtually always present.

The cornea is a 3-layered structure composed of a surface epithelium, and oligocellular collagenous multiple graft reactions in vascularized corneal beds. These antibody reactions are complement-dependent and attract polymorphonuclear leukocytes, which may form dense rings in the cornea at the sites of maximum deposition of immune complexes. In experimental animals, similar reactions have been produced by corneal xenografts, but the intensity of the reaction can be markedly reduced either by decomplementing the animal or by reducing its leukocyte population through mechlorethamine therapy.

Treatment

The mainstay of the treatment of corneal graft reactions is corticosteroid therapy. This medication is generally given in the form of frequently applied eye drops (eg, prednisolone acetate 1%, hourly) until the clinical signs abate. These clinical signs consist of conjunctival hyperemia in the perilimbal region, a cloudy cornea, cells and protein in the anterior chamber, and keratic precipitates on the corneal endothelium. The earlier that treatment is applied, the more effective it is likely to be. Neglected cases may require systemic or periocular corticosteroids in addition to local eye drop therapy. Occasionally, vascularization and opacification of the cornea occur so rapidly that corticosteroid therapy is useless, but even the most hopeless-appearing graft reactions have occasionally been reversed by corticosteroid therapy.

Patients known to have rejected many previous corneal grafts are managed somewhat differently, particularly if disease affects their only remaining eye. An attempt is made to find a close HLA match between donor and recipient. Pretreatment of the recipient with immunosuppressive agents such as azathioprine has also been resorted to in some cases. Although HLA testing of the recipient and the potential donor is indicated in cases of repeated corneal graft failure or in cases of severe corneal vascularization, such testing is not necessary or practicable in most cases requiring keratoplasty.

REFERENCES

Allansmith MR: *The Eye and Immunology.* Mosby, 1981.

Friedlaender MH: *Allergy and Immunology of the Eye.* Harper & Row, 1979.

Friedlaender MH (editor): Ocular allergy. *Int Ophthalmol Clin* 1988;**28**:261.

Friedlaender MH, Tabbara KF (editors): Immunological ocular disease. *Int Ophthalmol Clin* 1985;**25**:1.

Helmsen RJ et al: *Immunology of the Eye.* Workshop II: *Autoimmune Phenomena and Ocular Disorders.* Information Retrieval, 1981.

Kraus-Mackiw E, O'Connor GR (editors): *Uveitis: Pathophysiology and Therapy.* Thieme-Stratton, 1983.

O'Connor GR (editor): *Immunologic Diseases of the Mucous Membranes.* Masson, 1980.

O'Connor GR, Chandler JW (editors): *Advances in Immunology and Immunopathology of the Eye.* Masson, 1985.

Smith R, Nozik R: *Uveitis: A Clinical Approach to Diagnosis and Management.* Williams & Wilkins, 1983.

Smolin G, O'Connor GR: *Ocular Immunology.* Little, Brown, 1986.

Webb R, Friedlaender M: Immunology and uveitis. Pages 133–152 in: *Modern Management of Ocular Disease.* Spoor TC (editor). Slack, 1985.

45

Respiratory Diseases

Brian P. Zehr, MD, & Gary W. Hunninghake, MD

The lung, comprising both the tracheobronchial airways and the gas-exchanging parenchyma, is an immunologically competent organ, part of the mucosal immune system discussed in Chapter 15. This chapter will describe a variety of diseases, most of unknown origin but mediated by immunopathogenic mechanisms. Some of these diseases are restricted to the lungs, whereas others are multisystemic with prominent pulmonary involvement. Included are diseases involving the pathogenic effect of autoantibody (Goodpasture's syndrome), immune complex-meditated pulmonary tissue injury (idiopathic pulmonary fibrosis), granulomatous diseases, acute pulmonary injury from the effects of complement activation, injurious effects of eosinophilic infiltration in the lungs, and tissue destruction from pulmonary infection. Allergic and infectious diseases are discussed in other chapters.

The primary function of the lung is to facilitate the exchange of gases between ambient air and blood. There are 2 important consequences of this gas exchange function: (1) The lung is exposed to a wide variety of airborne environmental antigens, and (2) the lung must serve as a conduit and filter for the entire circulating blood volume. Therefore, the lung is continually exposed to a variety of air- and blood-borne substances that have the potential to trigger an inflammatory and immune process.

GOODPASTURE'S SYNDROME

Major Immunologic Features
- There are circulating anti-glomerular basement membrane (anti-GBM) antibodies.
- Immunoglobulin and complement are present as linear deposits in basement membranes of renal glomeruli and pulmonary alveoli.

General Considerations
Goodpasture's syndrome is a disease of unknown origin that occurs predominantly in young males and is characterized by the triad of pulmonary hemorrhage, glomerulonephritis, and antibody to basement membrane antigens. Intrapulmonary hemorrhage may be insignificant or may be severe and life-threatening; if prolonged, iron deficiency anemia may result. Renal involvement is commonly rapidly progressive, with oliguric renal failure occurring within weeks to months of the clinical onset of the disease (see Chapter 41).

Immunologic Pathogenesis
In more than 90% of cases, circulating antibodies (principally IgG) can be demonstrated early in the course of the disease. These antibodies are directed against renal tubular, renal glomerular, and pulmonary alveolar basement membranes. By immunofluorescence techniques, they can be demonstrated in these tissues in a characteristic linear deposition, where they are often accompanied by C3 deposition (see Fig 41–1). Antibody bound to basement membrane activates the complement cascade, resulting in the generation of chemotactic factors for various inflammatory cells. The inflammatory cells subsequently destroy the renal tubular, renal glomerular, and pulmonary alveolar basement membranes via the release of various reactive oxygen species and proteolytic enzymes. Recent studies demonstrate that the membrane antigenic site is probably within type IV collagen present in basement membranes throughout the body, but possibly it is more vulnerable to reaction with autoantibody within the lungs and kidneys owing to their unique filtration functions and blood flow characteristics.

Clinical Features
Pulmonary manifestations include pulmonary hemorrhage with or without hemoptysis and shortness of breath. The chest x-ray may reveal hilar infiltrates, which may fluctuate in intensity depending upon the degree of intra-alveolar hemorrhage (Fig 45–1). Bronchoalveolar lavage demonstrates hemosiderin-laden macrophages with or without erythrocytes. Gross or microscopic hematuria, proteinuria, increased blood urea nitrogen and serum creatinine, and decreased creatinine clearance are characteristic features of renal involvement.

Immunologic Diagnosis
The presence of circulating antibody to glomerular basement membrane (GBM) and the demonstration by tissue immunofluorescence of linear deposits of antibody, with or without C3, along the basement membrane of glomeruli or alveolar septa are diagnostic of the disease.

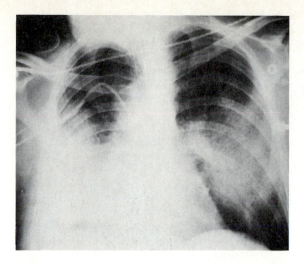

Figure 45–1. Chest x-ray of patient with Goodpasture's syndrome, showing extensive bilateral pulmonary infiltrates.

Differential Diagnosis

Pulmonary hemorrhage with renal failure may be seen in Wegener's granulomatosis, systemic lupus erythematosus, polyarteritis nodosa, and renal vein thrombosis with pulmonary embolism. These disorders lack the constellation of clinical, pathologic, and immunologic features on which the diagnosis of Goodpasture's syndrome is based.

Treatment & Prognosis

Since the disorder may be rapidly fatal, it is imperative that it be diagnosed and treated rapidly. For patients who are acutely ill, initial membrane plasma exchange to remove the anti-GBM antibodies is used, together with corticosteroids and cytotoxic drugs. This type of therapy frequently halts the progression of the disease and maintains renal function if instituted sufficiently early in the course of the disease. Bilateral nephrectomy, followed by renal transplantation after disappearance of the circulating anti-GBM antibodies, has also been used as therapy for this disease. Recurrences, however, have been reported following renal transplantation.

IDIOPATHIC PULMONARY FIBROSIS

Major Imunologic Features

- Immune complexes are present in blood and in the lungs.
- Nonspecific "autoimmune" antibodies are also present.

General Considerations

Idiopathic pulmonary fibrosis is an interstitial lung disease of unknown origin. The diagnosis is one of exclusion; ie, the patient must have no history of exposure to inhaled environmental agents known to cause interstitial lung disease or an underlying disease that is associated with the development of interstitial lung disease. Some patients show improvement after treatment with corticosteroid or cytotoxic drug therapy, and survival of 10–15 years following diagnosis has been documented; however, most patients die within 5 years.

Immunologic Pathogenesis

The trigger of this disorder is still unknown. It is known, however, that immune complexes are present in serum and in the lungs in the early, active phase of the disease. Although these immune complexes may trigger an inflammatory process in the lungs by activating the complement cascade, there is no evidence to date that this process occurs in the lungs of these patients. It has been shown, however, that immune complexes in the lungs stimulate alveolar macrophages to release various factors which appear to play an important role in the pathogenesis of this disorder. One such factor released by alveolar macrophages is leukotriene B_4, a lipid chemotactic factor that attracts neutrophils and eosinophils from blood into the lungs. The alveolar macrophages also release a variety of growth factors for fibroblasts, which increase the numbers of fibroblasts in the lungs and hence leads to the deposition of collagen. These observations are consistent with the pathologic features of the disease: increased numbers of polymorphonuclear leukocytes and a generalized fibrosis of the lung parenchyma.

Clinical Features

Patients commonly are first affected in the fifth to seventh decade of life; there is a history of gradually progressive exertional dyspnea and fatigability. Physical examination reveals dry bibasilar rales ("Velcro rales"), and there usually is clubbing of the digits. In advanced cases, cyanosis and evidence of cor pulmonale may be present. The chest x-ray shows interstitial fibrosis predominantly in the basilar areas of the lungs. Honeycombing of the lungs occurs in later stages. Pulmonary-function testing shows a restrictive defect with decreases in lung volumes and diffusing capacity. Arterial blood gases show normal or slightly decreased oxygen tension, which drops markedly with exertion.

Immunologic Diagnosis

Because this is a diagnosis of exclusion, there are no specific confirmatory tests. Serologic abnormalities may include positive tests for antinuclear antibodies or rheumatoid factor, increased amounts of immunoglobulins, and circulating immune complexes. Various immunologic tests are used primarily to exclude the presence of other interstitial lung disorders. The pathologic findings are also nonspecific and reveal a generalized inflammation and fibrosis of the alveolar capillary membrane and small airways of the lung. The primary use of lung biopsy is to exclude other disorders. Bronchoalveolar lavage reveals increased numbers of both alveolar macrophages and polymorphonuclear leukocytes; the most characteristic feature is an increased percentage of both neutrophils and eosinophils.

Differential Diagnosis

The differential diagnosis includes a lengthy list of interstitial lung diseases of both known and unknown origin. The principal considerations, however, include sarcoidosis, hypersensitivity pneumonitis, interstitial lung disease associated with collagen vascular diseases, and interstitial lung disease associated with certain inorganic dust exposures.

Treatment & Prognosis

Therapy is directed at suppressing active inflammation (alveolitis) and thus preventing further loss of function. High doses of corticosteroids may result in improvement and stabilization of pulmonary functions in some patients, but the treatment must be continued over a long period, usually indefinitely. Cytotoxic drugs have also been reported to benefit some patients. Supplemental oxygen, particularly during periods of exercise, allows a more active lifestyle.

SARCOIDOSIS

Major Immunologic Features

- There is circulating T lymphocytopenia.
- There is anergy to various skin test antigens.
- Polyclonal hypergammaglobulinemia is present.
- In early disease there are circulating immune complexes.
- There is an intense cellular immune response localized to sites of disease.

General Considerations

Sarcoidosis is a multisystem granulomatous disease of unknown origin. It is most common in young adults and is characterized by cutaneous, ocular, or pulmonary manifestations, although a significant number of asymptomatic patients are detected on the basis of an abnormal chest x-ray. More than 90% of patients have pulmonary manifestations; about one-quarter of these will develop permanent loss of pulmonary function. The disease is more prevalent in certain populations. For example, in the USA, the prevalence is much higher in the black than in the white population. The disease may also be more severe in blacks than in whites.

Immunologic Pathogenesis

The trigger of the disorder that we recognize as sarcoidosis is unknown. The earliest lesion is an accumulation of inflammatory cells in involved tissues. These are primarily monocyte-macrophages, and they form the cells that make up the granulomata.

The central core of the granuloma is made up of a number of activated mononuclear phagocytes including epithelioid cells, multinucleated giant cells, and macrophages. These cells are all derived from blood monocytes. Activated T cells are found at the periphery of the granuloma and play an important role in the pathogenesis of this disorder by releasing a variety of lymphokines. One of these, monocyte chemotactic factor, which has not been characterized chemically, attracts monocytes (the building blocks of the central core of the granulomata) to sites of disease. The activated T cells also release a variety of mediators, such as immune interferon, that are necessary for the activation of macrophages, a characteristic feature of this disorder. Interleukin-2, which is released by T cells, maintains the presence of large numbers of T cells at sites of disease by 2 mechanisms: (1) by acting as a specific chemotactic factor attracting T cells from blood to sites of granuloma formation, and (2) by stimulating T cells at sites of granuloma formation to proliferate.

The process of granuloma formation appears to be modulated by immunoregulatory T cells. In patients with active disease, the T cells are present in involved tissues in markedly increased numbers; they are primarily CD4 T cells. In contrast, fewer T cells are present in involved tissues in patients with inactive disease; they are primarily CD8 T cells.

The polyclonal hypergammaglobulinemia (increased levels of antibodies to a variety of agents including viruses and mycobacteria) of sarcoidosis is, at least in part, a by-product of granuloma formation. T cells at sites of granuloma formation release a variety of mediators that nonspecifically activate surrounding B cells to differentiate into immunoglobulin-secreting plasma cells.

Clinical Features

Acute sarcoidosis may present with fever, erythema nodosum, iritis, and polyarthritis; this combination of symptoms strongly suggests the presence of this disorder. Most often, however, patients note the insidious development of fatigue, weight loss, malaise, weakness, anorexia, fever, sweats, nonproductive cough, and progressive exertional dyspnea. Patients may also be asymptomatic, and the presence of the disorder is often suggested by a routine chest x-ray. In fact, the chest x-ray has been the most important means of detecting the disease (Fig 45–2). The chest x-ray demonstrates one of 4 types of involvement: type 0, normal; type I, bilateral hilar adenopathy alone; type II, hilar adenopathy and parenchymal abnormalities; and type III, parenchymal abnormalities without hilar adenopathy. These abnormalities are somewhat correlated with

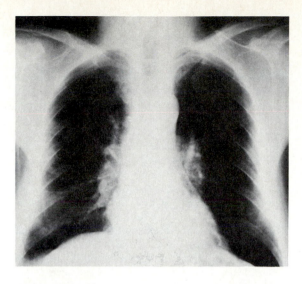

Figure 45–2. Chest x-ray of patient with sarcoidosis, showing bilateral hilar adenopathy and parenchymal granulomatous inflammatory infiltrates, particularly evident in the right lung.

the prognosis of the disease. Patients with a type 0 or I chest x-ray have a very good prognosis, whereas those with type III chest x-ray have a worse prognosis. Pulmonary-function studies may be normal or may reveal evidence of a restrictive lung disease characterized by a loss of lung volume, decreased diffusion capacity, and exercise-induced hypoxemia. Patients with advanced disease may also have an obstructive ventilatory defect.

Although the lung is the most commonly involved tissue, the disorder can affect any organ. All patients should be evaluated for the presence of granulomatous uveitis and heart disease because of the risk of blindness and death from cardiac arrhythmias, respectively.

Immunologic Diagnosis

The diagnosis can firmly be established only by the following criteria: (1) a compatible clinical picture; (2) histologic evidence of a systemic granulomatous disease compatible with sarcoidosis; and (3) no evidence of exposure to an agent that is known to cause granulomatous disease. The disorder is also frequently associated with a peripheral-blood T lymphocytopenia, anergy to a panel of skin tests for cellular immunity, hypergammaglobulinemia, circulating immune complexes, increased serum angiotensin-converting enzyme activity, and increased numbers of macrophages and CD4 T cells in bronchoalveolar lavage fluid; these findings suggest but are not specific for sarcoidosis. The Kveim test, a cutaneous hypersensitivity test associated with sarcoidosis, is largely of historical interest owing to the unavailability of antigen and availability of other diagnostic tests.

Differential Diagnosis

Sarcoidosis must be differentiated from a variety of granulomatous diseases, including various infectious diseases, hypersensitivity pneumonitis, berylliosis, drug reactions, and certain cancers. Type III sarcoidosis must also be distinguished from the other interstitial lung disorders.

Treatment & Prognosis

The presence of a progressive loss of lung function, cardiac disease, granulomatous uveitis, and central nervous system disease are absolute indications for corticosteroid therapy. Therapy should be continued as long as the disease is active. Corticosteroids may also be used to relieve many of the symptoms associated with sarcoidosis, such as joint involvement and erythema nodosum.

BERYLLIOSIS

Berylliosis is a systemic granulomatous disorder that primarily affects the lungs. It occurs as a response to the inhalation of metallic beryllium or beryllium salts, usually from occupational exposure. The spectrum of beryllium-induced lung disease includes 2 distinct but interrelated disease processes.

Acute berylliosis is a nonimmunologic inflammatory response to a large, intense exposure to metallic beryllium or other beryllium compounds. This process is the result of the irritant properties of beryllium, which induce histopathologic changes indistinguishable from those seen with chemical pneumonitis following exposure to any of a number of pulmonary irritants. In addition to these irritant effects, beryllium is unusual among toxic dusts in possessing antigenic properties. This can result in a chronic form of immune-mediated granulomatous disease. This usually occurs after chronic exposures, with a latency period ranging between several months and 25 years. Typically, noncaseating granulomas are present in the lungs, skin, skeletal muscle, bone, liver, spleen, lymph nodes, and myocardium.

Because of their small size, beryllium ions alone are not antigenic; therefore, it is postulated that they are haptens that bind to host carrier molecules to form hapten-carrier complexes. The lung macrophage is probably the source of the carrier molecule by ingesting beryllium and presenting it in an antigenic form to lymphocytes. This creates a population of sensitized T cells that produce the mediators for the subsequent formation of granulomas similar to those seen in sarcoidosis. In fact, the clinical features of chronic berylliosis strongly resemble those of pulmonary sarcoidosis.

BRONCHOCENTRIC GRANULOMATOSIS

Bronchocentric granulomatosis is characterized by a necrotizing granulomatous reaction centered around airways. There are no specific radiographic, clinical, immunologic, or physical findings. However, the disorder frequently presents as a solitary lesion on chest x-ray. Up to half the cases of bronchocentric granulomatosis occur in patients with chronic asthma. The nonasthmatic patient usually is asymptomatic but may have a chronic cough and some sputum production. The diagnosis is usually made after morphologic evaluation of tissue obtained at thoracotomy. Bronchocentric granulomatosis probably represents one of a limited number of ways that the bronchi can respond to an insult. The clinical features in bronchocentric granulomatosis patients with asthma are similar to those of allergic bronchopulmonary aspergillosis, which is the proper diagnosis when there is also a positive immediate skin response to *Aspergillus fumigatus,* increased total and specific IgE levels, presence of *A fumigatus* in the sputum, fragmented fungal elements in histologic sections, serum precipitins to *A fumigatus,* and blood and tissue eosinophilia (see Chapter 32). These findings suggest that in asthmatic patients, bronchocentric granulomatosis represents a hypersensitivity reaction to inhaled fungi or other microorganisms.

LYMPHOMATOID GRANULOMATOSIS

Lymphomatoid granulomatosis, as the name implies, is a disease with histologic findings of both an inflammatory granulomatous process and a lymphoproliferative disease. It is characterized by an angiocentric, angiodestructive pattern of granulomatous inflammation, as well as infiltration of tissues with a pleomorphic cellular process composed of atypical lymphocytes, plasmacytes, histiocytes, and other atypical lymphoreticular cells. Not infrequently, the disease will progress to malignant lymphoma. This has engendered debate about whether it represents a distinctive process or simply a point on the continuum from the more benign lymphocytic angiitis and granulomatosis to lymphomatoid granulomatosis to, finally, frank angiocentric malignant lymphoma.

Lymphomatoid granulomatosis is primarily a disease of the lungs, although other organ systems, most notably the skin, kidneys, and central nervous system, can also be involved. Laboratory and chest x-ray findings are nonspecific, and so diagnosis is dependent on the demonstration of characteristic histologic findings on biopsy. The disease is associated with a very poor prognosis, with a mortality rate of 65–90%. The disorder is usually treated with a combination of cyclophosphamide and prednisone or more aggressive chemotherapy.

BRONCHIECTASIS

Bronchiectasis is defined pathologically as a permanent dilatation of one or more subsegmental airways. The involved airways are distorted, leading to impaired clearance of secretions. As a consequence, there are recurrent infections, airway inflammation, and mucus hypersecretion. In the most severe cases, this results in the clinical findings of chronic cough, copious amounts of purulent sputum, recurrent pneumonia, hemoptysis, cyanosis, and digital clubbing.

Recurrent airway infections leading to bronchiectasis can occur in a variety of conditions, including cystic fibrosis, allergic bronchopulmonary aspergillosis, immotile cilia syndromes, airway occlusion by a foreign body, a variety of immunodeficiency states, and Kartagener's syndrome. Among the immunodeficiency states, the ones most commonly associated with bronchiectasis are those characterized by panhypogammaglobulinemia, eg, X-linked agammaglobulinemia and common variable hypogammaglobulinemia. Bronchiectasis has also been reported with selective IgA, IgM, and IgG4 deficiencies, although this is probably not a common manifestation of these disorders. Neutrophil and complement deficiencies can also lead to recurrent pulmonary infections and bronchiectasis.

PULMONARY INFILTRATES WITH EOSINOPHILIA

Pulmonary infiltrates with eosinophilia is a descriptive term for a number of distinct diseases characterized by eosinophilic pneumonia and, typically, peripheral-blood eosinophilia. These diseases may be considered examples of hypersensitivity lung disorders; however, they should not be confused with hypersensitivity pneumonitis, in which eosinophilia is not a feature.

Acute pulmonary eosinophilia (Löffler's syndrome), which is characterized by transient pulmonary infiltrates (Fig 45–3), can be caused by helminthic infections, by drugs, and probably by environmental antigens. Drug-induced eosinophilic lung disease can be caused by reactions to nitrofurantoin, sulfonamides, penicillin, chlorpropamide, thiazides, tricyclic antidepressants, hydralazine, isoniazid, *p*-aminosalicylic acid, nickel carbonyl vapors, gold salts, and others. In the drug-related disorders, therapy consists of withdrawal of the offending drug and treatment with corticosteroids, if necessary. Acute pulmonary eosinophilia associated with helminthic infection in the lungs (Löffler's syndrome) is a self-limited disorder; however, if ova are

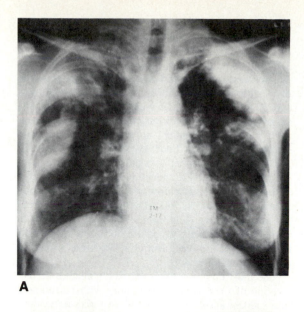

A

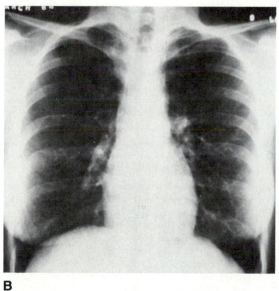

B

Figure 45–3. Acute pulmonary eosinophilia, showing pulmonary infiltrates during the clinically active phase of the disease (**A**) and resolution of the lesions (**B**).

present in the stool, appropriate antihelminthic therapy is required to prevent the extrapulmonary sequelae of parasitic infestation.

Tropical filarial eosinophilia is a disorder caused by infection with filarial worms such as *Wuchereria bancrofti* and *Brugia malayi*. It is characterized by cough with minimal sputum production, wheezing, and patchy infiltrates on chest x-rays. It occurs most commonly in southern Asia, Africa, and South America and is successfully treated with diethylcarbamazine.

Allergic bronchopulmonary aspergillosis occurs in a clinical setting of extrinsic asthma, pulmonary infiltrates, and eosinophilia. The major and minor diagnostic criteria for this disorder are listed in Table 45–1. It is probably initiated by *A fumigatus* colonization of the respiratory tract in atopic individuals. The bronchial asthma probably involves an IgE-mediated hypersensitivity, whereas the bronchiectasis associated with this disorder is thought to result from deposition of immune complexes (type III reaction) in the proximal airway. Long-term use of corticosteroids is usually required for adequate therapy (see Chapter 32).

Asthma is also a frequent, concurrent diagnosis in patients with **allergic angiitis and granulomatosis (Churg-Strauss syndrome).** This is a multisystem vasculitic disorder in which the predominant histologic features are eosinophilic infiltration of the vascular and perivascular tissues. In addition to the lungs, the skin, kidneys, and central and peripheral nervous systems may be involved. The illness carries a grave prognosis, which may be favorably altered by aggressive treatment with corticosteroids and immunosuppressive therapy (see Chapter 39).

Chronic eosinophilic pneumonia is characterized by fevers, night sweats, chills, weight loss, and anorexia. The chest x-ray findings have typically been described as the photographic negative of pulmonary edema with peripheral infiltrates predominating. Patients may have concurrent intrinsic bronchial asthma, but a specific etiologic antigen is not usually found. Treatment with corticosteroids will frequently result in dramatic clearing of the infiltrates and improvement in symptoms.

The **hypereosinophilic syndrome** is characterized by peripheral-blood and bone marrow eosinophilia with infiltration of multiple organs by mature eosinophils. In addition to the lungs, the heart, liver, spleen, and central nervous system are typically affected. In the proper clinical setting, the diagnosis should be considered after allergic, parasitic, and other known types of eosinophilia have been ruled out. Therapy consists of corticosteroids or hydrox-

Table 45–1. Diagnostic features of allergic bronchopulmonary aspergillosis

Main Diagnostic Criteria
1. Bronchial asthma
2. Pulmonary infiltrates
3. Peripheral eosinophilia (> 1000/mm³)
4. Immediate wheal-and-flare response to *A fumigatus*
5. Serum precipitins to *A fumigatus*
6. Elevated serum IgE
7. Central bronchiectasis

Other Diagnostic Features
1. History of brownish plugs in sputum
2. Culture of *A fumigatus* from sputum
3. Elevated IgE (and IgG)-class antibodies specific for *A fumigatus*

yurea or both. Cardiac dysfunction is frequently responsible for the majority of the morbidity and mortality associated with this syndrome.

PULMONARY VASCULAR LEUKOSTASIS

After the use of hemodialysis became widespread, a profound, transient neutropenia was noted to occur shortly after the beginning of the dialysis treatment. Subsequent studies demonstrated that this was related to exposure of patient plasma to dialyzer membranes and was caused by a complement-mediated aggregation of neutrophils and monocytes in the lungs. Exposure of serum to the membranes activates the alternative complement pathway, generating C3a and C5a. The generation of C5a has recently been shown to cause an increased expression of a granulocyte surface glycoprotein associated with increased aggregability. The reaction does not occur in granulocytopenic patients.

ADULT RESPIRATORY DISTRESS SYNDROME

The adult respiratory distress syndrome is a form of acute lung injury characterized by noncardiogenic pulmonary edema from increased vascular permeability. It can occur in the setting of a wide variety of clinical conditions including sepsis, gastric acid aspiration, pancreatitis, trauma, fat emboli syndrome, and central nervous system insult. In the proper clinical setting, a diagnosis of adult respiratory distress syndrome is made when there are diffuse, bilateral infiltrates on chest x-rays (consistent with pulmonary edema), no evidence of increased pulmonary capillary hydrostatic pressure (this usually requires placement of a pulmonary artery catheter), and refractory hypoxemia that cannot be corrected by high concentrations of oxygen. Despite recent improvements in supportive care, the mortality rate continues to remain as high as 60–70%. In most instances, mortality is not due solely to hypoxemia but instead results from the combined failure of multiple organ systems.

The most common etiologic mechanism is the activation of the complement system with recruitment and sequestration of neutrophils in pulmonary interstitial capillaries. In the capillaries, neutrophils can release a number of toxic products, including proteases and oxygen free radicals, which cause endothelial-cell damage, interstitial and intra-alveolar edema, hemorrhage, and fibrin deposition. The treatment of patients with adult respiratory distress syndrome is supportive.

REFERENCES

General

Crystal RG et al: Interstitial lung diseases of unknown cause: Disorders characterized by chronic inflammation of the lower respiratory tract. *N Engl J Med* 1984; **310**:154.

Hunninghake GW, Fauci AS: Pulmonary involvement in the collagen vascular diseases. *Am Rev Respir Dis* 1979; **119**:471.

Thomas PD, Hunninghake GW: State of the art: Current concepts of the pathogenesis of sarcoidosis. *Am Rev Respir Dis* 1987;**135**:747.

Bronchoalveolar Lavage

Daniele RP et al: Bronchoalveolar lavage: Role in the pathogenesis, diagnosis and management of interstitial lung disease. *Ann Intern Med* 1985;**102**:93.

Hunninghake GW et al: Inflammatory and immune processes in the human lung in health and disease: Evaluation by bronchoalveolar lavage. *Am J Pathol* 1979; **97**:149.

Goodpasture's Syndrome

Erickson SB et al: Use of combined plasmapheresis and immunosuppression in the treatment of Goodpasture's syndrome. *Mayo Clin Proc* 1979;**54**:714.

Idiopathic Pulmonary Fibrosis

Chapman JR et al: Definition and clinical relevance of antibodies to nuclear ribonucleoprotein and other nuclear antigens in patients with cryptogenic fibrosing alveolitis. *Am Rev Respir Dis* 1984;**130**:439.

Crystal RG et al: Idiopathic pulmonary fibrosis. *Ann Intern Med* 1976;**85**:769.

Gelb AF et al: Immune complexes, gallium lung scans, and bronchoalveolar lavage in idiopathic interstitial pneumonitis-fibrosis: A structure-function clinical study. *Chest* 1983;**84**:148.

Sarcoidosis

Hunninghake GW, Crystal RG: Mechanisms of hypergammaglobulinemia in pulmonary sarcoidosis: Site of increased antibody production and role of T-lymphocytes. *J Clin Invest* 1981;**67**:86.

Hunninghake GW, Crystal RG: Pulmonary sarcoidosis: A disorder mediated by excess helper T-lymphocyte activity at sites of disease activity. *N Engl J Med* 1981; **305**:429.

Hunninghake GW et al: Maintenance of granuloma formation in pulmonary sarcoidosis by T-lymphocytes within the lung. *N Engl J Med* 1980;**302**:594.

Berylliosis

Kriebel D et al: The pulmonary toxicity of beryllium. *Am Rev Respir Dis* 1988;**137**:464.

Stankus RP, Salvaggio JE: The organic dust pneumoconioses. *Clin Rev Allergy* 1985;**3**:235.

Bronchocentric Granulomatosis

Katzenstein A-L, Liebow AA, Friedman PJ: Bronchocentric granulomatosis, mucoid impaction, and hypersensitivity reactions to fungi. *Am Rev Respir Dis* 1975; **111:**497.

Koss MN, Robinson RG, Hockholzer L: Bronchocentric granulomatosis. *Hum Pathol* 1981;**12:**632.

Lymphomatoid Granulomatosis

Fauci AS et al: Lymphomatoid granulomatosis: Prospective clinical and therapeutic experience over 10 years. *N Engl J Med* 1982;**306:**68.

Liebow AA, Carrington CR, Friedman PJ: Lymphomatoid granulomatosis. *Hum Pathol* 1972;**3:**457.

Bronchiectasis

Barker AF, Bardana EJ: Bronchiectasis: Update of an orphan disease. *Am Rev Respir Dis* 1988;**137:**969.

Ellis DA et al: Present look at bronchiectasis: Clinical and social study and review of factors influencing prognosis. *Thorax* 1981;**36:**659.

Pulmonary Infiltrates with Eosinophilia

Schatz M, Wasserman S, Patterson R: The eosinophil and the lung. *Arch Intern Med* 1982;**142:**1515.

Slavin RG: Allergic bronchopulmonary aspergillosis. *Clin Rev Allergy* 1985;**3:**167.

Allergic Bronchopulmonary Aspergillosis

Patterson R et al: Allergic bronchopulmonary aspergillosis: Staging as an aid to management. *Ann Intern Med* 1982;**96:**286.

Rosenberg M et al: Clinical and immunologic criteria for the diagnosis of allergic bronchopulmonary aspergillosis. *Ann Intern Med* 1977;**86:**405.

Pulmonary Vascular Leukostasis

Craddock PR et al: Complement and leukocyte-mediated pulmonary dysfunction in hemodialysis. *N Engl J Med* 1977;**296:**769.

Adult Respiratory Distress Syndrome

Tate RM, Repine JE: Neutrophils and the adult respiratory distress syndrome. *Am Rev Respir Dis* 1983; **128:**552.

Ward PA, Johnson KS: Current concepts regarding adult respiratory distress syndrome. *Ann Emerg Med* 1985; **14:**724.

46

Mechanisms of Tumor Immunology

Philip D. Greenberg, MD

Tumor immunology is the study of (1) the antigenic properties of transformed cells, (2) the host immune responses to these tumor cells, (3) the immunologic consequences to the host of the growth of malignant cells, and (4) the means by which the immune system can be modulated to recognize tumor cells and promote tumor eradication. One potentially important function of the immune system is to provide protection from the outgrowth of malignant cells. This represents a formidable task because tumor cells have many similarities to normal cells, despite exhibiting abnormal propensities to proliferate, to spread throughout the host, and to interfere with normal organ functions. Thus, tumor cells present special problems to the host immune system beyond those presented by other self-replicating antigens such as bacteria, which can more easily be distinguished as foreign. Elucidating the processes that render a cancerous cell different from normal cells should aid in understanding how these transformed cells might be amenable to destruction and regulation by the immune system.

Normal cells have a variable capacity to proliferate and to express differentiated functions. These cell activities are tightly coordinated within an organ or tissue, so that the rate of cell loss due to the natural death of mature differentiated cells is equal to the rate of appearance of new cells from the less mature proliferating cell pool. If the stimulus for cell proliferation exceeds the requirement for cell replacement, as in some pathologic conditions, organ hypertrophy occurs with polyclonal expansion of cells from a pool that proliferates in response to growth signals. However, if the condition responsible for excess stimulation of cell growth is ablated, the rate of cell proliferation decreases and the organ hypertrophy resolves. In contrast to nonmalignant regulated polyclonal cell growth, an individual cell may undergo a transforming event and acquire the potential to produce daughter cells that proliferate independent of external growth signals. The autonomous growth of such transformed cells of monoclonal origin represents the basis of malignant disease. Many of the properties of tumor cells are summarized in Table 46–1. The protean effects of cancer reflect in large part the unrestrained growth of tumor cells that locally invade and disrupt normal

Table 46–1. Common properties of tumor cells.

1. Failure to respond to the regulatory signals responsible for normal growth and tissue repair.
2. Autonomous growth without an absolute requirement for exogenous growth signals.
3. Invasive growth through normal tissue boundaries.
4. Metastatic growth in distant organs following entry into blood and lymph channels.
5. Monoclonal origin, although genotypic and phenotypic heterogeneity may develop as tumor mass increases.
6. Differences in appearance and membrane antigenic display from nontransformed cells of the same tissue origin.

tissue as well as metastasize and grow in distant organs.

DEVELOPMENT OF TUMORS

The transformation of a normal cell to malignancy can result from a variety of different causes, the particular nature of which may help determine whether the immune system can control the outgrowth of the tumor cells. These transforming events may occur spontaneously by random mutations or gene rearrangements; alternatively, they may be induced by a chemical, physical, or viral carcinogen.

Tumors induced by chemical carcinogens were initially described in the 18th century, when chimney sweeps were observed to have an unusually high incidence of carcinoma of the scrotum. Polycyclic aromatic hydrocarbons in soot and tar have since been found to be a major class of carcinogens, and retention of tar in the wrinkles of the scrotum was apparently responsible for these tumors. In fact, painting tar on epithelial cells has become a useful experimental technique for inducing tumors in the laboratory. A second major class of carcinogens, the aromatic amines, was identified following the observation of a high frequency of bladder cancer among factory workers using aniline dyes. The precise mechanisms by which each chemical carcinogen induces neoplastic transformation have not been fully resolved, but they presumably reflect mutagenesis with altered function and expression of the cellular genome.

Evidence of tumor induction by physical carcinogens accrued rapidly following the discovery of x-rays and radioactivity in the late 19th century. Many of the early radiologists developed a radiodermatitis, which was followed by a long latency period and, eventually, skin cancer. The most dramatic evidence of radiation-induced carcinogenesis is in survivors of the atomic bomb explosions in Japan, who demonstrated an increased incidence of a wide range of tumors for more than 20 years after the nuclear holocaust. Ionizing radiation presumably directly injures cellular DNA, resulting in mutations, chromosomal breaks, and abnormal rearrangements, but the long latency period usually required for the appearance of tumors implies that the expression of malignancy in radiation-damaged cells may often require the presence of a promoter and additional genetic events. Another physical carcinogen, ultraviolet radiation, induces skin cancer on sun-exposed parts of the body, particularly in people with xeroderma pigmentosum, a disease in which there is a defective repair mechanism for UV-induced damage to DNA. The mechanisms of carcinogenesis by UV irradiation may be manifold, including production of carcinogenic oxide metabolites, induction of pyrimidine dimers, and, possibly, immunosuppression.

Viral oncogenesis is of particular interest in tumor immunology because of the great likelihood that cells transformed by the introduction of viral genes will express new virus-associated antigens that can be recognized by the immune system. Oncogenic viruses can be subdivided into either DNA or RNA types, depending on the genetic information carried by the intact virus. Most cells infected by the potentially oncogenic DNA viruses, which include papovaviruses, herpesviruses, and adenoviruses, permit viral replication with resulting cell lysis. However, infection of nonpermissive cells can result in integration of the viral DNA into the host genome and expression of only some of the viral genes, so that lytic virus particles are not formed. Transformation results either from direct triggering of host genes by the integrated viral DNA or from aberrant splicing of viral RNA messages by the host to produce new proteins that promote transformation. Although no DNA viruses with direct oncogenic potential have been isolated from human tumors, several cancers exhibit statistically significant linkage with particular viral infections. These include links between Epstein-Barr virus infection and both Burkitt's lymphoma and nasopharyngeal carcinoma, herpes simplex virus type II infection and cervical carcinoma, and hepatitis B virus infection and primary liver cancers.

Oncogenic RNA viruses contain genes for a polymerase called **reverse transcriptase,** which permits the use of the viral RNA as a template for transcription of a DNA copy, which can be integrated into the host genome. Because this is a reversal of the normal DNA-to-RNA transcription of genetic information, these viruses are often referred to as **retroviruses.** RNA tumor viruses were first discovered in chicken tumors and appear to be responsible for a large number of naturally occurring cancers in many species. Some of these viruses contain directly transforming oncogenes, whereas others must activate host genetic material. A class of human retroviruses, the human T cell leukemia viruses (HTLV), have now been identified as responsible for certain T cell leukemias and are related to human immunodeficiency virus (HIV), the cause of acquired immunodeficiency syndrome (AIDS). Many retroviruses, such as feline leukemia virus and HTLV, can spread horizontally from infected to normal hosts, and resistance to tumorigenesis appears to be partly dependent upon the generation of an immune response to virus-associated antigens in exposed resistant hosts.

Advances in molecular biology have provided the tools to better understand the events involved in transformation. Analogues to many of the viral oncogenes have been identified in the normal cellular genome, and in vitro studies have demonstrated that activation of these cellular oncogenes can transform normal cells under appropriate conditions. The role of cellular oncogenes in normal growth and development and the mechanism by which activation is normally regulated remain to be elucidated, but it is presumed that changes which result in maintaining these genes in a transcriptionally active state will result in transformation. This may occur by mutation, such as one that interferes with the function of a regulatory element; by a translocation that places the oncogene next to an active cellular gene, such as is observed in B cell tumors with the translocation of an oncogene next to an immunoglobulin V region gene; or by insertion of a promoter that enhances expression, such as may occur following integration of a slowly transforming retrovirus. Oncogenes code for a wide variety of products including membrane receptors, autocrine growth factors, and regulators of gene expression. The expression of at least some of these oncogene products should render malignant cells sufficiently disparate from normal cells for detection by immunologic methods and potentially for elimination by immunologically directed attack.

ANTIGENS ON TUMOR CELLS

The field of tumor immunology is based in large part on the supposition that tumors express antigens which permit immunologic separation of malignant from normal cells. Problems in the past demonstrating the immunogenicity of tumor cells to the host of origin led to a great deal of skepticism about the concept that tumors express distinct antigens. However, studies with experimental animal tumors as well as spontaneous human tumors have now convincingly demonstrated that many tumors do express antigens which can induce cellular and humoral responses in the host and have elucidated many of the reasons underlying the ineffective and often undetectable response in the primary host. The relevant tumor antigens fall into 2 major categories. **Unique tumor-specific antigens** are found only on tumor cells and therefore represent ideal targets for an immunologic attack. In contrast, **tumor-associated determinants** are found on tumor cells and also on some normal cells, but qualitative and quantitative differences in antigen expression permit the use of these antigens to distinguish tumor cells from normal cells. Host responses to tumor antigens are obviously much more likely with unique tumor-specific antigens.

A wide variety of tumor antigens have now been found on both spontaneous and experimentally induced tumors. Although the expression of these antigens must reflect a transformation-related heritable change in the genetic material of the cells, there are many distinct molecular mechanisms (Table 46–2) that may result in the production of a tumor antigen. The most straightforward mechanism is a transforming event that results in the production of a new protein, such as would occur following a retrovirus infection with the introduction of new genetic material and subsequent expression of viral proteins. Unique tumor antigens could also result from unique degradation products of abnormal cellular proteins that are aberrant owing to truncation, glycosylation, etc, such as reported for chemically induced tumors. Alternatively, altered expression of normal molecules could result from mutations that change protein structure, such as has been described for both major and minor histocompatibility antigens on tumors induced by chemical carcinogens. Some tumor antigens may result from the uncovering of normally nonexposed determinants, as observed with some of the complex branching glycolipid antigens in which deletion of a branch may expose a new antigenic determinant. Similarly, failure to correctly assemble multimeric membrane proteins, such as may occur following a mutation in one of the components, could result in immunogenic expression of previously undetected determinants on a normal component. Finally, tumor antigens may also result from the aberrant expression of fetal or differentiation antigens, such as observed with the expression on hu-

man gastric carcinoma cells of ABO blood group antigens disparate from the host ABO blood type.

Unique Tumor Antigens

These are antigens that can be detected only on tumor cells and not on other host cells. The best-studied unique tumor antigens are the new antigens expressed on tumors induced in inbred mice by oncogenic viruses and chemical carcinogens. Analysis of the presence of unique tumor antigens has been more difficult with tumors developing in outbred species because of the inability to perform tumor transplantation studies. Molecular techniques have now permitted the isolation of human retroviruses such as HTLV, the identification of viral proteins expressed in the tumor, and the demonstration that these unique viral antigens are potentially immunogenic. "Spontaneous" tumors, many of which may have actually been induced by exposure to environmental carcinogens, have no predictable antigenic markers and therefore have been harder to study. However, recent technologic advances have made it possible to expand low-frequency antigen-reactive T cells and antibody-forming B cells from tumor-bearing hosts. These measures have permitted the identification of tumor-specific T cells and antibodies derived from tumor-draining lymph nodes of patients with melanoma, breast cancer, leukemia, lymphoma, and lung cancer, as well as from lymph nodes following immunization with human colon carcinoma cells in association with an immunoadjuvant. Despite the presence of apparent tumor-specific lymphocytes, it has not yet been possible to isolate and characterize an unequivocal unique tumor antigen from human tumors.

Recent advances in molecular immunology, especially the elucidation of the pathways by which protein antigens are presented in association with major histocompatibility complex (MHC) molecules to T cells, have revolutionized our understanding of the potential origin of unique tumor-specific antigens. As previously perceived, T cells do not recognize integral membrane proteins that associate with membrane MHC molecules; rather, they recognize small peptides derived from intracellular degradation of proteins that are inserted into a peptide-binding cleft in the MHC molecule and are then transported with the MHC molecule to the cell surface (see Chapter 4). These insights are very enlightening, because any abnormal cellular protein, rather than just a protein detected on the membrane, is a potential immunogen. For example, analysis of an immunogenic chemically induced murine tumor demonstrated that the unique antigen was derived from a mutated intracellular protein. Thus, the presence in a tumor cell of a truncated or nonfunctional protein product of a mutated allele could result in the immunogenicity of that product. Moreover, these results suggest that the difficulties in detecting unique antigens on human

---

Table 46–2. Molecular mechanisms responsible for new tumor antigens.

1. Biosynthesis of a new molecule.
2. Unique degradation products of abnormal cellular proteins.
3. Alteration of the structure of a normal molecule.
4. Uncovering of normally protected molecules.
5. Incorrect assembly of multimeric antigens.
6. Aberrant expression of fetal or differentiation antigens.

tumors with monoclonal antibodies are predictable; they do not imply that these tumors do not express unique antigens but, rather, that new molecular approaches must be used in the future for their identification.

Tumor-Associated Antigens

Although it may not be possible to detect unique tumor antigens on all tumors, many tumors display antigens that distinguish them from normal cells. These tumor-associated antigens may be expressed on some normal cells at particular stages of differentiation, but the quantitative expression and/or the composite expression in association with other lineage or differentiation markers can be useful for identifying transformed cells. The identification of tumor-associated antigens has progressed rapidly with the advent of technology for generating and screening monoclonal antibodies. These monoclonal antibody reagents have permitted the isolation and biochemical characterization of the antigens and have been invaluable diagnostically for distinction of transformed from nontransformed cells and for definition of the cell lineage of transformed cells.

The best-characterized human tumor-associated antigens are the oncofetal antigens. These antigens are expressed during embryogenesis but are absent or very difficult to detect in normal adult tissue. The prototype antigen is **carcinoembryonic antigen (CEA),** a glycoprotein found on fetal gut and human colon cancer cells but not on normal adult colon cells. Since CEA is shed from colon carcinoma cells and found in the serum, it was originally thought that the presence of this antigen in the serum could be used to screen patients for colon cancer. However, it soon became apparent that patients with inflammatory lesions involving cells of endodermal origin, such as colitis or pancreatitis, as well as patients with other tumors, such as pancreatic and breast cancer, also had elevated serum levels of CEA. Despite these limitations, monitoring the fall and rise of CEA levels in colon cancer patients undergoing therapy has proven useful for predicting tumor progression and responses to treatment. Several other oncofetal antigens have been useful for diagnosing and monitoring human tumors. In particular, **alpha-fetoprotein,** an alpha-globulin normally secreted by fetal liver and yolk sac cells, is found in the serum of patients with liver and germinal cell tumors and can be used as a marker of disease status.

Differentiation and lineage-specific antigens, which are present on normal adult cells, may be aberrantly expressed on some tumor cells. For example, a T cell antigen, CD5, is commonly expressed on the malignant human B cells found in chronic lymphocytic leukemia, and an erythrocyte blood group antigen is frequently found on human stomach cancer cells. These inappropriately expressed antigens are very useful for identifying transformed cells, and their unexpected presence on tumor cells may ultimately aid in deciphering the regulation and function of such antigens on normally differentiated cells.

Many other tumor-associated antigens, which have unknown function but very limited tissue distribution on normal cells, have now been identified with monoclonal antibodies. Glycoprotein and glycolipid antigens isolated from malignant melanoma cells appear to be relatively specific for these tumors, although some expression on normal cells such as neuronal tissue has been detected. A glycoprotein found on human leukemia cells, called common acute lymphocytic leukemia antigen (CALLA or CD10), has been found to a minimal extent on other cells such as granulocytes and kidney cells. Many other similar examples exist, and the use of such antigenic markers for diagnostic and therapeutic purposes has great promise.

IMMUNOLOGIC EFFECTOR MECHANISMS POTENTIALLY OPERATIVE AGAINST TUMOR CELLS

Virtually all of the effector components of the immune system have the potential to contribute to the eradication of tumor cells. It is likely that each of these effector mechanisms plays a role in the control of tumor growth, but a particular mechanism may be more or less important, depending upon the tumor and setting. Thus, immunologically specific effector responses are probably most important with highly immunogenic tumors, and nonspecific effector responses are presumably of greater significance with less immunogenic tumors.

T Cells

The T cell response is unquestionably the most important host response for the control of growth of antigenic tumor cells; it is responsible for both the direct killing of tumor cells and the activation of other components of the immune system. T cell immunity to tumors reflects the function of the 2 T cell subsets: class II-restricted T cells, which largely represent CD4 helper T (T_H) cells that mediate their effect by the secretion of lymphokines to activate other effector cells and induce inflammatory responses, and class I-restricted T cells, which largely represent CD8 cytotoxic T (T_C) cells that can also secrete lymphokines but mediate their effect mostly by direct lysis of tumor cells.

The precise contribution of each T cell subset and T cell function to the antitumor response appears quite variable, but tumor-specific T cells from each subset are capable of mediating tumor eradication and have been detected in the peripheral blood of individual patients and in the cells infiltrating human tumors. Because most tumor cells express class I but not class II MHC molecules, the TH cell subset cannot directly recognize these tumor cells. Therefore, most TH cell responses are dependent upon antigen-presenting cells such as macrophages to present the relevant tumor antigens in the context of class II molecules for activation. After antigen-specific triggering, these T cells secrete lymphokines that activate TC cells, macrophages, NK cells, and B cells and can produce other lymphokines, such as lymphotoxin or tumor necrosis factor (TNF), which may be directly lytic to tumor cells (see Chapters 5 and 7). In contrast to TH cells, the TC cell subset is capable of directly recognizing and killing tumor targets by disrupting the target membrane and nucleus. However, only a minor fraction of class I-restricted T cells are capable of providing helper functions, and thus effective TC cell responses are generally dependent upon class II-restricted TH cell responses to provide the necessary helper factors to activate and promote the proliferation of TC cells.

B Cells & Antibody-Dependent Killing

A potential role for host antibody responses in human tumor immunity has been suggested by the occasional detection of tumor-reactive antibodies in the serum of patients. Moreover, recent studies in which hybridomas or B cell lines are formed from B cells derived from lymph nodes draining human tumors have suggested that human tumors may frequently elicit antibody responses to tumor-associated antigens. In addition to secreting antibodies that may contribute to the control of tumor growth, B cells with surface immunoglobulin reactive with tumor antigens may also play a role in binding, processing, and presenting tumor antigens for induction of T cell responses to the tumor.

There are 2 major mechanisms by which antibodies may mediate tumor cell lysis. Complement-fixing antibodies bind to the tumor cell membrane and promote attachment of complement components that create pores in the membrane, resulting in cell disruption due to loss of osmotic and biochemical integrity. An alternative mechanism is antibody-dependent cellular cytotoxicity (ADCC), in which antibodies, usually of the IgG class, form an intercellular bridge by binding via the variable region to a specific determinant on the target cell and via the Fc region to effector cells expressing Fc receptors. There are many potential effector cells that can mediate the lytic event, including natural killer (NK) and killer cells, macrophages, and granulocytes. ADCC is a more efficient in vitro lytic mechanism than is complement-mediated cytotoxicity, requiring fewer antibody molecules per cell to kill. Immunotherapy studies with monoclonal antibodies of different isotypes (and thus different capacities to fix complement or mediate ADCC) have also suggested that

ADCC may be the more important in vivo effector mechanism.

Natural Killer (NK) Cells

NK cells can kill a wide range of tumor targets in vitro (see also Chapter 5). Although the mechanism by which NK cells preferentially recognize and lyse transformed rather than normal targets is not well-defined, binding appears to reflect the usage of classes of cell surface adhesion molecules rather than reflect the presence of an antigen-specific receptor. Cytolysis by NK cells is mediated by the release of a cytotoxic factor(s) and the introduction of holes in the target cell membrane. The cytotoxic activity of NK cells can be augmented both in vitro and in vivo with the lymphokines interleukin-2 (IL-2) and interferon, and thus NK activity can be amplified by immune T cell responses. Recent studies have demonstrated that augmentation of NK activity in visceral organs enhances resistance to the growth of metastases. Therefore, NK cells may represent a first line of host defense against the growth of transformed cells at both the primary and metastatic sites, as well as providing an effector mechanism recruited by T cells to supplement specific antitumor responses.

Additional cytotoxic effector cells that bear many similarities to but can be distinguished from classic NK cells have also been identified. Natural cytotoxic (NC) cells kill a somewhat different spectrum of tumor targets than do NK cells, are resistant to glucocorticoids, and respond to IL-3. Lymphokine-activated killer (LAK) cells can be induced by very high doses of IL-2, are phenotypically heterogeneous (including both NK and other cell types), and kill a much broader spectrum of tumor targets than do NK cells, but their role during physiologic antitumor responses remains to be elucidated.

Macrophages

Macrophages are important in tumor immunity as antigen-presenting cells to initiate the immune response and as potential effector cells to mediate tumor lysis. Resting macrophages are not cytolytic to tumor cells in vitro, but they can become cytolytic if activated with macrophage-activating factors (MAF). MAF are commonly secreted by T cells following antigen-specific stimulation, and therefore the participation of macrophages as effector cells may be dependent upon T cell immunity. This is supported by studies showing that macrophages isolated from immunogenic tumors undergoing regression exhibit tumoricidal activity, whereas macrophages isolated from progressing or nonimmunogenic tumors generally show no cytotoxic activity. T cell lymphokines with MAF activity include gamma interferon, TNF, IL-4, and granulocyte-macrophage colony-stimulating factor (see Chapter 7).

The mechanisms by which macrophages recognize

tumor cells and mediate lysis are not fully defined. As with NK cells, activated macrophages bind to and lyse transformed cells in marked preference to normal cells. Binding by activated macrophages is an energy-dependent process that is also dependent upon trypsin-sensitive membrane structures. Several distinct mechanisms may be selectively elicited, dependent on the MAF by which macrophages can mediate lysis. These include intercellular transfer of lysosomal products, superoxide production, release of neutral proteases, and secretion of the monokine TNF.

POTENTIAL MECHANISMS BY WHICH TUMOR CELLS MAY ESCAPE FROM AN IMMUNE RESPONSE

The concept of host immune surveillance, with the immune system providing the function of surveying the body to recognize and destroy frequently developing immunogenic tumor cells, was formally proposed by Burnet. However, the failure to demonstrate an increased appearance of immunogenic tumors in immunodeficient hosts incapable of tumor rejection has modified current views of immune surveillance. Thus, effector populations, such as NK cells, rather than tumor antigen-specific immune responses are now believed to be important in the rejection of newly appearing tumor cells. It should be emphasized that antigen-specific responses may provide a surveillance function for the development of certain tumors, such as those induced by oncogenic DNA and RNA tumor viruses. Moreover, the failure of the immune system to prevent the emergence of other new tumors does not preclude the development of tumor-specific immune responses during the growth of established tumors. Indirect support for the presence of immunity to human tumors includes spontaneous regressions of tumors and regressions of metastatic lesions after removal of large primary tumors. Direct evidence of tumor-specific immunity has been provided by studies in which the use of in vitro technologies to selectively expand antigen-reactive T cells has permitted the detection of weak tumor-specific responses. Thus, it seems likely that even though the emergence of many tumors may reflect a failure of immune surveillance and the absence of an immune response during early tumor growth, a potentially detectable but unfortunately ineffective immune response may still be generated during progressive growth of the tumor. One important goal in tumor immunology is to determine why such responses are ineffective.

Many potential mechanisms permitting escape from immune destruction have been identified. Possible immunoselection of variant cells is suggested by analysis of the cells present in a tumor mass, which often reveals a heterogeneity with respect to morphology and surface phenotype. Some of these differences are cell cycle-dependent, but others result from random mutations in the proliferating cell population. Regardless of the underlying reason, if some of these differences result in a reduction in the expression of a tumor antigen being recognized by the immune system, the cells derived from this clone may have a selective advantage. Moreover, as growth of such a tumor variant proceeds, it will become the dominant population, which will make it increasingly difficult to identify that a host response to the tumor had been generated.

Antigenic modulation is similar to the immunoselection described above, in that an immune response to a tumor antigen results in the growth of antigen-negative cells. However, in this setting, antigen loss reflects only a phenotypic change in the tumor cell, and if the immune response is ablated, the antigen will be reexpressed. Antigenic modulation resulting from antibody responses has been extensively reported, but modulation from T cell responses has not yet been clearly identified.

Sera of hosts bearing progressive tumors have been shown in some instances to contain blocking factors that specifically inhibit both cell-mediated cytotoxicity and ADCC to the tumor. It is likely that there are many different types of blocking factors. For example, excess circulating antigen or antigen-antibody complexes may subvert immunity by occupying antigen-specific receptors and by attracting effector mechanisms to sites distal from the tumor. Some blocking factors may actually be suppressor factors released from suppressor T cells.

There are many mechanisms by which tumor cells can nonspecifically interfere with the expression of immunity in the host. Some tumor cells can release soluble factors that directly suppress immunologic reactivity. Perhaps the best-studied phenomenon is the inhibition of immune responses by macrophages obtained from hosts bearing progressive tumors. This appears to be mediated largely via the secretion of prostaglandins, and in vitro treatment of macrophages with the cyclooxygenase inhibitor indomethacin can overcome the inhibitory effects.

The presence of tumor-specific suppressor T (Ts) cells may represent a major reason for the difficulties in detecting tumor-specific immunity in cancer patients and for the impression that no response has been elicited. For example, even with many of the highly immunogenic animal tumors studied in the laboratory, the presence of Ts cells would prevent the detection of tumor-specific immunity in the host if the presence of immunity was not sought until the tumor had reached a stage comparable to that in which most cancer patients are studied. Moreover, recent studies with T cells cloned from patients with malignant melanoma have suggested that Ts cells specifically down-regulating the host response may be present in the lymphocytes infiltrating a tumor.

IMMUNOTHERAPY

Although the host immune system may often be inadequate for controlling tumor growth, the presence of identifiable tumor antigens on most tumor cells, the identification of a detectable but ineffective host response to many tumors, and an improved understanding of the mechanisms by which tumor cells evade immunity suggest that it may be possible to manipulate and amplify the immune system to promote tumor eradication. The recent technologic advances that permit isolation of lymphocyte subpopulations, identification and purification of tumor antigens, growth of selected antigen-specific T cells, amplification of immune responses with cytokines, and targeting of antibody-toxin conjugates to tumors have created a new potential and enthusiasm for the immunotherapy of tumors. Several distinct approaches to immunotherapy are being studied, and it seems likely that at least some of these approaches will soon be developed into important modalities for the treatment of tumors.

Immunization with Tumor Cells or Purified Antigens

Immunization of hosts bearing established progressing tumors with tumor cells or tumor antigen has generally been ineffective. It is now evident that such an approach is doomed to failure even with immunogenic tumors, since by this time the tumor is likely to have elicited a Ts cell response that inhibits tumor reactivity. Therefore, prior to attempting sensitization, it is mandatory that the host be depleted of Ts cells or that the tumor burden be decreased and time permitted for the Ts response to decay. Experimental models to examine the potential utility of immunization with killed tumor cells or purified antigens have now been developed, and significant therapeutic effects on residual micrometastatic tumors have been detected. Similar approaches are currently being studied in patients with colon cancer who have undergone resection of the primary lesion, and there is some preliminary evidence that a potentially beneficial antitumor response is being elicited.

Since many tumors are likely to be only weakly immunogenic, several methods are being explored to modify the tumor cell or tumor antigen to try to augment the response. In initial attempts, neuraminidase was used to alter the surface of human leukemia cells and potentially unmask new tumor determinants that might then be recognized on untreated targets, but this had only limited success. Modification of the tumor cell by binding a hapten such as trinitrophenyl or by infection with a virus such as vaccinia virus to provide a greater number of helper determinants has now yielded promising results in animal models. Another approach being explored in preclinical trials is the isolation and insertion of genes encoding tumor antigens into recombinant vectors, such as vaccinia viruses, that can be used to immunize animals to the tumor antigen by presenting it in an immunogenic context.

Adoptive Cellular Immunotherapy

Animal models have been developed in which hosts bearing advanced tumors can be treated by the transfer of tumor-specific syngeneic T cells. These models, in which syngeneic donor T cells immune to the tumor are used, have served as prototypes of what might be achievable if the host immune response to an autochthonous tumor could be selectively amplified, and they have been useful for elucidating the requirements for successful immunotherapy. A major obstacle to adoptive therapy of advanced tumors, as predicted from other studies, is the presence in the tumor-bearing host of Ts cells that must be eliminated prior to cell transfer to permit the expression of transferred immunity. Complete tumor elimination following adoptive therapy requires a long time, and the cells transferred must therefore be capable of persisting in the host to be effective. Noncytolytic lymphokine-producing class II-restricted Th cells, as well as directly lytic class I-restricted Tc cells, mediate antitumor effects in these models. Tumor-specific T cells expanded in vitro by culture with tumor and IL-2 are effective in adoptive therapy, and efficacy can be enhanced by infusing IL-2 after cell transfer, which has been shown to promote in vivo proliferation and survival of the transferred cultured T cells.

These studies are now being applied to the treatment of human cancers by isolating potentially tumor-reactive lymphocytes infiltrating solid tumors, expanding these cells in vitro by stimulation with tumor or IL-2 or both, and then reinfusing the cells into the patients. To enhance the efficacy of such therapy, patients are being treated with cyclophosphamide prior to cell transfer to deplete potential Ts cells; IL-2 is then administered after transfer. Preliminary results have suggested that these T cells can localize to sites of tumor and can mediate a significant therapeutic effect, particularly with some tumors such as melanoma. Although a great deal more must be learned to effectively and reproducibly detect and expand tumor-specific T cells from patients, these initial efforts at specific adoptive therapy are very encouraging.

While the in vitro effects of increasing doses of IL-2 on the generation of tumor-specific T cells were being examined, it was observed that a cytolytic effector cell lacking antigen specificity but displaying a marked preference for transformed cells was induced. These LAK cells, generated only in the presence of exceptionally high, nonphysiologic doses of IL-2, have now been extensively characterized and studied both in vitro and in vivo. LAK cells are phenotypically heterogeneous, but the major effector cell appears to be a non-T cell most similar to an activated NK cell. Administration of cytolytic LAK cells, particularly in association with IL-2, mediates substantial activity in the treatment of some human tumors. Although the efficacy of treatment with LAK cells and IL-2 appears to be limited by a lack of absolute specificity and toxicity to the host, there are many clinical settings, such as isolated pulmonary or liver metastases, in which it may be possible to utilize these effector cells to achieve a directed and potentially curative antitumor effect. Moreover, approaches are now being explored to improve the specificity of LAK cells by direct delivery of the lytic signal to the tumor through the use of bifunctional antibodies, ie, hybrid or conjugated monoclonal antibodies that have 2 specificities, one for an antigen that resides on the LAK cell and permits attachment to the effector cell and one for an antigen that resides on the tumor and promotes specific targeting.

Administration of Monoclonal Antibodies

The development of the technology for generating monoclonal antibodies has converted the previously unpromising field of tumor serotherapy into a form of treatment with enormous potential. Studies with antibodies of different isotypes have demonstrated that ADCC rather than complement-mediated cytotoxicity is the major in vivo effector mechanism following infusion of antibody. However, despite occasional reports of exciting clinical results, a large number of biologic problems still need to be overcome for this modality to be generally effective. Antibodies and the necessary ADCC effector cells do not appear to penetrate large tumor masses effectively, and tumor escape mechanisms, such as modulation of the target antigen from the tumor cell surface and selection of antigen loss variants, may frequently interfere with monoclonal antibody therapy.

Several approaches are being studied to augment the therapeutic activity of monoclonal antibodies. The most promising involve conjugation of cytotoxic drugs, toxins, or radioisotopes to the antibody to deliver a lethal hit directly to the tumor without requiring the participation of host effector cells. Antibody, drug, or toxin conjugates may be particularly useful in settings in which the antigen is rapidly endocytosed. In contrast, radioisotopes may be useful with large tumors or in the presence of immunoselection, because radioisotopes kill by emitting ionizing radiation and thus do not need to fully penetrate the tumor to kill all cells and can kill antigen-negative tumor variants in the tumor mass if they are in the proximity of antibody-binding tumor cells. Most of the tumor-reactive monoclonal antibodies being used in clinical trials recognize tumor-associated rather than tumor-specific antigens and thus are likely to recognize some normal tissues. Consequently, administration of some antibodies or antibody conjugates may prove to be unacceptably toxic to the host. However, in many instances, such as if the antibody recognizes a determinant on normal B cells and causes a transient depression of B cell number, this toxicity may be acceptable if a significant antitumor effect can be achieved. Future studies will need to carefully define the distribution of normal antigens recognized by each antibody to be used in therapy and the potential toxic complications, but it seems safe to predict that sufficient monoclonal antibodies with appropriate characteristics will be identified to permit the treatment of a wide variety of human tumors.

REFERENCES

Balman A, Brown K: Oncogene activation in chemical carcinogenesis. *Adv Cancer Res* 1988;**51**:147.

Bishop JM: The molecular genetics of cancer. *Science* 1987;**235**:305.

Burnet FM: Immunologic surveillance in neoplasia. *Transplant Rev* 1971;**7**:3.

Doherty PC, Kowles BB, Wettstein PJ: Immunological surveillance of tumors in the context of major histocompatibility restriction of T cell function. *Adv Cancer Res* 1984;**42**:1.

Greenberg PD et al: Therapy of disseminated tumors by adoptive transfer of specifically immune T cells. *Prog Exp Tumor Res* 1988;**32**:104.

Klein G: The approaching era of the tumor suppressor genes. *Science* 1987;**238**:1539.

Kripke ML: Immunoregulation of carcinogenesis: Past, present and future. *J Natl Cancer Inst* 1988;**80**:722.

North RJ: Down-regulation of the antitumor immune response. *Adv Cancer Res* 1985;**45**:1.

Reisfeld RA, Cheresh DA: Human tumor antigens. *Adv Immunol* 1987;**40**:323.

Rosenberg SA, Lotze MT, Mulé JJ: NIH Conference. New approaches to the immunotherapy of cancer using interleukin-2. *Ann Intern Med* 1988;**108**:853.

Rosenberg SA et al: Special Report: Use of tumor-infiltrating lymphocytes and interleukin-2 in the immunotherapy of patients with metastatic melanoma. *N Engl J Med* 1988;**319**:1676.

Sulitzeanu D: Human cancer-associated antigens: Present status and implications for immunodiagnosis. *Adv Cancer Res* 1985;**44**:1.

Urban JL, Schreiber H: Host-tumor interactions in immunosurveillance against cancer. *Prog Exp Tumor Res* 1988;**32**:17.

Vitetta ES, Uhr JW: Immunotoxins. *Annu Rev Immunol* 1985;**3**:197.

Weinberg RA: The genetic origins of human cancer. *Cancer* 1988;**61**:1963.

Weinstein JN et al: The pharmacology of monoclonal antibodies. *Ann NY Acad Sci* 1987;**507**:199.

Yuspa SH, Poirier MC: Chemical carcinogenesis: From animal models to molecular models in one decade. *Adv Cancer Res* 1988;**50**:25.

47

Cancer in the Immunocompromised Host

John L. Ziegler, MD

In the late 1950s, Sir McFarlane Burnet and Lewis Thomas proposed that the immune system maintains vigil over both alien microorganisms and altered somatic cells. When discovered, these undesirables are selectively eliminated. The logic of "immune surveillance," defined more explicitly by Burnet in 1970, finds support in the defense systems of lower organisms, which must resist fusion, invasion, or destructive parasitism to survive. Plants and prokaryotes maintain their integrity through highly conserved cell surface recognition systems. Multicellular eukaryotes evolved a more complex "adoptive" defense system, one impressive feature of which is the ability to discriminate between self and nonself. Other cognate functions, such as immunologic memory, regulatory networks, and a large repertoire of attack strategies, make the mammalian immune system comparable to the brain in complexity and function. Throughout phylogeny, the role of the immune system in ensuring the autonomy of the host is a basic tenet of evolutionary survival.

IMMUNE SURVEILLANCE

Inferential support for immune surveillance against neoplasia in humans comes from a variety of clinical observations. Patients with congenital immune deficiencies and patients with organ transplants who receive immunosuppressive therapy develop an excess incidence of some forms of cancer. Rare instances of "spontaneous" regression of tumors are ascribed to immune mechanisms. More recently, the discovery of tumor-specific antigens (see Chapter 46) and the observation of tumor-directed immune responses by using autologous lymphocytes and lymphokines provide further evidence for tumor immunity.

Studies of transplantable and spontaneous tumors in animals also lend support to the notion of tumor-directed immunity. For example, surgical removal of a growing tumor in mice renders them resistant to subsequent inocula of the same, but not a different, tumor. Such experiments are more successful when using transplantable tumors rather than spontaneous, autochthonous tumors. Aside from evidence of specific tumor immunity mediated by antibody and T cells, tumor cells can be killed nonspecifically by activated macrophages and natural killer (NK) cells. Finally, examples of "blocking factors" that prevent an immune response are evident in tumor-bearing hosts.

Criteria for Intrinsic Defense

An intrinsic defense against the development of neoplasia might be advantageous to the host. To be successful, it must meet at least 4 conditions. First, the tumor should express unique antigens that are accessible to the immune system. Second, the host must have a competent immune system and attack the tumor antigen with an appropriate tumor-directed cytotoxic response. Third, there should be no suppressive or blocking influences to obstruct the immune response. Finally, the number of tumor cells should be small enough for the immune attack to locate and eliminate the tumor entirely.

Immunotherapy Research

The 1970s saw an era of empirical immunotherapy, based on the assumptions listed above. The main objectives were to augment tumor cell antigenicity and to boost host immunity with various specific or nonspecific vaccines and stimulants. The results of these trials were disappointing, with only rare instances of clinical improvement. By the end of the decade, it was clear that most human tumors were at best only weakly antigenic. It was also obvious that immunotherapy was a "numbers game," with successful killing being dependent upon a high immunocyte-to-target cell ratio. Finally, successful therapeutic manipulation of the immune system demanded a much better appreciation of the intricacies of immunoregulation.

Advances in biotechnology have brought considerable enlightenment to the field of cancer immunology in the 1980s and 1990s. Antigens and separate cell populations can be defined by using monoclonal antibodies. The discovery, cloning, and production of purified growth factors permit experiments with high concentrations of purified immunocytes. Advances in molecular genetics provide techniques to identify tumor clonality. Progress in understanding immunoregulation, mechanisms of immune diversity, and the interactions of the various cellular members of the immune system has opened new doors to pharmacologic and biologic manipulation of the immune response. Finally, the identification of proto-oncogenes has enabled a better molecular and genetic understanding of oncogenesis, including the potential to identify tumor-specific oncogene products.

IMMUNOCOMPROMISE & CANCER

This chapter will focus on the phenomenon of cancer in the immunocompromised human host. **Immunocompromise** is a preferable term to "immunodeficiency" or "immunosuppression." The latter terms imply that the immune system is binary and capable of swaying, like a seesaw, between a normal "replete" state and a suppressed "deficient" state. This is clearly oversimplified, given our knowledge of the delicate and integrated nature of immune responses. Immunocompromise should be defined as a state of functional unresponsiveness, due in some circumstances to depletion of specific immune compartments and in others to dysfunction induced by drugs, physical agents, infections, cancer, or autoimmunity.

Oncogenesis

Experimentally, 3 processes lead to neoplasia: initiation, promotion, and progression (Fig 47–1). **Initiation** involves the alteration of DNA by a chemical, physical, or biologic agent that confers malignant potential onto the cell genotype. "Initiated" cells appear histologically normal but are rendered constitutively susceptible to malignant transformation. **Promotion** is thought to be a process by which the expression of genetic information is altered in the cell. **Progression** is the clonal evolution of established tumors that accounts for heterogeneity and varied phenotypic manifestations such as invasiveness, drug resistance, and metastatic potential. Thus, cancer is the end stage of a multistep process that evolves over long periods. Its development and behavior in the intact host are driven internally by the renegade genetic program and influenced externally by microenvironmental factors such as hormonal milieu, vascular supply, and immunity.

Function & Dysfunction of Proto-Oncogenes & Anti-Oncogenes

Proto-oncogenes are highly conserved genetic sequences that control cell growth and differentiation. More than 40 such genes have been described to date. These genes code for growth factors, receptors, and regulatory proteins that govern cell proliferation. They are normally inactive unless required for embryogenesis, replenishment of replicating tissues, or response to injury. They act in concert, instructing cell growth and differentiation in an orderly fashion.

Proto-oncogenes may be damaged or dysregulated by a variety of insults that result in mutation or translocation to another site in the genome. These accidents, if unrepaired, may cause qualitative or quantitative dysfunction such that the protein products are abnormal in configuration or become overproduced, leading the cell to an autonomous proliferative state.

Studies of heritable cancers have disclosed another set of regulatory genes that are recessive oncogenes (eg, retinoblastoma [RB] gene). These genes act to encourage differentiation or retard cell proliferation, hence their designation as anti-oncogenes. A structural deletion or mutation of one of the alleles of these genes (either inherited in the germ line or produced by somatic mutation), results in a cell that is highly susceptible to malignant transformation. A subsequent genetic accident in the hemizygote unmasks a lethal defect that results in cancer. The phenomenon of "recessive oncogene mutation" is noted in many human cancers such as retinoblastoma, small cell carcinoma of the lung, and cancer of the breast and colon.

Thus, 2 distinct genetic mishaps are presumably involved in oncogenesis (Fig 47–2). One produces aberrant proteins that induce a malignant phenotype. The other results in the loss or functional inactivity of regulatory restraints. Most experts agree that it is the combination of these genetic events that leads to neoplasia. As mentioned above, the environment of the cell also strongly influences the phenotypic expression of its genetic program. The stepwise progression of cancer noted clinically supports the notion that neoplastic transformation is not an "all-or-none" phenomenon.

Epithelial versus Immune System Tumors

Two distinct phenomena must be distinguished in the relationship between cancer and compromised immunity. The first is the high incidence of tumors of the immune system in the immunocompromised host. The immune system itself is programmed for replication upon antigenic exposure. Thus, immune dysfunction that causes unrestrained lymphocyte proliferation might be expected to predispose the host to neoplasia of rapidly dividing cells. The second phenomenon is the emergence of an excess of epithelial neoplasms, particularly among patients who survive a prolonged immunosuppressed state. These tumors may result from a true failure of immune surveillance to detect and eliminate strongly antigenic transformed cells.

Congenital Immunodeficiency & Neoplasia

Table 47–1 indicates the risk of cancer in children with congenital immunodeficiencies. Most of the

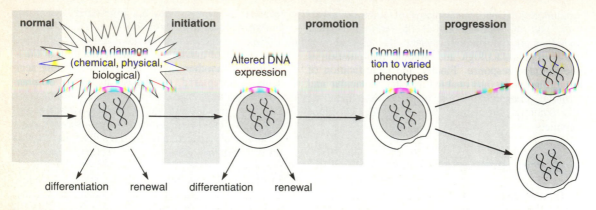

Figure 47–1. Pathogenesis of neoplasia. Normal cells have 2 choices upon division: differentiate or renew. When certain DNA mutations or chromosomal abnormalities occur, stem cells that are initiated may accumulate in a renewal cycle. These cells are more susceptible to a second genetic accident, and the chance of "promotion" to neoplastic transformation increases over time. As tumor develops, there is genetic drift in the cell renewal compartment, and clones of tumor cells "progress" in different phenotypic directions, producing tumor heterogeneity.

data that record these cancers are derived from 4 primary disorders: X-linked lymphoproliferative syndrome; Wiskott-Aldrich syndrome; ataxia-telangiectasia; and common variable immunodeficiency disease. Surveillance of malignant conditions in patients with other congenital immunodeficiencies is either lacking owing to the rarity of the disorder or not recorded. Two-thirds of the patients were younger than 20 years of age when the tumors were diagnosed. True risk assessment is difficult to measure because the accurate prevalence of the disease is unknown. Mild forms of these disorders may be undiagnosed, and many patients with more severe forms may die before cancer develops.

In the X-linked lymphoproliferative syndrome (Duncan's syndrome), a relationship exists between uncontrolled Epstein-Barr virus (EBV) infection of B lymphocytes and a progressive oligoclonal lymphoproliferation, leading to Burkitt-like non-Hodgkin lymphoma.

In the Wiskott-Aldrich syndrome, extranodal immunoblastic lymphoma occurs in up to 16% of patients. These tumors occur in the setting of generalized lymphadenopathy and do not appear to be of B cell origin. About half of these lymphomas are located in the brain, which may act as a "sanctuary" for lymphoproliferation. A role for an oncogenic virus (eg, papovavirus) has not been ruled out. In a

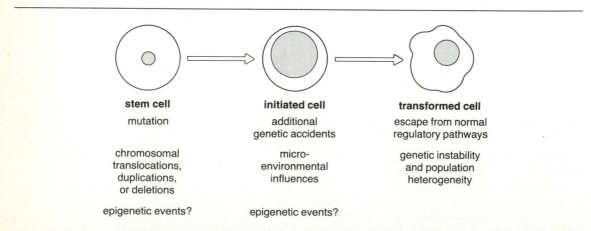

Figure 47–2. Molecular model of malignant transformation. Assuming that cancer is a disease of defective stem cells, there is consensus that the pathway to neoplasia involves multiple "hits" to stem cell DNA, such that the normal signals for self-renewal and differentiation become aberrant or misinterpreted. At the molecular level, these hits presumably alter the expression of regulatory proto-oncogenes that either stimulate or inhibit cell behavior.

Table 47–1. Risk of cancer in congenital immunodeficiency syndromes.[1]

Syndrome	Immune Defect	Malignant Tumors[2]	Percent Risk Overall	Median Age of Onset (years)
X-linked immunodeficiency syndrome	Impaired B cell responses to EBV antigens.		35%	10
Wiskott-Aldrich syndrome	Complex, multicompartmental defects.	NHL, AML HD	15–37%	6
Ataxia-telangiectasia	Complex, multicompartmental defects; defective DNA repair after gamma irradiation.	ALL, NHL, HD, nerve, ovarian, skin, stomach cancers	12%	9
Common variable immunodeficiency	Cellular and humoral defects.	NHL, stomach cancer	8%	16

[1]These data are drawn from the University of Minnesota registry on Immunodeficiency and Cancer and from elsewhere in the literature.
[2]Abbreviations: NHL, Non-Hodgkin lymphoma; AML, acute myeloid leukemia; HD, Hodgkin's disease; ALL, acute lymphoblastic leukemia.

minority of patients, Hodgkin's disease and acute myelocytic leukemia are also found.

In ataxia-telangiectasia, both Hodgkin's disease (the major subtype being lymphocyte depleted) and non-Hodgkin lymphoma occur, in a ratio of about 1:5. The latter cases are of histologic types associated with the 14q+ chromosomal abnormality characteristic of lymphocytes in patients with ataxia-telangiectasia. Patients with this disorder also manifest a defect in the repair of gamma radiation-induced DNA damage. Therefore, it is not surprising to encounter an excess of epithelial neoplasms (skin, ovarian, and stomach cancers) among older patients.

A small proportion of patients (2.5–8.5%, depending upon survival) with common variable immunodeficiency develop non-Hodgkin lymphoma. In longer-surviving patients, an excess incidence of stomach cancer is also found.

Lymphohematopoietic Cancers

The predominance of lymphoid and hematologic cancers in the setting of primary immune deficiency could be explained by the disruption of immune regulatory circuits. Lymphocytes replicate clonally in response to antigens. Their clonal expansion is dampened by a regulatory network (eg, anti-idiotypes, suppressor T cells) that prevents unlimited proliferation. It is possible that under circumstances of metabolic or cellular immune dysfunction, the regulatory network fails and normal restraints are lacking. Thus, under an unopposed barrage of paracrine and autocrine growth stimulation, clones of proliferating lymphocytes become susceptible to genetic accidents and malignant transformation. This process may be aided by concomitant viral infection (eg, with EBV) that aggravates dysregulation and provokes lymphoproliferation.

About 10% of lymphoid cancers recorded in patients with congenital immunodeficiency syndromes

are unclassified as to histologic type. By histologic and biologic criteria, these lymphomas reside on the border between reactive hyperplasia and true malignancy. Oligoclonal "cancers" probably represent a transitional state in the pathway of B cell neoplasia.

Cancer in Other Immunosuppressed Patients

In the last 3 decades, immunosuppressive treatment has been used for organ transplant recipients and for patients with autoimmune disorders, and cytotoxic and radiation therapy have been used for patients with cancer. A consequence of iatrogenic immunosuppression has been an excess occurrence of cancers among survivors of these conditions.

CANCER IN ORGAN TRANSPLANT RECIPIENTS

Thanks to a meticulously maintained registry of organ transplant recipients (the Cincinnati Transplant Tumor Registry), epidemiologic data on cancer incidence in this population are both up-to-date and reliable. More than 95% of registry participants received renal transplants.

Recipients of organ allografts must receive drugs to suppress the immune response to alloantigens in order to avoid graft rejection. Over the past 3 decades, various forms of immune suppression have been used. The earlier "broad-spectrum" regimens included both corticosteroids and azathioprine. The introduction of cyclosporine in the 1970s has led to more effective T cell-specific immunosuppression.

Cancer trends in allograft recipients are reminiscent of the experience in patients with primary immunodeficiency syndromes. In general, there is a 3-fold increase of neoplasms in this population compared with age-matched controls. The average time from transplantation to development of all tumors is 60 months; for lymphomas it is 37 months, and for Kaposi's sarcoma, 23 months.

Skin Cancer

The most common tumors are carcinomas of the skin, which account for 1238 (38%) of 3251 transplant-associated cancers (from the Cincinnati registry). This represents a 4- to 21-fold increase over the expected skin cancer incidence. These tumors are also unusual in the overrepresentation of squamous cell carcinomas compared with the more common basal cell type and with melanomas. Skin cancers were diagnosed with higher frequency in younger persons, and carcinomas often developed at multiple sites. Another feature was the increased clinical aggressiveness of these tumors and a mortality rate of 6%. This rate can be compared with the very low (1–2%) mortality rate in the general population, most of which is attributed to malignant melanoma.

Etiology and immunologic control of skin cancer in humans are incompletely understood. Of interest, however, is the demonstration that UV radiation-induced tumors in mice are antigenic in autochthonous hosts. Tumor-specific cytotoxic T cells are directed at the antigenic tumor cells. Failure of immunity has been attributed to antigen-specific suppressor T cells that inhibit tumor cell rejection. It is also know that UV light can alter the expression of class I major histocompatibility complex (MHC) antigens in the skin. Specific T cells bearing γ/δ T cell receptors recognize these antigens. Perhaps a failure of this surveillance system in immunocompromised patients is related to the emergence of excess skin cancers.

Anogenital Cancer

The second most common tumor in transplant recipients is carcinoma of the anogenital tract. Cervical carcinomas accounted for 16% of cancers (including 80% in situ lesions). Carcinoma of the vulva, perineum, scrotum, penis, and anus occurred in 3% of recipients with cancer. Taken together, anogenital tumors are increased more than 100-fold compared with the incidence in the age-matched general population.

A possible explanation for this excess is the association of anogenital neoplasia in general with human papillomavirus, especially with types 6, 11, 16, 18, 32, 35, and 37. Perhaps immunosuppression permits the activation of latent papillomavirus in anogenital tissues, and the resulting dysplastic epithelial lesions progress to neoplasia. Because these are virus-associated tumors, there may be some degree of immune surveillance in the immunocompetent host that is directed to virus-specific antigens of the epithelial cell surface. This response would normally identify and eliminate early papillomavirus-asso-

ciated tumors. In an immunocompromised host, such immunity would be impaired and a higher frequency of tumors might result.

Non-Hodgkin Lymphoma

Non-Hodgkin lymphoma constitutes 14% of cancers in transplant recipients. The major histologic types were diffuse large cell and immunoblastic. The majority of 100 tumors classified by modern immunologic techniques were of B cell origin; lymphomas of T cell origin accounted for 12%. As with lymphomas found in patients with primary immunodeficiencies, the majority were extranodal, with one-third involving the central nervous system. In addition, a small proportion of lymphomas defied classification. In individual transplant series, these are oligoclonal and are associated with EBV. They may regress upon withdrawal of immunosuppressive therapy, treatment with antiviral agents, or infusion of anti-B cell monoclonal antibodies.

Theories To Explain Posttransplant Lymphomas

Several hypotheses have been advanced to explain the lymphoproliferative syndromes associated with organ transplantation. These include (1) impaired immune surveillance, (2) chronic allostimulation from the engrafted tissue, (3) activation of endogenous viruses (particularly EBV), and (4) possible carcinogenic effects of immunosuppressive drugs.

A number of human studies have documented progressive cytogenetic and oncogene alterations that accompany phenotypic progression toward a more malignant state. The process may be reversed by withholding immunosuppressive therapy or by treatment with acyclovir. The statistical likelihood of lymphoma development probably depends on the proliferative rate, the total number of proliferating B cells, and the random chance of a genetic accident that confers growth advantage to a particular clone.

Although EBV has been associated with a majority of posttransplant lymphomas, perhaps 20–40% of tumors lack the EBV genome. It is possible that these tumors harbor another virus (such as human herpesvirus type 6 or a human retrovirus) or that they result from B cell proliferation driven by other mechanisms. For example, some B cell lymphoma lines produce an autocrine growth factor. Other lymphomas may be driven by an external source, such as a retrovirus or other antigenic stimulus.

A possible scenario, therefore, is that B cell lymphoproliferation is induced initially by activated EBV (or another virus), as a result of drug-induced impaired antiviral immunity (Fig 47–3). Continued B cell growth may be promoted by an abundance of B cell growth factors, unrestrained by the normal regulatory controls. Unopposed polyclonal B cell proliferation then progresses to oligoclonal "tu-

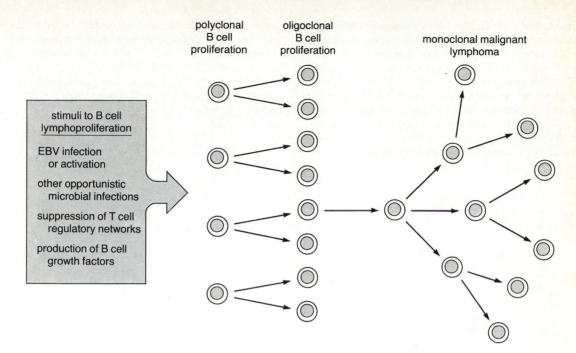

Figure 47–3. Suggested pathogenesis of B cell lymphoma in immunocompromised patients. Multiple pathways for B cell proliferation exist in the immunocompromised patient. These include direct viral activation (EBV) and indirect mitogenic stimuli from infecting microorganisms. In addition, the regulatory networks that normally hold B cell proliferation in check are impaired, and unrestrained B cell growth results. In this polyclonal population, the chances of autonomous growth of several clones increases over time, leading to oligoclonal and ultimately monoclonal lymphoma (see text).

mors," which evolve over time to a monoclonal malignant lymphoma.

Kaposi's Sarcoma

Kaposi's sarcoma is 400–500 times overrepresented among transplant recipients compared with the general population. This rare and unusual tumor is of endothelial origin and occurs sporadically in Caucasian men of eastern European descent. A polymorphic variety is endemic in certain central African countries. Like non-Hodgkin lymphomas, this tumor may regress when immunosuppressive therapy is stopped. Although spontaneous Kaposi's sarcoma usually appears on the skin and runs a benign course, transplant-associated tumors tend to involve internal organs, and the mortality rate is 25%.

In a large study of transplant recipients, no unusual epidemiologic features distinguished the subgroup with Kaposi's sarcoma, with the exception that one-third of the patients were women. Kaposi's sarcoma predominates among males, and women made up approximately one-third of the transplant series. (All received prednisone, and all but 2 received azathioprine.) Thus, the usual 9:1 male-to-female ratio became 2:1 in the transplant series.

There is an apparent absence of data on cancer in control populations, such as organ graft recipients

who are not immunosuppressed, or patients with organ failure who received immunosuppressive therapy but not allografts. A control group of otherwise healthy individuals who receive immunosuppressive treatment is obviously also lacking. Thus, the excess incidence of cancers in organ transplant recipients can be attributed to immunosuppression only by circumstantial inference, with some supporting evidence from experimental systems.

CANCER IN PATIENTS WITH AUTOIMMUNE DISORDERS

The true incidence of cancer in patients with autoimmune disorders is not known. Under certain conditions, chronic inflammation per se may predispose to neoplasia, possibly caused by the effects of free radicals produced at the site. Because autoimmune disorders are treated with immunosuppressive drugs, the additional effect of immunosuppression over a "baseline" of cancer susceptibility cannot be ascertained.

Most series of cancer incidence in patients with any particular autoimmune disease are small. There is an increased risk of lymphoma in patients with celiac disease and Sjögren's syndrome. Patients with rheumatoid arthritis are not at increased cancer risk unless treated chronically with cyclophosphamide or chlorambucil. One large series that includes patients with many autoimmune disorders treated chronically with immunosuppressive drugs disclosed a 12-fold increase of Hodgkin's disease, a 5-fold excess of squamous cell carcinoma of the skin, and a modest excess of other tumor types. Although limited in epidemiologic value, these series concur generally with the clinical experience in immunosuppressed organ transplant recipients.

SECOND TUMORS IN CANCER PATIENTS

Cancer patients, who are already partially immunocompromised by their tumors, may receive immunosuppressive anticancer therapy (ie, chemotherapy or radiotherapy or both) that worsens their immunocompromised state. Long-term follow-up of cancer survivors treated with cytotoxic drugs discloses a high incidence of second cancers. Most of these are acute leukemias of myeloid or monocytic origin and non-Hodgkin lymphomas. They occur an average of 4–6 years after treatment of the primary tumor. The most extensive follow-up has been performed in survivors of Hodgkin's disease. Their overall risk of a second cancer is sixfold, with an actuarial risk of approximately 1% per year up to 10 years, after which a plateau is reached. Alkylating agents contribute to the risk of leukemia, whereas radiation therapy is associated with the development of solid tumors.

Interpretation of the epidemiologic data in these groups is confounded by the direct carcinogenic effects of the anticancer treatment, the extent and duration of immunocompromise, and the possibility of a preexisting neoplastic diathesis. In contrast to the cancers in patients with autoimmune disorders that are similar to those in the transplant recipients, second cancers in cancer patients appear more closely related to direct carcinogenic effects of therapy.

HUMAN IMMUNODEFICIENCY VIRUS (HIV) INFECTION & THE DEVELOPMENT OF CANCER

Immunopathogenesis of AIDS

An understanding of acquired immunodeficiency syndrome (AIDS)-associated neoplasia emerges from a knowledge of AIDS immunopathogenesis. Although HIV in vitro is cytopathic to its target cell, the helper CD4 lymphocyte, in vivo effects of HIV on the immune system are not easily explained. One reason may be that only a very small proportion of circulating lymphocytes are infected and the virus is apparently latent in other lymphocytes and macrophages without cytopathic effects. Furthermore, there are noncytopathic strains of HIV. These observations have given rise to numerous theories that attempt to explain the early functional immune defects and the later depletion of various cell compartments in AIDS patients. Immunocompromise in patients with HIV infection is probably due both to direct viral effects and to many secondary events that occur as the immune system attempts to cope with the infection. In the latter category, evidence for "autoimmune" damage to HIV-infected lymphocytes and bystander damage to other immune cells is accumulating.

Kaposi's Sarcoma in AIDS Patients

In the early years of the AIDS epidemic, Kaposi's sarcoma predominated in homosexual men with AIDS, although in central Africa, where Kaposi's sarcoma is endemic, HIV-infected patients developed an aggressive, malignant form of the tumor. Inexplicably, the incidence of AIDS-associated Kaposi's sarcoma in the USA began to decline among homosexual men in the mid-1980s, from a frequency of 40% to about 20%, although the incidence of AIDS in this population remained unchanged.

The cause and pathogenesis of Kaposi's sarcoma are unknown. Epidemiologically, the tumor affects mostly men, with a suggestion of geographic or ethnic susceptibility. It has a widely varied natural history, usually starting as benign-appearing endothelial lesions that are multicentric and can regress spontaneously. Growing lesions may progress to more "sarcomatous" tumors, with local invasion and lymph node metastasis. Children tend to develop a more aggressive "lymphadenopathic" form. Patients with AIDS also have a varied course: Some very long-term survivors have cutaneous lesions that come and go spontaneously, whereas others have a rapid and malignant course with pulmonary and visceral tumors.

The histogenesis of Kaposi's sarcoma has been controversial. Although there is consensus that the tumor spindle cells are endothelial and neoplastic, an origin from both capillary venules and lymphatic endothelium has been claimed. Alternatively, the lesion might develop from lymphaticovenous anastomoses. A benign-appearing proliferation of endothelial cells in normal skin and lymph nodes suggests the existence of a premalignant condition. Clearly, however, Kaposi's sarcoma can invade tissues locally and metastasize.

Advances in Research

Recent experiments have advanced our understanding of the pathogenesis of Kaposi's sarcoma. The ability to grow Kaposi's sarcoma cells in vitro was enhanced by using conditioned media from a T lymphocyte line infected with HTLV-II. Other retroviruses, including HIV-1, also produced an angiogenic factor in smaller quantity, and certain avian retroviruses are associated with hemangiomatosis in fowl. Such cell lines later became autonomous and were shown to produce a variety of autocrine growth factors, including a fibroblast growth factor (FGF)-like substance. Coincidentally, an oncogene has been found in Kaposi's sarcoma DNA that codes for a new member of the FGF family. Upon inoculation into nude mice, these cell lines induce an intense angiogenic reaction of mouse origin.

Other studies on the HIV *tat* gene in transgenic mice showed that some of the male mice developed endothelial tumors indistinguishable from Kaposi's sarcoma. *tat* is a gene that transactivates HIV transcription and is responsible for turning an HIV-infected cell into a veritable virion factory. *tat* is under the control of both cellular and viral regulatory genes and appears to "turn on" viral production when the cell is coinfected with another virus, stimulated antigenically, or subjected to certain lymphokines. Interestingly, the *tat-1* gene of HTLV-I is also oncogenic in transgenic mice, producing transplantable mesenchymal tumors. The predilection for tumors in male mice is not understood.

Although epidemiologic evidence has implied that another virus acts as an etiologic cofactor, sensitive viral probes and culture techniques have thus far failed to disclose such an agent in Kaposi's sarcoma.

Host Immunity & Kaposi's Sarcoma

The relationship between host immunity and the natural history of Kaposi's sarcoma has been examined by many investigators. The conclusions to be drawn from these studies are as follows: (1) Kaposi's sarcoma may develop in persons with minimal immunocompromise; (2) the natural history of the tumor bears a close relationship to host immunity; (3) as host immune function declines, Kaposi's sarcoma lesions tend to become more aggressive; (4) conversely, lesions may regress spontaneously in patients whose immune systems remain stable or improve; (5) tumors will respond to chemotherapy, radiation, and various cytokines such as alpha interferon and tumor necrosis factor. There is a suggestion from some studies that specific human leukocyte antigen (HLA) genes may influence both susceptibility and prognosis.

In summary, the endothelial origin places Kaposi's sarcoma in the reticuloendothelial system, an immunoresponsive system. HIV infection (possibly through the activation of the retroviral *tat* gene) might provoke the production of local angiogenesis factors that act in a paracrine fashion on susceptible endothelial cells of lymphaticovenous origin. These cells proliferate and, in conjunction with cofactors, evolve clonally to more malignant lesions (Fig 47–4). The immune system fails to contain these

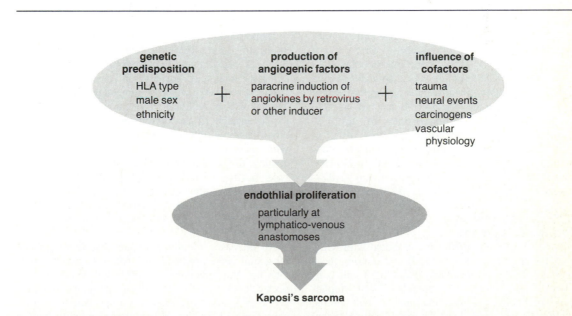

Figure 47–4. Suggested pathogenesis of Kaposi's sarcoma in immunocompromised patients. Kaposi's sarcoma is thought to begin as a vascular reaction to local angiokine production, which can be induced by a number of agents. The paracrine release of angiogenic factors (most probably those in the FGF family) causes endothelial cell proliferation and spindle cell formation. Initially, these proliferative lesions may respond to regulatory restraints, probably mediated by the immune system. With time, however, the lesions become autonomous and produce their own sustaining growth factors. Yet to be explained in this pathway are the roles of genetic predisposition and local cofactors (see text).

growths by either regulatory cytokines or appropriate surveillance of the malignant phenotype, and tumors appear. Cofactors yet to be explained are the male predominance (perhaps related to vascular physiology), genetic predisposition, and the unusual geographic distribution.

Non-Hodgkin Lymphoma in HIV-Infected Persons

Soon after the initial reports of AIDS-associated opportunistic infections and Kaposi's sarcoma, non-Hodgkin lymphoma was found in homosexual men with AIDS. As the AIDS epidemic progressed, the incidence of lymphoma rose commensurately, predominating in the homosexual and intravenous drug-abusing risk groups. The majority of well-characterized lymphomas are of B cell origin, about evenly divided between intermediate-grade large cell, high-grade immunoblastic, and small non-cleaved cell types.

Clinically, the lymphomas are extranodal in distribution, with a high frequency of central nervous system and bone marrow involvement. In addition, homosexual men have an excess of oral and rectal tumors. All series report a poor response to treatment and a high mortality rate. The major determinants of poor prognosis are a prior AIDS diagnosis, low CD4 lymphocyte counts, presence of extranodal tumor, aggressive cytotoxic chemotherapy regimens, and poor clinical condition.

AIDS-associated lymphomas are clinically and biologically heterogeneous. In a recent study of 24 specimens, all tumors primary in the brain were immunoblastic and monoclonal. At least half of non-central-nervous-system lymphomas were oligoclonal, and most of these were immunoblastic in histology. All B cell lymphomas displayed characteristic chromosome translocations that juxtapose the c-*myc* oncogene on the long arm of chromosome 8 to immunoglobulin loci on chromosomes 14, 22, or 2. c-*myc* internal rearrangements or mutations were frequent. Only 10 of 21 lymphoma specimens contained EBV DNA by dot-blot hybridization. No HIV proviral DNA has been detected in any AIDS-associated B or T cell lymphoma yet studied.

T Cell Lymphomas in HIV-Infected Persons

About 5% of the lymphomas associated with AIDS are of T cell origin. As with the B cell tumors, these lymphomas are heterogeneous, including T cell lymphoproliferative syndromes, cutaneous T cell lymphomas, lymphoblastic lymphoma, and T cell chronic lymphocytic leukemia. Thus far, only a single patient with a T cell lymphoproliferative syndrome has been shown to be dually infected with HIV-1 and HTLV-I. Because these 2 viruses may synergistically coinfect the same host, more T cell neoplasms may appear as the epidemic progresses, particularly among intrave-

nous drug abusers who are at high risk for HIV-1 and HTLV-I coinfection.

In a manner similar to the situation in immunosuppressed transplant recipients, AIDS-associated lymphoma is presumed to result from renegade growth of B cells, starting with polyclonal and progressing to oligoclonal proliferation. The latter condition may manifest clinically as malignant lymphoma, although most lymphomas are monoclonal by the time of clinical presentation.

Multiple factors conspire to stimulate polyclonal B cell proliferation in HIV-infected persons: HIV antigens, growth factors from T cells and macrophages, EBV infection, and antigenic stimulation from concomitant infections. Some investigators have described a "premalignant" condition of oligoclonal B cell hyperplasia and c-*myc* rearrangements followed by a stepwise progression to full-blown malignant lymphoma.

A definitive role for EBV cannot be confirmed at this time, even though experimental c-*myc* transfection into virus-infected B cells will produce frank malignant lymphoma. Presumably, EBV is one of several stimuli that induce B cell proliferation. Other candidates include another retrovirus or DNA virus (either exogenous or B cell tropic), activation of another oncogene such as the c-*ras* oncogene, or induction of autocrine B cell growth factors in selected lymphocyte clones.

Hodgkin's Disease & Other Neoplasms in HIV-Infected Persons

Demographic surveys of cancer rates in HIV-epidemic regions have disclosed only an excess of Kaposi's sarcoma and non-Hodgkin lymphoma. Oncologists who care for HIV-infected persons with Hodgkin's disease report a more aggressive natural history, with a predilection for tumor sites in unusual locations such as the rectum and parotid gland. A majority of patients have advanced stages of disease, with noncontiguous anatomic spread. Most patients display the mixed-cellularity histopathologic subtype, but the tumors are depleted of CD4 lymphocytes. Because the highest frequency of Hodgkin's disease occurs in the age group predominantly affected by HIV, an absolute excess incidence cannot yet be inferred.

An increased incidence of anal carcinoma in homosexual men predated the AIDS epidemic, and, thus far, the incidence has not risen above the expected level. Careful surveillance of anogenital cancer in HIV-infected persons is important for 2 reasons. First, these tumors are associated with human papillomavirus, as noted above, and this virus is prevalent and active in AIDS patients, particularly in the risk groups who transmit the virus sexually. Second, studies of HIV-infected men and women disclose an increase of papillomavirus-induced epithelial dysplasia in the anogenital tract, indicating viral activity and a high frequency of premalignant lesions.

Other Cancers in HIV-Infected Persons

Scattered reports have appeared of other cancers in AIDS patients. However, overall there is no epidemiologic evidence of an increase over expected rates. Some reported cancers, such as acute leukemia and skin, testicular, lung, colon, and pancreatic cancers, are relatively common in the HIV age groups at risk. Because HIV infection leads to endogenous virus activation, one might expect an excess of virus-associated tumors such as hepatocellular carcinoma, anal and cervical cancer, and, possibly, nasopharyngeal carcinoma. Although this is theoretically possible, these tumors probably require cofactors that may or may not be present in HIV-infected individuals. Furthermore, these tumors generally have a very long incubation period before malignant transformation. Nevertheless, continued surveillance of HIV risk groups for increased cancer incidence is important.

CONCLUSIONS

This survey of neoplasia in immunocompromised patients permits several general inferences about oncogenesis and the immune system. The first is that neoplasia of compartments of the lymphoreticular system (eg, non-Hodgkin lymphomas from lymphocytes, Kaposi's sarcoma from endothelial cells) predominates in all immunocompromised states. A plausible explanation is dysregulation of the natural proliferative program of these cells, induced stepwise by paracrine or autocrine growth factors, viruses, and genetic accidents.

Second, if a general theory of immune surveillance were correct, we might predict an excess of nonhematopoietic cancers in immunocompromised individuals. These would represent "escape" of nascent tumor cells from the expected immune response. With few exceptions, these cancers are not encountered, and the exceptions can be accounted for by the presence of codeterminants in the persons at risk. For example, epithelial carcinomas in ataxia-telangiectasia may reflect defective DNA repair of radiation-induced damage. Anogenital carcinomas in immunosuppressed transplant patients may reflect activation of papillomavirus infection.

To date, the experimental and clinical literature supports isolated specific instances of immune surveillance but does not validate a general theory. Thus, certain virus-associated tumors are antigenic to their host and evoke a tumor-directed immune response. Animals immunized to virus-induced tumors will resist implantation and successfully reject small transplanted tumors. Conversely, animals made tolerant to the tumor at birth will accept tumor implants. In humans, virus-associated tumors, such as the EBV-associated African Burkitt's lymphoma, evoke immune responses to viral antigens expressed on the tumor cell. These tumor-directed responses may be responsible in part for spontaneous remissions and long-term survival of treated patients.

Certain human tumors seem to be antigenic to their host. A tumor-specific antigen has been found in patients with melanoma, and evidence of specific T cell responses to transitional carcinoma of the bladder, malignant glioma, and carcinomas of the skin is reported. Carcinomas of the kidney and melanomas are particularly susceptible to nonspecific killing by activated NK cells. Other tumors express tumor-associated antigens of oncofetal origin, but these do not appear to evoke a protective immune response.

The majority of human cancers, however, are not strongly antigenic, presumably owing to such mechanisms as modification of histocompatibility antigens, cell surface glycosylation, or the production of blocking factors. Whatever the mechanism, the immune system fails to recognize most spontaneous tumors, not because of a recognized immune defect, but because the tumors themselves are relatively nonantigenic.

REFERENCES

Blattner WA, Hoover RN: Cancer in the immunosuppressed host. In: *Principles and Practice of Oncology*, 2nd ed. DeVita VT, Hellman S, Rosenberg SA (editors). McGraw-Hill, 1986.

Burnet FM: Immunologic surveillance in neoplasia. *Transplant Rev* 1971;**7**:3.

Delli Bovi P et al: An oncogene isolated by transfection of Kaposi's sarcoma DNA encodes a growth factor that is a member of the FGF family. *Cell* 1987;**50**:729.

Ensoli B et al: AIDS-Kaposi's sarcoma-derived cells express cytokines with autocrine and paracrine growth effects. *Science* 1989;**243**:223.

Frizzera G et al: Lymphoreticular disorders in primary immunodeficiencies. *Cancer* 1980;**46**:692.

Hanto DW et al: Epstein Barr virus (EBV) induced polyclonal and monoclonal B-cell lymphoproliferative diseases occurring after renal transplantation. *Ann Surg* 1983;**198**:356.

Janeway CA.: Frontiers of the immune system. (News and Views.) *Nature* 1988;**333**:804.

Kagan JM, Fahey JL: Tumor immunology. *JAMA* 1987;**258:**2988.

Kaplan LD et al: AIDS-related non-Hodgkin's lymphoma in San Francisco. *JAMA* 1989;**261:**719.

Kinlen LJ: Incidence of cancer in rheumatoid arthritis and other disorders after immunosuppressive treatment. *Ann Intern Med* 1985;**78 (Suppl):**44.

Knowles DM et al: Lymphoid neoplasia associated with the acquired immunodeficiency syndrome (AIDS). *Ann Intern Med* 1988;**108:**744.

Kripke ML: Immunoregulation of carcinogenesis: Past, present, and future. *J Natl Cancer Inst* 1988;**80:**722.

Levy JA, Ziegler JL: Hypothesis: Acquired immunodeficiency syndrome is an opportunistic infection and Kaposi's sarcoma results from secondary immune stimulation. *Lancet* 1983;**2:**78.

Lombardi I, Newcomb EW, Dalla-Favera R: Pathogenesis of Burkitt lymphoma: Expression on an activated c myc oncogene causes the tumorigenic conversion of EBV-infected human B lymphoblasts. *Cell* 1987;**49:**161.

Lymphoma in organ transplant recipients. (Editorial.) *Lancet* 1984;**1:**601.

Nakamura S: Kaposi's sarcoma cells: Long term culture with growth factor from retrovirus-infected CD4 + T cells. *Science* 1988;**242:**426.

Pelicci PG et al: Multiple monoclonal B cell expansions and c-*myc* oncogene rearrangements in acquired immune deficiency syndrome-related lymphoproliferative disorders. *J Exp Med* 1986;**164:**2049.

Penn I: Kaposi's sarcoma in immunosuppressed patients. *J Lab Clin Immunol* 1983;**12:**1.

Penn I: Tumors of the immunocompromised patient. *Annu Rev Med* 1988;**39:**63.

Purtilo DT: Opportunistic cancer in patients with immunodeficiency syndromes. *Arch Pathol Lab Med* 1987;**111:**1123.

Salahuddin SZ et al: Angiogenic properties of Kaposi's sarcoma-derived cells after long term culture in vivo. *Science* 1988;**242:**430.

Tucker MA et al: Risk of second cancers after treatment for Hodgkin's disease. *N Engl J Med* 1988;**318:**76.

Vogel J et al: The HIV tat gene induces dermal lesions resembling Kaposi's sarcoma in transgenic mice. *Nature* 1988;**335:**606.

Ziegler JL, Dorfman RK (editors): *Kaposi's Sarcoma. Pathophysiology and Clinical Management.* Marcel Dekker, 1988.

Neoplasms of the Immune System

48

John W. Parker, MD, & Robert J. Lukes, MD

Lymphomas and leukemias involving lymphocytes, plasma cells, monocytes, and natural killer (NK) cells are neoplasms of the immune system. The effects of these neoplasms upon immune function result primarily from loss or malfunction of the neoplastic cells. With increasing knowledge of the specific functions and immunophenotypes of normal cells of the immune system and evidence that lymphomas and leukemias reflect clonal expansions of cells at different stages of normal cell differentiation, immunophenotyping has become useful in identifying different types of lymphomas and leukemias. These tumors, which would not otherwise be detected by morphologic features alone, have different clinical behaviors and responses to therapy. Lymphomas and leukemias are frequently considered separate diseases, but most evidence indicates that they are essentially the same neoplasms, with different modes of onset, distribution, and spread.

CLASSIFICATION

Lymphomas and lymphocytic leukemias have traditionally been classified on the basis of morphologic and clinical features: leukemias as acute, subacute, or chronic, based on the onset and progression of disease, or according to morphologic characteristics as in the FAB (French-American-British) system, and lymphomas according to histologic features (Rappaport classification). Now that lymphoid neoplasms can be characterized immunologically as being of T or B lymphocyte origin, new, immunologically based classifications (Lukes-Collins and Kiel classifications) (Table 48–1) have been proposed. These recent classifications recognize lymphoid neoplasms as clonal expansions of single cells arrested at different stages of differentiation (Fig 48–1) and that they can be identified as such by both morphology and immunophenotype.

A working formulation of non-Hodgkin lymphomas was developed in 1982 for clinical use (Table 48–1). This classification is based on a combination of histologic and clinical features that characterize lymphomas according to clinical behavior, ie, low-, intermediate-, and high-grade lymphomas. However, it does not distinguish between T and B lymphocytic neoplasms, thereby ignoring the importance of immunophenotypes in diagnosis, prognosis, and therapy.

GENERAL CONSIDERATIONS

Neoplasms of the immune system may present locally, but are often widespread at the time of diagnosis, presumably because of the natural ability of the cells to circulate. Moreover, they frequently undergo changes in morphology and clinical behavior during the course of the disease; eg, well-differentiated cells transform into more rapidly proliferating, malignant cells. Some of these neoplasms are easily diagnosed from morphology on tissue sections or smears, but others are more subtle and require cytochemical, immunologic, ultrastructural, or karyotypic characterization for precise categorization. Even morphologically clear-cut cell types may be immunophenotypically heterogeneous and associated with differences in clinical behavior.

The morphologic appearance of neoplasms of immunopoietic cells is the result of several factors, including mixtures of neoplastic and normal cells, neoplastic and reactive cells at different stages of the cell cycle or transformation sequence, and differences in growth pattern. In early involvement of lymph nodes, the location of the lymphoma cells may help determine the cell of origin—B cell lymphomas arising in follicles and T cell neoplasms in the paracortical areas.

The clinical course of these neoplasms is related to the proportion of dividing and nondividing cells. Neoplasms such as chronic lymphocytic leukemia of the B cell type (B-CLL) are widespread but indolent, because of a predominant proportion of nondividing small lymphocytes. In contrast, Burkitt's lymphoma has a predominance of proliferating cells. The ability of an indolent process such as B-CLL to transform into a rapidly dividing immunoblastic lymphoma further illustrates the heterogeneity of these neoplasms. The stimuli or mechanisms for such

Table 48–1. Immunologically based lymphoma classifications and the "working formulation."[1]

Lukes-Collins Classification	Kiel Equivalent	Working Formulation
Undefined	U Cell Lymphoblastic, unclassified[2]	

B cell
  Small lymphocyte B-CLL
    Plasmacytoid lymphocyte
 	
  Mantle zone lymphoma
    Parafollicular (monocytoid) B cell
      lymphoma
    Marginal zone lymphoma
    Hairy cell leukemia
  Follicular center cell types
	B Cell
	  Lymphocytic, B-CLL
	  Lymphoplasmacytic/-cytoid (LP
	    immunocytoma)
		ML,[3] small lymphocytic (CLL)
		ML, small lymphocytic plasmacytoid

Small cleaved FCC
  Large cleaved FCC
 	
  Small noncleaved FCC
    Burkitt
    Non-Burkitt
  Large noncleaved FCC
  Immunoblastic sarcoma of B cell
    type
	Centrocytic
	Centroblastic-centrocytic[4]
	
	B lymphoblastic
	  Burkitt type
	  others
	Centroblastic
	B immunoblastic
		ML, follicular/diffuse, small cleaved
		ML, follicular/ diffuse, large cell or mixed
		    small cleaved and large cell
		ML, small noncleaved
		
		ML, Immunoblastic plasmacytoid

T cell
  Small lymphocyte T-CLL
  Convoluted lymphocyte
 	
  Cerebriform lymphocyte
 	
  Lymphoepithelioid lymphocyte
 	
  Immunoblastic sarcoma (T-cell) includ-
    ing node-based T-cell lymphoma
	T cell
	Lymphocytic, T-CLL
	T lymphoblastic (convoluted cell type
	  and others)
	Lymphocytic, mycosis fungoides and
	  Sézary's syndrome
	[Lymphoepithelioid][4]
	
	T immunoblastic
		ML, small lymphocyte
		ML, lymphoblastic convoluted or
		  nonconvoluted
		Mycosis fungoides
		
		ML, diffuse mixed and small and large
		  cell with epithelioid cells
		ML, large cell, immunoblastic, clear cell,
		  polymorphous

[1]Modified from Lukes RJ and Collins RD, *Tumors of the Hematopoietic System,* fascicle 28, AFIP, 1989.
[2]This category contains all lymphoblastic lymphomas that are immunologically undefined or cannot be typed for any of several reasons.
[3]ML, Malignant lymphoma.
[4]This category was not included in the Kiel classification, because at present many cases cannot be distinguished from Hodgkin's disease with a large number of T lymphocytes and very few Reed-Sternberg cells.

transformations are largely unknown but, in some instances, appear to be second mutational events. These transformations may be confusing diagnostically, but they are of extreme importance therapeutically. An additional complexity is the development of second, new neoplasms several years later, apparently the result of the chemotherapy or radiotherapy of the first neoplasm.

In summary, neoplasms of cells of the immune system are complex and may be difficult to diagnose. Nevertheless, recognition of morphologically distinct cell types and patterns of tissue involvement in conjunction with immunophenotyping, cytochemistry, karyotyping, and molecular biologic techniques make an orderly approach to diagnosis possible.

IMMUNOLOGIC FEATURES

The immunologic characteristics of neoplasms of the immune system reflect those of their cells of origin. Because each neoplasm is a clonal expansion of a normal immunopoietic cell type, and, because these clones may retain function, lose function, or malfunction, the immunologic end result varies considerably. Because most lymphocytic neoplasms are of the B cell type, the usual immunologic dysfunction relates to immunoglobulin production. T cell neoplasms may produce an excess of particular cytokines, but frequently they are not functional.

B cell lymphoma or leukemia cells generally do not respond to antigens or mitogens with in vitro transformation or immunoglobulin production, but the addition of healthy helper T cells or removal of suppressor T cells may partially correct this deficit.

Serum Immunoglobulins

Monoclonal serum immunoglobulins are important features of multiple myeloma and Waldenström's macroglobulinemia and, to a lesser degree, of some B cell lymphomas and leukemias. Concordance between serum and similar monoclonal surface immunoglobulins is an important feature of B cell lymphomas and leukemias. Hypogammaglobu-

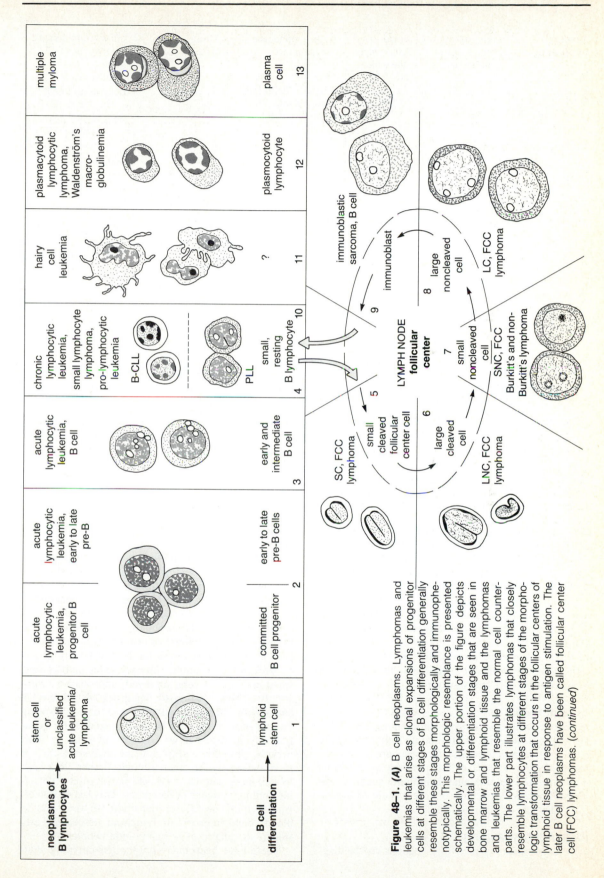

Figure 48–1. (A) B cell neoplasms. Lymphomas and leukemias that arise as clonal expansions of progenitor cells at different stages of B cell differentiation generally resemble these stages morphologically and immunophenotypically. This morphologic resemblance is presented schematically. The upper portion of the figure depicts developmental or differentiation stages that are seen in bone marrow and lymphoid tissue and the lymphomas and leukemias that resemble the normal cell counterparts. The lower part illustrates lymphomas that closely resemble lymphocytes at different stages of the morphologic transformation that occurs in the follicular centers of lymphoid tissue in response to antigen stimulation. The later B cell neoplasms have been called follicular center cell (FCC) lymphomas. *(continued)*

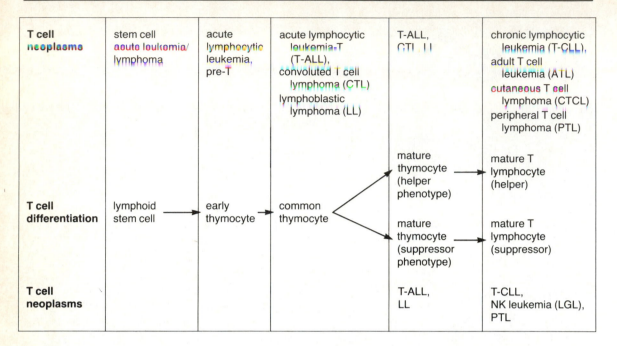

T cell neoplasms	stem cell acute leukemia/ lymphoma	acute lymphocytic leukemia, pre-T	acute lymphocytic leukemia-T (T-ALL), convoluted T cell lymphoma (CTL) lymphoblastic lymphoma (LL)	T-ALL, CTL, LL		chronic lymphocytic leukemia (T-CLL), adult T cell leukemia (ATL) cutaneous T cell lymphoma (CTCL) peripheral T cell lymphoma (PTL)
					mature thymocyte (helper phenotype)	mature T lymphocyte (helper)
T cell differentiation	lymphoid stem cell	early thymocyte	common thymocyte		mature thymocyte (suppressor phenotype)	mature T lymphocyte (suppressor)
T cell neoplasms				T-ALL, LL		T-CLL, NK leukemia (LGL), PTL

Figure 48–1. *(cont'd). (B)* As with B cell lymphomas and leukemias, there is morphologic and immunophenotypic resemblance between specific T cell neoplasms and cells at different stages of differentiation in the T cell system. However, the cytologic differences between stages in development and different lymphomas and leukemias are not as distinctive as for B cells. In addition, the stages in and location of antigen induced lymphocyte transformation of T cells are not as clearly apparent as for B cells. Because of this, morphologic stages in development are not presented here. Nevertheless, certain T cell neoplasms are morphologically distinctive, eg, convoluted T cell lymphoma-leukemia and Sézary cell lymphoma-leukemia. Small T lymphocytes in lymphoid tissue undergo morphologic transformation in response to antigens and give rise to T immunoblasts. Immunoblastic sarcomas (lymphomas) which phenotype as T cells closely resemble antigen-induced transformed lymphocytes.

linemia in B-CLL or B cell lymphoma may occur in advanced disease and lead to serious bacterial infections.

Cellular Immunity

T cell dysfunction may be manifested by delayed cutaneous anergy or defective in vitro responses to antigens and mitogens (see Chapter 19). Such indicators are most commonly but not necessarily seen in the late stages of disease. Infections with fungi, viruses, or opportunistic agents may be the clinical manifestation of T cell dysfunction.

Autoimmunity

Patients with a variety of autoimmune conditions (Sjögren's syndrome or Hashimoto's thyroditis) are at a higher than normal risk for lymphomas. In turn, some patients with B cell lymphoma or leukemia may develop autoimmune hemolytic anemia, immune thrombocytopenia, or rheumatoid diseases. (See Chapters 35, 36, and 38.)

Immunophenotyping

Cells in smears or histologic sections can be diag-

nostically typed by immunofluorescence or enzyme immunocytochemistry with specific antibodies, particularly monoclonal antibodies. Similar studies can be performed on cell suspensions of blood, bone marrow, or lymphoid tissues by using flow cytometry (FCM) (see Chapter 19). Immunocytochemistry has the advantage of visualizing cells in situ, associating antigens with morphology. This is useful in heterogeneous displays of normal and neoplastic cells in smears or sections, but has the disadvantages of background staining, interpretation ambiguities, small numbers of cells surveyed, and relative insensitivity in detecting small quantities of cell surface antigens. FCM has the disadvantage of not allowing visualization of the cells being analyzed, but it quantitatively analyzes large numbers of cells in short periods, provides multiparameter analysis with 2 or more antibodies or other biologic probes on a cell-by-cell basis, and has exquisite sensitivity for detecting cellular antigens or receptors. This last characteristic is quite useful for detection of rare cells in blood, bone marrow, or lymphoid tissues in early staging or relapse of hematopoietic neoplasms.

There have been many immunophenotyping studies of lymphomas and leukemias (Tables 48–2 to 48–4). Some are based on the analysis of cell suspensions by FCM, and others are based on the analysis of cells in smears or histologic sections by using immunocytochemistry procedures, particularly immunoperoxidase staining. Both involve the use of monoclonal antibodies directed against so-called differentiation antigens.

Flow cytometers examine individual cells passing through an exciting laser light beam simultaneously for size, nuclear irregularity, cytoplasmic granularity, and fluorochrome emission. Since multiple monoclonal antibodies, each labeled with a fluorochrome emitting a different color, and multiple color detectors are used, single cells can emit several colors and thus be characterized by multiple parameters.

As an example, a cell suspension prepared from a lymph node from a B cell lymphoma frequently shows 2 different populations based on cell size, nuclear shape, and cytoplasmic granularity (Fig 48–2). The large-cell population (L) generally contains most of the lymphoma cells, and the small-cell population consists primarily of small normal lymphocytes (S). These 2 populations can be examined separately by electronic gating. Presuming that the L gate contains lymphoma cells and that all the cells have been exposed to a panel of antibodies that distinguish T and B lymphocytes, a single-color and dual-color phenotype can be determined, the latter by labeling one antibody with fluorescein isothiocyanate, which emits green, and the other with phycoerythrin, which emits orange-red (Fig 48–2). It is clear from Fig 48–2 that the population of large cells is a homogeneous clone of B cells. The nonneoplastic small lymphocytes do not show this clonality, because they are primarily a mixture of normal or reactive T and B cells, with the B cells expressing combinations of heavy and light chains with both κ and λ present in a ratio of approximately 2.5:1 (eg, polyclonal or bitypic pattern).

In addition, one of the antigens that is present on most of the lymphoma cells can be used to select the lymphoma cells for DNA analysis. Thus, clonality and DNA cell cycle analysis can be performed simultaneously, analyzing several thousand cells per second. Phenotyping results can be available within 2–3 hours of receipt of the specimen. Although surface antigens on viable cells are most commonly examined, intracytoplasmic and nuclear antigens can also be detected in fixed cells.

The immunocytochemistry approach to immunophenotyping allows visualization of the morphology of the labeled cells, in situ, so that the architecture of the neoplasm is retained in histologic sections. Nuclear, cytoplasmic, and surface antigens are detected, although surface antigens of low density may be missed. This approach is somewhat slow, subjective, and semiquantitative, although automated image analysis resolves some of these problems and also allows for DNA analysis. Simultaneous multicolor analysis for more than one antigen per cell is generally not practical, and a complete panel of antibodies requires multiple sections, each stained for a different antigen.

DNA ANALYSIS

DNA cell cycle analysis by FCM has demonstrated a correlation of low-grade (favorable prognosis) and high-grade (unfavorable prognosis) lymphomas with the percentage of cells in S phase, high-grade lymphomas showing evidence of increased proliferative rate. Aneuploidy is detected, by single-color FCM, in 50% or less of all lymphomas, but this percentage is higher in intermediate- and high-grade lymphomas. The percentage of cells in S phase appears to help discriminate between intermediate- and high-grade lymphomas even better than aneuploidy does.

When only the neoplastic cells of a lymphoma that also contains normal and reactive T and B lymphocytes and histiocytes are analyzed, by using an antibody which will identify the neoplastic cells, the sensitivity of detecting aneuploid populations is increased (Fig 48–2). When only the cells bearing the restricted light chain of the B lymphoma cells are analyzed, the percentage of lymphomas that demonstrate aneuploidy increases to approximately 80%. Hyperdiploid B cell lymphomas tend to have higher S fractions and are intermediate- to high-grade lymphomas. Diploid lymphomas have low S fractions and are low-grade. Some may have 2 separate DNA clones, but both express the same light chain.

In acute lymphocytic leukemia (ALL) of childhood, aneuploidy is also relatively infrequent, but it is more frequent than in the nonlymphocytic leukemias. Changes in DNA content, as detected by FCM, correlate with changes in chromosome number, and stem lines can be detected with as few as 2 extra chromosomes.

Another use of FCM involves proliferation-associated nuclear antigens and DNA measurements. Such combinations help distinguish low-grade and high-grade lymphomas in both fresh and paraffin-embedded tissues (Fig 48–3).

Clonality

Lymphocytic neoplasms appear to be clonal expansions of cells at different stages of development, but 2 aspects tend to confuse the issue: the cells of origin may be stages in the normal sequence of T and B cell ontogeny and differentiation (Fig 48–1), or they may be stages in the normal T and B lymphocyte transformation process that occurs in response to antigens. Transformation results in increased numbers of effector cells, which give rise to cytokines (T) or antibodies (B). The morphology of

Table 48–2. Immunophenotypes: B cell tumor antigens, receptors, and enzymes.

B Cell Neoplasms	TdT	HLA-DR	CD 19 (B4)[1]	CD 24 (BA-1)	Heavy Chain Gene[2,3]	Light Chain Gene[2,4]	CD 10[5] (CALLA)	CD 20 (B1)[1]	CIg	SIg	Monoclonal CIg/SIg Light Chain	CD21 (B2)	CD5 (T1)	Complement Receptor	Fc Receptor	CD22 (HC-2)	PCA-1	Comments
Acute lymphocytic leukemia (non-T-ALL)																		
Stem cell (nonclassified) ALL	+	+	−	±[6]	γ	γ	−	−	−	−	−	−		−	−	−	−	
B progenitor cell ALL	+	+	−	±	γ	γ	−	−	−	−	−	−		−	−	−	−	
Early pre-B-ALL	+	+	+	±	R	γ	−	−	−	−	−	−		−	−	−	−	
Mid pre-B-ALL																		
1	+	+	+	±	R	γ/R	+	−	−	−	−	−		−	−	−	−	C ALL, FAB-L1,L2.
2	+	+	+	±	R	γ/R	+	+	−	−	−	−		−	−	−	−	C ALL, FAB-L1,L2.
Late pre-B-ALL	+	+	+	±	R	γ/R	+	+	+μ	−	−	−		−	−	−	−	
B-ALL	−	+	+	+	R	R	−	+	+μ	+	+	+		−	−	−	−	Small noncleaved FCC abdominal lymphoma frequent (Burkitt); FAB-L3.
Small lymphocytic leukemia or lymphoma (B-CLL)	−	+	±	+	R	R	−	±	+μ, μ/δ	+ weak μ, μ/δ	+	±	+	+	+	−	−	SIg Low intensity, CD5 common.
FCC lymphomas	−	+	±	±	R	R	±	±	+μ, γ, or α	+μ, γ, or α strong	+	±	±	+	+	±	−	SIg strong, T101 ±.
Prolymphocytic leukemia	−	+	±	+	R	R	±	+	+	+ strong	+	+	±	+	+	−	−	Differs from B-CLL because SIg strong; from hairy cell leukemia by no CD22.
Hairy cell leukemia	−	±	+	±	R	R	−	+	+μ, γ, or α	+ strong μ, γ or α	+	±	−	+	+	+	+	CD11(MO1) CD22(HC-2) monoclonal SIg and Ig gene rearrangement
Plasmacytoid lymphocytic lymphoma	−	+	+	+	R	R	−	+	+μ, γ or α	±	+	−	−	+	+	±	+	Ig nuclear inclusions (Dutcher bodies)
Multiple myeloma	−	±	−	−	R	R	−	−	+γ,α,δ, ε, or μ	±	+	−	−	−	−	−	+	Ig cytoplasmic inclusions (Russell bodies)

[1] B cell differentiation antigens (B1, B2, and B4) tend to be present on all B cell neoplasms, particularly on differentiated ones; but the presence of each varies from one lymphoma to another.
[2] R, Rearranged immunoglobulin genes; G, germ line immunoglobulin genes. G/R, germ line or rearranged immunoglobulin genes.
[3] Immunoglobulin heavy chain gene rearrangement is seen in some patients with precursor T-ALL (10–20%), immunoblastic lymphadenopathy (40%), and acute myelongenous leukemia (5%).
[4] Immunoglobulin κ gene rearrangement is seen in Hodgkin's disease (30–60%) and immunoblastic lymphadenopathy (40%).
[5] CALLA present on pre-B cells, but also on FCC.
[6] ±, Expressed on some tumors of this type, but not others.

Table 48–3. Immunophenotypes: T cell tumor antigens, receptors, and enzymes.

T Cell Neoplasms[1]	TdT	T Cell Receptor Gene Rearrangement		T9	T10	CD7 (Leu 9)	CD5 (Leu 1/ T1)	CD1 (T6)	CD2 (Leu 5/ T11)	CD3 (Leu 4/ T3)	CD4 (Leu3/ T4)	CD8 (Leu 2/ T8)	Comments
		β Chain	γ Chain[2]										
Early thymocyte (Pre-T-ALL)	+	+	+	+	+	+	+	−	±	−	−	−	
Common T thymocyte (T-ALL, CTL, LL)	+	+	...	−	+	+	+	+	+	±	±	±	
Late T thymocyte Helper differentiation (LL, T-ALL)	+	+	...	−	+	+	+	−	+	+	+	−	Phenotypic but not functional differentiation
Suppressor differentiation (T-ALL, LL)	+	+	...	−	+	+	+	−	+	+	−	+	
Mature T cell Helper differentiation (T-CLL, ATL, CTCL, PTL)	−	+	...	−	−	+	+	−	+	+	+	−	ATL phenotypes helper, but may show in vitro suppressor activity
Suppressor differentiation (T-CLL, T-gamma lymphoproliferative disorder [NK cell leukemia])	−	+	...	−	−	+	+	−	+	+	−	+	NK cell leukemia, Leu 7/HNK-1+, CD57

[1]Abbreviations: LL, lymphoplastic lymphoma; CTL, convoluted T cell lymphoma; CTCL, cutaneous T cell lymphoma; PTL, peripheral T cell lymphoma.
[2]..., Unknown.

Table 48–4. Phenotypic markers useful for lymphomas and lymphocytic leukemias.

Designation[1]	Monoclonal Antibody	Description
TdT		Nuclear enzyme present in immature hematopoietic cells. Originally thought to be a marker for T cell neoplasms, but found in poorly differentiated lymphocytic neoplasms of either T or B cell type.
HLA-DR (Ia)		Class II HLA. Surface antigen found on most B lymphocytes, monocytes, and activated T lymphocytes; frequently present on neoplastic cells of non–T-ALL, granulocytic leukemia, B-CLL, and B cell lymphomas.
Fc receptor		Receptor for Fc portion of IgG molecule. May make SIg clonality determination difficult because of binding of plasma immunoglobulin to cells via this receptor.
SIg		Immunoglobulin on surface of B lymphocytes which is synthesized by cells and transferred to cell membrane. When only one light chain type (κ or λ) is present on cells, indicates a clonally expanded population of neoplastic B cells. Monoclonal (restricted) light chain may be accompanied by one or 2 heavy chains (μ, γ, δ, or α).
CIg		Ig synthesized by B lymphocytes or plasma cells and present in cytoplasm. Restricted light and heavy chains (monoclonal) indicate neoplasm. CIg may be present in some B neoplastic cells when SIg is absent, particularly in plasmacytoid lymphocytic lymphomas and multiple myeloma.
B lymphocyte MAbs		
CD20	B1	Antigen present on essentially all B lymphocytes in blood, bone marrow, and lymphoid tissues. On most B lymphoma and B-CLL cells and about half of CALLA and ALLs. May be present in absence of SIg, and may be seen on some monocytes, but not on plasma cells.
CD21	B2	On a subset of B lymphocytes in blood, bone marrow, and lymphoid tissues (mantle zone and FCC). Is lost before B1 in differentiation to plasma cells. Also found on dendritic reticulum cells. Present on cells of some B cell lymphomas and B-CLL. May be present in absence of SIg. Antigen recognized is complement receptor (C3d).
CD19	B4	On early or pre-B cells after expression of Ia antigen. Is lost before plasma cell differentiation. Present on cells of almost all non–T ALL cases (common ALL), most B cell lymphomas, and B-CLL and essentially all CGL blast crisis cells. May be present on lymphoma cells when B1 and SIG are absent or of low density. The suggested sequence of B cell differentiation, ie, (1) Ia+, (2) Ia+ B4+, (3) Ia+ B4+ CALLA+, (4) Ia+ B4+ CALLA+ B1+, (5) Ia+ B4+ calla+ B1+ CIg+, is reflected in different B cell neoplasms.
CD24	BA-1	On B lymphocytes, monocytes, granulocytes, and some B lymphoma cells.
CD22	HC-2/ Leu 14/ SHCL-1	Found on hairy cell leukemia cells and other B cells. Many help distinguish from prolymphocytic leukemia.
–	PCA-1	On plasma cells and plasmacytoid lymphocytes, but also, weakly, on granulocytes, monocytes, and activated T cells. SIg may be absent, but CIg present. On cells of plasmacytoid lymphocytic lymphoma, multiple myeloma, plasma cell leukemia, and some hairy cell leukemias. Not on non–T-ALL, B-CLL, other B cell lymphomas, or T cell neoplasms. On some AML and CML cells.
CD10	J5/ CALLA	Although a marker for non–T-ALL (common ALL), is also present on normal and activated early B or pre-B cells in bone marrow, lymph nodes (FCC), and blood. Found in about 80% of cases of non–T-ALL and some B and T cell lymphomas, including FCC lymphomas (small noncleaved, Burkitt's), and T lymphoblastic lymphoma, but also on blast cells in 40–50% of cases of CGL in blast crisis. Present on small percentage of cells in normal bone marrow (higher in reactive marrows) and on FCC in lymph nodes.
T lymphocytes and related cells		
CD1	T6	On common thymocytes and Langerhans cells of the skin but on 0–1% of peripheral T cells. Frequently seen on cells of convoluted T cell lymphoma or leukemia (lymphoblastic lymphoma) and small percentage of T-ALL cells. Not on differentiated T cell neoplasms.
CD2	T11/Leu 5	On more than 95% of T lymphocytes including all E rosetting T cells. On cells from T-ALL, T-CLL, T cell lymphomas including lymphoblastic lymphomas and cutaneous T cell lymphomas (mycosis fungoides/Sézary syndrome).
CD3	T3/Leu 4	Essentially all mature T cells and 20–30% of thymocytes. Part of T cell receptor. Antigen tends to be on same neoplastic T cells as CD2, but there are occasional discrepancies.
CD4	T4/Leu 3	On most thymocytes and 60% of blood lymphocytes. Defines helper/inducer T lymphocytes. On T-ALL cells and identifies the predominant subset in mycosis fungoides/Sézary syndrome, but also in many cases of Hodgkin's disease and some reactive or infectious conditions such as tuberculosis.

Table 48–4 (cont'd.). Phelotypic markers useful for lymphomas and lymphocytic leukemias.

Designation[1]	Monoclonal Antibody	Description
CD8	T8/Leu 2	On 80% of thymocytes and 30–40% of blood lymphocytes. Suppressor/cytotoxic T lymphocytes. Found on cells in some cases of T-CLL, adult T cell lymphocytic leukemia, and T cell lymphomas.
CD5	T1/T101	Is a pan-T antigen, but also present on a small population of normal B cells in lymph nodes and tonsils and on medullary (high-density) and cortical (low-density) cortical thymocytes. On T-ALL, T lymphoblastic lymphoma cells, T-CLL, Sézary/mycosis fungoides cells. Also commonly on neoplastic cells of B-CLL and some B lymphoma cells. Useful in identifying a B cell neoplasm when other T cell markers or SIg are absent or of low intensity.
CD7	Leu 9	Pan-T cell antigen. On T-ALL cells and seen (rarely) in early acute myelogenous leukemia.
CD57	NKH-1/Leu 7	On LGL (4–10% of mononuclear cells). Marker for NK cells. Found in NK cell leukemia (LGL leukemia, T-gamma lymphoproliferative disorder).
Activated or proliferating cells		
–	T9	On erythroid progenitors (antigen is transferrin receptor), but also on T cell precursors and activated/proliferating T and B lymphocytes. On convoluted T lymphoma or leukemia cells.
–	T10	On activated and proliferating T and B lymphocytes. Common on proliferating T and B cell lymphoma or leukemia cells.

[1]IUIS, WHO Committee on Human Leukocyte Differentiation Antigen Classification.

cells at different stages in normal lymphoid transformation closely resembles that of specific lymphoma cells. An example is the follicular center cell (FCC) lymphomas, in which normal stages of transformation occurring in germinal centers are identical to the predominant cells in each of the types of FCC lymphoma. Nevertheless, clonal expansion arising from single progenitor cells in either ontogeny or transformation can be recognized morphologically, cytochemically, and immunophenotypically.

Immunophenotypic clonality in B cell lymphomas is usually straightforward, in that the majority of cells express one (2 at the most) heavy chain and one light chain (κ or λ) on the surface or in the cytoplasm. Thus, there is evidence of "monoclonality." With T cell lymphomas there is no such "gold standard" of monoclonality. Phenotypes using monoclonal antibodies against T cell differentiation antigens or receptors may be homogeneous, but since there is no comparable standard for monoclonality and because homogeneous phenotypes (eg, CD2, CD3, and CD4 T cells) can reflect either neoplasia or reactive hyperplasia, T cell phenotypes lack the precision provided by surface or cytoplasmic immunoglobulin clonality. Although a monoclonal expansion of B cells may occur in benign reactive hyperplasia, it is rare and may actually be a harbinger of a developing neoplasm.

CYTOGENETICS

With modern methods, karyotypic abnormalities can be detected in almost all malignant neoplasms. These are somatic genetic changes, which are not present in normal cells. Generally, all of the cells of a tumor show the same or related chromosome abnormalities. This evidence strongly supports the notion that most neoplasms arise from a single altered cell, with the somatic genetic changes represented by the chromosome abnormalities, providing a selective growth advantage for the progeny of the original "mutant" cell. However, although neoplasms represent clonal growth from a single cell of origin, they are frequently not homogeneous, since subpopulations evolve from the original clone by genetic instability of the neoplastic cells. Progression of the tumor may result from or produce chromosomal changes. Specific chromosomal changes associated with various types of tumors are particular rearrangements, gains, or losses of chromosomal segments. These changes probably point to sites in the genome where specific genes important in tumorigenesis are located.

Chromosomal changes are useful as adjunct diagnostic and prognostic tests in distinguishing neoplasia from reactive hyperplasia, particularly if the former is clonal in nature. Specific abnormalities such as trisomy 12 or translocation involving chromosome 14 may help to identify the particular neoplasm and may be useful in monitoring remission, relapse, and clinical progression. Examples of specific karyotypic abnormalities in lymphomas and leukemias are represented in Table 48–5. Common chromosomal rearrangements involving translocation to the terminal portions of the long arm of chromosome 14 (band 14q32), with the donor chromosome being number 8, 11, or 18, have been observed in Burkitt's lymphoma and other non-Hodgkin lymphomas, as well as in multiple myeloma and B-CLL.

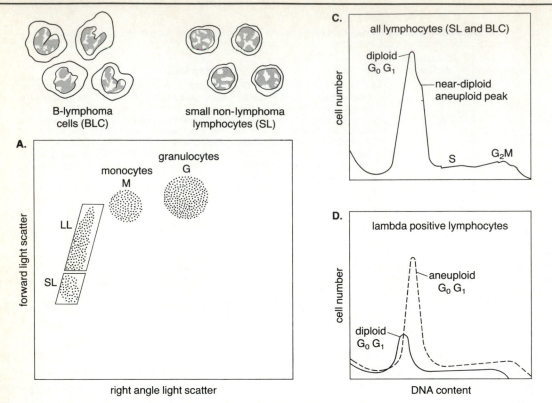

A.

B.

SINGLE COLOR

	CD2 (T11)	CD3 (T3)	CD4 (T4)	CD8 (T8)	CD5 (T1)	CD21 (B1)	CD19 (B4)	CD10 (CALLA)	HLA-DR	S Ig kappa	lambda
% large lymphocytes	10	8	5	3	87	88	92	85	90	2	89
% small lymphocytes	60	55	40	15	58	32	28	12	22	30	12

DUAL COLOR

	B4+/CALLA+ (green) (red)	SIg+/BI+ (green) (red)
% large lymphocytes	86	84
% small lymphocytes	5	29

Figure 48–2. Immunophenotype and DNA cell cycle of a B cell lymphoma. By using FCM, a lymphoid cell suspension can be immunophenotyped with monoclonal antibodies and also analyzed for DNA content. If all of the lymphoid cells, including both the lymphoma cells (LL), which in this example are larger than the residual normal (smaller) T and B lymphocytes (SL), and small lymphocytes are analyzed together, the phenotype and true ploidy of the lymphoma cells may be obscured. However, with FCM the large lymphoma cells can be analyzed separately from the small normal lymphocytes because of light scatter differences. In this example (**top**), the immunophenotype of the lymphoma cells is distinctly monoclonal (CD5+, CD21+, CD19+, CD10+, HLA-DR+, SIg lambda+), whereas the phenotype of the small lymphocytes is that of a mixture of normal T cells and polyclonal B cells. The lymphoma cells double mark for CD19 and CD10 and for SIg lambda and CD21. When the total lymphocyte population is analyzed for DNA content, the DNA cell cycle histogram shows a small shoulder on the right downslope of the diploid G_0G_1 peak (**Upper DNA histogram**). This can easily be missed as an aneuploid population. When the SIg lambda+ population is analyzed separately, there is a well-defined near-diploid (hyperdiploid) population, which can be separated from the diploid population. The latter may represent a small number of normal lymphocytes or a diploid lymphoma stemline, or both. This capacity for multiparameter analysis with identification of subpopulations by size and configurational differences and immunophenotype makes FCM exceedingly useful clinically.

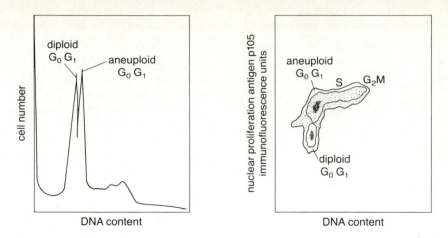

Figure 48–3. DNA cell cycle analysis in conjunction with quantitation of a nuclear proliferation antigen. A near-diploid lymphoma cell population may be partly or completely merged with diploid lymphocytes (***left***). By simultaneously analyzing for DNA content and the quality of nuclear antigen, which is increased in proliferating or activated cells, the two populations may be separated (***right***).

Cytogenetic information can help confirm a neoplastic or preneoplastic state, although the absence of a demonstrable karyotypic change does not rule out neoplasia. Certain nonrandom chromosomal abnormalities are so characteristic that they help establish a specific diagnosis [eg, the t(8;14) translocation of Burkitt's lymphoma; the trisomy 12 of B-CLL]. Prognostic value may also be provided as in ALL, in which the Ph-positive and t;11 subgroups have been shown to have a particularly poor prognosis, whereas cases with a normal karyotype or a chromosome count of 50–55 have a better than average prognosis.

Studies of Burkitt's lymphoma may explain the role of oncogenes in neoplasia and tumorigenesis. By a combination of cytogenetic and molecular genetic techniques, it has been demonstrated that translocations involving chromosomes 8 and 14, 8 and 22, or 2 and 8 result in a transcription of the active and rearranged immunoglobulin gene brought into juxtaposition with the so-called c-*myc* proto-oncogene, the human homolog of the retroviral v-*myc* oncogene. In the common t(8;14) translocation, the c-*myc* gene is translocated from its normal location on chromosome 8 to the immunoglobulin heavy chain locus on the long arm of chromosome 14 at band q32. In the other 2 translocations, 8 to 22 and 2 to 8, an immunoglobulin light chain locus is brought adjacent to c-*myc*. These rearrangements appear to bring the c-*myc* proto-oncogene under the influence of enhancers in or adjacent to the immunoglobulin loci, resulting in deregulation of expression of the *myc* gene and a presumed critical role in the altered growth of the neoplastic B cells. Studies in other patients have suggested that 2 new oncogenes on chromosomes 11 and 18 (*bcl-1* and *bcl-2*) may be activated in a manner similar to that of the c-*myc* gene in Burkitt's lymphoma.

Karyotypic studies indicating a clonal nature for T cell proliferations are less common, but occasionally they provide some prognostic or diagnostic information. Nonrandom karyotypic changes seem to be less frequent in T cell proliferations, but patterns are emerging. Some abnormalities are identical to those seen in B cell neoplasms (Table 48–5), including translocations to the terminal portion of the long arm of chromosome 14 (band q32) and deletions in the long arm of chromosome 6. In certain cases of T cell leukemia with a t(18;14) (q24;q11) translocation, a portion of the T cell receptor gene is brought into juxtaposition with the c-*myc* gene, with resultant deregulation similar to that seen in Burkitt's lymphoma involving the immunoglobulin genes.

MOLECULAR GENETICS

Many of the limitations of determining monoclonality of lymphoid neoplasms have been overcome by detection of rearrangements of DNA which assemble the antigen-specific receptor genes in B or T cells (see Chapters 6 and 10). The immunoglobulin and T cell receptor genes are composed of multiple, separated gene subsegments in their germ line or embryonic state. During development of the lymphoid system, this DNA recombination process assembles the components of the immunoglobulin genes in B cells and the T cell receptor genes in T cells. Much of what is known about these rearrangements was obtained from studies of lymphoid neoplasms. In turn, these studies have led to increased knowledge about the clonality, stage of development, and pathogenesis of leukemias and lymphomas.

Table 48–5. Common chromosomal translocation and other abnormalities in neoplasms.

Neoplasm	Translocation[1]
B cell neoplasms Burkitt's lymphoma	t(8;14) (q24;q32) t(8;22) (q24;q11) t(2;8) (p11;q24)
Multiple myeloma, B-CLL, small lympho- cytic lymphoma, dif- fuse large cell lymphoma	t(11;14) (q13;q32)
B-CLL	t(2;14) p11;q32) t(8;14) (q24;q11) t(14;17) (q32;q23)
Small cleaved FCC, diffuse and follicular large cell lymphoma	t(14;18) (q32;q21)
T cell neoplasms pre-T-ALL	t(11;14) (p13;q11)
T-CLL	t(14;14) (q11;q32) inv(14) (q11;q32)
ATL	inv(14) (q11;q32) t(9;21) (p24;q21) t(12;14) (q24;q11) del(6q)

**Acute lymphocytic
leukemia**
	Ph't(9,22) Philadelphia chromo-
	some
	t(10;14) (q24-5;q11)
	t(8q−;14q+)
	t(8;14) (q24;q11)
	14 q+
	t(11;14) (p13;q11)
	t(11;14) (q23;q32)
	t(4;11) (q21;q23)
	t(4q−;11q+)
	del(9p)
	del(6q)
	del(12p), t(12p)
	  Hypodiploidy (< 46 chromo-
	somes)
	  Pseudodiploidy (46 chromo-
	somes)
	  Hyperdiploidy (47–50 chromo-
	somes)
	  Hyperdiploidy (> 50 chromo-
	somes)

[1]t(8;14), Translocation from chromosome 8 to chromosome 14; (q24;q32), chromosome band q24 on chromosome 8 translocated to band q32 on chromosome 14.

Because there is a developmental order in the immunoglobulin and T cell receptor gene rearrangements during early B and T cell maturation, this information provides new means of categorizing neoplasms. Demonstration of clonality of a presumed tumor has been largely limited to the demonstration of the exclusive presence of one immunoglobulin light chain (κ or λ) in B cell neoplasms. No comparable marker of clonality has been available for T cell neoplasms. Normal or reactive B or T lymphocytes are polyclonal in origin and possess numerous immunoglobulin or T cell receptor gene rearrangements. A monoclonal neoplastic proliferation, however, represents the progeny of a single cell, so that all cells of the clone possess the same rearrangement. Therefore, it is possible to detect clonality for both B and T lymphocytes in a more sensitive manner then by immunophenotyping.

The developmental sequence of immunoglobulin and T cell receptor gene rearrangement has been derived from studies of fetal thymus and T- and B-ALL. So called non-T, non-B ALLs represent distinct stages of early B cell development, even though the cells lack expression of surface immunoglobulin. These tumors have a sequence of heavy chain rearrangement before light chains and κ light chain before λ. In T-ALL the β T cell receptor genes are rearranged early in intrathymic ontogeny before the α T cell receptor genes. Most T-ALLs have a rearranged β chain gene and express the β T cell receptor, but only half are mature enough to express the α T cell receptor. More mature ALLs express a complete CD3-Ti receptor complex.

Although these immunoglobulin and T cell receptor gene rearrangements are used to determine the lineage of a particular neoplasm, there is not complete lineage fidelity, because there is normal crossover of both immunoglobulin and T cell receptor gene rearrangements into the opposite lymphocyte lineage. This infidelity may represent remnants of an early process occurring before absolute lineage commitment. However, by combining immunoglobulin gene and T cell receptor gene rearrangements with immunophenotyping, almost all leukemias and lymphomas can be assigned to the correct lineage. Some neoplasms that arise from very early, uncommitted progenitor cells and have only germ line DNA may not be classifiable by these techniques.

Lineage Infidelity versus Promiscuity

Leukemias and lymphomas are neoplasms that have a monoclonal origin and represent maturation arrests or uncoupling of proliferation and differentiation. Nevertheless, examples of lineage infidelity in which leukemic cells simultaneously express markers of 2 different cell lines (T and B lymphocytes or lymphoid and myeloid cells) exist. Some of these cases of so-called lineage infidelity may be explained by technical or other limitations. The first limitation is inadequate evaluation of monoclonal antibodies for cell specificity. Very few antigens are cell type- or lineage-restricted, but the lack of an extensive initial screening of normal cells with the antibodies has resulted in initially incorrect reports of specificity (eg, CD5 antigen is present on normal T cells but also on a subset of normal B cells and on B-CLL cells; CD4 antigen is present not only on T cells but also on monocytes). The second is that monoclonal antibodies are not monospecific. As with other antibodies, they are potentially able to cross-react with a variety of antigenic determinants because specificity is the result of the relative affinity of antibody-combining sites, so that antigen specificity is never absolute. In addition, they may bind by their Fc rather than Fab regions. The third is that before a particular leukemic cell type can be related to a normal progenitor cell population, the immunophenotype of the latter must be known. This knowledge is relatively complete for known major subsets of differentiated cells, but small subsets have been recognized only retrospectively from comparison with leukemic phenotypes (eg, CD5$^+$ normal B cells recognized because of CD5$^+$ B-CLL cells). Information about phenotypes of stem or early progenitor cells is incomplete.

Nevertheless, these technical problems do not explain all of the examples of apparent infidelity, such as examples of immunoglobulin gene rearrangement in T cell and myeloid leukemias or T cell receptor gene rearrangement or expression in non-T cell leukemias. A proposed explanation by Greaves is that early, multipotential progenitor cells undergo simultaneous, incomplete gene rearrangements for immunoglobulin heavy chain, T cell receptor β gene, etc, so that if neoplastic clones arise from these cells, they may show similar mixed-gene rearrangements and expressions, not limited to immunoglobulin and T cell receptor. Greaves labeled this "lineage promiscuity," a transient phase of promiscuity of gene expression by bi- or multipotential progenitor cells, which may persist in leukemias and lymphomas arising from these precursor cells. Once cells are committed to a particular cell line, and this commitment may be influenced by external factors such as cytokines, they will express antigens, enzyme receptors, and other markers according to the lineage commitment, ie, lineage fidelity.

THERAPY

The therapy of neoplasms of the immune system is a combination of treating symptoms and signs (supportive) and administering cytotoxic therapy with multiple chemical agents in combination with radiation therapy and surgery. Most patients are treated on prescribed protocols, which vary somewhat from center to center and have different degrees of success depending on the type of neoplasm and associated organ and damage. Cytotoxic or other antitumor drugs in general affect DNA synthesis and are used in combination and in various delivery sequences to affect the maximum number of cells in the S phase. The fact that proliferating cells are more vulnerable to cytotoxic therapy may explain why cure rates may be better with aggressive neoplasms than with low-grade ones. The latter may have an indolent, prolonged course in which remission may be readily induced but is often short-lived.

Monoclonal Antibody Therapy

In principle, treating neoplasms with highly specific monoclonal antibodies directed at lymphoma or leukemia antigens has great appeal. However, attempts to treat lymphoma and lymphocytic leukemia patients with monoclonal antibodies have had variable results. Generally, there has been relatively little initial effect, with only transient improvement in lesions, but there have also been relatively minor side effects, less than might have been expected since the antibodies are of mouse origin. Inherent problems of monoclonal antibody therapy exist because (1) potential modulation of the cell surface antigen may be induced by exposure to the antibody; (2) circulating shed tumor antigen may bind antibody and prevent it from reaching the tumor cells; and (3) the production of antimouse antibodies may lead to antibody neutralization or allergic reactions. These drawbacks to immunotherapy are also a factor when monoclonal antibodies are conjugated to chemical toxins or radioisotopes in order to direct them to the neoplastic cells. Nevertheless, monoclonal antibodies conjugated to radioisotopes for tumor imaging have been used with some success.

An initially exciting approach to therapy is the use of monoclonal antibodies directed against an individual patient's own tumor immunoglobulin idiotype. Because lymphoma cells from some patients express more than one idiotype, and these may change over time, the necessity for using more than one anti-idiotype antibody is clear. Encouraging recent studies have demonstrated that monoclonal antibodies made against one patient's immunoglobulin idiotype may also recognize immunoglobulin idiotypes from other patients' neoplasms.

An area in which monoclonal antibodies against leukemia- and lymphoma-associated antigens are clearly useful is in the purging of bone marrow samples used for autologous bone marrow transplantion. Identification of the leukemia and lymphoma cells in the bone marrow of a patient in remission and their removal by the use of the same specific monoclonal antibodies (with complement or antibodies conjugated to toxins) allows tumor-free marrow to be reintroduced into the patient following total body irradiation. This approach has been used in patients with ALL, purging the marrow with combinations of antibodies to differentiation antigens or common acute lymphocytic leukemia antigen (CALLA) with complement. Patients with non-Hodgkin lymphoma have also been treated in this way, but it is important that the antibodies used to destroy the lymphoma and leukemia cells in bone marrow should not also destroy normal progenitor cells.

Some problems yet unresolved include localization of monoclonal antibodies exclusively in the neoplasm, the response of the host to his or her own tumor antigens, antigenic heterogeneity, and tumor modulation. Therefore, the ultimate value of this approach cannot be completely assessed. It would appear that the major use of these antibodies may lie in radioimaging, bone marrow purging, and combined treatment in which they are used to eliminate small residual neoplastic cells after chemotherapy or radiotherapy.

LYMPHOCYTIC NEOPLASMS OF B CELL ORIGIN

B cell neoplasms are much more common than T cell neoplasms in the USA and Europe. They arise in all lymphoid areas of normal B cell production (Table 48–6) and in some nonlymphoid tissues. Diagnosis is usually straightforward because of monoclonal immunoglobulins in serum or urine and on the surface or cytoplasm of the cells and because of the distinctive morphologic features of the FCC and plasmacytoid types. Because the majority of these B cell neoplasms arise from the follicular centers of lymphoid tissues, many retain a follicular growth pattern. The variation in morphology and clinical expression reflects the varying predominance of different stages of the cell cycle and transformation from small lymphocytes to large proliferating (transformed) lymphocytes. In most instances, patients

with B cell neoplasms are initially diagnosed with disease involving bone marrow or lymph nodes. When there is extensive bone marrow involvement, the cells frequently circulate in the peripheral blood and disseminate widely throughout lymphoid tissues. In B cell neoplasms such as multiple myeloma or plasmacytoid lymphocytic lymphomas, production of excessive quantities of immunoglobulins can be easily detected. Most patients with B cell neoplasms do not initially have splenomegaly or pancytopenia, and those who do usually have hairy cell leukemia.

Nonlymphoid tissue involvement by B cell lymphomas is common, particularly in the thyroid, gastrointestinal tract, salivary glands, and conjunctiva. Neoplasms of small lymphocytes and plasma cells can be morphologically identified, but less highly differentiated cells (pre-B-ALL) can be identified as B cells only by immunophenotyping. Small and transformed B lymphocytes cannot always be distinguished from small and transformed T lymphocytes cytologically, but they can be distinguished by immunophenotyping. Neoplasms such as small and large noncleaved FCC lymphomas and pre-B-ALL are predominantly actively dividing and show minimal differentiation. Cleaved FCC lymphomas, B-CLL, and hairy cell leukemia characteristically have few dividing cells and show minimal plasmacytic differentiation. Multiple myeloma and plasmacytoid lymphocytic lymphomas are predominantly differentiated, with small proliferating populations. Immunoblastic sarcomas of B cells are composed prima-

Table 48–6. Most common neoplasms of the immune system in different tissues.

Tissue	T Cell Neoplasm[1]	B Cell Neoplasm[1]	Mononuclear Phagocyte System[1]	Unknown[1]
Bone marrow	ALL	ALL, Small lymphocytic (B-CLL) multiple myeloma	ANLL	
Lymph nodes		SC FCC, LC FCC		Hodgkin's disease (LP, NS, MC)
Spleen		SC FCC, hairy cell leukemia	CML, ANLL	Hodgkin's disease (NS)
Thymus	HD, NS convoluted T-ALL			
Pharynx (Waldenström's myeloma)		SC FCC, LC FCC, LNC FCC		
Gonads		SNC FCC, IBS-B		
Lung		SC FCC, plasmacytoid		
Stomach and intestine		LNC FCC, IBS-B, plasmacytoid, SNC, LNC		
Skin	Cutaneous T cell lymphoma (cerebriform), MF, Sézary, IBS-T, Small T lymphocyte	Small B lymphocyte		
Conjunctiva		SC FCC, plasmacytoid		
Thyroid		LNC FCC, IBS-B, plasmacytoid		
Salivary gland		SC FCC		
Bone		SNC FCC (Burkitt), ALL		
Central nervous system	T-ALL	IBS-B, SNC FCC		

[1]Abbreviations: convoluted T, Convoluted T cell lymphoma or leukemia; ANLL, Acute nonlymphocytic leukemia; SC, small cleaved; LC, large cleaved; LNC, large noncleaved; SNC, small noncleaved; CML, chronic myelogenous leukemia; MF, mycosis fungoides; LP, lymphocyte predominance; NS, nodular sclerosis; MC, mixed cellularity; LD, lymphocyte depleted.

rily of transformed proliferating cells with various degrees of differentiation. The clinical features of B cell neoplasms relate to their proliferative rate, immunoglobulin production (hypo or hyper), and replacement of functioning cells in the bone marrow or other lymphoid tissues. Chromosomal abnormalities may also occur.

ACUTE LYMPHOCYTIC LEUKEMIA (ALL)

The etiology of acute leukemia in humans is still unknown, although implicating factors include RNA retroviruses, ionizing radiation, chemicals such as benzene, and genetic factors. Chromosomal abnormalities are detectable in some clinically healthy family members of patients with acute leukemia. Leukemic cells accumulate in bone marrow, blood, and other tissues, resulting in suppression of hematopoietic function with associated anemia, thrombocytopenia, and granulocytopenia. Infiltration of the central nervous system, liver, spleen, lungs, and other tissues adds to the expression and severity of the disease.

Improved understanding of the immunologic heterogeneity and biology of ALL has led to revisions in therapy. For example, the homing of normal T lymphocytes to tissues such as the central nervous system and testes has explained the frequent relapses involving these extramedullary sites in T-ALL and has shown the need for more focused and aggressive chemotherapy than is needed in "common ALL."

Common ALL or Pre-B-ALL

Most cases of ALL that do not type as T cells fall into this group—the most common neoplasm of childhood. Onset is typically between the ages of 2 and 10 years; however, the disease may occur in individuals in their 30s and 40s. The incidence is higher in males than in females.

A. Clinical Features: Patients present with weakness, fatigue, bleeding, bruising, fever, chills, and infections. Bone and joint pain are common, and central nervous system symptoms due to increased intracranial pressure may be present. Pronounced leukocytosis, anemia, and thrombocytopenia are usual.

B. Pathology: This leukemia is characterized by massive marrow infiltration with blast cells, and massive marrow necrosis may be present. Hepatosplenomegaly and lymphadenopathy are common. Nuclei are round with fine nuclear chromatin and indistinct nucleoli. Relapses in the marrow are usually focal, but the testes may be involved.

C. Immunologic Features: Patients with acute leukemia may have decreased delayed hypersensitivity and variable immunoglobulin levels. Infections are common and life-threatening. Prognosis may re-

late in part to abnormalities in immune function as indicated by decreased lymphocyte phytohemagglutinin responses in vitro and depressed delayed hypersensitivity skin test reactions, both of which are reflections of poor cellular immunity. In both T and B cell acute leukemias, immune cell functions may be suppressed because of replacement of normal lymphocytes, an imbalance in regulatory cells, or production of immunosuppressive factors (Tables 48–2 and 48–4).

D. Differential Diagnosis: This includes granulocytic leukemia, other types of ALL, and metastatic neuroblastoma.

E. Therapy: Current multiagent therapy produces remission in 90–95% of childhood patients, with most achieving prolonged remission and apparent cure. Poor prognosis is associated with an onset at younger than 2 years or older than 10 years of age, leukocytosis in excess of 200,000/μL, and involvement of the central nervous system at diagnosis; black patients also have a poor prognosis.

B-ALL

A. Clinical Features: B-ALL is the least common and most aggressive form of ALL. Incidence is greater in males than in females. The median age of onset is 13 years, older than for common ALL of childhood. Extensive marrow involvement and leukemia in cases of small noncleaved FCC lymphoma, Burkitt's type, may be diagnosed as B-ALL. Marrow failure from infiltration and systemic symptoms is common. Lymphadenopathy, hepatosplenomegaly, bone involvement, neurologic abnormalities due to central nervous system infiltration, and abdominal masses are frequent. Circulating leukemia cells may account for 80% of leukocytes of 20,000–30,000/μL. Anemia, thrombocytopenia, and uricacidemia are common.

B. Pathology: In sections of involved tissues and in peripheral blood, blast cells are similar to those seen in other forms of ALL.

C. Immunologic Features: See Tables 48–2 and 48–4.

D. Differential Diagnosis: This includes small noncleaved FCC lymphoma (Burkitt's type), other types of ALL, and acute granulocytic leukemia.

E. Therapy: Combination chemotherapy may result in complete remission but is usually followed by rapid relapse, so survival is usually less than 6 months from diagnosis.

SMALL LYMPHOCYTIC LYMPHOMAS & LEUKEMIAS

A. Clinical Features: The onset is generally in elderly individuals (older than 55 years) and occurs more often in males than in females. Initial manifestations are lymphadenopathy or B-CLL. Patients may be initially asymptomatic or may present with fatigue, weakness, thrombocytopenia, hemolytic anemia, and hypogammaglobulinemia. Although most have disseminated disease at diagnosis, the course is usually indolent and prolonged, with survival for 7–10 years with no initial therapy and only conservative therapy thereafter. The staging of B-CLL correlates with survival: stage 0, lymphocytosis in blood and marrow; stage 1, lymphocytosis and lymphadenopathy; stage 2, lymphocytosis and hepatomegaly with or without splenomegaly; stage 3, lymphocytosis with anemia; stage 4, lymphocytosis with thrombocytopenia. Approximately 1% of patients transform to immunoblastic sarcoma of B cell type (Richter's syndrome), and aggressive terminal infection is common.

B. Pathology: There is diffuse involvement of superficial lymph nodes, bone marrow, spleen, liver, other tissues, and blood. Neoplastic cells are small, round lymphocytes with dense chromatin and scanty cytoplasm. Transformed lymphocytes and mitotic figures are seen in the pale, so-called proliferation centers.

C. Immunologic Features: See Tables 48–2 and 48–4.

D. Differential Diagnosis: This includes small cleaved FCC lymphoma, plasmacytoid lymphocytic lymphoma, small T cell lymphocytic lymphoma (T-CLL), hairy cell leukemia, and Hodgkin's disease.

E. Therapy: Because of the indolent course, aggressive multiagent therapy is contraindicated. Patients managed conservatively survive 7–10 years or more.

PROLYMPHOCYTIC LEUKEMIA

Prolymphocytic leukemia is an uncommon variant of CLL. It differs from small cell CLL in that the leukemic cells are larger with more cytoplasm and a prominent nucleolus, and response to therapy is poor. Approximately two-thirds have the phenotype of B cells and one-third have that of T cells. Surface immunoglobulin staining is more intense than is seen in B-CLL, but the cells generally express HLA-DR, CD20, and CD19, as do B-CLL cells, but they do not form rosettes with mouse erythrocytes and are CD5 negative. Most cases of T prolymphocytic leukemia are CD4 but not CD8. A small number of patients with B-CLL develop prolymphocytic leukemia after 1–5 years; this is followed by a more aggressive course.

FOLLICULAR CENTER CELL (FCC) LYMPHOMAS

These lymphomas usually arise from follicular centers in lymph nodes, spleen, tonsils, or intestines. They usually develop in superficial or retroperitoneal lymph nodes, but occasionally in other tissues such as thyroid or stomach. The predominant cell may be a dormant small lymphocyte (cleaved) or transformed lymphocyte (noncleaved). The majority of non-Hodgkin lymphomas are FCC in origin. However, histologically, they may have a follicular or diffuse pattern, and they often change from follicular to diffuse over time. The indolent disease associated with the small cleaved type frequently changes to more rapidly proliferating aggressive disease. Although the cells all arise in the lymphoid follicles, there is a great range of expressions so that the different cell types closely resemble the stages in lymphocyte transformation that occur in the germinal centers of the follicles in response to antigen. Partial lymph node involvement occurs early in the disease, and the size and shape of the cells vary according to cell type or stage in transformation.

1. SMALL CLEAVED FCC LYMPHOMAS

A. Clinical Features: These lymphomas make up 20–30% of the lymphomas in the USA and most commonly occur in males 50–60 years of age. Asymptomatic peripheral lymphadenopathy is a common initial finding, and disseminated disease is usually present at diagnosis. However, the course is indolent, with survivals of 7–10 years with little or no therapy. About half of the cases progress to an aggressive noncleaved FCC lymphoma, which responds poorly to current therapy.

B. Pathology: A follicular growth pattern is seen in most cases, but there is interfollicular infiltration by the small cleaved cells, and perinodal extension is common. Lymph node, bone marrow, spleen, and hepatic portal areas are often involved, with occasional massive necrosis. Other tissue involvement is uncommon. Homogeneous infiltrates of small cells with irregular nuclear indentions, deep cleavage planes, and scanty cytoplasm are characteristic and distinctive.

C. Immunologic Features: See Tables 48–2 and 48–4.

D. Differential Diagnosis: This includes follicular hyperplasia, small lymphocytic lymphoma (T or B cell), plasmacytoid lymphocytic lymphoma, and large cleaved FCC lymphomas.

E. Therapy: Little or no therapy is necessary in asymptomatic individuals for 3–4 years, but after that time chemotherapy may be indicated as the disease progresses.

2. LARGE CLEAVED FCC LYMPHOMAS

A. Clinical Features: These lymphomas account for approximately 5% of lymphoid neoplasms and 10% of FCC lymphomas in the USA. They are more common in males, and the mean age of onset is 50 years. There is peripheral and retroperitoneal lymphadenopathy, splenomegaly, hepatomegaly, and involvement of the gastrointestinal tract and bone marrow. Widely disseminated disease is common at diagnosis, and systemic symptoms are common. The disease is indolent or moderate in its rate of progression.

B. Pathology: There is follicular or diffuse involvement of peripheral, mesenteric, and retroperitoneal lymph nodes. Sclerosis is common in involved tissues, including extranodal masses. The nuclei vary widely in size and configuration, but are frequently large and irregular with deep cleavage planes. They may be hyperlobated and mistaken for Reed-Sternberg cells. The cytoplasm is indistinct but methyl green-pyronine (MGP)-positive, and there may be occasional cases with cytoplasmic immunoglobulin inclusions. Small cleaved cells and reactive plasma cells are variably present.

C. Immunologic Features: See Tables 48–2 and 48–4.

D. Differential Diagnosis: This include small cleaved FCC lymphoma, large noncleaved FCC lymphoma, Hodgkin's disease, nodular sclerosis, and metastatic carcinoma with sclerosis.

E. Therapy: Optimal therapy is yet to be determined, and the disease may be more indolent than was initially thought.

3. SMALL NONCLEAVED FCC LYMPHOMAS

Small noncleaved FCC lymphomas are characterized by rapidly enlarging lymph nodes or extradonal masses, and occasionally there is leukemia resembling B-ALL. Most show a diffuse pattern of involvement, and tumor masses obliterate the normal architecture of lymph nodes and other tissues. Necrosis may be pronounced. The cells are small transformed lymphocytes with variable nuclear size and many mitoses. A "starry-sky" appearance is present in most cases, owing to large, pale "tingible-body" macrophages.

Burkitt Type
A. Clinical Features: This disease is endemic in equatorial Africa, but the incidence in the USA and Europe is low. The African disease is associated with Epstein-Barr virus (EBV) as a probable cause. These lymphomas are more common in males than females, with an average age at onset of 7 years. There is prominent, massive involvement of the jaw, ovaries, kidneys, liver, mesentery, and central nervous system.

Cases in the USA are not associated with EBV and arise in slightly older children (11 years), again more commonly in males than in females. Common involvement of the ileocecal region results in intussusception and obstruction. Peripheral lymph nodes, kidneys, ovaries, mesentery, bone marrow, and central nervous system are less frequently involved. Children older than 13 years at onset have a poorer prognosis than younger children.

B. Pathology: The lymphoma cells are uniform in size with small nuclei and MGP-positive cytoplasm containing lipid vacuoles.

C. Immunologic Features: See Tables 48–2 and 48–4.

D. Differential Diagnosis: This includes large noncleaved FCC lymphoma, immunoblastic sarcoma (B cell), convoluted T cell lymphoma and leukemia, granulocytic sarcoma, and carcinoma with "starry-sky" appearance.

E. Therapy: Response to cyclophosphamide therapy may be dramatic, but depends upon the size of the tumor and the age of the patient, with older children having a poorer prognosis.

Non-Burkitt Type
A. Clinical Features: This type makes up approximately 6% of lymphomas in the USA, with a median onset at 50 years of age (range, 10–70 years). Males and females are equally involved. There is peripheral lymphadenopathy and widespread disease in the great majority of cases, with bone marrow, central nervous system, gastrointestinal tract, and liver involvement. A B-ALL-like leukemia is seen occasionally.

B. Pathology: The non-Burkitt type is distinguished from the Burkitt type by the variable nuclear size and shape. Large noncleaved cells are infrequently present.

C. Immunologic Features: See Tables 48–2 and 48–4.

D. Differential Diagnosis: This is the same as for the Burkitt type (above).

E. Therapy: Multiagent chemotherapy is generally ineffective, with a median survival time of approximately 1 year.

4. LARGE NONCLEAVED FCC LYMPHOMAS

A. Clinical Features: Approximately 6% of lymphoid neoplasms and 12% of FCC lymphomas in the USA are of this cell type. Males are more frequently affected than are females; the median age of onset is 54 years (range, 18–90 years). Three-quarters of the patients present with lymphadenopathy, pain, and systemic symptoms. The gastrointestinal tract, particularly the small intestine, is commonly involved. Fewer patients have central nervous system disease with masses or lymphomatous meningitis. Bone marrow involvement is relatively infrequent.

B. Pathology: Lymph nodes are diffusely involved in most cases, but there is extranodal involvement also. The cells are homogeneous with generally round nuclei, but occasional binuclear and multinuclear cells may be confused with Reed-Sternberg cells. Nuclei have fine dispersed chromatin, and nucleoli are prominent. MGP-positive cytoplasm is abundant.

C. Immunologic Features: See Tables 48–2 and 48–4.

D. Differential Diagnosis: This includes small noncleaved FCC lymphoma, large cleaved FCC lymphoma, immunoblastic sarcoma (B or T cell), granulocytic sarcoma, and carcinoma.

E. Therapy: Multiagent chemotherapy (bleomycin, doxorubicin, cyclophosphamide, vincristine, and prednisone) produces remission in approximately three-quarters of patients with disseminated disease. Complete response is generally followed by disease-free survival, but relapses may occur months or years later.

IMMUNOBLASTIC SARCOMA OF THE B CELL TYPE (IBS-B)

A. Clinical Features: This disease often arises from small lymphocytic neoplasms or from chronic immune disorders and accounts for 3–4% of lymphoid neoplasms in the USA. The onset is commonly in the fifth decade, with equal incidence in males and females. Approximately one-third of patients have a history of prior immune disease, such as congenital immune deficiency syndrome and autoimmune disease (Wiskott-Aldrich syndrome, X-linked immunoproliferative disease, acquired autoimmune disease, Sjögren's syndrome, rheumatoid arthritis, AIDS, immune deficiency related to organ transplant, and immunoblastic lymphadenopathy). Other patients have histories of other lymphocytic neoplasms, including B-CLL and plasmacytoid lymphocytic lymphoma. Initial presenting features include peripheral lymphadenopathy and, to a lesser extent, involvement of the gastrointestinal tract, lungs, and brain. Systemic symptoms, including fever, night sweats, and weight loss, are present in more than half of patients at the time of diagnosis. There is mild anemia and absolute lymphocytopenia, and some patients have bone marrow involvement. Occasional patients have monoclonal paraproteinemia or hypogammaglobulinemia.

B. Pathology: Involved organs show diffuse homogeneous populations of large transformed lymphocytes, plasmacytoid immunoblasts, and plasma cells. The cytoplasm is MGP-positive as a result of abundant RNA.

C. Immunologic Features: See Tables 48–2 and 48–4.

D. Differential Diagnosis: This includes immunoblastic sarcoma (T cell), large noncleaved FCC (diffuse), small noncleaved FCC (diffuse), large cleaved FCC (diffuse), granulocytic sarcoma, carcinoma, and benign immunoblastic proliferations in abnormal immune responses.

E. Therapy: Multiagent chemotherapy produces complete remission in about half of all patients, but the overall median survival time is only about 2 years.

HAIRY CELL LEUKEMIA (Leukemic Reticuloendotheliosis)

A. Clinical Features: Approximately 3% of lymphoid neoplasms in the USA and 2% of all leukemias are hairy cell leukemia. Four times as many males as females are affected. The disease is most common in the fifth decade, but the age range is 20–80 years. Commonly, patients present with marrow failure, granulocytopenia and infection, thrombocytopenia and bleeding, and anemia with weakness and fatigue. Splenomegaly occurs in most patients, with pain in the left upper quadrant, and hepatomegaly and lymphadenopathy are common. Occasionally, paraproteinemia and osteolytic lesions are seen. The course of disease varies from a slow, chronic progression to rapid deterioration. Median survival is 5–6 years, with patients most commonly dying from bacterial, fungal, or mycobacterial infections. Circulating hairy cells are not common, and marrow biopsy is used for diagnosis because marrow is difficult to aspirate in this disease.

B. Pathology: There is focal or diffuse involvement of the bone marrow, spleen (red pulp), lymph node (interfollicular), and liver. Cells in bone marrow, spleen, and other organs are larger than lymphocytes, with abundant eosinophilic or clear cytoplasm and oval or dumbbell-shaped nuclei containing fine, even chromatin. Nucleoli are not prominent, and mitotic figures are rare. These cells are closely packed in tissues, so that microvilli are not easily seen, although there is electron-microscopic evidence of interdigitating cytoplasmic processes. Electron microscopy also demonstrates "ribosomal lamellar complexes." Hairy cells in peripheral blood are so called because of hairlike microvillar projections of the cytoplasm, but this feature is not always easily seen and is not specific for these cells. The most useful cytochemical marker is the presence of tartrate-resistant acid phosphatase in the cytoplasm.

C. Immunologic Features: See Tables 48–2 and 48–4.

D. Differential Diagnosis: This includes small lymphocytic lymphoma and leukemia (B or T cell), plasmacytoid lymphocytic lymphoma, multiple myeloma, and mast cell proliferations.

E. Therapy: Splenectomy may produce temporary remissions. Chemotherapy produces variable results.

PLASMACYTOID LYMPHOCYTIC LYMPHOMA

A. Clinical Features: Patients with plasmacytoid lymphocytic lymphoma may or may not have Waldenström's macroglobulinemia. The usual onset of this lymphoma is in the sixth to seventh decade, and males are slightly more commonly affected. Patients with Waldenström's macroglobulinemia show increased plasma viscosity and sometimes the hyperviscosity syndrome caused by an excess of monoclonal IgM. Clinical features are weakness, fatigue, malaise, and anorexia; congestive heart failure; neurologic symptoms such as vertigo, nystagmus, and stupor; and hematologic symptoms such as mucosal hemorrhage and anemia. There may be visual loss as a result of retinal hemorrhages and papilledema. Lymphadenopathy and hepatosplenomegaly are common, but unlike the symptoms of multiple myeloma, bone lesions, pain, and renal failure are rare, although Bence Jones proteinuria occurs in some patients. Lung, skin, or conjunctival infiltrates may be present in patients with plasmacytoid lymphocytic lymphomas. Some of these patients may have no IgM paraproteinemia and no hyperviscosity syndrome, but they may have anemia, fever, night sweats, lymphadenopathy, and extranodal masses. This disease is relatively indolent, and survival for 3–7 years is common with nonaggressive therapy. Some patients may progress to IBS-B.

B. Pathology: Diffuse or focal involvement of lymph node, spleen, bone marrow, and other tissues is common. Small round lymphocytes and plasmacytoid cells with pyroninophylic, periodic acid–Schiff (PAS)-positive cytoplasm are characteristic. PAS-positive immunoglobulin inclusions may be seen in the nucleus (Dutcher bodies) or cytoplasm (Russell bodies). Pale pseudofollicles similar to those seen in B-CLL and plasmacytoid immunoblasts are typically present.

C. Immunologic Features: See Tables 48–2 and 48–4.

D. Differential Diagnosis: This includes small lymphocytic lymphoma (B-CLL), small cleaved FCC lymphoma (diffuse), and reactive lymphocytosis.

E. Therapy: The severe hyperviscosity may occur as a medical emergency, requiring prompt hydration and plasma exchange. The hyperviscosity is due to the high serum concentration of monoclonal IgM, polymer or aggregate formation, cryoprecipitation, antibodies active against serum protein, and erythrocyte abnormalities. Plasmapheresis is effective in removing circulating IgM and offers immediate relief of the symptoms and signs of hyperviscosity. It may be performed on a maintenance schedule until chemotherapy is effective. Oral chlorambucil in low doses is given daily, but if there is no response, intermittent high-dose chlorambucil and prednisone may improve the average life expectancy.

PLASMA CELL NEOPLASMS & DYSCRASIAS

Neoplasms of plasma cells are considered neoplasms of the B lymphocyte system, since they appear to arise from plasmacytoid B lymphocytes. Because these cells are responsible for secreting immunoglobulins, malfunctions of this system result in the excessive production of abnormal immunoglobulins or portions of immunoglobulin molecules. The abnormal immunoglobulin is a product of a single clone of lymphoid cells (plasmacytoid lymphocytes or plasma cells) and is called a paraprotein or myeloma protein; the disease is referred to as a monoclonal gammopathy. These abnormal proteins have typical serum electrophoretic and immunoelectrophoretic patterns (see Chapter 18) and may be associated with neoplastic plasma cells or be secondary to other conditions, such as nonhematopoietic neoplasms, rheumatoid disorders, and chronic inflammatory states. Plasma cell dyscrasias therefore encompass a somewhat confusing spectrum of diseases in that there is evidence that patients may have paraproteins many years before the onset of clinical disease, with no progression to a neoplasm and no clinical evidence associated with the paraprotein. This period may be relatively short in multiple myeloma (2–3 years) or quite long in benign monoclonal gammopathy (25–30 years).

If the disease is suspected on clinical grounds, a complete clinical work-up includes routine laboratory tests, measurements for serum viscosity, radiologic examination, hematologic profile, and renal function tests. Specific immunologic laboratory tests should be performed. The most important of these are serum protein electrophoresis, immunoelectrophoresis, and immunofixation electrophoresis (see Chapter 18), which demonstrate diagnostic, quantifiable patterns of paraproteins. Because some patients may produce cryoglobulins, which will precipitate at low temperatures, serum should be separated at 37 °C. In immunoelectrophoresis, antibodies against the major heavy and light chains are used. One heavy chain class and one light chain type are detected (see Chapter 18). In almost all cases there will be an immunoelectrophoretic precipitin arc for κ and λ light chains similar in electrophoretic mobility to the heavy chain, except in "heavy chain disease," in which κ and λ light chains are not present. Monoclonal κ or λ light chains are excreted in the urine of some patients with multiple myeloma and are designated Bence Jones protein. They may be detected by immunoelectrophoresis or immunofixation electrophoresis of concentrated urine.

MULTIPLE MYELOMA

A. Clinical Features: Diagnosis is based on finding large numbers of cytologically malignant plasma cells in the bone marrow, characteristic lytic bone lesions, and an associated serum or urine monoclonal protein. Approximately 80% of patients have serum paraprotein and 50% have urinary protein. There are reduced levels of nonmyeloma immunoglobulins, and patients have recurrent infections, anemia, and, occasionally, renal failure or hypercalcemia. X-rays show characteristic punched-out lytic bone lesions throughout the skeleton in most patients. Generalized osteoporosis is also common, and spontaneous fractures occur.

Recurrent bacterial infections with pneumococci and gram-negative bacteria are common, particularly terminally. Hypercalcemia may be associated with vomiting, dehydration, uremia, and cardiac arrhythmias and requires rapid rehydration and other therapy. Multiple factors may cause renal failure, including precipitation of paraprotein in the tubules, amyloidosis, hypercalcemia, hyperuricemia, invasion of the kidneys by the neoplastic plasma cells, precipitation of cryoproteins, and, occasionally, the hyperviscosity syndrome and pyelonephritis. Renal disease is most frequent and severe in patients with Bence Jones proteinuria, possibly owing to the toxicity of Bence Jones proteins for renal tubular cells or precipitation at low pH. Hemodialysis or plasmapheresis may maintain the patient until chemotherapy is effective. Acute leukemia, usually monocytic or myelomonocytic, may occur 1–10 years after the diagnosis. Life expectancy following diagnosis of this acute leukemia is short (6 months). Possible etiologies include chromosomal or other abnormalities induced by the cytotoxic chemotherapy or a second neoplasm arising as part of the natural history of the disease. Plasma cell leukemia occurs in a few patients with neoplastic plasma cells in the peripheral blood. If it occurs early in the disease, it may be mistaken for ALL, acute myelogenous leukemia, or mast cell leukemia, but it is recognized by the paraprotein in blood and urine, the lytic bone lesions, the severe hypercalcemia, or renal failure. It may also be a terminal event in multiple myeloma.

B. Pathology: The bone marrow is usually infiltrated with nodules of myeloma cells, although diffuse involvement is occasionally seen. The cells are abnormal plasma cells with abundant MGP- and PAS-positive cytoplasm and nuclei with fine chromatin and single large nucleoli. Mitoses are rare, but patients may develop more malignant disease with mitoses, eg, IBS-B.

C. Immunologic Features: See Tables 48–2 and 48–4.

D. Differential Diagnosis: This includes metastatic cancer to breast, prostate, thyroid, and kidney, as well as other benign or malignant monoclonal gammopathies.

E. Therapy: Therapy is largely supportive, but local radiation therapy may relieve pain and reduce tumor masses. Extensive radiation of multiple sites may produce pancytopenia. About 70% of patients respond to cytotoxic chemotherapy, with increased median survival and improved quality of life. Melphalan, with or without prednisone, is the usual regimen, but cyclophosphamide is also used effectively and, although it has adverse side effects, is less toxic to bone marrow stem cells. Multiple drugs are also used in various combinations as initial therapy for certain patients and for patients in relapse.

SOLITARY PLASMACYTOMA

A solitary plasmacytoma may be found on routine x-ray or in patients who complain of bone pain or pressure on surrounding structures. The disease appears to represent an isolated malignant plasma cell neoplasm that can occur in bone or soft tissues. Bone and extramedullary plasmacytomas are probably different diseases. The former has a higher prevalence of paraproteins and is associated with a poorer prognosis with after progression to multiple myeloma; it may be an early form of multiple myeloma. Extramedullary soft tissue plasmacytomas tend to have a more indolent course, usually show no paraprotein, and only occasionally progress to multiple myeloma. Treatment is generally by surgical excision or local radiotherapy. Recurrence is common and may occur as generalized multiple myeloma.

AMYLOIDOSIS

Deposits of amyloid may be associated with plasma cell neoplasms and dyscrasias. Amyloid is a complex substance. It contains fragments of an immunoglobulin light chain, especially the V region; antibodies directed against this light chain may react with Bence Jones proteins. A nonimmunoglobulin component has a molecular weight of approximately 8000, with 76 amino acids, and is of unknown origin. Another component is a glycoprotein related antigenically to an α_1 globulin present in small amounts in normal human plasma.

Amyloid may arise from (1) the catabolism by macrophages of antigen-antibody complexes; (2) synthesis in situ of whole immunoglobulins or of light chains with reduced solubility; (3) genetic deletions of the light chain gene, producing an anomolous protein with reduced solubility; or (4) separate synthesis of discrete regions of the light chain. Amyloid deposits may be detected in tissues by light microscopy as eosinophilic material on hematoxylin-eosin-stained sections. These deposits are birefringent with polarized light, and electron microscopy shows nonbranching fibrils, 8.5 nm wide and of various lengths. Special stains will selectively stain the material.

A suggested classification is present in Table 48–7.

HEAVY CHAIN DISEASES

Patients with this rare disease complex have paraproteins of one of the 3 major types of heavy chain (γ, μ, or α) in blood and urine; α chain disease is the most common. Immunoelectrophoresis demonstrates that heavy chains, but not light chains, are present. There may be partial deletion of the Fc portion of the heavy chain, deletion in the hinge region, or a combination of the two.

α Chain Disease

Patients commonly present with a severe malabsorption syndrome with chronic diarrhea, steatorrhea, weight loss, and hypocalcemia, and they may have lymphadenopathy. The small intestine is infiltrated with plasma cells, lymphocytes, and histiocytes; these may appear to be benign initially, but as the disease progresses the plasmacytoid cells appear cytologically less mature and extend beyond the lamina propria. α chain disease is associated with abdominal lymphomas in patients living in the Mediterranean area, but the disease may occur in other geographic areas as well. Rare cases of involvement of the respiratory tract instead of the gastrointestinal tract have been reported.

γ Chain Disease

Some patients with this disease may die within weeks of onset, and others may survive for more than 20 years. Commonly, the patients have a lymphoproliferative disorder with hepatosplenomegaly, lymphadenopathy, and uvular and palatal edema. Infection is common and is the usual cause of death. The patients have recurrent fevers, anemia, leukopenia, and atypical circulating lymphocytes.

μ Chain Disease

IgM heavy chain disease is seen in patients with long-standing B-CLL with progressive hepatosplenomegaly.

BENIGN MONOCLONAL GAMMOPATHY

A small percentage of elderly people may have monoclonal serum or urine paraproteins without other evidence of neoplastic disease. Some may later develop multiple myeloma, but the majority do not. The presence of high and increasing serum levels of paraproteins, low serum levels of normal immunoglobulins, and significant amounts of Bence Jones protein in the serum and urine indicate an increased likelihood of developing multiple myeloma within a short period. Although patients with benign uncomplicated monoclonal gammopathy tend to remain asymptomatic, prolonged follow-up is necessary because some of them may develop multiple myeloma or other plasma cell neoplasms many years later.

CRYOGLOBULINEMIA

A variety of serum and plasma proteins precipitate at low temperature. Some of these are nonimmunoglobulin cyroproteins such as cryofibrinogen, C-reactive protein-albumin complex, and heparin-precipitable protein. The cryoimmunoglobulins may precipitate at temperatures as high as 35 °C, so that during collection of blood, the specimen must be maintained at 37 °C to avoid loss of a cryoprecipitated globulin (see Chapter 18). The rate at which the cryoglobulins precipitate may vary from minutes to days. Therefore, detection of cryoglobulins requires observation of the serum at 4 °C for at least 72 hours (see Chapter 18).

Small amounts of polyclonal serum cryoglobulin is normally present in healthy individuals. Three

Table 48–7. Classification of amyloidosis.

	Clinical Type	Sites of Deposition
Familial	Amyloid polyneuropathy (Portuguese, dominant inheritance)	Peripheral nerves, viscera
	Familial Mediterranean fever (recessive)	Liver, spleen, kidneys, adrenals
Generalized	Primary	Tongue, heart, gut, skeletal and smooth muscles, nerves, skin, ligaments
	Associated with plasma cell dyscrasia	Liver, spleen, kidneys, adrenals
	Secondary (infection, inflammation)	Any site
Localized	Lichen amyloidosis	Skin
	Endocrine-related (eg, thyroid carcinoma)	Endocrine organ (thyroid)
Senile		Heart, brain

types of pathologic cryoglobulins have been identified: Type I (25%) includes IgM and occasionally IgG and rarely IgA or Bence Jones protein; type II (25%) includes mixed cryoglobulins with a monoclonal IgM or occasionally IgG or IgA complexed with autologous normal IgG; and type III (50%) includes mixtures of polyclonal IgM and IgG. Patients with monoclonal type I cryoglobulins usually suffer from the symptoms of their underlying disease (eg, multiple myeloma or Waldenström's macroglobulinemia). Patients with type II or III cryoglobulins may have immune complex disease with purpura, arthritis, and nephritis. These immune complexes often fix complement in vivo and in vitro.

Treatment is generally directed against the underlying disease, but avoidance of cold may be necessary to avoid vascular symptoms. Cytotoxic drugs directed against the plasmacytoid cells producing the globulins, with or without prednisone, sometimes produce remissions. Serious complications, such as vascular occlusion and hemorrhage, can be acutely treated by plasmapheresis.

BENIGN HYPERGAMMAGLOBULINEMIC PURPURA

This is a rare disease usually seen in young and middle-aged women. It is characterized by a dependent purpuric rash brought on by exercise or alcohol. Some of these patients have autoimmune disorders, particularly systemic lupus erythematosus or Sjögren's syndrome. The patients characteristically have a monoclonal IgG-κ paraprotein that acts as a rheumatoid factor, forming complexes with circulating IgG. Serum levels of IgA and IgM are normal or increased, and there are no findings of multiple myeloma. Treatment is directed at prevention and correction of the underlying autoimmune disorder. Severe symptoms may warrant plasmapheresis.

LYMPHOCYTIC NEOPLASMS OF T CELL ORIGIN

Evidence for the T cell origin of certain lymphomas and leukemias comes from their location in the thymus and paracortical areas of lymph nodes and from their immunophenotyping as T lymphocytes. Approximately 20% of non-Hodgkin lymphomas and acute lymphocytic leukemias have T cell features. This is a complex group of diseases with marked biologic and clinical heterogeneity. Certain T cell lymphomas, including the cutaneous T cell lymphomas and convoluted T cell lymphoma, are distinct clinical and pathologic entities with defined diagnostic criteria and clinical expressions, but so-called peripheral or nodal T cell neoplasms are heterogeneous. Immunophenotypes of some T cell neoplasms may reflect fetal stages of T cell development, whereas others, such as the cutaneous T cell lymphomas and leukemias, have more differentiated phenotypes (Table 48–3). Still other T cell neoplasms have phenotypes that differ from those of known normal T cell populations and may reflect the neoplastic state of the affected T cells.

T cell lymphomas and leukemias usually arise in bone marrow, thymus, lymph nodes, or skin (Table 48–6). Clinical and pathological distinction between the convoluted T cell lymphomas and the acute lymphoblastic leukemias of T cell type may be difficult, suggesting that they are essentially the same disease. T cell lymphomas arising in lymph nodes are usually diffuse but vary in histology and phenotype. They may be comparable to the FCC lymphomas and IBS-B, in which there are various predominant cell types and transitions to more primitive cells or differentiated cells. In B cell lymphomas, effector B cells (plasmacytoid lymphocytes) are easy to recognize, whereas in T cell neoplasms, dormant resting T cells cannot be distinguished from effector cells other than by functional assays.

A subset of T cell neoplasms involve primarily the skin. The neoplastic cells are characteristic because of their highly irregular (cerebriform) nuclei. However, the diseases produced are frequently disseminated, with involvement of blood, lymph nodes, bone marrow, and viscera, and it appears that the neoplastic cells originate in lymphoid tissues and migrate from the blood to the skin.

T cell neoplasms are generally more aggressive and grow more rapidly than their B cell counterparts. T-ALL and convoluted T cell lymphomas are quite aggressive, disseminating early and widely. The cutaneous T cell lymphomas frequently are indolent initially, but later they transform into aggressive immunoblastic sarcomas. The small T lymphocyte neoplasms (T-CLL) are more aggressive than their B cell counterparts. The more aggressive T cell neoplasms, particularly convoluted T cell lymphomas, are quite sensitive to chemotherapeutic agents, but therapeutically resistant relapses are common.

ACUTE LYMPHOCYTIC LEUKEMIA OF T CELL TYPE (T-ALL)

A. Clinical Features: This leukemia arises from bone marrow and constitutes approximately 20% of childhood ALL in the USA. Males are affected 2–3 times more frequently than females, and the median age at diagnosis is approximately 12 years. Clinical, pathologic, and immunologic features are similar to those of convoluted T cell lymphomas. Early symptoms and signs are of bone marrow failure with anemia, bleeding, thrombocytopenia, and infection.

Mediastinal masses are present in about 50% of patients and produce the superior vena cava syndrome, pleural and pericardial effusions, and cardiac decompensation. Central nervous system involvement, hepatosplenomegaly, peripheral lymphadenopathy, and marked leukocytosis are common; bone tenderness may be present; and serum terminal deoxyribonucleotidyl (TDT) transferase is elevated.

B. Pathology: Tissues show diffuse involvement by cells that typically contain irregular convoluted nuclei with granular, finely stippled nuclear chromatin. The cytoplasm is scant, and there is a wide range in nucleus and cell size. Focal cytoplasmic acid phosphatase activity and coarse granular or blocklike PAS positivity is present in about one-third of cases.

C. Immunologic Features: See Tables 48–3 and 48–4.

D. Differential Diagnosis: This includes convoluted T cell lymphoma, common ALL, "stem cell" leukemia, acute granulocytic leukemia, and neuroblastoma.

E. Therapy: Combination chemotherapy produces complete remission in most patients, and a significant number may achieve long-term disease-free survival; however, because of the predilection for central nervous system involvement, cranial irradiation and intrathecal chemotherapy are important.

CONVOLUTED T CELL LYMPHOMA

These neoplasms appear to be of thymic origin and usually are associated with mediastinal masses. Dissemination is frequent, as is development of a leukemic phase quite similar to T-ALL.

A. Clinical Features: This lymphoma makes up about 10% of all lymphoid neoplasms seen in the USA. It is typically a disease of teenagers and young adults and of males more often than females. A large mediastinal mass with associated symptoms requiring immediate therapy is common. However, it may present as leukemia with a lymphocytosis of greater than 100,000/μL associated with anemia and thrombocytopenia. Peripheral nodes and the central nervous system are commonly involved, the latter in the form of leukemic meningitis or masses. Other tissues may be involved.

B. Pathology: The cells that diffusely infiltrate the various tissues are characterized by nuclear irregularities or convolutions with scalloped nuclear borders or linear subdivisions. The chromatin is dispersed and granular, and nucleoli are inconspicuous. Cytoplasm is scant and typically contains prominent focal acid phosphatase activity. There is a high mitotic rate.

C. Immunologic Features: See Tables 48–3 and 48–4.

D. Differential Diagnosis: This includes small noncleaved FCC lymphoma, T-ALL, and thymoma.

E. Therapy: Emergency radiation therapy is indicated for the mediastinal mass and results in rapid tumor regression. Relapse usually occurs. In the past, survival was approximately 1 year, but therapy comparable to that for childhood ALL with cranial irradiation and intrathecal chemotherapy has produced long-term disease-free survival in approximately half of all patients.

SMALL T LYMPHOCYTE NEOPLASMS (T-CLL)

Adult T Cell Leukemia (ATL)

This disease is common in Japan and is endemic in the southwestern parts of that country. It also occurs in the Caribbean. ATL is associated with the human T cell leukemia virus type I (HTLV-I). Anti-HLTV-I antibodies are found in more than 90% of Japanese patients with ATL in endemic regions, but 10–20% of healthy individuals also have antibodies. Antibodies have also been found in patients in the West Indies and, sporadically, in the USA. ATL occurs primarily in the fifth decade in Japan, although there is a wide age span. Males and females are affected equally. Lymphadenopathy, hepatomegaly, and splenomegaly are common, as are skin lesions. Leukocytosis ranges from 6000 to 480,000/μL. Marrow involvment is minor, but hypercalcemia is common. Response to therapy is poor, with a median survival of less than 1 year.

In the USA the age of onset is earlier than in Japan (mean, 33 years), and males are more commonly affected than females. Peripheral and retroperitoneal but not mediastinal lymphadenopathy is common. Other organs may be involved. Osteoporosis is accompanied by hypercalcemia, but parathormone levels are normal. Multiagent chemotherapy is generally unsuccessful, with a median survival of less than 1 year.

Prolymphocytic Leukemia of T Cell Type (T-PLL)

Elderly males are the most commonly affected by this disease. Splenomegaly is prominent, but hepatomegaly and peripheral lymphadenopathy are less common. CLL therapy is inadequate, as is splenic radiotherapy, with a median survival of less than 6 months.

T-CLL with Cytoplasmic Azurophilic Granules

A. Clinical Features: This is an indolent and protracted disease, with survivals of 10–20 years. Patients are generally in their mid 50s at diagnosis, although there is a wide age distribution. Splenomegaly may be prominent, but hepatomegaly, lymphadenopathy, and skin involvement are uncommon. A lymphocytosis of less than 50,000/μL is common, but neutropenia may result in recurrent infections. This is probably the same disease as large granular lymphocyte/natural killer (NK) cell leukemias (see below).

B. Pathology: The distinction between the more aggressive ATL and T-PLL, on the one hand, and T-CLL, on the other hand, with azurophilic granules is important. ATL cells have irregular (knotty or indented) nuclei. T-PLL cell nuclei have acidophilic chromatin and prominent nucleoli. The T-CLL cells with azurophilic granules are Downey-like cells with prominent azurophilic granules and basophilic nuclear chromatin. Although cytology helps distinguish among the 3 types, a diffuse tissue distribution may occur in all 3 types.

C. Immunologic Features: See Tables 48–3 and 48–4.

D. Differential Diagnosis: This includes small B lymphocytic neoplasms, especially B-CLL.

E. Therapy: Therapy is the same minimal therapy used for B-CLL, and prolonged survival in the absence or limited use of specific therapy is common.

PERIPHERAL T CELL LYMPHOMAS

A. Clinical Features: Neoplasms in this heterogeneous group, which tend to involve lymph nodes, are relatively uncommon. The patients are generally adults presenting with regional or generalized lymphadenopathy, and frequently they have advanced disease at presentation. Retroperitoneal and mediastinal adenopathy is common.

B. Pathology: Involvement of tissues by the neoplastic cells is usually diffuse and uniform. Follicular centers are generally absent in involved lymph nodes. The cell infiltrates contain small and large lymphocytes with abundant clear cytoplasm, mixed with varying numbers of T immunoblasts. The small lymphocytes have irregular twisted nuclei with little cytoplasm, but in immunoblastic sarcoma of T cell type, transformed cells with indented irregular nuclei and conspicuous nucleoli are present. The cytoplasm of the immunoblasts is MGP-positive.

C. Immunologic Features: See Tables 48–3 and 48–4.

D. Differential Diagnosis: This includes IBS-B, large noncleaved FCC lymphoma, and Hodgkin's disease (mixed cellularity).

E. Therapy: The remission rate with multiagent chemotherapy is low, and survival is usually less than 1 year. However, better responses have been observed.

LYMPHOEPITHELIOID LYMPHOCYTIC LYMPHOMA OF T CELL TYPE
(Lennert's Lymphoma)

A. Clinical Features: This is a disease primarily of adult males, with cervical lymphadenopathy and tonsil involvement. It frequently evolves to IBS-T.

B. Pathology: Lymph nodes or tonsils are diffusely infiltrated with small lymphocytes having twisted irregular nuclei. There are clusters of epithelioid macrophages, which are distinct from the scattered individual epithelioid macrophages of the peripheral T cell lymphomas. There may be focal or multifocal immunoblasts. Skin and splenic white pulp are occasionally involved.

C. Immunologic Features: See Tables 48–3 and 48–4.

D. Differential Diagnosis: This includes abnormal immune reactions, Hodgkin's disease (lymphocytic and histiocytic, diffuse), IBS-T, and immunoblastic lymphadenopathy.

E. Therapy: There is some question about whether this is a true lymphoma or a premalignant lymphocytic proliferation that may progress to IBS. Therefore, therapy may be withheld until there is evidence of progression to IBS-T. Because there is resemblance to Hodgkin's disease, some patients have been treated with Hodgkin's disease therapy.

CUTANEOUS T CELL LYMPHOMAS

These include cerebriform T cell lymphomas, mycosis fungoides, and Sézary syndrome.

A. Clinical Features: These neoplasms tend to be initially indolent but may evolve into widespread aggressive lymphomas. The disease occurs in middle age, with males affected more commonly than females. The first manifestation of disease is on the skin. In mycosis fungoides early skin involvement is nonspecific, but in time localized or generalized skin tumors develop. Peripheral and visceral lymphadenopathy and hepatosplenomegaly occur as the skin tumors develop. In the Sézary syndrome there is a generalized pruritic erythroderma with hyperpigmentation and exfoliation. Scaling and fissuring of the skin on the palms and soles are common. Even when the disease appears to be limited to the skin, the characteristic cerebriform cells present in the peripheral blood and lymph nodes provide evidence of more widespread disease.

B. Pathology: The skin is densely infiltrated with leukocytes and other cells, particularly in the epidermis. Characteristic clusters of cells in the epidermis are called Pautrier's abscesses. Lymph nodes may be diffusely infiltrated, but involvement is usually interfollicular and is mixed with the dermatopathic changes associated with skin disease. The predominant cell is usually small, with a "cerebriform" nuclear shape, so called because of extensive convolutions, which give the nuclei the 3-dimensional appearance of brain tissue. Larger dysplastic cells with condensed chromatin are also present, and although transformed T cells are not common in early disease, there may be a transformation in late disease to T immunoblasts. Mitoses are not common until the late, aggressive phase of the disease.

C. Immunologic Features: See Tables 48–3 and 48–4.

D. Differential Diagnosis: This includes inflammatory reactive lymphocytoses of the skin and lymph nodes, small lymphocytic B neoplasms of the skin, other T cell lymphomas involving the skin, and psoriasiform dermatoses.

E. Therapy: During the first 5–10 years of disease, local skin therapy with superficial electron beam irradiation may be helpful for cosmetic improvement of the skin. However, the disease ultimately progresses. With advanced disease, multiagent chemotherapy may produce complete remissions, but survival averages only 1–2 years. Progression to an aggressive lymphoma of the skin or other tissues, which occurs in about 20% of patients, is associated with a poor prognosis.

HODGKIN'S DISEASE

Hodgkin's disease comprises a group of neoplasms initially affecting lymph nodes and later affecting the liver, spleen, bone marrow, and lungs. The neoplastic cells appear to be the Reed-Sternberg cells. Some are mononuclear, but the diagnostic Reed-Sternberg cells are binucleate with huge eosinophilic nuclear inclusions. Hodgkin's disease is quite heterogeneous, with various degrees of expression of the Reed-Sternberg cell component and reacting lymphocytes and histiocytes.

The cell of origin of the Reed-Sternberg cells is still debated among those who favor the monocyte-macrophage, a transformed B or T lymphocyte, or the granulocyte. For many years the disease was considered to be infectious rather than neoplastic because of the clinical course and pathology. However, an infectious etiology has never been proven. It is now considered to be a neoplastic disease. The proliferating cells occasionally show aneuploidy and chromosomal abnormalities, indicating a clonal proliferation.

The pathologic diagnosis of Hodgkin's disease is made on the basis of a distinctive lymphoid tissue reaction, which in some ways resembles a cellular immune response, and the demonstration of the diagnostic Reed-Sternberg cells. Whether the apparent immunologic reaction is directed against T or B lymphocytes, macrophages, or the Reed-Sternberg cells is not clear. On occasion, the extraordinarily reactive lymphocytic component seen in Hodgkin's disease leads to confusion with non-Hodgkin lymphomas. This distinction may be artificial if the Reed-Sternberg cells ultimately prove to be of lymphocytic origin.

A. Clinical Features: There are different histologic and clinical types of Hodgkin's disease, but the most common symptom in all is painless peripheral lymphadenopathy. Cervical and supraclavicular nodes are most commonly involved, and axillary and inguinal node involvement is less common. Systemic symptoms are prominent, particularly in older patients, and imply a worse prognosis. Pruritus and pain in enlarged lymph nodes following alcohol ingestion may occur but do not imply a poor prognosis. Extranodal presentation is not common, and splenomegaly is present in less than 20% of patients. The progression of disease is predictable, spreading from initially involved lymph nodes to contiguous lymphoid tissues, either antegrade or retrograde. There is ultimate dissemination into parenchymal organs, with the liver and lungs most commonly involved. Bone marrow involvement is uncommon. Staging is by physical examination, laboratory analysis, chest x-ray, lymphangiogram, abdominal computed tomogram (CT scan), and liver-spleen scan. The clinical stages (Table 48–8) determine specific treatment.

B. Pathology: The Rye classification divides the histopathology into 4 types: lymphocyte predominance, nodular sclerosis, mixed cellularity, and lymphocyte depletion (Table 48–8). The histopathologic differences reflect the immunologic reaction to the neoplasm and the types of Reed-Sternberg cells. The lymphocyte-predominance, mixed-cellularity, and lymphocyte-depletion types are related, and progression from lymphocyte predominance to depletion occurs in individual patients. The nodular sclerosis type appears to be a different entity. In the lymphocyte-predominance type, the lymphocytosis may be diffuse or nodular, with the diffuse form being more likely to progress to lymphocyte depletion. Some patients initially present with the mixed-cellularity or lymphocyte-depletion type.

C. Immunologic Features: Patients commonly have frequent bacterial infections (*Pneumococcus* or *Haemophilus influenzae*) related to an underlying secondary immunodeficiency involving defective phagocytosis and chemotaxis, as well as a decreased antibody response to certain antigens, although immunoglobulin levels are normal or increased. They are also frequently anergic to delayed hypersensitivity skin test antigens, particularly when lymphocytopenia is severe.

The cellular origin of the diagnostic cell of Hodgkin's disease, the Reed-Sternberg cell, remains a mystery. Other cells (lymphocytes, histiocytes, eosinophils) appear to be reactive components of the lesions, whereas the Reed-Sternberg cell and its mononuclear variants are the true neoplastic cells. A variety of evidence has suggested derivation from B or T lymphocytes, histiocytes, interdigitating reticulum cells, or granulocytes. Recent immunoperoxidase staining with monoclonal antibodies shows

Table 48–8. RYE classification of Hodgkin's disease.

Histologic Subtype	Percentage of US Cases	Predominant Features	Prognosis
Lymphocyte predominance	10	Young adult males, stage 1 or 2 at diagnosis; few Reed-Sternberg cells, good lymphocyte host response, connective tissue bands minimal.	Excellent
Nodular sclerosis	60	Young females, stage 1 or 2 at diagnosis; predominant nodules due to wide bands or birefringent collgen, mediastinal mass, "lacunar" variants of Reed-Sternberg cells.	Excellent
Mixed cellularity	20	Majority with stage 3 or 4 at diagnosis; abdominal involvement common, lymphocytes, plasma cells, eosinophils mixed with Reed-Sternberg cells, diffuse involvement of nodes.	Good
Lymphocyte depletion	10	Older males, stage 3 or 4 at diagnosis; systemic symptoms, prolonged fever of unknown origin, abdominal and bone marrow involvement, numerous Reed-Sternberg cells, diffuse fibrosis, and few lymphocytes, indicating poor host response.	Relatively poor

staining patterns that do not answer the question other than to suggest an origin from the interdigitating reticulum cell or from an unrecognized cell precursor. The diagnostic Reed-Sternberg cells are binucleated with huge inclusionlike nucleoli and pale cytoplasm. They are rarely seen in the lymphocyte-predominance type of disease, but are often present in the nodular-sclerosis type and in some cases of lymphocyte depletion. They are required for diagnosis in the mixed-cellularity type because of lack of other distinctive features. The lymphocytes in Hodgkin's disease show variable immunophenotypic patterns but are generally predominantly T cells and most frequently CD4 T cells. The latter may be so prominent in peripheral blood or lymph nodes as to suggest the neoplastic clonal expansion of CD4 T cells seen in mycosis fungoides and Sézary syndrome, but in Hodgkin's disease they are present because of reactive clonal expansion. Reed-Sternberg cells may also be seen in benign conditions such as infectious mononucleosis, other benign reactive states, and some non-Hodgkin lymphomas. Thus, they are diagnostic of Hodgkin's disease only in the appropriate histological setting.

D. Differential Diagnosis: Lymphocyte-prodominance Hodgkin's disease may be confused with small cleaved FCC lymphomas, toxoplasmosis, and other reactive lymphocytoses. Nodular sclerosis may resemble nodular mixed-cellularity or lymphocyte-depletion Hodgkin's disease, or metastatic carcinoma. The differential diagnosis of mixed-cellularity Hodgkin's disease includes the other types of Hodgkin's disease, immunoblastic lymphadenopathy, lymphoepithelial lymphocytic lymphomas, granulomotous reactions, nodal T cell lymphomas, and reactive lymph node hyperplasia. The lymphocyte-depletion type of Hodgkin's disease must be differentiated from the changes seen in lymph nodes from patients receiving chemotherapy

and immune-deficient states including advanced AIDS. In some cases of lymphocyte depletion, lymph nodes may be replaced by pleomorphic Reed-Sternberg cells, so that the pathology suggests IBS-T, IBS-B, or other pleomorphic neoplasms including carcinomas.

E. Therapy: The clinical prognosis is excellent for the lymphocyte-predominance and nodular sclerosis types of Hodgkin's disease, good for the mixed-cellularity type, and relatively poor for the lymphocyte-depletion type. Therapy in all instances depends upon the histologic type and clinical stage. Staging to determine the extent of disease involves the presence or absence of systemic symptoms such as fever, night sweats, weight loss; blood work including leukocyte, renal, and liver function studies, erythrocyte sedimentation rate, serum copper, and fibrinogen; radiologic examination including lymphangiography and CT scan; biopsy; laparotomy; and splenectomy. After a complete workup, the patient is staged according to the modified Ann Arbor Staging System: stage I, involvement of a single lymph node region; stage II, 2 or more lymph node regions on the same side of the diaphragm; stage IIIa, lymph node regions on both sides of the diaphragm and abdominal disease limited to the upper abdomen, abdomen, colon, spleen, splenic hilar node, celiac node, and hepatic portal node; stage IIIb, lymph node regions on both sides of the diaphragm and abdominal disease including para-aortic, mesenteric, iliac, or inguinal involvement with or without disease in the upper abdomen; stage IV, diffuse or disseminated involvement of one or more extralymphatic organs or tissues, with or without associated lymph node enlargement.

Treatment consists of radiotherapy for localized disease, with the addition of multiagent chemotherapy for disseminated disease, using MOPP (mechlorethamine, vincristine [Oncovin], procarbazine, prednisone). Approximately 75% of all patients with Hodgkin's disease are cured by appropriate therapy. However, because of the long-term survival that ensues, second neoplasms may appear later. These include acute granulocytic leukemia (7%) and non-Hodgkin lymphoma (15%). There is also male and female infertility secondary to chemotherapy, as well as hypothyroidism and bone marrow depression.

NEOPLASMS OF THE MONONUCLEAR PHAGOCYTE SYSTEM

Neoplasms of the mononuclear phagocyte system include acute and chronic monocytic leukemia and the various types of malignant histiocytoses. The latter are a confusing group, because so many different histiocytic processes are usually included. Further confusion is caused by the fact that for many years the Rappaport classification of lymphomas has included a large category of histiocytic lymphomas. Current evidence indicates that true histiocytic neoplasms are rare. To call them "histiocytic lymphomas" is a misnomer, since "lymphoma" by definition means a neoplasm of lymphocytes. Nevertheless, there are true malignant neoplasms of histiocytes, and they have some distinctive morphologic, cytochemical, ultrastructural, and immunophenotypic features. If tumor masses or infiltrates of dysplastic or cytologically malignant histiocytes (mononuclear phagocytes) are present, a diagnosis of true histiocytic lymphoma may be made. However, these proliferations must be distinguished from reactive macrophage infiltrates, benign histiocytes seen in the lipid storage diseases, granulomatous diseases, and metastatic carcinoma cells that may be phagocytic.

HISTIOCYTIC MEDULLARY RETICULOSIS

This is a rare disorder seen primarily in males in their 30s. Clinically, there is wasting, severe hemolytic anemia, fever, weakness, and short-duration weight loss. Peripheral lymphadenopathy, splenomegaly, and hepatomegaly are common, as are nodules and papules of the skin. The hemolytic anemia is apparently due to erythrophagocytosis by the malignant histiocytes, and there is also thrombocytopenia, apparently from splenic sequestration. Leukopenia is common, and, rarely, there is a leukemic phase. Median survival is approximately 6 months, although complete remission has occurred with combination chemotherapy. Central nervous system relapse is common. Three types of histiocytes are seen; all 3 types are found in lymph node sinuses,

splenic red pulp, and the marrow. These include immunoblastlike cells, pleomorphic histiocytes showing erythrophagocytosis, and normal-appearing histiocytes with quite prominent erythrophagocytosis. Lymph nodes frequently show complete filling of the medullary and subcapsular sinuses with neoplastic histiocytes. The cells typically are α-naphthyl acetate esterase-positive and stain by immunoperoxidase techniques with α1-antichymotrypsin and α1-antitrypsin.

The differential diagnosis includes other malignant histiocytoses and virus-associated hemophagocytic syndrome.

OTHER MALIGNANT HISTIOCYTOSES

Very few patients have true histiocytic cancers; however, the clinical disease is very similar to lymphocytic lymphomas. Most patients are males with an average age of onset of 50–60 years, although younger patients have been described. Splenomegaly, peripheral lymphadenopathy, and skin lesions are common, the skin lesions being multiple, rapidly growing, bluish-red nodules. There may be a mild anemia, but laboratory work is generally normal and the bone marrow is only rarely involved. Information about prognosis and therapy is of little use because of the rareness of the disease and the inconsistently applied diagnostic criteria.

Lymph nodes show extensive accumulations of neoplastic histiocytes with abundant eosinophilic cytoplasm and atypical nuclei. Sinusoidal involvement is the usual prominent pattern of growth. In some cases the pattern makes it difficult to distinguish from metastatic carcinoma. Prominent vascular proliferation is common. Individually the cells are indistinguishable from the atypical histiocytes in histiocytic medullary reticulosis. Phagocytic activity is not always a prominent feature, and cytochemical and ultrastructural studies may be necessary to indicate that the neoplastic cells are histiocytes. The cells may be PAS-positive and show nonspecific esterase activity. Muramidase activity may be detected by immunocytochemistry, but this is frequently not helpful. Some of the cells are labeled by α1-antichymotrypsin, but ultrastructural examination is frequently required for diagnosis of the more primitive neoplasms.

A. Differential Diagnosis: This includes IBS-B, IBS-T, soft tissue sarcomas, metastatic carcinoma, histiocytic medullary reticulosis, and a range of non-neoplastic histiocytoses (histiocytosis X).

B. Immunologic Features: The well-differentiated histiocytic tumors generally stain with the antibodies Leu M1,CD11c (Leu M5), CD14 (My4), CD13 (My7), My8, CD33 (My9), CD11b (OKM1), Leu M3; however, they are negative with CD15 (Leu M1) and Ki-1. Intermediately differentiated tumors may show Leu M1 staining and are generally CD15

(Leu M3), CD11c (Leu M5), CD14 (My4), CD13 (My7), My8 and CD11b (OKM1)-positive; but are Ki-1-negative and show a mixed pattern with My9. The undifferentiated types are quite rare and have not been completely phenotyped; however, they may be Leu M1-positive.

ACUTE MYELOMONOCYTIC LEUKEMIA

Acute myelomonocytic leukemia accounts for about 20–30% of the acute myeloid leukemias in the USA. Males and females are affected equally, with an average age of onset of 55 years. The disease is quite rare in children. Patients present with bone marrow failure and anemia, thrombocytopenia, hemorrhage, and infection. Some complain of bone and joint pain. Up to 50% will have hepatosplenomegaly and adenopathy. Leukocyte counts tend to be in the range of 55,000/μL, with a high proportion of blast cells. The response to multiagent chemotherapy is generally poor, with a median duration of complete response of 10 months.

The bone marrow is generally heavily infiltrated with immature granulocytes and monocytes. Monocyte progenitors, myeloblasts, and promyelocytes are all present, and Auer rods may be seen.

The neoplastic cells are Sudan black-positive and PAS-positive. The monocyte progenitor cells stain for α-naphthyl acetate (or butyrate) esterase, and the granulocyte precursors are chloroacetate esterase-positive. Examination by electron microscopy shows the distinctive filaments and nuclei of monocytic and granulocytic cells.

ACUTE MONOCYTIC LEUKEMIA

A. Clinical Features: Acute monocytic leukemia is very rare in the USA and affects males and females equally. It affects 2 age groups: those younger than 10 years and those older than 40 years (mean, 58 years). The clinical features are generally similar to those of acute granulocytic leukemia, including bone marrow failure with anemia, thrombocytopenia, bleeding, and infection. Hepatosplenomegaly and lymphadenopathy are present in approximately half of all patients. The leukocyte count is high (above 100,000/dL in about 50% of patients). Monoblasts are frequent, and the cells show various degrees of staining for esterase, Sudan black, and PAS. Rearrangements of chromosome 11 have been reported.

B. Pathology: The bone marrow is diffusely and homogeneously involved. The neoplastic cells show the nuclear folding and abundant cytoplasm of monocytes. Some are large blasts with weak or negative cytochemical staining, and others are Sudan black-, PAS-, and esterase-positive promonocytes.

Granulocytic components usually make up less than 10% of the cells.

C. Immunologic Features: Acute myelomonocytic leukemia and acute monocytic leukemia have been characterized with monoclonal antibodies FABM4 and FABM5, respectively. Both cell types generally stain with monoclonal antibodies that recognize myeloid and monocyte differentiation antigens. These include CD14 (My4), CD13 (My7), My8, CD33 (My9), CD11b (MO1/OKM1), and MO5.

D. Differential Diagnosis: This includes acute and chronic myelomonocytic leukemias.

E. Therapy: The response to combination chemotherapy is similar to that of acute granulocytic leukemia, with complete remission in approximately 40–60% of patients for less than 1 year. Central nervous system relapse is common.

INTERRELATION OF GRANULOCYTIC & LYMPHOCYTIC LEUKEMIAS

Patients with chronic myelogenous leukemia frequently, after an average of approximately 3 years, develop an acute phase of the disease called blast crisis. Because the blast cells may show a lineage different from myeloid cells, immunophenotyping of these cells is important for therapeutic decisions. The blast cells may express antigens and enzymes characteristic of B lymphoblasts, T lymphoblasts, erythroblasts, myeloblasts, or megakaryoblasts. The cells of approximately one-third of patients with blast crisis have the phenotype of B immunoblasts (TdT$^+$, CD10 [CALLA]$^+$, Ia$^+$, CD20$^+$, cytoplasmic IgM$^+$, with rearrangements of immunoglobulin heavy and light chain genes). Rarely do the blasts have the phenotype of T lymphoblasts (TdT$^+$, CD5$^+$, CD3$^+$, CD2$^+$). Patients with lymphoid blast crisis may respond to vincristine and prednisone chemotherapy, whereas patients with myeloid blast do less well with this combination. Myeloid blast cells tend to be positive for CD13 (My7), CD33 (My9), CD11b (MO1/OKM1). All of the blast cells, no matter what the differentiation, retain the Philadelphia chromosome.

NATURAL KILLER (NK) CELL/LARGE GRANULAR LYMPHOCYTE (LGL) LEUKEMIA (T-Gamma Lymphoproliferative Disease)

A subset of T lymphocytes with Fc receptor for IgG, the so-called T-gamma lymphocytes, contains a population of cells with large cytoplasmic granules, called large granular lymphocytes (LGL). These cells seem to be largely responsible for NK activity. In a small number of patients with leukemia, the phenotype and morphology of the cells indicate that they are proliferations of large granular lymphocytes. Patients are generally elderly males, and the LGL infiltrate bone marrow and spleen and are present in peripheral blood. The patients typically have chronic neutropenia. The cells may have the phenotype of cytotoxic/suppressor T cells or NK cells, or both. Some investigators consider this to be a nonneoplastic lymphoproliferation, whereas others believe it is a type of T-CLL.

Recently, clonal chromosomal abnormalities have been observed, indicating that the condition is a true neoplasm. The phenotype and reduced NK activity suggest that the LGL are immature. The cells usually are acid phosphatase-positive and β-glucoronidase-positive, and express CD3, CD2, CD8, and the NK-associated antigen CD57 (Leu 7 or HNK1). They are generally sheep erythrocyte rosette-positive. Trisomy 14 (47xy, + 14) and trisomy 8 (47xy, + 8) have been reported, and there is clonal rearrangement of the gene for the β-chain of the T cell receptor.

The rather indolent course of this leukemia suggests that it may be an early stage of disease similar to B-CLL, which slowly evolves to a more aggressive disease.

Although most of the patients have a chronically progressive disease, others may have a more aggressive course, with a lymphoma of LGL. In these patients the disease progresses rapidly, and high-dose chemotherapy is needed. In addition, some patients with T-ALL may have cells with characteristics of NK cells.

Not only do the cells from patients with LGL leukemia demonstrate in vitro NK activity, but they also show antibody-dependent cellular cytotoxicity (ADCC). They also suppress T cell proliferation and immunoglobulin synthesis in vitro, but most produce erythroid colony-forming units and burst-forming units. Most of the patients with chronic disease do not require cytotoxic chemotherapy, but they must be treated with antibiotic therapy because of repeated bacterial infections related to their neutropenia.

BENIGN CONDITIONS MIMICKING OR ASSOCIATED WITH NEOPLASMS OF THE IMMUNE SYSTEM

There are several conditions of proliferation of cells of the immune system that may be confused with lymphomas or leukemias or, in some cases,

may evolve into true neoplasms. Confusion in diagnosis may lead to nonmalignant disease being diagnosed as malignant neoplasms. Many of these conditions are associated with aberrant immune responses. Immunophenotyping may help to distinguish reactive from neoplastic processes by virtue of identifying monoclonality with or without gene rearrangement confirmation. These conditions include the following:

(1) **Benign follicular hyperplasia:** This may be so severe as to mimic FCC lymphomas and the follicular hyperplasia seen in the AIDS-related complex (ARC). It may occur in certain infections, rheumatoid arthritis, drug reactions, and, rarely, immunodeficiencies, but frequently there is no apparent underlying primary disease. The cells have a B cell phenotype, but are polyclonal.

(2) **Angiofollicular hyperplasia:** Follicular centers are enlarged, but there is also an increase in interfollicular plasmacytoid cells. These cells have a polyclonal B cell phenotype but bear CD4. Large asymptomatic mediastinal masses may be present. Patients have anemia, polyclonal hypergammaglobulinemia, thrombocytopenia, and marrow plasmacytosis. Some may progress to malignant lymphoma or Kaposi's sarcoma.

(3) **Sjögren's syndrome (see Chapter 36):** This is characterized by inflamation of the salivary glands (sialadenitis) with proliferations of lymphocytes, plasmacytoid cells, and immunoblasts, which may progress to lymphoma. There is an increased risk of developing IBS-B and plasmacytoid lymphocytic lymphomas.

(4) **Hashimoto's thyroiditis (see Chapter 37):** The thyroid contains lymphoid follicles with hyperplastic follicular centers. The frequency of lymphomas is 1% or less, but most of the lymphomas that do arise in the thyroid (FCC lymphomas) are in elderly female patients with Hashimoto's thyroiditis.

(5) **Systemic lupus erythematosus (see Chapter 36):** This disease usually affects young women with cervical or generalized lymphadenopathy who have follicular hyperplasia and interfollicular expansion of plasma cells and immunoblasts. These patients rarely develop IBS-B.

(6) **Immunoblastic reactions in infectious mononucleosis, vaccinations, and herpes zoster:** Following stimulation of the immune system by certain infections or vaccinations, lymph nodes may enlarge and show clusters of small and transformed lymphocytes (immunoblasts) in the interfollicular areas, with focal necrosis and occasional Reed-Sternberg-like cells. Atypical lymphocytes are seen in the peripheral blood. The resemblance to IBS-B and Hodgkin's disease may create diagnostic problems. However, the cells are phenotypically polyclonal.

(7) **Drug reactions:** Drugs, particularly phenytoin (Dilantin), may produce a follicular hyperplasia and

lymphadenopathy with areas of focal necrosis. Lymph nodes contain eosinophils, and the pathology may suggest Hodgkin's disease. Rarely do lymphomas develop in these patients.

(8) Abnormal immune reactions, including immunoblastic lymphadenopathy (IBL) (angioimmunoblastic lymphadenopathy): IBL is a diffuse involvement of the lymph node characterized by the presence of plasmacytoid immunoblasts and plasma cells, branching small vessels with PAS-positive walls, and general hypocellularity due to an overall decrease in the number of lymphocytes. Deposits of granular pale acidophilic interstitial material separate these cells. Phenotypically, the B cells and plasma cells are polyclonal and T cells appear to be benign. However, T cell receptor β-chain gene rearrangements have been reported in cases of angioimmunoblastic lymphadenopathy, suggesting clonal T cell proliferations. Some patients also show T cell receptor γ-chain and immunoglobulin heavy chain gene rearrangements. Approximately 10–20% of patients with this condition develop IBS-B, and others develop T cell neoplasms.

(9) Gluten-sensitive enteropathy (see Chapter 40): These patients with malabsorption show small bowel atrophy with increased numbers of lymphocytes and plasma cells. The incidence of malignant lymphoma is increased, but with insidious onset. Most patients have IBS-B with monoclonal cytoplasmic IgM.

(10) X-linked lymphoproliferative syndrome (Duncan's syndrome) (see Chapter 24): Lymph nodes and the spleen show excessive immunoblastic infiltrates, separating and replacing the lymphoid follicles and associated with a marked plasmacytosis and decreased T cell numbers. The liver and bone marrow may be involved. This syndrome is rare; it usually affects males between 5 months and 23 years of age. Most die of infectious mononucleosis, aplastic anemia, or hypogammaglobulinemia, but some develop malignant lymphomas. The latter are usually monoclonal B cell lymphomas, although the initial B cell immunoblastic proliferation is polyclonal. Even if progression to IBS-B has not occurred, the immunoblastic proliferation may be confused with this lymphoma.

(11) Immunosuppressed patients: These include organ transplant patients (see Chapters 47 and 60) and AIDS patients with B cell lymphomas (see Chapter 55). The risk for lymphoma in patients receiving transplants following or during immunosuppression is approximately 40 times that of the normal population. The lymphoproliferative disorder may occur in the transplanted organ, particularly the heart, or in other organs. Multiple allotransplants increase the risk even more. Lymphomas that arise are almost always B cell in origin, but they may not have surface immunoglobulin or be monoclonal or polyclonal for surface and cytoplasmic immunoglob-

ulin. Heavy and light chain gene rearrangements have been reported, even when the phenotype is polyclonal. A role for EBV in the etiology has been proposed, but the constant antigenic stimulation of the graft in conjunction with the suppressed immune response has suggested that the neoplastic clones of B cells arise by somatic mutation.

Since the early 1980s, it has been clear that patients with AIDS and ARC have a high incidence of lymphomas, almost all of which are B cell lymphomas. Since the majority of individuals with asymptomatic HIV infection will eventually progress to ARC and then to AIDS, and because there are an estimated 1–1.5 million individuals in the USA who are currently infected but asymptomatic and another estimated 250,000 who have ARC, the number of patients with AIDS and thus with AIDS-related lymphoma will continue to increase. Immunophenotyping studies on these lymphomas have demonstrated that most are of B cell origin, with the majority showing monoclonal surface immunoglobulin staining for κ or λ (κ predominating), expression of a variety of B cell differentiation antigens, and immunoglobulin gene rearrangements. Some lymphomas, however, have polyclonal immunoglobulin patterns and others lack surface immunoglobulin. Initially, certain lymphomas appear as a multiclonal B cell expansion followed by evolution to a monoclonal phenotype. The similarity to the lymphomas arising in immunosuppressed organ-transplant patients is striking.

The great majority of the AIDS-related lymphomas are high-grade, IBS-B, or small noncleaved FCC lymphomas, Burkitt or non-Burkitt in type. Discrepancies between reported histologic types and the course and response to therapy in different centers are explained by differences in histologic classification. However, most agree that they are high-grade lymphomas and have distinctive features which include a high incidence of central nervous system involvement by the lymphomas, particularly by IBS-B. In addition, almost all patients present with disseminated disease and systemic symptoms at time of diagnosis. An unusual generalized involvement by lymphomas occurs in the myocardium, adrenals, ear lobes, maxillae, popliteal foci, gallbladder, orbit, and rectum.

The chromosomal abnormalities in the AIDS-related lymphomas are the same as those commonly reported in Burkitt's lymphoma, ie, translocations between chromosomes 8 and 14 and between 8 and 22. The survival time of AIDS patients with lymphomas is extremely short with or without therapy. Various centers have reported median survivals ranging from 5 to 28 months for patients on therapy. Various multiagent combinations and radiation therapy have been attempted, generally with poor results.

REFERENCES

General

Lennert K: *Malignant Lymphomas Other than Hodgkin's Disease. Histology, Cytology, Ultrastructure, Immunology.* Springer-Verlag, 1978.

Lennert K, Collins RD, Lukes RJ: Concordance of the Kiel and Lukes/Collins classifications of non-Hodgkin lymphomas. *Histopathology* 1983;**7**:549.

Lennert KA et al: The histopathology of malignant lymphoma. *Br J Cancer* 1975;**31(Suppl)**:193.

Lukes RJ, Collins RD: Immunologic characterization of human malignant lymphomas. *Cancer* 1974;**34**:1488.

Lukes RJ, Collins RD: Tumors of the hematopoietic system. In: *Atlas of Tumor Pathology,* Second Series, fascicle 28. US Armed Forces Institute of Pathology, 1989.

Lukes RJ et al: A morphologic and immunologic surface marker study of 299 cases of non-Hodgkin's lymphomas and related leukemias. *Am J Pathol* 1978;**90**:461.

Mann RB, Jaffe ES, Berard CW: Malignant lymphoma: A conceptual understanding of morphologic diversity. *Am J Pathol* 1979;**94**:105.

National Cancer Institute Sponsored Study of Classifications of Non-Hodgkin's Lymphomas: *Cancer* 1982;**49**:2112.

Immunologic Features, Immunophenotyping

Anderson KC et al: Expression of human B cell associated antigens on leukemias and lymphomas: A model of human B cell differentiation. *Blood* 1984;**63**:1424.

Borowitz MJ et al: Monoclonal antibody phenotyping of B cell non-Hodgkin lymphomas. The Southeastern Cancer Study Group experience. *Am J Pathol* 1985;**121**:514.

Borowitz MJ et al: The phenotypic diversity of peripheral T-cell lymphomas. *Hum Pathol* 1986;**17**:567.

Bray RA, Landay AL: Identification and functional characterization of mononuclear cells by flow cytometry. *Arch Pathol Lab Med* 1989;**113**:579.

Braylan RC, Benson NA: Cell surface markers and cell cycle analysis of lymphomas. *Cytometry* (Suppl) 1988;**3**:73.

Coon JS, Landay AL, Weinstein RS: Advances in flow cytometry for diagnostic pathology. *Lab Invest* 1987; **57(5)**:453.

Deegan MJ: Membrane antigen analysis in the diagnosis of lymphoid leukemias and lymphomas. *Arch Pathol Lab Med* 1989;**113**:606.

Foon KA, Todd RF III: Immunologic classification of leukemia and lymphoma. *Blood* 1986;**68**:1.

Friedman AS, Nadler LN: Cell surface markers in hematologic malignancies. *Semin Oncol* 1987;**14**:193.

Greaves NF et al: Lineage promiscuity in hemopoietic differentiation and leukemia. *Blood* 1986;**67**:1.

Horning SJ et al: Clinical and phenotypic diversity of T cell lymphomas. *Blood* 1986;**67**:1578.

Janssen J et al: Prognostic significance of immunologic phenotype in hairy cell leukemia. *Blood* 1984; **63**:1241.

Knowles DN II: Lymphoid cell markers: Their distribution and usefulness in the immunophenotypic analysis of lymphoid neoplasms. *Am J Surg Pathol* 1985; **9(Suppl)**:85.

LeBien TW, McCormack RT: The common acute lymphoblastic leukemia antigen (CD10): Emancipation from a functional enigma. *Blood* 1989;**73**:625.

Lukes RJ et al: Immunologic approach to non-Hodgkin lymphomas and related leukemias. Analysis of the results of multiparameter studies of 425 cases. *Semin Hematol* 1978;**15**:322.

Parker JW: Flow cytometry in the diagnosis of lymphomas. *Cytometry* (Suppl) 1988;**3**:38.

Parker JW: Immunological basis for the redefinition of malignant lymphomas. *Am J Clin Pathol* 1979; **72(Suppl)**:679.

Picker LJ et al: Immunophenotypic criteria for the diagnosis of non-Hodgkin's lymphoma. *Am J Pathol* 1987; **128**:181.

Roholl PJM et al: Immunologic marker analysis of normal and malignant histiocytes. *Am J Clin Pathol* 1988; **89**:187.

Tubbs RR et al: Immunohistological cellular phenotypes of lymphoproliferative disorders: Comprehensive evaluation of 564 cases including 256 non-Hodgkin lymphomas classified by the International Working Formulation. *Am J Pathol* 1983;**113**:207.

Schuurman HJ et al: Immunophenotyping of non-Hodgkin's lymphoma: Correlation with relapse-free survival. *Am J Pathol* 1988;**131**:102.

Strauchen JA, Dimitriu-Bona A: Immunopathology of Hodgkin's disease: Characterization of Reed-Sternberg cells with monoclonal antibodies. *Am J Pathol* 1986;**123**:293.

Turner RR et al: Flow cytometric measurements of proliferation-associated nuclear antigen p105 and DNA content in non-Hodgkin's lymphomas. *Arch Pathol Lab Med* 1989;**153**:907.

Willman CL, Stewart CC: General principles of multiparameter flow cytometric analysis. Applications of flow cytometry in the diagnostic pathology laboratory. *Semin Diagn Pathol* 1989;**6**:3.

DNA Content & Cell Proliferation

Braylan RC: Flow cytometric analysis in lymphomas. *Arch Pathol Lab Med* 1989;**113**:627.

Bauer KD et al: Prognostic implications of ploidy and proliferative activity in diffuse large cell lymphomas. *Cancer Res* 1986;**46**:3173.

Christensson B et al: Cell proliferation and DNA content in non-Hodgkin lymphoma. *Cancer* 1986; **58**:1295.

Look AT: Aneuploidy and percentage of S phase cells determined by flow cytometry correlate with cell phenotype in childhood acute leukemia. *Blood* 1982;**60**:959.

Roos G et al: Prognostic significance of DNA analysis by flow cytometry in non-Hodgkin's lymphoma. *Hematol Oncol* 1985;**3**:233.

Shackney SE et al: The biology of tumor growth in the non-Hodgkin's lymphomas. A dual parameter flow cytometry study of 220 cases. *J Clin Invest* 1984; **3**:1201.

Tomer A et al: Flow cytometric analysis of megakaryocytes from patients with abnormal platelet counts. *Blood* 1989;**74**:594.

Wain SL, Braylan C, Borowitz MJ: Correlation of monoclonal antibody phenotyping and cellular DNA content in non-Hodgkin's lymphoma. *Cancer* 1987; **60**:2403.

Weiss LM et al: Proliferative rates of non-Hodgkin's lymphomas as assessed by Ki-67 antibody. *Human Pathol* 1987;**18**:1155.

Cytomolecular Genetics

Berliner N et al: Detection of clonal excess in lymphoproliferative disease by kappa/lambda analysis: Correlation with immunoglobulin gene DNA rearrangement. *Blood* 1986;**67**:80.

Cossman J et al: Molecular genetics in the diagnosis of lymphoma. *Arch Pathol Lab Med* 1988;**112**:117.

Korsmeyer SJ: Antigen receptor genes as molecular markers of lymphoid neoplasms. *Clin Invest* 1987; **79**:1291.

Korsmeyer SJ: Immunoglobulin and T cell receptor genes reveal the clonality, lineage, and translocations of lymphoid neoplasms. In: *Important Advances in Oncology*, V DeVita (editor). Lippincott, 1987.

Kristoffersson U et al: Prognostic implication of cytogenetic findings in 106 patients with non-Hodgkin lymphoma. *Cancer Genet Cytogenet* 1987;**25**:55.

Lebeau M, Rowley J: Recurring chromosomal abnormalities in leukemia and lymphoma. *Cancer Surv* 1984;**3**:372.

Nowell PC, Croce CM: Chromosomes, genes and cancer. *Am J Pathol* 1986;**125**:8.

Nowell PC et al: The most common chromosome change in 86 chronic B cell or T cell tumors: A 14q32 translocation. *Cancer Genet Cytogenet* 1986; **19**:219.

Sklar J, Weiss LM: Application of antigen receptor gene rearrangement to the diagnosis and characterization of lymphoid neoplasms. *Annu Rev Med* 1988;**39**:315.

Stewart CC: Flow cytometric analysis of oncogene expression in human neoplasias. *Arch Pathol Lab Med* 1989;**113**:634.

Waldmann TA: The arrangement of immunoglobulin and T cell receptor gene in human lymphoproliferative disorders. *Adv Immunol* 1987;**40**:247.

B Cell Neoplasms

Anderson LG, Talal N: The spectrum of benign to malignant lymphoproliferation in Sjogren's syndrome. *Clin Exp Immunol* 1972;**10**:199.

Bartl R et al: Histologic classification and staging of multiple myeloma: A retrospective and prospective study of 674 cases. *Am J Clin Pathol* 1987;**87**:342.

Blattner WA, Blair A, Mason TJ: Multiple myeloma in the United States, 1950–1975. *Cancer* 1981; **48**:2547.

Browman GP, Neame PB, Soamboonsrup P: The contribution of cytochemistry and immunophenotyping to the reproducibility of the FAB classification of acute leukemia. *Blood* 1986;**68**:900.

de Martini RM et al: Lymphocyte immunophenotyping of B-cell lymphomas: A flow cytometric analysis of neoplastic and non-neoplastic cells in 271 cases. *Clin Immunol Immunopathol* 1988;**49**:365.

Deutcher TF, Fahey JL: The histopathology of the macroglobulinemia of Waldenstrom. *J Natl Cancer Inst* 1959;**22**:887.

Greaves MF et al: Immunologically defined subclasses of acute lymphoblastic leukemia in children: The relation to presentation features and prognosis. *Br J Haematol* 1981;**48**:179.

Harris NL, Bhan AK: B cell neoplasms of the lymphocytic, lymphoplasmacytoid and plasma cell types: Immunohistologic analysis and clinical correlation. *Hum Pathol* 1985;**16**:829.

Horning SJ, Rosenberg SA: The natural history of initially untreated low-grade non-Hodgkin's lymphomas. *N Engl J Med* 1984;**311**:1471.

Jansen J et al: Cell markers in hairy cell leukemia studied in cells from 51 patients. *Blood* 1982;**59**:52.

Kubagawa H et al: Studies on the clonal origin of multiple myeloma. Use of individually specific (idiotype) antibodies to trace the oncogenic event to its earliest point of expression in B cell differentiation. *J Exp Med* 1979;**150**:792.

Levine AM et al: Immunoblastic sarcoma of T cell versus B cell origin. I. Clinical features. *Blood* 1981;**58**:52.

Nadler LM et al: B cell origin of non-T cell acute lymphoblastic leukemia. A model for discrete stages of neoplastic and normal pre-B cell differentiation. *J Clin Invest* 1984;**74**:332.

Rai R et al: Clinical staging of chronic lymphocytic leukemia. *Blood* 1975;**46**:219.

Robinson DSF et al: Normal counterparts of hairy cells and B lymphocytes in the peripheral blood. An ultrastructural study with monoclonal antibodies and the immunogold method. *Leuk Res* 1985;**9**:335.

Schwartz RS, Beldotti L: Malignant lymphomas following allogenic disease: Transition from an immunological to a neoplastic disorder. *Science* 1965;**149**:1511.

VanCamp B, Reynaert P, Broodtaerts L: Studies on the origin of the precursor cells in multiple myeloma, Waldenstrom's macroglobulinemia and benign monoclonal gammopathy. I. Cytoplasmic isotype and idiotype distribution in peripheral blood and bone marrow. *Clin Exp Immunol* 1981;**44**:82.

York JC et al: Changes in the appearance of hematopoietic and lymphoid neoplasms: Clinical, pathologic and biologic implications. *Hum Pathol* 1984;**15**:11.

T Cell Neoplasms

Barcos MP, Lukes RJ: Malignant lymphoma of convoluted lymphocytes: A new entity of possible T cell type. Pages 147–178. In: *Conflicts in Childhood Cancer: An Evaluation of Current Management*. Vol 4. Sinks LF, Godden JE (editors). Alan R Liss, 1975.

Bernard A et al: Cell surface characterization of malignant T cells from lymphoblastic lymphoma using monoclonal antibodies: Evidence for phenotypic differences between malignant T cells from patients with acute lymphoblastic leukemia and lymphoblastic lymphoma. *Blood* 1981;**57**:1105.

Bertness V et al: T cell receptor gene rearrangements as clinical markers of human T cell lymphomas. *N Engl J Med* 1985;**313**:534.

Borowitz MJ et al: The phenotypic diversity of peripheral T cell lymphomas: A Southeastern Cancer Study Group experience. *Hum Pathol* 1986;**17**:567.

Bunn PA et al: Clinical course of retrovirus associated acute T cell lymphoma in the United States. *N Engl J Med* 1983;**309**:257.

Chan WC et al: Heterogeneity of large granular lymphocyte proliferations: Delineation of two major subtypes. *Blood* 1986;**68**:1142.

Greer JP et al: Peripheral T cell lymphoma: A clinicopathologic study of 42 cases. *J Clin Oncol* 1984;**2**:788.

Hinuma Y et al: Antibodies to adult T cell leukemiavirus-associated antigen (ATLA) in sera from patients with ATL and controls in Japan: A nationwide seroepidemiologic study. *Int J Cancer* 1982;**29**:631.

Horning SJ et al: Clinical and phenotypic diversity of T cell lymphomas. *Blood* 1986;**67**:1578.

Knowles DN, Pelicci PG, Dalla-Favera R: T cell receptor beta chain gene rearrangements: Genetic markers of T cell lineage and clonality. *Hum Pathol* 1986;**17**:546.

Lutzner M et al: Cutaneous T cell lymphomas: The Sezary syndrome, mycosis fungoides, and related disorders. *Ann Intern Med* 1979;**83**:534.

Nasu K et al: Immunopathology of cutaneous T cell lymphomas. *Am J Pathol* 1985;**119**:436.

Reinherz EL et al: Discrete stages of human intrathymic differentiation: Analysis of normal thymocytes and leukemic lymphoblasts of T cell lineage. *Proc Natl Acad Sci USA* 1980;**77**:1588.

Sausville EA et al: Histologic assessment of lymph nodes in mycosis fungoides/Sezary syndrome (cutaneous T cell lymphoma). Clinical correlations and prognostic import of a new classification system. *Hum Pathol* 1985;**16**:1098.

Waldmann TA et al: Rearrangements of genes for the antigen receptor on T cells as markers of lineage and clonality in human lymphoid neoplasms. *N Engl J Med* 1985;**313**:776.

Watanabe S: Pathology of peripheral T cell lymphomas and leukemias. *Hematol Oncol* 1986;**4**:45.

Weiss LM et al: Clonal rearrangements of T cell receptor genes in mycosis fungoides and dermatopathic lymphadenopathy. *N Engl J Med* 1985;**313**:539.

Weiss LM et al: Morphologic and immunologic characterization of 50 peripheral T cell lymphomas. *Am J Pathol* 1985;**118**:316.

Hodgkin's Disease

Coleman CN et al: Hematologic neoplasia in patients treated for Hodgkin's disease. *N Engl J Med* 1977;**297**:1249.

Drexler HG et al: Is the Hodgkin cell a T- or B-lymphocyte? Recent evidence from geno- and immunophenotypic analysis and in vitro cell lines. *Hematol Oncol* 1989;**7**:95.

Forni M et al: B and T lymphocytes in Hodgkin's disease: An immunohistochemical study utilizing heterologous and monoclonal antibodies. *Cancer* 1985;**55**:728.

Hsu S, Yang K, Jaffe ES: Phenotypic expression of Hodgkin and Reed-Sternberg cells in Hodgkin's disease. *Am J Pathol* 1985;**118**:209.

Kant JA et al: The pathologic and clinical heterogeneity of lymphocyte depleted Hodgkin's disease. *J Clin Oncol* 1986;**4**:284.

Lukes RJ: Criteria for involvement of lymph node, bone marrow, spleen, and liver in Hodgkin's disease. *Cancer Res* 1971;**31**:1755.

Lukes RJ, Butler JJ: The pathology and nomenclature of Hodgkin's disease. *Cancer Res* 1966;**26**:1063.

Lukes RJ et al: Report of the nomenclature committee. *Cancer Res* 1966;**26(Part 1)**:1311.

Mononuclear Phagocyte Neoplasms

Roholl PMJ et al: Immunologic marker analysis of normal and malignant histiocytes. *Am J Clin Pathol* 1988; **89**:187.

Conditions Mimicking Neoplasms or Associated with a High Incidence of Neoplasms of the Immune System

Butler JJ: Nonneoplastic lesions of lymph nodes of man to be differentiated from lymphomas. *Natl Cancer Inst Monogr* 1969;**32**:233.

Childs CC, Parham DM, Berard CW: Infectious mononucleosis. The spectrum of morphologic changes simulating lymphoma in lymph nodes and tonsils. *Am J Surg Pathol* 1987;**11**:122.

Cleary ML, Warnke R, Sklar J: Monoclonality of lymphoproliferative lesions in cardiac transplant recipients: Clonal analysis based on Ig-gene rearrangements. *N Engl J Med* 1984;**310**:477.

Dorfman RF, Warnke R: Lymphadenopathy simulating the malignant lymphomas. *Hum Pathol* 1974;**5**:519.

Hartsock RJ: Reactive lesions in lymph nodes. Chap 9, p 196, in: *The Reticuloendothelial System*. Monograph 16.

Holmes GKT et al: Coeliac disease, gluten-free diet, and malignancy. *Gut* 1976;**17**:612.

Lukes RJ, Tindle BH: Immunoblastic lymphadenopathy: A prelymphomatous state of immunoblastic sarcoma. *Recent Results Cancer Res* 1978;**64**:241.

Purtilo DT: X-linked lymphoproliferative syndrome: an immunodeficiency disorder with acquired agammaglobulinemia, fatal infectious mononucleosis, or malignant lymphoma. *Arch Pathol Lab Med* 1981; **105**:119.

Symmers WS: Drug-induced lymphoma-like lymphadenopathies and their relation to lymphomas. Pages 696–701 in: *Systemic Pathology*. Vol 2. Churchill Livingstone, 1978.

49

Mechanisms of Immunity to Infection

John Mills, MD, & David J. Drutz, MD

The environment in which we live is populated by microorganisms, many of which are capable of causing disease. The immune system probably evolved primarily as a defense against infection by these omnipresent pathogenic microorganisms. However, nonimmunologic defenses against infectious disease (Table 49–1) are at least as important as immunologic defenses, especially in preventing early stages of infection. Collectively, these immunologic and nonimmunologic defense mechanisms are responsible for maintaining our internal milieu free of microorganisms. In some instances, normal host defense mechanisms may be able to maintain the sterility of distal portions of the "external" portions of the host despite continuous exposure to contamination. The best example of this is the respiratory tract, in which the tracheobronchial tree distal to the carina is normally sterile.

As our understanding of the immune system has improved, the boundary between specific and nonspecific immune resistance to infection has blurred. For example, natural killer (NK) cells and macrophages function in nonspecific immune defense mechanisms, but they may be activated by lymphokines produced as a result of the specific interaction between immune lymphocytes and antigens. These cells may also become specific effectors through cooperation with antibody.

Host defenses against infection—whether specific or nonspecific—are also characterized by considerable redundancy. This may explain why profound defects in one sector of host defenses ordinarily result in only a minimal increase in the overall susceptibility to infection.

NONIMMUNOLOGIC DEFENSES AGAINST INFECTION

Host Defenses at Body Surfaces

For an invading pathogen to produce infection, it must first slip through an impressive barrier of surface defenses that operate wherever intact body tissues interface with the environment. These barriers—the skin, the respiratory epithelium, the gastrointestinal epithelium, etc—are largely nonspecific and nonimmunologic, but they constitute a vital component of host defense.

Many pathogens initiate infection by attaching to mucosal epithelial cells. All epithelial cells are covered with a mucus layer, which serves in part to prevent microorganisms from attaching to the cell surface. Coordinated movement of the underlying cilia sweeps organisms entrapped in the mucus layer out of the body. This process may be assisted by coordinated movements of these organs, such as coughing or peristalsis. Intestinal epithelial cells have a short (30-hour) half-life, which also limits the efficiency of infection. If the invading microorganism happens to attach to a desquamating epithelial cell, infection is prevented.

Many substances coating body surfaces serve as local disinfectants and antimicrobial substances. The skin has a high content of fatty acids, which are inhibitory to bacteria and fungi. The stomach serves as the guardian of the gastrointestinal tract, as it secretes hydrochloric acid with a pH between 1 and 2, which is sufficient to kill most gastrointestinal pathogens. Factors that reduce gastric acidity, such as treatment with antacids or H_2 blockers, can increase the susceptibility of the host to enteric pathogens. A number of specific bactericidal or fungicidal proteins are formed on body surfaces. For example, the enzyme lysozyme, which is present in tears and many other mucosal secretions, is bactericidal for many gram-positive bacteria. Most of the bacteria suscep-

Table 49–1. Nonimmunologic host defense mechanisms.

Surface defenses
Mucus
Coughing/peristalsis
Epithelial-cell turnover
Local disinfectants (gastric acid, skin lipids)
Normal microbial flora
Inflammatory reaction
Cells
  Phagocytic cells
    PMN
    Monocyte-macrophages
  NK cells
Complement (alternative pathway)
Prostaglandins and leukotrienes
Cytokines (interferons, IL-1, etc)

tible to lysozyme are classified as nonpathogens, but it may be that they are nonpathogenic because of the large amounts of lysozyme in secretions. Many other mucosal proteins with specific activity against microorganisms, eg, lactoferrin, have been described. Lactoferrin is an iron-binding protein that maintains the concentration of free iron necessary for bacterial replication below levels at which most bacteria grow.

Most animal and human surfaces that are exposed to the environment are colonized by nonpathogenic (or weakly pathogenic) bacteria and fungi collectively known as the normal flora. Sites populated by the normal flora include the mouth, skin, and gastrointestinal tract (Table 49–2). The composition of the normal flora varies with the site. However, anaerobic bacteria are important components at all sites. The density of the normal flora also varies greatly depending on the location; for example, the gastrointestinal tract at the stomach and proximal small bowel is virtually sterile, whereas the contents of the distal colon may contain 10^{11} bacteria/g of contents.

The normal flora clearly serves a protective role. For example, elimination of the anaerobic component of the gastrointestinal normal flora by antimicrobial therapy has been shown to increase the susceptibility of patients to infection by enteric pathogens such as *Shigella* and *Salmonella*. However, the extent to which the normal flora participates in host defense and the mechanisms by which it prevents colonization or infection by pathogens are incompletely defined. Some mechanisms that have been identified include stimulation of antibodies and T cells cross-reactive with pathogenic microorganisms, competition for nutrients, competition for receptor sites on epithelial cells, and secretion of substances toxic to pathogens (eg, secretion of

bactericidal short-chain fatty acids by intestinal anaerobes).

Inflammation

Immunoglobulins and phagocytic cells play a major role in host defenses at external surfaces; they are also critical to host defenses within the body.

Cells whose major function is phagocytosis of foreign materials and killing of microorganisms are frequently referred to as "professional phagocytes," to differentiate them from other cells, including epithelial cells, that have some capacity to ingest foreign material (Table 49–3). These cells include neutrophils, basophils, eosinophils, and cells of the monocyte-macrophages series, including blood monocytes and tissue macrophages such as Kupffer's cells and alveolar macrophages. Professional phagocytes also have surface Fc and complement receptors that facilitate phagocytosis, and they contain enzymes in lysosomal granules that will kill eukaryotic and prokaryotic cells. NK cells are lymphoid cells that have surface Fc receptors, but they are nonphagocytic and do not contain microbicidal systems such as lysosomes. They primarily mediate lysis of virus-infected cells (see below and Chapter 51).

Invasion of a host by a pathogen that is able to evade the surface defenses described above usually results in an inflammatory response. The components of this response include phagocytic cells, soluble factors (eg, complement, arachidonic acid metabolites), and the response of local host tissues and organs (eg, the vascular tree; see Chapters 11–14). In viral infections, NK cells and interferons (see Chapters 7 and 11) are probably important in early nonspecific defense mechanisms. Invasion by microorganisms produces changes in the host that attract phagocytic cells (especially PMN); in addition, some substances produced by pathogens (eg, the N-formyl peptides produced by bacteria) are chemotactic (attractive for phagocytic cells) in themselves. The PMN, which are usually the first cells at the site of infection, attack the invading pathogen and simultaneously produce chemoattractants to call in additional phagocytic cells, both PMN and monocyte-macrophages. PMN products also produce important changes in host tissues (eg, vasodilatation). Monocyte-macrophages and other cells produce cytokines such as interleukin-1 (IL-1), tumor necrosis factor

Table 49–2. The normal flora.

Site	Representative Organisms
Oral mucosa	Viridans streptococci Anaerobic streptococci
Vagina	Anaerobic streptococci *Lactobacillus*
Dental plaque	*Fusobacterium* (anaerobes) *Veillonella* (anaerobes) Actinomycetes (anaerobes) Spirochetes (anaerobes)
Colonic mucosa	*Bacteroides* (anaerobes) *Fusobacterium* (anaerobes) *Escherichia coli* (anaerobes) *Clostridium* (anaerobes) *Lactobacillus* Anaerobic streptococci and staphylococci
Skin	*Propionibacterium* (anaerobes) *Staphylococcus epidermidis* *Corynebacterium* *Pityrosporum, Malassezia*

Table 49–3. Phagocytic cells.

Neutrophilic leukocytes
Eosinophilic leukocytes
Basophilic leukocytes
Blood monocytes
Tissue macrophages
Kupffer's cells of the liver
Alveolar macrophages
Astroglial cells

(TNF), and interferons. These cause fever and further augment the inflammatory reaction by attracting additional cells, augmenting the activity of these cells, and inducing vasodilatation (see Chapter 7).

Fever

Elevation of body temperature (fever) in response to infection is nearly universal in humans and other animals; this response has been highly conserved during evolution. It is therefore reasonable to conclude that fever is an important host defense mechanism. However, this contention has been difficult to prove, except for poikilothermic animals such as lizards. The main problem in proving the role of fever in antimicrobial defense in homoiothermic animals has been in dissociating the effects of the endogenous pyrogens (IL-1, TNF) that produce fever from the complex effects of fever per se. Fever has a salutory effect on the course of infection, whereas hypothermia has deleterious effects. Although these data would argue for not reducing fever in patients with infections (eg, through tepid sponging or antipyretic drugs such as aspirin), high fever itself may be deleterious. In addition, the role of fever as a host defense mechanism is probably adjunctive rather than central, and it becomes insignificant if effective antimicrobial chemotherapy is being administered.

IMMUNOLOGIC DEFENSES AGAINST INFECTION

Immunologic defenses are, by definition, those host defense mechanisms which have specificity toward the invading pathogen and which are augmented on second and subsequent exposures. The specificity of the host response to invading microorganisms is determined primarily by immunoglobulins and T lymphocytes. However, the response frequently requires recruitment of otherwise nonspecific components such as complement and phagocytic cells.

Antibody-Mediated Host Defenses

Antibodies serve a variety of important host defense functions, both alone and in conjunction with nonspecific effectors (Table 49–4) (see Chapter 9). Functions of antibodies include neutralization of the biologic activity of bacterial toxins (the mechanism by which tetanus and diphtheria toxoid vaccines protect against disease), inhibition of enzyme activity (eg, the neuraminidase of influenza virus), blocking of the adherence of bacteria to mucosal surfaces, and inhibition of the growth of some prokaryotes such as *Mycoplasma*. Viruses may be neutralized in the presence of antibody alone, but many enveloped viruses are neutralized more efficiently if complement is also present. Although in vitro lysis of virus-infected cells by specific antibody and complement has been documented, the overall role of this phenomenon in host defense is unclear. Opsonization—preparing material for ingestion by phagocytic cells—also may occur with antibody alone, although the combination of antibody and complement usually increases the efficiency of ingestion. Killing of gram-negative bacteria by IgM antibody has an absolute requirement for complement.

T Lymphocyte-Mediated Host Defenses

Although T lymphocytes play a central and critical role in the generation of the immune response to invading microorganisms (see also Chapter 5), their role is predominantly one of recruiting, facilitating, and augmenting other effectors, rather than of directly attacking the pathogens themselves. Viruses are the major exception to this generalization, as the T lymphocyte-mediated attack on virus-infected cells constitutes a major host defense against established viral infection. The specific T cell response to virus-

Table 49–4. Principal antibody-mediated host defense.

Immunologic Function	Pathogens Affected[1]	Principal Antibody Classes Involved	Nonspecific Cofactors Required
Opsonization	V, B, F	IgG, IgM	Phagocytic cells and complement (in some cases)
Neutralization	V, B[2]	IgG, IgM, IgA	Complement (in some cases)
Inhibition of binding	B, F(?)	IgA	None
Bacteriolysis	B	IgM	Complement
Toxin neutralization	B	IgG	None
Enzyme inhibition	V, B(?)	IgG	None
(ADCC)	V, ?F, ?P	IgG	None
Growth inhibition	*Mycoplasma*	IgG, IgA	None
	B[3]	IgA	Lactoferrin

[1]V, viruses; B, bacteria; F, fungi.
[2]Bacterial toxins only.
[3]IgA against bacterial nonbinding proteins synergistically inhibits growth with lactoferrin.

infected cells is mediated by CD8 cytotoxic T lymphocytes (CTLs); in addition, for some viral infections (eg, by herpes simplex virus) NK cells and macrophages are important in recovery from infection. Secretion of lymphokines, especially gamma interferon, by immune lymphocytes is responsible for augmented NK and CTL activity. Lymphokines also activate macrophages, which constitute a major host defense against many bacterial, fungal, and parasitic infections. Interferons produced by virus-infected cells that are not a part of the immune system (eg, alpha interferon from fibroblasts) have a direct antiviral effect, but they also augment NK cell and macrophage function. A possible direct role for T cells in antibacterial defense has been suggested by recent studies showing specific lysis of *Listeria monocytogenes*-infected macrophages by sensitized T lymphocytes.

Complement

Complement acts by inactivating microorganisms and by facilitating phagocytosis (opsonization); in both roles it is often assisted by antibody (Table 49–4) (see Chapter 14). In addition, complement breakdown products induce vasodilation and are chemoattractants. The alternative complement pathway alone can be stimulated to kill some gram-negative bacteria and inactivate some viruses in the absence of antibodies. Specific antibody, however, is required for activation of the classic complement pathway, which plays an important role in host defenses to bacterial and other infections (Table 49–4). Early in infection, prior to synthesis of specific antibodies, the ability of the alternative complement pathway to nonspecifically opsonize or kill certain bacteria may be critical to recovery from infections.

Phagocytic Cells

Phagocytic cells fulfill a number of important functions in host defense (Table 49–5) (see Chapter 12). They subserve nonspecific roles such as phagocytosis and secretion of monokines and enzymes, but these functions are often augmented by lymphokines

Table 49–5. Functions of phagocytic cells thought to be important in host defenses.

Chemotaxis
Phagocytosis
  Nonfacilitated
  Facilitated (opsonization)
Killing
  Intracellular
    Oxygen-dependent
    Oxygen-independent
  Extracellular
    Nonfacilitated
    Antibody-facilitated (ADCC)
Secretion
  Monokines (IL-1, TNF, etc)
  Enzymes (proteases, etc)

secreted as the result of a specific immune response, as described above. Many organisms have extracellular products (eg, the polysaccharide capsule on pneumococci) that inhibit phagocytosis. Once ingested by phagocytic cells, the microorganisms are attacked by a variety of microbicidal systems (Table 49–5). Organisms that can survive and replicate within the professional phagocyte are termed "facultative intracellular pathogens."

In addition, Fc-bearing phagocytic cells and NK cells may have immunologic specificity imposed upon them by antibody: the so-called antibody-dependent cellular cytotoxicity (ADCC) reaction (Table 49–4). When coated with specific IgG antibody, virus-infected cells and perhaps fungi and other eukaryotic pathogens become susceptible to killing by these NK cells and macrophages (and perhaps by PMN in some cases). The immunologic specificity of this reaction is wholly imparted by the antibody. The importance of the ADCC mechanism has been demonstrated conclusively in some experimental viral infections (eg, adult and neonatal murine herpes simplex virus infection), but it is thought to play some role in many other infections.

IMMUNOPATHOLOGY OF INFECTION

Disease may result directly from injury induced by a pathogen, for example, the paralysis and death caused by secretion of tetanus toxin by *Clostridium tetani*. However, in other cases the host response to the pathogen may contribute to the resulting disease and, in a few instances, may be solely responsible for the resulting clinical findings. In addition, the host immune response may facilitate or augment infection in some cases, such as the antibody-mediated enhancement of dengue virus and human immunodeficiency virus (HIV) infection of Fc-bearing cells such as macrophages. Lastly, some pathogens, particularly viruses, may injure the immune system itself, producing transient or even longstanding immunosuppression. Infection with HIV is the most important example of this type of host–parasite interaction (see Chapter 55).

Nonspecific host immune responses to invading pathogens, ie, the inflammatory response or some component of it, may be injurious in many cases. Release of inflammatory mediators causes pain and swelling, and the enzymes secreted by PMN and macrophages may produce permanent tissue damage. In most instances the beneficial effects of the local inflammatory response far outweigh any deleterious ones. However, for the patient suffering from the discomfort of a large staphylococcal abscess, this may be a difficult point to make!

Endotoxin-mediated host injury, which clinically results in the sepsis syndrome or septic shock, is usually consequent to severe infection by gram-negative bacteria such as meningococci. In this instance, much of the resulting disease is attributable to the host response to the endotoxin, not to direct injury by the endotoxin itself. Although endotoxin has many effects, including triggering of the complement and coagulation systems, the major events from the standpoint of the pathogenesis of the sepsis syndrome are stimulation of IL-1 and TNF synthesis by macrophages. Pretreatment of animals with antibodies specific for TNF reduces the mortality rate associated with experimental administration of endotoxin.

There are many examples of host injury secondary to the humoral immune response to a pathogen. The most important examples occur in immune complex disease (see Chapter 32). Poststreptococcal glomerulonephritis results from formation of complexes between streptococcal antigens and host IgG antibody, which are deposited in the kidney, attracting complement and inflammatory cells. Chronic antigen-antibody complex disease may occur in hepatitis B virus infection, with a clinical syndrome of polyarteritis nodosa. Infection by *Mycoplasma pneumoniae* induces antibody to the I blood group antigen on erythrocytes, even though the I antigen is not found on the organisms. In some patients who develop high titers of this antibody, hemolytic anemia may develop.

Clear examples of host injury secondary to the cellular immune response are more difficult to identify. It is likely that some of the clinical features of tuberculosis are attributable to delayed hypersensitivity to the proteins of *M tuberculosis,* but as the organism itself produces injury, this has been difficult to prove. Liver cell damage by hepatitis B virus is probably due wholly or partly to the CTL response to viral antigens, but direct proof of this point is also lacking.

REFERENCES

Dinarello CA, Cannon JG, Wolff SM: New concepts on the pathogenesis of fever. *Rev. Infect Dis* 1988;**10**:168.

Kilian M, Mestecky J, Russel MW: Defense mechanisms involving Fc-dependent functions of IgA and their subversion by bacterial IgA proteases. *Microbiol Rev* 1988;**52**:296.

Mims CA: *The Pathogenesis of Infectious Diseases,* 3rd ed. Academic Press, 1986.

Neighbor PA, Bloom PR: Natural resistance to virus infections. *Semin Infect Dis* 1980;**3**:272.

Notkins A, Oldstone MBA (editors): *Concepts in Viral Pathogenesis.* Springer Verlag, 1984.

Roth JA (editor): *Virulence Mechanisms of Bacterial Pathogens.* Am Soc Microbiol, 1988.

Sanders WE, Sanders CC: Microbial antagonism: A potent defense against infection. *Clin Microbiol News* 1982;**4**:127.

Southern P, Oldstone MB: Medical consequences of persistent viral infection. *N Engl J Med* 1986;**314**:359.

Sprunt K, Leidy G: The use of bacterial interference to prevent infection. *Can J Microbiol* 1988;**34**:332.

Taylor PW: Bactericidal and bacteriolytic activity of serum against gram-negative bacteria. *Microbiol Rev* 1983;**47**:46.

Tramont EC: General or nonspecific host defense mechanisms. Chapter 4 in: *Principles and Practice of Infectious Diseases,* 2nd ed. Mandell GL, Douglas RG Jr, Bennett JE (editors). Wiley, 1985.

Urbaschek B (editor). Perspectives on bacterial pathogenesis and host defense: Proceedings of a Symposium. *Rev Infect Dis* 1987;**9**:S431.

Bacterial Diseases

50

John L. Ryan, PhD, MD

Immunity to bacterial infections is mediated by both cellular and humoral mechanisms. Bacteria express many different surface antigens and secrete a variety of virulence factors (eg, toxins) that may trigger immune responses. Since the topic of bacterial immunity is vast, attention in this chapter will be focused on 3 principal types of immunity to bacteria, with examples for which pathogenesis and host responses are well characterized.

(1) The first is immunity to **toxigenic bacterial infections**. Bacterial exotoxins and endotoxins are important in the pathogenesis of specific diseases. Exotoxins are the sole virulence factor in certain toxigenic bacterial infections, and immunity directed against these toxins can completely prevent disease.

(2) The second is immunity to **encapsulated bacteria**. These organisms evade phagocytosis by coating themselves with innocuous polysaccharide. Encapsulated bacteria may be gram-positive or gram-negative, and vaccines containing purified capsular antigens generate protective immunity.

(3) The third is immunity to **intracellular bacteria**. These bacteria avoid the host immune response because they grow inside cells, particularly phagocytes. The same evasive mechanism is utilized by many fungal and parasitic pathogens. Cellular immunity mediated by macrophages that are activated by specific lymphocytes and their products is the critical mode of host defense against this group of bacteria.

SERODIAGNOSIS

Serodiagnosis of bacterial diseases is of value only in specific circumstances. IgG antibody is long-lived, and its presence, although indicative of exposure to antigenic stimulation from previous infection or immunization, gives little or no information on current bacterial infection. IgM antibody is usually produced within days to a few weeks after exposure to antigen, and thus its presence suggests recent exposure in most cases. As with viral diseases, serial determinations of antibody levels with rising titers are of greater diagnostic value, but because of the time intervals required, they are usually of little clinical value.

In general, culture of specific pathogens is required to confirm the diagnosis of a bacterial disease. Serologic tests may aid in diagnosis when diseases are caused by bacteria that are difficult to grow. *Brucella* is one such species. These organisms are difficult to culture from patients' specimens, and there is no useful delayed hypersensitivity skin test. Even though many mycobacteria are also difficult to grow, antibody titers are not helpful in diagnosis. Thus, in contrast to viral and fungal pathogens, the serologic tests in bacterial infections remain primarily a tool for epidemiologic studies rather than for clinical diagnosis in individual cases. Nevertheless, most bacteria induce specific antibody responses, which, in most cases, can be easily measured in serum. As discussed below, these antibody responses are often critical in determining the host response to an infecting agent.

EXOTOXINS & ENDOTOXINS

Exotoxins are noxious proteins that are secreted by many bacteria. These toxins are often heat-labile and thus can be heat-inactivated for use as vaccines to prevent toxigenic bacterial disease. Many bacteria produce more than one protein exotoxin, making vaccine development more difficult. Endotoxins are somatic lipopolysaccharide-protein complexes. These complex antigens are located in the outer membrane of all gram-negative bacteria. Toxicologic activity is associated with the lipid A component of the endotoxin, whereas the serologic determinants are polysaccharides. Antibody directed against specific polysaccharides can be protective both by enhancing phagocytosis directly and by fixing complement for lysis. Unfortunately, from an immune standpoint, there are usually antigenic differences in the polysaccharide components of endotoxins among strains of bacteria. Thus, in general, infection with one strain does not generate protective immunity to reinfection with a different strain of the same species. IgM and IgG antibodies directed against the lipid A component of lipopolysaccharide have different capacities to neutralize the infectivity of gram-negative bacteria. It appears that IgM is a more potent neutralizing antibody than IgG. This is particularly true for cross-reacting antibody directed against core polysaccharide or lipid A determinants of gram-negative bacteria.

TOXIGENIC BACTERIAL DISEASES

In this section, 2 groups of toxigenic diseases will be considered. In the first group, an exotoxin is the sole virulence determinant, and vaccines directed at the exotoxin can generate effective immunity. In the second group, toxins are major virulence factors, but other pathogenic factors exist, making specific immune responses less effective in disease prevention (Fig 50–1). Antibody to toxins can neutralize the toxin by several mechanisms, including enhancing clearance by macrophages or blocking binding sites on toxin for its cellular receptors.

Clostridium Species

Clostridia are obligate anaerobic, sporeforming gram-positive rods, which cause a variety of clinical diseases. *Clostridium tetani* is the cause of tetanus. Disease occurs when spores are introduced into wounds from contaminated soil or foreign bodies. After these spores germinate, a potent neurotoxin called tetanospasmin is produced. Tetanospasmin binds to specific glycolipids in nerve cells in the peripheral nervous system and ascends to the spinal cord from nerves in the periphery. The toxin blocks normal postsynaptic inhibition of spinal reflexes, leading to generalized muscular spasms, or "tetany." A vaccine prepared from the inactivated

toxin, termed "toxoid," prevents disease by generating antibodies that neutralize the toxin. It is recommended that all children be immunized with tetanus toxoid soon after birth (see Chapter 58). Subsequent boosts of immunity to toxoid are required every 10 years during adult life to maintain a protective level of antibody. There does not appear to be significant antigenic variation in tetanus toxins, since the single vaccine is protective.

Clostridium botulinum is another exotoxin-producing species for which immunity requires neutralizing antibodies to the toxin (antitoxin). *C botulinum* causes botulism, which is primarily a food-borne disease, occurring when spores or toxin are ingested from contaminated food. The botulinum toxin acts by inhibiting the release of acetylcholine neurotransmitter at the neuromuscular junctions. This produces diplopia, dysphagia, and, in severe cases, respiratory arrest. Botulism is treated with antitoxin, which is equine antiserum directed against the 3 most common toxin serotypes: A, B, and E. A pentavalent toxoid (A, B, C, D, E) is distributed by the Centers for Disease Control. This toxoid is prepared from formalin-treated toxins, which are adsorbed to aluminum phosphate to enhance immunogenicity. Natural immunity does not occur, because immunogenic doses of these toxins are lethal.

Several other *Clostridium* strains cause pyogenic infections that are mediated, in part, by cytopathic exotoxins. The most common are soft tissue infections caused by *Clostridium perfringens,* which releases a potent lecithinase called α toxin. This toxin

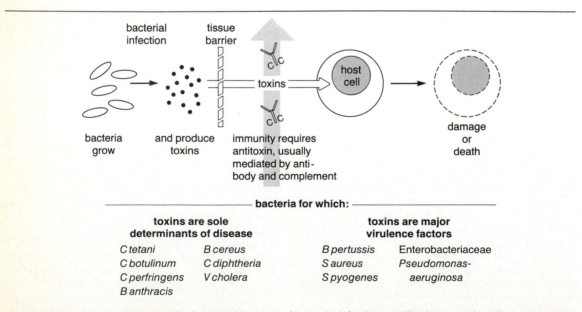

Figure 50–1. Toxigenic bacterial infections. In this group of bacterial infections, antibody to protein toxins and complement play a protective role in enhancing survival.

has been associated with massive intravascular hemolysis in uncontrolled infection. *C perfringens* also secretes several other toxins, including an enterotoxin that is an important cause of food poisoning. Therapy with antitoxins has not been useful in treating diseases caused by *C perfringens,* because the organism secretes such a wide variety of toxins.

Bacillus Species

Bacillus species are facultative anaerobic gram-positive rods that can form spores. They are similar to clostridia, except for their facultative anaerobic metabolism. One of the first pathogenic bacteria to be studied was *Bacillus anthracis,* the only nonmotile species in the genus. The disease anthrax is caused by human contact with animal products contaminated by *B anthracis.* Animals are infected by ingestion of the bacteria or spores in the environment. Pathogenicity depends on toxin production, and the disease can be prevented by vaccination against attenuated bacteria. Pasteur was the first to show that vaccination could prevent anthrax in animals. The anthrax exotoxin is complex, consisting of at least 3 components: protective antigen, edema factor, and lethal factor. The protective antigen, which is not toxic alone, induces immunity and is the major component of current vaccines. *B anthracis* has also been shown to have a polysaccharide capsule, which may contribute to the virulence of this organism.

Bacillus cereus, the other toxigenic *Bacillus* species, is a common cause of food poisoning. Several toxins, including a pyogenic toxin and enterotoxins, are produced. Little is known about protective immunity to these bacteria.

Corynebacterium diphtheriae

Corynebacteria are facultative anaerobic gram-positive rods that do not form spores. The most important species is *Corynebacteria diphtheriae,* the cause of diphtheria. This organism colonizes the mucous membranes of the posterior pharynx and elaborates a potent exotoxin. The toxin kills cells by covalently linking adenosine diphosphoribose to elongation factor 2, which is required for cellular protein biosynthesis. Immunity to diphtheria depends on the presence of antibody to the toxin. Diphtheria toxoid, a formalin-inactivated toxin preparation, is currently used worldwide to vaccinate infants against diphtheria. Immunity to diphtheria is assessed by using the Schick test. In this test, small amounts of toxin and toxoid are injected intradermally at different sites. If no response is observed at either site after 48 hours, the patient is immune to the toxin (has circulating antitoxin) and is not hypersensitive to the toxoid. If there is necrosis at the toxin site and response at the toxoid site, the patient does not have protective antibody. An immediate reaction at both sites indicates allergy to the proteins. A delayed reaction at one or both sites indicates cellular immunity to the proteins. The Schick test has been very useful in assessing immunity to *C diphtheriae.* It is no longer used very often, and has been replaced with antibody titers. Nevertheless, it has provided insight into the importance of maintaining adequate circulating antibody to toxin to ameliorate or prevent clinical infection.

Vibrio cholerae

The vibrios are curved, gram-negative bacilli with polar flagellae. Infection with *Vibrio cholerae,* the agent of cholera, occurs after ingestion of contaminated water. Organisms multiply in the gut and release an enterotoxin, which binds to epithelial cells and triggers massive secretion of fluid and electrolytes. Severe diarrhea may occur within hours after infection, and the fluid loss is often life-threatening, particularly in infants and young children. Cholera is unique among the toxigenic diseases in that antibody to the toxin does not fully prevent disease. Infection with *V cholerae* induces systemic and mucosal antibody. Mucosal IgA, which prevents attachment of the bacteria in the gut, may be the most important form of immunity. Cholera vaccines induce short-term protection and elicit only IgM and IgG responses unless administered orally. Neither IgM nor IgG functions well in the intestinal lumen. Further research is needed to develop cholera vaccines that confer life-long immunity.

Bordetella pertussis

Pertussis (whooping cough) is caused by mucosal infection with *Bordetella pertussis,* a small, gram-negative coccobacillary organism that replicates in bronchial mucosa. Infection is characterized by paroxysmal coughing, which can result in significant morbidity in young children. *B pertussis* contains several antigens that may elicit immune responses, but the critical factors in immunity to this organism are not fully understood. Killed whole bacteria are currently used as a vaccine, but acellular vaccines are under active development. Pertussis vaccine is given in combination with diphtheria toxoid and tetanus toxoid (DPT) to infants at 2, 4, and 6 months of age, with boosters usually given 1 year later and again before the children begin to attend school. Immunity to pertussis is relatively short-lived, lasting only 3 years after completion of primary immunization or boosting. Antibody that prevents attachment of the bacteria to respiratory epithelium appears to be the first line of defense, with antitoxin providing further protection against a protein exotoxin produced by the bacteria.

The presence of *B pertussis* in the DPT combination vaccine may enhance the antibody response to both protein toxoids (DT). The lipopolysaccharide in the outer membrane of *B pertussis* is a potent immune adjuvant. Thus, it is advantageous as well as convenient to use the combined vaccine.

Staphylococcus aureus

Staphylococci are facultative anaerobic, nonmotile gram-positive cocci that are most often seen as clusters in gram-stained specimens. *Staphylococcus aureus* is probably the single most prevalent pathogen in skin and soft tissue infections. Its virulence has been studied intensively, but the mechanism remains obscure. The primary line of defense against staphylococci is the polymorphonuclear leukocyte, which phagocytoses and kills the bacteria. *S aureus* produces a vast number of virulence factors, including toxins, which may contribute to its pathogenicity. Production of coagulase, a factor that can bind and activate fibrinogen, defines the species *S aureus*. At least 4 separate hemolysins are also produced. A nonhemolytic leukocidin is cytotoxic for granulocytes. In addition, *S aureus* secretes several enterotoxins, an exfoliative toxin associated with epidermal necrolysis, and an exotoxin associated with the toxic shock syndrome.

The immune response to *S aureus* infections is inadequate in that previous infection does not protect the host from reinfection. The few strains of *S aureus* that have capsules do generate protective antibody, but these strains are not commonly pathogenic. Similarly, antibodies to the toxic shock exotoxin and to the exfoliative exotoxins seem to prevent the specific clinical syndromes caused by these toxins. Pyogenic *S aureus* infections occur, however, despite the presence of multiple antibodies against cellular components in the host. Only the number and functional capacity of granulocytes are critically important in the defense against *S aureus*.

Another *Staphylococcus* strain associated with human disease is *Staphylococcus epidermidis*. This strain produces few toxins and is associated primarily with bacteremias in patients with plastic catheters or other foreign objects in the bloodstream. *S epidermidis,* as the name implies, is one of the most common bacteria of the skin flora. It adheres to catheters or other materials by means of an extracellular polysaccharide slime, which inhibits the ability of granulocytes to function properly. Protective immunity to this organism does not appear to develop, since repeated infections may occur in susceptible hosts.

Streptococcus Species

Streptococci are a diverse group of catalase-negative, facultatively anaerobic gram-positive cocci, which cause a variety of toxigenic and pyogenic infections in humans. *Streptococcus pyogenes* is the most important bacterial cause of pharyngitis. Late sequelae, such as rheumatic fever and glomerulonephritis, may follow infection with certain strains of this species.

Most streptococcal infections do not confer immunity unless the syndrome is mediated by toxins, such as the streptococcal pyogenic exotoxins associated with scarlet fever. The antigenic composition of streptococci is complex, with approximately 18 group-specific carbohydrate antigens lettered A–R. These antigens are useful for classifying streptococci, but they do not elicit protective immunity. Group A streptococci contain another set of type-specific M antigens, known as M proteins (more than 80 types exist). These proteins are antiphagocytic factors and enhance the virulence of group A streptococci. The M proteins do generate protective IgG antibody, but since there are many serotypes of M protein, reinfection with another strain is common.

Streptococci of groups A, B, C, F, and G produce many extracellular products that may elicit protective immunity. Streptolysins O and S are cytopathic proteins that inhibit phagocytosis and killing by leukocytes. A variety of proteinases exist, including streptokinase and other degradative enzymes such as hyaluronidase and deoxyribonuclease, which enhance the pathogenicity of the organism. Antibodies may be produced to all of these factors during infection. The widely used Streptozyme test is a hemagglutination procedure that detects a variety of antibodies against streptococcal enzymes.

Group D streptococci have recently been reclassified as enterococci and are antigenically distinct from other streptococci in that they do not possess a group-specific carbohydrate antigen, but they do have a group-specific glycerol teichoic acid antigen.

Most of the streptococci that normally colonize the human oropharynx do not possess group-specific antigens and are classified in the viridans group. Many individual strains may be defined by biochemical tests, but none of these streptococci are prominent toxin producers. They are active in causing periodontal diseases and are the most common causes of infective endocarditis. Little is known about protective immunity to this diverse group of organisms.

Gram-Negative Rods

Gram-negative rods produce a variety of toxins and are responsible for many infectious diseases. The family Enterobacteriaceae is composed of 5 major genera: *Escherichia, Klebsiella, Proteus, Yersinia,* and *Erwinia*. These are all glucose-fermenting, nonsporeforming bacilli. All members of the family Enterobacteriaceae, but particularly *Escherichia* and *Salmonella,* have undergone extensive immunologic analyses. They are serotyped on the basis of O antigens (polysaccharides associated with the lipopolysaccharide component of the outer membrane), K antigens (polysaccharide capsular components), and H antigens (proteins associated with flagellae).

Some of these organisms are partially responsible for contributing to the immune pathogenesis of the spondyloarthropathies. The well-known association of the class I molecule HLA-B27 and ankylosing spondylitis, as well the association of the disease with preceding enteric infection, has stimulated a search for molecular mimicry, ie, identity between epitopes on a bacterium and one in the human host. The immune response to *Klebsiella pneumoniae* elicits antibody that can bind to HLA-B27 on the surface of synovial lining cells. Similar molecular mimicry has been shown for *Shigella flexneri,* which produces an arthritogenic epitope that is shared by HLA-B27 antigen. Thus, the immune response to certain members of the Enterobacteriaceae may result in autoimmune disease in selected hosts.

Each member of the family Enterobacteriaceae contains an endotoxin. This endotoxin is a lipopolysaccharide-protein complex in the outer membrane and contains the O-specific serologic group. The biologically active components of the endotoxin are the lipid A and certain lipoproteins associated with the lipopolysaccharide.

Enterotoxins are also produced by many members of the Enterobacteriaceae, particularly *Escherichia coli. E coli* has at least 2 enterotoxins, an immunogenic heat-labile toxin and a nonimmunogenic heat-stable toxin. More typical exotoxins are also related to certain strains of *E coli, Shigella,* and *Yersinia.*

Immunity to the Enterobacteriaceae is achieved early in life after colonization of the gut with *E coli.* Antibodies against K and O antigens are generated and are protective against autologous serotypes. Prior to the development of antibody, the neonate is susceptible to systemic and particularly to central nervous system infection by *E coli.* In adult life, these bacteria cause opportunistic as well as enteric diseases. Attempts to transfer passive immunity with antiserum to *E coli* have proved effective in both animal and some human studies. Antibodies directed against the endotoxin component may be able to exert antitoxic activity and prevent the morbidity and mortality associated with sepsis. Studies using monoclonal antibodies directed against the lipid A subunit of endotoxin are currently in progress in an attempt to improve the rate of survival from gram-negative septicemia.

Pseudomonas aeruginosa is the most clinically important nonfermenting gram-negative rod and has been the subject of extensive immunologic analysis. It characteristically produces exotoxin A, a cytolytic factor with a similar mechanism of action to diphtheria toxin. Antibodies directed against exotoxin A as well as the lipopolysaccharide appear to be important in immunity to infection with *P aeruginosa.* Different serotyping schemes have been used to define *P aeruginosa* for epidemiologic purposes. Multivalent vaccines containing several serotypes to protect immunocompromised patients from invasive *Pseudomonas* infection are under investigation. *Pseudomonas* is a virulent opportunistic pathogen that commonly invades immunocompromised pa-

tients. The role of antibody to endotoxin in ameliorating human disease has been shown in animals by using homologous and heterologous antisera to protect them against lethal *P aeruginosa* infections.

ENCAPSULATED BACTERIA

Bacteria that express capsular polysaccharide present a unique problem for the immune system. Capsular polysaccharide inhibits phagocytosis by both macrophages and polymorphonuclear leukocytes. Effective phagocytosis requires functional leukocyte receptors for the Fc region of immunoglobulin and C3b or C3bi (Fig 50–2). Opsonization of encapsulated bacteria with antibody and complement is necessary for phagocytes to efficiently ingest and kill these pathogens. The charge and hydrophilicity of unopsonized encapsulated bacteria inhibit phagocytosis by interfering with attachment of leukocytes and bacteria. Immaturity of humoral immunity in the very young and decline of humoral immunity in the elderly probably account for the susceptibility of individuals at these stages of life to invasive disease by encapsulated bacteria.

Bacterial vaccines hold great promise for enhancing immunity against encapsulated bacteria. Since polysaccharides are relatively poor immunogens, complexes of protein with polysaccharides may represent more effective vaccine candidates. Coupling of weak antigens with other types of adjuvants may also improve the efficacy of vaccines.

Streptococcus pneumoniae

Streptococcus pneumoniae strains, commonly called pneumococci, differ from other streptococci in that they contain complex polysaccharide capsules that determine the major virulence determinant in the species. Pneumococci are respiratory pathogens that colonize upper airways and cause bronchitis or pneumonia after aspiration of respiratory secretions. The capsule inhibits alveolar macrophage phagocytosis and allows the pneumococcus to multiply in the lung. Patients with abnormal mucocillary reflexes or decreased alveolar macrophage function are more susceptible to infection. Patients with decreased systemic clearance of bacteria are susceptible to disseminated disease.

Type-specific antibody is elicited and is protective, but there are more than 80 serotypes of pneumococci. Thus, reinfection with a different serotype is common in susceptible persons. The polysaccharide capsule is sometimes cross-reactive with the capsular polysaccharides of different genera, including *Haemophilus* and *Klebsiella.* A vaccine containing capsular polysaccharide from the 23 most prevalent or virulent serotypes is available for adult patients at high risk for pneumococcal disease.

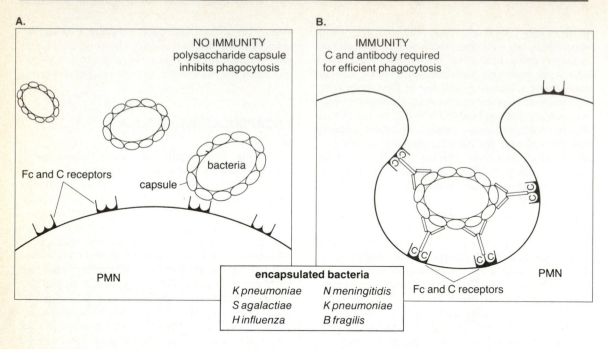

Figure 50–2. Encapsulated bacteria. Polysaccharide capsules allow bacterial multiplication by avoiding receptor-mediated phagocytosis. If specific antibody to the capsule is present, both antibody and complement serve as opsonins to enhance the uptake of bacteria by host phagocytes.

Streptococcus agalactiae (Group B)

The group B streptococci are a leading cause of neonatal meningitis. Most disease occurs because of colonization of the infant from vaginal flora during parturition. Group B organisms contain 4 major capsular serotypes. Sialic acid, one of the carbohydrate components of group B streptococcal capsular polysaccharide, can block complement activation. This prevents a key nonspecific defense mechanism in infants who are without adequate antibody levels. Type-specific antibodies are protective for group B streptococcal disease. Both passive immunization with IgG antibody to capsular polysaccharides and active immunization with polysaccharides to prevent group B streptococcal disease in the neonatal period are under investigation.

Haemophilus influenzae

Of the several species of *Haemophilus* that are known, *Haemophilus influenzae* is the most prevalent pathogen. Several distinct capsular serotypes have been defined, but type b *H influenzae* is responsible for most clinical disease. *H influenzae* is a respiratory pathogen that colonizes the oropharynx and causes bronchitis, pneumonia, or disseminated infection when local or systemic host defense factors are compromised. The type b capsule is a polyribitol phosphate. The susceptibility of a given host to infection is directly related to serum levels of bactericidal antibody. Maternal IgG is lost within a few

months after birth, and natural antibody is acquired by 3–4 years of age. The development of natural antibody may be related to colonization and subsequent immunization with nonpathogenic members of the family Enterobacteriaceae that contain cross-reactive capsular polysaccharides. *H influenzae* type b capsular polysaccharide (PRP) is a weak immunogen, and vaccines have not been effective in children younger than 2 years. Recently, conjugate vaccines with diphtheria toxin and outer membrane proteins linked to PRP have shown promise of effective immunization of children between 1 and 2 years of age. There are few bacterial diseases in which the protective role of antibody has been so clearly demonstrated as in *H influenzae* type b disease.

Neisseria Species

These are gram-negative cocci containing high levels of cytochrome c oxidase. The 2 pathogenic species are *Neisseria gonorrhoeae* (gonococcus) and *Neisseria meningitidis* (meningococcus). There is no definite role of anticapsular antibody in immunity to gonococcus. Repeated infections with gonococci are quite common. Mucosal antibody directed against surface proteins appears to have some protective value, and the complement system is particularly important in the maintenance of bactericidal activity. The meningococcus normally inhabits the pharynx without producing disease. This provides a reservoir for outbreaks and produces some immunity in the host. The critical antigenic components of the meningococcus are capsular polysaccharides, and 9 distinct serotypes can elicit group-specific protective antibody. IgM antibody appears to be more protective than does IgG, perhaps because of its more potent complement-fixing activity. Patients deficient in the terminal complement components C6, 7, 8 or properdin are susceptible to recurrent neisserial infections. Vaccines are available to both group A and group C *N meningitidis*. Group B capsular polysaccharides are cross-reactive with *E coli* capsular polysaccharides (K1 antigens), and no vaccine is available against this strain. The importance of antibody in protection against meningococcal disease is underscored by the peak incidence of disease, which occurs at about 1 year of age, when maternal antibody has waned and acquired antibody has not yet been produced.

Klebsiella pneumoniae

Klebsiella species are members of the family Enterobacteriaceae that are characterized by polysaccharide capsules with more than 70 serotypes. Although they are predominantly intestinal organisms that cause opportunistic infections, they are also associated with primary pneumonias. This is probably related to the ability of these bacteria to avoid phagocytosis in the absence of antibody. The capsular polysaccharides found in *Klebsiella* are related to those in *Streptococcus* and *Haemophilus*. The role of specific anticapsular antibodies in *Klebsiella* has not been elucidated. Immunity appears to be multifactorial, with disease most commonly occurring in debilitated patients with depressed host defenses.

Bacteroides fragilis

Bacteroides fragilis and closely related species are obligate anaerobic nonsporeforming gram-negative rods, which colonize the intestinal tract and are often associated with intra-abdominal abscess formation. Unless the mucous membrane barrier of the gastrointestinal or respiratory tract is damaged, *B fragilis* represent harmless normal flora. In the presence of tissue necrosis or trauma, *B fragilis* may be released into a relatively low-oxygen environment, allowing growth and elaboration of several enzymes that potentiate tissue damage. *B fragilis* also contains a capsular polysaccharide that is a key virulence factor in animal models of infection. The capsule mediates resistance to phagocytosis, and capsular antibody enhances the phagocytic killing of these bacteria.

INTRACELLULAR BACTERIAL PATHOGENS

Many bacteria have developed the ability to avoid host defense systems by invading cells so that serum antibody and complement cannot harm them and granulocytes cannot recognize them (Fig 50–3). These bacteria induce T cell-mediated immunity in the same fashion as fungi, parasites, and viruses. Serum antibody and complement are not markers of resistance for these bacteria. The presence of sensitized T lymphocytes and activated macrophages is the key factor in immunity. Microbial antigens are expressed on the surface of macrophages after the antigens are processed, in conjunction with products of the major histocompatibility complex. In this configuration, macrophages interact with T lymphocytes to produce macrophage-activating factors such as gamma interferon. This complex series of events is required for the expression of effective immunity to intracellular pathogens.

Salmonella Species

Salmonella species are members of the family Enterobacteriaceae and cause a significant proportion of enteric disease. Three major species (*Salmonella typhi*, *Salmonella choleraesuis,* and *Salmonella enteritidis*) exist. Based on serologic reactions, there are more than 1700 types of *S enteritidis*. Most invasive disease, such as typhoid fever, is caused by *S typhi*, and it is of great interest that this is the only species of *Salmonella* with a surface capsular antigen. This capsule, therefore, is a key virulence factor for *S typhi*. Antibody against the capsule is not protective, and many typhoid carriers have circulating antibody. This reflects the ability of salmonellae to reside within cells of the reticuloendothelial system. Salmonellae usually enter the body by ingestion and cause enterocolitis if they are present in sufficient numbers to survive the acidic environment of the stomach. If they invade mucosal tissues, they can cause disseminated disease. Immunity to *Salmonella* involves activation of macrophages by sensitized T lymphocytes through lymphokine secretion. Circulating antibodies do not penetrate the cell to eradicate intracellular bacteria. Thus circulating antibody represents a marker of infection, but not of immunity.

Other Intracellular Bacterial Pathogens

Bacterial strains other than *Salmonella* that are intracellular pathogens include *Legionella, Listeria,* and *Brucella. Legionella pneumophila* and related strains are obligate intracellular parasites of macrophages. These bacteria exhibit optimal growth only within cells. Antibodies to serogroup-specific antigens are produced and are useful for diagnostic or epidemiologic studies, but they have not proved to be protective. Antigen-specific T lymphocyte activation with release of gamma interferon and other macrophage-activating factors enhances immunity to *Legionella*.

Listeria monocytogenes is a gram-positive rod

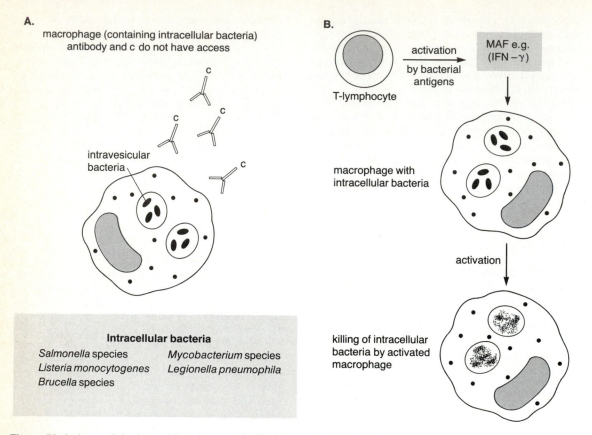

A.

macrophage (containing intracellular bacteria)
antibody and c do not have access

intravesicular
bacteria

Intracellular bacteria

Salmonella species   *Mycobacterium* species
Listeria monocytogenes   *Legionella pneumophila*
Brucella species

B.

T-lymphocyte

activation
by bacterial
antigens

MAF e.g.
(IFN−γ)

macrophage with
intracellular bacteria

activation

killing of intracellular
bacteria by activated
macrophage

Figure 50–3. Intracellular bacterial pathogens. Antibody and complement have no access to intracellular pathogens. Lymphokines mediate macrophage activation, which allows the killing of these bacteria by both oxidative and nonoxidative mechanisms.

similar to *Corynebacterium;* it causes meningeal infections or sepsis in adults and a variety of infections in neonates. Although antibody may play some role in preventing invasion, it is clear that the macrophage is the primary mode of defense against these bacteria. Investigations in animal models have demonstrated that T lymphocyte function is important in macrophage activation for immunity to *Listeria*.

Brucella species are small coccobacillary gram-negative bacteria that resemble *Haemophilus* in appearance and are spread to humans through contact with animals (zoonosis). Three strains are pathogenic for humans and cause systemic disease that may be chronic or subacute. The first is *Brucella abortus* from cattle, the second is *Brucella suis* from pigs, and the third is *Brucella melitensis,* usually from goats and sheep. Diagnosis is often made by serology, but antibody does not confer immunity. Immunity to *Brucella* species is conferred by activated macrophages produced by specifically sensitized T lymphocytes and lymphokines derived from them. The specific antigens that elicit cellular immunity to brucellosis have not been defined.

Mycobacterium Species

The genus *Mycobacterium* comprises a unique group of bacteria characterized by a lipid-rich cell wall that contains N-glycolylneuraminic acid. The major pathogenic strain is *Mycobacterium tuberculosis,* although *Mycobacterium intracellulare* has emerged as a significant pathogen in patients with acquired immunodeficiency syndrome (AIDS). Tuberculosis has been one of the great infectious scourges of mankind throughout history and remains a major world health problem today. One reason is that despite decades of excellent research into the immune mechanisms relating to tuberculosis, an effective vaccine has not been found. Bacillus Calmette-Guérin (BCG), an attenuated *Mycobacterium bovis* strain, has been used for more than 60 years and is able to confer delayed cutaneous hypersensitivity but no clear-cut cellular immunity. Serum antibody plays no role in immunity to mycobacterial diseases. Sensitized T lymphocytes and activated macrophages are the critical factors in immunity. The components of the cell wall of *M tuberculosis* that may confer immunity have been analyzed in detail. Both proteins and polysaccharides have immunogenic potential, and there are data supporting a substantive role for the polysaccharide components as the key epitopes for cellular immunity. A purified protein derivative is used as an intradermal antigen to measure delayed hypersensitivity to *M tuberculosis*. A positive delayed skin test demonstrates previous exposure to the bacteria and is often correlated with immunity. There is not a one-to-one correlation between a positive skin test and immunity, however, and further definition of the protective antigens in the tubercle bacillus is needed before immunity to *M tuberculosis* can be understood.

Immunity to mycobacteria such as *M intracellulare* and *Mycobacterium leprae* (the agent of Hansen's disease, ie, leprosy) is also mediated by cellular immunity, with serum components playing an insignificant role. The occurrence of *M. intracellulare* infections in AIDS patients suggests that T cell immunity is important in resistance to mycobacterial infections.

CONCLUSIONS

Immunity to bacterial infections is extremely complex because of the diverse virulence factors used by bacteria to enhance their survival. Primary nonspecific defense against bacterial infections is afforded by granulocytes, which ingest and kill most potential pathogens. Specific immunity is needed for protection against encapsulated or intracellular bacteria. This requires the development either of antibody, which can enhance killing by its opsonic or complement-fixing activity, or of T cell immunity, which can activate the microbicidal activity of macrophages. In many infections, a complex interaction of immune mechanisms is required to achieve protective immunity. Thus, antibody, complement, granulocytes, lymphocytes, and macrophages are all needed to permit the development of protective immunity to many bacterial pathogens.

REFERENCES

General

Braude AI (editor): *Infectious Diseases and Medical Microbiology*, 2nd ed. Saunders, 1986.

Sherris JC (editor): *Medical Microbiology: An Introduction to Infectious Diseases*. Elsevier, 1984.

Specific

Daniel DM. Antibody and antigen detection for the immunodiagnosis of tuberculosis: Why not? What more is needed? Where do we stand today? *J Infect Dis* 1988; **158:**678.

Densen P et al: Familial properdin deficiency and fatal meningococcemia. *N Engl J Med* 1987;**316:**922.

Dezfulian M, Bitar RA, Bartlett JG: Kinetics study of immunologic response to *Clostridium botulinum* toxin. *J Clin Microbiol* 1987;**25:**1336.

Fierer J: *Pseudomonas* and *Flavobacterium*. Chap 33, pp 314–320, in: *Infectious Diseases and Medical Microbiology*, 2nd ed. Braude AI (editor). Saunders, 1986.

Gazapo E et al: Changes in IgM and IgG antibody concentrations in brucellosis over time: Importance for diagnosis and follow-up. *J Infect Dis* 1989;**159:**219.

Griffiss JM et al: Vaccines against encapsulated bacteria: A global agenda. *Rev Infect Dis* 1987;**9:**176.

Harriman GR et al: The role of C9 in complement-mediated killing of *Neisseria*. *J Immunol* 1981; **127:**2386.

Johnston RB: Recurrent bacterial infections in children. *N Engl J Med* 1984;**310:**1237.

Kasper DL: The polysaccharide capsule of *Bacteroides fragilis* subspecies *fragilis:* Immunochemical and morphologic definition. *J Infect Dis* 1976;**133:**79.

McCabe WR et al: Immunization with rough mutants of *Salmonella minnesota:* Protective activity of IgM and IgG antibody to the R595 (Re Chemotype) mutant. *J Infect Dis* 1988;**158:**291.

Orskov F, Orskov I: Enterobacteriaceae. Chap 31, pp 292–303, in: *Infectious Diseases and Medical Microbiology*, 2nd ed. Braude AI (editor). Saunders, 1986.

Ryan KJ: *Corynebacteria and Other Non-Spore Forming Microbiology. An Introduction to Infectious Diseases*. Sherris JC (editor). Elsevier, 1984.

Schwimmbeck MD, Oldstone MBA: Molecular mimicry between human leucocyte antigens B27 and *Klebsiella. Am J Med* 1988;**85(Suppl 6A):**51.

51

Viral Infections

John Mills, MD

The interactions between viruses and the host immune system are not only complex and fascinating but also critical in determining the outcome of infection and strategies for its prevention. Viruses share the qualities of being complex immunogens with other pathogens that replicate in the host. They can stimulate both cellular and humoral immune responses, which then have a major influence on the outcome of infection. However, because viruses parasitize cellular metabolic processes during their own replication, they have a unique capacity to directly alter cell structure and function. This chapter considers some representative viral diseases of humans, selected either because of their clinical relevance or because they illustrate important facets of the interaction between virus infection and host immunity. Viruses that chiefly infect cells of the immune system are considered in Chapter 55.

Viruses are obligate intracellular parasites. Thus, clinical features of infection by a specific virus are determined by which cells are infected and whether the virus itself produces cellular pathology. In addition, for many viruses, the host immune response to viral antigens induces additional injuries, called **immunopathic effects,** which are qualitatively different from viropathic effects. Most of the disease morbidity associated with some viruses is, in fact, secondary to the host response. The outcome of virus infection may be broadly classified into those in which the virus is eliminated (eg, influenza virus and poliovirus) and those in which the virus remains latent (herpes simplex virus and human immunodeficiency virus). Other infections have late immunologic sequelae (Table 51–1). For some viruses, the host immune response is one determinant of whether the infection becomes latent.

INFLUENZA VIRUS

Major Immunologic Features
- Virus undergoes marked antigenic variation.
- Cellular immune response to infection eliminates virus.
- Postinfectious immunologic complications occur frequently.
- Humoral immunity induced by vaccines is partially protective.

General Considerations
Influenza is a respiratory infection with systemic manifestations; it is caused by influenza viruses. The disease occurs chiefly in epidemics, predominantly during the winter months. Although all age groups are affected, the severity of the illness is greatest at the extremes of age, and the mortality rate is highest in the elderly and in individuals with underlying chronic cardiorespiratory disease. Recurrent epidemics of influenza contribute significantly to the premature death of patients in these risk groups.

Virology
Influenza virus has an envelope and an RNA genome that is segmented (7–8 pieces) rather than the continuous strand characteristic of most viruses. The virus has several important structural proteins (Table 51–2), and, in general, each genome segment specifies one protein.

Three types of influenza virus, A, B, and C, are known; the classification is based on the antigenic characteristics of the ribonucleoprotein and matrix proteins, as well as other features. Influenza A virus is unique in part because it infects both humans and other animals (pigs, horses, fowl, and seals) and be-

Table 51–1. Viral infections with immunologic sequelae.

Acute Viral Infection	Late Immunologic Sequelae
Measles virus	Subacute sclerosing panencephalitis (SSPE)
Influenza virus	Guillain-Barré syndrome
Rubella virus	Rubella encephalopathy
Hepatitis B virus	Polyarteritis nodosa
Respiratory syncytial virus	Asthma (unproved association)
Epstein-Barr virus	Guillain-Barré syndrome

Table 51–2. Major structural proteins of influenza virus.

Protein	Location	Function
Hemagglutinin	Surface (envelope)	Acts as ligand for cell receptor acetylneuraminic acids
Neuraminidase	Surface (envelope)	Releases progeny virus from cell
Matrix protein	Internal	Stabilizes virus coat
RNA polymerase	Internal	Replicates RNA genome
Nucleoprotein	Internal	Stabilizes RNA within virion

cause it is the principal cause of pandemic influenza. When a cell is infected by 2 different influenza A viruses, the segmented RNA genomes of the 2 parental virus types mix during replication, so that virions of the progeny may contain RNA and protein from both parents (so-called ''recombinants,'' even though they are really reassortants). Influenza A virus thereby varies its surface hemagglutinin and neuraminidase molecules by recombining with other strains (including animal strains) as well as by using the mutational mechanisms common to all pathogens. These phenomena result in new epidemic strains (Fig 51–1). Influenza B virus does not have an animal reservoir to select novel hemagglutinin types, and thus the range of antigenic variation observed is narrower than that for influenza A virus. Influenza C virus appears to have only one serotype and differs from types A and B in some other features as well.

The principal targets for influenza virus infection are the ciliated epithelial cells of the upper and lower respiratory tract. Influenza virus infection kills these cells, which regenerate slowly during convalescence. Virus shedding terminates with recovery from infection, and neither chronic nor latent infection occurs.

Clinical Features

Influenza is spread primarily via aerosols; fomites do not appear to play a significant role. The clinical features of influenza are fever, cough, myalgia, headache, and malaise. Mild pharyngeal or conjunctival irritation is common, and gastrointestinal symptoms may occur as well, especially in children. There are no characteristic abnormalities on routine laboratory testing. Influenza may be diagnosed by culture of the virus from nasopharyngeal or pulmonary secretions, by direct detection of viral antigens on desquamated respiratory epithelial cells with fluorescently labeled monoclonal antibodies, or by demonstration of an antibody response to the virus in convalescent-phase sera.

Immunologic Pathogenesis

Although influenza virus stimulates a vigorous host immune response, including specific antibodies and cytotoxic T cells, most of the clinical findings are probably due directly to the cytopathic effects of this virus. In animal models of influenza, immunosuppression has a variable effect on the course of the infection, depending on the experimental details; however, virus replication is invariably prolonged. Nonetheless, patients with a wide variety of immunodeficiency disorders do not clearly show increased susceptibility to influenza virus infection. Patients who have underlying chronic cardiorespiratory disease have much higher morbidity and mortality rates than do otherwise healthy patients.

Cellular immunity, measured by either skin test reactivity or in vitro lymphocyte activation to antigens, is slightly depressed during acute influenza. The mechanism of this effect is uncertain, although it may be related to production of inhibitors of interleukin-1 (IL-1). This brief period of cellular immunosuppression appears to have no adverse clinical sequelae and does not interfere with the antiviral immune response. In contrast, influenza virus infection suppresses normal pulmonary antibacterial defenses, so that patients recovering from influenza have a greatly increased risk of developing bacterial pneumonia. The mechanism of this effect is unknown, but it may be the disruption of the mucociliary escalator combined with impaired function of pulmonary alveolar macrophages or neutrophils.

Influenza is associated with a number of postinfectious disorders, which are probably mediated by immune mechanisms. These include encephalitis (Chapter 43), myopericarditis (Chapter 39), and Goodpasture's syndrome (Chapters 41 and 46). The pathogenesis of these complications is unknown.

Antibodies directed against hemagglutinin and

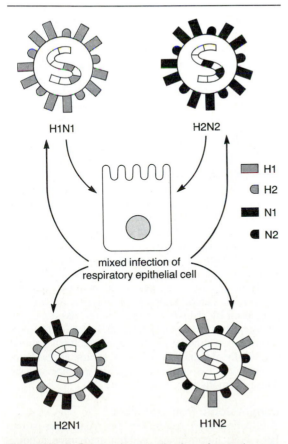

Figure 51–1. Schematic reproduction of genetic reassortment in influenza viruses. Shown are the major surface proteins and their corresponding gene segments.

neuraminidase surface proteins are critical determinants of host resistance to influenza virus. Antibodies to the hemagglutinin prevent the virus from attaching to cells and neutralize infectivity. Alone, they can prevent infection. Antibodies to neuraminidase inhibit the release of virus from cells and its subsequent spread to other cells within the host or to other people. Although antineuraminidase antibodies do not prevent infection, they ameliorate disease.

Treatment

Amantadine and rimantadine are cyclic amines that arrest influenza A virus replication in vitro and are active clinically. If started shortly after the onset of symptoms, treatment with either drug will shorten the duration of disease by about 50%. These drugs are also effective prophylactically, reducing the incidence of severe disease by more than 80%. However, their utility is limited by a relatively high incidence of adverse reactions, their limited antiviral spectrum, and the propensity of influenza A virus to become resistant.

Prevention

Vaccines against influenza virus were developed within a few years after identification of the virus in 1933. They were prepared by growing the virus in embryonated eggs and then inactivating its infectivity with chemical disinfectants. Currently, vaccines are made from egg-grown virus inactivated with β-propiolactone, but the viral antigens are separated from egg proteins by zonal centrifugation to avoid sensitization or reaction to egg proteins. The vaccine is standardized by hemagglutinin content, which is the only viral antigen found in significant amounts in the vaccine. The strains of influenza A and B viruses used for vaccine production (influenza C virus is not included because of its minor public health importance) are changed annually to reflect the antigenic characteristics of current isolates, on the recommendations of the Centers for Disease Control.

When given annually, influenza vaccines induce protection against both severe and mild influenza. Protection against infection per se is usually minimal or nonexistent. Protection is due entirely to the stimulation of antibodies directed against the hemagglutinin protein (see Table 51–2). The efficacy of the vaccine is limited by continuing antigenic variation in influenza A and B viruses, especially the extreme antigenic changes that occur in influenza A virus.

Influenza vaccines are relatively free of serious side effects, although painful local reactions are relatively common. At least one type of influenza virus—the swine influenza virus—has been associated with production of Guillain-Barré syndrome when administered as a vaccine. No other influenza virus type has yet been associated with this complication.

Research on improving influenza vaccines centers on development of live attenuated vaccines, insertion of hemagglutinin and neuraminidase genes into other vectors such as vaccinia virus, and attempts to find protective epitopes on molecules that are not subject to antigenic variation.

RESPIRATORY SYNCYTIAL VIRUS

Major Immunologic Features

- Repeated infection by an antigenically stable virus occurs throughout life.
- Infection in infancy is associated with bronchospasm, possibly related to production of IgE antibodies to the virus.
- An experimental vaccine worsened the clinical manifestations of infection.

General Considerations

Respiratory syncytial virus causes respiratory infections in children and adults. Infections occur in annual epidemics, commonly during the winter or rainy months. The disease causes severe pneumonia and bronchiolitis in infants, whereas upper respiratory infection predominates in adults.

Virology

Respiratory syncytial virus is an enveloped virus with a continuous, single-stranded RNA genome. There is only one serotype, although minor antigenic variation in envelope proteins are detected with monoclonal antibodies or nucleic acid sequencing. The virus infects respiratory epithelium and causes extensive cytopathology, including characteristic syncytia. Recovery from infection is complete, and neither latent nor chronic infection occurs.

Clinical Features

The virus is spread through airborne droplets, by interpersonal contact, and through fomites. In infants 4–24 months of age, respiratory syncytial virus infection is frequent and is often associated with lower respiratory tract disease. It is the most common cause of bronchiolitis—pneumonia associated with bronchospasm and air trapping (Fig 51–2). The severity of disease is greatest in infants with underlying chronic cardiorespiratory conditions. Infection is diagnosed by recovery of the virus in tissue culture, by identification of viral antigens from desquamated respiratory epithelial cells with monoclonal antibodies, or by documentation of a serum antibody response. Precise virologic diagnosis is important because chemotherapy is available.

Immunologic Pathogenesis

Infection with respiratory syncytial virus stimulates both humoral and cellular immunity. Control and elimination of established infection are primarily functions of intact cellular immunity, since patients

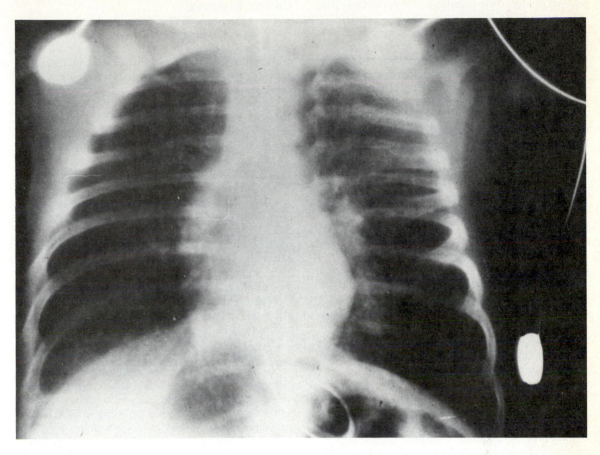

Figure 51–2. Chest x-ray of 1-year-old child with bronchiolitis due to respiratory syncytial virus, showing diffuse hyper-inflation and air trapping with a left upper lobe infiltrate.

with defective cellular immunity may become persistently infected with the virus. Antibody appears to partially protect against reinfection and disease, and maternal IgG antibody transferred transplacentally to the fetus confers some protection against disease early in life. Similar passive-transfer experiments with cotton rats have confirmed the protective role of serum antibody. Resistance to infection is also attributable to respiratory IgA antibody, although the shorter half-life of IgA limits its effectiveness.

The pathogenesis of the wheezing and air trapping associated with respiratory syncytial virus infection in infancy is not fully understood. Allergy to the virus is one possibility, since infection stimulates virus-specific IgE antibody, which can result in mast cell degranulation. The severity of bronchiolitis is directly proportionate to the quantity of mast cell products in respiratory secretions. Although immunopathogenic mechanisms may explain some of the pathogenesis of respiratory syncytial virus bronchiolitis, direct viral cytopathic effects are almost certainly responsible for a significant component of the disease.

Treatment

A nucleotide analog, ribavirin, has been shown to accelerate the recovery of children with respiratory syncytial virus infection, and is licensed for this indication in the USA. The drug is aerosolized and administered by inhalation. Because of the high cost of the drug, it is generally used only for children with underlying chronic cardiorespiratory disease who are at risk for severe morbidity or mortality from respiratory syncytial virus infection.

Prevention

Many efforts to produce a vaccine have been made because of the morbidity and mortality rates associated with respiratory syncytial virus infection in infants. An immunogenic, formalin-inactivated whole respiratory syncytial virus vaccine was field-tested in the 1960s. In a placebo-controlled trial, the vaccine produced the paradoxical effect of increasing the susceptibility to infection. There is no clear explanation for these results. Respiratory syncytial virus shares some similarities with measles virus, and the augmented pulmonary disease following immunization with inactivated respiratory syncytial virus may be due to a selected response to viral antigens that occur in inactivated measles vaccine (see the discussion of measles virus, below). There has been considerable reluctance to undertake further clinical trials of candidate respiratory syncytial virus vaccines because of the adverse reactions to this experimental vaccine.

MEASLES VIRUS

Major Immunologic Features

- Rash results from host cellular immune response to virus.
- Infection depresses cellular immunity.
- Either infection or immunization results in long-lasting immunity.
- Unbalanced immune response from immunization may result in atypically severe disease following subsequent infection.

General Considerations

Measles virus causes an important acute exanthem of childhood and a chronic, slowly progressive neurologic disease, subacute sclerosing panencephalitis (SSPE), which may follow decades after an acute infection. The highly infectious virus is spread primarily by the respiratory route. Acute infection is associated with significant morbidity and mortality rates, especially in individuals in developing countries. An effective live, attenuated vaccine is available; if used widely, it could prevent nearly all cases.

Virology

Measles virus is a paramyxovirus with an envelope and a single-stranded RNA genome. Only one clinically important strain exists, with only minor antigenic variations. The virus has 3 internal proteins, including a ribonucleoprotein and an RNA-dependent RNA polymerase, and 3 envelope proteins, the matrix and fusion proteins and a hemagglutinin. A protective immune response is directed primarily against the fusion and hemagglutinin proteins. Acute infection of cells results in their death, commonly accompanied by syncytial giant cell formation. The selective pressure of host immune responses may result in the selection of virus variants that cause chronic infection. Acute infection by measles virus is well controlled in most patients with a normal immune response, but it results in a latent state of infection in most individuals.

Clinical Features

The virus is spread primarily via the airborne route, through the upper respiratory tract. After an incubation period of 9–11 days, during which the virus undergoes subclinical replication at unknown sites, patients develop fever, cough, coryza, and conjunctivitis. Within 1 or 2 days, an erythematous, maculopapular rash develops, which quickly spreads over the entire body. In malnourished children, enteritis is prominent. The main complications are bacterial superinfections, such as otitis media and pneumonia, and a postviral encephalitis.

Decades after the primary infection, a small proportion of individuals develop SSPE, a chronic, progressive neurologic disorder due to persistent infection of the central nervous system; this condition is caused by defective variants of measles virus. It is particularly common in those who acquired measles before the age of 2 years.

In children who are vaccinated with inactivated measles virus vaccine, an "atypical" form of measles can occur, with acute infection, characterized by pleomorphic skin eruptions, including a vesicular rash, and pneumonitis. This condition is thought to be due to an unbalanced immune response to the virus (see below).

The diagnosis of measles can be made clinically in most cases. Lymphopenia is a characteristic laboratory abnormality in acute cases. The diagnosis may be confirmed by recovering the virus from blood or oropharyngeal secretions in tissue culture, by demonstrating viral antigen on leukocytes or respiratory epithelium, or by documenting the development of IgG antibodies to the virus during convalescence. The presence of IgM antibody to measles virus during the illness also confirms the diagnosis.

Immunologic Pathogenesis

Acute infection with measles virus markedly depresses cellular immunity, as measured by delayed hypersensitivity, skin test reactivity, or lymphocyte activation in vitro (see Chapter 19). In some cases, this immunosuppression is associated with reactivation of infections such as tuberculosis. Some suppression of antibody responses also occurs. The mechanism of the immunosuppression is unclear but is probably related to a direct effect of the virus on B and T lymphocytes. Control of measles virus replication is a function of cellular immunity, and patients with defects in cellular immunity often develop progressive, fatal infections. Immunodeficient patients usually fail to develop a rash, suggesting its dependence on T cell immunity. Resistance to infection is primarily due to humoral immunity, specifically to antibodies to the viral envelope proteins. Evidence for this is that resistance to measles virus may be conferred by passive administration of human IgG containing antibodies to the virus. Protective antibodies elicited by infection persist for life.

Antibodies that develop in response to immunization may not persist as long, particularly if the vaccine was administered before 1–2 years of age.

The first measles vaccines were made from inactivated virus. Natural infection following such vaccination often resulted in severe disease, but with very atypical clinical features such as pneumonitis and vesicular skin rash. These early vaccines stimulated antibody to the viral hemagglutinin, but not to the fusion protein—in contrast to live virus vaccines or natural infection, in which a vigorous antibody response occurs to both proteins. This "unbalanced" immune response may be responsible for the atypical disease. Because the inactivated vaccine has not been used for decades, cases of atypical measles should now be rare.

Prevention

Resistance to disease following measles virus infection is predominantly a function of serum antibody, which results from natural infection, infection with attenuated vaccine strains of measles virus, or passive immunization. Passive administration of pooled human IgG (immune serum globulin [ISG] or intravenous immunoglobulins [IVIG]) is not a long-term control measure, but is useful for postexposure prophylaxis of nonimmune subjects. It will prevent measles even if given up to 1 week after exposure.

Measles vaccines are currently live, attenuated viruses given parenterally. They are extremely effective and prevent disease in more than 95% of those immunized. However, because measles virus is extremely infectious and highly communicable, herd immunity is negligible and epidemics can still occur even if more than 95% of the population has protective antibodies (ie, less than 5% of the population is susceptible). Thus, control of the disease requires high compliance with immunization guidelines. All children should be immunized unless they have a congenital or acquired defect in cellular immunity contraindicating live virus vaccination (see Chapter 58). Current cases of measles in the USA are largely attributable to immigration of unvaccinated individuals or poor vaccination of the indigenous population. Some recent cases have occurred in vaccinated individuals with subprotective antibody titers.

HEPATITIS B VIRUS

Major Immunologic Features

- It is transmitted in blood products or by sexual contact.
- Liver damage is secondary to antiviral cellular immune response.
- Acute and chronic immune complex disease may occur.
- Infection and immunization result in long-lasting, solid resistance.

- Perinatal transmission can be prevented by passive antibody administration followed by active immunization.

General Considerations

Hepatitis B virus (HBV) is a major cause of acute and chronic hepatitis as well as hepatic carcinoma. The virus causes either acute, self-limited infection or a chronic infection that persists for the life of the host. Chronic carriers may remain infectious for life and are the major reservoir for the virus. It is estimated that there are more than 100 million chronic hepatitis B carriers worldwide.

Virology

HBV is a nonenveloped DNA virus with a unique structure and mode of replication. It is related to several other animal hepatitis viruses, which collectively are known as hepadnaviruses. They contain double-stranded DNA with a nicked or single-stranded region, and they replicate via a DNA intermediate encoded by virus-associated DNA-dependent DNA polymerases. These enzymes are structurally closely related to the reverse transcriptases of retroviruses, which are enveloped viruses with an RNA genome. The major proteins of HBV are the surface antigen (HBsAg) and core antigen (HBcAg). Although subtypes of the virus are recognized, this distinction is not clinically important. Following infection, the virus replicates primarily in hepatocytes, with production of large amounts of excess surface antigen, HBsAg, which then circulates in the blood. Acute infection may resolve, with complete elimination of the virus, or may be followed by chronic persistent infection in which viral cDNA is integrated into the host genome. Persistent infection is associated with a high risk of hepatic carcinoma.

A defective RNA virus, hepatitis delta virus (HDV), can replicate only in HBV-infected cells, and thus causes infection only in patients with HBV infection. The delta virus genome codes for only one protein, delta antigen, and following replication, genomes of the progeny are packaged in HBsAg. HDV may be cotransmitted with HBV or may superinfect patients with chronic HBV infection.

Clinical Features

HBV is transmitted almost exclusively by sexual contact; parenteral inoculation of blood or blood products through transfusion, parenteral drug abuse, tattooing, or acupuncture; and from infected mothers to their infants during birth (perinatal transmission). The incubation period varies from 3–4 weeks to nearly 6 months; however, it is generally 1–2 months. The majority of infections are asymptomatic, although laboratory testing reveals "chemical" hepatitis with elevated transaminase levels and the presence of HBV infection (see below). Some 10–

20% of infected patients will have symptomatic hepatitis, and about 1% of those will develop fatal fulminant hepatitis. A proportion of patients who recover from acute infection will then go on to chronic infection, which, in turn, may be asymptomatic or associated with chronic hepatitis. Chronic infection is a major risk factor for the development of hepatoma; the incubation period may be up to 40 years.

Age and ethnicity are major variables in determining the outcome of HBV infection. Infection of the neonate during birth is rarely associated with acute hepatitis, but more than half of those children will become lifelong carriers of HBV. In contrast, although hepatitis occurs in 10–20% of HBV infections acquired in adult life, chronic carriage occurs in fewer than 5% of cases. Asians appear to be at higher risk than whites for developing chronic carriage.

HDV is transmitted primarily by intravenous drug use, although some infections have been transmitted by sexual contact, particularly between homosexual men. HDV coinfection with HBV usually results in more severe disease than HBV infection alone; in some instances, the course of the disease may be bimodal. HDV superinfection of patients chronically infected with HBV often results in marked worsening of the chronic hepatitis.

HBV infection was initially recognized and now is most frequently diagnosed by detection of the excess HBsAg present in serum during both acute and chronic infection. This antigen can be detected by a variety of methods; currently, radioimmunoassay (RIA) and enzyme-linked immunosorbent assay (ELISA) are the most commonly used, and both are highly sensitive and specific. More than 95% of patients with acute and chronic infection will have antigen detected by these techniques. Screening of blood donors for HBsAg, as well as exclusion of paid donors, has dramatically reduced the incidence of HBV infection among recipients of blood and blood products.

Another useful test for the diagnosis of acute HBV infection is detection of the IgM antibody to core antigen (IgM anti-HBcAg), which, unlike HBsAg, is present only in patients with acute HBV infection. This test is useful for differentiating acute and chronic HBV infection and non-A, non-B hepatitis (Table 51–3). The antibody response to HBsAg tends to be delayed for several months following infection and hence is seldom used for diagnosis. However, the presence of either anti-HBsAg or anti-HBcAg indicates past infection. Fig 51–3 shows the time course of HBV serologic markers and the resulting host immune response in relation to infection.

Immunologic Pathogenesis

Hepatic damage following HBV infection is attributable primarily to the cellular immune response to the virus. HBV infection of hepatocytes by itself is noninjurious, and the clinical and laboratory findings of hepatitis do not appear unless cytotoxic T lymphocytes directed against the virus are generated. Thus, infection in patients with reduced cellular immunity (eg, neonates) tends to be asymptomatic. However, resolution of the acute infection and elimination of the virus also depend upon the same cellular immune response; hence, immunodeficient patients also have a much higher incidence of chronic persistent infection.

HBV infection is associated with overproduction (occasionally massive) of HBsAg. In some patients with acute HBV infection, simultaneous synthesis of anti-HBsAg results in immune-complex disease, manifested by fever, skin rashes, arthralgia, and arthritis. Glomerulonephritis is rare. These findings wane as HBsAg antibody levels increase and HBsAg levels fall, resulting from control of the infection by the cellular immune response. A small proportion of patients with chronic HBV infection develop polyarteritis, which is probably also due to HBsAg immune complexes.

Treatment

Chronic HBV infection is associated with considerable morbidity and mortality, and there is no established drug treatment. However, several studies have

Table 51–3. Use of HBV markers for the diagnosis of hepatitis.

Markers Present in Serum			Diagnosis
HBsAg	IgM Anti-HBcAg	Anti-HBsAg	
+	+	−	Acute HBV infection.
−	+	−	Acute HBV infection (after HBsAg has disappeared).
+	−	±	Chronic HBV infection; may have non-A, non-B virus superinfection.
−	−	+[1]	Past HBV infection; HBV vaccination. Indicates immunity.

[1]IgG-class anti-HBcAg also present if infection has occurred (not present following immunization).

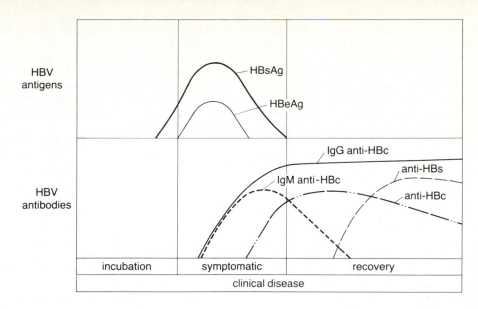

Figure 51–3. Schematic diagram showing temporal pattern of viral markers, illness, and antibody response in HBV infection. The solid lines show the expected response in acute, self-limited infection, whereas the dotted lines show the response in chronic infection. Illness includes symptoms, signs, and chemical evidence of hepatitis.

shown promising results from the combination of recombinant alpha interferon and a nucleoside analog, vidarabine. More recently, interferon has been used because of the toxicity of vidarabine. With one or more courses of treatment, about 50% of patients temporarily clear HBsAg and up to 25% appear to be cured. A brief course of corticosteroids given prior to the interferon appears to improve the outcome. Although the vidarabine acts to inhibit HBV replication, the mechanism of action of the interferon and the glucocorticoids is less clear. Glucocorticoid pretreatment may augment virus replication and increase concomitant expression of viral antigens on the surface of the chronically infected hepatocytes. Subsequently, interferon would augment cellular immune response mechanisms by natural killer (NK) cells or cytotoxic T lymphocytes, which then kill the virus-infected cells. Interferon may also increase expression of class I HLA antigens on the surface of the hepatocytes, which facilitates their recognition by cytotoxic T lymphocytes.

Prevention

Cytotoxic T lymphocytes are critical to recovery from HBV infection and elimination of the virus. In contrast, resistance to HBV infection is mediated effectively by antibody to HBsAg alone. Administration of antibody to HBsAg prevents infection, and eliciting anti-HBsAg by immunization with inactivated or recombinant HBsAg confers resistance as well.

Preventive measures for HBV infection employ either pooled human immune serum globulin with high titers of antibody to HBsAg (hepatitis B immune globulin [HBIG]) or HBV vaccine. The latter consists of HBsAg, either purified from the plasma of chronic carriers or prepared by recombinant DNA techniques. Both types of vaccines are extremely safe and induce protective antibodies in more than 95% of individuals immunized.

Control measures may be implemented either in anticipation of infection or after infection has already occurred; the latter is known as "postexposure prophylaxis." Postexposure prophylaxis is indicated when a susceptible individual has been exposed to someone with active infection (ie, a patient with HBsAg in the blood), for example through sexual contact or a needle-stick injury. It is also administered postpartum to infants born to mothers with HBV infection. Passive immunity is achieved immediately by administration of HBIG. Then active immunity is stimulated by administration of HBV vaccine. Postexposure prophylaxis is highly effective, particularly if it is initiated within a few days of the exposure.

Preexposure immunization against HBV infection is indicated for individuals who are at high risk of infection and who lack protective HBsAg in the blood. Candidates for vaccination include health care workers, parenteral drug abusers, and individuals with multiple sexual partners. HBIG has no role in preexposure prophylaxis.

HEPATITIS A VIRUS

Hepatitis A virus (HAV) is an enteroviruslike poliovirus with a different cell receptor and tissue tropism from other enteroviruses. However, like many other enteroviruses, it is transmitted primarily by the fecal-oral route. Following ingestion, the virus travels via the bloodstream to the liver, the exclusive site of virus replication. Replication in the liver results in a brief period of viremia (5–10 days) and shedding of virus in the stools for 1–2 weeks. The infection resolves completely in all cases, except for rare instances of fatal infection. In contrast to HBV, chronic or latent infection does not occur. Resolution of infection is dependent on intact cellular immunity, since patients with cellular immunodeficiency may experience prolonged virus shedding and disease, similar to the case with other enteroviruses (see the section below on poliovirus).

The incubation period of HAV infection averages 30 days and ranges from 10 to 50 days. Most infections, especially those in children, are asymptomatic, although evidence of "chemical" hepatitis is usually found on laboratory testing. The mortality rate during acute infection is about 0.1% overall, but it is lower in children and increases with increasing age.

HAV infection generates a vigorous antibody response, which protects against reinfection and serves as the basis for diagnosis. Detection of the transient anti-HAV IgM response is the single most useful test for acute infection, whereas detection of the long-lasting anti-HAV IgG response is the best marker for past infection and resistance to subsequent infection. Infection may also be documented by demonstrating the development of IgG antibody response by comparing acute- and convalescent-phase serum specimens. However, this approach is cumbersome and may yield false-negative results, especially if the acute-phase serum specimen was obtained too long after the initial antibody response; thus, it is little used today. Unlike HBV, there is no serologic test for HAV antigen.

Resistance to HAV infection is mediated solely by serum antibody to the virus. This has been demonstrated by studies showing passive transfer of protection by immune globulin that contains antibody to HAV. Protection from HAV infection can be achieved with pooled human ISG given every 3–6 months. The intramuscular preparation is usually used, although intravenous immune globulin is also effective. Protection from illness may also be achieved by administration of ISG within 1 week following exposure to HAV. An effective vaccine is theoretically possible, since the viral structural proteins are highly immunogenic and only one viral serotype is known, but to date none is currently available.

RABIES VIRUS

Rabies virus infection is enzootic in many wild animal species, including foxes, skunks, and bats. It can infect many domestic animals (dogs are the most commonly infected), although infection of domestic animals is unusual in developed countries because of the widespread application of control measures. When rabies virus infects humans, generally as the result of an animal bite, the resulting disease is virtually 100% fatal. Hence, preventive measures are of paramount importance.

Rabies virus is an enveloped RNA virus that is related to several other animal viruses. Although only one serotype is detectable by the usual clinical criteria, studies with monoclonal antibodies have identified strains with differing geographic and host ranges. Following a bite wound, the virus replicates in muscles and nerves, extends centripetally along peripheral nerves over a period of days to months, and finally reaches the spinal cord and central nervous system. At this stage the infection is associated with the hyperexcitability and hydrophobia characteristic of rabies. There are no effective antiviral drugs, and even with maximum supportive care, virtually every affected individual dies.

Because of the tremendous epidemiologic and public health implications of a case of rabies, the clinical diagnosis of rabies must be supported by laboratory data. Viral antigens can be detected by immunofluorescence with specific antisera or monoclonal antibodies in the brains of animals and humans and in corneal epithelial cells of humans. This technique is more sensitive than the histopathologic demonstration of Negri bodies. A diagnosis can also be made by demonstrating a rise in antibody titer following infection, although this is less useful clinically.

Animal data support a role for the host immune response in the pathogenesis of rabies. Although immunosuppression of animals prior to infection shortens the latency period and increases the mortality rate, immunosuppression after infection may delay mortality, even though brain virus titers are increased. In immunosuppressed animals with high brain virus titers, administration of rabies hyperimmune serum markedly worsens disease, further supporting the role of the immune system in production of illness.

Antibody to the virus is protective. Individuals with serum antibody elicited by immunization are resistant to infection, and protection from disease can be achieved even after infection by administration of hyperimmune animal or human antibodies. These antibodies are effective only if given shortly after infection, and their efficacy is increased by local administration around the site of the bite wound, suggesting that they act by local neutralization of the virus.

The first rabies vaccines were prepared by Pasteur, who used virus that had been adapted to growth in rabbit neural tissue and then inactivated by heating and drying. Currently, many rabies vaccines are available; however, the only one used widely in developed countries is inactivated virus grown in human fibroblasts. This vaccine is highly immunogenic, protective if given either before or immediately after infection, and relatively free of serious side effects. Although animal-derived vaccines from rabbit or monkey brain or embryonated egg are effective in preventing rabies and are still available in many developing countries, the nervous-tissue antigens present in these products may cause allergic encephalitis in the vaccine recipients.

POLIOVIRUS

Poliovirus is the cause of poliomyelitis, an acute encephalomyelitis that results in asymmetric paralysis with muscle atrophy. Although cases of paralysis almost certainly due to poliovirus have been recognized for thousands of years, the 20th century has seen a marked increase in the incidence of the disease and a change from endemic to epidemic spread. Development of poliovirus vaccine in the middle of the twentieth century and its widespread application in developed countries have resulted in the virtual elimination of the disease in vaccinated populations.

Poliovirus is an enterovirus and is a member of the family of small, nonenveloped RNA viruses that includes the echoviruses, coxsackieviruses, hepatitis A virus, and rhinoviruses. Although closely related by structure, mode of replication, and RNA sequence homology, these viruses exhibit tremendous antigenic diversity, and there is little or no serologic relatedness or cross-resistance among them. Poliovirus has 3 non-cross-reactive serotypes, serotypes 1, 2, and 3. Infection generates a vigorous cellular and humoral immune response to the coat proteins of the virus.

Patients infected with poliovirus and the other enteroviruses shed large amounts of virus in the feces, often for periods of weeks or months. Infection is transmitted when a susceptible individual ingests food or water contaminated by infected feces. The virus replicates in the intestinal tract, and viremia occurs; this is followed by seeding of the spinal cord and central nervous system. Although most patients (> 99%) recover without sequelae, the remainder suffer some degree of motor nerve dysfunction,

which varies from minimal weakness of an extremity to severe paralysis of all major muscle groups. Partial or complete recovery may occur after the acute illness.

Resolution of infection and elimination of the virus appear to require intact cellular immune mechanisms, since patients with defective cellular immunity continue to shed poliovirus as well as other enteroviruses for months or years after infection. However, resistance to infection is mediated by serum neutralizing antibody. Administration of pooled human ISG containing antibodies to poliovirus will prevent the disease, even if given a few days after exposure. In addition, inactivated vaccines that stimulate humoral but not cellular immunity are also highly protective. Intestinal infection can still occur in the presence of serum antibodies; however, viremia with seeding of the central nervous system, the cause of morbidity and mortality, does not occur.

The first poliovirus vaccine consisted of tissue-culture-grown suspensions of poliovirus types 1–3, which were inactivated with formalin. Although inactivated (Salk) vaccine is highly effective for preventing paralytic poliomyelitis, it has several disadvantages. It requires parenteral injection (hence, there is an increased cost for needles and syringes); booster doses are required to maintain immunity; and it does not displace wild-type poliovirus circulating in the community. Live, attenuated (Sabin) vaccine can be given orally; it does not routinely require booster doses; and when immunization is widespread in a community, the vaccine virus displaces the wild-type virus in the environment, thus reducing the risk of paralytic disease among the unimmunized. However, live poliovirus may revert to virulence, producing paralytic disease in vaccinees or their contacts.

Both inactivated and live attenuated poliovirus vaccines are manufactured and used today, although either one or the other is usually selected by national vaccination programs. For example, the live attenuated virus is used in the USA; inactivated virus is used in Scandinavia. Although the choice between live and inactivated virus vaccine is often the subject of heated debate, either type of vaccine will virtually eliminate paralytic poliomyelitis if used correctly. Active investigation is under way to improve both the live attenuated and inactivated vaccines.

REFERENCES

General

Ennis FA (editor): *Human Immunity to Viruses.* Academic Press, 1983.

Hirsch RL: The complement system: Its importance in the host response to viral infections. *Microbiol Rev* 1982;**46**:71.

Kauffman RS, Fields BN: Pathogenesis of viral infections. Chapter 10 in: *Virology.* Fields BN et al (editors). Raven Press, 1985.

Notkins AL, Oldstone MB: *Concepts in Viral Pathogenesis.* Springer Verlag, 1984.

Oldstone MB: Distortion of cell functions by noncytotoxic viruses. *Hosp Pract* (July) 1986;**15**:82.

Quinnan GV Jr: Immunology of viral infections. Chapter 5 in: *Textbook of Human Virology*. Belshe RB (editor). PSG Publishing Co, 1984.

Sissons JG, Oldstone MB: Host response to viral infections. Chapter 14 in: *Virology*. Fields BN et al (editors). Raven Press, 1985.

Influenza Virus

Ada GL, Jones PD: The immune response to influenza infection. *Curr Top Microbiol Immunol* 1986;**128**:1.

Air GM, Laver WG, Webster RG: Antigenic variation in influenza viruses. *Contrib Microbiol Immunol* 1987;**8**:20.

Askonas BA, Taylor PM, Esquivel F: Cytotoxic T cells in influenza infection. *Ann NY Acad Sci* 1988;**532**:230.

Cohen JP, Macauley C: Susceptibility to influenza A in HIV-positive patients. (Letter.) *J Am Med Assoc* 1989;**261**:245.

Klenk HD, Rott, R: The molecular biology of influenza virus pathogenicity. *Adv Virus Res* 1988;**34**:247.

Murphy BR, Webster RG. Influenza viruses. Chapter 51 in: *Virology*. Fields BN et al (editors). Raven Press, 1985.

Townsend AR: Recognition of influenza virus proteins by cytotoxic T lymphocytes. *Immunol Res* 1987;**6**:80.

Respiratory Syncytial Virus

Josephs S et al: Parainfluenza 3 virus and other common respiratory pathogens in children with human immunodeficiency virus infection. *Pediatr Infect Dis J* 1988;**7**:207.

McIntosh K, Chanock RM: Respiratory syncytial virus. Chapter 54 in: *Virology*. Fields BN et al (editors). Raven Press, 1985.

Murphy BR et al: Current approaches to the development of vaccines effective against parainfluenza and respiratory syncytial viruses. *Virus Res* 1988;**11**:1.

Stott EJ, Taylor G: Respiratory syncytial virus. Brief review. *Arch Virol* 1985;**84**:1.

Welliver RC: Detection, pathogenesis, and therapy of respiratory syncytial virus infections. *Clin Microbiol Rev* 1988;**1**:27.

Measles Virus

Johnson RT, Griffin DE, Moench TR: Pathogenesis of measles immunodeficiency and encephalomyelitis: Parallels to AIDS. *Microb Pathog* 1988;**4**:169.

Norrby E: Measles. Chapter 55 in: *Virology*. Fields BN et al (editors). Raven Press, 1985.

ter Meulen V: Autoimmune reactions against myelin basic protein induced by corona and measles viruses. *Ann NY Acad Sci* 1988;**540**:202.

ter Meulen V, Carter MJ: Measles virus persistence and disease. *Prog Med Virol* 1984;**30**:44.

Hepatitis B Virus

Chatzinoff M, Friedman LS: Delta agent hepatitis. *Infect Dis Clin North Am* 1987;**1**:529.

Perillo RP et al: Prednisone withdrawal followed by recombinant alpha interferon in the treatment of chronic hepatitis B. *Ann Intern Med* 1988;**109**:95.

Sherlock S: The natural history of hepatitis B. *Postgrad Med J* 1987;**63 (Suppl 2)**:7.

Thomas HC et al: Virus-host interactions in chronic hepatitis B virus infection. *Semin Liver Dis* 1988;**8**:342.

Wilson B, Wanda J: Recent advances in the biology and immunology of hepatitis B. *Baillieres Clin Gastroenterol* 1987;**1**:623.

Hepatitis A Virus

Coulepsis AG, Anderson BN, Gust ID: Hepatitis A. *Adv Virus Res* 1987;**32**:129.

Rabies Virus

Baer GM: Rabies Virus. Chapter 49 in: *Virology*. Fields BN et al (editors). Raven Press, 1985.

Fungal Diseases

52

David J. Drutz, MD

Infectious diseases caused by fungi are called **mycoses.** Fungi, like mammalian cells, are eukaryotes, ie, they possess a true nucleus containing several chromosomes, bounded by a nuclear membrane. In contrast, bacteria are prokaryotes, with a single linear chromosome and no true nucleus. The principal sterol of the mammalian cell membrane is cholesterol; that of fungi is ergosterol. Ergosterol is the target of amphotericin B and the antifungal azoles. Fungal cell walls have no counterpart in mammalian cells, and they differ from those of bacteria by lacking peptidoglycans, teichoic acids, and lipopolysaccharides (endotoxin). In their place are the external and antigenic **peptidomannans** embedded in matrices of α- and β-**glucans;** structural rigidity is provided by sheets, disks, or fibrils of chitin (poly-β-1,4-N-acetylglucosamine).

Although there are thousands of fungi in nature, relatively few are pathogenic for normal humans. Table 52–1 lists common mycoses according to the usual sites of infection. Superficial mycoses usually occur on the body external to common immunologic influences. Cutaneous mycoses produce delayed hypersensitivity responses to the local presence of keratinolytic fungi. Subcutaneous and systemic mycoses represent successful challenges to major immunologic host defense mechanisms. Some systemic mycoses (eg, blastomycosis, coccidioidomycosis, histoplasmosis, and paracoccidiodomycosis) are due to primary pathogens, theoretically capable of infecting anyone present in an endemic area. Others (eg, candidiasis, cryptococcosis, aspergillosis, and zygomycosis) are due to opportunistic pathogens, which seldom cause life-threatening tissue invasion in the absence of impaired host defenses. *Pneumocystis carinii* has traditionally been considered a protozoon. However, recent RNA studies and electron-microscopic analysis suggest that it may be related to fungi. Except for *Malassezia* and *Pityrosporum* spp, *Candida albicans, C tropicalis,* and *C glabrata,* most fungi reach the body from the external environment. Most primary invasive mycoses are acquired by the inhalation of specialized forms (conidia and spores) that are progeny of filamentous soil forms of the fungi. Once inhaled, some fungi reproduce in the body in the original filamentous (mycelial, hyphal) form. Others adopt specialized forms (yeasts, spherules, and endospores) more suit-

able for host survival and tissue invasion. The latter fungi are referred to as **dimorphic fungi.** Table 52–1 indicates the forms assumed by common fungi when invading host tissues. A major attribute of all opportunistic filamentous fungi is the tendency to invade blood vessels (**angioinvasion**), with resultant tissue infarction (Table 52–2).

Immunity to the mycoses is principally cellular, involving neutrophils, macrophages, lymphocytes, and probably natural killer (NK) cells. With the possible exception of the dermatophytes and *Rhizopus arrhizus,* the principal etiologic agent of zygomycosis, fungi are not susceptible to direct killing by antibody and complement. It has been proposed that in vitro susceptibility of fungi to inhibition or killing by neutrophils discriminates between primary pathogenicity and opportunism. Patients with neutropenia or defective neutrophil function appear predisposed to hematogenously disseminated candidiasis or filamentous mycoses (eg, aspergillosis and zygomycosis). Patients with defective cell-mediated immunity (CMI) (eg, acquired immunodeficiency syndrome [AIDS] sufferers) are predisposed to mucosal candidiasis or hematogenously disseminated cryptococcosis, histoplasmosis and coccidioidomycosis (Table 52–3). Allergy to fungi is discussed in Chapters 29–33.

Salient features of the superficial, cutaneous, and subcutaneous mycoses may be found in Tables 52–1 to 52–4. The major systemic invasive mycoses found in the Western hemisphere are described below.

SYSTEMIC INVASIVE MYCOSES: PRIMARY PATHOGENS

BLASTOMYCOSIS

Major Immunologic Features
- Yeasts are large and singly-budding and commonly exceed the size of phagocytes.
- Islands of suppuration (microabscesses) amid granulomas are produced.
- It may be more severe in patients with defective CMI.

Table 52–1. Common mycoses according to usual sites of disease production.

Site and Disease	Etiologic Agents	Origin	Invasive Form	Pathophysiologic Basis	Principal Clinical Features
Superficial mycoses Pityriasis (tinea) versicolor	*Malassezia* and *Pityrosporum* spp	Hair follicle (yeasts)	Yeasts and/or mycelia	Decreased epithelial turnover allows normal flora to produce disease.	Flat, branny skin lesions; variously pigmented or non-pigmented.
Pityrosporum folliculitis	*Malassezia/ Pityrosporum* spp	Hair follicle (yeasts)	Yeasts	Obstructed hair follicles are damaged by follicular flora.	Acneiform folliculitis.
Tinea nigra	*Phaeoannelomyces werneckii*	Soil (mycelia)	Mycelia	Hyperhidrosis permits infection from environment.	Brown-black nonscaly macules (especially on palms).
White piedra	*Trichosporon beigelii*	Soil, skin (mycelia)	Mycelia and yeasts	Poor personal hygiene permits infection from environment or by normal flora.	Soft whitish nodules on hair shaft.
Black piedra	*Piedraia hortai*	Soil (mycelia)	Mycelia	Poor personal hygiene permits infection from environment.	Hard gritty black nodules on hair shaft.
Cutaneous mycoses Dermatophytosis	*Epidermophyton, Trichophyton,* and *Microsporum* spp	Soil and animal fur (mycelia)	Mycelia	Etiologic agents are keratinolytic; infection is potentiated by warmth, moisture, and occlusion; cutaneous inflammation is due to delayed-hypersensitivity reaction.	Tinea pedis (scaly, vesicular, ulcerative), tinea cruris (dry, red, scalloped, expanding), tinea corporis (ringworm), tinea barbae (suppuration, beard), tinea capitis (scalp; resembles seborrhea), tinea unguium (nails).
Subcutaneous mycoses Chromoblastomycosis	*A Cladosporium Fonsecaea, Phialophora,* and *Rhinocladiella* spp	Soil (mycelia)	Mycelia and sclerotic bodies	Traumatic implantation.	Papules, warty tumors, plaques, cauliflowerlike growths.
Mycetoma	*Acremonium, Exophiala, Leptosphaeria, Madurella, Microsporum, Neotestudina,* and *Pseudallescheria* spp	Soil (mycelia)	Mycelia and grains	Traumatic implantation.	Swelling, draining fistulae, pus, and grains.
Sporotrichosis	*Sporothrix schenckii*	Vegetation (mycelia)	Yeasts	Traumatic implantation.	Subcutaneous nodules along lymphatics.
Systemic Invasive Mycoses Primary pathogens Blastomycosis	*Blastomyces dermatitidis*	Soil (mycelia)	Yeasts	Inhalation of conidia.	Pulmonary, spreading to skin, bones, male reproductive tract.
Coccidioidomycosis	*Coccidioides immitis*	Soil (mycelia)	Spherules and endospores	Inhalation of arthroconidia.	Pulmonary, spreading to skin, bones, joints, meninges.
Histoplasmosis	*Histoplasma capsulatum*	Soil (mycelia)	Yeasts	Inhalation of microconidia.	Pulmonary, spreading to reticuloendothelial system, mucous membranes, adrenals.
Paracoccidioidomycosis	*Paracoccidioides brasiliensis*	Soil (mycelia)	Yeasts	Inhalation of conidia.	Pulmonary, spreading to reticuloendothelial system, skin, mucous membranes, adrenals.
Opportunistic pathogens Candidiasis	Principally *Candida albicans, C tropicalis,* and *T glabrata*	Mucosal surfaces (yeasts, pseudomycelia)	Yeasts, pseudomycelia, mycelia	Local extension; bloodstream invasion from colonization sites (mucosal disruption).	Mucosal site, spreading to eyes, skin, kidneys, myocardium, other sites.
Cryptococcosis	*Cryptococcus neoformans*	Soil (yeast, possibly mycelia)	Yeasts	Inhalation of desiccated yeasts or basidiospores.	Pulmonary, spreading to meninges, brain, bone, skin.

(continued)

Table 52–1 (cont'd). Common mycoses according to usual sites of disease production.

Site and Disease	Etiologic Agents	Origin	Invasive Form	Pathophysiologic Basis	Principal Clinical Features
Aspergillosis	*Aspergillus fumigatus, A flavus, and A niger,* principally	Soil (mycelia)	Mycelia	Inhalation of conidia.	Invasive pulmonary or sinus disease, leading to hematogenous dissemination.
Zygomycosis	*Rhizopus, Absidia, Cunninghamella, Mortierella,* and *Saksenaea* spp	Soil (mycelia)	Mycelia	Inhalation of spores.	Invasive sinus or pulmonary disease, leading to hematogenous dissemination.
Pneumocystosis	*Pneumocystis carinii*	Unknown	Cysts and trophozoites	Inhalation of infective particles or arousal from latency.	Progressive interstitial lung disease with or without cysts, pneumothorax.
Phaeohyphomycosis	Approximately 40 genera of pigmented fungi (eg, *Alternaria, Bipolaris Cladosporium, Exserohilum, Phialophora, Wangiella*)	Soil (mycelia)	Mycelia	Inhalation or implantation of common environmental fungi (pigmented; dematiaceous).	Invasive sinus or pulmonary disease, leading to hematogenous dissemination.
Hyalohyphomycosis	Diverse nonpigmented fungi (eg, *Fusarium, Paecilomyces, Pseudallescheria, Scopulariopsis*)	Soil (mycelia)	Mycelia	Inhalation or implantation of common environmental fungi (nonpigmented)	Invasive sinus or pulmonary disease, leading to hematogenous dissemination.

General Considerations

Blastomycosis is an inhalation-acquired mycosis that can produce primary pulmonary infection or hematogenously disseminated disease involving predominantly skin, bones, and the male genitourinary tract. *Blastomyces dermatitidis,* the cause of this disease, is a spherical multinucleated yeast with thick walls and single broad-based buds. The mycelial form of *B dermatitidis* is a soil organism found on river banks predominantly in the south-central USA and around the Great Lakes. A closely related fungus occurs in Africa. Infection occurs by inhalation of fungal microconidia in endemic areas (eg, by hunters, trappers, campers, or boaters). Hunters and their dogs have been simultaneously infected. There are sporadic and occasionally common-source outbreaks. Endemic areas are defined by the occurrence of cases, since there is no reliable skin test to gauge population exposures. No convincing sex or age prevalence is apparent in common-source outbreaks. Men are more susceptible than women to progressive pulmonary or hematogenous disease. There is no known genetic predisposition.

Pathology

See Table 52–2.

Clinical Features

A. Signs and Symptoms: Primary exposure may be asymptomatic, or it may produce an influenzalike syndrome. Pneumonia, pleuritis, pulmonary cavitation, and mediastinal adenopathy may occur. Hematogenous dissemination may occur in the presence or absence of apparent pulmonary disease. Favored sites of metastatic infection include skin (papules, pustules, or verrucous granulomas that heal centrally and extend peripherally); bone (lytic lesions, especially vertebrae and long bones, with or without draining sinuses); and prostate, testis, and epididymis. Central nervous system infection occurs in about 5% of cases. Gastrointestinal tract involvement almost never occurs.

B. Laboratory Findings: These include leukocytosis, abnormal chest x-ray, and evidence of specific organ dysfunction at metastatic loci. Diagnosis is established by finding large budding yeasts on smears or histologic sections and by recovering the fungus in culture.

C. Immunologic Diagnosis: See Table 52–4. With the possible exception of antibody directed against the A antigen, immunologic tests lack either sensitivity or specificity.

D. Differential Diagnosis: This includes diverse granulomatous infectious diseases (eg, other mycoses and tuberculosis), sarcoidosis, and pulmonary cancer.

E. Treatment: Ketoconazole may be equivalent to amphotericin B, except in severely ill or immunocompromised patients, for whom intravenous amphotericin B is preferable.

F. Prevention: No vaccine is available.

G. Complications and Prognosis: Untreated extrapulmonary blastomycosis carries a 20–90% mortality rate, depending on the individual series. The mortality rate with therapy is less than 10%. Most relapses occur within 1 year of treatment, but they have been documented after as long as 9 years.

Table 52–2. Pathologic features of subcutaneous and systemic mycoses.

Mycosis	Predominant Location of Fungi	Suppuration	Granulomas	Caseation	Fibrosis	Calcification	Other
Subcutaneous							
Chromomycosis	Extracellular (sclerotic bodies)	Dominant	Dominant	Rare	Dominant	Rare	PH[1]; transdermal elimination.
Mycetoma	Extracellular (grains)	Dominant	Dominant	Rare	Dominant	Rare	Grain color varies by etiologic agent; grains surrounded by amorphous material reflecting immune complex deposition (Hoeppli-Splendore phenomenon).
Sporotrichosis	Intracellular and extracellular (yeasts)	Dominant	Dominant	Occasional	Occasional	Rare	Asteroid bodies with Hoeppli-Splendore phenomenon.
Systemic							
Primary pathogens							
Blastomycosis[2]	Extracellular (yeasts)	Dominant	Dominant	Rare	Occasional	Occasional	PH.
Coccidioidomycosis[2]	Extracellular (spherules)	Dominant (endospores)	Dominant (spherules)	Rare	Occasional	Occasional	PH.
Histoplasmosis	Intracellular (yeasts)	Rare	Dominant	Occasional	Dominant	Dominant	Proliferative endarteritis (lungs).
Paracoccidioidomycosis[2]	Extracellular (yeasts)	Dominant	Dominant	Rare	Dominant	Occasional	PH.
Opportunistic pathogens							
Cryptococcosis[2]	Extracellular (yeasts)	Rare	Dominant	Rare	Rare	Rare	Extensive accumulation of extracellular capsular material may produce local anatomic distortions.
Candidiasis[3]	Intracellular (yeasts), extracellular (pseudomycelia, mycelia)	Dominant	Rare	Rare	Rare	Rare	Granuloma formation common only with CMCC.
Aspergillosis[3]	Extracellular (mycelia)	Dominant	Rare	Rare	Rare	Rare	Angioinvasion and infarction.
Zygomycosis[3]	Extracellular (mycelia)	Dominant	Rare	Rare	Rare	Rare	Angioinvasion and infarction.
Pneumocystosis	Extracellular (trophozoites, cysts)	Rare	Rare		Occasional		Foamy intra-alveolar infiltrate and alveolar epithelial damage.

[1]PH, Pseudoepitheliomatous hyperplasia of skin and mucosal lesions.
[2]Severely depressed CMI is often associated with poor granuloma formation and increased suppuration with increased numbers of microorganisms (blastomycosis, coccidioidomycosis, paracoccidioidomycosis) or with gelatinous masses of encapsulated fungi (cryptococcosis).
[3]Severe neutropenia is often associated with loss of suppurative tissue response.

COCCIDIOIDOMYCOSIS

Major Immunologic Features
- Inhaled arthroconidia have an antiphagocytic surface.
- Spherules exceed the size of phagocytes and have an antiphagocytic surface.
- Endospores are released in packets that exceed the size of phagocytes.
- Mixed granulomas and suppuration occur.
- Primary infections may be signaled by erythema nodosum or erythema multiforme.
- Negative skin test (coccidioidin, spherulin) and high complement fixation antibody titer suggest hematogenous dissemination.

Table 52–3. Effect of common immunologic abnormalities on disease course of common mycoses.

Mycosis	Reduction in PMN[1]	Reduction in CMI	Other
Superficial			
Pityriasis (tinea) versicolor	None	None	Lipid hyperalimentation therapy is associated with *Malassezia* and *Pityrosporum* fungemia and pulmonary vasculitis, especially in infants[2]
Pityrosporum folliculitis	None	None	Treatment with corticosteroids predisposes to folliculitis
Tinea nigra	None	None	
White piedra	Hematogenous dissemination of *T beigelii*[3]	None	
Black piedra	None	None	
Cutaneous			
Dermatophytosis	None	Increased severity and chronicity of *T rubrum* infection	
Subcutaneous			
Chromomycosis	None	None	
Mycetoma	None	None	
Sporotrichosis	None	Probable increase in severity or likelihood of dissemination	
Systemic, Invasive			
Primary pathogens			
Blastomycosis	None	Probable increase in severity or likelihood of dissemination	
Coccidioidomycosis	None	Definite increase in severity	Definite increase in severity and dissemination in AIDS; possible increase in severity and dissemination in second and third trimesters of pregnancy
Histoplasmosis	None	Definite increase in severity	Definite increase in severity and dissemination in AIDS
Paracoccidioidomycosis	None	Probable increase in severity or likelihood of dissemination	
Opportunistic pathogens			
Candidiasis	Hematogenous dissemination	Increased severity of mucosal disease	
Cryptococcosis	None	Definite increase in severity	Drastic increase in severity and dissemination in AIDS
Aspergillosis	Invasive paranasal sinus and respiratory infection, and hematogenous dissemination	Possible increase in severity	
Zygomycosis	Invasive paranasal sinus and respiratory infection, and hematogenous dissemination	Possible increase in severity	Diabetic ketoacidosis predisposes to invasive paranasal sinus infection
Pneumocystosis	None	Decreased CMI is a prerequisite for infection	Drastic increase in incidence and severity in AIDS
Phaeohyphomycosis	Invasive paranasal sinus infection and hematogenous dissemination	None	
Hyalohyphomycoses	Invasive paranasal sinus infection and hematogenous dissemination	None	

[1] < 500 PMN/dL.
[2] *Malassezia* and *Pityrosporum* are lipophilic fungi. Lipid hyperalimentation therapy allows them to gain access to the bloodstream. Patients with *Malassezia* and *Pityrosporum* fungemia do not have tinea versicolor or folliculitis.
[3] Patients with *T beigelii* sepsis do not necessarily have white piedra.

Table 52–4. Immunologic diagnosis of subcutaneous and systemic mycoses.

Mycosis	Serologic Tests[1]		Delayed Hypersensitivity Skin Test[1,2]	Comments[1,3]
	Antibody	Antigen		
Subcutaneous Chromoblasto-mycosis	None	None	None	Chromoblastomycosis is diagnosed by its characteristic clinical appearance (warty plaques, nodules, and cauliflowerlike excrescences), together with the demonstration of characteristic pigmented sclerotic bodies in histologic sections. Specific etiologic diagnoses must be established by culture.
Mycetoma	None	None	None	Mycetoma is diagnosed by its characteristic clinical picture (sinuses discharging pus and grains). Specific etiologic diagnosis rests upon microscopic examination of grains and cultures of grains and biopsy material.
Sporotrichosis	LPA, YCA, ID, CF	None	Investigational only	Serologic tests are generally valuable only in extracutaneous and disseminated infection. A slide latex agglutination titer of $\geq$ 1:8 is presumptive evidence of disseminated or systemic infection.
Systemic Primary pathogens Blastomycosis	ID, CF (blastomycin as antigen); ID, CF EIA (A antigen)	None	Blastomycin (mycelial phase), BASWS (investigational only)	The blastomycin skin test and serologic tests lack sensitivity and specificity; there is major cross-reactivity with histoplasmosis. Tests for antibody to A antigen are more specific (especially ID and EIA).
Coccidioido-mycosis	IgM (TP, IDTP, LPA); IgG (CF, IDCF) (coccidioidin as antigen)	Experimental only	Coccidioidin (mycelial phase), spherulin (spherule phase)	IgM tests are positive early and transiently; IgG tests are positive later and more persistently. A CF antibody titer in blood > 1:32 suggests hematogenous dissemination, especially if skin tests are negative. A positive CF titer in the cerebrospinal fluid is virtually diagnostic of meningitis.
Histoplasmosis	CF (whole yeast cells as antigen); CF (histoplasmin as antigen); ID (histoplasmin as antigen); LPA (histoplasmin as antigen)	Experimental only	Histoplasmin (mycelial phase), histolyn CYL (yeast phase)	A positive histoplasmin skin test can artificially elevate CF antibody titers and produce a positive ID test ("m" band). Histolyn CYL is less likely to do this. An ID antibody "h" band suggests active infection. An LPA antibody titer $\geq$ 1:32 suggests active infection. A CF antibody titer $\geq$ 1:32 or a fourfold titer rise suggests active infection.
Paracoccidioido-mycosis	IgG (precipitins; CF)	None	Various "paracoccidioidins" (mycelial phase), investigational only	Elevated precipitin titers (transient) precede elevated CF titers (more persistent). The number and duration of precipitin bands are directly proportional to disease activity. The CF titer is directly proportional to the severity of illness. The skin test is commonly negative with active disease.

(continued)

Table 52–4 (cont'd.). Immunologic diagnosis of subcutaneous and systemic mycoses.

Mycosis	Serologic Tests[1]		Delayed Hypersensitivity Skin Test[1,2]	Comments[1,3]
	Antibody	Antigen		
Opportunistic pathogens				
Cryptococcosis	YCA, IFA, CF, BF, PHA, EIA, and others (diverse antigen preparations)	Capsular polysaccharide (LPA)	"Cryptococcin" (investigational only)	Cryptococcal skin tests and tests for antibody lack sensitivity and specificity. The LPA for cryptococcal antigen is highly sensitive and specific. Rare (low-titer) cross-reactivity with *T beigelii*. A positive cerebrospinal fluid test is diagnostic of cryptococcal meningitis.
Candidiasis	Multiple, diverse serologic tests (precipitins, agglutinins most common; CIE, IHA, IFA, RIA)	Mannan (heat stable; RIA, EIA, LPA) Heat-labile antigen (LPA); mannose (GLC); arabinitol (GLC)	Oidiomycin	Skin tests lack diagnostic value (healthy persons are positive). Antibody tests lack sensitivity and specificity, especially in immunosuppressed patients. Mannan antigen tests are positive in low titer, generally too late in the course of illness to be useful diagnostically. Heat-labile antigen lacks sensitivity and specificity in immunocompromised patients. Tests for mannose and arabinitol are not of proven diagnostic efficacy.
Aspergillosis	Multiple, diverse serologic tests (precipitins most common)	Galactomannan (RIA, EIA)	"Aspergillin"	More than 90% of patients with ABPA have positive *Aspergillus* skin tests and precipitin titer elevation. More than 90% of patients with aspergilloma have precipitin titer elevation. Serologic tests for antibody lack sensitivity and are without value in patients with invasive aspergillosis. Galactomannan antigen detection (experimental) is not of proven efficacy in diagnosis.
Zygomycosis	None	None	None	Serologic tests for zygomycosis have been unsuccessful owing to poor antibody response to the antigens that have been tested. The disease moves with such rapidity that death may occur before characteristic antibody uses can be documented.

[1]Abbreviations: BASWS, an alkali-soluble, water-soluble blastomycosis skin test preparation; BF, bentonite flocculation; CIE, counterimmunoelectrophoresis; CF, complement fixation; EIA, enzyme immunoassay; ID, immunodiffusion; IDCF, immunodiffusion with the CF antigen; IDTP, immunodiffusion with the TP antigen; IFA, indirect immunofluorescence assay; IHA, indirect hemagglutination; GLC, gas-liquid chromatography; LPA, latex particle agglutination; PHA, passive hemagglutination; RIA, radioimmunoassay; TP, tube precipitin; YCA, whole yeast cell agglutination.

[2]Skin tests are predominantly of epidemiologic importance, defining loci of endemicity. A positive skin test indicates only that infection has occurred in the past. Some skin tests (especially histoplasmin) can influence serologic test results.

[3]In vitro correlates of CMI (eg, lymphocyte blastogenesis and migration inhibition) have been studied extensively, but are insufficiently standardized for routine diagnostic use.

- Disease is much more severe with defective CMI (including AIDS).
- Infection confers solid immunity.

General Considerations

Coccidioidomycosis is an inhalation-acquired mycosis that can produce primary pulmonary infection, progressive pulmonary disease, or hematogenously disseminated disease involving predominantly skin, subcutaneous tissues, bones, joints, and meninges. It is caused by *Coccidiodes immitis,* a fungus characterized uniquely by large spherules that rupture to release hundreds of endospores which mature, in turn, to more spherules. The mycelial form of *C immitis* is a soil organism found in semidesert areas of the USA (eg, California, Arizona, and Texas), contiguous areas of Mexico, and scattered areas of Central and South America. Infection occurs by inhalation of arthroconidia in endemic areas (eg, by tourists, travelers, farmers, archeologists, or construction engineers).

Sporadic and, occasionally, common-source outbreaks occur (eg, dust storm in central California). Endemic areas are defined by skin test (coccidioidin, spherulin) reactivity. Susceptibility to hematogenous dissemination is greatest at the extremes of age. It is also positively correlated with male sex, race (blacks and Filipinos are the commonest victims), deficient CMI, and hormonal status (it occurs more often in the second and third trimesters of pregnancy than in the first). The growth of *C. immitis* is stimulated by estrogen. There is a Suspected HLA-related susceptibility to infection (HLA-A9).

Pathology

See Table 52–2.

Clinical Features

A. Signs and Symptoms: Primary exposure may be asymptomatic (60%) or associated with an influenzalike syndrome. In some patients (especially white women) there may be transient arthralgias, erythema nodosum, or erythema multiforme (also known as valley fever, and desert rheumatism). Similar immunologic phenomena have been observed with histoplasmosis and blastomycosis. Pneumonia, pleuritis, and pulmonary cavitation may occur; cavitary lung disease may be chronic or progressive. Hematogenous dissemination usually occurs in the absence of apparent pulmonary disease. Among the usual manifestations of metastatic infection are skin lesions including nodules, ulcers, sinus tracts from deeper loci, and verrucous granulomas. Also involved are bones, joints, tendon sheaths, and meninges. Meningitis may be the sole apparent locus of metastasis. The gastrointestinal tract is rarely involved.

B. Laboratory Findings: These include leukocytosis, eosinophilia (including cerebrospinal fluid), abnormal chest x-ray, and evidence of specific organ dysfunction at metastatic loci. Diagnosis is established by demonstrating endosporulating spherules on smears and histologic sections and by recovering the fungus in cultures.

C. Immunologic Diagnoses: See Table 52–4. Immunologic tests are useful in diagnosis and prognosis. Negative delayed-hypersensitivity skin tests and an elevated (or rising) complement fixation (CF) titer suggests hematogenous dissemination. An elevated CF titer in the cerebrospinal fluid is virtually diagnostic of coccidioidal meningitis, which is often culture-negative. Coccidioidin (and presumably spherulin) skin testing in a patient with active erythema nodosum may produce a violent, necrotic skin test reaction.

D. Differential Diagnosis: This includes diverse granulomatous infectious diseases (eg, mycoses, tuberculosis), sarcoidosis, and cancers.

E. Treatment: Amphotericin B is the drug of choice in patients with hematogenous dissemination; it must be given intrathecally for meningitis. Ketoconazole is ameliorative and useful for long-term maintenance therapy of nonmeningeal disease.

F. Prevention: A recently tested spherule vaccine failed to demonstrate effective protection. No other vaccine is available.

G. Complications and Prognosis: Most patients recover spontaneously from primary infection. Erythema nodosum and erythema multiforme are considered particularly good prognostic signs. Some 2–4% of primary infections go on to progressive cavitary lung disease (poorly responsive to antifungal drugs; extirpative surgery may be required) or hematogenously disseminated disease. Meningitis is fatal without therapy.

HISTOPLASMOSIS

Major Immunologic Features

- It is a reticuloendothelial system disease in which tiny yeasts reside in macrophages.
- Granulomas with or without caseation are present.
- Cavitary lung disease may have a partial immunologic basis (subintimal arterial proliferation; pulmonary infarction).
- Progressive ocular histoplasmosis syndrome is probably immunologic in origin.
- The disease is more severe in patients with defective CMI (including AIDS).
- Prominent calcification and fibrosis occur during healing.
- Immunity to reinfection occasionally wanes.

General Considerations

Histoplasmosis is an inhalation-acquired mycosis that can produce primary pulmonary infection, progressive pulmonary disease, or hematogenously disseminated disease involving predominantly the reticuloendothelial system, mucosal surfaces, and adrenal glands. It is caused by *Histoplasma capsulatum*, a tiny intracellular yeast. *H capsulatum* is a soil saprobe (mycelial form) that is found worldwide. In the USA it is particularly common in river valleys of the southeastern and central states. It grows particularly well in soil fertilized by bird droppings and bat guano, especially in caves. Infection occurs by inhalation of microconidia in endemic areas eg, by farmers, cave explorers, tourists, or construction workers. Sporadic and, occasionally, common-source outbreaks occur (eg, construction in Indianapolis). A positive delayed-hypersensitivity skin test is extremely common in endemic areas. Hematogenous dissemination is especially common at the extremes of age. Progressive pulmonary disease, strongly resembling tuberculosis, is especially common in white men with chronic obstructive pulmonary disease. There is no known genetic predisposition.

Pathology
See Table 52–2.

Clinical Features
A. Signs and Symptoms: Primary exposure may be asymptomatic or associated with a flulike syndrome. Pneumonia, pleuritis, pulmonary cavitation, and mediastinal adenopathy may occur. Except in infants, hematogenous dissemination usually occurs in the absence of apparent pulmonary disease. Favored sites of metastatic infection include the reticuloendothelial system (hepatosplenomegaly; lymphadenopathy; bone marrow involvement with anemia, leukopenia, and thrombocytopenia); mucous membranes (oronasopharyngeal ulcerations); gastrointestinal tract (malabsorption); and adrenals (adrenal insufficiency). An intense fibrotic response during healing may lead to fibrous mediastinitis. Calcification is common at healed loci (''buckshot'' granulomas of the lungs; splenic calcifications). The progressive ocular histoplasmosis syndrome may represent an immunologic response to fungi that otherwise are found without symptoms at the posterior pole of the eye.

B. Laboratory Findings: These include leukocytosis or leukopenia, thrombocytopenia, and anemia. There is evidence of specific organ dysfunction at metastatic loci. Diagnosis is established by the presence of intracellular yeasts on smears (eg, buffy coat smears in AIDS patients); histologic specimens (eg, mucosal biopsies); or cultures of sputum, blood, bone marrow, and liver biopsy material.

C. Immunologic Diagnoses: See Table 52–4. Serologic tests may be useful in assessing disease activity and, less frequently, in establishing the diagnosis. A positive histoplasmin skin test may spuriously elevate antibody titers detected serologically.

D. Differential Diagnosis: This includes diverse granulomatous infectious diseases (eg, mycoses, tuberculosis, leishmaniasis, and toxoplasmosis), sarcoidosis, Whipple's disease and other causes of malabsorption, and lymphohematogenous cancer.

E. Treatment: Ketoconazole is probably equivalent to amphotericin B, except in severely ill or immunocompromised patients, for whom amphotericin B is the drug of choice.

F. Prevention: No vaccine is available.

G. Complications and Prognosis: Most primary infections resolve spontaneously. Progressive cavitary pulmonary disease is difficult to treat and may contribute to death from underlying pulmonary insufficiency. Hematogenous dissemination is generally fatal in the absence of therapy. Relapses are common in those with severe underlying immunode-

ficiency. Adrenal insufficiency may occur years after the original disease is quiescent.

PARACOCCIDIOIDOMYCOSIS

Major Immunologic Features
- Large, multiply budding yeasts may exceed the size of phagocytes.
- Mixed granulomas and suppuration occur.
- It may be more severe with defective CMI.

General Considerations
Paracoccidioidomycosis is an inhalation-acquired mycosis that can produce primary pulmonary infection or hematogenously disseminated disease involving predominantly the skin, mucous membranes, reticuloendothelial system, and adrenals. It is caused by *Paracoccidioides brasiliensis*, a large, spherical, uninucleate yeast with highly characteristic multiple buds attached by narrow necks. The mycelial form of *P brasiliensis* is a soil saprobe that has only rarely been recovered from the environment in its endemic area in tropical and subtropical forests of Latin America, particularly Brazil, Venezuela, and Colombia. Paracoccidioidomycosis is the most common systemic mycosis in South America. Infection occurs by inhalation of conidia and is most common among agricultural workers. The disease is sporadic. Skin test surveys suggest that men and women are equally susceptible. However, men are 12–48 times as likely to experience hematogenous dissemination as women, perhaps because physiologic concentrations of estrogen can prevent the conversion of conidia to invasive yeasts. In Brazilians, HLA-B40 antigen is more common in patients than controls; in Colombians, HLA-A9 and -B13 are more common.

Pathology
See Table 52–2.

Clinical Features
A. Signs and Symptoms: Primary exposure may be asymptomatic, or pneumonia, pleuritis, pulmonary cavitation, and mediastinal adenopathy may occur. Hematogenously disseminated disease occurs in 2 main forms, juvenile and adult. In the juvenile pattern, the primary pulmonary infection disseminates rapidly, with predominant reticuloendothelial system involvement. In the adult form, fungi, presumably aroused from latency, give rise to progressive localized lung disease, skin lesions, mucocutaneous lesions, reticuloendothelial system infection, and adrenal involvement. Oropharyngeal mucosal invasion is characteristic, with ulcerating lesions that involve most of the oral adventitia. Lesions are so painful that eating is difficult; tooth loss is common. Involvement of the gastrointestinal tract may lead to malabsorption; adrenal involvement can produce adrenal insufficiency.

B. Laboratory Findings: These include leukocytosis and evidence of specific organ dysfunction at metastatic loci. Diagnosis is established by demonstrating multiple-budding yeasts on smears or histologic sections and by recovering the fungi in culture.

C. Immunologic Diagnosis: See Table 52–4. Serologic tests are of use in monitoring the course of established disease.

D. Differential Diagnosis: This includes diverse granulomatous infectious diseases (eg, mycoses, tuberculosis, leishmaniasis, yaws, and syphilis), sarcoidosis, and cancer.

E. Treatment: Ketoconazole is the drug of choice.

F. Prevention: No vaccine is available.

G. Complications and Prognosis: Disseminated paracoccidioidomycosis is generally fatal in the absence of therapy. Disease that was originally acquired asymptomatically may present as disseminated infection years after the infected individual has emigrated from the endemic area.

SYSTEMIC INVASIVE MYCOSES: OPPORTUNISTIC PATHOGENS

CANDIDIASIS

Major Immunologic Features

- The source of the infection is usually normal host flora.
- Intact mucosal barriers represent the major nonspecific host defense mechanism.
- Phagocytes ingest yeasts but attack pseudomycelia and mycelia by extracellular apposition.
- Neutropenia predisposes to hematogenous dissemination.
- Defective CMI predisposes to invasive mucosal disease.
- Thrush and esophagitis are major presenting features of AIDS.
- Chronic mucocutaneous candidiasis is a specific syndrome in patients with defective immunoregulation.

General Considerations

Candidiasis is a general term for diseases produced by *Candida* species and encompasses colonization, superficial infection (eg, thrush, vaginitis, cystitis, and intertrigo), deep local invasion (eg, esophagitis), and hematogenous dissemination (eg, to the eyes, skin, kidneys, and brain). The species that most commonly cause candidiasis are *C albicans* (yeasts, pseudomycelia, and mycelia), *C tropicalis* (yeasts and pseudomycelia), and *Torulopsis glabrata* (yeasts only). *Candida* species are found in nature, but human infection usually arises from normal flora. *C albicans*, *C tropicalis*, and *T glabrata* are commonly found on mucous membranes (eg, vagina, and gastrointestinal tract), but rarely on the skin. Vaginal colonization is increased by diabetes mellitus, pregnancy, and the use of oral contraceptive agents. Carriage at all sites is increased by antibiotics. Hematogenous dissemination occurs most commonly in a setting of neutropenia or gastrointestinal mucosal disruption after repeated abdominal surgery. Neonates may be colonized or infected by passage through a colonized birth canal; premature infants in intensive care units are at particularly high risk of life-threatening *Candida* sepsis. Vaginal colonization occurs after menarche. Disseminated infection occurs in both sexes and at all ages as a function of immunologic impairment. Chronic mucocutaneous candidiasis (CMCC) shows a familial tendency in about 20% of cases. In about 50% of cases there is associated endocrinopathy (eg, hypoparathyroidism, hypoadrenalism, hypothyroidism, or diabetes mellitus). The cause of this association is not known.

Pathology

See Table 52–2.

Clinical Features

A. Signs and Symptoms: Mucosal *candidiasis* is characterized by thrush, laryngitis, esophagitis, gastritis (especially in patients with drug-induced hypochlorhydria), vaginitis, cystitis, and intestinal candidiasis (the assumed source of hematogenous dissemination in most neutropenic patients). Vulvovaginitis is probably the most common overall manifestation of *Candida* infection. CMCC is manifested by persistent infection of skin, scalp, nails, and mucous membranes and is often accompanied by chronic dermatophyte infections. Associated findings include alopecia, depigmentation, cheilosis, blepharitis, keraconjunctivitis, corneal ulcers, and cutaneous horn formation. Hematogenously disseminated candidiasis results in metastatic involvement, particularly of the eyes (chorioretinitis), muscles (myalgias), skin (macronodular skin lesions), and kidneys (parenchymal destruction, papillary necrosis, and bezoar formation). Hematogenous (miliary) pulmonary infection is common, but *Candida* aspiration pneumonia is rare. Other manifestations include myocardial abscesses, meningitis, cerebral abscesses, and arthritis. The "hepatosplenic candidiasis syndrome" is manifested by *Candida* abscesses in the liver and spleen and reflects an apparent isolated portal vein fungemia occurring consequent to heavy intestinal colonization or infection.

B. Laboratory Findings: These include leukopenia or leukocytosis and evidence of specific organ dysfunction at metastatic loci. Diagnosis is established by direct histologic demonstration of fungal tissue invasion and/or recovery of fungi in culture from normally sterile areas. Candidemia may reflect the presence of a contaminated intravascular line and does not always indicate progressive infection. Candiduria indicates cystitis more frequently than it indicates progressive renal infection.

C. Immunologic Diagnosis: See Table 52–4. Serologic tests are not helpful in neutropenic patients.

D. Differential Diagnosis: This includes diverse septicemic syndromes (eg, *Staphylococcus aureus* and *Pseudomonas aeruginosa* infections) and diverse opportunistic infectious diseases of neutropenic patients, including mycoses.

E. Treatment: Topical imidizoles are used for thrush and vaginitis, ketoconazole for vaginitis or progressive mucocutaneous infection, amphotericin B for deep local invasive infection or hematogenous dissemination, and amphotericin B plus flucytosine (depending on renal function) for disseminated infections that involve the eyes or central nervous system. Candiduria can usually be cured by removal of a urinary catheter plus a short course of amphotericin B or flucytosine.

F. Prevention: Prophylactic administration of nystatin or ketoconazole to immunocompromised patients has not been clearly shown to prevent *Candida* infections. Ketoconazole may actually predispose to infection by *C tropicalis* or *T glabrata,* which are less susceptible than *C albicans* to ketoconazole, or to infection by *Aspergillus,* which is completely resistant to ketoconazole.

G. Complications and Prognosis: CMCC can be ameliorated but not cured by chronic ketoconazole therapy. *Candida* endocarditis is essentially incurable without valve replacement. Empirical amphotericin B therapy in febrile neutropenic patients has led to an improved prognosis for recovery in these patients, who are otherwise extremely difficult to diagnose and often die untreated. Reversal of neutropenia is the most important single predictor of recovery from infection.

CRYPTOCOCCOSIS

Major Immunologic Features

- Unencapsulated environmental yeasts acquire a capsule in the lungs.
- Encapsulated yeasts evade phagocytosis.
- Free capsular polysaccharide triggers suppressor cells, down-regulating host defenses.
- Disease is much more common and severe in patients with defective CMI, particularly AIDS sufferers.
- Detection of free capsular polysaccharide is extremely helpful in diagnosis.

General Considerations

Cryptococcosis is an inhalation-acquired mycosis that is initiated by symptomatic or asymptomatic pulmonary infection. It most commonly presents with meningitis. Less common sites of hematogenous dissemination include skin, bones, eyes, and prostate. It is caused by *Cryptococcus neoformans,* an encapsulated yeast with 4 serotypes (A, B, C, and D) based on antigenic differences in the capsular polysaccharide. Virulence is linked to encapsulation and the capacity to synthesize melanin. Cryptococci are ubiquitous, and the disease occurs worldwide. Serotypes A and D are most commonly found in avian habitats (eg, in pigeon dung); serotypes B and C have an unknown ecologic niche. Serotype A causes most disease worldwide; serotype D is common only in Europe. Disease caused by serotypes B and C is found predominantly in subtropical areas (including Southern California). Serotypes A and D are the most common causes of cryptococcal infection in immunocompromised patients and are overwhelmingly the most common serotypes recovered from patients with AIDS. Studies with poorly standardized ''cryptococcin'' skin tests suggest that asymptomatic infection may be common. Immunosuppression (including AIDS) causes the disease to emerge from apparent latency. Some 6–13% of AIDS patients will develop a *C neoformans* infection. Cryptococcosis is more common in males, even excluding the current AIDS population. Infection is rare in children. The disease is sporadic. There is no known genetic predisposition.

Pathology

See Table 52–2.

Clinical Features

A. Signs and Symptoms: Cryptococcal infection commonly presents as isolated meningitis. Disease of the lungs is generally not apparent, even though this is the site of fungal entry. However, in patients who do present with pulmonary infection, meningeal involvement may be inapparent or absent. The most common manifestations of pulmonary cryptococcosis are solitary or multiple infiltrates or nodules. In severely immunocompromised patients (eg, AIDS sufferers), there may be miliary nodules and an acute respiratory distress syndrome that leads rapidly to death. Cryptococcal meningitis is commonly a subtle or subacute process characterized by headache, impaired mentation, optic neuritis or papilledema, cranial nerve palsies, and seizures. Hydrocephalus may lead to progressive mental deterioration. Manifestations of meningeal involvement in AIDS patients may also be subtle, despite disproportionately huge numbers of fungi in the cerebrospinal fluid. Other sites of hematogenous dissemination include the skin (particularly prominent in AIDS patients), bones, prostate, kidneys, and liver.

B. Laboratory Findings: Meningitis is usually low-grade, with lymphocytosis and low sugar levels in cerebrospinal fluid. The diagnosis is usually established by India ink stains, cryptococcal antigen detection, and positive cultures of the cerebrospinal fluid. Organisms may also be cultured from blood, skin lesions, urine, and prostatic secretions.

C. Immunologic Diagnosis: See Table 52–4. Demonstration of cryptococcal antigen in cerebrospinal fluid or blood is extremely helpful in establishing the diagnosis. In AIDS patients, antigen titers are extremely high.

D. Differential Diagnosis: The differential diagnosis of pulmonary cryptococcosis includes diverse infections and cancers. Cryptococcal meningitis may be confused with diverse chronic hypoglycorrhachic syndromes, including tuberculosis or coccidioidomycosis. Symptoms may be erroneously attributed to a primary psychiatric disorder. In AIDS patients the differential diagnosis includes the gamut of opportunistic infections commonly encountered in this disorder.

E. Treatment: Amphotericin B is used with or without flucytosine. The experimental drug fluconazole shows promise in the long-term maintenance therapy of infected AIDS patients, who cannot be cured definitively of this mycosis. Prostatic foci of infection may be particularly difficult to eradicate.

F. Prevention: No vaccine is available.

G. Complications and Prognosis: The likelihood of cure is inversely proportional to the severity of underlying immunosuppression. Although the cryptococcal antigen test is very helpful in establishing a diagnosis, the decrease in antigen titer may not be proportionate to the extent of clinical therapeutic response. Thus, disappearance of antigen from cerebrospinal fluid may not be a realistic therapeutic goal.

ASPERGILLOSIS

Major Immunologic Features

- Infection is caused by inhalation of conidia (common environmental contaminants).
- Conidia are ingested and killed by alveolar macrophages.
- Phagocytes attack mycelia by extracellular apposition.
- Neutropenia or neutrophil dysfunction predisposes to respiratory tract invasion, angioinvasion, and hematogenous dissemination.
- Balls of fungi may colonize previously damaged respiratory tissues (aspergilloma).
- Allergy may develop to inhaled conidia or to fungi colonizing the bronchial tree (atopic asthma, extrinsic allergic alveolitis, allergic bronchopulmonary aspergillosis).

General Considerations

Aspergillosis is a poorly descriptive term, which includes disease processes characterized by colonization, allergy, or tissue invasion. In addition, *Aspergillus* spp produce mycotoxins. Aflatoxin (*A flavus*) is linked epidemiologically to hepatocellular carcinoma; gliotoxin (*A fumigatus*) is toxic to macrophages and cytotoxic T cells. The focus of this section is on invasive aspergillosis. Allergic bronchopulmonary aspergillosis (ABPA) is discussed elsewhere (see chapter 33). *Aspergillus* spp are among the most common environmental saprophytic fungi. Only a few thermotolerant species are pathogenic for humans, most notably *A fumigatus, A flavus,* and *A niger. Aspergillus* infections occur worldwide. Outbreaks of invasive aspergillosis have followed exposure to conidia released by hospital construction, contaminated air-conditioning ducts and filters, and fireproofing materials above false ceilings. Invasive infection occurs in both sexes at all ages, as a function of immunologic impairment. There is no known genetic predisposition.

Pathology

See Table 52–2.

Clinical Features

A. Signs and Symptoms: Invasive pulmonary aspergillosis occurs characteristically in immunosuppressed, neutropenic patients. Widespread bronchial ulceration, parenchymal invasion, and angioinvasion lead to patchy necrotizing pneumonia, thrombosis, and infarction. Widespread metastatic infection may occur. Infarcted lung tissue may contain necrotic sequestrae that resemble aspergillomas. A similar process may take place in the paranasal sinuses, resulting in a clinical picture identical to that of rhinocerebral mucormycosis (see below). An indolent, semi-invasive pulmonary infection occasionally occurs in immunocompetent patients with underlying chronic obstructive pulmonary disease.

B. Laboratory Findings: These include neutropenia, abnormal chest or sinus x-rays, and evidence of specific organ dysfunction at metastatic loci. Diagnosis depends on histologic demonstration of tissue invasion by an exclusively mycelial fungus. Cultivation of *Aspergillus* spp from respiratory secretions may reflect only transient colonization; blood cultures are virtually never positive.

C. Immunologic Diagnosis: See Table 52–4. Serologic tests for antibody are not useful in diagnosis of invasive aspergillosis; antigen tests are promising, but still experimental. Delayed-hypersensitivity skin tests and precipitin titers may be quite helpful in the diagnosis of ABPA.

D. Differential Diagnosis: This includes diverse opportunistic pulmonary infections (bacterial and fungal), pulmonary infarction, diverse septicemic syndromes, and rhinocerebral mucormycosis.

E. Treatment: Amphotericin B is the only drug of proven therapeutic value. It must be used early and aggressively if the patient is to survive.

F. Prevention: Hospital rooms with enclosed filtered ventilation systems provide some degree of protection from environmental fungi.

G. Complications and Prognosis: Invasive aspergillosis is commonly fatal. An aggressive approach to diagnosis and treatment is essential. Empirical amphotericin B therapy in febrile neutropenic patients who are not responding to broad-spectrum antibacterial agents is commonly used in an attempt to prevent this and other opportunistic mycoses. Reversal of neutropenia is the single most important predictor of recovery from this infection.

ZYGOMYCOSIS

Major Immunologic Features
- Infection is caused by inhalation of spores.
- Spores are ingested and prevented from germinating by alveolar macrophages.
- Phagocytes attack mycelia by extracellular apposition.
- Acidotic states predispose to invasive paranasal sinus infection.
- Neutropenia predisposes to paranasal sinus, pulmonary, and disseminated infection.

General Considerations
Zygomycosis is the preferred term for mucormycosis, a suppurative opportunistic mycosis that produces predominantly paranasal sinus (rhinocerebral) disease in patients with acidosis and rhinocerebral, pulmonary, or disseminated disease in patients with neutropenia. The most common etiologic agent is *Rhizopus arrhizus;* others include *Absidia, Cunninghamella, Mortierella,* and *Saksenaea* spp. These are all common environmental contaminants. Colonization and infection are uncommon in healthy persons; zygomycosis is less common than invasive aspergillosis in immunocompromised patients. Infection occurs sporadically; clusters of infection are rare. Invasive infection occurs in both sexes and at all ages as a function of acidosis or immunosuppression. There is no known genetic predisposition.

Pathology
See Table 52–2.

Clinical Features
A. Signs and Symptoms: These are virtually identical to those of invasive aspergillosis. Rhinocerebral mucormycosis accounts for about 50% of all cases of mucormycosis; more than 75% of cases occur in patients with acidosis, especially diabetic ketoacidosis. However, increasing numbers of cases are being seen in association with neutropenia and immunosuppression. Early clinical features include nasal stuffiness, bloody nasal discharge, facial swelling, and facial and orbital pain. Later manifestations include orbital cellulitis, proptosis, endophthalmitis, orbital apex syndrome, cranial nerve palsies, and cerebral extension.

B. Laboratory Findings: These include acidosis (principally diabetic ketoacidosis), neutropenia, abnormal paranasal sinus or chest x-rays, and evidence of specific organ dysfunction at sites of local extension (central nervous system) or metastatic loci. Diagnosis depends on histologic demonstration of tissue invasion by an exclusively mycelial fungus. Cultures are positive in fewer than 20% of patients, and even positive cultures may represent the presence of fungal contaminants.

C. Immunologic Diagnosis: See Table 52–4. There are no useful tests available.

D. Differential Diagnosis: This includes diverse opportunistic paranasal sinus infections (aspergillosis, phaeohyphomycosis, hyalohyphomycosis) and diverse opportunistic pulmonary bacterial and fungal infections.

E. Treatment: Amphotericin B is the only drug of proven value. Aggressive surgical debridement is required for paranasal sinusitis or rhinocerebral mucormycosis.

F. Prevention: No effective preventive measures are known.

G. Complications and Prognosis: Rhinocerebral mucormycosis advances at an extremely rapid rate; an aggressive approach to diagnosis and treatment is essential. Survival is more likely in the setting of diabetic ketoacidosis than that of neutropenia.

PNEUMOCYTOSIS

The cause of pneumocytosis (*Pneumocystis carinii*) is tentatively classified as a fungus. However, there is considerable evidence that the microorganism is a protozoan.

Major Immunologic Features
- Infection is apparent only in patients with impaired CMI or in infants with severe protein-calorie malnutrition (marasmus).
- It is the most common index diagnosis for AIDS.
- Disease is predominantly alveolar and interstitial; extrapulmonary spread is distinctly rare.

General Considerations
Pneumocystis carinii pneumonia (PCP) is an apparently inhalation-acquired disease, but the environmental form of the pathogen has never been identified. PCP occurs predominantly in patients with impaired CMI and is the defining opportunistic infection for AIDS. *P carinii* is a unicellular eukaryote with a proposed life cycle consisting of trophozoites and cysts. It can be maintained transiently in cell culture but has never been cultivated independently in cell-free media. Electron-microscopic studies and

more recent RNA studies, suggest that *P carinii* may be more closely related to fungi than to other protozoa. Seroepidemiologic studies indicate that over more than two-thirds of normal children have acquired antibody to *P carinii* by 3–4 years of age. Clinical attributes of the presumed infecting event are unknown, and autopsy studies have failed to provide evidence of residual pulmonary microorganisms in persons who have died of unrelated causes. The occurrence of PCP in immunocompromised adults could represent either new infection or arousal of inapparent disease from latency. When PCP occurs in infants with AIDS or marasmus, it is assumed to represent primary infection. Common-source outbreaks of PCP have occurred, suggesting that infection may be spread by aerosol. Most cases, however, appear to be sporadic. Diverse animal species harbor *P carinii,* as evidenced by spontaneous occurrence of PCP in response to immunosuppression. There is no evidence of spread from animals to humans; there are antigenic differences among human and animal strains. Prevalence is directly related to the occurrence of marasmus or impaired CMI. Neutropenia is not a risk factor. There is no independent age or sex-related susceptibility. Of reported patients with AIDS, 65% have PCP either alone (60%) or in combination with Kaposi's sarcoma as the index diagnosis; another 20% develop the disease later in the course of illness. There is no known genetic predisposition.

Pathology

See Table 52–2.

Clinical Features

A. Signs and Symptoms: These include fever, cough, and shortness of breath, especially in patients with prolonged fatigue and weight loss.

B. Laboratory Findings: These include CD4 T cell counts of generally less than 200/μL; elevated nonspecific serum lactic dehydrogenase level; and diffuse alveolointerstitial infiltrates on chest x-ray, sometimes with cystic changes or pneumatoceles. Hypoxemia and alveolar-to-arterial O_2 tension differences are common, especially in response to exercise. Gallium lung scanning is sensitive, but not specific. Diagnosis is established by visualizing characteristic organisms in expectorated sputum, induced sputum, bronchoalveolar lavage specimens, or lung biopsy specimens obtained transbronchially or by open thoracotomy.

C. Immunologic Diagnosis: See Table 52–4. There are several experimental techniques for detecting an antibody response to *P carinii* or free *P carinii* antigen. However, these are not of current clinical value. It is not clear whether a direct fluorescent-antibody technique now available to identify *P carinii* in respiratory specimens is superior to simpler staining techniques (Giemsa and fast silver stains).

D. Differential Diagnosis: This includes the gamut of diseases caused by opportunistic pulmonary pathogens in patients with AIDS or profoundly depressed CMI. Among these are tuberculosis, histoplasmosis, cryptococcosis, toxoplasmosis, cytomegalovirus infection, bacterial pneumonia, lymphomas, and Kaposi's sarcoma.

E. Treatment: Standard therapies include oral or intravenous trimethoprim-sulfamethoxazole and intramuscular or intravenous pentamidine isethionate. A variety of experimental therapies are under evaluation (including dapsone, difluoromethylornithine, trimetrexate, clindamycin plus primaquine; erythromycin, and aerosolized pentamidine). Corticosteroids are useful both in the prevention and in the treatment of PCP-induced acute respiratory failure. *P carinii* is not susceptible to common antifungal drugs (eg, amphotericin B and ketoconazole).

F. Prevention: PCP prophylaxis has prolonged the life expectancy of AIDS patients who are receiving zidovudine. Effective regimens include oral trimethoprim-sulfamethoxazole, aerosolized pentamidine, intramuscular pentamidine, oral pyrimethamine-sulfadoxine (Fansidar), and others. No vaccine is available.

G. Complications and Prognosis: Aggressive use of prophylaxis in AIDS patients is decreasing the frequency of PCP as an index diagnosis. Aerosolized pentamidine may delay or change the presentation of PCP to less easily recognized forms (eg, apical cystic disease and hematogenously disseminated disease, both of which are extremely rare at present). Pneumothorax is a late but important complication of PCP.

REFERENCES

GENERAL

Chandler FW: Pathology of the mycoses in patients with the acquired immunodeficiency syndrome (AIDS). *Curr Top Med Mycol* 1985;**1**:1.

Chandler FW, Kaplan W, Ajello L: *Histopathology of Mycotic Diseases.* Year Book, 1980.

Chandler FW, Watts JC: *Pathologic Diagnosis of Fungal Infections.* ASCP Press, 1987.

Cox RA: *Immunology of the Fungal Diseases.* CRC Press, 1989.

Drutz DJ: Chapter 32 Fungal diseases. Page 863, in: *Immunological Diseases,* 4th ed. Samter M et al (editors). Little, Brown, 1988.

Musial CE, Cockerill FR III, Roberts GD: Fungal infections of the immunocompromised host: Clinical and laboratory aspects. *Clin Microbiol Rev* 1988;**1**:349.

Reiss E: *Molecular Immunology of Mycotic and Actino-mycotic Infections.* Elsevier, 1986.

Rippon JW: *Medical Mycology,* 3rd ed. Saunders, 1988.

SUPERFICIAL MYCOSES

Pityrosporum and *Malassezia*

Danker WM et al: *Malassezia* fungemia in neonates and adults: Complication of hyperalimentation. *Rev Infect Dis* 1987;**9**:743.

Klotz SA: *Malassezia furfur. Infect Dis Clin N Am* 1989;**3**:53.

Marcon MJ, Powell DA: Epidemiology, diagnosis, and management of *Malassezia furfur* systemic infection. *Diagn Microbiol Infect Dis* 1987;**1**:161.

White Piedra; *Trichosporon beigelii*

Steinman HK, Papenfort RB: White piedra—A case report and review of the literature. *Clin Exp Dermatol* 1984;**9**:591.

Walling DM et al: Disseminated infection with *Trichosporon beigelii. Rev Infect Dis* 1987;**9**:1013.

Walsh TJ: Trichosporonosis. *Infect Dis Clin N Am* 1989;**3**:43.

SUBCUTANEOUS MYCOSES

Dermatophytosis

Feingold DS: What the infectious disease subspecialist should know about dermatophytes. Page 154 in: *Current Clinical Topics in Infectious Diseases.* Vol 8. Remington JS, Swartz MN (editors). McGraw-Hill, 1987.

Chromomycosis

Fader RC, McGinnis MR: Infections caused by dematiaceous fungi: Chromoblastomycosis and phaeohyphomycosis. *Infect Dis Clin N Am* 1988;**2**:925.

Mycetoma

McGinnis MR, Fader RC: Mycetoma: A contemporary concept. *Infect Dis Clin N Am* 1988;**2**:939.

Sporotrichosis

Winn RE: Sporotrichosis. *Infect Dis Clin N Am* 1988;**2**:899.

SYSTEMIC INVASIVE MYCOSES

Blastomycosis

Bradsher RW: Blastomycosis. *Infect Dis Clin N Am* 1988;**2**:877.

Coccidioidomycosis

Knoper SR, Galgiani JN: Coccidioidomycosis. *Infect Dis Clin N Am* 1988;**2**:861.

Drutz DJ: Coccidioidal pneumonia. Page 472 in: *Respiratory Infections: Diagnosis and Management.* Pennington JE (editor). Raven Press, 1989.

Histoplasmosis

Alsip SG, Dismukes WE: Approach to the patient with suspected histoplasmosis. Page 254 in: *Current Clinical Topics in Infectious Disease.* Vol 7. Remington JS, Swartz MN (editors). McGraw-Hill, 1986.

Graybill JR: Histoplasmosis and AIDS. *J Infect Dis* 1988;**158**:623.

Wheat LJ: Histoplasmosis. *Infect Dis Clin N Am* 1988;**2**:841.

Paracoccidioidomycosis

Restrepo A: Immune response to Paracoccidioidis brasilienses in human and animal hosts. *Curr Top Med Mycol* 1988;**2**:239.

Sugar AM: Paracoccidioidomycosis. *Infect Dis Clin N Am* 1988;**2**:913.

Candidiasis

Crislip MA, Edwards JE Jr: Candidiasis. *Infect Dis Clin N Am* 1989;**3**:103.

Odds FC: *Candida and Candidosis,* 2nd ed. Saunders, 1988.

Cryptococcosis

Perfect JR: Cryptococcosis. *Infec Dis Clin N Am* 1989;**3**:77.

Aspergillosis

Bossche HV, Mackenzie DWR, Cauwenbergh G (editors): *Aspergillus and Aspergillosis.* Plenum, 1987.

Levitz SM: Aspergillosis. *Infect Dis Clin N Am* 1989;**3**:1.

Zygomycosis

Rinaldi MG: Zygomycosis. *Infect Dis Clin N Am* 1989;**3**:19.

Pneumocystosis

Edman JC et al: Ribosomal RNA sequence shows *Pneumocystis carinii* to be a member of the fungi. *Nature* 1988;**334**:519.

Hopewell PC: *Pneumocystis carinii* pneumonia: Diagnosis. *J Infect Dis* 1988;**157**:1115.

Hughes WT: *Pneumocystis carinii Pneumonitis.* 2 vol. CRC Press, 1987.

ul Haque A et al: *Pneumocystis carinii:* Taxonomy as viewed by electron microscopy. *Am J Clin Pathol* 1987;**87**:504.

Phaeohyphomycosis and Hyalohyphomycosis

McGinnis MR, Hilger AE: Infections caused by black fungi. *Arch Dermatol* 1987;**123**:1300.

53

Parasitic Diseases

Donald Heyneman, PhD, & James H. McKerrow, MD, PhD

Parasitic diseases such as malaria, schistosomiasis, and leishmaniasis are among the most important health problems in developing countries. Not only is understanding of the immunology of parasitic disease essential to control these diseases by immunization—the study of the host response to parasites continues to lead to important discoveries about the immune response itself. For example, the response to schistosome eggs by infected mice represents one of the best experimental models for studying the formation and regulation of granulomatous inflammation. Immature schistosomes (schistosomula) and eggs have also provided an in vitro experimental model for elucidating the function of the eosinophil.

Immune responses to the complex antigenic structures of parasites have diverse manifestations and do not always lead to complete protective immunity. For example, immunity with specific protection to reinfection occurs after primary infection with cutaneous leishmaniasis; in falciparum malaria, partial protection against recurrent infection results from persistently low levels of parasitemia, which stimulates production of protective antibody (concomitant immunity or premunition) (see below).

Unfortunately, as is the case with other infectious diseases also, the immune response to parasites can produce more serious disease than the parasite itself. Examples are the hepatic granulomas of schistosomiasis, antigen-antibody complex glomerulonephritis in quartan malaria, and antibody-mediated anaphylactic shock from a ruptured hydatid cyst or from too-rapid killing of filarial microfilariae.

Some of the most fascinating and perplexing aspects of parasitic disease are the variety of mechanisms by which the parasite evades the immune response (Fig 53–1). A parasite can "hide" within a host's own cells, as in leishmaniasis; disguise itself as "self" with host antigens, as in schistosomiasis; or produce successive waves of progeny with different surface antigens, as in African trypanosomiasis. Nonspecific immunosuppression, due to a variety of stimuli, is characteristic of a number of parasitic infections. The ability of parasites to adapt to the host environment is the essence of successful parasitism, and it increases immeasurably the difficulty of developing immunization procedures against parasitic infection.

Major worldwide efforts are under way to produce vaccines against malaria and schistosomiasis. Improved serodiagnostic antigen detection and diagnostic DNA probes are becoming available. The serodiagnostic procedures available at the Centers for Disease Control (CDC), Atlanta, Ga, can be found in the CDC *Reference and Disease Surveillance Manual.*

THE IMMUNE RESPONSE TO PROTOZOA

Protozoa are important agents of worldwide disease. Falciparum malaria, for example, is still one of the most lethal diseases in humans in spite of massive efforts at eradication and control. In developing countries, especially in Africa, malaria and trypanosomiasis take enormous tolls of life and are significant barriers to economic development, survival of domestic animals, and human occupation of vast grazing lands. Amebiasis, giardiasis, and toxoplasmosis are widespread even in highly developed countries. The use of immunosuppressive drugs to treat cancer and to prevent rejection of transplanted organs has resulted in activation of otherwise subclinical infections with protozoa such as *Toxoplasma* or has induced an overwhelming systemic infection with the nematode *Strongyloides stercoralis*. In some instances, deaths have been caused by these infections rather than by the underlying illness for which treatment was being given. Cryptosporidiosis is a common complication of acquired immunodeficiency syndrome (AIDS).

MALARIA

Major Immunologic Features
- Complex partial humoral and cellular immunity occurs with multiple exposure.
- Nonimmune individuals in endemic areas have significantly higher mortality rates from cerebral malaria.

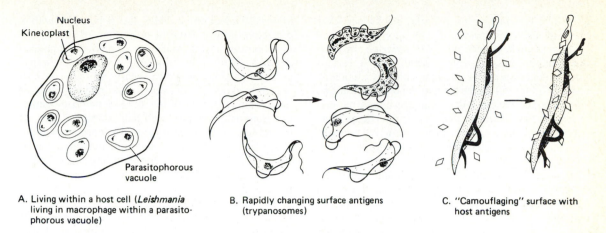

A. Living within a host cell (*Leishmania* living in macrophage within a parasitophorous vacuole)

B. Rapidly changing surface antigens (trypanosomes)

C. "Camouflaging" surface with host antigens

Figure 53–1. Some of the devious ways in which parasites evade the host immune response.

- Immunity to sporozoites can be induced by using tandemly repeated peptides from the parasite's surface.
- Species-specific protective IgG antibody is produced against merozoites after multiple infections.
- Immunosuppression of other antibodies occurs during the course of disease.
- Parasites display antigenic variation.
- T-cell activation, as well as humoral antibody response, is probably the key to development of a vaccine.

General Considerations

Human malaria is caused by species of *Plasmodium*. It is transmitted by female anopheline mosquitoes that ingest the sexual forms of the parasite in blood meals. The infective sporozoites develop in the mosquito and are injected into the definitive (human) host when bitten by the insect. In the human, the parasites first develop in an exoerythrocytic form, multiplying within hepatic cells without inducing an inflammatory reaction. The progeny, or merozoites, invade host erythrocytes to begin the erythrocytic cycle and initiate the earliest phase of clinical malaria. The gametocyte is the sexual stage taken up by the mosquito.

Destruction of erythrocytes occurs on a 48-hour cycle with *Plasmodium vivax* and *Plasmodium ovale* and every 72 hours with *Plasmodium malariae*. The characteristic chills-fever-sweat malarial syndrome follows this cyclic pattern, being induced by synchronous rupture of infected erythrocytes by the mature asexual forms (schizonts), releasing merozoites that quickly invade new erythrocytes. *Plasmodium falciparum*, although classically thought to use a 48-hour cycle, is, in fact, frequently not synchronous. In contrast to the exoerythrocytic stage, the erythrocytic merozoites induce an array of humoral responses in the host, as demonstrated by complement fixation, precipitation, agglutination, and fluorescent antibody reactions.

In *P vivax* and *P ovale* infections, relapse after a period of dormancy may result from periodic release of infective merozoites from the liver, which lacks an immune response to the intracellular parasites. This is apparently determined by the genetic constitution of the invading parasite sporozoites. When the erythrocytic cellular and humoral protection is deficient (from concurrent infection, age, trauma, or other debilitating factors), the reappearing blood-stage forms induce a new round of clinical malaria until the erythrocytic cycle is again controlled by a humoral and T cell host response. True relapse, as opposed to delayed exoerythrocytic cycle or a recrudescence of erythrocytic infection, generally will occur for up to 5 years with some strains of *P vivax* and possibly 2–3 years for *P ovale*. *P malariae* appears to recur only as a recrudescent erythrocytic infection, sometimes lasting 30 or more years after the primary infection. *P falciparum* may have a short-term recrudescence but does not develop a true relapse from liver-developed merozoites.

Blackwater fever, formerly a common and rapidly fatal form of falciparum malaria among colonists in Africa, has declined in frequency with reduction in quinine therapy. It is associated with repeated falciparum infection, inadequate quinine therapy, and possibly genetic factors more frequently found in whites. The resulting rapid, massive hemolysis of both infected and uninfected erythrocytes is thought to result from autoantibodies from previous infections that react with autoantigens (perhaps an erythrocyte-parasite-quinine combination) derived from a new infection with the same falciparum strain. With increased use of quinine to prevent or treat chloroquine-resistant falciparum malaria, blackwater fever may increase in frequency in coming years.

Quartan malaria, caused by *P malariae,* in African children has been associated with a serious complement-dependent antigen-antibody immune complex glomerulonephritis and nephrosis, resulting in edema and severe kidney damage unless the disease is arrested early. After loss of the edema, persistent symptomless proteinuria or slowly deteriorating renal function is common. Stable remission with corticosteroid therapy occurs when proteinuria is restricted to only a few classes of protein and histologic changes are minimal. However, patients with poorly controlled generalized proteinuria are probably not benefited by antimalarial or immunosuppressive therapy. Chronic *P malariae* infection probably triggers an autoimmunity perpetuating the immune complex glomerulonephritis, but the antigen involved is not yet identified.

Innate, nonacquired immunity to malaria is well demonstrated. African or American blacks lacking Duffy blood group antigen Fy(a-b-) are immune to *P vivax,* as this genetic factor appears to be necessary for successful merozoite penetration of the human erythrocyte by this plasmodial species. Intracellular growth of the malaria parasites is also affected by the hemoglobin molecular structure. Sickle cell (SS) hemoglobin inhibits growth of *P falciparum.* This genetic factor is widespread in areas of Africa hyperendemic for falciparum malaria. Though prevalence of infection appears unaffected by the sickling trait, *severe* infections in individuals with hemoglobin A/S (sickle cell trait) are very much reduced compared with those in non-sickling homozygote individuals. Similarly, *P falciparum* growth is retarded in erythrocytes with the fetal hemoglobin (F)—hence the selective advantage of β-thalassemia heterozygotes, in whom postnatal hemoglobin F declines at a lower than normal rate. Other red cell abnormalities such as glucose-6-phosphate dehydrogenase deficiency appear to be protective of the erythrocyte and reduce the severity of plasmodial infection.

Both acquired and innate specific or nonspecific resistance to malaria is influenced by a number of genetic traits that reflect strong selective pressure in areas with specific mosquito-human-*Plasmodium* combinations. A very gradual long-term resistance to hyperendemic falciparum malaria is acquired in African populations. The resistance develops years after the onset of severe disease among nearly all children over 3 months of age. Initial passive protection is present owing to transplacental maternal IgG. There are estimates of a million malaria deaths a year in Africa, chiefly among children under 5 years of age. Nonetheless, even after surviving this, a large proportion of adults remain susceptible to infection and show periodic parasitemia, while their serum contains antiplasmodial antibodies, some with demonstrated protective action. Susceptibility to low-level infection provides the population with a protective **premunition** or prevention of subsequent infection during the course of a chronic asymptomatic current infection. It is believed that in these hyperendemic areas of Africa, nearly all residents harbor throughout their lives a continuous series of falciparum infections of low to moderate pathogenicity. Antibodies are produced that inhibit the entry of merozoites into erythrocytes. All immunoglobulin classes are elevated in the serum of malaria patients, but IgG levels appear to correlate best with the degree of malaria protection (or control of acute manifestations).

By various protective adaptations (eg, antigenic variability), the parasites survive and—by reason of a limited level of erythrocyte destruction—elicit only a mild host response. Therefore, innate and acquired protective host responses (specific and nonspecific) and parasite counteradaptations to these host characteristics occur. In addition, vector biology and population fluctuation, as well as the parasite's response to varied ecologic conditions (such as a required ambient temperature for successful development of the sporogonic cycle in the mosquito), add to the vagaries of differential host/parasite survival. Immunity to *P falciparum* malaria, for example, is species- and strain-specific. If immune individuals migrate to other, geographically distinct endemic areas, they may acquire new disease.

Immunization has become a major focus of malaria research, accelerating with Trager and Jensen's breakthrough in 1976 of a continuous-culture method for producing erythrocyte asexual stages in vitro.

Recent research has been directed toward developing a nonliving vaccine. If sporozoites are incubated in vitro with sera from vaccinated animals, a taillike immune precipitate is formed called the circumsporozoite reaction. This reaction is correlated with loss of parasite infectivity. The target antigens of this reaction were first identified by using monoclonal antibodies. These were found to be polypeptides that cover the entire surface membrane of the parasite, are species-specific, and contain repeating epitopes.

Subsequently, using recombinant DNA techniques, the genes encoding the circumsporozoite epitopes have been cloned and sequenced. An important finding was that the immunodominant epitope consisted of tandem repeated sequences of amino acids (asparagine-alanine-asparagine-proline in *P falciparum*). This discovery implied that a very simple vaccine antigen might be developed. In fact, synthetic peptides based on these sequences can elicit polyclonal antibodies that neutralize sporozoite infectivity in vitro and in animals. Unfortunately, human trials have demonstrated genetic diversity in the ability to respond to antigens in the vaccine. Because an antisporozoite vaccine would have to be 100% effective to be practical (one sporozoite escaping could initiate a new cycle), development of a multistage vaccine (sporozoite, merozoite, or gametocyte) is now the goal.

The second approach to vaccine development—a killed or inactivated merozoite vaccine—induces an antibody that reacts with the red cell surface and selectively agglutinates infected erythrocytes to produce a strain- and species-specific clinical cure. New infections can still develop, since there is no protection against sporozoites or the exoerythrocytic cycle. So long as the humoral titer is high, however, merozoites (but not gametocytes) will be destroyed, and symptoms will not develop. Rhesus monkeys, which normally are quickly killed by monkey malaria (*Plasmodium knowlesi*), were fully protected for 18 months when vaccinated with *Plasmodium knowlesi* merozoites. Freund's complete adjuvant is required—a major deterrent to development of a human vaccine. The synthetic adjuvant muramyl dipeptide is now used instead of Freund's adjuvant in rhesus monkey immunization studies. Helper T cells, other cell-mediated effector mechanisms, and humoral antibody are all involved. Extracellular merozoites are specifically inhibited by IgG and IgM in the absence of complement. Immunization in rhesus monkeys induces complete elimination of parasites after 1–3 weeks, whereas natural immunity following repeated infection and drug cure is associated with chronic relapsing parasitemia. Immunization probably is associated with far fewer soluble circulating antigens than occur in natural infection, which preferentially stimulates suppressor cells or lymphocyte mitogens, all of which favor parasite survival. Difficulties of immunization with a merozoite vaccine even with a nontoxic adjuvant include the risk of contamination of the merozoite vaccine with blood group substances acquired during its cultivation, and substantial potential problems of vaccine delivery, cost, and acceptance. Nonetheless, the possibility of a prophylactic or therapeutic merozoite vaccine is most promising.

TOXOPLASMOSIS

Major Immunologic Features
- Specific antibody is present.
- There is a nonspecific increase in serum immunoglobulins.
- Natural acquired immunity is widespread; cell-mediated immunity is probably the major means.

General Considerations

Toxoplasma infection in humans is generally asymptomatic; it has been estimated that as much as 40% of the adult population in the world is infected, as well as all species of mammals that have been tested for the presence of this ubiquitous parasite. Clinical disease, which develops in only a small fraction of those infected, ranges from benign lymphadenopathy to an acute and often fatal infection of the central nervous system. The developing fetus and the aged or otherwise immunologically compromised host are most vulnerable to the pathologic expression of massive infection and resulting encystation in the eye or brain. Damage to the fetus is greatest during the first trimester, when the central nervous system is being organized, and nearly all such instances end in fetal death. Infection of the mother during the second trimester may produce hydrocephaly, blindness, or varying lesser degrees of neurologic damage in the fetus. Most cases of fetal infection occur during the third trimester, resulting in chorioretinitis or other ophthalmic damage, reduced learning capacity or other expression of central nervous system deficit, or asymptomatic latent infection that may become clinically apparent years later. Women exposed *before* pregnancy—as indicated by a positive indirect immunofluorescent or Sabin-Feldman dye test—are thought to be unable to transmit the infection in utero.

Many potential sources of infection have been suggested, including tissue cysts in raw or partially cooked pork or mutton and oocysts passed in feces of infected cats (the true final hosts). Yet these sources seem insufficient to account for such large numbers of infections. The major reservoirs of infection are as yet unknown. *Toxoplasma* infection usually occurs through the gastrointestinal tract, and the protozoa can apparently penetrate and proliferate in virtually every cell in the body, though very rarely in mature red cells, forming cysts that remain viable for long periods. Following a cellular and humoral immune response, only encysted parasites can survive.

In most cases, the diagnosis of toxoplasmosis is made by serology. The diagnosis of acute infections by the indirect fluorescent-antibody (IFA) technique for IgM or IgG is most commonly used. A positive test for IgM appears approximately 5 days after infection, and IgG approximately 1–2 weeks. Because an IgG reaction may persist for months to years, IgM IFA is diagnostically more useful, since a single high titer is indicative of acute infection. For confirmation, 2 specimens are generally drawn at a 3-week interval and tested simultaneously. A serial rise in titer is a reliable indication of recent infection.

In ocular toxoplasmosis, no rise in titer is observed, but a negative serology can be used to rule out chorioretinitis. The IgM IFA test can also be used during pregnancy and on cord blood, but serologic positivity may be suppressed by immunosuppresive therapy or AIDS.

The ability of macrophages to kill infective trophozoites is greatly increased if the parasites are first exposed to antibody and complement. This mechanism may be one way that parasite numbers are reduced in the infected host. The parasite can multiply only to a certain number within macrophages before the host cells are destroyed. When this occurs, extracellular trophozoites come into contact with antibody and may be more efficiently killed by macrophages than before.

Cell-mediated immunity is also involved in protection against *Toxoplasma* because delayed hypersensitivity and its in vitro correlates such as production of migration inhibitory factor (MIF) develop early in toxoplasmosis, and protection results only from infection with *living* organisms. Interferon is also produced, and activated macrophages can be demonstrated that kill or inhibit multiplication of the parasite, which would effectively reduce the parasite burden. In such cellular immunity, macrophage activation is probably affected by the action of antigen upon specifically sensitized T lymphocytes, which in turn produce lymphokines that activate the macrophages.

An intact immune system is necessary for protection against *Toxoplasma;* thus, immunosuppression to control transplant rejection or malignancies or infection with HIV may result in active toxoplasmosis. This phenomenon may result either from the elimination of sensitized lymphocytes previously limiting an inapparent infection or from inability of the immunosuppressed host to mount an adequate protective response to new infection.

Vaccination of the population with strains of low virulence would probably be effective in establishing protection to *Toxoplasma,* but most persons develop adequate protection after natural infection. Although no such vaccine is available, the procedure probably would not be worthwhile, except for previously uninfected women of childbearing age to prevent intrauterine transmission.

AMEBIASIS

Major Immunologic Features
- Specific antibody is detectable following tissue invasion by virulent strains.
- Skin tests for immediate and delayed hypersensitivity are positive following recovery from hepatic abscess.

General Considerations
Understanding the immune response to *Entamoeba histolytica,* the agent of amebiasis, is complicated by the fact that there are 2 distinct levels of disease. In most cases, infection appears to be by relatively nonpathogenic strains, which produce mild symptoms or more often an asymptomatic infection identified only by the passage of cysts in the stool.

A smaller percentage of infections, which nevertheless can be quite common in certain endemic areas, are due to more virulent, "pathogenic" strains. In these infections, colitis with ulceration of the intestinal mucosa and extraintestinal dissemination can produce very serious disease. The most common manifestation of extraintestinal "metastasis" of *E histolytica* trophozoites is liver abscess. *E histolytica* infections that are confined to the intestinal lumen may elicit an antibody response as a result of secretion of amebic proteins, but T lymphocytes are unresponsive to the amebic antigens. Invasive disease, however, produces more profound effects on the immune system with both specific IgG and IgM antibodies detectable by the enzyme-linked immunosorbent assay (ELISA). Serodiagnosis is very useful in documenting extraintestinal amebiasis, with a 92–98% positive rate. There is an 80–90% positive rate in patients with ulcerations and colitis of the intestine but no extraintestinal disease. Although this antibody reaction can be used for diagnosis of invasive or extraintestinal disease, it does not necessarily indicate active acute infection but may instead be due to prior exposure to the organism.

Cell-mediated immunity to *E histolytica* antigens can be demonstrated by delayed hypersensitivity skin tests in many patients who do not have clinically evident disease. Recent evidence indicates that patients with amebic abscess of the liver have depressed cell-mediated immunity to amebic antigens while retaining their ability to respond to other skin test antigens. Macrophages from animals with amebic liver abscesses are deficient in their release of reactive oxygen intermediates, are unresponsive to lymphokines, and are not cytotoxic to the *E histolytica* trophozoites in vitro. Trophozoites from pathogenic strains are also able to lyse neutrophils. Nevertheless, when lymphocyte activation can occur, CD8 lymphocytes can kill amebae on contact. Cell-mediated immunity returns after treatment for liver abscesses, and there is usually no recurrence of infection. It is not known whether this is due to protective immunity.

Other normally nonpathogenic amebas such as *Naegleria* or *Acanthamoeba* can invade the central nervous system and cause rapid death due to meningoencephalitis (*Naegleria*) or local lesions in the throat or on the skin which may finally involve the central nervous system and produce death (*Acanthamoeba*). Probably little immune response to *Naegleria* occurs, owing to the brief survival of infected patients; however, *Acanthamoeba* may induce an immune response because of the duration of infection. No protective immune mechanisms to these parasites have been demonstrated.

LEISHMANIASIS

Leishmania is a genus of obligate intracellular parasites that infect macrophages of the skin and viscera to produce disease in both animals and humans. Sandflies, the principal vector, introduce the parasites into the host while taking blood meals.

A range of host responses interact with a number of parasite leishmanial species and strains to produce a panoply of pathologic and immunologic responses. Leishmania represents an important lesson in how different species or strains of the same parasite can produce drastically different diseases.

1. CUTANEOUS LEISHMANIASIS

Major Immunologic Features
- Cell-mediated immunity is a critical factor.
- Delayed hypersensitivity is present.
- There is little or no specific serum antibody.

General Considerations
Old World cutaneous leishmaniasis, or tropical sore, is caused chiefly by various forms of *Leishmania-Leishmania tropica, Leishmania major,* and *Leishmania aethiopica*. These agents induce an immune response characterized by nonprotective antibody but strong cell-mediated immunity. In cutaneous leishmaniasis, it is chiefly the patient's immune response to the infection that determines the form taken by the clinical disease; however, the strain of parasite may also determine part of the host response. If the patient mounts an adequate but not excessive cell-mediated immune response to the parasite, healing of the ulcerative lesions and specific protection result. However, if cell-mediated immunity to the parasite is inadequate or suppressed, the result may be diffuse cutaneous disease, in which there is little chance of spontaneous cure. In the Old World, this condition is due chiefly to *L aethiopica* in East Africa. A similar form, caused by *L mexicana* subsp *pifanoi*, occurs in Venezuela, again in specifically anergic patients. The cause of the specific anergy and whether it is host- or parasite-induced are unknown. On the other hand, an excessive cell-mediated immune response produces lupoid or recidiva leishmaniasis, caused by *L tropica,* in which nonulcerated lymphoid nodules form at the edge of the primary lesion; these lesions persist indefinitely, although parasites are not easily demonstrated. Recidiva leishmaniasis may occur from 2 to 10 years after the initial lesion. Thus, a spectrum of host responses to cutaneous leishmaniasis exists, ranging from multiple disseminated parasite-filled ulcers or nodules (anergic response) to single, spontaneously cured immunizing sores, to recidiva hyperactive host responses with few or no parasites (allergic response). Parasite strain differences in virulence and other factors add to the complexity of the host-parasite interaction, resulting in prolonged disease or cure with immunity. The variability in cutaneous leishmaniasis may be related to variable susceptibility of *Leishmania* strains to intracellular killing by macrophages.

Delayed hypersensitivity ordinarily occurs early during the course of cutaneous leishmaniasis; nevertheless, new lesions can develop for several months. Secondary lesions quickly assume the histologic picture of the early lesions (the isophasic reaction) and usually heal at the same time as the primary lesion or shortly thereafter. Protection appears to be permanent after a primary infection has terminated naturally, although immunosuppressive treatment of patients residing in endemic areas has resulted in reinfection in previously protected individuals. It is not known whether this is due to new infection or to recrudescence of the old disease. If excision is used to terminate the primary infection before spontaneous healing has taken place, protection against reinfection may not occur. Animal experiments indicate that sensitized lymphocytes are widely distributed when the lesion heals. Thereafter, new disease presumably cannot occur, because immune lymphocytes are generally distributed in lymph nodes and spleen. Reinfection is usually manifested by a prolonged delayed hypersensitivity response at the site of the sandfly bite, but ulceration does not follow. Vaccination with virulent strains of the parasite is a common practice for cosmetic protection and to ensure uninterrupted work in highly endemic areas, as in parts of southern USSR and Israel. "Vaccination" against *L major* is a full, lesion-producing infection in a selected skin area. Avirulent, modified, or dead parasites will not induce a protective response. In fact, only the most virulent strains will protect against the same and other strains; less virulent forms protect only against reexposure to the same strain. It appears that specific T cell clones can confer immunity.

Cell-mediated and humoral immune responses may act together to produce protection after initial infection.

2. VISCERAL LEISHMANIASIS

Major Immunologic Features
- Delayed hypersensitivity only after spontaneous recovery or chemotherapy.
- Increased nonspecific immunoglobulin levels.
- Cases polyclonal B cell hypergammaglobulinemia.
- Parasites in cells throughout body produce systemic disease with release of cachectin, characterized by leukopenia and splenomegaly.

General Considerations
The immune response to visceral leishmaniasis (kala-azar)—caused by various subspecies of *Leishmania donovani* (considered separate species by some authors)—is remarkably different from that of cutaneous leishmaniasis, although the parasites are essentially indistinguishable. Massive polyclonal hypergammaglobulinemia with little or no evidence of

cell-mediated immunity is the rule in visceral leishmaniasis. There is no quantitative relationship between the elevated serum immunoglobulin and antiparasite antibodies, which are, moreover, not species-specific. The elevated immunoglobulin diminishes rapidly when treatment begins. Delayed cutaneous hypersensitivity to parasite antigens becomes demonstrable only after spontaneous recovery or treatment, which suggests that cell-mediated mechanisms play a role in the resolution of the infectious process. Under certain circumstances, post-kala-azar dermal "leishmanoid" occurs. Nodules containing many parasites form papules as a result of incomplete or defective cell-mediated immunity, or a persistent allergic reaction to parasite antigens. Most cases have been reported from India, developing 6 months to 2 years after cure of kala-azar. Insufficient data are available at this time to establish exact correlation between delayed hypersensitivity and protection. Serodiagnosis is readily available by indirect hemagglutination, immunofluorescence, complement fixation, direct agglutination, and ELISA.

3. AMERICAN LEISHMANIASIS

Major Immunologic Features
- Positive delayed hypersensitivity occurs.
- There is no specific serodiagnosis.

General Considerations
Cutaneous leishmaniasis of the New World is caused by a number of leishmanial pathogens now divided into 2 species complexes: *Leishmania mexicana* (subdivided into 4 or more subspecies) and *Leishmania braziliensis* (subdivided into 4 or more subspecies). The parasite subspecies are distinguished on the basis of growth characteristics in the vector and in culture, isoenzyme electrophoresis patterns, kinetoplast DNA analysis, lectin-binding specificities, excreted factor serotyping, and monoclonal antibody probes. Geographic factors, hosts, and the character of the disease produced in humans are also important.

The most significant clinical distinction in the *L mexicana* complex is the high frequency of ear cartilage lesions (chiclero ulcer) and rare diffuse cutaneous leishmaniasis. In the *L braziliensis* complex, metastatic lesions develop, usually within 5 years of healing of the initial ulcer, which itself may be large, persistent, and disfiguring. Nasal cartilage and other nasopharyngeal tissues are attacked and destroyed by this subsequent massive ulceration (espundia), which may erode away much of the face and cause death by septic bronchopneumonia, asphyxiation, or starvation. This manifestation of American leishmaniasis is frequently nonresponsive to treatment. Parasites are abundant in the early stages of espundia but subsequently are rare,

whereas persistent infiltration of giant cells, plasma cells, and lymphocytes is characteristic. Delayed and perhaps immediate hypersensitivity and circulating antibody levels are higher in espundia than in cases of the primary lesion alone. The mucocutaneous form is thought to be an allergic or abnormal immunologic manifestation of infection with the type subspecies *L braziliensis*.

A skin test (Montenegro test) is rapidly positive with cutaneous leishmaniasis, particularly the New World forms. Assays for lymphocyte proliferation or production of lymphokines such as gamma interferon are also positive. Dermal response to kala-azar is slower, becoming positive only after cure of the visceral infection. Serodiagnosis of cutaneous leishmaniasis is still unsatisfactory because of low serum antibody levels and, in Latin America, because of cross-reactions with Chagas' disease antibodies.

Greatly increased levels of immunoglobulins, especially of the IgM class, are regularly present in infected humans and animals. The increased immunoglobulin levels do not correlate with protection but, rather, are nonspecific. The Montenegro test is very useful in the diagnosis of cutaneous disease; it is positive in visceral leishmaniasis after treatment. This test is negative in the anergic phase of disease. IFA tests using promastigotes and ELISA are available, but cross-reactivity with antigens of other infections (leprosy, trypanosomiasis, etc.), has been noted in one study with ELISA.

An exciting recent advance in field analysis of species (*L mexicana* versus *L braziliensis* complexes) is the use of nonradioactive species-specific DNA probes. The *Leishmania* species infecting a patient can be determined from a small amount of parasite material in a cutaneous lesion.

TRYPANOSOMIASIS

1. AFRICAN TRYPANOSOMIASIS

Major Immunologic Features
- Increase in nonspecific IgM.
- Succession of parasite populations in bloodstream, each with a different antigenic coating.

General Considerations
Trypanosoma brucei subsp *gambiense,* also called *T gambiense,* is the agent of chronic Gambian or West African sleeping sickness. *Trypanosoma brucei* subsp *rhodesiense,* also called *T rhodesiense,* is the agent of acute Rhodesian or East African sleeping sickness. Both cause human disease, and the Rhodesian form is most responsible for denying vast areas of Africa to human occupation, chiefly in the flybelt regions where the tsetse fly vectors are found. Tsetse-borne trypanosomes (*Trypanosoma brucei* as

well as several other species) infect domestic animals with similar or even greater virulence. The impact of this dual threat—one to humans and the other to domestic animals, especially cattle—has had an enormous effect on human history in Africa. The great herds of wild herbivores, once abundant everywhere, have survived in this region because of their natural tolerance to heavy infections. The trypanosomes multiply extracellularly in successive waves in the human and animal bloodstream but produce very little disease in spite of their numbers. Only when the parasites enter the central nervous system does the ravaging disease sleeping sickness develop. It is this pathologic phase of an otherwise harmless chronic or recurrent infection to which humans and domestic animals succumb and which most native antelope and other herbivores resist.

Greatly increased levels of immunoglobulins, especially of the IgM class, are regularly present in infected humans and animals. The increased immunoglobulin levels, which do not correlate positively with protection, may result from B cell stimulants produced by the trypanosomes themselves or by the increased IgG production by helper T cells, which act nonspecifically to increase immunoglobulin levels. A large proportion of the immunoglobulin in infected hosts is nonspecific in nature.

Although trypanosomes are continually exposed to the host immune system in the bloodstream, they evade the host's defenses. The first hint of how this is accomplished was noted in 1910, when the periodicity of fever in patients with trypanosomiasis was correlated with a sharp rise and fall in the number of trypanosomes found in the blood. More recently, it was discovered that when individual organisms are cloned in culture, each clone displays a unique antigenic surface protein. When organisms first enter the host (Fig 53–2), the host immune system generates antibodies against the predominant surface antigen (variable surface glycoprotein [VSG]). Antibodies can kill over 90% of the original infecting trypanosome population. The reason not all of the trypanosomes are killed is that some have switched on a different VSG antigen not recognized by the initial immune response. This switch occurs spontaneously and can be detected in immune-deficient mice. It is therefore not dependent upon the host immune response. The switch occurs very rapidly, so that by 5 days into an infection, parasites with more than one antigen type can be detected. By 6 days, as few as 15% of the trypanosomes may still have the initial surface VSG. This switching from one VSG to another explains the waves of parasitemia and periodicity of the fever characteristic of trypanosomiasis. The potential VSG repertoire is not known, although parasites derived from a single parent trypanosome have been found with more than 100 distinct VSGs.

What is the mechanism by which the trypanosome can so quickly switch its surface coat? Recombinant DNA techniques have been used to unravel part of the mystery.

One copy of the VSG gene is located on a specific trypanosome chromosome (Fig 53–3). If that VSG is to be expressed, a copy is made of the gene, and it is translocated to another chromosome close to the telomere. In this new location—and only in the new location—it is transcribed into messenger RNA to which a 35-nucleotide sequence is added. This small

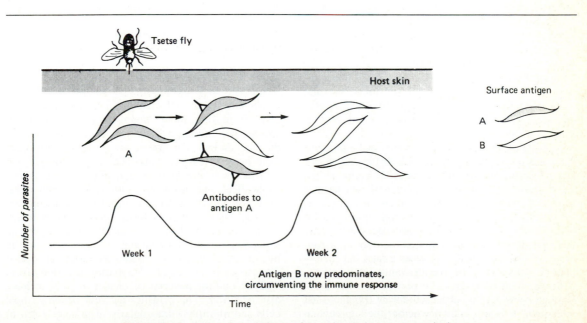

Figure 53–2. Antigenic variation and parasitemia in trypanosomiasis.

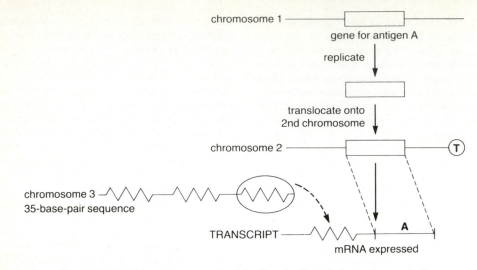

Figure 53–3. Molecular mechanism of antigenic diversity in trypanosomiasis.

35-nucleotide sequence has been transcribed from yet another site where many of these small sequences are found closely linked to each other. Most trypanosome proteins have this small sequence at the beginning of their message. Therefore, it is assumed that it is necessary for expression of the messenger RNA. However, some of the VSGs come from genes that are already near the telomere and therefore do not translocate before expression. Although the mechanism of "gene jumping" and subsequent expression has been elucidated, the exact mechanism by which one VSG is switched to another is still unclear. Understanding of this switching mechanism might provide a means of interrupting the ability of trypanosomes to change their antigenic disguises.

Serodiagnosis of trypanosomiasis is possible by using indirect immunofluorescence, ELISA, indirect hemagglutination, direct agglutination, gel precipitation for IgM titration, and gel precipitation using trypanosomal antigen. However, none of these methods are yet suitable for field studies or surveys in Africa.

Specific antibodies to trypanosomes can either lyse the parasites or clump them. Clumping allows for more efficient removal of the parasites by the reticuloendothelial system. It is controversial whether humans or domestic animals living in endemic areas develop resistance to infection, although epidemiologic observations suggest that resistance does arise. The fact that there are healthy human carriers of *T rhodesiense*—which usually produces a fatal infection—implies that some protective mechanism must exist.

Suppression of immune responses to other unrelated antigens may be observed during trypanosomal infections. It is not known whether the suppression results from exhaustion of B cells, the presence of suppressor T cells, a lack of helper T cells, or the availability of fewer T cells to interact with new antigens.

The multiplicity of antigenic variants observed during field studies in bovines makes vaccination an unlikely solution to trypanosomiasis unless common antigens can be found.

2. AMERICAN TRYPANOSOMIASIS

Major Immunologic Features
- Specific antibody not necessarily indicative of active infection.
- Delayed hypersensitivity present.
- No antigenic variation.

General Considerations

An estimated 24 million people in Central and South America are infected with *Trypanosoma cruzi*, and 50 million more are at risk. The resulting chronic debilitating affliction, Chagas' disease, has no cure and is a major factor in premature death from heart disease in Latin America—especially in rural areas where housing and nutrition are inadequate. The disease is transmitted to humans when fecal contamination from infected bloodsucking triatomine bugs occurs in fresh bites, mucous membranes, or abraded skin, frequently from nighttime scratching that rubs the vector's liquid feces into the bite or causes it to be taken into the mouth or rubbed into the eyes. Accidental laboratory infections from sprayed culture material or chance injections have also occurred. The parasites actively penetrate host cells and multiply intracellularly. The acute form of the disease is characterized by myocardiopathy, lymphadenopathy, hepatosplenomegaly, parasitemia, fever, and malaise. Colonies of intracellular amastigotes develop in striated muscles, smooth muscles, and the reticuloendothelial system. The disease is often fatal in infants or children, but in adults a chronic form usually follows the initial infection, sometimes after a considerable interval, producing a disease characterized by cardiac enlargement with megacolon, megaesophagus, and degeneration of the peripheral and central nervous systems; this is found in parts of Brazil. In chronic disease, nests of intracellular parasites can be found, but parasitemia accompanied by fever is infrequent.

Serologic tests include complement fixation (still the test of choice), latex agglutination (for rapid screening), indirect hemagglutination (for epidemiologic studies using samples collected on filter paper, which is also suitable for ELISA), and the direct agglutination test (sensitive for congenital infection). All have some cross-reactions, especially with *Leishmania*. Antibody may persist after infection and therefore does not indicate active disease. High titers of antibody do not appear to limit the infection in humans; however, complement-dependent lysis of the parasites can be demonstrated in vitro with sera from experimentally infected hosts. This lysis may be an important mechanism for parasite control in vivo. However, lytic antibody does not afford complete protection against reinfection, since passive transfer of hyperimmune serum is not always effective. The lytic action of antibody may need cooperation with cells such as macrophages to eliminate or lower the parasite burden. Animals can be protected against virulent strains of the organism by infection with avirulent or partially virulent strains or by passive transfer of sensitized lymphocytes. Acquired resistance to virulent strains is probably the result of previous inapparent infection with strains of low virulence.

Activated macrophages can be demonstrated in *T cruzi* animal infections and may play the major role in protection against this infection. Delayed hypersensitivity, lymphocyte activation, and MIF production can be documented during infection, but the role of cell-mediated immunity has not been fully elucidated. Cardiac damage may be the result of an immune response to cross-reacting antigens of *T cruzi* and rabbit cardiac muscle, since *T cruzi*-sensitized lymphocytes are cytotoxic for unparasitized cardiac muscle cells in vitro as well as for parasitized cells. Antibody may also participate in immune destruction of normal cells. Attempts to vaccinate against disease might do more harm than good if such sensitized lymphocytes against shared antigens should develop.

THE IMMUNE RESPONSE TO HELMINTHS

Multicellular parasites, by reason of their size, more complex tissue and organ structure, and varied and active metabolism, induce very complex host responses. Further complicating the picture is the fact that several forms of the parasite may be present in the host, each eliciting a unique immune response.

The primary antigens of helminths may often be metabolic by-products, enzymes, or other secretory products. For example, the eggs of *Schistosoma mansoni* have been shown to secrete unique antigens that induce granuloma formation; the various stages of developing nematodes have stage-specific antigens, often molting fluids, to which the host responds in various ways; and the granules in the stichocytes, special cells located in the "neck" of *Trichuris trichiura,* elicit specific antibody.

Trematodes, cestodes, and nematodes, probably all share common antigens. The 2 most frequent responses to helminths—eosinophilia and reaginic antibody (IgE)—are both T cell-dependent. Moreover, certain helminths have been shown to potentiate the immune response to other antigens, perhaps by common metabolic by-products acting as nonspecific adjuvants. In addition, helminthic infection often induces strong and sometimes self-destructive immunopathologic reactions, such as the excessive granulomatous response to schistosome eggs caught in host tissues.

TREMATODES

Trematodes are important pathogens of humans and domestic animals. Fascioliasis debilitates and kills domestic animals in large numbers and renders the livers unfit for human consumption. Schistosomiasis is a major disease of humans. The lung flukes of the genus *Paragonimus* cause central nervous system complications in humans if they encyst in the brain. In the lung, considerable mechanical damage results. *Clonorchis sinensis,* the fish-borne Chinese liver fluke, causes much morbidity both in the Orient and among recent emigrants from endemic areas, producing infection that may last the lifetime of the host.

1. SCHISTOSOMIASIS

Major Immunologic Features
■ Response to invading worms is both humoral (IgE, IgM, IgG) and cellular (eosinophils, macrophages).

- A serum sickness-like acute disease may develop (Katayama fever).
- Chronic disease occurs owing to granulomatous reaction to eggs with subsequent fibrosis.
- Developing larvae and adult worms evade immune response by camouflaging their surface with host antigens.

General Considerations

Schistosomiasis in humans is caused by *Schistosoma mansoni, Schistosoma japonicum, Schistosoma haematobium,* and *Schistosoma mekongi.* The advent of new high dams in many areas of the world, especially Africa, has increased the prevalence of schistosomiasis, because the additional irrigation made possible by the dams has vastly enlarged the habitat of the freshwater snails that serve as intermediate hosts to the worms. The life cycle of this parasite depends upon skin penetration of the definitive host by infective larvae produced in large numbers in the snail. Because attempts to reduce snail populations have largely failed, infection has become rampant in these areas. *S mansoni,* now widespread in Africa and the Middle East, has also spread extensively in South America. *S haematobium* is found in all watered areas of Africa and the Arabian peninsula. *S japonicum* is found in the Yangtze River watershed in China, where it has been subjected to a vast control effort but is still common in Szechwan province and may be returning to the main river valley. It is also common in the central Philippines. A purely animal-infecting (zoophilic) form is found in Taiwan. *S mekongi,* a newly described species similar to *S japonicum,* causes human disease in Thailand, Laos, and Cambodia, with a scattering of cases in Malaysia, recently described as *S malaysiensis.* There is also a focus of *S japonicum* in Sulawesi (Celebes) that may prove to be a distinct species.

In brief, the life cycle of the schistosomes that infect humans is as follows: Infected humans and animals excrete eggs that hatch in water, releasing miracidia; these actively penetrate snails in which several generations of multiplying larvae (sporocysts) develop. These in turn produce great numbers of fork-tailed cercariae, the stage infective for humans, which leave the host snail at the rate of 300–3000 per day. The cercariae penetrate the skin of the definitive host, leaving the tail outside, and enter the bloodstream as minute motile immature schistosomula, which migrate in 3–8 days to the lungs and eventually to the liver. Further development and adult worm pairing take place about 5 weeks after skin penetration. The paired mature schistosomes then migrate against the venous flow into the mesenteric or vesical venules, where eggs are deposited. The embryo (miracidium) within the egg secretes proteases to facilitate passage through the blood vessel and adjacent tissue into the lumen of the intestine (or bladder in the case of *S haematobium*). Egg movement is probably aided by peristalsis of the intestine or contractions of the bladder.

Unfortunately, not all the eggs reach the lumen of the intestine or bladder. Some become trapped in the submucosa, and others do not leave the bloodstream but instead are carried with the portal venous flow to the liver, or by collateral circulation to other organs of the body. Because of their size, eggs reaching the liver become trapped in the portal venules and do not enter into the sinusoids. When eggs are trapped in the liver, the wall of the intestine, or the bladder, they elicit a granulomatous inflammation that is the hallmark of the chronic stage of schistosomiasis. An early infiltrate of neutrophils and lymphocytes may be seen around eggs, but distinctive granulomas containing a core of macrophages and eosinophils, surrounded by a cuff of lymphocytes, appear shortly. The early stages of inflammation may be seen by 6 weeks, but granulomas reach their maximal cellularity within 9–12 weeks. Later, an increasing number of fibroblasts can be seen in association with the granulomas, and the cellular lesion becomes slowly replaced by collagen. In the liver, older lesions become periportal scars. Since numerous eggs are deposited, a circumferential periportal fibrosis called Symmer's clay pipestem fibrosis develops. This fibrosis blocks normal blood flow from the portal venous system to the sinusoids, resulting in portal hypertension and its complications.

The factors that initiate granuloma formation are soluble proteins secreted through pores in the eggshell by the embryonic miracidium. These soluble egg products, some of which have been purified, are used in one serodiagnostic test for schistosomiasis. As might be expected from the complex group of cells comprising the granuloma, the mechanisms of granuloma formation, modulation, and subsequent fibrosis are complex. Interleukins and lymphokines have been identified, as well as factors from the egg itself that may be both chemotactic and mitogenic for fibroblasts. Nevertheless, the importance of cellular immunity in granuloma formation has been underscored by the observation that both the granulomatous reaction to schistosome eggs and subsequent periportial fibrosis are absent or significantly diminished in thymic-deficient ("nude") mice and in mice with severe combined immunodeficiency (SCID).

While the immune response to schistosome eggs is the central immunopathologic mechanism in chronic schistosomiasis, it is not the only immune response of importance in schistosome infection. In some previously infected individuals, invading cercariae may elicit a dermatitis with features of both immediate and delayed hypersensitivity. This is similar to the "swimmers' itch" produced by nonhuman schistosomes. Some schistosome species may produce an acute form of schistosomiasis (Katayama fever) characterized by fever, eosinophilia, lymphadenopathy, diarrhea, splenomegaly, and urticaria. This appears to be an anaphylactic (IgE) or serum sickness (IgG) reaction. In fact, cases of glomerulonephritis secondary to schistosome antigen-antibody complexes have been reported.

An important unresolved question is whether protective immunity to schistosomiasis develops in humans after infection. Studies in Kenya and Gambia have shown that schistosome-infected individuals in an endemic area who had been treated with antischistosome drugs showed an age-dependent resistance to reinfection. Children were much more easily reinfected than were adults, suggesting that true human immunity can be acquired with age. However, these conclusions remain controversial because the studies were retrospective and because it is difficult in field studies to control for important factors such as the amount of water contact. Nevertheless, identification of "resistant" groups of children may help to identify important parasite antigens. Augmentation of the response to these antigens would be one rational approach to vaccine development.

The question of immunity to reinfection has been studied intensively in animal models. Two models in particular have been used. In the first of these, called the **concomitant immunity model,** mice are infected with 20–30 normal *S mansoni* cercariae 6 weeks prior to challenge. In the second, called the **attenuated vaccine model,** mice are immunized by 400–500 cercariae attenuated by 20–50 kilorads of gamma radiation 2 weeks before challenge.

By comparing normal with various immune-deficient mouse strains, the cellular and antibody requirements of vaccine immunity have been investigated. Vaccinated mice with T lymphocyte deficiencies, as well as mice immunosuppressed from birth, have a sharply diminished resistance to a challenge infection. On the other hand, mice deficient in complement, mast cells, natural killer (NK) lymphocytes, and IgE show no difference in resistance compared with normal controls. Macrophages appear to be key effector cells in the resistance of vaccinated mice to challenge infection.

The exact site of killing of schistosomula in vaccinated mice remains controversial. Some evidence exists for immune killing in the skin, while other studies indicate that most killing occurs in the lungs.

Immunodiagnosis of schistosome infection in the absence of egg excretion by the host can be accomplished in various ways, both humoral and cellular. Stage-specific humoral responses can be used to produce circumoval precipitation, schistosomule growth inhibition or death; and complement fixation, hemagglutination, and various precipitation reactions. None of these reactions can be positively correlated with protection. Immediate and delayed cutaneous hypersensitivity develop in most individuals during the course of the disease, although the specificity of these reactions is often suspect, owing to antigens that cross-react with those of other worms. However, the purification of novel antigenic fractions and sensitive ELISA or radioimmunoassays may improve the specificity of these responses.

Major efforts are now under way to develop a nonliving vaccine for schistosomiasis. This goal is being approached in a variety of ways. Some laboratories are identifying antigens recognized by serum from patients infected with schistosomes and then attempting to clone the genes coding for these antigens. This would allow unlimited production of polypeptide antigen for augmentation of the immune response. Another approach involves identifying groups of individuals in endemic areas who appear to show heightened resistance to the disease. Antigens unique to these groups are then searched for and characterized. A third approach involves purification of proteins critical for the metabolism and development of the parasite within the host and testing purified protein for immunogenicity. All of these studies are still very early but represent one of our best hopes for control of the disease.

2. CERCARIAL DERMATITIS (Swimmers' Itch)

The invasion of a previously sensitized host by the cercariae of schistosomes, particularly those of avian origin, can cause severe 2-stage reactions in the skin. The first stage begins within minutes of contact and consists of a wheal-and-flare reaction. The second stage becomes evident 16–24 hours after contact, with development of papules which are essentially delayed-hypersensitivity reactions. These reactions have been shown to be very specific in that persons infected with *S mansoni* did not react to cercariae of an avian schistosome known to cause violent reactions in persons with swimmers' itch.

CESTODES

There are 2 types of immune response to cestodes. One is directed against the intestinal lumen-dwelling adult tapeworms such as *Diphyllobothrium latum* and *Taenia saginata,* which have restricted, nonhumoral immunogenic contact. The response is chiefly cell-mediated, is induced primarily by the scolex, affects growth and strobilation of challenge worms, and varies considerably with the host species. The other is directed against migratory tissue-encysting larval tapeworms such as *Hymenolepis nana* (in its intravillous larval phase), *Echinococcus granulosus* (hydatid cyst), and *Taenia solium* (cysticercosis), which have intimate and continuous tissue contact and induce a strong parenteral host response detectable as serum antibody and strongly protective against reinfection. Serodiagnostic tests are available only for the larval tissue cestode parasites, and humoral responses that protect the challenged host have only recently been described for this form of cestode parasitism. ELISA for serodiagnosis of cysticercosis—with some cross-reactivity—has been developed.

1. ECHINOCOCCOSIS

Major Immunologic Features
- IgE is elevated.
- Anaphylaxis occurs owing to ruptured cyst fluids.
- Casoni skin test is of questionable use.
- Diagnostic antibody is present.

General Considerations

The most serious human cestode infection is that caused by *Echinococcus.* These tiny tapeworms do not produce pathologic lesions in the definitive host, the dog, but severe complications occur when their eggs are ingested by humans and other animals. The larval form of the tapeworm hatches from the egg in the intestine of the intermediate host, eg, humans, and then claws its way through the intestinal mucosa and is transported through the lymphatic and blood vessels to sites in which it grows to enormous proportions, although it is enclosed by a heavy cyst wall laid down by both the host and the parasite. In humans, *Echinococcus* normally forms fluid-filled cysts in the liver, but these can also occur in the lungs, brain, kidneys, and other parts of the body. Hydatid cysts are highly immunogenic and result in production of high titers of IgE and other immunoglobulins. If a cyst is ruptured, anaphylactic response to the cyst fluid can cause death. Little or no protection seems to be elicited by this highly immunogenic cestode, because the hydatid cysts remain alive for years and, in animals, can be shown to increase in number as the host ages. Humans are usually a dead-end host, for the cysts must be eaten by a canid to become sexually mature. There is some evidence that complement-mediated lysis of protoscoleces (the numerous future scoleces in hydatid fluid or "hydatid sand") might be protective in the infected human or other intermediate host.

The Casoni skin test indicates past or present echinococcosis. It consists of intradermal injection of hydatid cyst fluid, resulting in both immediate and delayed hypersensitivity. The specificity of this test is in doubt because of cross-reactions with other helminths. Heating the cyst fluid slightly increases the specificity of the test. Serodiagnosis can be made by hemagglutination, complement fixation, and flocculation tests, ELISA, and radioimmunoassay, using serum from the patient and specially fractionated antigenic components made from cyst fluid. These tests are not species-specific.

NEMATODES

Nematodes are the commonest, most varied, and most widely distributed helminths infecting humans. As with other parasites, immunogenicity is a reflection of the degree and duration of parasite contact with the host's tissues. Even with the intestinal lumen dwellers such as *Ascaris,* there is a migratory larval phase in which such contact is made—in most cases, in the pulmonary capillaries and alveolar spaces. The hookworms of humans (*Ancylostoma duodenale* and *Necator americanus*) also undergo a migration, except that the infective larvae enter via the skin or buccal mucosa rather than as hatchlings in the small bowel. *Strongyloides stercoralis,* the small intestinal roundworm of humans, undergoes a similar hookwormlike migration (as well as a stage of internal autoreinfection or reinvasion via the mucosa of the large intestine).

The immature stages are particularly immunogenic, probably because of their high production of antigens from secretory glands and of enzymes or other products from these metabolically active stages. Commercially prepared vaccines are available only for nematodes, and all are living larval worms, irradiated to arrest their development but not their immunogenicity. These are the cattle and sheep lungworms *Dictyocaulus viviparus* and *Dictyocaulus filaria* and the dog hookworm *Ancylostoma caninum.* Another important group of human parasites are the filariae (chiefly *Wuchereria bancrofti, Brugia malayi, Loa loa, Onchocerca volvulus,* and the related guinea worm, *Dracunculus medinensis*). Diagnosis of these infections is often difficult, in part because of the presence of common antigens that preclude highly specific immunologic tests. Hypersensitivity reactions may occur after drug treatment (such as with diethylcarbamizine for *Onchocerca*) where large numbers of dead or dying microfilariae produce severe skin reactions and edema or (with *Loa*) where dead adult worms may induce severe central nervous system reactions.

1. TRICHINOSIS

Major Immunologic Features
- Skin tests for immediate and delayed hypersensitivity are positive.
- Diagnostic antibody is present.

General Considerations

Trichinosis is acquired by ingestion of the infective larvae of *Trichinella spiralis* in uncooked or partially cooked meat. Pork is the primary source of infection in humans. The larvae are released from their cysts in the meat during digestion and rapidly develop into adults in the mucosa of the host's small intestine. After copulation in the lumen, the males die and the females return to the intestinal mucosa, where for about 5–6 weeks they produce 1000–1500 larvae per female, which migrate through the lymphatic system to the bloodstream. These larvae travel in the blood to all parts of the body and develop in voluntary muscles, especially in the diaphragm, tongue, masticatory and intercostal muscles, larynx, and the eye. Within the sarcolemma of striated muscle fibers, the larvae coil up into cysts whose outer walls are rapidly laid down by host histiocytes. Larvae may remain viable and infective for as long as 24 years, even though the cysts calcify. The encysted larvae apparently do not yield protection. The migrating larvae and adult forms of the parasite excrete antigens that appear to be responsible for protection from subsequent challenge infections. An important expression of host resistance is active expulsion of developing or adult worms from the gut of a parasitized host—the so-called self-cure phenomenon. This occurs when a new infection initiates a host response, resulting in elimination of the old one—the opposite of concomitant immunity.

The expulsion of *T spiralis* in humans appears to follow the mechanism proposed by Ogilvie and coworkers for the *Nippostrongylus brasiliensis* rodent hookworm. A 2-step mechanism is proposed: antibody-induced metabolic damage that blocks feeding by the worms followed by worm expulsion by activated lymphocytes. Active infection initiates a far stronger response than is possible when either lymph node cells or serum is passively transferred. Both antibodies and cells are probably required for full expression of intestinal resistance, and the effect is synergistic rather than additive.

Trichinella infection sometimes presents characteristic clinical symptoms such as edema of the eyelids and face but often presents less specific clinical signs such as eosinophilia, which can be suggestive of several other parasitic infections. Specific immunodiagnostic tests may thus be of great importance. The bentonite flocculation test for human trichinosis is of value because of its high degree of specificity. A skin test (Bachman intradermal test) produces both immediate and delayed responses.

In humans, infection with *Trichinella* initially elicits IgM antibody followed by an IgG response. IgA antibody has been reported, which is not surprising, because the female worms are in the intestinal mucosa, though the locally produced protective gut antibodies probably are IgG1 rather than IgA or IgM. This antibody reaction against the feeding worms is complement-independent and, as noted, precedes the rapid expulsion of the antibody-damaged worms by T lymphocytes.

Although *Trichinella* is extremely immunogenic in its hosts, it can also exert an immunosuppressive action. Certain viral infections are more severe during infection with this parasite, and skin grafts show delayed rejection. On the other hand, cellular immu-

nity to BCG seems to be potentiated when *T spiralis* is present, and *T spiralis*-infected mice are less susceptible to *Listeria* infections.

2. ASCARIASIS

Major Immunologic Features
- Specific antibody detectable.
- Elevated IgE.

General Considerations

Ascaris, the giant roundworm of humans, is a lumen-dwelling parasite as an adult and causes little inconvenience to the host except in the heaviest infections, though even single adult worms may produce mechanical damage by entering the bile or pancreatic ducts or penetrating a weakened gut wall. For example, worm penetration through an amebiasis intestinal lesion produces peritonitis. Ingestion of eggs results in larvae that migrate through the intestinal wall to eventually reach the lung via the bloodstream. In a previously infected host, hypersensitivity reactions in the lung resulting from high levels of IgE can cause serious pneumonitis. Acute hypersensitivity to *Ascaris* antigens often develops in laboratory workers and makes it virtually impossible for them to continue working with the nematode.

Cases of sudden death in Nigeria have been ascribed to *Ascaris*-induced anaphylactic shock, part of what has been termed ''a helminth anaphylactic syndrome'' heretofore rarely diagnosed or recognized. Death probably resulted from release of a mast cell degranulator by the worms, since degranulated mast cells were found throughout the body tissues in these children, or from a reagin-*Ascaris* allergen interaction at the mast cell surface. Allergy to ascariasis may underlie many of the symptoms of *Ascaris* infection, including abdominal pain.

Antibodies to *Ascaris* are of no diagnostic or protective value, although they are formed during infection; however, hemagglutination tests can be of epidemiologic value.

3. TOXOCARA INFECTIONS

Toxocara canis, the dog ascarid, is now known to infect small children who ingest its eggs in dirt. *Toxocara* eggs produce a population of migrating larvae that are immobilized in the tissues of humans and consequently never produce worms in the intestinal tract. Visceral larva migrans is characterized by high peripheral eosinophilia and chronic granulomatous lesions associated with the migrating larvae; such larvae in the eyes of infected children have been confused with retinoblastoma and diagnosed only after enucleation of the affected eyeball. Immunodiagnostic tests for visceral larva migrans have therefore been eagerly sought. Initially, lack of specificity for *T canis* was a great problem, but specific immunodiagnostic methods have been developed that should allow prompt diagnosis, and a sensitive ELISA for antibody to this parasite is in common use in the USA. Visceral larva migrans can also be caused by larvae of other nematodes such as the common ascarids of cats (*Toxocara mystax, Toxascaris leonina*)

and also some members of the genus *Capillaria*, which migrate in human tissue but do not develop further. Dog and cat hookworms (*Ancylostoma brasiliense, Ancylostoma caninum, Ancylostoma ceylonicum*) produce a similar "lost larva" condition in which skin-invading larvae from pet-contaminated sandy soil tunnel into the skin, where they produce serpiginous, pruritic, tracklike lesions, a condition called **cutaneous larva migrans.**

REFERENCES

General

Cohen S, Warren KS (editors): *Immunology of Parasitic Infections*. Blackwell, 1982.

Ellner JJ, Mahmoud AF: Phagocytes and worms: David and Goliath revisited. *Rev Infect Dis* 1982;**4**:698.

Kagan IG, Maddison SE: Immunology of parasites: General aspects. Pages 315–325, in: *Immunology of Human Infection,* Part 2, *Viruses and Parasites,* of: *Immunodiagnosis and Prevention of Infectious Diseases.* Nahmias AJ, O'Reilly RH (editors). Plenum, 1982.

Kay AB et al: Leukocyte activation initiated by IgE-dependent mechanisms in relation to helminthic parasitic disease and clinical models of asthma. *Int Arch Allergy Appl Immunol* 1985;**77**:69.

Klesius PH: Immunopotentiation against internal parasites. *Vet Parasitol* 1982;**10**:239.

Lobel HO, Kagan IG: Seroepidemiology of parasitic diseases. *Annu Rev Microbiol* 1978;**32**:329.

Mauel J: In vitro induction of intracellular killing of parasitic protozoa by macrophages. *Immunobiology* 1982; **161**:392.

Mitchell GF et al: Examination of strategies for vaccination against parasitic infection or disease using mouse models. Pages 323–328 in: *Contemporary Topics in Immunobiology,* Vol 12. Marchalonis JJ (editor). Plenum, 1984.

Nussenzweig R: Parasitic disease as a cause of immunosuppression. *N Engl J Med* 1982;**306**:423.

Soulsby EJL (editor): *Immune Responses in Parasitic Infections: Immunology, Immunopathology, and Immunoprophylaxis.* Vol 1: *Nematodes.* Vol 2: *Trematodes and Cestodes.* Vol 3: *Protozoa.* Vol 4: *Protozoa, Arthropods, and Invertebrates.* CRC Press, 1987.

Voller A, De Savigny D: Diagnostic serology of tropical parasitic diseases. *J Immunol Methods* 1981;**46**:1.

Wakelin D: Immunity to parasites. In: *How Animals Control Parasitic Infection.* Arnold, 1984.

Wakelin D: Genetic control of immunity to helminth infections. *Parasitol Today* 1985;**1**:17.

Serodiagnostic Tests

Desowitz RS: *Ova and Parasites. Medical Parasitology for the Laboratory Technologist.* Harper & Row, 1980.

Kagan IG, Norman LG: Immune response to infection: parasitic. in: *CRC Handbook Series in Clinical Laboratory Science.* Section F. Vol 1, Part 2. Seligson D (editor). CRC Press, 1979.

Reference and Disease Surveillance. Center for Infectious Diseases, CDC, 1985.

Sun, T: *Pathology and Clinical Features of Parasitic Diseases.* Masson Monograph in Diagnostic Pathology. Vol 5. Masson, 1982.

Amebiasis

Denis M, Chadee K: Immunopathology of *Entamoeba histolytica* infections. *Parasitol Today* 1988;**4**:247.

Patterson M et al: Serological testing for amoebiasis. *Gasteroenterology* 1980;**78**:136.

Trissl D: Immunology of *Entamoeba histolytica* in human and animal hosts. *Rev Infect Dis* 1982;**4**:1154.

Cestodiases

Chemtal AK et al: Evaluation of five immunodiagnostic techniques in *Echinococcus* patients. *Bull WHO* 1981; **59**:767.

Diwan AR et al: Enzyme-linked immunosorbent assay (ELISA) for the detection of antibody to cysticerci of *Taenia solium. Am J Trop Med Hyg* 1982;**31**:364.

Grogl M et al: Antigen-antibody analyses in neurocysticercosis. *J Parasitol* 1985;**71**:433.

Hopkins CA, Barr IF: The source of antigen in an adult tapeworm. *Int J Parasitol* 1982;**12**:327.

Schantz PM, Kagan IG: Echinococcosis (hydatidosis). Chap 8, pp 104–129 in: *Immunological Investigation of Tropical Parasitic Diseases.* Houba V (editor). Churchill Livingstone, 1980.

Williams JF: Recent advances in the immunology of cestode infections. *J Parasitol* 1979;**65**:337.

Leishmaniasis

Louis JA et al: The in vitro generation and functional analysis of murine T cell populations and clones specific for a protozoan parasite, *Leishmania tropica. Immunol Rev* 1982;**61**:215.

Reed SG: Immunology of *Leishmania* infections. Pages 291–314 in: *Parasitic Diseases: The Immunology,* Vol 1. Dekker, 1981.

Scott P, Sacks D, Sher A: Resistance to macrophage-mediated killing as a factor influencing the pathogenesis of chronic cutaneous leishmaniasis. *J Immunol* 1983; **131**:966.

Malaria

Jensen JB et al: Induction of crisis forms in cultured *Plasmodium falciparum* with human immune serum from Sudan. *Science* 1982;**216**:1230.

Kreier JP (editor): *Immunology and Immunization.* Vol 3. Academic Press, 1980.

Miller LH et al: The resistance factor to *Plasmodium vivax* in blacks: The Duffy-blood-group genotype, *FyFy. N Engl J Med* 1976;**295**:302.

Nussenzweig RJ, Nussenzweig V: Development of sporozoite vaccines. *Philos Trans R Soc Lond [Biol]* 1984;**307**:117.

WHO Scientific Working Group on the Immunology of Malaria: Development of malaria vaccines: Memorandum from a USAID/WHO meeting. *Bull WHO* 1983;**61**:81.

Zavala F et al: Rationale for development of a synthetic vaccine against *Plasmodium falciparum* malaria. *Science* 1985;**228**:1436.

Nematodiases

Denham DA: Vaccination against filarial worms using radiation-attenuated vaccines. *Int J Nucl Med Biol* 1980;**7**:105.

DesMoutis I et al: *Onchocerca volvulus:* Detection of circulating antigen by monoclonal antibodies in human onchocerciasis. *Am J Trop Med Hyg* 1983;**32**:533.

Gamble HR: *Trichinella spiralis:* Immunization of mice using monoclonal antibody affinity-isolated antigens. *Exp Parasitol* 1985;**59**:398.

Hayashi Y et al: Vaccination of BALB/c mice against *Brugia malayi* and *B pahangi* with larvae attenuated by gamma irradiation. *Jpn J Exp Med* 1984;**54**:177.

Ogilvie BM et al: *Nippostrongylus brasiliensis* infection in rats: The cellular requirement for worm expulsion. *Immunology* 1977;**32**:521.

Pneumocystiasis

Furuta T et al: Detection of antibodies in *Pneumocystis carinii* by enzyme-linked immunosorbent assay in experimentally infected mice. *J Parasitol* 1985;**71**:522.

Schistosomiasis

Butterworth AE et al: Studies on the mechanism of immunity in human schistosomiasis. *Immunol Rev* 1982;**61**:5.

Capron A et al: Mechanisms of immunity to schistosomes and their regulation. *Immunol Rev* 1982;**61**:41.

Damian RT et al: *Schistosoma mansoni:* Parasitology and immunology of baboons vaccinated with irradiated cryopreserved schistosomula. *Int J Parasitol* 1985;**15**:333.

Deelder AM, Kornelis D: Immunodiagnosis of recently acquired *Schistosoma mansoni* infection: A comparison of various immunological techniques. *Trop Geogr Med* 1981;**33**:36.

Harn DA et al: Anti-egg monoclonal antibodies protect against cercarial challenge in vivo. *J Exp Med* 1984;**159**:1371.

McLaren DJ: The role of eosinophils in tropical disease. *Semin Hematol* 1982;**19**:100.

Mitchell GF et al: Analysis of infection characteristics and antiparasite immune responses in resistant compared with susceptible hosts. *Immunol Rev* 1982; **61**:137.

Nogueira-Machado JA et al: *Schistosoma mansoni:* Cell-mediated immunity evaluated by antigen-induced leukocyte adherence inhibition assay. *Immunol Lett* 1985;**9**:39.

Phillips SM, Colley DG: Immunologic aspects of host responses to schistosomiasis: Resistance, immunopathology, and eosinophil involvement. *Prog Allergy* 1978;**24**:49.

Sher FA et al: Mechanisms of protective immunity against *Schistosoma mansoni* infection in mice vaccinated with irradiated cercariae. 6. Influence of the major histocompatibility complex. *Parasite Immunol* 1984;**6**:319.

Taylor DW et al: Genetic engineering and a schistosome vaccine. *Vet Parasitol* 1984;**14**:285.

Von Lichtenberg F: Conference on contended issues of immunity to schistosomes. *Am J Trop Med Hyg* 1985;**34**:78.

Warren KS: Immunology. In: *Schistosomiasis: Epidemiology, Treatment, Control.* Jordan P, Webbe G (editors). Pitman, 1982.

Wyler DJ et al: Fibroblast stimulation in schistosomiasis. 5. Egg granuloma macrophages spontaneously secrete a fibroblast-stimulating factor. *J Immunol* 1984;**132**:3142.

Trematodiases

Feldheim W, Knobloch J: Serodiagnosis of *Opisthorchis viverrini* by an enzyme immuno-assay. *Trop Med Parasitol* 1982;**33**:8.

Levine DM et al: Comparison of counterelectrophoresis, the enzyme-linked immunosorbent assay, and Kato fecal examination for the diagnosis of fascioliasis in infected mice and rabbits. *Am J Trop Med Hyg* 1981;**29**:602.

Trypanosomiasis

Araujo FG et al: Monoclonal antibodies to stages of *Trypanosoma cruzi:* Characterization and use for antigen detection. *Infect Immun* 1982;**37**:344.

Donelson JE, Turner MJ: How the trypanosome changes its coat. *Sci Am* (Feb) 1985;**252**:44.

Esser KL, Schornblecher MJ: Expression of two variant surface glycoproteins on individual African trypanosomes during antigen switching. *Science* 1985; **229**:290.

Hudson L: Immunobiology of *Trypanosoma cruzi* infection and Chagas' disease. *Trans R Soc Trop Med Hyg* 1981;**75**:493.

Kagan IG: American trypanosomiasis (Chagas' disease). Pages 49–64 in: *Immunological Investigation of Tropical Parasitic Diseases.* Houba V (editor). Churchill Livingstone, 1980.

Nilsson L-A, Voller A: A comparison of thin layer immunoassay (TIA) and enzyme-linked immunosorbent assay (ELISA) for the detection of antibodies to *Trypanosoma cruzi. Trans R Soc Trop Med Hyg* 1982;**76**:95.

Parsons M et al: Antigenic variation in African trypanosomes: DNA rearrangements program immune evasion. *Immunol Today* 1984;**5**:43.

Snary D: Cell surface glycoproteins of *Trypanosoma cruzi:* Protective immunity in mice and antibody levels in human chagasic sera. *Trans R Soc Trop Med Hyg* 1983;**77**:126.

54

Spirochetal Diseases

Charles S. Pavia, PhD, & David J. Drutz, MD

Spirochetes are a highly specialized group of motile gram-negative bacteria, with a slender and tightly helically coiled structure. They range from 0.1 to 0.5 μm in width and from 10 to 50 μm in length. One of the unique features of spirochetes is their motility by rapidly drifting rotation, often associated with a flexing or undulating movement along the helical path. These bacteria belong to the order Spirochaetales, which includes 2 families: Spirochaetaceae and Leptospiraceae. Important members of these groups include *Treponema, Borrelia,* and *Leptospira.*

Spirochetal infections leading to such diseases as syphilis and the other treponematoses, Lyme disease, relapsing fever borreliosis, and leptospirosis are important worldwide health problems. A better understanding of the immunobiology of the disease-causing spirochetes has become crucial in efforts to develop effective vaccines, because there has been no significant modification in excessive sexual activity, personal hygiene practices, or vector control. Further knowledge of immune responses to spirochetes is essential for their eventual control by immunization, and studies of the host–spirochete relationship have led to important new insights into the immune system itself. Serologic techniques have now become indispensable diagnostic tools for detection of many of the spirochetal diseases, especially syphilis and Lyme disease (Fig 54–1). The response of rabbits and guinea pigs to *Treponema pallidum* infection is an excellent experimental model for studying the development of resistance to syphilitic reinfection and the relative roles of humoral versus and immunity in protection against syphilis. Unfortunately, the immune response to spirochetal infections, as in other infections, may paradoxically cause immunologically induced disease in the host, such as aortitis, immune-complex glomerulonephritis, the gummatous lesions of syphilis, and the arthritis of Lyme disease.

SYPHILIS

Major Immunologic Features

- Both nonspecific, anticardiolipin, and specific antitreponemal antibodies are detectable following primary infection.

- Cell-mediated immunity becomes activated during or after the late secondary stage.
- Immunosuppression occurs during various phases of the disease.
- A complex state of partial immunity develops late following an untreated primary infection.

General Considerations

T pallidum is the spirochetal bacterium responsible for the sexually transmitted disease syphilis, which can have severe pathologic consequences if untreated and for which there is no vaccine. The organism is noncultivable, highly motile, and infectious, and it replicates extracellularly in vivo.

With the institution of antibiotic therapy in the mid-1940s, the incidence of syphilis fell sharply from a high of 72 cases per 100,000 in 1943 to about 4 per 100,000 in 1956. The Centers for Disease Control, however, recently reported a significant increase in primary and secondary syphilis cases, which can be attributed, in part, to changing lifestyles, sexual practices, and other factors such as an unusually high prevalence and resistance to antibiotics in patients with acquired immunodeficiency syndrome (AIDS). The estimated annual rate per 100,000 increased nationwide from 10.9 cases in 1986 to 13.3 cases in 1987. This represents the largest rise in more than 10 years. Syphilis continues to rank annually as the third or fourth most frequently reported communicable disease in the USA.

The course of syphilis in humans is marked by several interesting phenomena. Without treatment the disease will usually progress through several well-defined stages. This is unlike most other infectious diseases, which are ultimately eliminated by the host's immune system or, in severe cases, result in death. The relatively slow generation time of treponemes, which is estimated at 30–33 hours, contributes to this unique course. During the first 2 stages (primary and secondary syphilis) there is almost unimpeded rapid growth of *T pallidum,* leading to an early infectious spirochetemic phase of disease. The third stage (tertiary syphilis) occurs much later, following a prolonged latency period. Alterations in this stage are due primarily to tissue-damaging immune responses elicited by small numbers of previously deposited or disseminated spirochetes.

Syphilis activates both humoral and cell-mediated

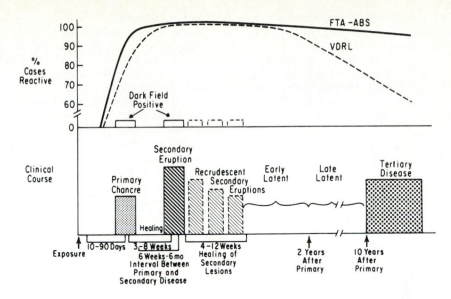

Figure 54–1. The course of untreated syphilis. (Reproduced, with permission, from Joklik WK et al (editors), *Zinsser Microbiology,* 19th ed. Appleton-Century-Crofts, 1988.)

immunity, but this protection is only partial. The relative importance of each type of immune response is not fully known. Protective immunity against re-exposure is incomplete, especially during early stages, when it develops relatively slowly. Evidence for the participation of humoral immunity in syphilis is as follows:

(1) A variety of nonspecific "reaginic" or Wassermann cardiolipin and specific antibodies are routinely present in the sera of patients with syphilis.

(2) *T pallidum*-immobilizing antibodies (TPIA) are regularly present in the sera of syphilitic patients.

(3) The frequency with which TPIA are found increases as syphilis progresses to latent and tertiary infection.

(4) Partial immunity can be conferred in experimentally infected laboratory animals by passive transfer of serum from syphilis-immune donors. This protection is apparent when treponemes are injected intradermally into these animal hosts. Chancres may be either prevented or delayed, and dissemination of treponemes from the primary focus of infection may be reduced by passive immunization.

Interestingly, humans who have been experimentally infected with *T pallidum* also develop increased local resistance to rechallenge at a cutaneous site. This local resistance is referred to as **chancre immunity.** Chancre immunity persists if primary infection remains untreated and syphilis progresses to a latent stage. Although chancre immunity is indicative of heightened local resistance, it does not prevent the systemic spread of *T pallidum* from the site of initial challenge. Chancre immunity may be at-

tributable to antibody, because both the immunity and reaginic antibodies wane after treatment of primary syphilis. The time required depends on the titer of antibody and the severity of the illness. For several reasons, it is not likely that the antibodies are completely protective:

(1) Treponemes from the initial infection persist systemically during latent syphilis, even though there is resistance to a second challenge. This suggests that the organism has found sanctuary in some sort of privileged residence, where it resists or is unaffected by host defenses.

(2) Some antibodies are nonspecific and are found in other diseases such as systemic lupus erythematosus. They might even be directed against host rather than treponemal antigens.

(3) By preventing the attachment of treponemes to cells in tissue culture, antibodies might, in fact, aid the organisms in escaping host defense mechanisms.

(4) Circulating immune complexes are formed during infection with *T pallidum*. They are demonstrable in sera of both rabbits and patients with syphilis. They may be composed of cardiolipin-anticardiolipin as well as of treponemal antigen-antitreponemal antibody. They may act to depress the synthesis of IgG against independent antigens, such as sheep erythrocytes. It is conceivable that circulating immune complexes prevent the host from synthesizing treponemicidal antibody during primary syphilis or from synthesizing antitreponemal antibody that might act in concert with cell-mediated immunity against *T pallidum.*

(5) The patterns of antibody production change

during the course of untreated syphilis. Patients with secondary syphilis have antitreponemal antibody as well as anticardiolipin antibody. These antibodies are of both IgG and IgM classes. As the disease enters latency, antitreponemal IgM antibody production ceases and patients are left with antitreponemal IgG and anticardiolipin IgM and IgG. The clinical significance of this sequence of events is uncertain.

Recent investigations in animal models have increasingly implicated cell-mediated immunity as a critical element in host response to *T pallidum*. Evidence for the participation of cell-mediated immunity in syphilis is as follows:

(1) Passive transfer of syphilis immune serum is only partially protective and does not follow classic models of humoral immunity.

(2) Syphilis progresses through the primary and secondary stages despite the presence of antibodies that immobilize the infecting organism.

(3) Delayed hypersensitivity to treponemal antigens is absent in primary and early secondary syphilis but develops late in secondary infection and is regularly present in latent and tertiary syphilis.

(4) Granulomatous lesions characterize tertiary syphilis.

(5) Immunization with killed microorganisms is usually unsuccessful, whereas immunization with live attenuated organisms has produced immunity.

(6) In vitro lymphocyte reactivity to treponemal and nontreponemal antigens and T lymphocyte counts are suppressed during primary and secondary syphilis.

(7) Infecting rabbits with *T pallidum* stimulates acquired cellular resistance to *Listeria;* this reaction is mediated by T lymphocytes.

(8) Both T and B cells are effective in conferring antisyphilis immunity when transferred from nonimmune recipients to normal challenged recipients.

It is puzzling why so much time is required for patients to develop humoral and cellular immunity to syphilis. One theory holds that the mucoid envelope of *T pallidum* renders it highly resistant to phagocytosis; only after the treponemes have remained in the host for some time is the mucoid coat broken down sufficiently for phagocytosis to occur. (Treponemal mucopolysaccharides also suppress lymphocyte blastogenic response to concanavalin A.) As a result, treponemal proliferation outstrips the rate of antigenic processing for stimulation of humoral and cellular immune mechanisms; a condition of "antigen overload" then occurs, with production of secondary immunosuppression. An alternative explanation is that sensitization with treponemal antigen leads primarily to generation of antibodies that then block antigenic sites, thereby inhibiting an appropriate cell-mediated immune response.

The proposed immunologic mechanisms are highly speculative.

Clinical Features

The severe late manifestations or complications of syphilis occur in the blood vessels and perivascular areas. However, sexual contact is the common mode of transmission, with inoculation on the mucous membranes of genital organs.

The first clinically apparent manifestation of syphilis (primary syphilis) is an indurated, circumscribed, relatively avascular and painless ulcer (chancre) at the site of treponemal inoculation. Spirochetemia with secondary metastatic distribution of microorganisms occurs within a few days after onset of local infection, but clinically apparent secondary lesions may not be observed for 2–4 weeks. The chancre lasts 10–14 days before healing spontaneously.

The presence of metastatic infection (secondary syphilis) is manifested by highly infectious mucocutaneous lesions of extraordinarily diverse description as well as headache, low-grade fever, diffuse lymphadenopathy, and a variety of more sporadic phenomena. The lesions of secondary syphilis ordinarily go on to apparent spontaneous resolution in the absence of treatment. However, until solid immunity develops—a matter of about 4 years—25% of untreated syphilitic patients may be susceptible to repeated episodes of spirochetemia and metastatic infection.

Following the resolution of secondary syphilis, the disease enters a period of latency, with only abnormal serologic tests to indicate the presence of infection. During this time, persistent or progressive focal infection is presumably taking place, but the precise site remains unknown in the absence of specific symptoms and signs. One site of potential latency, the central nervous system, can be evaluated by examining the cerebrospinal fluid, in which pleocytosis, elevated protein levels, and a positive serologic test for syphilis are indicative of asymptomatic neurosyphilis.

Only about 15% of patients with untreated latent syphilis go on to develop symptomatic tertiary syphilis. Serious or fatal tertiary syphilis in adults is virtually limited to disease of the aorta (aortitis with aneurysm formation and secondary aortic valve insufficiency), the central nervous system (tabes dorsalis, general paresis), the eyes (interstitial keratitis), or the ears (nerve deafness). Less frequently, the disease becomes apparent as localized single or multiple granulomas known as "gummas." These lesions are typically found in skin, bones, liver, testes, or larynx. The histopathologic features of the gumma resemble those of earlier syphilitic lesions, except that the vasculitis is associated with increased tissue necrosis and often frank caseation.

Immunologic Diagnosis

In its primary and secondary stages, syphilis is best diagnosed by dark-field microscopic examination of material from suspected lesions. Diagnostic serologic changes do not begin to occur until 14–21 days following acquisition of infection. Serologic tests provide important confirmatory evidence for secondary syphilis but are the only means of diagnosing latent infection (Fig 54–1; Table 54–1). Many forms of tertiary syphilis can be suspected on clinical grounds, but serologic tests are important in confirming the diagnosis. Spirochetes are notoriously difficult to demonstrate in the late stages of syphilis.

Two main categories of serologic tests for syphilis (STS) are available: tests for reaginic antibody and tests for treponemal antibody.

A. Tests for Reaginic Antibody: This is an unfortunate and confusing designation; there is no relationship between this antibody and IgE reaginic antibody. Patients with syphilis develop an antibody response to a tissue-derived substance (from beef heart) that is thought to be a component of mitochondrial membranes and is called "cardiolipin." Antibody to cardiolipin antigen is known as Wassermann, or reaginic, antibody. Numerous variations (and names) are associated with tests for this antigen. The simplest and most practical of these are the VDRL test (Venereal Disease Research Laboratory of the US Public Health Service), which involves a slide microflocculation technique and can provide qualitative and quantitative data, and the rapid plasma reagin (RPR) circle card test. Positive tests are considered to be diagnostic of syphilis when there is a high or increasing titer or when the medical history is compatible with primary or secondary syphilis. The tests may also be of prognostic aid in following response to therapy, because the antibody titer will revert to negative within 1 year of treatment for seropositive primary syphilis or within 2 years of that for secondary syphilis. Because cardiolipin antigen is found in the mitochondrial membranes of many mammalian tissues as well as in diverse microorganisms, it is not surprising that antibody to this antigen should appear during other diseases. A positive VDRL test may be encountered, for example, in patients with infectious mononucleosis, leprosy, hepatitis, and systemic lupus erythematosus. Al-

though the VDRL test lacks specificity for syphilis, its great sensitivity makes it extremely useful.

B. Tests for Treponemal Antibody: The first test used for detecting specific antitreponemal antibody was the *T pallidum* immobilization (TPI) test. Although highly reliable, it proved to be too cumbersome for routine use. A major test used until recently was the fluorescent *T pallidum* antibody (FTA) test. If virulent *T pallidum* from an infected rabbit testicle is placed on a slide and overlaid with serum from a patient with antibody to treponemes, an antigen-antibody reaction will occur. The bound antibody can then be detected by means of a fluoresceinated anti-human immunoglobulin antibody. The specificity of the test for *T pallidum* is enhanced by first absorbing the serum with nonpathogenic treponemal strains. This modification is referred to as the FTA-ABS test. (If specific anti-IgM antibody to human gamma globulin is used, the acuteness of the infection or the occurrence of congenital syphilis can be assessed. However, this test may sometimes be falsely positive or negative in babies born of mothers with syphilis.)

The FTA-ABS test is reactive in approximately 80% of patients with primary syphilis (versus 50% for the VDRL test). Both tests are positive in virtually 100% of patients with secondary syphilis. Whereas the VDRL test shows a tendency to decline in titer after successful treatment, the FTA-ABS test may remain positive for years. It is especially useful in confirming or ruling out a diagnosis of syphilis in patients with suspected biologic false-positive reactions to the VDRL test. However, even the FTA-ABS test may be susceptible to false-positive reactions, especially in the presence of lupus erythematosus.

The microhemagglutination-*T pallidum* (MHA-TP) test, a simple passive hemagglutination test, is a satisfactory substitute for the FTA-ABS test. Its principal advantages are economy of technician time and money. Its results correlate closely with those of the FTA-ABS test, except during primary and early secondary syphilis, when both the VDRL and FTA-ABS are more likely to show reactivity. The VDRL test is

Table 54–1. Serologic tests for syphilis.[1]

Antigen	Antigen Source	Tests[2]	Percent Reactivity During		
			Primary Stage	Secondary Stage	Tertiary Stage
Nontreponemal	Extracts of tissue (cardiolipin-lecithin-cholesterol	Complement fixation (Wassermann, Kolmer) Flocculation (VDRL, Hinton, Kann)	78	90	77
Treponemal	*T pallidum* Reiter strain *T pallidum*	RPCF TPI FTA-ABS MHA-TP	61 56 85 85	85 94 99 98	72 92 96 95

[1]Reproduced, with permission, from Joklik WK et al (editors), *Zinsser Microbiology,* 19th ed. Appleton-Century-Crofts, 1988.
[2]FTA-ABS, Fluorescent treponemal antibody-absorption; MHA-TP, microhemagglutination assay for *T pallidum;* RPCF. Reiter protein complement fixation; TPI, *T pallidum* immobilization.

the only one that can be used with reliability in the evaluation of cerebrospinal fluid.

The interpretation of serologic data from patients with syphilis may be extremely complex in some cases. For example, a prozone phenomenon may be encountered in secondary syphilis; serofastness may characterize late syphilis; and the VDRL test may be negative in up to one-third of patients with late latent syphilis.

Differential Diagnosis

Syphilis produces sufficiently diverse clinical manifestations that a textbook of general internal medicine should be consulted for a discussion of the differential diagnosis.

Prevention

If used properly, condoms can be an effective barrier against the sexual transmission of syphilis. Promising results with antigen produced by recombinant DNA technology may soon lead to a syphilis vaccine. Early treatment with antibiotics is the only way known to prevent the later ravages of syphilis.

Treatment

Penicillin is the drug of choice for syphilis in all its stages. Because the lesions of tertiary syphilis may be irreversible, it is crucial to identify and treat the disease before tertiary lesions begin. AIDS patients with syphilis must be treated more intensively with penicillin. This reinforces the notion that curing syphilis depends on interactions between an intact immune system and the treponemicidal effects of antibiotics.

Complications & Prognosis

The most frequent complication of treatment is the **Jarisch-Herxheimer reaction,** which occurs in up to half of patients with early syphilis and is manifested by fever, headache, myalgias, and exacerbation of cutaneous lesions. The intensity of a Jarisch-Herxheimer reaction reflects the intensity of local inflammation prior to treatment and is thought to result from the release of antigenic material from dying microorganisms. The reaction is of short duration (2–4 hours) and is generally not harmful, although shock and death have been attributed to this reaction in tertiary forms of the disease. (The Jarisch-Herxheimer reaction has also been described in the treatment of louse-borne borreliosis, brucellosis, and typhoid fever.)

Other immunologic complications of syphilis include paroxysmal cold hemoglobinuria and nephrotic syndrome.

It is estimated that one in 13 patients who receive no treatment for syphilis will develop cardiovascular disease, one in 25 will become crippled or incapacitated, one in 44 will develop irreversible damage to the central nervous system, and one in 200 will become blind.

NONVENEREAL TREPONEMATOSES

The causes of yaws (*T pallidum subsp pertenue*), pinta (*Treponema carateum*), and bejel (*T pallidum subsp endemicum*) are human pathogens responsible for this group of contagious diseases, which are endemic among rural populations in tropical and subtropical countries. Unlike syphilis, these diseases are not transmitted by sexual activity but arise when treponemes are transmitted primarily by direct contact, mostly among children living under poor hygienic conditions. These 3 treponemal species are morphologically and antigenically similar to *T pallidum*, yet give rise to slightly different disease manifestations. Pinta causes skin lesions only; yaws causes skin and bone lesions; and bejel (so-called endemic syphilis) affects the mucous membranes, skin, and bones. They do resemble venereal syphilis by virtue of the self-limiting primary and secondary lesions, a latency period with clinically dormant disease, and late lesions that are frequently highly destructive. The serologic responses for all 3 diseases are indistinguishable from one another and from that of venereal syphilis, and there is the same degree of slow development of protective immunity associated with prolonged, untreated infection.

LYME DISEASE

Major Immunologic Features
- Multisystem spirochetal disease involves inflammation of skin, joints, and nervous system.
- Specific antibody is diagnostic following infection.
- Cell-mediated immunity is activated during or shortly after the early stage of disease.

General Considerations

In the mid-1970s a geographic clustering of an unusual rheumatoid arthritis-like condition involving mostly children and young adults occurred in northeastern Connecticut. This condition proved to be a newly discovered disease, named Lyme disease after the town of its origin. The arthritis is characterized by intermittent attacks of asymmetric pain and swelling primarily in the large joints (especially the knees) over a period of a few years. Epidemiologic and clinical research showed that the onset of symptoms was preceded by an insect bite and unique skin rash probably identical to that of an illness following a tick bite, first described in Europe at the turn of the century. The beneficial effects of penicillin or tetracycline in early cases suggested a microbial origin for what was initially called Lyme arthritis.

Lyme disease is now the most common tick-transmitted illness, and it has been reported in at least 36 states. However, it occurs primarily in 3 geographic regions: the coastal areas of the Northeast from Maine to Maryland, the Midwest in Wisconsin and Minnesota, and the far West in parts of California and Oregon. These geographic areas parallel the location of the primary tick vector of Lyme disease in the USA—*Ixodes dammini* in the east and midwest and *Ixodes pacificus* in the far west. Lyme disease has been reported in many other countries, especially in western Europe, corresponding to the distribution of *Ixodes ricinus* ticks. The greatest concentration of cases is in the northeastern USA, particularly in New York state, where the disease is endemic on Long Island and just north of New York City in neighboring Westchester County.

In the early 1980s spirochetal organisms were isolated and cultured from the midguts of *Ixodes* ticks taken from Shelter Island, NY (an endemic focus), and shortly thereafter they were cultured from the skin rash site, blood, and cerebrospinal fluid of patients with Lyme disease. This newly discovered spirochete, called *Borrelia burgdorferi*, is microaerophilic, resembles other spirochetes morphologically, and is slightly larger than the treponemes. Unlike the pathogenic treponemes, *B burgdorferi* can be readily cultivated in vitro in a highly fortified growth media.

Clinical Features

Lyme disease is an illness having protean manifestations with symptoms that include (1) an erythematous expanding red annular rash with central clearing; (2) fever, headache, stiff neck, nausea, and vomiting; (3) neurologic complications such as facial nerve (Bell's) palsy and meningitis; and (4) arthritis in about 50% of untreated patients. These symptoms occur most frequently from May to November, when ticks are active and numerous and people are engaged in many outdoor activities. The most characteristic feature of early Lyme disease is a skin rash, often referred to as erythema chronicum migrans (ECM), which appears shortly (3–32 days) after a bite from an infected tick. The lesion typically expands almost uniformly from the center of the bite and is usually flat or slightly indurated with central clearing and reddening at the periphery. It is noteworthy, however, that many Lyme disease victims do not recall being bitten by a tick or do not develop classic ECM. On the other hand, at various intervals after the initial rash, some patients develop similar but smaller multiple secondary annular skin lesions that last for several weeks to months. Biopsy of these skin lesions reveals a lymphocytic and plasmacytic infiltrate. Various flulike symptoms such as malaise, fever, headache, stiff neck, and arthralgias are often associated with ECM. The late manifestations of Lyme disease may include migratory and polyarticular arthritis, neurologic and cardiac in-

volvement with cranial nerve palsies and radiculopathy, myocarditis, and arrhythmias. Lyme arthritis typically involves a knee or other large joint. It may enter a chronic phase, leading to destruction of bone and joints if left untreated. Interestingly, Lyme arthritis is less common in Europe than in the USA, but neurologic complications are more prevalent in Europe. Unique strain variations expressing antigenic subtypes between European and North American isolates of *B burgdorferi* probably explain these dissimilarities.

In most cases, humoral and cell-mediated immune responses are activated during borrelial infection. Antibody, mostly of the IgM class, can be detected shortly after the appearance of ECM; thereafter, there is a gradual increase in overall titer and a switch to predominant IgG antibody response for the duration of an untreated infection. Most notably, very high levels of antibody have been found in serum and joint fluid taken from patients with moderate to severe arthritis. Although the presence of such high antibody titers against *B burgdorferi* may reduce the spirochete load somewhat, they appear not to ameliorate the disease process completely and, indeed, may actually contribute to some of the pathologic changes. These serologic responses form the basis of laboratory tests to aid in the diagnosis of Lyme borreliosis. On the basis of lymphocyte transformation assays, peripheral blood T cells from Lyme disease patients respond to borrelial antigens primarily after early infection and following successful treatment. Also, addition of antigens to synovial cells in vitro from infected patients triggers the production of interleukin-1, which could account for many of the harmful inflammatory reactions associated with this disease. Human mononuclear and polymorphonuclear phagocytes can both ingest and presumably destroy *Borrelia*. Thus, borrelial antigen-stimulated T cells or their products may activate macrophages, limiting dissemination and resulting in enhanced phagocytic activity and the eventual clearance of spirochetes from the primary lesion.

Immunologic Diagnosis

Successful isolation and culture of *B burgdorferi* from skin lesions, blood, and joint and cerebrospinal fluid in suspected cases of Lyme disease is rare. Antibody responses important in diagnosis typically begin to occur 3–5 weeks after the onset of ECM, but they can be obliterated by early antibiotic therapy. Serologic tests provide important confirmatory evidence for all stages of Lyme disease and may be the only way of diagnosing atypical cases. There is some evidence that a small percentage of untreated patients with Lyme disease produce few or no detectable antibodies throughout the course of infection. The most commonly used serologic tests are the enzyme-linked immunosorbent assay (ELISA) and indirect fluorescent-antibody assay (IFA). Because of its sensitivity, adaptability to automation, and ease of quantitation, the ELISA is probably the preferred method. Standard indirect IFA and newer quantitative solid-phase IFAs are available. An indirect hemagglutination antibody test, patterned after a similar test for syphilis but using borrelial antigens, is currently being evaluated and may prove to be an inexpensive and reliable alternative to other antibody detection systems. These tests are designed to detect total serum antibody to *Borrelia* without differentiating between IgG or IgM antibodies. The availability of IgM tests would be of great utility, because this class of antibody usually shows preferentially elevated levels early in primary infection or relapse and in sera of newborn infants following transplacentally acquired infections. For all these assays, false-positive reactions are relatively rare but can occur if a patient has syphilis, infectious mononucleosis, systemic lupus erythematosus, or rheumatoid arthritis. Serum from Lyme disease patients can sometimes be reactive in specific treponemal antibody tests, but is consistently negative for the nontreponemal (VDRL) tests.

Differential Diagnosis

Like syphilis, Lyme disease produces such a diverse number of clinical symptoms that a textbook of general internal medicine should be consulted for a detailed account of differential diagnosis. Patients with Lyme disease are usually distinguished by their characteristic skin lesions and diagnostic serologic changes. Distinctions must be made from syphilis, rheumatoid arthritis, and chronic fatigue syndrome, which produce similar symptoms.

Prevention

Avoiding *Borrelia*-infected ticks or tick-infested areas will guarantee protection against Lyme disease. For those living in endemic areas, a few simple precautions will help minimize possible exposure. These include wearing clothing that fully protects the body and using repellents that contain DEET (diethyltoluamide). If a tick does attach to the skin, careful removal with tweezers shortly after it attaches followed by application of alcohol or another suitable disinfectant will make borrelial transmission unlikely.

Treatment & Prognosis

Early disease is adequately treated with a 2–3-week course of penicillin or tetracycline. Later complications such as arthritis and the neuropathies may require more intense and prolonged antibiotic therapy. There are, however, some concerns regarding the universal efficacy of treatment. Despite the use of very aggressive and repeated antibiotic therapy, there are reports of some patients with persisting Lyme disease-like symptoms, indicating that irreversible damage may have occurred in a manner analogous to late-stage syphilis. It is unclear whether this phenomenon is due at least in part to persistence of pathogenic *Borrelia,* possibly because of antibiotic resistance.

RELAPSING-FEVER BORRELIOSIS

Relapsing fever is an acute febrile disease of worldwide distribution and is caused by arthropod-borne spirochetes belonging to the genus *Borrelia*. Two major forms of this illness are louse-borne relapsing fever (for which humans are the reservoir and the body louse, *Pediculus humanus,* is the vector) and tick-borne relapsing fever (for which rodents and other small animals are the major reservoirs and ticks of the genus *Ornithodorus* are the vectors). *B recurrentis* causes louse-borne relapsing fever and is transmitted from human to human following the ingestion of infected human blood by the louse and release of newly acquired organisms onto the skin or mucous membranes of a new host. The disease is endemic in parts of central and east Africa and South America. The causative organisms of tick-borne relapsing fever are numerous and include *B hermsii, B turicatae,* and *B parkeri* in North America, *B hispanica* in Spain, *B duttonii* in east Africa, and *B persica* in Asia. Ticks become infectious by biting and sucking blood from a spirochetemic animal. The infection is transmitted to humans or animals when saliva is released by a feeding tick through bites or penetration of intact skin.

After an individual has been exposed to an infected louse or tick, *Borrelia* penetrate the skin and enter the bloodstream and lymphatic system. After a 1–3-week incubation period, spirochetes replicate in the blood and there is an acute onset of shaking chills, fever, headache, and fatigue. Concentrations of *Borrelia* can reach as high as 10^8 spirochetes/mL of blood, and these are clearly visible after staining blood smears with Giemsa or Wright's stain. During febrile disease, *Borrelia* are present in the patient's blood but disappear prior to afebrile episodes and subsequently return to the bloodstream during the next febrile period. Jaundice can develop in some severely ill patients as a result of intrahepatic obstruction of bile flow and hepatocellular inflammation; if left untreated, patients can die from damage to the liver, spleen, or brain. The majority of untreated patients, however, recover spontaneously. They produce borrelial antibodies that have agglutinating, complement-fixing, borreliacidal, and immobilizing capabilities and that render patients immune to reinfection with the same *Borrelia* serotype. Serologic tests designed to measure these antibodies are of limited diagnostic value because of antigenic variation among strains and the coexistence of mixed populations of *Borrelia* within a given host during the course of a single infection. Diagnosis in the majority of cases requires demonstration of spirochetemia in febrile patients.

LEPTOSPIROSIS

Leptospirosis is an acute, febrile disease caused by various serotypes of *Leptospira*. Often referred to as Weil's disease, infection with *Leptospira interrogans* causes diseases that are extremely varied in their clinical presentations and that are also found in a variety of wild and domestic animals. Transmission to humans occurs primarily after contact with contaminated urine from leptospiruric animals. In the USA, dogs are the major reservoir for exposure of humans to this disease. After entering the body through the mucosal surface or breaks in the skin, leptospiral bacteria cause an acute illness characterized by fever, chills, myalgias, severe headaches, conjunctival suffuseness, and gastrointestinal problems. Most human infections are mild and anicteric, although in a small proportion of victims, severe icteric disease can occur and be fatal, primarily owing to renal failure and damage to small blood vessels. After infection of the kidneys, leptospiras are excreted in the urine. Liver dysfunction with hepatocellular damage and jaundice is common. Antibiotic treatment is curative if begun during early disease, but its value thereafter is questionable.

Diagnosis of leptospirosis depends upon either seroconversion or the demonstration of spirochetes in clinical specimens. The macroscopic slide agglutination test, which uses formalized antigen, offers safe and rapid antibody screening. Measurement of antibody for a specific serotype, however, is performed with the very sensitive microscopic agglutination test involving live organisms. This method provides the most specific reaction with the highest titer and fewer cross-reactions. Agglutinating IgM-class-specific antibodies are produced during early infection and persist in high titers for many months. Protective and agglutinating antibodies often persist in sera of convalescent patients and may be associated with resistance to future infections.

REFERENCES

General

Barbour AG: Laboratory aspects of Lyme borreliosis. *Clin Microbiol Rev* 1988;**1**:399.

Benach JL, Bosler EM (editors): Lyme disease and related disorders. *Ann NY Acad Sci* 1988;**539**:1.

Fitzgerald TJ: Pathogenesis and immunology of *Treponema pallidum*. *Annu Rev Microbiol* 1981;**35**:29.

Schell RF, Musher DM (editors): *Pathogenesis and Immunology of Treponemal Infections*. Marcel Dekker, 1983.

Syphilis

Baseman JB et al: Virulence determinants among the spirochetes. Page 203 in: *Microbiology—1979*. Schlessinger D (editor). American Society for Microbiology, 1979.

Baughn RE, Tung KS, Musher DM: Detection of circulating immune complexes in the sera of rabbits with experimental syphilis: Possible role in immunoregulation. *Infect Immun* 1980;**29**:575.

Bryceson AD: Clinical pathology of the Jarisch-Herxheimer reaction. *J Infect Dis* 1976;**133**:696.

Hanff PA et al: Humoral immune response in human syphilis to polypeptides of *Treponema pallidum*. *J Immunol* 1982;**129**:1287.

Lukehart SA et al: Invasion of the central nervous system by *Treponema pallidum*: Implications for diagnosis and treatment. *Ann Intern Med* 1988;**109**:855.

Pavia CS, Niederbuhl CJ: Acquired resistance and expression of a protective humoral immune response in guinea pigs infected with *Treponema pallidum* Nichols. *Infect Immun* 1985;**50**:66.

Pavia CS, Niederbuhl CJ: Adoptive transfer of antisyphilis immunity with lymphocytes from *Treponema pallidum*-infected guinea pigs. *J Immunol* 1985;**135**:2829.

Pavia CS, Folds JD, Baseman JB: Cell-mediated immunity during syphilis: A review. *Br J Vener Dis* 1978;**54**:144.

Schell RF, Chan JK, Le Frock JL: Endemic syphilis: Passive transfer of resistance with serum and cells in hamsters. *J Infect Dis* 1979;**140**:378.

Lyme Disease

Barbour AG, Heiland RA, Howe TR: Heterogeneity of major proteins of Lyme disease borreliae: A molecular analysis of North American and European isolates. *J Infect Dis* 1985;**152**:478.

Barbour AG, Tessier SL, Hayes SF: Variation in a major surface protein of Lyme disease spirochetes. *Infect Immun* 1984;**45**:94.

Benach JL et al: Interactions of phagocytes with the Lyme disease spirochete: Role of the Fc receptor. *J Infect Dis* 1984;**150**:497.

Burgdorfer W et al: Lyme disease: A tick-borne spirochetosis? *Science* 1982;**216**:1317.

Craft JE, Grodzicki RL, Steere AC: Antibody response in Lyme disease: Evaluation of diagnostic tests. *J Infect Dis* 1984;**149**:789.

Dattwyler RJ et al: Seronegative Lyme disease: Dissociation of specific T- and B-lymphocyte responses to *Borrelia burgdorferi*. *N Engl J Med* 1988;**319**:1441.

Magnarelli LA, Anderson JF, Johnson RC: Cross-reactivity in serological tests for Lyme disease and other spirochetal infections. *J Infect Dis* 1987;**156**:183.

Steere AC et al: The spirochetal etiology of Lyme disease. *N Engl J Med* 1983;**308:**733.

Leptospirosis
Adler B, Faine S: The antibodies involved in the human immune response to leptospiral infection. *J Med Microbiol* 1978;**11:**387.

Alexander AD: Serological diagnosis of leptospirosis. Chap 69, pp 435–439, in: *Manual of Clinical Laboratory Immunology,* 3rd ed. Rose NR, Friedman H, Fahey JL (editors). American Society for Microbiology, 1986.

Relapsing Fever Borreliosis
Meier JT, Simon MI, Barbour AG: Antigenic variation is associated with DNA rearrangements in a relapsing fever *Borrelia. Cell* 1985;**41:**403.

Southern PM, Sanford JP: Relapsing fever: A clinical and microbiological review. *Medicine* 1969;**48:**129.

Infections of the Immune System

55

Suzanne Crowe, MBBS, & John Mills, MD

Although measles virus infection has been recognized for decades as a cause of immunosuppression, Epstein-Barr virus (EBV) was the first pathogen shown to cause immune dysfunction as a result of directly infecting cells of the immune system. Since then, other viruses, especially herpesviruses and retroviruses, have been identified that can infect cells of the immune system and produce immune suppression, immune stimulation, or both. The discovery of the human immunodeficiency virus (HIV), which primarily infects immune cells, has provided additional impetus for understanding the mechanisms by which virus infection results in immune dysfunction.

HUMAN IMMUNODEFICIENCY VIRUS

Major Immunologic Features

- CD4 cells of the immune system, including T lymphocytes, monocyte-macrophages, follicular dendritic cells, and Langerhans' cells, are infected.
- There are progressive global defects of humoral and cell-mediated immunity.
- CD4 (helper/inducer) T lymphocytes are depleted.
- There is polyclonal activation of B lymphocytes with increased immunoglobulin production.
- Disease progresses despite vigorous humoral and cell-mediated responses to the virus.

General Considerations

The acquired immunodeficiency syndrome (AIDS) was first recognized in 1981. The identification of HIV as the causative agent of AIDS in 1984 was rapidly followed by characterization of this virus and the target cells that it infects and by elucidation of the multiple consequences of infection. Epidemiologic studies have identified the major populations at risk of acquiring infection and the routes by which the virus can be transmitted. The clinical illnesses associated with HIV infection have been classified, and therapeutic strategies to treat or suppress them have been designed. By 1985, diagnostic kits had been developed for the detection of antibody to HIV, potentially therapeutic compounds were being screened for in vitro activity against this virus, and clinical trials for safety and efficacy of these potential drugs had begun. In 1987, only 6 years after the initial recognition of the AIDS epidemic and 3 years after identification of the etiologic agent, zidovudine (2'-azido-3'-deoxythymidine [AZT]), the first antiretroviral agent, was licensed by the US Food and Drug Administration for treatment of HIV infection.

Infection with HIV results in an acquired defect in immune function, especially involving cell-mediated immunity. Infected individuals may be asymptomatic or have progressive disease associated with recurrent opportunistic infections, certain cancers, severe weight loss, and central nervous system degeneration.

The recognition of the viral etiology of AIDS has stimulated immunologists to investigate the pathogenesis of the disease. Rational development of effective antiretroviral compounds can be aided by knowledge of the mechanisms by which HIV can damage the immune system. Although research on HIV has probably provided us with more pathogenetic information than we have on any other virus, the genesis of the characteristic and profound immune dysfunction caused by HIV still remains incompletely understood.

Etiology

A. Virology: HIV is a member of the retrovirus family, a group of enveloped viruses possessing the enzyme reverse transcriptase. This enzyme allows the virus to synthesize a DNA copy of its RNA genome. HIV was previously termed "human T lymphotrophic virus type III (HTLV-III)," "lymphadenopathy-associated virus (LAV)," and "AIDS-related virus (ARV)." However, molecular characterization of these retroviruses demonstrated their relatedness, and they are regarded as variants of the same virus. HIV has been subclassified within the lentivirus family, a group of nontransforming retroviruses with a long latency period from infection to the onset of clinical features and similar morphologic features and nucleotide sequence homology. Other members of the lentivirus family include visna and caprine arthritis-encephalitis viruses, which cause chronic, progressive neurodegenerative disease in sheep and goats, respectively. The clinical picture of lentivirus infection in sheep and goats is similar to that resulting from HIV infection in humans and is characterized by a slow and progressive disorder of the immune system and the brain. HIV is also closely related to simian immunodeficiency virus (SIV), which causes an AIDS-like illness in macaque monkeys, and to HIV-2, a human retrovirus that is most prevalent in West Africans and also causes AIDS (Table 55–1; Fig 55–1).

B. Genomic Organization: HIV consists of an inner core, containing an RNA genome, surrounded by a lipid envelope. The HIV genome (Fig 55–2) contains the standard retroviral structural genes, *env, gag,* and *pol,* encoding the viral envelope proteins, core protein, and reverse transcriptase, respectively. Many of these gene products are made as precursor proteins, which require cleavage by viral proteases or cellular enzymes later in the replicative cycle.

The virus possesses at least 6 other genes, a feature that makes HIV unique among retroviruses. The first of these additional genes to be recognized was *tat,* a positive feedback regulator of HIV replication, which can accelerate viral protein production by several thousandfold. *rev (trs/art)* encodes proteins that inhibit the transcription of the regulatory genes. However, this negative regulatory effect may be overcome to permit expression of viral proteins by binding of the *rev* protein to a *cis*-acting antirepressive sequence (CAR). The product of the virion infectivity gene, *vif (sor),* increases viral infectivity and may be responsible for the efficient cell-to-cell transmission observed with HIV. *nef (3′ orf)* is a negative regulatory factor whose protein product inhibits viral replication. Recently, 2 new genes have been described: the *vpr* (viral protein R) gene, whose function is not yet known, and the *vpu* (viral protein

Table 55–1. Classification of retroviruses.

Oncoviruses	Lentiviruses	Spumiviruses
Avian retroviruses	Visna/maedi virus	Human foamy virus
Bovine leukemia virus	Caprine arthritis encephalitis virus	Simian foamy virus
Murine retroviruses	Equine infectious anemia virus	
Feline leukemia virus HTLV-I and HTLV-II	HIV-1 and HIV-2 Simian immuno-deficiency virus	

U) gene, whose protein product is thought to negatively regulate viral replication (Fig 55–2).

C. Pathogenesis of Infection: HIV infection affects predominantly the immune system and the brain. The dominant immunologic feature of HIV infection is progressive depletion of the CD4 (helper/inducer) subset of T lymphocytes, thereby reversing the normal CD4:CD8 ratio and inexorably worsening immunodeficiency. The depletion of CD4 lymphocytes is predominantly due to the tropism of HIV for these and other CD4-bearing cells because the CD4 cell surface molecule functions as a receptor for the virus. The CD4 lymphocyte is necessary for the proper functioning of the immune system. It interacts with antigen-presenting cells, B cells, cytotoxic T cells, and natural killer (NK) cells (see Chapter 5). Thus, it is easy to see that infection and depletion of this cell population could induce profound immunodeficiency. However, in situ hybridization studies suggest that only very few (about 1 in 10,000) CD4

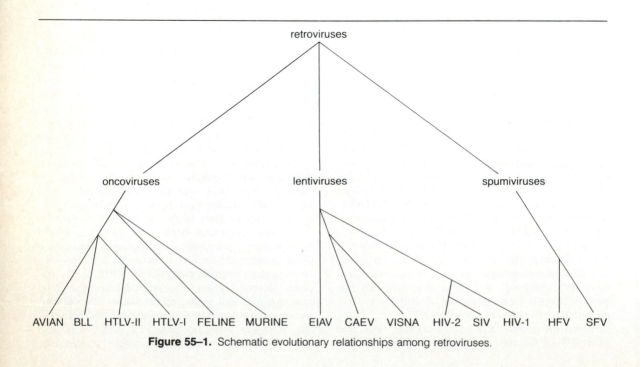

Figure 55–1. Schematic evolutionary relationships among retroviruses.

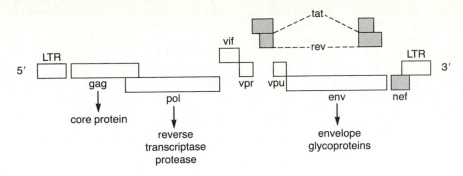

Figure 55–2. Genomic organization of HIV. The 9.6-kb genome of HIV consists of both structural and regulatory sequences (see text for details). HIV has a far more complex genome than other retroviruses do.

lymphocytes contain replicating HIV. Thus, it is hard to explain the pathogenesis of the immunologic dysfunction of AIDS and profound loss of circulating CD4 cells by infection of this cell population alone.

The finding that the CD4 molecule is present on cells other than helper/inducer T lymphocytes was accompanied by evidence that HIV could infect other cell populations which expressed this molecule on their surface. Other cells susceptible to HIV infection include monocyte-macrophages, microglial cells, Langerhans' cells, follicular dendritic cells, immortalized B cells, retinal cells, and colonic mucosal cells (Table 55–2). Monocyte-macrophages are thought to provide a major reservoir for HIV in vivo and may contribute to the pathogenesis of the immune deficiency by functioning abnormally. For example, HIV-infected monocyte-macrophages secrete an inhibitor of interleukin-1 (IL-1), a cytokine of major importance in T cell proliferative responses (see Chapter 7). Although the pathogenesis of immune dysfunction associated with HIV infection is incompletely understood, it is likely that the process occurs through collective dysfunction of both antigen-presenting cells, such as macrophages, and T lymphocytes, especially the CD4 subset.

What is the likely sequence of events following HIV infection? The first cell population to come in contact with HIV is postulated to be the monocyte-macrophage. These cells ingest HIV and can process the virus into a form that is recognized by T cells.

Table 55–2. Cells infected by HIV.

CD4 T lymphocytes
Monocyte-macrophages
Follicular dendritic cells
Langerhans' cells
Microglial cells
Immortalized B cells
Retinal cells
Colonic mucosal cells
Endothelial cells

Viral antigens are presented to the CD4 lymphocytes in conjunction with class II major histocompatibility complex (MHC) molecules. Upon recognition of the displayed viral antigen and MHC protein, T cells bind to the complex and become activated. Following infection with HIV, the virus replicates within these CD4 lymphocytes until the cells undergo cytolysis, a process that may be mediated by HIV envelope glycoprotein, other toxic viral products, or autoreactive CD8 cells. HIV replication within monocyte-macrophages occurs at a leisurely pace compared with that within lymphocytes, with little cytopathology. Monocyte-macrophages may also harbor the virus in a latent state. The factors that trigger latently infected cells to produce virus are not completely known and may involve both cellular activating factors such as the transcriptional activator NF kappa B or alteration in HIV regulatory genes such as a decrease in *nef*.

The other major feature of HIV infection is involvement of the central nervous system. The clinical findings range from minor memory defects to personality changes to progressive, fatal dementia. The mechanism of brain damage is obscure. As there is no evidence to support direct neuronal infection with HIV, it is more likely that soluble factors secreted by other infected cells (for example, infected monocytes that transport the virus to the brain) may alter the function of neurons and contribute to the dementia. In infected brain tissue, HIV has been detected in multinucleated giant cells composed predominantly of monocyte-macrophages, suggesting a major pathogenetic role for these cells. An alternative hypothesis is that HIV may competitively inhibit neuroleukin from binding to neurons. This neurotrophic factor shares homology with a conserved region of the HIV envelope glycoprotein, gp120.

Epidemiology

By mid-1989, there were approximately 85,000 reported cases of AIDS in the USA. The disease is recognized as a global health problem, with cases of

AIDS being reported in more than 170 countries and an estimated 5 million HIV-infected people worldwide. In the USA, Europe, and Australia, transmission of HIV has been documented to occur via sexual contact, administration of infected blood or blood products, artificial insemination with infected semen, exposure to blood-containing needles or syringes, or transmission from an infected mother to her fetus or to the infant during or after birth. Homosexual activity accounts for the majority of sexually transmitted cases in these countries. Male-to-female transmission is more commonly reported than female-to-male transmission; whether this is secondary to epidemiologic factors (a larger number of infected males) or to greater efficacy of transmission is not known. Transmission from mother to offspring usually occurs by transplacental passage of the virus, with estimates for the incidence of transmission of HIV from an infected mother to her child varying from 20 to 70%. Following the introduction of programs to exclude blood donors who are members of high-risk groups and the serologic testing of donated blood, the risk of acquiring HIV from infected blood or blood products has been virtually eliminated. Thus, the groups presently at highest risk are homosexual and bisexual men, intravenous drug abusers who share needles or syringes, sexual partners of people in high-risk groups, and children born to infected mothers (Table 55–3). Health care workers are at risk of HIV infection, but this risk is considered to be very low. Epidemiologic data do not support transmission of HIV by casual contact, insects, or sharing of utensils (tableware, toothbrushes, etc). There are no data to suggest aerosolized transmission of the virus.

In Central and Western Africa, cases of AIDS are equally distributed among men and women, and heterosexual transmission (especially from infected female prostitutes to their clients) is thought to account for the majority of cases. In Africa, risk factors associated with HIV infection in heterosexuals include large numbers of sexual partners, prostitution, sex with prostitutes, a history of sexually transmitted disease such as gonorrhea or syphilis, or genital ulceration of any cause. There does not appear to be any increased risk of acquisition of infection from anal intercourse. Other risk factors of uncertain overall significance include multiple use of needles or syringes in health clinics and ritualistic practices in which unsterilized instruments are used; these include scarification, tattooing, ear-piercing, and male and female circumcision.

Exposure to HIV does not always result in infection. However, one exposure may be sufficient to cause infection, depending on inoculum size, route of entry, and, perhaps, host factors. The dose to infect 50% of exposed individuals (ID50) is not known for humans, but it is presumed to be low (less than 10–100 virions). It is likely that both cell-free and cell-associated viruses are infectious. It is estimated that about 30% of HIV-infected individuals will contract AIDS over a 3-year period from the time of infection. Although it is not known what proportion of infected individuals will ultimately develop AIDS, mathematical models predict that most persons infected with the virus will eventually develop the disease. The latency period (from time of infection to onset of disease) may vary according to viral inoculum, route of entry, and age of the patient.

Clinical Features

A. Acute HIV mononucleosis: Following infection with HIV, an individual may remain asymptomatic or develop an acute illness that resembles infectious mononucleosis. This syndrome usually occurs within 2–6 weeks following infection, with reported periods ranging from 5 days to 3 months. The predominant symptoms are fever, headache, sore throat, malaise, and rash. Clinical findings include pharyngitis (which may be exudative and may be accompanied by mucosal ulceration); generalized lymphadenopathy; a macular or urticarial rash on the face, trunk, and limbs; and hepatosplenomegaly (Table 55–4). During the acute illness, antibodies to HIV are generally undetectable. Although the illness is often severely incapacitating, requiring bed rest or even hospitalization, some individuals experience only mild symptoms and do not seek medical attention.

Acute infection with HIV has also been associated with neurologic disease, including meningitis, encephalitis, cranial nerve palsies, myopathy, and peripheral neuropathy. These findings are usually accompanied by features of the acute HIV mononucleosis syndrome.

B. AIDS-related complex (ARC): This poorly defined condition basically encompasses patients in-

---

Table 55–3. Individuals at risk of HIV infection.

High risk
  Homosexual and bisexual men
  Intravenous drug abusers who share needles or syringes
  Sexual partners of people in high-risk groups
  Children born to infected mothers
Low risk
  Health care workers, including nurses, doctors, dentists,
    and laboratory staff

Table 55–4. Clinical features of acute HIV infection.

Fever and sweats
Myalgia and arthralgia
Malaise and lethargy
Lymphadenopathy
Pharyngitis
Anorexia, nausea, and vomiting
Headaches and photophobia
Macular rash

fected with HIV but not with acute mononucleosis who have clinical findings short of those fulfilling the Centers for Disease Control (CDC) criteria for AIDS. The condition is regarded as evidence of progressive immune dysfunction. Constitutional symptoms and signs include persistent fever, night sweats, weight loss, unexplained chronic diarrhea, eczema, psoriasis, seborrheic dermatitis, generalized lymphadenopathy, herpes zoster, oral candidiasis, and oral hairy leukoplakia. The last 3 conditions are regarded as poor prognostic indicators and herald progression to AIDS. HIV-related thrombocytopenia (defined as a platelet count of < 50,000/μL without other known causes) is found in less than 10% of individuals and usually does not result in a bleeding diathesis.

C. AIDS: The criteria for diagnosis of AIDS have been defined by the CDC and comprise certain opportunistic infections and cancers, HIV-related encephalopathy, and HIV-induced wasting syndrome.

The most common opportunistic infections encountered are *Pneumocystis carinii* pneumonitis (which is the presenting illness in more than 60% of patients newly diagnosed with AIDS in developed countries); disseminated cryptococcosis; toxoplasmosis; mycobacterial disease (both *Mycobacterium avium* complex and tuberculosis); chronic, ulcerative, recurrent herpes simplex virus infection; disseminated cytomegalovirus infection; and histoplasmosis (Table 55–5). Patients with AIDS also have a higher incidence of *Salmonella* bacteremia, staphylococcal infections, and pneumococcal pneumonia. Children with AIDS may develop opportunistic infections such as *P carinii* pneumonia, but they have a higher incidence of lymphocytic interstitial pneumonitis and recurrent bacterial infections than adults do.

The most common cancer diagnosed in AIDS patients is Kaposi's sarcoma, a neoplasm or neoplasm-like disease involving endothelia and mesenchymal stroma. Once common, this tumor is now less frequently seen as a presenting illness. The reason for this is obscure. Late in the course of immune dysfunction, high-grade B cell lymphomas are encountered; these are generally resistant to therapy.

The CDC has recently revised the definition of AIDS to include HIV-related encephalopathy and HIV wasting syndrome and a broader range of AIDS-indicative diseases in individuals who have laboratory evidence of HIV infection. Thus, the oc-

casional patients who die of HIV-related dementia without related opportunistic infections are now classified as having AIDS.

Laboratory Diagnosis
A. Serology:
1. Seroconversion–During the primary illness, antibodies to HIV are not detected in the serum; they generally appear 2–12 weeks after the onset of illness. In rare instances, antibodies may remain undetectable for as long as 3 years following infection, although HIV may be demonstrated by viral culture or DNA amplification techniques such as the polymerase chain reaction (PCR). IgM antibodies, detected by immunofluorescence, generally precede IgG antibody detection by Western immunoblot. During seroconversion, antibodies directed against the various viral proteins do not develop simultaneously. Those directed against HIV p24 (core) and gp41 (transmembrane) proteins can be detected before those directed at the *pol* gene products on Western blot. There may be a "window" period during which time the screening enzyme-linked immunosorbent assay (ELISA) is negative but antibodies can be demonstrated by Western blot. HIV antigenemia (predominantly HIV p24, measured by enzyme immunoassay) usually precedes seroconversion. Following the appearance of antibodies (specifically anti-HIV p24), HIV p24 antigen levels decline. They may later reappear, coincident with a loss of anti-HIV p24 antibody (Fig 55–3). Whereas about 70% of AIDS patients have detectable HIV antigen in their sera, the HIV antigen test is positive in fewer than 20% of asymptomatic individuals. African pa-

Table 55–5. Common opportunistic infections encountered in AIDS patients.

Pneumocystis carinii pneumonia
Toxoplasmosis
Mycobacterium avium complex disease
Disseminated *Mycobacterium tuberculosis* infection
Persistent, ulcerative herpes simplex virus infection
Disseminated cytomegalovirus infection

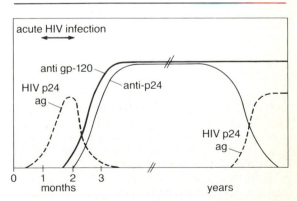

Figure 55–3. Common pattern of serologic response following HIV infection. P24 antigen (P24 ag) may be first detected during the acute HIV mononucleosis phase of infection. The initial antibody to appear in the serum is usually that directed against the HIV envelope glycoprotein gp120 (anti-gp120), and its level remains elevated throughout the course of the disease. Antibody directed against the core protein (anti-p24) appears in the serum coincident with the decline in p24 antigen levels.

tients rarely have detectable HIV antigenemia, perhaps owing to higher antibody levels. Persistence of HIV antigen following the acute infection in an asymptomatic carrier is probably associated with a more rapid progression to symptomatic disease.

2. Screening for HIV–ELISA is the basic screening test currently used to detect antibodies to HIV. Purified whole virus is disrupted, and viral proteins are then immobilized on plastic beads or multiwell trays. Test serum containing antibodies to HIV will bind to these viral proteins. An enzyme-linked anti-human antibody added to the reaction will bind to the complex and be detected calorimetrically. The ELISA is both highly sensitive (> 99%) and highly specific (> 99% in high-risk populations).

3. Confirmatory Tests–A repeatedly reactive ELISA should be confirmed by either a Western blot or, less commonly, a radioimmune precipitation assay, immunofluorescence assay, or ELISA with recombinant antigens. Because of its high sensitivity, a negative ELISA does not usually warrant confirmatory testing. The Western blot detects specific antibodies directed against the various HIV proteins. Purified viral proteins are run on a polyacrylamide gel, transferred to a nitrocellulose membrane, and then reacted with the test serum. Antibodies to HIV present in the serum will bind to the specific viral protein (Fig 55–4).

B. Neonatal Diagnosis: Neonates with HIV infection pose a difficult serodiagnostic problem because maternal IgG antibody crosses the placenta. Thus, the infant will passively acquire anti-HIV antibody, which may persist for up to 15 months. The predictive value of specific IgM antibodies in the diagnosis of neonatal and perinatal infection awaits clarification. Culture of the virus from peripheral blood or tissue or demonstration of HIV antigen is therefore necessary to be confident of the diagnosis of HIV infection in asymptomatic infants born to HIV-infected mothers. The PCR, which amplifies HIV genome present in cells or serum, may provide a useful adjunct to diagnosis in the future.

Immunologic Findings

A. CD4 Lymphocyte Depletion: The immunologic hallmark of AIDS is a defect in cell-mediated immunity, characteristically associated with a decrease in the number and function of the CD4 T lymphocytes. The decrease in CD4 lymphocytes is due initially to a selective loss of the Leu 8$^+$ (TQ$^+$) subset or suppressor-inducer subset. Later in the disease the Leu 8$^-$ subset, which subserves the helper function for antigen-driven antibody responses, is also decreased. In individuals with advanced disease and opportunistic infections, the total CD4 lymphocyte count is often less than 100/μL (the normal value being more than 400/μL). Persistently and markedly depressed CD4 lymphocyte counts are virtually diagnostic of HIV infection.

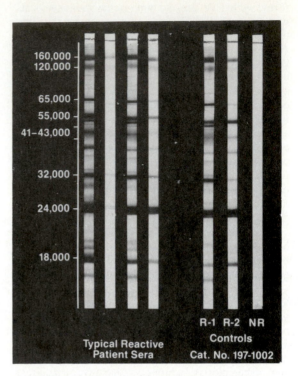

Figure 55–4. Western blot analysis. Reactive sera typically contain demonstrable antibodies to envelope proteins gp160, gp120, and gp41, as well as to core proteins p55 and p24 and to reverse transcriptase p32. Detection of antibody to p24 alone is insufficient to meet the diagnostic criteria for a positive Western blot and may be due to a nonspecific reaction. Alternatively, a reactive band at 24,000 may represent an early serologic response during seroconversion. (Photograph courtesy of Bio-Rad Laboratories, Richmond, Calif.)

There is a spectrum of CD4 cell numbers in all clinical stages of HIV infection: Some asymptomatic individuals have very low counts, whereas occasionally the values are normal in individuals with AIDS. Individuals who present with Kaposi's sarcoma frequently have higher CD4 cell counts than those who initially present with AIDS-defining opportunistic infections. This suggests that patients who present with opportunistic infections have more severe immunologic dysfunction than those with Kaposi's sarcoma. CD4 cell levels are of prognostic value: The risk of progression to AIDS in a given time interval increases as the CD4 count declines.

The CD4:CD8 ratio invariably becomes inverted primarily as a consequence of CD4 lymphocyte depletion. However, a variety of other conditions, including infection with EBV, hepatitis B virus, and cytomegalovirus (CMV) can cause inversion of the CD4:CD8 ratio, primarily owing to an increase in the CD8 subset. Thus, this ratio is of no diagnostic value.

B. Abnormal Delayed-Type Hypersensitivity Responses: Delayed-type hypersensitivity responses are usually decreased in HIV-infected subjects but are of little value in monitoring disease progression.

C. T Cell Proliferative Responses: The normal in vitro proliferative responses of CD4 T lymphocytes to soluble antigens (such as tetanus toxoid) and mitogens (such as concanavalin A, phytohemagglutinin, or pokeweed mitogen) are impaired in HIV-infected individuals, especially AIDS patients. This abnormality may be due to a selective loss of a subset of CD4 lymphocytes, to defective antigen presentation by monocyte-macrophages, or to direct viral suppression of CD4 lymphocyte function. Current evidence favors a functional defect of this cell population rather than an abnormality of antigen-presenting cells. Responses to mitogens tend to vary and are less severely impaired than responses to antigen. Antigen responses but not mitogen responses strictly require the interaction of the CD4 molecule on the surface of the lymphocyte with the class II MHC molecule. The HIV envelope glycoprotein (gp120) binds to the CD4 molecule, and its presence could interfere with the interaction with the class II MHC molecule, thus explaining why mitogen responses are less impaired than antigen responses.

D. Cytotoxic Lymphocyte Responses: Cells infected with HIV provide a target for lysis by the various types of cytotoxic cells, including MHC-restricted cytotoxic lymphocytes, MHC-nonrestricted NK cells, and lymphokine-activated cells. Cytotoxic T lymphocyte (CD8 or CD4) responses and NK cell activity are present but quantitatively defective in cells from HIV-infected individuals with ARC and AIDS. Although the number of NK cells is relatively normal when compared with uninfected controls, and binding of these cells to their target is unimpaired, their cytotoxic capacity is moderately diminished.

E. B Cell Responses:

(1) Polyclonal B cell activation resulting in hypergammaglobulinemia is commonly found in HIV-infected individuals, resulting predominantly in increases in serum IgG1, IgG3, and IgM levels. This spontaneous secretion of immunoglobulin by B cells is not always present, and in HIV-infected infants panhypogammaglobulinemia may occur.

(2) Autoantibodies directed against erythrocytes, platelets, lymphocytes, neutrophils, nuclear proteins, and myelin have been found in patients infected with HIV. In some instances these have been associated with disease (eg, HIV-associated thrombocytopenia).

(3) Antibody capable of neutralizing HIV in vitro is present in low titer in the sera of infected individuals. However, there is no evidence that this antibody has a protective role. Neutralizing antibody is directed against gp120 and possibly p24.

(4) B cell proliferative responses to T cell-independent specific B cell mitogens (such as formalinized *Staphylococcus aureus* Cowan strain 1) are impaired.

(5) Despite depression of helper T cell function and abnormalities of humoral immunity, HIV-infected individuals can often mount appropriate antibody responses to commonly used vaccines. However, a decrease in response is generally found as HIV disease progresses.

F. Monocyte-Macrophage Responses: The HIV-infected monocyte-macrophage is probably the major reservoir for HIV in vivo. There are conflicting data about the degree of monocyte-macrophage dysfunction and the specific functions that are altered as a result of HIV infection. It is likely, balancing the weight of current evidence, that phagocytosis, antigen presentation, and chemotaxis are moderately impaired. Infected macrophages produce an inhibitor of IL-1 termed contra-IL-1, which may contribute to the impairment of T cell proliferative responses observed in HIV-infected individuals (Table 55–6).

G. Other Immunologic Responses: Other abnormal immunologic parameters include decreased lymphokine production (in particular, interleukin-2 [IL-2] and gamma interferon), decreased expression of IL-2 receptors, and an increase in the level of circulating immune complexes. Elevated serum levels of β_2-microglobulin are of some prognostic importance in predicting progression to AIDS.

H. Hematologic Findings: Subjects with acute HIV mononucleosis generally have leukopenia with an atypical lymphocytosis. Transient thrombocytopenia occurs in some patients. With disease progression, the total leukocyte count falls, with an associated lymphopenia, reflecting depletion of CD4 lymphocytes. The hemoglobin and hematocrit decrease as a result of anemia due to chronic disease. Mild thrombocytopenia is common.

Differential Diagnosis

Acute HIV mononucleosis must be distinguished from infectious mononucleosis caused by EBV, CMV infection, and, less commonly, rubella, secondary syphilis, hepatitis B, and toxoplasmosis (Table 55–7). Once there is evidence of immunodefi-

Table 55–6. Potential role of macrophages in the pathogenesis of AIDS.

Act as target for HIV
Provide reservoir for HIV
Contribute to immune deficiency through abnormal function
  Defective phagocytosis
  Defective chemotaxis
  Defective antigen presentation
  Production of an interleukin-1 inhibitor
Contribute to T cell depletion through a cell fusion process[1]

[1]Shown in vitro only.

Table 55–7. Differential diagnosis of acute HIV infection.

EBV infectious mononucleosis
CMV infection
Rubella
Secondary syphilis
Hepatitis B
Toxoplasmosis

ciency, it should be ascertained that this is an acquired rather than a congenital defect and that there is no other underlying explanation for the clinical and immunologic manifestations, such as hematologic cancer or tissue transplantation. However, any individual with laboratory-confirmed HIV infection and a definitively diagnosed disease that meets the CDC criteria for AIDS is considered to have AIDS, regardless of the presence of other potential causes of immune deficiency.

Treatment

A. Life Cycle of HIV: The initial phase of the replicative cycle of HIV involves binding of specific epitopes of the CD4 molecule on the surface of the target cell to defined regions of gp120. Following this, HIV enters the cell and is uncoated. Viral RNA is then used as a template by reverse transcriptase to make a minus-strand DNA copy, thus forming an RNA–DNA hybrid. Soon thereafter, the RNA strand is degraded by the ribonuclease H activity of reverse transcriptase. A positive DNA strand is synthesized, and the linear double-stranded DNA molecule changes conformation to become circular. Some of this DNA migrates to the nucleus and subsequently becomes integrated into the cellular DNA. Further replication of HIV depends on poorly understood changes within the cell. Then, cellular RNA polymerases transcribe the viral DNA to form viral genomic RNA and messenger RNA, which directs the synthesis of viral proteins. These proteins undergo posttranslational protein cleavage and glycosylation. Within the cytoplasm the final stage of assembly of viral proteins occurs and is followed by the budding of the mature virion through the cell membrane, with simultaneous acquisition of envelope (Fig 55–5).

B. Antiretroviral Therapy: The complicated machinery used by HIV in its replicative cycle has provided many specific target sites for potential intervention (Table 55–8). Because reverse transcriptase is not normally present in human cells, selective inhibitors of this enzyme have been a major focus of drug development. Zidovudine (AZT) is a thymidine analogue that requires phosphorylation by host nucleoside kinases to the triphosphate derivative within the infected cell for it to be active. Once phosphorylated, the drug inhibits the virus-encoded reverse transcriptase enzyme, since it has about 100 times the affinity for this enzyme as it does for the

host DNA polymerase. Zidovudine further prevents HIV replication by becoming incorporated into the transcribed DNA strand and thus preventing further HIV DNA synthesis. In clinical trials, individuals treated with zidovudine have had lower mortality rates and less frequent opportunistic infections than those receiving placebo. During zidovudine therapy, CD4 lymphocytes initially increase in number but usually return to baseline levels within 6 months of the start of therapy. There has been a recent report of zidovudine resistance developing over a similar period, but the clinical significance of this observation is uncertain. Other reverse transcriptase inhibitors, such as the pyrophosphate analogue foscarnet, do not require cellular phosphorylation for activity and act directly on the enzyme. Agents acting at other sites in the replicative cycle are in preclinical or clinical trials.

C. Immunorestorative Therapy: Attempts to restore the defective immune system have to date generally been ineffective. Treatment with IL-2 has not been shown to alter the course of HIV infection; the alleged immune stimulator inosine pranobex (Isoprinosine) has been associated with only transitory immunologic benefit; bone marrow and peripheral blood lymphocyte transplantation is not regarded as useful, because the transplanted cells also become infected with HIV. It is possible that combinated therapy with an immunomodulatory agent together with one or more antiretroviral agents may be more effective than either alone. In certain patients with Kaposi's sarcoma, administration of high-dose alpha interferon has been beneficial. Interferon inducers such as the mismatched double-stranded RNA compound Ampligen are effective in vitro in inhibiting HIV replication. Early clinical trials with this drug suggested temporary clinical improvement with restoration of immune responses, but these studies have not been confirmed. Granulocyte-macrophage colony-stimulating factor (GM-CSF) has been used in clinical trials following in vitro reports of its antiviral efficacy. However, recent data suggest that in vitro, this compound may in fact increase viral replication within monocyte-macrophages. Clinical studies have not documented a striking augmentation

Table 55–8. Targets for antiretroviral therapy.

Target	Therapy
HIV binding and cell entry	Soluble recombinant CD4, dextran sulfate, castanospermine, heparin
Reverse transcription	Zidovudine, Foscarnet, HPA-23
Regulatory proteins	*tat* inhibitors
HIV translation and protein assembly	Ribavirin, protease inhibitors
Budding from cell	Interferons

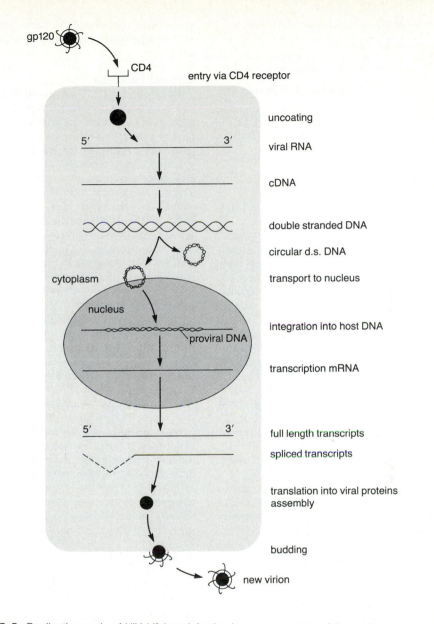

Figure 55–5. Replicative cycle of HIV. Lifelong infection is a consequence of the viral replicative cycle.

of viral replication. On the other hand, hematopoietic growth factors such as GM-CSF may be useful for treating cytopenias occurring in AIDS patients, whether they are due to drugs, opportunistic infections, or HIV itself.

Prevention

A. Vaccines: Although much information has accumulated regarding the biology of HIV, this has not provided even a promising candidate vaccine (Table 55–9). Strains of HIV vary in their nucleic acid sequence by up to 20% as a result of high-frequency point mutations that occur during the rep-

lication of the virus. This variation is most evident in the envelope region of HIV. Of interest, certain regions are conserved between different isolates (for example, the region of gp120 that interacts with CD4), and other regions of the gene are highly variable. Unfortunately, the major antigenic epitopes (and therefore, predictably, the major protective epitopes) are in the regions associated with the highest degree of strain-to-strain variation. This genomic diversity is one of the many major obstacles hampering vaccine development, as an effective vaccine should provide protection against all strains of HIV. Another impediment to vaccine development is the

Table 55–9. Obstacles to development of HIV vaccine.

Genomic diversity of HIV strains
Progression of infection despite vigorous immune response
Transmission of HIV in vivo by cell fusion as well as by cell-free virus
Unacceptability of attenuated or inactivated whole-virus vaccines
Failure of all protection studies in chimpanzees to date
Lack of a good animal model
Potential enhancement of HIV replication by neutralizing antibody

fact that HIV is spread from cell to cell via a fusion process as well as by cell-free virus.

Vaccines containing attenuated virus or inactivated whole virus would meet with serious ethical concerns because of difficulty in guaranteeing their safety. Recombinant HIV envelope glycoproteins expressed in a cell culture system (eg, mammalian cells, bacteria, or yeasts) and HIV genes inserted into an attenuated vector (eg, vaccinia virus) are currently undergoing trials in chimpanzees. Neutralizing antibodies have been produced to these viral proteins in vaccinated animals. Thus far, these vaccines have had minimal success in providing protection against subsequent challenge with strains of HIV. Because chimpanzees are not an ideal animal model for human HIV infection, and because of the shortage of supply of these animals, trial vaccination of humans is now under way. Other strategies in vaccine development include production of anti-idiotype vaccines and construction of synthetic peptides.

B. Education: The major thrust of strategies to prevent HIV infection lies in education of individuals about practicing safe sex, in which the transmission of bodily fluids (specifically semen, vaginal secretions, and blood) is prevented, and not sharing needles or syringes, or at least thoroughly washing these items with bleach if they must be shared.

CYTOMEGALOVIRUS

Major Immunologic Features

- CD8 lymphocyte numbers increase and CD4 lymphocyte numbers transiently decrease.
- Cell-mediated immunity is depressed.

General Considerations

Cytomegalovirus (CMV) is a member of the herpesvirus family, a group that includes the human pathogens EBV, herpes simplex virus types 1 and 2, varicella-zoster virus, and human herpesvirus type 6, as well as many animal pathogens. Similar to other herpesviruses, CMV is associated with persistent, latent, and recurrent infection, the last being due to reactivation of latent virus.

The prevalence of infection within a community varies with socioeconomic status, being as low as 40% in upper strata and approaching 100% in lower groups.

Clinical Features

Infection with CMV can result in a variety of clinical syndromes, depending partially on the immune state of the infected individual (Table 55–10). In healthy subjects, infection is usually subclinical, occasionally causing an infectious mononucleosis-like syndrome resembling that due to EBV or primary HIV infections (however, pharyngitis is unusual). There is a tendency to develop allergic skin rashes to antibiotics, similar to that observed during acute EBV infection. If infection is acquired in utero, following primary maternal infection, the infant may be born with cytomegalic inclusion disease (CID), with features of hepatosplenomegaly, microcephaly, chorioretinitis, thrombocytopenia, and jaundice. Although only about 5–10% of infants with prenatal infection are born with CID, another 2–5% develop abnormalities such as deafness, spasticity, intellectual retardation, and dental defects within the first 2 years of life. Asymptomatic perinatal infection may be acquired as a result of exposure to CMV in the birth canal or through breast-feeding.

Immunocompromised patients, such as those with AIDS or those being treated with immunosuppressive drugs, are prone to disseminated CMV infection. In this instance, the infection involves predominantly the retinas, gastrointestinal tract (especially the colon, esophagus, and liver), and lungs. Such individuals often have progressive disease, despite high levels of serum-neutralizing antibody. Organ transplant recipients develop generalized and occasionally fatal CMV disease more commonly following primary than reactivated infection.

Immunologic Findings

A. CMV Serology: IgM antibodies are produced following initial infection and generally persist for 3–4 months. IgG antibodies appear at the same time, peak about 2 or 3 months after infection, and persist for many years and often for life. However, complement-fixing IgG antibody levels may fluctuate and even disappear within a few years of infection. Reactivation of infection generally fails to produce an IgM response.

B. Cellular Immunity: Primary infection is fol-

Table 55–10. Clinical manifestations of CMV infection.

Prenatal infection
  Cytomegalic inclusion disease
Immunocompetent host
  Subclinical infection
  CMV mononucleosis
Immunocompromised host
  Disseminated CMV: retinitis, esophagitis, colitis, pneumonitis, other sites

lowed by activation of both MHC-restricted cyto-toxic CD8 T lymphocytes, whose function is to specifically destroy CMV-infected cells, and MHC-nonrestricted NK cells. Both the humoral and cellular responses that occur following infection develop relatively slowly. The cell-mediated response, specifically directed against CMV intermediate-early (IE) antigens, is the most important aspect of host defense. However, CMV infection results in a general impairment of cellular immunity, characterized by impaired blastogenic responses to nonspecific mitogens and specific CMV antigens, diminished cytotoxic ability, and elevation of the CD8 lymphocyte subset with a moderate but transient decrease in the number of CD4 lymphocytes. Thus, there is a delicately balanced relationship between the CMV-mediated immune dysfunction and the ability of the host to control the virologic response. This balance is in part temporal: Initially, viral replication and cell-mediated immunopathology occur unhindered, with the immune function being restored during convalescence. Furthermore, the underlying immune status of the infected individual is of major prognostic importance.

In the immunocompetent individual, specific defects in the cell-mediated immune response are restored within a few months following infection. However, seropositive individuals may intermittently excrete CMV for many years or perhaps for life, owing to low-grade chronic infection or reactivation of latent infection.

The immune response following primary CMV infection in transplant recipients is usually severely impaired; there is usually marked depression of cytotoxic T cell and NK cell responses, diminished antibody-dependent cellular cytotoxicity, depressed proliferative responses to CMV and nonspecific antigens and mitogens, and decrease or loss of delayed-hypersensitivity reactions. Although an IgM and IgG antibody response is usually detected, occasionally there may be failure to mount an antibody response following primary infection in these patients. Transplant recipients who were previously seropositive for CMV invariably undergo reactivation of latent virus following transplantation. Patients with AIDS who develop reactivation of latent CMV infection do not mount an IgM response.

The immaturity of the immune response in infants with congenital or perinatal infection results in chronic excretion of CMV in nasopharyngeal secretions and urine. Blastogenic responses of lymphocytes in response to CMV is impaired in these chronically infected children. This defect, the major feature of cell-mediated dysfunction in these children, is eventually restored coincident with cessation of viral excretion.

Treatment

There are 2 antiviral agents effective against CMV: foscarnet and gancyclovir. Treatment with these agents is limited to immunocompromised individuals. Combination therapy with gancyclovir plus high-dose intravenous immunoglobulin has been successful in treating interstitial pneumonitis due to CMV following allogeneic bone marrow transplantation.

EPSTEIN-BARR VIRUS

Major Immunologic Features

- B lymphocytes are target cells.
- There is atypical T cell lymphocytosis.
- Heterophil antibodies are produced.
- There is in vitro transformation of B lymphocytes.
- There is an active specific humoral immune response.

General Considerations

EBV is a member of the herpesvirus family and, as such, shares certain features with the other members, including the ability to establish persistent and latent infection. EBV can transform B lymphocytes and has clinically relevant oncogenic potential. Primary infection, which may be subclinical, results in a lifelong carrier state.

Pathogenesis

The virus initially replicates within the pharyngeal epithelium, with subsequent infection of B lymphocytes in subjacent lymphoid tissue. Circulating lymphocytes are responsible for generalized infection. Following the acute infection, EBV remains latent within the B lymphocyte population; these cells most probably provide a lifelong reservoir of the virus. Intermittent seeding of the pharyngeal epithelia, with low-level replication within these cells, allows potential transmission of infection to susceptible members of the community.

Clinical Features

In 1964, Epstein, Achong, and Barr described the presence of viral particles in cultured fibroblasts from tissue from a patient with Burkitt's lymphoma. Since then, this DNA virus has been causally associated with acute infectious mononucleosis, nasopharyngeal carcinoma, lymphomas in immunocompromised individuals, X-linked lymphoproliferative syndrome (Duncan's syndrome), and 2 HIV-related conditions, oral hairy leukoplakia and lymphocytic interstitial pneumonitis (Table 55–11). EBV has been proposed as the cause of the chronic fatigue syndrome. At this time there is substantial evidence against this causal association.

Infectious mononucleosis is the most common illness caused by EBV. This disease occurs most frequently in young adults. Typical features include fe-

Table 55–11. Diseases associated with EBV.

Infectious mononucleosis
Burkitt's lymphoma
Nasopharyngeal carcinoma
Lymphomas in immunocompromised host
X-linked lymphoproliferative syndrome
Oral hairy leukoplakia[1]
Lymphocytic interstitial pneumonitis[1]

[1]In HIV-infected individuals.

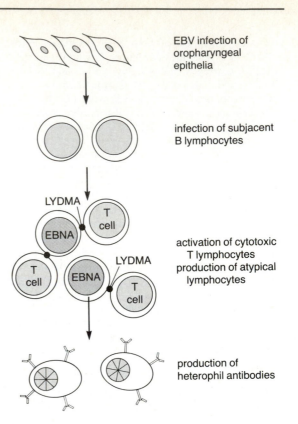

Figure 55–6. Pathogenesis of infectious mononucleosis. Following infection of oropharyngeal epithelia, EBV infection spreads to the subjacent B lymphocytes. Activation of cytotoxic T lymphocytes by EBV antigens results in the appearance of atypical lymphocytes in the peripheral blood.

ver; sore throat, often with exudate; generalized lymphadenopathy; and splenomegaly. Chemical hepatitis is present in most patients, and a few develop frank jaundice. About 10% of patients develop a macular rash; therapy with amoxicillin or ampicillin frequently produces an eruption.

Laboratory Diagnosis of Infectious Mononucleosis

Usually a mild leukopenia precedes the development of a leukocytosis (and absolute lymphocytosis) during the second to third week of illness. Up to 50–70% of the lymphocytes are atypical. IgM heterophil antibodies, which agglutinate sheep erythrocytes, are present. These antibodies must be distinguished from Forssman's antibodies present in patients with serum sickness, which also agglutinate sheep erythrocytes. Differentiation of the various heterophil antibodies is based on absorption techniques, with guinea pig kidney and bovine erythrocytes. EBV-associated heterophil antibodies are found in the sera of more than 90% of individuals with infectious mononucleosis. They persist for 3–6 months.

The pattern of antibody response to EBV initially reflects the synthesis of viral antigens involved in cell lysis, notably the early antigen (EA), viral capsid antigen (VCA), and EBV-induced membrane antigen (MA). VCA and MA are classified as late antigens, since their expression is suppressed in the presence of inhibitors of DNA synthesis. The appearance of antibody directed against the EBV nuclear antigen (EBNA) usually occurs weeks to months after infection. EBNA is present in all cells containing the viral genome, whether latently or productively infected (Fig. 55–6).

Immunologic Features of EBV Infection

The host immune response plays a critical role in restricting the primary infection. The importance of the immune system can be observed following infection of individuals with normal versus depressed immune function. Subjects with severe cellular immunodeficiency, such as renal transplant recipients, may develop fulminant mononucleosis or monoclonal B cell malignancy. The X-linked lymphoproliferative syndrome occurs in males who have an inherited immune defect that predisposes them to a severe, often fatal form of infectious mononucleosis. Uncontrolled EBV replication within the pharyngeal epithelia may be central to the development of EBV-associated nasopharyngeal carcinomas and lymphomas. By comparison, individuals with intact immune function can control the proliferative potential of EBV-infected lymphocytes and regulate replication within pharyngeal epithelia, thus preventing the emergence of lymphoproliferative disorders and cancer.

EBV infects B lymphocytes through binding to the C3d receptor on the cell surface. Following infection, large numbers of atypical lymphocytes appear within the circulation which are not, in fact, virus-infected B cells but result from polyclonal activation of cytotoxic/suppressor (CD8) cells (Fig 55–7). The importance of suppressor T cells in limiting primary infection has not been established, although these cells may be responsible for the generalized impairment of cell-mediated immunity associated with acute infection. Virus-specific cytotoxic T cells can be detected in peripheral blood early after infection. Of interest, these cells appear to specifically recog-

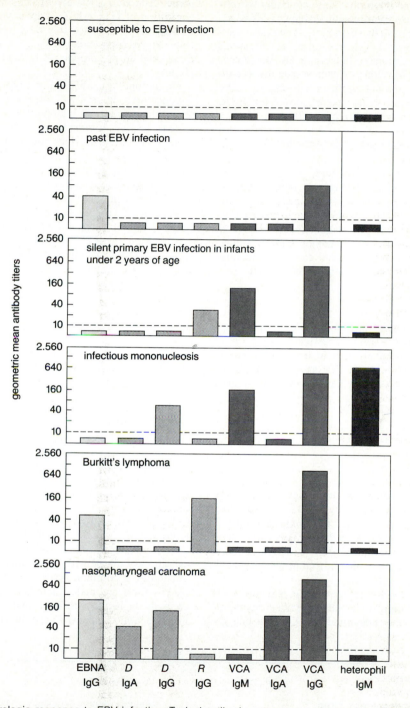

Figure 55–7. Serologic response to EBV infection. Typical antibody patterns are observed in different clinical conditions caused by EBV. Abbreviations: D, diffuse; R; restricted.

nize virus-infected B lymphocytes expressing **lymphocyte-determined membrane antigen (LYDMA),** without requiring MHC restriction. The true specificity of cytotoxic T cell responses in infectious mononucleosis remains to be completely elucidated. The mechanism for viral persistence may involve inhibition of the normal replicative cycle of EBV within B cells prior to the expression of LYDMA, the target antigen for cytotoxic T cells.

Differential Diagnosis of Infectious Mononucleosis

Streptococcal pharyngitis and, less commonly, diphtheria may resemble infectious mononucleosis. In individuals who present with jaundice, hepatitis A, B, non-A, non-B hepatitis, and delta hepatitis should be considered. The hematologic changes in infectious mononucleosis, together with serology, generally clarify the issue. Other causes of mononucleosislike illnesses are discussed under the HIV section in this chapter.

Treatment

Therapy for infectious mononucleosis is symptomatic. Although EBV is sensitive to acyclovir in vitro, the drug is of no clinical benefit. However, oral hairy leukoplakia (an HIV-associated EBV infection) responds clinically and virologically to acyclovir.

HUMAN T CELL LEUKEMIA VIRUS TYPE I (HTLV-I)

The field of human retrovirology is relatively young: The first human retrovirus was isolated from the T lymphocytes of 2 black men with aggressive T cell cancers in the USA in 1980. This virus, now called HTLV-I, has since been causatively linked with adult T cell leukemia and, more recently, with tropical spastic paraparesis.

Molecular studies have shown that leukemic cells from patients with adult T cell leukemia contain provirus, that is, virus integrated into the host cell genome. Although a variety of cells will support the replication of HTLV-I, T lymphocytes are the preferential target cells for this virus. HTLV-I-infected cells express high levels of IL-2 receptors; however, these cells do not produce IL-2, and IL-2 mRNA is absent.

On morphology, HTLV-I is a type C retrovirus of the oncovirus subfamily (Table 55–1). This virus can transform normal T lymphocytes, allowing these cells to become immortalized. This can occur even though this retrovirus does not possess an *onc* gene. It is not clear by what mechanism HTLV-I transforms cells; integration of the provirus in proximity to the c-*myc* gene (a cellular *onc* gene) may result in subsequent expression of this gene.

Endemic HTLV-I infection exists in parts of the Caribbean region, Japan, and Africa. The modes of transmission of HTLV-I are virtually identical to those for HIV: via infected blood, through sexual contact, and from mother to child. There is no direct evidence for transplacental transmission of HTLV-I; however, transmission to the infant commonly occurs via the mother's milk, analogous to transmission of bovine leukemia virus.

HUMAN HERPESVIRUS TYPE 6 (HHV-6)

The T lymphotropic HHV-6 is the most recent addition to the human herpesvirus family. Although this virus replicates primarily in T cells, the virus was initially called "human B lymphotropic virus (HBLV)" because it was isolated from B cells of 6 individuals with lymphoproliferative disorders. Molecular studies indicate that HBLV and HHV-6 are different strains of the same human herpesvirus. Cells infected with HHV-6 develop nuclear and cytoplasmic inclusions, with electron-microscopic features typical of other herpesviruses. HHV-6 has been causally associated with exanthema subitum (roseola infantum), a common disease of infancy characterized by fever and rash. There is a high prevalence of antibody in healthy children and adults, indicating that infection is acquired early in life.

REFERENCES

Human Immunodeficiency Virus

Centers for Disease Control: Revision of the CDC surveillance case definition for acquired immunodeficiency syndrome. *MMWR* 1987;**36(Suppl):**1S.

Haseltine WA: Replication and pathogenesis of the AIDS virus. *J AIDS* 1988;**1:**217.

Ho DD, Pomerantz RJ, Kaplan JC: Pathogenesis of infection with human immunodeficiency virus. *N Engl J Med* 1987;**317:**278.

Lane HC, Fauci AS: Immunologic abnormalities in the acquired immunodeficiency syndrome. *Annu Rev Immunol* 1985;**3:**477.

Mitsuya H, Broder S: Strategies for antiviral therapy in AIDS. *Nature* 1987;**325:**773.

Oberg B: Antiviral therapy. *J AIDS* 1988;**1:**257.

Pahwa S: Human immunodeficiency virus in children: Nature of immunodeficiency, clinical spectrum and management. *Pediatr Infect Dis J* (May 7) 1988; **(Suppl):**S61.

Seligmann M et al: Immunology of human immunodeficiency virus infection and the acquired immunodeficiency syndrome. An update. *Ann Intern Med* 1987;**107**:234.

Spickett GP, Dalgleish AG: Cellular immunology of HIV-infection. *Clin Exp Immunol* 1988;**71**:1.

Tindall B et al: Primary HIV infection: Clinical and serological aspects. In: *Infectious Diseases Clinics of North America: Medical Management of AIDS*. Vol 2. Moellering RC, Sande MA, Volberding PA (editors). Saunders, 1988.

Cytomegalovirus

Onorato IM et al: Epidemiology of cytomegalovirus infections: Recommendations for prevention and control. *Rev Infect Dis* 1985;**7**:479.

Stagno S et al: Congenital and perinatal cytomegalovirus infections: Clinical characteristics and pathogenic factors. Pages 65–85 In: *CMV: Pathogenesis and Prevention of Human Infection. Birth Defects: Original Article Series*. Vol 20, no. 1. Plotkin SA et al (editors). March of Dimes Birth Defects Foundation, 1984.

Epstein-Barr Virus

Rickinson AB: Cellular immunological responses to EBV infection. In: *The Epstein-Barr Virus: Recent Advances*. Epstein MA, Achong BG (editors). Wiley, 1986.

Human T Lymphotropic Virus Type I

Minamoto GY et al: Infection with human T cell leukemia virus type I in patients with leukemia. *N Engl J Med* 1988;**318**:219.

Viola MV: Human T cell virus. *Clin Microbiol Newsl* 1984;**6**:1. [Entire issue.]

Human Herpesvirus Type 6

Niederman JC, et al: Clinical and serological features of human herpesvirus-6 infection in three adults. *Lancet* 1988;**2**:817.

56

Opportunistic Infections in the Compromised Host

Lowell S. Young, MD

"Compromised host" is a term that refers to a patient who either has an underlying immunologic defect which predisposes to infection or is being treated with medication or therapy (eg, radiation) which impairs host resistance to infection. Mechanisms responsible for immunodeficiency are discussed in Chapter 23. Typical examples of patients with compromised host defenses are those who have a hematologic cancer, those who are being treated with pharmacologic doses of corticosteroids, or those who have had organ transplants and are receiving immunosuppressants. The immunosuppression that accompanies many forms of treatment has created a large and growing population of patients who must be considered immunocompromised (see Chapter 61).

The term "opportunistic" relates to the ability of organisms of relatively low virulence to cause disease in the setting of altered immunity. Most of these microorganisms are part of the human normal gastrointestinal or skin flora or are usually harmless components of the environment. More virulent organisms such as staphylococci or pneumococci (see Chapter 50), which cause infection even in normal hosts, can cause as serious or even more serious clinical syndromes of infection in the setting of impaired host resistance.

HOST DEFECTS PREDISPOSING TO INFECTION

Mechanical barriers to microorganisms play an important role in limiting the access of potentially invasive organisms to the host. These are nonspecific barriers and represent a first line of defense. Beyond these barriers are the components of host defense, which are summarized in Table 56–1. Specific immunity is the functional effect of antibodies or cell-mediated immune responses. Mobile (eg, neutrophils) or fixed (eg, Kupffer's cells) phagocytes function more efficiently after antibody binding to microorganisms, a process known as opsonization. Table 56–1 summarizes the important host defenses and shows that certain forms of therapy, usually drugs or radiation, may result in defects that mimic those present in disease states.

Table 56–1 also suggests typical infecting pathogens that may complicate disease states. These associations are by no means absolute, but summarize patterns that have been repeatedly observed in such patients. For instance, mycobacterial, pneumocystic, and cryptococcal infections are those against which the bulwark of host defense is considered to be the cell-mediated immune system. These opportunistic infections do not occur in the typical patient with acute myelocytic leukemia, a disease characterized by a defect in the absolute number of circulating neutrophils. Patients with leukemia are more typically prone to infections caused by aerobic gram-negative bacteria and staphylococci (so-called "pyogenic" bacteria). Thus, gram-negative bacillary infections are less common in patients with acquired immunodeficiency syndrome (AIDS) or Hodgkin's disease than in those with leukemia, but the associations are not absolute. Noteworthy is that medical treatment, such as immunosuppressive therapy, can blur these associations. Radiation that results in pan-

Table 56–1. Impaired host defenses, therapy mimicking disease states, and infectious complications.

Host Defense Element	Disease State	Therapy Mimicking Disease State	Infectious Complications
Polymorphonuclear neutrophil	Acute myelocytic leukemia	Cyclophosphamide, cytarabine	Staphylococci, gram-negative bacteria, *Aspergillus* spp, *Candida* spp
Monocyte-macrophage, lymphocyte	Hodgkin's disease, AIDS	Corticosteroids, cyclosporine, Antithymocyte globulin	Mycobacteria, *Nocardia* spp, *Pneumocystis* spp, *Candida* spp
Circulating antibody	Multiple myeloma, chronic lymphatic leukemia	Corticosteroids, antimetabolites	Pneumococci, other encapsulated bacteria

cytopenia can cause functional defects or a reduction in the number of circulating neutrophils and thus predisposes to acute bacterial infection. Deficiencies in specific antibodies are common in chronic lymphatic leukemia and multiple myeloma. Impaired synthesis of antibodies results in less efficient opsonization and impaired clearance of microorganisms.

APPROACH TO THE IMMUNOCOMPROMISED PATIENT

Although an underlying disease may suggest an association with an opportunistic pathogen, the converse is also true. Detection of *Pneumocystis carinii* in lung sections or pulmonary secretions suggests a disorder such as lymphoma or AIDS. What these introductory concepts have emphasized is there are, indeed, 3 approaches to patients with opportunistic infection in the setting of compromised host defenses. One is the immunologic approach; this involves considering the nature of the defect that predisposes to infection. The second is the syndrome-oriented approach; this involves considering the presentation of a cluster of signs and symptoms (eg, meningitis, diarrhea, or pneumonia) and hence inferring the most likely causative organisms in the process known as differential diagnosis. Finally, there is the organism-oriented approach; this involves considering the likely sites of infection and the type of immunologic defect when a specific pathogen is isolated from body fluids like blood. The clinician should integrate these 3 approaches in diagnosing and treating the patient with suspected opportunistic infection.

DISEASE ASSOCIATIONS

Table 56–1 suggests specific host defects that are associated with opportunistic infection. There are additional patterns derived from clinical experience. These are discussed below.

Leukemia & Lymphoma
These diseases (see Chapter 48) often represent the more dramatic examples of compromised host defense. Patients with acute leukemia, by virtue of their functional neutropenia, are at risk of developing precipitous, overwhelming opportunistic bacterial and fungal infection. The same is true of recipients of bone marrow transplants who are treated with immunosuppressants. As soon as neutrophil function is reconstituted, (circulating cells $\geq$ 500/mL), serious infections may abate.

Splenectomy
It has long been recognized that the spleen serves an important function, both as a site of antibody synthesis and as a reservoir of phagocytic cells capable of filtering out organisms that are circulating in the bloodstream. Splenectomized patients are particularly prone to infections caused by *Streptococcus pneumoniae*, *Haemophilus influenzae*, meningococci, and staphylococci.

Sickle Cell Anemia
This disorder has been associated with pneumococcal sepsis, meningitis, and *Salmonella* osteomyelitis.

Diabetes Mellitus
Diabetes (see Chapter 37) has been clinically associated with increased susceptibility to infection, but the specific mechanisms are multifactorial. At high blood glucose concentrations (high osmolarity) and during ketoacidosis, phagocytic and bactericidal activity is reduced. A leukocyte chemotactic defect has been reported at elevated blood glucose levels.

Chronic renal failure
Decreased movement of neutrophils rather than impaired killing has been reported to occur in this condition.

Alcoholism & Hepatic Cirrhosis
In liver disease, the role of the liver as filter for microorganisms may be impaired and organisms can "bypass" this filter. Antibody responses are normal, but leukocyte mobilization may be impaired. Alcohol has a direct inhibitory effect on leukocyte proliferation.

Rheumatic Diseases
Complement deficiencies have been reported to occur in systemic lupus erythematosus (see Chapter 36). Circulating immune complexes present in hypersensitivity states per se have been postulated to impair particle clearance in vivo. Some rheumatoid disorders are associated with neutropenia and lymphopenia.

Hypocomplementemia
This has also been postulated to be a factor in increased susceptibility to infection (see Chapter 28). Low complement levels (particularly of the terminal lytic components) have been associated with meningococcal disease.

Infections
In certain immunodeficiency disorders, amplification of infections may in fact be related to factors elaborated by the organisms themselves. Such factors are the production of toxins or the ability to secrete factors that enhance intracellular survival even within host tissues.

APPROPRIATE DIAGNOSIS

A high index of suspicion for unusual pathogens and an appreciation of the causes of a specific clinical syndrome form the cornerstone of the clinical approach to the immunocompromised patient. It is important that appropriate cultures of all body fluids or sites suspected of being infected are taken prior to the initiation of treatment. Proper diagnosis may involve invasive studies, such as lumbar puncture and lung biopsy, and noninvasive imaging, such as magnetic resonance imaging or radionuclide scans. Table 56–2 is a summary of the clinical syndromes and the organisms that should be suspected in specific settings.

A useful clinical approach is to work backward from the clinical presentation to the organisms that have been associated with infections in specific body sites and in patients with specific immunologic defects. For instance, central nervous system infection in patients with impaired cellular immunity is most likely to be due to listerias or cryptococci. In patients with leukemia or neutropenia, infection that spreads by vascular routes and is caused by pseudomonads or staphylococci is relatively more common.

DIAGNOSTIC TESTS

Although treatment will clearly have to be initiated in the acute stages of any opportunistic infection, immunologic screening tests may be of some use in determining the nature of the underlying defect when an unusual infection appears (see Chapters 18, 19, and 22). As mentioned above, patients with known defects in immune function are prone to the types of infections summarized in Table 56–1.

Conversely, the question may arise at the bedside about the potential underlying defect in a patient with an unusual infection. The tests that are summarized in Table 56–3 may not be available in some medical centers. Some, such as quantitation of total antibody classes, total and differential leukocyte counts, and lymphocyte subsets, may be used as initial screening procedures to ascertain immunologic defects. More sophisticated tests are necessary in certain circumstances to elucidate the exact mechanism of the defect in host defense. This is particularly true in the phagocyte disorders, in which a variety of specific enzymatic defects exist. Screening for some of the neutrophil disorders is possible by using the Nitro Blue Tetrazolium dye test or other measures of oxidative killing.

TREATMENT

The specifics of treatments of opportunistic infection are clearly beyond the scope of this chapter. Currently, a wide variety of broad-spectrum antibacterial agents are available, and this is the area in which the greatest progress has been made. Treatment of fulminating bacterial infections with broad-spectrum antibiotics has resulted in a significant decrease in mortality and morbidity rates, particularly

Table 56–2. Infectious syndromes and differential diagnoses.

Syndrome	Potential Causative Agent			
	Bacteria	**Fungi**	**Viruses**	**Parasites**
Fever, suspected septicemia, skin lesions	*Staphylococcus aureus,* gram-negative bacilli, *Nocardia* spp	*Candida* spp, *Aspergillus* spp, *Cryptococcus* spp, *Trichosporon* spp, zygomycetes	Herpes simplex virus	(May be significant in tropics)
Central nervous system infection	*Listeria* spp, *Nocardia* spp, *Staphylococcus aureus, Pseudomonas aeruginosa, Mycobacterium tuberculosis*	Cryptococcus spp, Aspergillus spp, zygomycetes, *Candida* spp	Varicella-zoster virus, herpes simplex virus, human immuno-deficiency virus	*Strongyloides* spp
Pulmonary infection	Gram-positive (pneumococci, staphylococci, nocardias, mycobacteria); gram-negative (enteric bacilli, legionellas, pseudomonads)	*Aspergillus* spp, *Coccidioides* spp, *Histoplasma* spp, *Petriellidium* spp, *Cryptococcus* spp, *Candida* spp, *Pneumocystis* spp	Cytomegalovirus, adenovirus, herpes simplex virus, varicella-zoster virus	*Toxoplasma* spp, *Strongyloides* spp
Oroesophageal ulceration or Inflammation	Anaerobic bacteria, streptococci, gram-negative bacilli (especially pseudomonads)	*Candida* spp, *Aspergillus* spp, zygomycetes, *Histoplasma* spp	Herpes simplex virus, cytomegalovirus	
Diarrhea	*Clostridium difficile, Salmonella* spp, *Shigella* spp, *Campylobacter* spp		Rotavirus, enteroviruses, Norwalk virus	*Giardia* spp, *Cryptosporidium* spp, *Entameba histolytica*

Table 56–3. Immunologic screening tests[1].

Immune System Component	Tests
Antibody response	Quantitative levels of IgG, IgM, IgA; Isohemagglutinin titers; Rubella titer, diphtheria-tetanus titer; response to *Haemophilus influenzae* type B or other nonattenuated or live vaccines.
Complement level	Total hemolytic complement; C3, C4, C5, factor B.
Phagocyte function	Leukocyte and differential cell count; Nitro Blue Tetrozolium (NBT) test; other tests for oxidative burst of phagocytosis.
Cell-mediated immunity	PMN chemotaxis; skin tests (*Candida albicans*, purified protein derivative, diphtheria-tetanus, mumps); total T cells and T cell subsets; mitogen responses.

[1]See Chapters 18, 19, and 22.

from infections due to gram-negative bacteria, in the past 20 years. Persistence of infection is often associated with persistence of the immunologic defect, but other factors, such as a foreign body (eg, an indwelling vascular catheter), must be considered. The treatment of parasitic, fungal, and viral infections has been more frustrating because there are fewer effective antimicrobial drugs for these organisms.

REVERSAL OF UNDERLYING IMMUNOLOGIC DEFECTS

Although antibiotics have definitely prolonged life and reduced morbidity, the ultimate ability to control and prevent such infections rests on the ability to correct the immunologic impairment. When the defect that predisposes to infection is caused by essential drug therapy, the clinical dilemma is obvious. Sometimes, reducing immunosuppression will have a major role in the control of an opportunistic infection. With some congenital neutrophil disorders, a variety of investigational therapies have been tried, eg, gamma interferon for chronic granulomatosis disease (see Chapter 27).

Realistically, neutrophil replacement has not been a practical approach, simply because of the enormous requirements for adequate quantities of leukocytes for transfusion. Investigative approaches for stimulating the neutrophil pool, such as the use of colony-stimulating factors, may ultimately prove useful. Immunoglobulin for replacement therapy in hypogammaglobulinemia has long been available, but more recent advances in the technology allow the delivery of large quantities of more specific antibodies that have been modified for intravenous infusion (see Chapter 24).

In the future, monoclonal antibodies may make it possible to deliver even larger amounts of specific antibodies for prophylaxis and treatment. Treatment of disorders of cell-mediated immunity has not yet responded to attempts at cell replacement (see Chapters 25–27). Theoretically, immune modulators such as interleukins or interferons could help reconstitute these important components of the immune system (see Chapters 57 and 62). More controversial approaches include plasma exchange for removal of immune complexes, toxins, and other factors.

PROPHYLAXIS

Since organisms that cause significant infection in the opportunistic host are often part of the normal flora or are abundant in the environment, attempts to suppress these potentially infectious agents have met with variable success. Isolation of the patient is controversial and expensive, but may in fact limit exposure of selected patients to some important disease-causing microorganisms (eg, *Legionella pneumophila* or *Aspergillus* spp). Organisms that are part of the normal flora are clearly more difficult to suppress or eliminate. Prophylactic antimicrobial drugs have a limited role, but they have been successful against *Pneumocystis* infection and gram-negative bacteremia in immunocompromised cancer patients. Prophylaxis of infection may be achieved by immunization or passive administration of antibodies.

REFERENCES

EORTC International Antimicrobial Therapy Cooperative Group: Ceftazidime combined with a short or long course of amikacin for empirical therapy of gram-negative bacteremia in cancer patients with granulocytopenia. *N Engl J Med* 1987;**317**:1692.

Gallin JI, Fauci AS (editors): *Advances in Host Defense Mechanisms.* Raven Press, 1985.

Pizzo PA et al: Empiric antibiotic and antifungal therapy for cancer patients with prolonged fever or granulocytopenia. *Am J Med* 1982;**72**:101.

Ross SC, Densen P: Complement deficiency states and infection: Epidemiology, pathogenesis and consequences of neisserial and other infections in an immune deficiency. *Medicine* 1984;**63**:243.

Rubin RH, Young LS: *Clinical Approach to Infection in the Compromised Host,* 2nd ed. Plenum Press, 1988.

Young LS: Nosocomial infections in the immunocompromised adult. *Am J Med* 1981;**70**:398.

Section IV.
Immunologic Therapy

Approaches to Immune Response Modulation

57

William Seaman, MD

The chapters in Section IV address clinical methods for altering the immune response and its consequences. This topic requires an understanding of the normal mechanisms for the regulation of immunity, which are reviewed in detail in Section I and are briefly summarized here as an introduction to considerations of therapy.

NORMAL MECHANISMS FOR IMMUNE RESPONSE REGULATION

The immune system is self-regulatory. The response to antigen is specific and finite. If the antigen is removed, the immune response declines, but it establishes "memory" for itself, so that subsequent exposure to the same antigen triggers a more vigorous immune response. Normally, there is no response to self antigens; each individual has immunologic "tolerance" to his or her own antigens.

Fig 57–1 presents a simplified view of the cellular requirements for the normal induction of antibody by most antigens. Antibody is produced by **B lymphocytes** (B cells) and plasma cells. The primary signal for antibody production is recognition of the antigen by cell surface immunoglobulin (IgM or IgD) receptors on the B cell membranes. The cell surface immunoglobulin can bind to antigen that is free in solution; that is, the antigen does not have to be attached to another cell.

The response of B cells to specific antigen can be mimicked in vitro by anti-IgM or anti-IgD antibody; such antibodies also bind to surface immunoglobulins. They thereby stimulate resting B cells (B cells in G_0) to increase their cytoplasmic volume, to enter the early G_1 phase of cell cycling, and to become more sensitive to other signals that are required for further activation of the B cells.

The "secondary" signals that promote full B cell activation include a variety of molecules produced

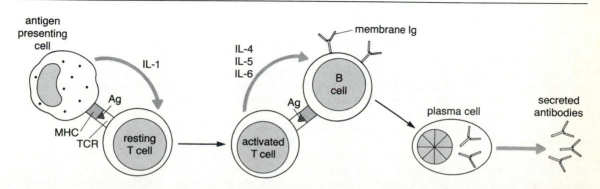

Figure 57–1. Cellular pathways for the humoral immune response to T cell-dependent antigens. Resting helper T cells respond to antigen presented by specialized APC (usually macrophages). Antigen (Ag) is recognized by T cells in the context of MHC antigens. T cells activated by this pathway can then stimulate B cells to produce antibody. The interaction between T cells and B cells also involves recognition by T cells of antigen that is associated with MHC antigens.

by **T lymphocytes** (T cells), including interleukin-4 (IL-4), IL-5, and IL-6. These signals are provided when the activated T cell recognizes antigen on the surface of the B cell. Unlike B cells, T cells do not respond to antigen that is free in solution. Instead, they respond to antigen on B cells or **antigen-presenting cells** (APC) when the antigens or antigen fragments are bound to molecules of the class II major histocompatibility complex (MHC) on the cell surface. These include the HLA-DP, HLA-DQ, and HLA-DR antigens.

A single T cell can provide IL-4, IL-5, and IL-6. The T cells that produce these interleukins express the surface marker **CD4.** The CD4 molecule binds to class II MHC molecules and appears to play a role in promoting the T cell response to antigens that are bound to class II MHC antigens.

There are at least 2 major subsets of CD4 T cells. One makes factors that primarily promote B cell activation, including IL-4, IL-5, and IL-6. The other primarily makes factors, such as IL-2 and gamma interferon, whose effects include the activation of other T cells. Thus, CD4 cells can provide "help" for both humoral immunity (B cells) and cellular immunity (T cells) and are therefore sometimes called helper T cells. CD4 T cells normally make up about 60–70% of circulating T cells.

Most of the remaining T cells express CD8. CD8 T cells, like CD4 T cells, respond to antigen only when it is bound to MHC, but CD8 T cells respond to antigen that is bound to class I MHC. These include the HLA-A, HLA-B, and HLA-C antigen or molecules. CD8 T cells do not provide help for B cell activation. They include cells that can promote T cell activation, but they also include cytotoxic T cells and cells that actively suppress immunity (possibly by killing other immune cells). CD8 T cells are therefore sometimes called cytotoxic/suppressor T cells. CD8 T cells are not shown in Fig 57–1, but they present another possible target for immunoregulation.

For CD4 T cells to provide the signals for B cell activation, they must themselves first be activated by responding to antigen on specialized APC, usually macrophages (Fig 57–1). The T cells recognize antigen on APC in the same manner as they do on B cells; they respond only to antigen that is associated with class II MHC. Macrophages and other specialized APC, however, not only present antigen but also provide stimuli, particularly IL-1, that are required to activate resting T cells. Thus, the recognition of antigen by T cells, like B cells, is itself not sufficient to stimulate the full activation of resting cells. Instead, "secondary" activation signals are required. Once the T cell is activated, it can respond to antigen on any cell, provided that the cell expresses class II MHC and presents the antigen in association with class II MHC. Moreover, just as the recognition of antigen by B cells can be mimicked

by anti-IgM or anti-IgD antibody, the recognition of antigen by T cells can be mimicked by antibodies to the T cell antigen receptor or by anti-CD3 antibodies.

IMMUNOMODULATION

Mechanisms for immunomodulation could be directed at any of the cells in the pathway outlined in Fig 57–1. They could be directed at B cells, T cells, or APC. Mechanisms that specifically recognize antigens and that attempt antigen-specific immune regulation would involve B cells or T cells, or both. Because T cells are central to the regulation of both humoral and cellular immunity, they are a central target for antigen-specific immunomodulation.

Attempts at immunomodulation have recently focused in particular on the interleukins, which provide activation signals for cells of the immune system. Now that many of these interleukins have been produced by gene cloning, it is possible to obtain purified interleukins in quantities that permit their use in vivo, as discussed in Chapters 7 and 62. Combinations of interleukins are currently being used in clinical trials, as are combinations of interleukins with antimetabolites or tumor necrosis factors or both.

Because there are specific receptors on cell surfaces for most of the interleukins, it is also possible, when the receptors have been identified, to examine the effects of **monoclonal antibodies** directed against the receptors. Such antibodies may either mimic or inhibit the effects of the interleukin. The use of monoclonal antibodies against these and other molecules on the surface of lymphocytes is discussed further below.

With these cellular and molecular pathways in mind, approaches to immunomodulation can be further simplified by considering whether immunity is to be stimulated or suppressed. When immune stimulation is desired, it may be either antigen-specific or, for the treatment of generalized immune deficiency, nonspecific. When immune inhibition is desired, as in allergy, autoimmunity, or transplantation, the goal is virtually always antigen-specific immune suppression. Unfortunately, most of the currently available techniques for immune suppression are not antigen-specific.

Stimulation of Immunity to Known Antigens

Vaccination and other forms of immunization have been in use for more than 2 centuries in Western society and even longer in China. Immunization remains the most successful clinical approach to immunomodulation. The topic is addressed in detail in Chapter 58. Immunization may include the use of **adjuvants** to promote immunity. Some adjuvants affect the way in which antigen is presented. For example, the immune response is increased when protein antigens are precipitated by alum or are presented on the surface of liposomes (membrane-bound vesicles). Emulsification of antigens prolongs the duration of antigen presentation. Other adjuvants act on the host rather than on the antigen. The immunization of animals, for example, is potentiated by mixing the antigen with certain organic molecules obtained from bacteria. An example is muramyl dipeptide (N-acetylmuramyl-L-alanyl-D-isoglutamine [MDP]), a bacterial peptidoglycan. The effects of MDP, as with most adjuvants, are not fully understood. MDP stimulates macrophages but also appears to stimulate B cells directly. The effects of adjuvants, therefore, are not antigen-specific. Because they are administered together with antigen, however, they selectively promote the response to the antigen.

Stimulation of Immunity to Unknown (or All) Antigens

Adjuvants have been used experimentally to promote a generalized increase in immunity against unknown antigens. This has been attempted particularly in the treatment of cancer; for many cancers, there is compelling evidence that the immune system participates in host defense against the tumor cells, but the identity of the tumor-specific antigens has proved elusive. The results of this treatment have not been sufficiently successful to justify its widespread application for this purpose.

With an increase in our understanding of lymphocyte activation (Fig 57–1), it has recently been possible to consider the clinical use of cytokines that act as **secondary signals** for the activation of B cells or T cells. They themselves are not sufficient to activate B cells or T cells, but, instead, a combination of antigen and secondary signals is required. This offers the potential for antigen-specific immune stimulation even when the antigen is not known, by supplying or mimicking the secondary activation signals, which can activate only the cells that also recognize the antigen. This approach is discussed in Chapters 7 and 62. Most cytokines that provide secondary activation signals to B cells or T cells, or both, have more widespread and complex effects than are provided in the simplistic view given in Fig 57–1. Nonetheless, they may have significant effects on immunity, and a variety of clinical trials of cytokines are in progress.

A related approach to immune stimulation derives from in vitro studies of lymphocyte activation. Monoclonal antibodies to certain T cell surface molecules (eg, CD5 and CD28) potentiate the antigen-specific activation of T cells. Presumably, these T cell surface molecules normally serve as receptors for unknown physiologic activation signals, either soluble molecules or molecules on the surface of other cells, such as APC. Even though the physiologic activation signals are not identified, monoclonal antibodies directed against these T cell antigens might promote the T cell response to antigen in vivo by increasing the activation of T cells that encounter antigen but not other T cells. Of course, it would be necessary to use such antibodies in a manner that did not deplete the T cells. A possible approach to this issue, although largely speculative, is to design peptides that will have the same effect as the anti-T cell antibody.

It is also possible to provide activation signals for all T cells by treatment with monoclonal antibody to the T cell antigen receptor (TCR) or to the associated molecular complex, CD3. Anti-CD3 monoclonal antibody has been used extensively to deplete T cells in the treatment of allograft rejection. The administration of anti-CD3 antibody, however, causes systemic symptoms of fever, myalgias, and vasodilation, probably secondary to T cell activation and release of lymphokines by T cells that have not yet been destroyed. It is possible to administer antilymphocyte monoclonal antibody in a manner that does not deplete the target lymphocytes, by removing or inactivating the Fc portion of the antibody or by giving low doses of antibody. This offers the potential for using antibodies such as anti-CD3 as agents of immune potentiation rather than suppression. The use of anti-CD3 in low doses in mice has been shown to enhance tumor rejection. A variation on this approach is to make a "hybrid" antibody that recognizes both CD3 and tumor cells (Fig 57–2). The hybrid antibody could thus link T cells to tumor cells at the same time that the T cells are activated.

Another approach to cancer therapy that is not antigen-specific is the administration of a combina-

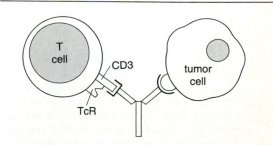

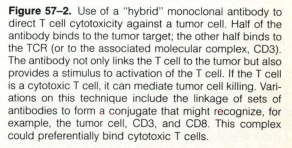

Figure 57–2. Use of a "hybrid" monoclonal antibody to direct T cell cytotoxicity against a tumor cell. Half of the antibody binds to the tumor target; the other half binds to the TCR (or to the associated molecular complex, CD3). The antibody not only links the T cell to the tumor but also provides a stimulus to activation of the T cell. If the T cell is a cytotoxic T cell, it can mediate tumor cell killing. Variations on this technique include the linkage of sets of antibodies to form a conjugate that might recognize, for example, the tumor cell, CD3, and CD8. This complex could preferentially bind cytotoxic T cells.

tion of IL-2 and **lymphokine-activated killer (LAK) cells,** which are lymphocytes that have been activated to kill a broad range of tumor cells by incubation in vitro with IL-2. Although LAK cells can be generated from T cells, the majority appear to derive from **natural killer (NK) cells.** NK cells are large granular lymphocytes that spontaneously kill a limited range of tumors. When NK cells are incubated with IL-2, they are stimulated to kill a much wider range of tumors. The mechanism by which LAK cells recognize the tumor cells is not known.

A recent refinement of this technique is to isolate lymphocytes that are infiltrating rejected tumors, expand these cells by culture in IL-2, and then administer these **tumor-infiltrating lymphocytes (TIL)** together with IL-2. TIL have greater specificity for the tumor than do LAK cells. The nature of TIL is not well-defined. As with the administration of LAK cells, the concomitant use of IL-2 causes severe and extensive toxicity. Whether the benefits of therapy outweigh these effects remains to be established. Regardless, it is clear that LAK cells preferentially kill tumor cells, and this ability to discriminate malignant from normal cells is of great interest in considering approaches to the therapy of cancer.

IMMUNE SUPPRESSION

Antigen-Specific Immune Suppression

The ability to induce antigen-specific immune suppression is the goal in the treatment of allergies, autoimmunity, and allograft rejection. This goal has proved elusive. Desensitization of patients who have allergic rhinitis, asthma, or anaphylaxis to insect venom appears to work primarily by shifting the immune response from IgE to IgG antibody and therefore can be considered a combination of immunosuppressive therapy and immunization (see Chapter 59).

It is theoretically possible to induce long-lasting antigen-specific immune tolerance in patients, since tolerance to self antigens is induced during maturation of the immune system and is sustained throughout life. It is now clear that self-tolerance is regulated at the level of T cells; although some self-reactive B cells appear to be eliminated during ontogeny, others survive. Moreover, somatic mutation of immunoglobulin genes offers the constant potential for developing autoantibodies. The TCR, on the other hand, undergoes little, if any, somatic mutation. Thus, deletion of autoreactive T cells, which occurs in the thymus during embryogenesis, is permanent. Although deletion of autoreactive T cells in the thymus is clearly an important mechanism for achieving self-tolerance, it cannot be the only one; not all self antigens can be presented in the thymus, and there is a need to regulate potentially autoreactive T cells that escape deletion in the thymus. There is strong evidence that self-tolerance is sustained in part by "suppressor" T cells, which inactivate or delete autoreactive T cells.

The ability of the immune system to sustain antigen-specific immune tolerance is thus as potent as the ability to respond to foreign antigens. If the mechanisms by which tolerance is induced and sustained can be established, it may be possible to manipulate or adapt this process therapeutically.

Even though we lack a full understanding of normal mechanisms for self-tolerance, there are a variety of methods for inducing antigen-specific immune tolerance in animals; some of these methods are being tested in humans. One of these is the use of monoclonal antibodies to CD4, on T cells. Treatment with anti-CD4 suppresses humoral and, to a lesser extent, cellular immunity in mice and has been used successfully to treat a variety of experimental autoimmune diseases. Interestingly, during treatment with anti-CD4 antibody, exposure to certain antigens, such as foreign immunoglobulin, is followed by long-lasting antigen-specific immune tolerance to the foreign antigen. This is sustained even after therapy with anti-CD4 antibody is stopped. Immune tolerance can also be induced by the use of $F(ab)'_2$ anti-CD4 antibody, which lacks the Fc fragment of immunoglobulin and therefore does not deplete the CD4 T cells.

In other animal studies, immune tolerance has been induced by coupling antigen to autologous (self) blood or spleen cells. The mechanism by which this approach permits the induction of immune tolerance is not known. In vitro, exposure to antigen in this manner renders the antigen-specific T cells unresponsive to future exposure to antigen, even antigen that is presented on macrophages.

Therapy Directed Against Antigen-Specific Cells

Attempts at induction of antigen-specific immune tolerance rely on manipulation of the immune system during exposure to antigen so that the antigen-specific response is shifted from immunity to tolerance. An alternative approach is to identify and eliminate the subset of antigen-responding cells. This approach could be directed either at B cells or at T cells. Most attempts to date have been directed at B cells. Different B cells recognizing different antigens have different surface immunoglobulins, which can be detected not only by their specificity for antigen but also by structural differences between the immunoglobulins themselves. These structural differences render each immunoglobulin antigenically distinct, so that it is possible to develop sera or monoclonal antibodies that react with a unique, very limited range of surface immunoglobulins. Such sera or monoclonal antibodies recognize **idiotypes,** or antigenic determinants on immunoglobulins, usually in the variable region, that distinguish one immunoglobulin from another. This offers the potential for using anti-idiotype monoclonal antibodies to delete a specific subset of B lymphocytes, thereby deleting a specific immune response.

This approach is hampered by the fact that most antigens are complex and immune responses are directed against many different sites (epitopes) on the same molecule. Despite this complexity, there are many examples, both in animals and in humans, in which the humoral immune response to antigen—even complex antigens—is highly restricted to immunoglobulins expressing a limited range of idiotypes. This is the case in autoimmune responses, notably the response to DNA in patients with systemic lupus erythematosus (SLE). In NZB/NZW mice, which develop a disease that closely resembles SLE, there is a similar restriction of the autoimmune response, and treatment with anti-idiotype monoclonal antibody has been used to retard the development of autoimmunity. Even when this treatment has depleted more than 90% of the autoimmune response, however, the effect is temporary; the autoimmune response returns, using antibodies that have a different idiotype. Thus, at least in this situation, the elasticity of the immune response prevents successful long-term therapy with anti-idiotype antibodies.

A similar approach has been used with limited success in the treatment of B cell cancers that express surface immunoglobulin. In this situation, monoclonal antibodies can be administered that selectively react with idiotypic determinants on the malignant cells. Although the first patient treated in this manner had a dramatic and long-term response to therapy, subsequent attempts at therapy have generally met with much less success, in part owing to the emergence of malignant cells that no longer express the idiotype.

Recently, it has been shown that antigen recognition by T lymphocytes may also rely on a limited range of TCR genes. Antibodies directed against the products of these genes may therefore identify subsets of T cells that are antigen-specific. In certain animal models for autoimmune disease, monoclonal antibodies to subsets of TCR have been used to prevent an autoimmune response. An example is the development of experimental allergic encephalitis in mice following immunization with myelin basic protein; this disease has been used as a model for multiple sclerosis. To date, however, a search for highly restricted TCR in human autoimmune disease has not proved successful.

Use of Monoclonal Antibodies Against MHC Antigens

Because T cells always recognize antigen in association with an MHC molecule expressed on the surface of the APC (referred to here as MHCM), another potential method for immune suppression is the blockade of antigen presentation by a specific MHCM. If presentation of an antigen were restricted to one MHCM, the immune response to this antigen would be inhibited while the immune response to antigens presented by another MHCM would not be inhibited. This might also work for certain autoantigens. One possible (but unproven) explanation for the association of certain autoimmune diseases with only one allele of the MHC system is the specific presentation of an antigen or autoantigen by that allele. Rheumatoid arthritis, for example, occurs more frequently in individuals expressing HLA-DR4. Possibly, blockade of HLA-DR4 would inhibit this disease, while the normal immune response could still be initiated by another MHCM, including the other allele of HLA-DR.

It has been difficult to test this hypothesis for practical reasons. In vitro, monoclonal antibodies to an MHCM can be used to block its ability to present antigen. In vivo, such monoclonal antibodies deplete the target cells. For monoclonal antibodies directed against class II MHC antigens, this includes all B cells as well as monocytes and macrophages. In addition, class II MHC antigens are expressed by certain nonlymphoid cells, including vascular endothelial cells. This may account for episodes of thrombosis in primates treated with monoclonal antibodies to class II MHC antigens.

Although it is possible to overcome this problem (for example, by the use of the $F(ab)'_2$ fragment of the monoclonal antibody, which does not deplete cells), the long-term effectiveness of monoclonal antibody therapy is reduced or eliminated by a host immune response to the monoclonal antibody itself. Until this can be overcome, it will be difficult to evaluate the potential for this approach to immune suppression.

Therapy Directed Against Activated (Antigen-Responsive) Cells

When lymphocytes respond to antigen, they alter the expression of molecules on their cell surface. Activated T cells, for example, increase the expression of the receptor for IL-2 (IL-2R). Selective elimination of antigen-responsive T cells, identified by the expression of IL-2R, would thus impair an ongoing immune response without destroying the potential for future immune responses to different antigens. Antibodies to IL-2R have been used with this intent, either unmodified or coupled to toxins (such as ricin) that facilitate cell destruction. Such therapy has been impaired by the host immune response to the monoclonal antibodies. Therefore, an alternative approach has been tried in which IL-2 itself, coupled to toxin, is used to identify and destroy activated T cells. The coupling of IL-2 to toxin, however, renders it immunogenic, preventing long-term therapy. If tolerance could be induced to an agent such as this, it might be possible to sustain therapy in a manner that would selectively impair an ongoing immune response.

Nonspecific Immune Suppression

Methods of immune suppression that are currently in clinical use are detailed in Chapter 61. Most methods of immune suppression are not antigen-specific. Rather, they suppress the entire immune response and often inflammatory responses as well. Their effects, moreover, are not usually limited to the immune system. Antimetabolites kill all dividing cells. Their effect on the immune system is only partially selective, in that antigen-responding cells are stimulated to proliferate. The use of cyclosporine provides a potent means of immune suppression, but its clinical use is limited by its toxicity, particularly its renal toxicity. In contrast, the reactivity of anti-lymphocyte antibodies, although not antigen-specific, is at least limited to cells of the immune system.

Despite their disadvantages, current methods for immune suppression are important in the treatment of autoimmunity and transplant rejection. It is hoped that more potent and more specific therapies will be available in the near future.

REFERENCES

General

Dean JH, Thurmond LM: Immunotoxicology: An overview. *Toxicol Pathol* 1988;**15**:265.

Fauci AS et al: NIH Conference. Immunomodulation in clinical medicine. *Ann Intern Med* 1987;**106**:421.

Hadden JW: Immunopharmocology. Immunomodulation and immunotherapy. *JAMA* 1987;**258**:3005.

Schrieber L: Immunomodulators. *Agents Actions* 1988; **24(Suppl)**:254.

Waldmann H: Immunosuppression with monoclonal antibodies: Some speculations about tolerance in the context of tissue grafting. *Transplant Proc* 1988; **20(Suppl 8)**:46.

Lymphocyte Surface Molecules Providing Secondary Activation Signals

Ledbetter JA et al: Antibody binding to CD5 (Tp67) and Tp44 T cell surface molecules: Effects on cyclic nucleotides, cytoplasmic free calcium, and cAMP-mediated suppression. *J Immunol* 1986;**137**:3299.

Lymphokine-Activated Killer (LAK) Cells & Tumor-Infiltrating Lymphocytes (TIL)

Rosenberg SA: Immunotherapy of patients with advanced cancer using interleukin-2 alone or in combination with lymphokine activated killer cells. *Important Adv Oncol* 1988(Review);217.

Rosenberg SA et al: Use of tumor-infiltrating lymphocytes and interleukin-2 in the immunotherapy of patients with metastatic melanoma. A preliminary report. *N Engl J Med* 1988;**319**:1676.

Therapy with Antibodies Directed Against Immunoglobulin Idiotypes

Hahn BH, Ebling FM: Suppression of NZB/NZW murine nephritis by administration of a syngeneic monoclonal antibody to DNA. Possible role of anti-idiotypic antibodies. *J Clin Invest* 1983;**71**:1728.

Miller RA et al: Treatment of B cell lymphoma with monoclonal anti-idiotypic antibody. *N Engl J Med* 1982; **306**:517.

Therapy with Antibodies Directed Against the T Cell Receptor or the Associated CD3 Complex

Acha-Orbea H et al: Limited heterogeneity of T cell receptors from lymphocytes mediating autoimmune encephalomyelitis allows specific immune intervention. *Cell* 1988;**54**:263.

Jaffers GJ et al: Monoclonal antibody therapy. Anti-idiotypic and non-anti-idiotypic antibodies to OKT3 arising despite intense immunosuppression. *Transplantation* 1986;**41**:572.

Norman DJ: An overview of the use of the monoclonal antibody OKT3 in renal transplantation. *Transplant Proc* 1988;**20**:1248.

Therapy with Antibodies to T Cell Activation Antigens

Diamantstein T et al: Interleukin 2 receptor—a target for immunosuppressive therapy. *Transplant Rev* 1987; **1**:177.

Preijers FW et al: Human T lymphocyte differentiation antigens as targets for immunotoxins or complement-mediated cytotoxicity. *Scand J Immunol* 1988; **28**:185.

Therapy with Antibodies to Class II Major Histocompatibility Antigens

McDevitt HO, Perry R, Steinman LA: Monoclonal anti-Ia antibody therapy in animal models of autoimmune disease. *Ciba Found Symp* 1987;**129**:184.

Immunization

58

Moses Grossman, MD, & Stephen N. Cohen, MD

The goal of immunization in any one individual is the prevention of disease. The goal of immunization of population groups is the eradication of disease. Immunization has accounted for some spectacular advances in health around the world. Childhood immunizations have been accepted as part of routine health care; in the USA, the federal government has financed the purchase of vaccines for the public sector and all states have passed legislation requiring proof of immunization as a condition for school entry. As a result, poliomyelitis, diphtheria, and tetanus have all but disappeared in developed nations; measles, rubella, and pertussis have become rare. Smallpox has been eradicated, and the World Health Organization has made poliomyelitis the next target for eradication.

HISTORICAL OVERVIEW

It has been recognized for centuries that individuals who recover from certain diseases are protected from recurrences. The moderately successful but hazardous introduction of small quantities of fluid from the pustules of smallpox into the skin of uninfected persons (variolation) was an effort to imitate this natural phenomenon. Jenner's introduction of vaccination with cowpox virus (1796) to protect against smallpox was the first documented use of a live, attenuated viral vaccine and the beginning of modern immunization. Koch demonstrated the specific bacterial cause of anthrax in 1876, and the causes of several common illnesses were rapidly identified thereafter. Attempts to develop immunizing agents followed (Table 58–1).

TYPES OF IMMUNIZATION

Immunization may be active, in which an antigen (usually a modified infectious agent or toxin) is ad-

ministered, resulting in an active production of immunity, or passive, in which antibody-containing serum or sensitized cells are administered to provide passive protection for the recipient.

ACTIVE IMMUNIZATION

Active immunization results in the production of antibodies directed against the infecting agent or its toxic products; it may also initiate cellular responses mediated by lymphocytes and macrophages. The most important protective antibodies include those that inactivate soluble toxic protein products of bacteria (antitoxins), facilitate phagocytosis and intracellular digestion of bacteria (opsonins), interact with the components of serum complement to damage the bacterial membrane and hence cause bacteriolysis (lysins), or prevent the proliferation of infectious virus (neutralizing antibodies). Newly appreciated are the antibodies that interact with components of the bacterial surface to prevent adhesion to mucosal surfaces (antiadhesins). Some antibodies may not be protective and, by "blocking" the reaction of protective antibodies with the pathogen, may actually depress the body's defenses.

Table 58–1. Historical milestones in immunization.

Variolation	1721
Vaccination	1795
Rabies vaccine	1885
Diphtheria toxoid	1925
Tetanus toxoid	1925
Pertussis vaccine	1925
Viral culture in chick embryo	1931
Yellow fever vaccine	1937
Influenza vaccine	1943
Viral tissue culture	1949
Poliovaccine, inactivated (Salk)	1954
Poliovaccine, live, attenuated (Sabin)	1956
Measles vaccine	1960
Tetanus immune globulin (human)	1962
Rubella vaccine	1966
Mumps vaccine	1967
Hepatitis B vaccine	1975
First recombinant vaccine (hepatitis B)	1986
Conjugate polysaccharide vaccine for *H influenzae* B	1988

Antigens react with antibodies in the bloodstream and extracellular fluid and at mucosal surfaces. Antibodies cannot readily reach intracellular sites of infection, where viral replication occurs. However, they are effective against many viral diseases in 2 ways: (1) by interacting with the virus before initial intracellular penetration occurs and (2) by preventing locally replicating virus from disseminating from the site of entry to an important target organ, as in the spread of poliovirus from the gastrointestinal tract to the central nervous system or of rabies virus from a puncture wound to peripheral neural tissue. Lymphocytes acting alone and antibody interacting with lymphoid or monocytic effector K cells may also recognize surface changes in virus-infected cells and destroy these infected "foreign" cells.

Types of Vaccines

The agent used for active immunization is loosely termed "antigen" or "vaccine." It may consist of live, attenuated viruses (measles virus) or bacteria (Bacillus Calmette-Guérin [BCG]) or killed microorganisms (*Vibrio cholerae*). It may also be an inactivated bacterial product (tetanus toxoid) or a specific single component of bacteria (polysaccharide of *Haemophilus influenzae*. It may be a recombinant DNA segment (hepatitis B virus), in which case it would be expressed in another living cell (yeasts, *Escherichia coli*). In each case, it usually contains—in addition to the desired antigen—other ingredients including other antigens, suspending fluids that may be complex and may contain protein ingredients of their own (tissue culture, egg yolk), preservatives, and adjuvants for enhanced immunogenicity (aluminum, protein conjugate). Undesirable reactions may occur not only to the antigen itself but also to these added components.

Active immunization with living organisms is generally superior to immunization with killed vaccines in inducing a long-lived immune response. A single dose of a live, attenuated virus vaccine often suffices for reliable immunization. Multiple immunizations are recommended for poliovirus in case intercurrent enteroviral infection or interference among 3 simultaneously administered virus types in the trivalent vaccine prevents completely successful primary immunization. The persistence of immunity to many viral infections may be explained by repeated natural reexposure to new cases in the community, the unusually large antigenic stimulus provided by infection with a living agent, or other mechanisms such as the persistence of latent virus.

All immunizing materials—live organisms in particular—must be properly stored to retain effectiveness. Serious failures of smallpox and measles immunization have resulted from inadequate refrigeration prior to use. Agents presently licensed for active immunization are listed in Table 58–2.

Factors in Immunization

Primary active immunization develops more slowly than the incubation period of most infections and must therefore be induced prior to exposure to the etiologic agent. By contrast, "booster" reimmunization in a previously immune individual provides a rapid secondary (anamnestic) increase in immunity.

Previous infection can also substantially alter the response to an inactivated vaccine. For example, volunteers who have recovered from cholera or who live in a cholera-endemic area respond to parenteral immunization with an increase in anticholera secretory IgA, which is not seen in immunized control subjects.

The route of immunization may be an important determinant of successful vaccination, particularly if nonreplicating immunogens are used. Thus, immunization intranasally or by aerosol, which stimulates mucosal immunity (see Chapter 15), often appears to be more successful than parenteral injection against viral or bacterial respiratory challenges.

The route of administration recommended by the manufacturer and approved by the FDA should be used. Vaccines containing adjuvants such as aluminum hydroxide should always be given deep into the muscle and not subcutaneously. The ideal intramuscular injection site is the anterolateral portion of the upper thigh.

The timing of primary immunization, the interval between doses, and the timing of booster injections are based on both theoretic considerations and vaccine trials. The resulting recommendations should be followed closely. Many factors are involved. For instance, the age at which measles immunization is administered in the USA was changed from 12 to 15 months because the persistent maternal antibody, although present in small amounts only, was shown to interfere with active antibody formation by the child. Ironically, now that most mothers have induced immunity rather than naturally acquired measles antibody, their lower antibody titer may require that childhood immunization be changed back to 12 months of age.

Because of the clonal nature of immunity, it is possible—and, in fact, routine practice—to give many different antigens simultaneously. Some antigens are premixed (measles, mumps, rubella [MMR] and diphtheria, tetanus, pertussis [DPT]), whereas others may be given on the same day at different sites (DTP and *Haemophilus*). However, live virus vaccines that are not given on the same day should be given at least 1 month apart.

Splenectomy may markedly impair the primary antibody response to thymus-independent antigens such as bacterial polysaccharides, although many splenectomized patients respond normally to polysaccharide antigens because of priming by natural exposure prior to splenectomy.

Table 58–2. Materials available for active immunization.[1]

Disease	Product (Source)	Type of Agent	Route of Adminis-tration	Primary Immunization	Duration of Effect	Comments
Cholera	Cholera vaccine.	Killed bacteria	SC, IM, ID	2 doses 1 week or more apart.	6 months[2]	50% protective; International Certificate may be required for travel.
Diphtheria	DTP, DT (adsorbed for child under age 7; Td (adsorbed) for all others.	Toxoid	IM	3 doses 4 weeks or more apart, with an additional dose 1 year later for a child under age 7. (Can be given at same time as polio vaccine if doses at least 8 weeks apart.) A fifth dose before entering school is recommended if the fourth dose was given before the fourth birthday.	10 years[3]	Regular booster injections are recommended every 10 years. After the seventh birthday use the adult-type tetanus-diphtheria toxoid (Td). This product has a lower antigenic content and is less likely to produce reactions in older individuals.
Haemophilus influenzae influenza	Haemophilus b polysaccharide vaccine.	Polysaccharide	IM	1 dose.	1½–3½ years	As of 1988, the PRP-D conjugate vaccine is recommended for all children between 18 and 60 months of age. It should be given at 18 months to all children. Children who have received the old PRP vaccine between 18 and 24 months of age should receive a booster dose of the conjugate after a 2-month interval. The vaccine can be given at the same time as DPT.
Hepatitis B	Hepatitis B vaccine (human carriers). (Recombinant DNA, produced in yeast. Human carrier— derived vaccine is no longer being manufactured in the USA but is still available commercially.)	Formalin-treated purified viral antigen	IM	2 doses 1 month apart, followed by a booster given 6 months later. *Do not freeze vaccine*; this causes aggregation and loss of potency. The simultaneous administration of HBIG in a separate syringe at a separate site does not appear to impair the effectiveness of the vaccine.	Variable, about 5 years	A stable, adjuvant-supplemented vaccine from highly purified formalin-activated HBsAg harvested from human carriers. Recommended for all individuals at high risk of exposure to HBV infection, including health care personnel such as surgeons, anesthesiologists, autopsy staff, phlebotomists, operating room and dialysis nurses, medical technologists, dentists, and other staff exposed to patients with a high rate of HBV carriage; for patients undergoing chronic hemodialysis or repeatedly receiving plasma or clotting factor concentrates for clotting disorders; in the first week of life for newborn children of carrier mothers; for sexual and household contacts of HBV carriers (families accepting children from countries with high endemic rates of HBV infection should have the child screened and should be vaccinated if the child is HBsAg-positive); for male homosexuals, intravenous drug abusers, and prison populations with problems of homosexuality and drug use; for clients and staff of institutions for the mentally retarded, and classroom contacts of aggressively behaving deinstitutionalized mentally retarded HBV carriers; for heterosexually active persons with multiple partners; for travelers to areas endemic for HBV for more than 6 months (begin series at least 6 months prior to departure), especially if sexual contacts are anticipated in these areas; and for morticians. Anti-HBs titers in individuals repeatedly exposed to the risk of HBV infection should be checked at intervals of 2–3 years as well as at the time of definite exposure to blood or saliva suspected of being HBsAg-positive, if *(continued)*

Table 58–2 (cont'd). Materials available for active immunization.[1]

Disease	Product (Source)	Type of Agent	Route of Administration	Primary Immunization	Duration of Effect	Comments
Hepatitis B (cont'd.)						not measured within the previous year. A single booster dose should be given if a nonprotective level of anti-HBs is found. There is no evidence that the vaccine can transmit acquired immunodeficiency syndrome (AIDS).
Influenza	Influenza virus vaccine, monovalent or bivalent (chick embryo). Composition of the vaccine is varied depending upon epidemiologic circumstances.	Killed whole or split virus types A and B	IM	1 dose. (Two doses 4 weeks or more apart are recommended in individuals who have not previously received the current antigenic components or been otherwise exposed to the current strain of virus. Two doses of the split virus products should be used in persons 12 years of age or under because of fewer side effects.)	1 year	Give immunization by November. Recommended annually for individuals with chronic cardiovascular or pulmonary disease, for residents of nursing homes and other chronic care facilities, for medical personnel who may spread infection to high-risk patients, and for healthy individuals over 65 years of age, as well as for patients with chronic metabolic disorders, renal dysfunction, anemia, immunosuppression, or asthma. Patients receiving chemotherapy for malignant disease are likely to respond better if immunized between courses of treatment.
Measles[4]	Measles virus vaccine, live (chick embryo).	Live virus	SC	1 dose at age 15 months.	Permanent	Reimmunize if given before 15 months of age; may prevent natural disease if given less than 48 hours after exposure.
Meningococcus	Meningococcal polysaccharide vaccine (combination vaccine against groups A, C, Y, and W135).	Polysaccharide	SC	1 dose. Since primary antibody response requires at least 5 days, antibiotic prophylaxis with rifampin (600 mg or 10 mg/kg every 12 h for 4 doses) should be given to household contacts.	?Permanent in older children and adults; transient in children < 2 years.	Recommended in epidemic situations, for use by the military to prevent outbreaks in recruits, for patients with anatomic or functional asplenia, for individuals with a congenital deficiency of terminal components of the complement cascade, and possibly as an adjunct to antibiotic prophylaxis in preventing secondary cases in family contacts. Not reliably effective in infants, who require booster injections if antibody is to last for a year (especially antibody to group C). Revaccination may be indicated for individuals at high risk of infection, particularly if first immunized before age 4. The need to reimmunize adults and older children is unknown.
Mumps[4]	Mumps virus vaccine, live (chick embryo).	Live virus	SC	1 dose.	Permanent	Reimmunize if given before 1 year of age.
Pertussis	DTP.	Killed bacteria	IM	As for DTP.	Up to 5 years[3]	Not generally recommended after the seventh birthday. Contraindications to beginning or continuing pertussis immunization include a history of seizures or the development of seizures before the 4-dose primary series is completed. Immunization of these children should be deferred until it can be determined whether an evolving neurologic illness is present. For infants who have received fewer than 3 doses of DTP, the decision to pursue immunization should be made before 1 year of age; children with seizures have a higher risk of adverse outcome from pertussis itself and are at increased risk of exposure as they

Disease	Vaccine	Type	Route	Dosage	Duration	Comments
Pertussis (cont'd.)						grow older and contact other children. If the neurologic condition is stable and seizures are well controlled, the benefits of immunization outweight the hazards, although the parents should be warned of an 8-fold increased risk of postimmunization convulsions if febrile convulsions have occurred previously. Definitive contraindications to further administration of DTP include hypersensitivity to the vaccine, an evolving neurologic disorder, or history of a severe reaction. The latter usually occurs within 48 hours of vaccination and is characterized by collapse in a shocklike state, persistent uncontrolled screaming for 3 hours or more, a temperature of 40.5 °C (105 °F) or higher, convulsions or a severely altered state of consciousness, general or local neurologic signs, or a systemic allergic reaction. An acellular pertussis vaccine producing fewer local reactions is in use in Japan and is undergoing clinical trials in the USA.
Plague	Plague vaccine.	Killed bacteria	IM	3 doses 4 weeks or more apart.	6 months[3]	Recommended only for occupational exposure and not for residents of endemic area in the southwest USA.
Pneumococcus	Pneumococcal polysaccharide vaccine, polyvalent.	Polysaccharide	SC, IM	0.5 mL, if possible before splenectomy or before instituting chemotherapy.	Uncertain—probably at least 5 years in adults, but erratic in children under age 5	Recommended for patients with cardiorespiratory disease or other chronic illness, for patients with sickle cell disease, for patients with functional, congenital, or postsurgical asplenia, and for patients with nephrotic syndrome or with cerebrospinal fluid leakage. Also suggested for immunosuppressed or alcoholic patients and for patients aged 65 or older. Only the 23 most common serotypes are incorporated in the vaccine. Children up to age 2, splenectomized children, and some chronically ill patients respond unreliably. *Caution:* Because of a marked increase in adverse reactions following revaccination, booster doses should generally *not* be given, even to recipients of the earlier less comprehensive and less immunogenic vaccine. However, a booster is warranted after 3–5 years for high-risk children and is recommended after 3–4 months off chemotherapy for children first immunized while receiving it. Can be given at the same time as influenza or DTP vaccines.
Poliomyelitis	Poliovirus vaccine, live, oral, trivalent (monkey kidney, human diploid).	Live virus types I, II, III	Oral	2 doses 6–8 weeks or more apart, followed by a third dose 8–12 months later. (Can be given at the same time as primary DTP immunization.) A fourth dose before entering school is recommended if the third dose was given before age 4.	Permanent	Recommended for adults only if at increased risk by travel to epidemic or highly endemic areas or occupational contact. Individuals who have completed a primary series may take a single booster dose if the risk of exposure is high.

(continued)

Table 58–2 (cont'd.). Materials available for active immunization.[1]

Disease	Product (Source)	Type of Agent	Route of Administration	Primary Immunization	Duration of Effect	Comments
Poliomyelitis (cont'd.)	Poliomyelitis vaccine, inactivated.	Killed virus types I, II, III	IM	3 doses 4–8 weeks apart, followed by a fourth dose 6–12 months later. A fifth dose before entering school is recommended if the fourth dose was given before age 4. A single booster dose should be given every 5 years until age 18, after which the need is uncertain.	5 years[3]	Killed virus vaccines are preferred for immunologically deficient patients and their household contacts. Adults who have not previously received oral polio vaccine and who are at risk because of travel or, minimally, from immunization of their children should receive the inactivated vaccine. A new "enhanced" inactivated vaccine contains more antigenic material and is more immunogenic.
Rabies	Rabies vaccine (human diploid).	Killed virus	IM or (preexposure only) ID	**Preexposure:** 2 doses 1 week apart, followed by a third dose 2–3 weeks later. **Postexposure:** Always give rabies immune globulin as well. If not previously immunized, give a total of 5 doses, on days 0, 3, 7, 14, and 28 (WHO recommends a sixth dose 90 days after the first dose). If the vaccinee is immunocompromised (or if only DEV is available), a serum specimen should be collected on day 28 or 2–3 weeks after the last dose and tested for rabies antibody.[5] If the antibody level is insufficient, a booster should be given and the titer remeasured 2–3 weeks later. *If previously immunized* with diploid vaccine, do not give serum therapy. Give 2 booster doses, one immediately and one 3 days later. **Note:** Unexplained immediate-type (anaphylactic) hypersensitivity reactions have occurred during primary rabies immunization with vaccine from different manufacturers. Immunization of such individuals should be discontinued unless there is actual exposure to rabies virus or inapparent or unavoidable rabies contact is truly likely to occur. In the later situations, the serologic response to rabies should be checked and booster doses omitted if protective titers have already been attained; vaccination should be continued only under careful supervision. Rabies vaccine, Adsorbed (RVA Michigan Department of Public Health) a newly licensed vaccine can be used for both preexposure and postexposure prophylaxis. There is limited experience with and limited availability of this vaccine, but it appears to have a far decreased incidence of hypersensitivity reactions.	2 years[3] if titer < 1:16	Preexposure immunization only for occupational or avocational risk or residence in hyperendemic area. For animal bite, consider antitetanus and other antibacterial measures as well. **Caution:** Several reports document unexpectedly poor response to intradermal immunization. If the intradermal route is used, rabies antibody must be measured 2–3 weeks after the third dose of vaccine. If the antibody titer is < 1:16, an additional dose should be given and the antibody level retested 2–3 weeks later. If the antibody response of an individual who has received intradermal vaccine within the past 12 months is unknown, the level should be checked; if more than 12 months have elapsed, a booster should be given and the titer tested 2–3 weeks later. If a rabies exposure takes place following preexposure immunization by the intradermal route and there is no documentation of an adequate antibody level, a full course of HRIG and IM rabies vaccine should be given. Serologic testing does not appear to be necessary if preexposure prophylaxis was given by the IM route.
Rubella[4]	Rubella virus vaccine, live (human diploid).	Live virus	SC	1 dose (to ensure successful immunization, some experts recommend that a second dose be given to children no later than the fourth or fifth grade).	Permanent	Give after 15 months of age. Because a history of rubella is unreliable and because the vaccine is innocuous in immune recipients, unimmunized women of childbearing age should be vaccinated without serologic testing. Vaccination should be

	Type	Route	Dosage[1]	Duration of Immunity[2]	Comments
Rubella[4] (cont'd.)					avoided during pregnancy on theoretical grounds unless there is a risk of exposure due to an outbreak; however, there is no evidence of vaccine-induced fetal damage in over 200 recipients. Vaccination is contraindicated for those receiving systemic corticosteroids for more than 2 weeks; for leukemic or immunosuppressed patients for at least 3 months after chemotherapy has been discontinued; for recipients of immune globulin treatment other than anti-Rh therapy within the following 2 weeks or prior 3 months; and for individuals with allergy to neomycin but not to eggs or penicillin. If a female is immunized postpartum and has received blood products or Rh immune globulin, serologic testing should be done 6–8 weeks later to confirm successful immunization. Viremia can occur if antibody has fallen to low levels; the frequency and thus the clinical importance of this phenomenon are unknown.
Smallpox	Smallpox vaccine (calf lymph, chick embryo). Available from CDC[7].	Live vaccinia virus	ID	1 dose.	3 years	Smallpox has been eradicated, and smallpox vaccine is no longer available to civilian populations.
Tetanus	DTP, DT (adsorbed) for children under age 7; Td, T (adsorbed) for all others.	Toxoid	IM	3 doses 4 weeks or more apart.	10 years[3,5]	Recipients aged 7 or above should be given a third dose 6–12 months after second. (See Table 58-5 regarding use of hyperimmune globulin.)
Tuberculosis	BCG vaccine.	Live attenuated Mycobacterium bovis	ID, SC	1 dose.	?Permanent[6]	Recommended in USA only for PPD-negative contacts of ineffectively treated or persistently untreated cases and for other unusually high risk groups.
Typhoid	Typhoid vaccine.	Killed bacteria	SC	2 doses 4 weeks or more apart, or 3 doses 1 week apart (less desirable).	3 years[3]	70% protective. Recommended only for exposure from travel, epidemic, or household carrier and not, for example because of floods.
Yellow fever	Yellow fever vaccine (chick embryo).	Live virus	SC	1 dose	10 years[2]	Certificate may be required for travel. Recommended for residence or travel to endemic areas of Africa and South America. Avoid administration to an immunologically incompetent host or an individual on long-term (> 2 weeks) corticosteroid therapy.

[1] Dosages for the specific product, including variations for age, are best obtained from the manufacturer's package insert. Immunizations should be given by the route suggested for the product.
[2] Revaccination interval required by international regulations.
[3] A single dose is a sufficient booster at any time after the effective duration of primary immunization has passed.
[4] Combination vaccines available.
[5] For contaminated or severe wounds, give booster if more than 5 years have elapsed since full immunization or last booster. A single booster any time after primary immunization is effective.
[6] Test for PPD conversion 2 months later, and reimmunize if there is no conversion.
[7] Drug Immunobiologic and Vaccine Service, Center for Infectious Diseases. Telephone: (404) 329-3311 (main switchboard, day) or (404) 329-3644 (nights and weekends).

Technique of Immunization

When administering vaccines intended for subcutaneous or intramuscular deposition, it is essential to pull back on the syringe before depressing the plunger to make certain that the product will not be injected intravenously, resulting in lessened immunizing effect and increased untoward reactions. It is particularly important to use a sufficiently long needle (usually >1 in) for intramuscular delivery of adjuvant-containing (eg, alum or aluminum phosphate-adsorbed) vaccines; subcutaneous inoculation of adjuvants may result in tissue necrosis.

Recent studies of injection techniques suggest that the anterolateral thigh or deltoid site is preferable to the buttocks. Even with the usual precautions, use of the latter site occasionally leads to sciatic nerve damage, and in adults most injections meant for intramuscular delivery are instead delivered into fat.

The intradermal route of immunization is under intensive study as a means of obtaining an earlier or greater immune response with the same amount of antigen or of inducing a satisfactory immune response with a smaller quantity of expensive immunogens such as the hepatitis B and rabies vaccines.

Adverse Reactions & the Risk:Benefit Ratio

All vaccines approved and licensed in the USA have been shown to be safe and effective. However, each of them has also been shown to cause adverse reactions. Sometimes these are minimal in occurrence rate and severity, as in tetanus toxoid. Historically, some immunizing agents produced adverse reactions that were so severe they would be unacceptable today; variolation and the original rabies vaccine made from spinal cord material are 2 examples. Smallpox vaccination with vaccinia virus carried a very acceptable risk at a time when smallpox posed an imminent and serious threat. However, as the risk of smallpox declined to the point at which the disease was eradicated, the risk:benefit ratio of the vaccine has increased and is now infinite. At present, the most controversial vaccine in routine use is the whole-cell pertussis vaccine. It is only about 70% effective for protection, causes very frequent minor reaction, and occasionally results in serious neurologic reactions. However, it is still used because the risk:benefit ratio is acceptably low. Japan, the United Kingdom, and Sweden have experienced a significant rise in the fatality rate from pertussis since the use of the vaccine was discontinued. An acellular pertussis vaccine is expected to be available soon.

Unique Hazards of Live Vaccines

Because of their potential for infection of the fetus, live vaccines should *not* be given to a pregnant woman unless there is a high immediate risk (eg, a poliomyelitis epidemic). A pregnant woman traveling in an area endemic for yellow fever *should* be immunized because the risk of infection exceeds the small theoretic hazard to fetus and mother. If yellow fever vaccination is being performed solely to comply with a legal requirement for international travel, however, the woman should seek a waiver with a letter from her physician. Live vaccines, furthermore, can cause serious or even fatal illness in an immunologically incompetent host. They generally should not be given to patients receiving corticosteroids, alkylating drugs, radiation, or other immunosuppressive agents or to individuals with known or suspected congenital or acquired defects in cell-mediated immunity (eg, severe combined immunodeficiency disease, leukemias, lymphomas, Hodgkin's disease, and acquired immunodeficiency syndrome [AIDS]). Patients with pure hypogammaglobulinemia but no defect in cell-mediated immunity usually tolerate viral infections and vaccines well but have a 10,000-fold excess of paralytic complications over the usual one case per million recipients, in part because of the frequent reversion of attenuated poliovirus strains to virulence in the intestinal tract. Since live poliovirus is shed by recipients, it should not be given to household contacts of these patients either.

Even in immunocompetent hosts, live vaccines may result in mild or, rarely, severe disease.

The early measles vaccines caused high fever and rash in a significant proportion of recipients. Subacute sclerosing panencephalitis, a rare complication of natural infection, has occurred following administration of live, attenuated measles vaccine (see Chapter 43), but the rate of about one case per million is one-tenth to one-fifth the rate following natural measles, and the number of cases of measles encephalitis has fallen 100-fold since the introduction of the vaccine. The mild, recurrent arthralgia or arthritis that can follow rubella immunization may represent the consequences of a secondary rather than a primary infection in an individual who has low levels of antibodies not detected by all assays and who has in vitro evidence of cell-mediated immunity.

Because passage through the human intestinal tract occasionally results in reversion of oral attenuated poliovirus vaccine (particularly type III) to neurovirulence, paralytic illness has occurred in recipients or, rarely, their nonimmune contacts, especially adults. The success of live polio vaccines in preventing widespread natural infection has resulted in the paradox that the vaccine itself now accounts for a large fraction of the few cases of paralytic poliomyelitis seen each year in the USA. Killed (Salk) vaccine also appears to be effective in abolishing polio, and the major advantages of live (Sabin) vaccine, which sustain its use despite the small risk of paralysis (5 cases per million doses in nonimmune recipients), are its ease of administration and more durable immune response.

Live vaccines may contain undetected and undesirable contaminants. Epidemic hepatitis resulted in the past from vaccinia and yellow fever vaccines containing human serum. More recently, millions of people received SV40, a simian papovavirus contained in live or inactivated poliovirus vaccine prepared in monkey kidney tissue culture. Although a virus closely related to SV40 has been isolated from the brains of patients with progressive multifocal leukoencephalopathy, a lethal degenerative disease, there is no known history of polio immunization in these cases. An increased incidence of cancer in children of mothers who received inactivated polio vaccine during pregnancy was suggested in 2 studies but not in a 20-year follow-up of a large number of childhood recipients. SV40 can now be detected and excluded from human viral vaccines, but other undetected viruses might be transmitted by vaccines grown in nonhuman cell lines. Yellow fever vaccine has been reported to be probably contaminated with avian leukosis virus. Bacteriophages and probably bacterial endotoxins have also been shown to contaminate live virus vaccines, although without known hazard thus far.

Live viral vaccines probably do not interfere with tuberculin skin testing, although they depress some measurements of lymphocyte function.

Unlike live vaccines, inactivated vaccines may safely be given to immunocompromised hosts. They may not, however, dependably elicit an adequately protective immune response.

The risk:benefit ratio of live measles vaccine is sufficiently low to recommend its use in patients with human immunodeficiency virus (HIV) infection—even immunocompromised patients.

Other Adverse Effects

Allergic reactions may occur on exposure to egg protein (in measles, mumps, influenza, and yellow fever vaccines) or antibiotics or preservatives (eg, neomycin or mercurials) in viral vaccines. Patients with known IgE-mediated sensitivity to a vaccine component (eg, egg albumin in yellow fever vaccine grown in eggs) should not receive the vaccine unless successfully desensitized (in cases when immunization is essential). Occasionally, the product of a different manufacturer does not contain the offending allergen. Improvements in antigenicity and better purification procedures in vaccine production decrease the amount and number of foreign substances injected and result in fewer side effects.

Reporting Adverse Effects & Legal Liability

Lawsuits arising out of adverse reaction to vaccines have led to steep increases in the cost of vaccines in recent years. The 1988 costs of vaccines in the public sector are shown in Fig 58–1. Because of the high costs of litigation and liability insurance,

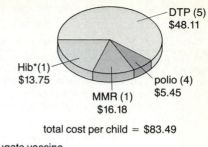

total cost per child = $83.49

*conjugate vaccine

Figure 58–1. Vaccine costs for immunizing one child in public health programs, 1988.

the threat to development and production of new vaccines prompted the passage of the National Childhood Vaccine Injury Act of 1986. This Act provides for compensation of those injured by adverse reactions and at the same time mandates that certain events following vaccination be reported. These new requirements are summarized in Tables 58–3 and 58–4.

This new federal compensation plan to assume responsibility for unavoidable adverse reactions is still untried. Preventable adverse effects can be minimized by reading vaccine labels, storing vaccines carefully, using the correct method of administration at the proper site, and being aware of contraindications, particularly by identifying immunocompromised hosts.

PASSIVE IMMUNIZATION

Immunization may be accomplished passively by administering either preformed immunoreactive serum or cells.

Antibody, either as whole serum or as fractionated, concentrated immune (gamma) globulin that is predominantly IgG, may be obtained from human or animal donors who have recovered from an infectious disease or have been immunized. These antibodies may provide immediate protection to an antibody-deficient individual. Passive immunization is thus useful for individuals who cannot form antibodies or for the nonimmunocompromised host who might develop disease before active immunization could stimulate antibody production, which usually requires at least 7–10 days.

Additionally, passive immunization is useful when no active immunization is available, when passive immunization is used in conjunction with vaccine administration (eg, in rabies vaccination), in the management of specific effects of certain toxins and venoms, and, finally, as an immunosuppressant.

Antibody may be obtained from humans or ani-

Table 58–3. Reportable events following vaccination.

Vaccine/Toxoid	Event	Interval from Vaccination
DTP.P, DTP/polio combined	Anaphylaxis or anaphylactic shock	immediate
	Encephalopathy (or encephalitis)[1]	7 days
	Shock-collapse or hypotonic-hyporesponsive collapse[1]	7 days
	Residual seizure disorder[1]	Variable[1]
	Any acute complication or sequela (including death) of above events	No limit
	Events (such as convulsions) described in manufacturer's package insert as contraindications to additional doses of vaccine[2]	See package insert
Measles, mumps, and rubella; Td, tetanus toxoid	Anaphylaxis or anaphylatic shock.	immediate
	Encephalopathy (or encephalitis)[1]	15 days for measles, mumps, and rubella vaccines; 7 days for DT, Td, and T toxoids
	Residual seizure disorder[1]	Variable[1]
	Any acute complication or sequela (including death) of above events.	No limit
	Events described in manufacturer's package insert as contraindications to additional doses of vaccine[2]	See package insert
Oral polio vaccine	Paralytic poliomyelitis	
	in a nonimmunodeficient recipient	30 days
	in an immunodeficient recipient	6 months
	in a vaccine-associated community case	No limit
	Any acute complication or sequela (including death) of above events	No limit
	Events described in manufacturer's package insert as contraindications to additional doses of vaccine[2]	See package insert
Inactivated polio vaccine	Anaphylaxis or anaphylactic shock	immediate
	Any acute complication or sequela (including death) of above event	No limit
	Events described in manufacturer's package insert as contraindications to additional doses of vaccine[2]	See package insert

[1]Aids to interpretation: Shock-collapse or hypotonic-hyporesponsive collapse may be evidenced by signs or symptoms such as decrease in or loss of muscle tone, paralysis (partial or complete), hemiplegia, hemiparesis, loss of color or turning pale, white, or blue, unresponsiveness to environmental stimuli, depression of or loss of consciousness, prolonged sleeping with difficulty arousing, or cardiovascular or respiratory arrest. Residual seizure disorder may be considered to have occurred if no other seizure or convulsion unaccompanied by fever or accompanied by a fever of less than 102 °F occurred before the first seizure or convulsion after the administration of the vaccine involved. AND, if in the case of measles, mumps, or rubella-containing vaccines, the first seizure or convulsion occurred within 15 days after vaccination OR in the case of any other vaccine, the first seizure or convulsion occurred within 3 days after vaccination. AND, if 2 or more seizures or convulsions unaccompanied by fever or accompanied by a fever of less than 102 °F occurred within 1 year after vaccination. The terms "seizure" and "convulsion" include grand mal, petit mal, absence, myoclonic, tonic-clonic, and focal motor seizures and signs. "Encephalopathy" means any significant acquired abnormality of, injury to, or impairment of function of the brain. Among the frequent manifestations of encephalopathy are focal and diffuse neurologic signs, increased intracranial pressure, or changes lasting at least 6 hours in the level of consciousness, with or without convulsions. The neurologic signs and symptoms of encephalopathy may be temporary with complete recovery, or they may result in various degrees of permanent impairment. Signs and symptoms such as high-pitched and unusual screaming, persistent unconsolable crying, and bulging fontane are compatible with an encephalopathy but, in and of themselves, are not conclusive evidence of encephalopathy. Encephalopathy usually can be documented by slow wave activity on an electroencephalogram.
[2]The health care provider must refer to the Contraindication section of the manufacturer's package insert for each vaccine.

mals, but animal sera give rise to an immune response that leads to rapid clearance of the protective molecules from the circulation of the recipient and the risk of allergic reactions, particularly serum sickness or anaphylaxis (see below). Thus, to obtain a similar protective effect, much more animal antiserum must be injected compared with human antiserum (eg, 3000 units of equine tetanus antitoxin versus 300 units of human tetanus immune globulin).

Human Immune Globulin

This preparation is derived from alcohol fractionation of pooled plasma. The antibody content of im-

mune globulin is almost all of the IgG isotype and reflects the infection and immunization experience of the donor pool. Three types of preparations are available: standard immune gamma globulin for intramuscular use (IGIM), standard immune globulin adapted for intravenous use (IGIV), and special immune globulins with a known high content of antibody against a particular antigen; the last may be available for intravenous or intramuscular use.

Immune globulin should be given only when its efficacy has been established. Although its side effects are minimal, the administration is painful and rare anaphylactoid reactions have been described. It

Table 58–4. Reporting of events occurring after vaccination.

Reporting	Vaccine Purchased with Public Money[1]	Vaccine Purchased with Private Money[1]
Who reports	Health care provider who administered the vaccine.	Health care provider who administered the vaccine.
What products to report	DTP, P, measles, mumps, rubella, DT, Td, T, OPV, IPV, and DTP/polio combined.	DTP, P, measles, mumps, rubella, DT, Td, T, OPV, IPV, and DTP/polio combined.
What reactions to report	Events listed in Table 58–3 including contraindicating reactions specified in manufacturer's package inserts.	Events listed in Table 58–3 including contraindicating reactions specified in manufacturer's package inserts.
How to report	Initial report taken by local, county, or state health department. State health department completes CDC form 71.19.	Health care provider completes Adverse Reaction Report-FDA form 1639 (include interval from vaccination, manufacturer, and lot number on form).

Where to report	State health departments send CDC form 71.19 to:
	    MSAEFI/IM (E05)
	    Centers for Disease Control
	    Atlanta, GA 30333.
		Send completed FDA form 1639 to:
		    Food and Drug Administration (HFN-730)
		    Rockville, MD 20857

Where to obtain forms	State health department.	FDA and publications such as *FDA Drug Bulletin*.

[1]D, Diphtheria toxoid; P, pertussis vaccine; T, tetanus toxoid; d, diphtheria toxoid (adult type); OPV, oral polio vaccine; IPV, inactivated polio vaccine.

is not useful for the immunologically normal child or adult with frequent viral infections. There is no evidence that HIV infections can be transmitted by the administration of immune globulin. *Caution:* The intramuscular form should *never* be given intravenously; very serious systemic reactions may result from the presence of high-molecular-weight aggregated immunoglobulins.

IGIV is derived from the same pool of adult donors and also consists almost solely of IgG antibodies. The immune globulin has been adapted to intravenous use by eliminating high-molecular-weight complexes that may activate complement in the recipient. The advantages of the intravenous route are the ability to administer large doses of immune globulin, the more rapid onset of action, and the avoidance of intramuscular injections, which are painful and may be contraindicated because of a tendency to bleed. IGIV is particularly valuable as replacement therapy for antibody deficiency disorders and for the management of idiopathic thrombocytopenic purpura. The cost, however, is approximately 5 times the cost of IGIM. Approximately 2.5% of patients receiving IGIV will experience side effects of fever or vasoactive phenomena (usually vasodilatation), but these reactions can usually be prevented by slow administration of the material.

Special Preparations of Human Immune Globulin

Many preparations with a high titer of a specific antibody are available. These are prepared either by hyperimmunizing adult donors or by selecting lots of plasma tested for a high specific antibody content. Most of these are available in the intramuscular form; a few are currently being made available for intravenous use.

Animal Sera & Antitoxins

These preparations are used only when human globulin is not available, because they carry a much higher risk of anaphylactic reactions. They are usually prepared from hyperimmunized horses or rabbits.

No antiserum of animal origin should be given without carefully inquiring about prior exposure or allergic response to any product of the specific animal source. Whenever a foreign antiserum is administered, a syringe containing aqueous epinephrine, 1:1000, should be available. If allergy is suspected by history or shown by skin testing and no alternative to serum therapy is possible, desensitization may be attempted as outlined in Chapter 59.

The various materials available for passive immunization, of both human and animal origin, are detailed in Table 58–5.

Passive Immunization in Noninfectious Diseases

A. Prevention of Rh Isoimmunization: Rh-negative women are at hazard of developing anti-Rh antibodies when Rh-positive erythrocytes enter their circulation. This occurs regularly during pregnancy with an Rh-positive fetus, whether the pregnancy ends in a term or preterm delivery or in abortion. It may also occur with other events listed below. The development of anti-Rh antibodies threatens all subsequent Rh-positive fetuses with erythroblastosis. This can be prevented by administration of Rh immune globulin to the mother.

Rh-negative females who have not already developed anti-Rh antibodies should receive 300 μg of Rh immune globulin within 72 hours after obstetric delivery, abortion, accidental transfusion with Rh-positive blood, chorionic villus biopsy, and, proba-

Table 58–5. Materials available for passive immunization. (All are of human origin unless otherwise stated.)

Disease	Product	Dosage	Comments
Black widow spider bite	Antivenin widow spider, equine.	1 vial IM or IV.	A second dose may be given if symptoms do not subside in 3 hours.
Botulism	ABE polyvalent antitoxin, equine.	1 vial IV and 1 vial IM; repeat after 2–4 hours if symptoms worsen, and after 12–24 hours.	Available from CDC.[1] A 20% incidence of serum reactions. Only type E antitoxin has been shown to affect outcome of illness. Prophylaxis is not routinely recommended but may be given to asymptomatic exposed persons.
Diphtheria	Diphtheria antitoxin, equine.	20,000–120,000 units IM depending on severity and duration of illness.	Active immunization and perhaps erythromycin prophylaxis, rather than antitoxin prophylaxis, should be given to nonimmune contacts of active cases. Contacts should be observed for signs of illness so that antitoxin may be administered if needed.
Hepatitis A	Immune globulin.	0.02 mL/μg IM as soon as possible after exposure up to 2 weeks. A protective effect lasts about 2 months.	Modifies but does not prevent infection. Recommended for sexual and household contacts of infected persons including diapered children and their staff contacts in a child care center if one case occurs among them or if cases are recognized in the households with more than 2 children. (If cases occur in more than 3 homes, consider prophylaxis for all households with diapered children attending the center.) In centers without diapered children, prophylaxis is recommended only for classroom contacts of an index case. Prophylaxis is also suggested for coworkers of an infected food handler (but not generally for patrons) and for persons exposed to a common source *if* cases have not yet begun to occur. Prophylaxis is not recommended for personal contacts at offices, schools, hospitals, or institutions for custodial care *except* in an outbreak centered in these areas.
		For continuous risk of exposure, a dose of 0.05 mL/kg is recommended every 5 months.	Personnel of mental institutions, facilities for retarded children, and prisons appear to be at chronic risk of acquiring hepatitis A, as are those who work with nonhuman primates. Also recommended for travelers who will remain in endemic areas for more than 2 months.
Hepatitis B	Hepatitis B immune globulin (HBIG).	0.06 mL/kg IM up to a maximum of 5 mL as soon as possible after exposure, preferably within 24 hours, but up to 14 days for sexual exposure. HBV vaccination begun within 7 days of exposure is recommended in preference to a second HBIG injection 25–30 days after the first.	Administer to nonimmune individuals as postexposure prophylaxis following sexual contact with HBsAg-positive individuals (one dose of HBIG appears to be as effective as 2 doses for sexual exposure). For percutaneous or mucosal exposure to known HBsAg-positive or high-risk material, prophylactic strategy depends upon testing the source and upon the vaccination history of the exposed person (see Table 58–2). Of no value for persons already demonstrating anti-HBsAg antibody. Administration of various live virus vaccines should be delayed for at least 2 months after this concentrated immune globulin has been given. Pregnant women should be screened before delivery or as soon as possible thereafter, and newborn infants of all carriers should be given HBIG, 0.5 mL, within 12 hours of birth. Immunization with HBV vaccine should be started within the first week of life (see Table 58–2). High-risk mothers include women of Asian, Pacific island, or Alaskan Eskimo descent, whether immigrant or US-born; women born in Haiti or sub-Saharan Africa; and women with a history of acute or chronic liver disease, work or treatment in a hemodialysis unit, work or residence in an institution for the mentally retarded, repeated blood transfusions, frequent occupational exposure to blood in a medicodental setting, rejection as a blood donor, household exposure to an HBV carrier or a hemodialysis patient, multiple episode of sexually transmitted disease, or percutaneous use of illicit drugs. HBIG has no effect upon non-A,non-B hepatitis.
Hypogamma-globulinemia	Immune globulin.	0.6 mL/kg IM every 3–4 weeks.	Give double dose at onset of therapy. Immune globulin is of no value in the prevention of frequent respiratory infections in the absence of demonstrable hypogammaglobulinemia.
	Immune globulin IV.	100–150 mg/kg IV about once a month, depending on maintenance of serum IgG levels.	Ordinary immune globulin cannot safely be given intravenously because of complement-activating aggregates. It is difficult to administer sufficient IM globulin to maintain normal IgG levels in immunodeficient children or to passively protect acutely infected individuals who lack a specific antibody. This material contains a very small amount of IgA and can cause an allergic reaction in a sensitive IgA-deficient recipient. The IgE in some preparations may cause some reactions; although one product causes symptoms, particularly if confirmed by skin testing, another preparation may not.

(continued)

Table 58–5. (cont'd.). Materials available for passive immunization. (All are of human origin unless otherwise stated.)

Disease	Product	Dosage	Comments
Measles	Immune globulin.	0.25 mL/kg IM as soon as possible after exposure. This dose may be ineffective in immunoincompetent patients, who should receive 20–30 mL.	Live measles vaccine will usually prevent natural infection if given within 48 hours following exposure. If immune globulin is administered, delay immunization with live virus for 3 months. Do not vaccinate infants under age 15 months.
Rabies	Rabies immune globulin.[2]	20 IU/kg, 50% of which is infiltrated locally at the wound site if anatomically feasible, and the remainder given IM. (See also rabies vaccine in Table 58–2.) If the equine product is used, the dose is 40 IU/kg.	Give as soon as possible after exposure. Recommended for all bite or scratch exposures to carnivores, especially bat, skunk, fox, coyote, or raccoon, despite animal's apparent health, if the brain cannot be immediately examined and found rabies-free. Give also even for abrasion exposure to known or suspected rabid animals as well as for bite (skin penetration by teeth) of escaped dogs and cats whose health cannot be determined. Not recommended for individuals with demonstrated antibody response from preexposure prophylaxis.
Rh isoimmunization (erythroblastosis fetalis)	Rh_o (D) immune globulin.	1 dose IM within 12 hours of abortion, amniocentesis or chorionic villus biopsy, obstetric delivery of an Rh-positive infant, or transfusion of Rh-positive blood in an Rh_o (D)-negative female.	For nonimmune females only. May be effective at much greater postexposure interval. Give even if more than 72 hours have elapsed. One vial contains 300 µg of antibody and can reliably inhibit the immune response to a fetomaternal bleed of 7.5–8 mL as estimated by the Betke-Kleihauer smear technique. Some groups also recommend administration of 100 µg of antibody at 28 and 34 weeks of pregnancy to prevent prepartum isoimmunization. Transient seropositivity for anti-HAV and anti-HBV antibodies may follow the administration of large doses.
Snakebite	Antivenin coral snake, equine. Antivenin rattlesnake, copperhead, and moccasin, equine.	At least 3–5 vials IV.	Dose should be sufficient to reverse symptoms of envenomation. Consider antitetanus measures as well.
Tetanus	Tetanus immune globulin.[3]	Prophylaxis: 250–500 units IM. Therapy: 3000–5000 units IM.	Give in separate syringe at separate site from simultaneously administered toxoid. Recommended only for major contaminated wounds in individuals who have had fewer than 2 doses of toxoid at any time in the past (fewer than 3 doses if wound is more than 24 hours old). (See tetanus toxoid in Table 58–2.) There is some evidence that 250 units given intrathecally to mildly affected patients prevents progression to severe disease and death, but intrathecal therapy is not effective in severe cases with generalized repeated spasms.
Vaccinia	Vaccinia immune globulin. (Available from CDC.[1])	Prophylaxis: 0.3 mL/kg IM. Therapy: 0.6 mL/kg IM. VIG may be repeated as necessary for treatment and at intervals of 1 week for prophylaxis.	Give at a different site if used to prevent dissemination in a patient with skin disease who must undergo vaccination. May be useful in treatment of vaccinia of the eye, eczema vaccinatum, generalized vaccinia, and vaccinia necrosum and in the prevention of such complications in exposed patients with skin disorders such as eczema or impetigo. Also recommended to prevent fetal vaccinia when a pregnant woman must be vaccinated. VIG should rarely be needed, since smallpox vaccination is now limited to military personnel and at-risk laboratory workers.
Varicella	Varicella-zoster immune globulin (VZIG).	1 vial/10 kg or fraction thereof, up to a maximum of 5 vials, given IM within 96 hours of exposure.	It should be administered to nonimmune leukemic, lymphomatous, or immunosuppressed children, children receiving prednisone at ≥2 mg/kg/d for any reason, or other immunoincompetent children <15years of age who have had household, hospital (same room containing ≤4 beds or adjacent beds in large ward), or playmate (>1 hour play indoors) contact with a known case of varicella-zoster. Should also be given to exposed bone marrow transplant patients regardless of immune history of donor, to exposed infants born before 28 weeks of gestation, and to neonates whose mothers have developed varicella <5 days before or 48 hours after delivery or who are exposed postnatally and whose mothers have uncertain or negative histories of varicella. VZIG should be considered for adults—especially pregnant women and immunocompromised patients—having close contact with a case of varicella-zoster as defined above for children and whose history suggests suscepti-

(continued)

Table 58–5. (cont'd.). Materials available for passive immunization. (All are of human origin unless otherwise stated.)

Disease	Product	Dosage	Comments
			bility. A negative history for varicella is extremely unreliable (only about 8% of adults who believe they are nonimmune become infected after household exposure) and should if possible be checked by a serologic test such as the fluorescent-antibody test against membrane antigen, because of the high cost of VZIG. Protective antibody levels can be attained using immune globulin IV in a dose of 6 mL/kg if VZIG is unavailable.

[1]Available from the Centers for Disease Control. Telephone: (404) 329-3311 (main switchboard, day) or (404) 329-3644 (night).
[2]Antirabies serum, equine, may be available but is much less desirable.
[3]Bovine and equine antitoxins may be available but are not recommended. They are used at 10 times the dose of tetanus immune globulin.
[4]Contact the regional blood center of the American Red Cross.
Note: Passive immunotherapy or immunoprophylaxis should always be administered as soon as possible after exposure to the offending agent. Immune antisera and globulin are always given intramuscularly unless otherwise noted. Always question carefully and test for hypersensitivity before administering animal sera.

bly, amniocentesis, especially if the needle passes through the placenta. This passive immunization suppresses the mother's normal immune response to any Rh-positive fetal cells that may enter her circulation, thus avoiding erythroblastosis fetalis in future Rh-positive fetuses; it may protect in a nonspecific manner as well, analogous to the "blocking" effect of high-dose IgG in ameliorating autoimmune diseases such as idiopathic thrombocytopenic purpura. Even if more than 72 hours has elapsed after the exposures listed above, Rh immune globulin should be administered, since it will be effective in at least some cases. Three of 6 subjects were protected from the immunogenic effect of 1 mL of intravenous Rh-positive erythrocytes by 100 μg of anti-Rh globulin given 13 days later. Some workers have also suggested the administration of anti-Rh globulin to Rh-negative newborn female offspring of Rh-positive mothers to prevent possible sensitization from maternal-fetal transfusion.

A significant number of Rh isoimmunizations occur during pregnancy rather than at the time of delivery. This can be almost completely prevented by administration of anti-Rh globulin at 28 weeks of gestation. The American College of Obstetricians and Gynecologists recommends routine administration of 300 μg of Rh immune globulin at 28 weeks of gestation and again at delivery as soon as it is determined that the infant is Rh-positive. Prior to 28 weeks of gestation, any condition associated with fetomaternal hemorrhage (abortion, amniocentesis, ruptured ectopic pregnancy) should be treated with Rh immune globulin (a 50-μg "minidose" is used before 12 weeks and a standard 300-μg dose is used thereafter). A larger dose is necessary when a significant fetomaternal hemorrhage (more than 25 μg/mL of incompatible cells) has taken place.

B. Serum Therapy of Poisonous Bites: The toxicity of the bite of the black widow spider, the coral snake, and crotalid snakes (rattlesnakes and other pit vipers) may be lessened by the administration of commercially available antivenins. These are of equine origin, so the risk of serum sickness is high and the possibility of anaphylaxis must always be considered.

Antisera for scorpion stings and rarer poisonous bites, especially of species foreign to North America, may also be available.

Information on the use and availability of antivenins is often available from Poison Control Centers, particularly those in cities having large zoos, such as New York and San Diego. A Snakebite Trauma Center has been established at Jacobi Hospital in New York ([212] 430-8183). In addition, an antivenin index listing the availability of all such products is maintained by the Poison Control Center in Tucson, Arizona ([602] 626-6016 or 626-6000).

C. Kawasaki Syndrome: This severe disease, a form of generalized vasculitis, produces coronary artery aneurysms that may result in myocardial infarction in a significant number of cases. There is a large and convincing body of evidence that IGIV given during the acute phase of the disease substantially improves the outcome. The dose and duration that have been successful in clinical trials are 400 mg daily for 5 days given as early as possible during the acute phase.

D. Thrombocytopenic Purpura: In this disease, IGIV is given because it presumably prolongs platelet survival by blocking Fc receptors for IgG on macrophages that ingest antibody-coated platelets.

Hazards of Passive Immunization

Illness may arise from a single injection of foreign serum but more commonly occurs in patients who have previously been injected with proteins from the same or a related species. Reactions range in severity from serum sickness arising days to weeks following treatment to acute anaphylaxis with hives, dyspnea, cardiovascular collapse, and even death (see Chapter 31). Typical manifestations of serum sickness include adenopathy, urticaria, arthritis, and fever (see Chapter 32). Demyelinating encephalopathy has been reported.

Rarely, the administration of human immune globulin is attended by similar allergic reactions, particularly in patients with selective IgA deficiency (see Chapter 24). Viral hepatitis may be transmitted by whole human plasma or serum but not by the purified γ globulin fraction.

The administration of intact lymphocytes to promote cell-mediated immunity is hazardous if the recipient is immunologically depressed. The engrafted donor cells may "reject" the recipient by the graft-versus-host reaction, producing rash, pancytopenia, fever, diarrhea, hepatosplenomegaly, and death (see Chapter 60).

COMBINED PASSIVE-ACTIVE IMMUNIZATION

Passive and active immunization are often simultaneously undertaken to provide both immediate, transient protection and slowly developing, durable protection against rabies or tetanus. The immune response to the active agent may or may not be impaired by the passively administered antibodies if the injections are given at separate sites. Tetanus toxoid plus tetanus immune globulin may give a response superior to that generated by the toxoid alone, but after antiserum has been given for rabies, the course of immunization is usually extended to ensure an adequate response.

Parenterally administered live virus vaccines such as measles or rubella virus should not be given until at least 6 (and preferably 12) weeks after the administration of immune globulin.

CLINICAL INDICATIONS FOR IMMUNIZATION

Immunizing procedures are among the most effective and economical measures available for preservation and protection of health. The decision to immunize a specific person against a specific pathogen is a complex judgment based upon an assessment of the risk of infection, the consequences of natural unmodified illness, the availability of a safe and effective immunogen, and the duration of its effect.

HERD IMMUNITY

The organisms that cause diphtheria and tetanus are ubiquitous, and the vaccines have few side effects and are highly effective, but only the immunized individual is protected. Thus, immunization

must be universal. By contrast, a nonimmune individual who resides in a community that has been well immunized against poliovirus and who does not travel has little opportunity to encounter wild (virulent) virus. Here the immunity of the "herd" protects the unimmunized person since the intestinal tracts of recipients of oral polio vaccine fail to become colonized by or transmit wild virus. If, however, a substantial portion of the community is not immune, introduced wild virus can circulate and cause disease among the nonimmune group. Thus, focal outbreaks of poliomyelitis have occurred in religious communities objecting to immunization.

The present controversy over pertussis immunization is discussed above.

ANTIGENIC SHIFT & ANTIGENIC VARIATION

Each immunologically distinct viral subtype requires a specific antigenic stimulus for effective protection. Immunization against adenovirus infection has not benefited civilian populations subject to many differing types of adenovirus, in contrast to the demonstrated value of vaccine directed against a few epidemic adenovirus types in military recruits. Similarly, immunity to type A influenza virus is transient because of major mutations in surface chemistry of the virus every few years (antigenic shifts). These changes render previously developed vaccines obsolete and may not permit sufficient production, distribution, and utilization of new antigen in time to prevent epidemic spread of the altered strain. Antigenic variation may also be an important impediment to immunization against HIV infection.

SPECIFIC DISEASES

Pertussis

Several acellular vaccines used in Japan for the past 8 years are saline suspensions of 2 antigens: formalin-treated lymphocyte proliferative factor (pertussis toxin) and filamentous hemagglutinin. The degree of protection afforded by acellular vaccine appears to be about the same (70%) as that for the whole-cell product, and minor reactions (fever, pain) are less frequent. Because the acellular vaccine is administered at the age of 2 years, it is not yet known whether it is free of neurologic sequelae when used in infants.

Poliomyelitis

Two forms of polio vaccine are available. The live, attenuated oral (Sabin) vaccine, used in the USA and many parts of the world, is cheap, effective, and easily administered. Infection causing paralysis occurs in only one per 7 million immunodeficient recipients or members of their households. The killed virus vaccine (Salk) is also effective, particularly in the new "enhanced" form. It requires injection and gives a shorter duration of immunity, but is free of the danger of producing paralysis in the recipient or household members. Immunodeficient individuals should receive the killed vaccine. Adults who have never been immunized are protected by herd immunity in developed countries and should therefore be immunized with the killed (Salk) vaccine prior to travel to areas endemic for polio.

Smallpox

Smallpox vaccine is effective and usually safe, but the immunity it confers is of relatively short duration, declining after about 3 years. The last known case of naturally occurring smallpox was reported from Somalia in October 1977, and the risk from even the low rate of complications significantly exceeds the benefits of vaccination. Thus, vaccination against smallpox is no longer recommended.

Rabies

Previously available rabies vaccines did, if only rarely, give rise to severe reactions. The risk of exposure is low, and preexposure immunization is thus reserved for travelers to hyperendemic areas and for persons with occupational or avocational hazard. Human diploid vaccine may change this risk:benefit assessment. Approximately 30,000 courses of antirabies treatment are given annually in the USA, and perhaps only 20% of these are necessary when the recommended treatment guidelines are carefully followed.

Cholera

Cholera immunization offers only temporary and incomplete protection. It is of little use to travelers and should be given only when the risk of exposure is high or in fulfillment of local regulations.

AGE AT IMMUNIZATION

The natural history of a disease determines the age at which immunization is best undertaken. Pertussis, polio, and diphtheria often infect infants; immunization against these diseases is therefore begun shortly after birth. Serious consequences of pertussis are uncommon beyond early childhood, and pertussis vaccination is not usually recommended after 6 years of age. Since the major hazard of rubella is the congenital rubella syndrome, and since nearly half of congenital rubella cases occur with the first pregnancy, it is very important to immunize as many females as possible prior to puberty. In this way the theoretic hazard of vaccinating a pregnant female and endangering the fetus is avoided, although inadvertently immunized fetuses have thus far not been reported to

be damaged by their exposure to the attenuated virus.

The efficacy of immunization may also be age-related. Failure may occur because of the presence of interfering antibodies or an undeveloped responsiveness of the immune system. Infants cannot be reliably protected with live measles, mumps, or rubella vaccines until maternally derived antibody has disappeared. Because a proportion of children immunized as late as 1 year of age fail to develop antibody after measles vaccination, the age recommended for measles vaccine administration has been changed to 15 months (see above), and some workers have made the same suggestion for rubella vaccine administration. Most of the children without antibody, however, may actually have been protected, based on the lack of an IgM response to reimmunization and in vitro evidence of cell-mediated immunity. Furthermore, delay in immunization is attended by a decrease in the number of children actually immunized, which approximates the improved rate of seroconversion. Individuals who were vaccinated at an earlier age in accordance with recommendations in effect at that time should be revaccinated. Infants frequently develop severe infections with *H influenzae* type b, pneumococci, or meningococci, but injecting them with purified capsular polysaccharide has failed to reliably yield a good antibody response, despite the excellent activity of the same antigen in older children and adults. Indeed, one study has shown that several children with early severe disease due to *H influenzae* did not develop active immunity and also failed to show a good antibody response to vaccine administered after 2 years of age. This failure to respond raises the question of a possible immune defect in the patients most in need of protection.

Recommendations for Childhood Immunization

Despite the extraordinary impact of immunization in the developed world, WHO estimates that of every 1000 children born today, 5 are crippled by poliomyelitis, 10 die of neonatal tetanus, 20 die of pertussis, and 30 die of measles and its complications. A rational program of immunization against infectious diseases begins in childhood, when many of the most damaging and preventable infections normally appear. Table 58–6 summarizes the current guidelines for immunization in childhood as compiled by the Expert Committee on Infectious Diseases of the American Academy of Pediatrics. The need for childhood immunization has increased because unimmunized individuals in a partially immune population will be less exposed to such childhood diseases as measles and mumps and will therefore develop them later than they otherwise would. When these illnesses do occur in adolescence or adulthood, they are often diagnostically bewilder-

Table 58–6. Guidelines for routine immunization of normal infants and children.

Diseases	Vaccine	Schedule of Doses				
		First	**Second**	**Third**	**Fourth**	**Fifth**
Diphtheria-tetanus-pertussis	DTP, adsorbed	2 mo	4 mo	6 mo	18 mo	4–6 yr[1]
Poliovirus I, II, and III	Oral trivalent	2 mo	4 mo	6 mo[2]	18 mo	4–6 yr[3]
Measles-mumps-rubella	MMR or singly	15 mo				
H influenzae	Conjugated PRP vaccine	18 mo				

[1]Adult-type combined tetanus-diphtheria toxoid (Td) is recommended at 10-year intervals thereafter.
[2]Optional in nonendemic areas.
[3]Only 3 doses are necessary if the third dose is given after the fourth birthday.

ing to the physician unprepared for such illnesses in this age group. Epidemic measles is now occurring in college students.

The physician should provide the patient with a clear and up-to-date record of all immunizations, which is useful in future medical encounters and in fulfilling school registration and other institutional requirements. Physicians can improve immunization rates by developing recall systems to identify children who are due for immunizations and by using the occasion of a visit for intercurrent illness to investigate and augment a patient's immune status. It is *not* necessary to restart an interrupted series of vaccinations or to add extra doses. If the vaccine history is unknown and there are no obvious contraindications, the child or adult should be fully immunized appropriately for his or her age. Reimmunization poses no significant risk.

For developing nations in which much preventable serious infection occurs in the first few years of life, WHO recommends an accelerated immunization program: at birth, oral poliovirus and BCG; at ages 6, 10, and 14 weeks, oral poliovirus and DTP; at age 9 months, measles (to be repeated in the second year of life if given before age 9 months).

Immunization of Adults & the Elderly

Childhood immunization programs have significantly decreased the incidence of preventable infections in developed countries. However, optimal immunization of adult populations has not yet been achieved. Much disease preventable by immunization continues to exist. Table 58–7 lists the most important immunizations for the adult and elderly population.

SIMULTANEOUS IMMUNIZATION WITH MULTIPLE ANTIGENS

The simultaneous inoculation of the nonliving antigens of diphtheria, tetanus, and pertussis (DTP) gives a response equal to that seen with their sepa-

Table 58–7. Immunizations recommended for adults 18 years of age and older.

Immunobiologic	Major Indications	Major Precautions
Influenza vaccine	Adults with high-risk conditions, residents of nursing homes or other chronic-care personnel, healthy persons age 65 years or older.	History of anaphylactic hypersensitivity to egg ingestion.
Pneumococcal polysaccharide vaccine (23-valent)	Adults who are at increased risk of pneumococcal disease and its complications because of underlying health conditions; healthy older adults, especially those age 65 years or older.	Vaccine safety in pregnant women has not been evaluated. Revaccination is not recommended.
Hepatitis B vaccine	Adults at increased risk of occupational, environmental, social, or family exposure to hepatitis B.	Pregnancy should not be considered a contraindication if the woman is otherwise eligible.
Tetanus-diphtheria toxoid	All adults at mid-decade ages.	History of a neurologic or hypersensitivity reaction after a previous dose.
Measles vaccine	Adults born after 1956 without verification of live measles vaccine on or after first birthday, physician-diagnosed measles, or laboratory evidence of immunity; susceptible travelers to foreign countries.	Pregnancy; history of anaphylactic reaction following egg ingestion or receipt of neomycin; immunosuppression.
Rubella vaccine	Adults without verification of live vaccine on or after first birthday or laboratory evidence of immunity; susceptible travelers to foreign countries.	Pregnancy; history of anaphylactic reaction following receipt of neomycin; immunosuppression.

rate injection; the endotoxic components of *Bordetella pertussis* may even act as an adjuvant, providing a superior immune response against the other antigens.

Similarly, the single injection of a mixture of live, attenuated measles, rubella, and mumps viruses or the simultaneous administration of live measles, smallpox, and yellow fever vaccines gives good responses to each component of the mixture. However, between 2 and 14 days following the administration of one live virus vaccine, there is a period of suboptimal response to a subsequently injected live virus vaccine. Live vaccines that are not given simultaneously should be given at least 4 weeks apart if time permits. The administration of cholera and yellow fever vaccines within 1–3 weeks of each other decreases the antibody response to both agents. Therefore, these immunizations also should be given at the same time or at least 4 weeks apart.

IMMUNIZATION FOR FOREIGN TRAVEL

National health authorities may require an International Certificate of Vaccination against cholera or yellow fever from travelers, usually depending upon the presence of these diseases in countries on their itinerary. Cholera vaccination may be given by any licensed physician; because it is not very effective, it is not generally recommended except when required. The certificate must be completed in all details and then validated with an officially approved stamp. Yellow fever vaccination may be administered and the certificate validated only at an officially designated center, which may be located by contacting the state or local health department. In addition to these legal requirements, all adults are advised to be adequately immunized against measles, tetanus, and diphtheria and to undergo additional immunizations (against poliomyelitis, typhoid, hepatitis A, and meningococcal meningitis) if they are visiting areas where the frequency of illness in the population or the level of sanitation increases the risk of infection. Travelers should be immunized against plague if contact with wild rodents or rabbits in an endemic rural area is anticipated and to hepatitis B if sexual contacts are anticipated in Southeast Asia or sub-Saharan Africa. A formalin-inactivated vaccine against Japanese B encephalitis, not licensed in the USA, may be available in several Asian countries where the infection is endemic; long-term travelers to areas with a significant risk of infection (China, India, Japan, Korea, Nepal, and Thailand) should ask at their embassies how vaccine may be obtained.

Travelers to malaria-endemic areas should be specifically advised to use mosquito repellents, malaria chemoprophylaxis, and acute therapy of presumptive infections.

No special immunizations are generally recommended for persons traveling from the USA to Western Europe, Canada, Australia, or Japan. Detailed suggestions of the USPHS are given country by country in its *Health Information for International Travel Supplement* (see References).

VACCINES FOR SPECIAL POPULATIONS

The greatest application of vaccines is in routine immunization of children and adults in large population groups. However, some vaccines are used only for population groups at greater hazard of disease by virtue of geography, occupation, or special exposure. The armed forces continue to vaccinate military personnel with vaccinia virus. They also use an oral adenovirus vaccine containing types 4 and 7, as well as a polyvalent meningococcal vaccine, for all recruits.

Veterinarians and animal handlers usually receive preexposure rabies vaccination, whereas postexposure rabies immunization is appropriate for the general public. Hepatitis B vaccine is recommended for those with increased occupation, household, or lifestyle risks.

VACCINES CURRENTLY IN DEVELOPMENT

Many vaccines are currently in various stages of development. New ones produced by recombinant DNA technology can be anticipated. The first of these to be licensed and marketed is hepatitis B recombinant vaccine; many others are in various stages of design and production. Synthetic analogs of antigen and possibly anti-idiotype antibodies may be developed in the future.

Varicella vaccine is almost ready for licensing and marketing. Vaccines against cytomegalovirus, herpes simplex virus, gonococci, *Plasmodium, Pseudomonas aeruginosa,* respiratory syncytial virus, rotavirus, *Shigella,* and many other pathogens are undergoing active development in the laboratory and in clinical trials. An effort is under way to conjugate the polysaccharide capsule of pneumococci to protein in a manner analogous to what has been accomplished with *H influenzae.*

Special immunoglobulin pools high in specific antibodies are being developed. The use of monoclonal antibodies in clinical practice is discussed in Chapter 62.

H INFLUENZAE TYPE B

The polysaccharide vaccine against *Haemophilus* (PRP) was licensed in 1985. It was known at that time that the vaccine was not effective before the age of 2 years; by that age, 50–75% of children who were going to acquire an invasive infection with this organism had already acquired it. In 1988 *Haemophilus* polysaccharide conjugated to diphtheria toxoid (PRP-D) was licensed. This vaccine is more antigenic than PRP and can be used at an earlier age; it is currently licensed for use at 18 months of age. PRP vaccines with other conjugates (tetanus toxoid, the outer member of the meningococcus organism) are also undergoing clinical trial. Validation of a conjugate vaccine that could be used at 2 months of age would significantly reduce the morbidity and mortality rates associated with this important bacterial pathogen.

HIV INFECTION

Active efforts are under way to develop a recombinant DNA vaccine utilizing HIV viral components, but its success will depend upon the rapidity of antigenic shift by the virus (see Chapter 55). The current recommendation for HIV-infected children is that they receive all the normal childhood immunizations (Table 58–5), with the exception that polio immunization be restricted to the inactivated form (Salk). This is principally to protect other adult members of the household who may be seriously immunocompromised. Live measles vaccine is recommended, despite the theoretic hazard, because of the severe form of measles infection that occurs in HIV-infected children.

REFERENCES

ACIP (Immunization Practices Advisory Committee): Immunization of children infected with human immunodeficiency virus. *MMWR* 1988;**37**:181.

Advice for travelers. *Med Lett* 1987;**29**:53.

American College of Obstetrics and Gynecology: *The Selective Use of Rh (D) Immune Globulin (Rh IG)*. ACOG Technical Bulletin No. 61, 1983.

Cherry JD et al: Report of the task force on pertussis and pertussis immunization, 1988. *Pediatrics* 1988;**81**:939.

Committee on Immunization, Council of Medical Societies: *Guide for Adult Immunization*. American College of Physicians, 1985.

Dwyer JM: Intravenous therapy with gamma globulin. *Adv Intern Med* 1987;**32**:111.

Fedson DS: Adult immunization: Protocols and problems. *Hosp Pract* (July) 1986;**21(7)**:143.

Health Information for International Travel, 1990. HHS Publication No (CDC) 86-8280. [Revised annually.]

Immunization Practices Advisory Committee: Prevention and control of influenza. *MMWR* 1988;**37**:361.

La Force MF: ,Immunizations, immunoprophylaxis, and chemoprophylaxis to prevent selective infections. *JAMA* 1987;**275**:2464.

National Childhood Vaccine Injury Act: Requirements for permanent vaccination records and for reporting of selected events after vaccination. *MMWR* 1988;**37**:197.

Pennington JE: Properties and characteristics of immunoglobulin G intravenous preparation. *Rev Infect Dis* 1986;**8**:S371.

Rutledge SL, Snead OC: Neurologic complications of immunizations. *J Pediatr* 1986;**109**:917.

Smith MH: National childhood vaccine injury compensation act. *Pediatrics* 1988;**82**:264.

Summary of the second national forum on adult immunization. *MMWR* 1987;**36**:677.

Williams WW et al: Immunization policies and vaccine coverage among adults. *Ann Intern Med* 1988;**108**:616.

59

Allergy Desensitization

Abba I. Terr, MD

Allergy **desensitization** is a form of treatment in which the patient is deliberately exposed to low doses of allergens for the purpose of reducing or eliminating the allergic response. It is also called allergen immunotherapy, hyposensitization, or allergy injection therapy. The procedure consists of frequent repeated injections of increasing amounts of allergen until the patient achieves increased tolerance to that specific allergen on natural exposure. It is most often used in IgE antibody-mediated diseases, but it has been used in other forms of allergy as well. Ideally, the treatment goal is complete abolition of the sensitivity, but in practice the result is usually only a diminution in symptoms. It is an adjunct to allergen avoidance and symptomatic drug therapy, not the primary mode of treatment or a substitute for avoidance of allergens. Nevertheless, it is usually effective in situations where allergen avoidance is not possible.

Noon published the first report of desensitization for hay fever in England in 1911. Since then it has been extensively used in allergy practice to treat hay fever and allergic asthma. Since the early 1960s a sufficient number of controlled clinical trials have been completed to clearly establish its effectiveness in allergic rhinitis and Hymenoptera venom anaphylaxis. So far there have been too few definitive studies of its use in asthma to draw firm conclusions. Short-term desensitization has been accomplished in some cases of penicillin and insulin allergy. Successful oral desensitization has been reported for some drug-induced cutaneous eruptions, but these findings are uncontrolled. It is often attempted in *Rhus* contact dermatitis (poison ivy or poison oak), but to date it has not been shown to be effective in this disease. The mechanism of desensitization is still uncertain, but it is thought to be immunologic. A variety of specific immunologic responses are induced during desensitization treatment. Promising improvements in the procedure are currently under study.

METHODS

The general procedure for desensitization in allergic rhinitis used today is similar to the method used originally by Noon. Sterile allergen extracts are administered subcutaneously in increasing doses once or twice a week until a dose is reached that produces a transient small local area of inflammation at the injection site. This dose is then given as a maintenance dose once every 2–4 weeks. Originally the course of treatment was preseasonal for a single-season pollen allergy, beginning 3–6 months before the expected onset of the season and terminating at the onset of the season. Because most patients with allergic rhinitis have allergies to different pollens at different times of the year as well as year-round dust or mold allergy, perennial (year-round) injection therapy is the most common schedule used by allergists today. The injections include a mixture of all relevant inhalant allergens, and after the maximum dose of the mixture is reached, the maintenance dose is continued for several years.

The injections are given subcutaneously. Oral, sublingual, and inhaled methods of desensitization have been tried, but none has been shown to be effective in preventing diseases caused by IgE antibodies. Local nasal immunotherapy, in which allergen extract is administered by nasal spray, is currently under active investigation, but results to date show only marginal efficacy.

Extracts used in immunotherapy are the same as those used for testing (see Chapter 30). In most cases they are crude aqueous extracts of the common inhalant allergens. Some are now standardized for content of the major allergen to ensure uniformity among different batches of extracts. Purified major allergens, such as ragweed antigen E, have been used in clinical studies and may be effective in treatment of certain patients with restricted sensitivity to that allergen. Many allergic patients, however, have multiple sensitivities and therefore require the multiple allergens present in crude allergen extracts.

Injection Technique

Details of administering therapeutic allergen injections to patients with atopic or anaphylactic disease are important for the success and safety of the treatment. Because of possible risk of systemic reactions, facilities must be available to treat systemic reactions. Such potentially fatal reactions usually begin within 30 minutes after the injection. Treatment should be withheld on a day when the patient is experiencing acute asthma or a fever. Small local swelling with itching at the injection site is acceptable. Excessive local swelling or any systemic reaction requires a reduction in dose. The dose should also be reduced if there has been a lapse in treatment.

Duration of Treatment

There are insufficient data to set guidelines for the overall length of desensitization in atopy. The variability in the natural course of disease, the vagaries of environmental exposures for the many different indoor (dust, molds, animals) and outdoor (pollens, molds) allergens, and the effect of nonallergic factors (weather, pollution, infections, stress) make definitive controlled long-term studies technically difficult. The immunologic changes induced by desensitization (see below), either singly or in combination, do not correlate sufficiently with symptomatic relief to be used to determine the duration of therapy. However, there is a progressive reduction of symptoms of pollen allergy for the first 3 or 4 years of preseasonal ragweed injections, after which the therapeutic effect levels off. There are no data on recurrence after the injections are stopped. Some allergists recommend that treatment be discontinued after 2 successive symptomless years.

Hymenoptera venom desensitization for anaphylaxis has been shown to be highly effective in reducing the risk of reactions from spontaneous stings throughout the period of active treatment at the maintenance dosage. Studies are now being conducted to assess the effects of discontinuing treatment, but until results are available, patients with life-threatening reactions should continue venom desensitization indefinitely.

Clinical Results

The results of the first controlled clinical trial of desensitization were published in the early 1960s, 50 years after the first use of this form of therapy for atopic disease. Since then, results from approximately 30 placebo-controlled double-blind studies show that desensitization is effective in seasonal and perennial allergic rhinitis when sufficient allergen is given to induce an immunologic response. The effect is immunologically specific. Fig 59–1 shows the results of one such study on patients with seasonal ragweed hay fever. On average, symptoms are considerably reduced, especially at the peak of the pollen season. Similar efficacy has been shown for other pollens and for molds, house dust, and dust mites.

Controlled trials on patients with allergic asthma are more difficult to perform because the disease is exacerbated by so many nonallergic factors such as respiratory infections, atmospheric irritants, and emotions. Nevertheless, one study showed that desensitization treatment of asthma caused by allergy to cats reduced the bronchoprovocation response to cat allergen inhalation.

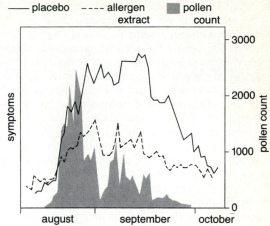

Figure 59–1. Desensitization therapy in patients with allergic rhitis. Results of a placebo-controlled double-blind trial of ragweed allergen injections on the allergic symptoms of patients with ragweed hay fever during the ragweed pollinating season. (Adapted, with permission, from Norman PS, Winkenwerder WL, Lichtenstein LM: Trials of alum-precipitated pollen extracts in the treatment of hay fever. *J Allergy Clin Immunol* 1972;**50:**31.)

Hymenoptera insect venom anaphylaxis responds exceedingly well to desensitization: 95% of treated patients are protected from reactions to deliberate or unintentional stings, whereas about 50% of untreated or placebo-treated controls continue to experience systemic reactions to insect stings. Venom desensitization also appears to be effective in patients who respond to insect stings with urticaria or with consistently large local swellings at the sting site, but these conditions are not considered serious enough to warrant the treatment.

Desensitization has not been evaluated as a treatment for atopic dermatitis because exacerbations of the skin lesions usually do not correlate with inhalant allergen exposure. Food allergen injection therapy has not been evaluated for efficacy against any of the clinical manifestations of food allergy.

IMMUNOLOGIC EFFECTS

Several different immunologic effects are induced in allergic patients by desensitization therapy.

Hyposensitization

The term "desensitization" implies an absence of the preexisting allergen-specific IgE antibody, conversion of the wheal-and-erythema skin test to negative, loss of the target organ response to the allergen by provocative-dose testing, and a cure of the disease. In practice, desensitization is rare, being achieved in only about 5% of patients on an adequate course of therapy. Most treated atopic patients are hyposensitized. Immunologic and clinical measures of the specific IgE-mediated allergy are significantly lessened but not eliminated, even after many years of the injection treatment. The level of circulating IgE antibody falls below pretreatment levels only after many months of treatment (Fig 59–2). It is important to note that IgE antibody production is enhanced transiently during the first few months of low-dose allergen injections, and some patients experience a corresponding temporary worsening of symptoms during that time.

Immunization

An allergen-specific IgG antibody is induced by treatment (Fig 59–2). The antibody is often called "blocking antibody," because it inhibits the effect of IgE antibody in the passive-transfer (Prausnitz-Küstner) skin test and in the passive-transfer in vitro histamine release assay. Blocking antibodies of the IgA isotype may also be demonstrated in the serum of treated patients, but blocking activity in secretions does not occur to a significant extent. Recent studies suggest that blocking antibody of the IgG4 subclass may correlate better with clinical improvement than that of other IgG subclasses. The presence of block-

ing antibody in serum is sustained as long as the maintenance injections are continued; the level then drops off gradually after treatment is stopped.

Regulation of IgE Antibody Production

There is limited evidence from a few studies that desensitization therapy alters regulatory factors in the production of allergen-specific IgE antibody. Some in vitro experiments indicate that treatment generates specific T cells with suppressor activity on IgE antibody production.

Combination Effects

It is likely that the beneficial effect of desensitization treatment in allergic diseases may derive from an optimal combination of each of the immunologic changes described above—and perhaps others—since no single effect, such as the quantity of blocking antibody, correlates well with clinical improvement. Regardless of the precise mechanism, desensitization is specific for the allergens injected, is dose-related, and requires repeated and prolonged parenteral administration.

ADVERSE EFFECTS

The possible adverse effects of desensitization are both immediate and long-term. The immediate hazard is a systemic anaphylactic reaction. The risk is greatest both during the early weeks or months of treatment while the dose is being increased before a significant level of blocking antibody has been achieved and again when the dose is at or near the maintenance dose. Systemic reactions are unpredictable and may occur after years of uneventful injections. They are more likely to happen during the patient's pollen allergy season than during the off-season. Fever and physical exercise increase blood flow, causing more rapid absorption of the injected allergen and hence enhancing the risk of reaction.

The prevalence of systemic reactions is unknown. A recent study showed that on average, about one death occurs each year in the USA from allergy injection treatment or skin testing, some because of dosage errors. About half occur in patients with active asthma.

Other immediate adverse effects are the same as for any subcutaneous injection, such as vasovagal reactions, infections, or injury from injecting the needle into the wrong tissue.

There appear to be no late or long-term ill effects from immunotherapy. With the use of aqueous allergen extracts, there is no evidence that repeated injections induce de novo allergic sensitization to components to which the patient was not previously sensitive. There are no proven instances in which allergen desensitization produces systemic immune-complex disease or other late sequelae.

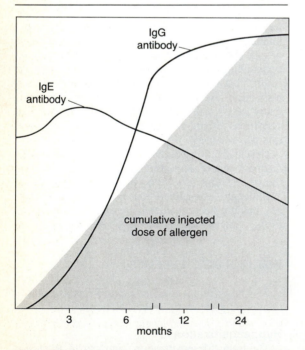

Figure 59–2. Immunologic changes during prolonged desensitization therapy for IgE-mediated diseases. The level of circulating IgE antibody is initially increased and later decreased below pretreatment levels. IgG antibody appears rapidly after the start of treatment, and its level is sustained while treatment continues.

INDICATIONS

Atopy

Desensitization has been used for almost 80 years to treat allergic rhinitis, and today it is widely accepted as beneficial. It is indicated for patients who are allergic to unavoidable inhalant allergens such as pollens and fungi and whose symptomatic periods are severe, prolonged, and not well controlled by antihistamines or other symptomatic medications. House dust and dust mite desensitization is used in conjunction with a program of dust and mite elimination, since the latter is rarely completely effective. Allergists are currently divided in their opinion about injections of animal dander extracts for treatment of allergy to pets in the home or for occupational animal allergy. Opponents point out the paucity of controlled studies, presumed excessive risk of systemic reactions, and concern about unknown long-term effects of immunization with animal protein. Although there are insufficient controlled clinical trials, the indications for desensitization of allergic asthma parallel those for allergic rhinitis. Desensitization is not indicated for treatment of atopic dermatitis or allergic gastroenteropathy. Patients with atopic dermatitis may receive injections for concomitant allergic rhinitis or asthma if indicated, but starting doses should be low and the buildup in dosage should be slow, because injected allergens may cause a flare of the dermatitis. Desensitization is not indicated for food allergy.

Anaphylaxis

Desensitization is indicated for any patient with a history of anaphylaxis from a Hymenoptera insect sting who has a positive skin test to one or more Hymenoptera venoms. Many authorities exclude from treatment those patients whose reaction to the sting was limited to urticaria, regardless of the skin test results, because such patients generally do not have an excessive risk of systemic anaphylaxis on future stings. There is no indication for desensitization treatment of localized swelling from an insect sting, no matter how large the swelling, since these also do not predict future anaphylaxis. The injected allergens for treatment of anaphylaxis should include all of the venoms that give a positive skin test, since identification of the stinging insect under usual conditions of a spontaneous sting is usually unreliable.

Desensitization for anaphylaxis to drugs has been successful for selected cases of penicillin and insulin allergy. In those instances, injection of increasing doses at intervals of approximately 30 minutes achieves a clinical state of desensitization permitting therapeutic use of the drug on a regular basis. If the drug is withdrawn, the patient may again become allergic.

Urticaria

Desensitization has never been shown to be effec-

tive therapy for urticaria, and it is not indicated for this condition.

Immune-Complex Allergies

Desensitization is not necessary for treatment of cutaneous Arthus reactions or for serum sickness. These are self-limited reactions, which subside when the allergen has been eliminated.

Allergic Contact Dermatitis

Oral and subcutaneous desensitization with extracts of *Rhus* oil has been used for many years, but there is no evidence for its effectiveness in prevention of *Rhus* allergic dermatitis (from poison ivy and poison oak), and therefore it is not indicated for these conditions.

Hypersensitivity Pneumonitis

Desensitization is not indicated for this disease.

Others

Injections of bacterial extracts were fashionable at one time for treatment of nonallergic (instrinsic) asthma and other diseases. There is no immunologically sound rationale for such treatment. Injections of staphylococcal extracts for recurrent furunculosis has been advocated but not evaluated.

MONITORING DESENSITIZATION

Desensitization of atopy is a treatment that continues for years. Indications for starting this long-term process are usually clear, but selection of allergens, dosages and frequency of injections, and duration of therapy must be individualized. The beneficial and adverse responses are difficult to predict in advance. It is therefore important to establish a long-term goal and program for monitoring treatment at the outset.

Changes in serum levels of specific IgE antibody and induced IgG blocking antibody correlate statistically with clinical improvement, but these are not useful monitors of progress in individual cases. Some allergists repeat skin testing at regular intervals, but clinical improvement can occur without change in skin test reactivity. The principal reason for retesting is to diagnose new sensitivities when symptoms worsen or appear at new seasons.

At present, assessing desensitization for effectiveness requires monitoring of symptoms and physical signs of illness, as well as performing objective tests such as pulmonary functions when applicable. It is reasonable to discontinue the injections after 2 or 3 successive disease-free years.

DESENSITIZATION WITH MODIFIED ALLERGENS

There has been a continuing effort to improve the effectiveness of specific injection therapy and reduce the risk of reactions and the number of injections through the use of adjuvants and chemical alteration, modification, and polymerization of the allergen.

Adjuvants

Incomplete Freund's adjuvant—emulsification of aqueous antigen in mineral oil—enhances the immune response by providing an insoluble lipid depot in the subcutaneous tissue from which droplets of allergen are gradually released, thereby simulating repeated injections of allergen over time. It is commonly used in research to generate large quantities of antibodies in animals. In the early 1960s this method of "one-shot" desensitization given preseasonally underwent extensive clinical trials. The treatment was probably similar in effectiveness to conventional multi-injection desensitization, but mineral oil persists indefinitely in tissues and causes long-lasting nodules, cysts, and sterile abscesses that might require surgical removal. This form of therapy was abandoned because of concern about potential carcinogenicity.

Adsorption of allergens onto alum produces an insoluble antigen that is more efficiently phagocytosed by macrophages. Alum-adsorbed allergens have had limited acceptance in practice for many years. The hoped-for advantages over aqueous allergens—fewer injections and improved efficacy—have never been demonstrated.

Allergoids

Formalin treatment of toxic antigens such as tetanus toxin yields a toxoid, a molecule without toxicity that retains antigenicity, thereby permitting complete and safe active immunity. The same principle has been exploited with allergens for desensitization, but to date attempts to modify allergens with formalin, propylene glycol, urea, and other chemicals to eliminate or reduce allergenicity and risk of systemic reactions while preserving immunogenicity to the native allergen have been unsuccessful.

Polymerized Allergens

The most promising method to date for improving desensitization is the technique of polymerizing protein allergens with glutaraldehyde. Covalently linked allergen monomers provide a molecule with low allergenicity in proportion to the degree of polymerization. Theoretically, monomeric and polymeric molecules are equally effective in bridging IgE antibodies for (undesired) allergy-producing mediator release, whereas the polymer, when phagocytosed and processed by the antigen-presenting macrophage, presents many more antigenic epitopes for the (desired) protective immune response. Although not yet released for clinical practice, several different polymerized inhalant allergens have been confirmed by therapeutic trials to have the theoretic advantages of this form of desensitization.

REFERENCES

American Academy of Allergy and Immunology Executive Committee: Personnel and equipment to treat systemic reactions caused by immunotherapy with allergenic extracts. (Position statement.) *J Allergy Clin Immunol* 1986; **77**:271.

Grammer LC, Shaughnessy MA, Patterson R: Modified forms of allergen immunotherapy. *J Allergy Clin Immunol* 1985;**76**:397.

Johnstone DE, Dutton A: The value of hyposensitization therapy for bronchial asthma in children: A 14-year study. *Pediatrics* 1968;**47**:793.

Lichtenstein LM, Norman PS, Winkenwerder WL: Clinical and in vitro studies on the role of immunotherapy in ragweed hay fever. *Am J Med* 1968;**44**:514.

Lowell FC, Franklin W: A double-blind study of the effectiveness and specificity of injection therapy in ragweed hay fever. *N Engl J Med* 1965;**273**:675.

Noon L: Prophylactic inoculation against hay fever. *Lancet* 1911;**1**:1572.

Norman PS: Immunotherapy for nasal allergy. *J Allergy Clin Immunol* 1988;**81**:992.

Norman PS: An overview of immunotherapy: Implications for the future. *J Allergy Clin Immunol* 1980;**65**:87.

Ohman JL: Allergen immunotherapy in asthma: Evidence for efficacy. *J Allergy Clin Immunol* 1989;**84**:133.

Rocklin RE: Clinical and immunologic aspects of allergen-specific immunotherapy in patients with seasonal allergic rhinitis and/or allergic asthma. *J Allergy Clin Immunol* 1983;**73**:323.

Sherman WB, Connell JT: Changes in skin-sensitizing antibody titer (SSAT) following two to four years of injection (aqueous) therapy. *J Allergy Clin Immunol* 1966; **37**:123.

Terr AI: Immunologic basis for injection therapy of allergic diseases. *Med Clin N Am* 1969;**53**:1257.

Clinical Transplantation 60

Marvin R. Garovoy, MD, Juliet S. Melzer, MD, Nancy Ascher, MD, PhD, Don Magilligan, Jr, MD, & Marek Bozdech, MD

Transplantation of organs is becoming increasingly successful. What was once an experimental and life-saving emergency procedure is being transformed into a life-enhancing and technologically advanced form of therapy.

The first successful renal transplant was performed in 1954. Subsequently, advances in histocompatibility testing and immunosuppressive drug therapy made renal transplantation a clinical reality in the 1960s. Improved skills and handling of immunosuppressive drugs (prednisone and azathioprine) resulted in a decline in infectious complications and marked reduction in mortality rates. The 1970s witnessed the beneficial effects of blood transfusions and antilymphocyte globulin (ALG) as graft-enhancing treatments. The 1980s may be characterized as the era of cyclosporine and the advent of monoclonal antibody therapy—immunosuppressive agents that have greatly improved the success rate of kidney transplants and have also made possible heart, liver, and pancreas engraftment with better results than before. Transplant outcome has become so promising that it is now being offered early in the care of many patients with chronic and debilitating diseases.

KIDNEY TRANSPLANTATION

Patients with end-state renal disease can be considered for renal transplantation. Absolute contraindications are conditions that would interfere with the safe administration of anesthesia or immunosuppressive therapy. These include debilitating cardiopulmonary disease, cancer, and active peptic ulcer disease or infection. Preoperative immunologic evaluation includes erythrocyte ABO blood grouping, histocompatibility testing (determination of the patient's and potential donor's human leukocyte antigens (HLA antigens) and the degree of haplotype matching), and state of presensitization to HLA antigens (see Chapter 21). Medical evaluation to rule out contraindications to transplantation frequently includes intestinal x-rays, voiding cystourethrography, dental and pulmonary evaluations, and assessment of cardiac status.

ABO Testing

Erythrocyte ABO testing is performed on all recipients and potential donors. The ABO system is present not only on erythrocytes but also on the vascular endothelium of the graft, with the result that renal transplants are performed only between ABO-compatible pairs. The danger of transplanting across the ABO barrier is the production of very rapid graft rejection owing to preformed isohemagglutinins that injure the vascular endothelium and elicit a coagulation reaction in situ. The same rules that apply to blood transfusion compatibility also apply to renal transplantation: For a type O recipient the donor should be type O; for a type A recipient the donor may be type A or O; for a type B recipient the donor may be type B or O; and for a type AB recipient the donor may be type A, B, or O. It is possible to overcome the ABO barrier by plasmapheresis to lower the natural titer of anti-A or anti-B antibodies and by administration of cyclophosphamide to prevent new antibody formation, but the long-term safety and efficacy of this experimental approach are unknown.

Living Related Donor Transplantation

All recipients and their potential donors should have complete testing for HLA-A, -B, -C, -DR, and -DQ antigens (see Chapter 21). On the basis of family typings, it is usually possible to determine the genotype or haplotype (chromosome) assignment for each identified antigen. The value of haplotype matching (zero, one, or 2) was established clinically: 2-haplotype-matched siblings can be expected to achieve 90% graft survival at 1 year; one-haplotype-matched (sibling or parent) pairs achieve 75–85% survival at 1 year, and zero-haplotype-matched family members achieve only 50–60% survival at 1 year without further conditioning of the immune status of the recipient.

A common clinical dilemma is the need to choose among several available compatible donors. Cellular immune assay of the mixed lymphocyte culture (MLC) (see Chapters 19 and 21) is used for this purpose in several centers. Each donor who is a one-haplotype match with the patient shares only a single set of HLA-DR, -DQ genes. The MLC test evaluates the recipient's in vitro proliferative response to the single set of mismatched HLA-DR, -DQ genes. One-haplotype-matched pairs with low or weak MLC responses are associated with excellent (90%) graft survival, whereas comparably matched pairs with strong MLC responses historically have poorer (60%) graft survival. In some centers, the low rate of graft survival among one-haplotype-matched pairs with strong MLC responses led to the cessation of this type of transplantation until a solution was found (see Blood Transfusion, below).

Presensitization

Prior exposure to transplantation antigens can lead to sensitization manifested by the development of cytotoxic antibodies against HLA antigens. Patients who have antibodies to HLA antigens may have a poorer graft outcome. Moreover, patients who are sensitized and receive second and subsequent transplants are more likely to reject these grafts than are those who receive a primary graft. This likelihood is especially increased in patients who rapidly rejected their first graft (in < 3 months). Whether repeated rejection is caused by specific sensitization to transplantation antigens or reflects a high immune reactivity of the recipient is under investigation.

Cross-Matching

The cross-match test is used to determine the presence of any preformed antibodies (presensitization) to donor HLA antigens. A cross-match typically is performed by using the patient's most recent serum and donor lymphocytes (either peripheral blood mononuclear cells or isolated T or B lymphocytes) (see Chapter 21). Positive cross-matches are a contraindication to transplantation, since they are associated with very early and uncontrollable rejection episodes, leading to irreversible graft loss.

Cadaveric Transplantation

In circumstance when the recipient has no family members as potential donors, the opportunity exists to receive a kidney from a recently deceased individual (cadaveric transplantation). Recipients referred for this type of treatment undergo comparable immunologic evaluation of ABO grouping, HLA typing, and antibody screening and are then placed on a waiting list. While waiting, these patients often receive random blood transfusions both to treat anemia and to increase graft survival. This exposure increases the likelihood of producing anti-HLA antibodies in response to the leukocytes or leukocyte fragments contained in each unit of blood. Other likely causes of formation of anti-HLA antibodies include pregnancy and previously rejected grafts. To monitor the extent of anti-HLA antibodies produced, serum from each recipient is collected monthly and tested in a manner known as screening. The patient's serum is cross-matched against a panel of lymphocytes obtained from many individuals. The number of individuals whose cells are killed is often expressed as a percentage of the panel (eg, 10% panel-reactive antibody). By this procedure, it is possible to determine the extent of presensitization, ie, how often the patient is likely to have a positive cross-match, assuming that the transplant organ is taken from the same genetic pool of donors as the lympho-

cyte panel. In addition, knowing the HLA antigens on the lymphocyte panel cells that have been lysed makes it possible to analyze the specificities of the antibodies present in the serum and responsible for the positive reactions. For example, if 4 of the cells that were injured on the panel have antigen B8 in common, the antibody is considered to be anti-B8. Knowing the HLA antibody specificities in a recipient's serum allows the transplant team to avoid donors bearing those transplant antigens. Typically, in choosing a cell panel, 40–50 cells are chosen; this allows each HLA antigen to be represented approximately twice.

Donor Selection

When a potential cadaveric donor's organs are harvested, a section of spleen, some lymph nodes, and some peripheral blood are collected. The donor ABO blood group and HLA antigens are determined from these samples. The waiting list of recipients can then be cross-matched against the donor tissues, using the patient's current serum and the recipient's highest-reacting serum within the past 2 years to exclude the possibility of a positive cross-match. Recipients who are ABO-compatible and cross-match-negative become available for further consideration. Often, there may be a second round of cross-match testing among this smaller pool of recipients, in which additional past sera are chosen to be certain of no hidden presensitization. From among the ABO-compatible, cross-match-negative recipients, the best-matched recipients may then be selected. In programs in which a large enough choice of recipients is not available to find a perfectly matched recipient, additional criteria such as length of time on the waiting list, urgency of medical condition, and whether this is a first or second transplant are considered in recipient selection.

Donor Evaluation

Family studies conducted to evaluate a potential family donor include a complete medical evaluation. There is no long-term change in survival or life-style of individuals who have undergone uninephrectomy for donation. Because of increased success rates of related-donor transplantation, owing to improved immunosuppression and preoperative conditioning, it is now possible to consider living donors who share 2, one, or no haplotypes with the recipient. Limited studies indicate that living unrelated donors can be considered, with appropriate preoperative conditioning procedures. Evaluation of donor motivation and psychologic factors is necessary.

Cadaveric donors can be considered when determined to be neurologically dead following spontaneous intracerebral hemorrhage or head trauma. Cadaveric donors must be free from metastasizing tumors, kidney dysfunction, or active infection (particularly with hepatitis viruses or HIV). Hemodynamic stabilization with volume expansion and the conservative use of vasopressors maintain optimal organ function. The use of corticosteroids in cadaveric donors is controversial. The living-donor nephrectomy procedure includes a flank incision through which the kidney is removed, preserving all renal arteries and veins. The ureter is removed with all periureteral soft tissue in order to include the ureteral blood supply and prevent distal ureteral avascular necrosis. Organ recovery from cadaveric donors includes removal of both kidneys with renal arteries and veins frequently left en bloc with the donor aorta and vena cava. Both ureters are removed, including all periureteral soft tissue, in order to include the ureteral blood supply and prevent distal ureteral avascular necrosis. Samples of spleen and lymph nodes are also removed for donor tissue typing and cross-matching against potential recipients.

Once removed, the kidney is flushed with mixed-electrolyte solutions to remove all donor blood and to be cooled. Cadaveric kidneys can be stored by either of 2 methods. Cold storage involves packing in ice to maintain subphysiologic temperatures. Alternatively, the aorta or renal arteries are cannulated, and a cold mixed-electrolyte solution is instilled by continuous cold pulsatile perfusion. Cadaver renal transplantation within the first 48 hours after donor nephrectomy is preferred.

Blood Transfusion

Recipient preconditioning can include a variety of measures. For patients awaiting cadaveric transplantation, it has been found that preoperative random blood transfusion is correlated with improved allograft survival. Untransfused patients have approximately 40–50% graft function after 2 years, whereas patients who have received blood transfusions have a 60–80% chance of long-term cadaver graft function. Although as little as 1 unit of random blood has been correlated with improved results, the larger the number of transfusions, the better the graft survival. Mechanisms for the transfusion effect include elimination of immunologic responders who will demonstrate cytotoxic antibodies contraindicating transplantation, development of specific and nonspecific suppressor T cells, and generation of blocking or anti-idiotypic antibodies.

For individuals awaiting related-donor transplantation, improved allograft success in one- and zero-haplotype-matched donor-recipient pairs has come through experiments involving the transfusion of donor-specific blood. These protocols call for multiple transfusions (usually 3) of small amounts of blood (100–200 mL) over several weeks during which the development of cytotoxic antidonor antibodies in the recipient is monitored. In 10–30% of recipients, cytotoxic antidonor antibodies develop, contraindicating transplantation. This antidonor sensitization can be reduced to less than 10% in the majority of one-haplotype-matched pairs by the simultaneous administration of azathioprine (1–2 mg/kg/d) during donor-specific transfusion. In the remaining 70–90% who do not become sensitized, 1-haplotype-matched allograft results have improved from approximately 65% (without donor-specific transfusion) to 95% allograft survival after 2 years with pretransplant donor-specific transfusion. In limited studies of zero-haplotype-matched donor-recipient pairs and unrelated living donor-recipient pairs, excellent allograft survival (> 90% at 2 years) has been achieved with donor-specific transfusion. In 2-haplotype-matched donor-recipient pairs, random blood transfusions or donor-specific transfusion also correlates with an improved posttransplant course and allograft success (> 90% at 2 years). Mechanisms of the donor-specific transfusion effect may include selection of immunologic nonresponders, induction of specific and nonspecific suppressor T cells, development of blocking or possibly anti-idiotypic antibodies, and clonal deletion.

Transplant Surgery

The operative procedure for the recipient includes an iliac incision through which the graft is placed in the retroperitoneal position against the psoas muscle (Fig 60–1). A renal artery anastomosis to either the internal or external iliac artery and renal vein anastomosis to the external iliac vein are standard. Ureteroneocystotomy involving anastomosis of the ureter to bladder mucosa through an anterior cystot-

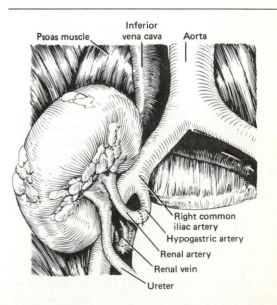

Figure 60–1. Technique of renal transplantation. (Reproduced, with permission, from Way LW (editor): *Current Surgical Diagnosis & Treatment,* 7th ed. Lange, 1985.)

omy incision is a usual approach. The ureter is often passed through a short submucosal tunnel in the bladder wall to prevent vesicoureteral reflux.

Postoperatively, hemodynamic stability is achieved with fluids to optimize renal perfusion and renal function. Careful monitoring of electrolytes, blood urea nitrogen, and creatinine to evaluate renal function is mandatory. All cadaveric kidneys have some degree of acute tubular necrosis, ranging from very mild to very severe. Dialysis is required in 13–50% of cadaveric renal transplant recipients during the period of acute tubular necrosis (usually 5–10 days). Acute tubular necrosis is rare in patients receiving related-donor transplants since donor nephrectomy and recipient transplant are performed simultaneously, precluding the need for renal storage.

Postoperative Immunosuppression

Postoperative immunosuppression is the most variable aspect of recipient care. Standard immunosuppression to prevent rejection includes corticosteroids, and additional immunosuppression is chosen depending upon the type of allograft and tissue match (see Chapters 61 and 63). The use of cyclosporine (5–15 mg/kg/d) has clearly improved long-term allograft success in recipients of cadaveric and some related-donor transplants. Cyclosporine is definitely nephrotoxic, and monitoring of drug dosages and drug levels (100–400 μg/mL) is required.

Azathoprine, an antimetabolite that interferes with new DNA formation in proliferating cells, is frequently used (2–5 mg/kg/d) in combination with prednisone and cyclosporine. Azathioprine is potentially hepatotoxic, whereas cyclophosphamide is a nonheptotoxic alternative. ALG (10–20 mg/kg) or antithymocyte globulin (ATG), a heterologous serum prepared in animals immunized with human lymphocytes or thymocytes, respectively, is a potent immunosuppressive reagent and acts through antilymphocytic properties. This heterologous animal protein can be made in horses, sheep, goats, or rabbits. Monoclonal antibodies against specific T cell subsets are also in clinical use. Lymphoplasmapheresis occasionally is used to remove recipient lymphocytes and immunoglobulin while immunosuppressive drugs are concurrently administered. Local graft irradiation has been utilized but has not provided reliable immunosuppression.

Rejection

Classic signs and symptoms of acute rejection include swelling and tenderness over the allograft and decrease in renal function. Systemic manifestations such as temperature elevation, malaise, poor appetite, and generalized myalgia can be seen. Decrease in renal function is diagnosed by a decrease in urine volume, by increasing blood urea nitrogen and creatinine levels, and radiographically by ultrasonogra-

phy (blurring of corticomedullary junctions) and by radionuclide renal scans showing decreased blood flow. In the presence of a decline in renal function, however, the differential diagnosis includes prerenal azotemia and obstruction, acute tubular necrosis, pyelonephritis, and other drug-induced toxicity. In addition, recurrence of the primary renal disease and de novo glomerulonephritis can be late causes of decreased renal function. Renal biopsy is frequently performed to histologically diagnose the cause of graft dysfunction.

Mechanisms of Rejection

A. Acute: Evidence suggests that blood-borne antigen-presenting cells (''passenger cells'') in grafts provide the primary stimulus. These are dendritic cells and monocytes expressing class II HLA molecules. These cells are necessary to present antigen in a form that lymphocytes can recognize. The antigen-presenting cells also provide a second signal, interleukin-1 (IL-1), and IL-2, which aid in triggering lymphocyte activation (Fig 60–2). IL-1 not only is involved in the activation of helper/inducer CD4 T cells but probably also is important for the activation of unprimed cytotoxic CD8 T cells and B lymphocytes. The activation of helper/inducer T cells by alloantigen is pivotal to the development of cell immune responses against the graft. Once activated, these cells release IL-2, which is an essential cofactor in the activation of both CD8 T cells and B cells. As a consequence of exposure to antigen plus the interleukins, there is clonal proliferation and maturation of alloantigen-reactive cells. This leads to the development of effector T cells, which migrate from lymphoid tissue via the blood to all tissues, including the graft, where they mediate damage at antigen-containing sites, and antibody, which is released into the blood or locally within the graft, where it has access to these antigens.

The precise mechanism by which T cells destroy the graft is still under study. Effector T cells that can destroy graft tissue develop from both CD8 and CD4 subclasses (Fig 60–3). The results are similar except that CD8 T cells recognize HLA-A, -B antigen-bearing cells, whereas CD4 T cells recognize HLA-DR antigen-bearing cells. Both CD4 and CD8 subclasses of effector cells probably can directly destroy graft cells by classic cytotoxic T cell mechanisms. However, another important consequence of T cell activation is their release of other lymphokines, especially gamma interferon (IFN γ), which can produce 2 important effects. First, IFN γ induces increased expression of HLA-A, -B, and -DR on graft tissue, which potentially makes the graft more vulnerable to effector mechanisms. Second, it activates monocytes to mediate a destructive delayed hypersensitivity response against the graft.

Hence, T cells can directly cause target cell injury or activate macrophages into nonspecific destruc-

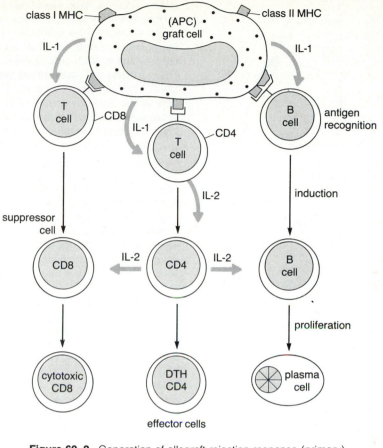

Figure 60–2. Generation of allograft rejection response (primary).

tion. Lymphokines in addition to IL-2 and IFN γ are released from activated T cells; they include IL-4 and IL-5, which play a role in directing B cell production of antibody. Antibody-mediated damage may then take place directly through complement activation or by recruitment of antibody-dependent cell-mediated cytotoxic (ADCC) effector cells (Fig 60–2). Most of the cells that arrive in the graft early after transplantation are lymphocytes, which migrate out of the capillary and venous beds, but after 4–7 days a remarkably heterogeneous collection of cell types appears. Those of the lymphocytic series predominate over the monocyte/macrophage and include also a few polymorphonuclear neutrophils. Although a variety of cell types are present, there is some evidence that early rejection of solid-tissue allografts is associated with T lymphocytes having direct cytotoxic activity against donor target cells. A significant number of B lymphocytes, null cells, and monocytes also appear in the early infiltrate, and although cytotoxic T cell activity is easily demonstrated at first, later stages of rejection may involve a non-T killer cell. In all phases, the presence of

antibodies and ADCC effector cells makes this mechanism an additional possibility. Macrophages appear to play an effector and suppressor role, whereas some B lymphocytes become activated and begin immunoglobulin synthesis in situ. When the host has been primed to donor antigens before transplantation, an accelerated process, often marked by antibody-mediated vasculitis, may result.

Recent applications of anti-T cell monoclonal antibodies in staining biopsies and in vivo as therapy add considerable support to the key role of T lymphocytes in most cases of rejection. When immunofluorescence or immunoperoxidase techniques are used with renal graft biopsies, 50–90% of the infiltrating cells generally express CD3 and CD6, with varying proportions of CD4 and CD8 cells. Although the peripheral blood often shows an increased proportion of CD4 cells in association with acute rejection episodes, many investigators relate rejection in the kidney to a preponderance of CD8 cells. More precisely, there is a preponderance of CD8 cells in the blood and perivascular areas in the grafts of patients experiencing irreversible rejection (ratio

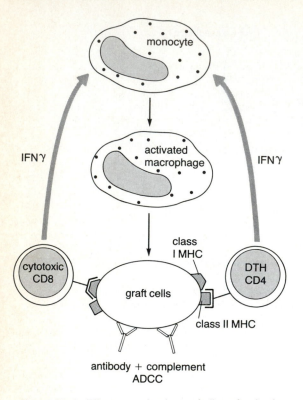

Figure 60–3. Effector mechanisms of allograft rejection.

of CD4 to CD8 cells < 1.0). When peripheral blood CD4:CD8 ratios are higher, perivascular ratios are also higher, and rejection usually is reversible with therapy. High-dose corticosteroids, given either intravenously (methylprednisolone, 1 g/d for 3 days) or orally (prednisone, 5–10 mg/kg/d for 5 days), are often used to treat acute rejection. Corticosteroids function through several pathways. They reduce the capacity of antigen-presenting cells to express class II antigens and to release IL-1. They also inhibit the alloactivation of T cells and consequently the release of IL-2. Their effect on migration and function of effector cells, as well as their capacity to release IFN γ, may explain their efficacy in reversing acute rejection. In this regard, they are known to produce lymphocytopenia, especially of CD4 T cells, by delaying transit of the lymphocytes through marrow and lymphoid tissues.

If there is no response or only a partial response to corticosteroids, ALG may be given (10–20 mg/kg/d for 5–14 days). ALG lyses lymphocytes, especially T cells, making it an excellent agent for treatment of acute rejection. ALG, however, is associated with anaphylaxis, serum sickness, and fever. Biologic effects also vary, since there is no effective measure for standardization.

Monoclonal antibodies (OKT 3 antibodies) recently have been introduced as specific therapy. A mouse IgG2, a monoclonal antibody to the T cell surface molecule CD3, is used for the treatment of rejection. Not only is it effective for the treatment of initial bouts of rejection, but rejection episodes that are resistant to high-dose steroids usually respond to OKT 3 therapy (5 mg/d intravenously for 10 days). OKT 3 initially causes an acute T lymphocyte depletion as the antibody-coated T lymphocytes are opsonized by the reticuloendothelial system. After 48 hours of therapy, there is a slow return of T lymphocytes to the circulation; however, the T cell receptor-CD3 complex is modulated (cleared) from the cell surface. Without a sufficient number of CD3 molecules present, T cell activation is impaired. One side effect of therapy with this foreign protein may be the production of antimouse antibodies in a small percentage of patients; this can limit the effectiveness of a subsequent course of therapy. In the future, monoclonal antibodies against lymphokine receptors such as IL-2 or other markers of activation may be tested.

B. Hyperacute: Preformed anti-ABO isohemagglutinins or anti-class I HLA antibodies, when present in sufficient quantity, will bind to the vascular endothelium and trigger a cascade of immunologic events. Initially, fixation of complement components and complement activation ensues, followed by activation of the clotting pathway. This series of events, if severe enough, can result in microthrombi within glomerular capillary loops and arterioles, leading to severe ischemia and necrosis of the graft. At present, there are no effective means of treating this lesion once it begins. Emphasis is therefore placed on prevention by careful assessment of ABO blood type and donor-specific sensitization to HLA antigens by cross-match testing prior to transplantation.

C. Chronic: Chronic rejection, which can occur months to years after transplantation, is characterized by a narrowing of the vascular arterial lumen owing to growth of endothelial cells that line the vascular bed. The actual control mechanisms for this response are unknown but may include immunologic injury signals, monocyte release of IL-1, and platelet and endothelial cell release of platelet-derived growth factor. Initially, the proliferating endothelial cell lesion is reversible, but once it progresses to fibrotic changes within the blood vessel wall itself, it is unresponsive to current modes of immunosuppression and progresses to graft ischemia, extensive interstitial fibrosis, and ultimate loss of renal function. Since there is no specific therapy for this form of rejection, emphasis is again placed on minimizing chronic immunologic stimuli by seeking the greatest possible degree of histocompatibility between recipients and donors.

Outcome

Survival of patients after renal transplantation is

not significantly different from that of patients undergoing dialysis. In most series, patient survival at 2 years is 90–95%. Graft survival, defined as allograft function adequate to maintain life without dialytic treatment, is 75–80% at 2 years in cadaveric renal allograft recipients treated with corticosteroids and either cyclosporine or ALG/OKT 3. Related-donor transplants have greater than 90% success at 2 years.

Surviving renal allografts have normal function, with mean creatinine levels of less than 2 mg/dL in most series. A functioning allograft therefore affords the recipient an optimal chance for normalization of health and is associated with minimal morbidity and mortality rates.

LIVER TRANSPLANTATION

Extensive experimental work in the field of liver transplantation has been performed since the early 1950s. Early investigators, using a variety of animal models, demonstrated that liver transplantation was feasible. The use of large-animal models indicated potential problem areas such as control of the splanchnic circulation during cross-clamping (the predecessor of the venovenous bypass) and rejection in grafts progressing to liver failure in animals untreated with immunosuppressive agents. The first human liver transplant was performed in 1963. Although this and the next several transplants were all unsuccessful, liver transplantation later became a successful procedure because of improved methods of immunosuppression. In 1987, more than 1100 liver transplants were performed in the USA, and nearly 100 liver transplant centers exist throughout the world at this time.

Although liver grafts were initially thought to be immunologically privileged, subsequent data from experimental liver transplantation has indicated that this is not the case. In certain strains of pigs and rats, liver grafts between the same donor and recipient combination have prolonged survival even though allogeneic kidney allografts are rejected within a short time. In addition, animals tolerate subsequent skin grafts from the same donor for prolonged periods but promptly reject third-party skin grafts. These effects are specific to only limited strains. There is, however, evidence that liver transplant rejection occurs by substantially different mechanisms from kidney transplant rejection. As a consequence of these different mechanisms and the difference of expression of major histocompatibility complex (MHC) antigens on the surface of liver cells and bile duct cells, the rejection response of the liver is distinctly different from that of other whole organs.

Indications

The indication for liver transplantation is the cer-

tainty that an individual's disease process is likely to progress to death within 2 years or that the compromise in life-style is so severe as to merit the risk of transplant. Although some diseases are known to be fatal in the long term, it is only recently that the use of longitudinal studies in primary biliary cirrhosis and sclerosing cholangitis has elucidated specific factors that can predict for short-term survival. Liver transplantation is usually not indicated until the life expectancy of the individual is expected to be less than 2 years. Hepatic dysfunction may be manifested by alterations in either synthetic or regulatory ability.

Signs and symptoms of progressive liver deficiency include malaise, weight loss, encephalopathy, ascites, coagulopathy, hypoalbuminemia, hyperbilirubinemia, and renal insufficiency. At present, many potential liver transplant recipients (particularly children) die before a suitable organ becomes available. The most common indication for liver transplant in the adult population to date has been non-A, non-B viral postnecrotic cirrhosis or chronic active hepatitis. Other diagnoses for which liver transplantation has been performed include primary biliary cirrhosis, sclerosing cholangitis, hepatitis B, cirrhosis, and inborn errors of metabolism. Some patients with hepatocellular tumors or cholangiocarcinomas have received transplants, and a few patients have survived long term (3–5 years), but in the vast majority of patients the tumor has recurred with fatal consequences. Similarly, patients with hepatitis B antigen-positive chronic active hepatitis frequently have recurrent hepatitis B antigenemia following transplantation. A large number of these patients have developed recurrent hepatitis and cirrhosis, although the rapidity of progression of chronic active hepatitis leading to cirrhosis and liver failure has been questioned. Techniques to decrease hepatitis B antigenemia, such as the use of hepatitis B hyperimmune globulin, may prove useful. There is renewed interest in liver transplantation in patients with alcohol-related liver failure because there is increasing evidence that these patients have results comparable to that of patients with other causes of liver failure. Most transplant centers require that these patients remain abstinent from alcohol for 3–12 months and that they can comply with posttransplant treatment regimens.

The most common diagnosis for which liver transplantation is performed in infants and children is extrahepatic biliary atresia. This disease occurs in between 1:8,000 and 1:12,000 live births in the USA. Children commonly undergo the Kasai procedure, which has long-term effectiveness in one-third to one-half of all patients. For patients with failed hepaticojejunostomy, liver transplantation is the only viable solution. Other indications for liver transplants in children are inborn errors of metabolism such as α_1-antitrypsin deficiency, tyrosinemia, and

Wilson's disease. As outcome has improved, liver replacement has been used to treat liver-based inborn errors of metabolism that result in extrahepatic organ system failure. For example, one patient with homozygous familial hypercholesterolemia has received a heart-liver transplant, and several patients with α_1-antitrypsin deficiency and renal involvement have received combination liver-kidney transplants.

Procedure

Orthotopic liver transplantation is the most commonly used method to date. This involves the removal of the host liver and replacement with the transplanted liver in the orthotopic position. Heterotopic transplantation is less frequently performed, as the clinical results have been less successful than with orthotopic transplantation. In heterotopic transplantation, the native liver is left in place and the transplanted liver is placed at an ectopic site. After removal from the donor, the donor liver is flushed with heparinized lactated Ringer's solution and then preserved in preservation solution and stored in the cold. The recently developed UW solution enables the liver to be preserved for more than 24 hours in some cases. This has greatly expanded the ability to transport organs long distances and to use back-up recipients if the first recipient proves unacceptable for transplantation. The recipient hepatectomy is technically the most difficult phase of the transplant operation because of frequent portal hypertension, previous surgery, and coagulopathy. Often there is excessive bleeding due to numerous adhesions at the operative site. The liver is mobilized although not removed until the donor organ is brought into the operative field and examined. The anhepatic phase is the time of greatest physiologic stress, because at this point the liver is removed and clamping of the portal vein and vena cava results in decreased venous return to the heart. This may in part be overcome by the use of venovenous bypass, which serves to bypass the splanchnic circulation and the infrahepatic vena caval circulation. The anhepatic phase lasts from the time when the host liver is removed until the vascular clamps are released, reperfusing the new liver. The revascularization phase requires attention to hemostasis. Revascularization involves supply to the liver via either the portal vein or the hepatic artery, or both, depending on the individual's anatomy and stability on venovenous bypass. The specific type of arterial revascularization depends on the blood supply to the donor organ. Complex revascularization may be required if multiple arteries are supplying the donor liver. The bile duct is reconstructed by using a choledochocholedochostomy, preferably when the recipient common duct is of good quality, or a choledochojejunostomy if the recipient duct is poor quality (eg, in biliary atresia) or of marked unequal size compared with the donor's common bile duct (Fig 60–4). Improvements

in surgical technique, new technologic advances such as the venovenous bypass, the availability of the UW solution, and the ability to control coagulation have decreased operative mortality rates and expanded the preservation time.

Outcome

Early graft failure, also known as primary nonfunction, may be a devastating complication if the patient does not receive a second transplant. Primary nonfunction is really a spectrum of diseases that range from no graft function (and certain death without retransplantation) to a liver whose function is mildly impaired at the outset but regains function within the first few days or weeks after transplantation. Factors related to primary nonfunction include the nature of the donor injury, the donor retrieval operation, the preservation solution, the length of preservation, host immunologic factors, the transplant operation, and host cardiovascular factors. Infectious complications after transplantation are frequent. Survival after infection relates to the type of offending organisms. Bacterial infections from pulmonary, bladder, and vascular sites usually respond to antibiotics, but fungal or viral infections may be associated with higher mortality and morbidity rates. Rejection is common after liver transplantation and may be seen in 75% of patients when defined by histologic means alone (see below). Rejection can be readily diagnosed (see below) by frequent percutaneous biopsies and is easily and successfully treated when diagnosed early. Late failure is due to chronic rejection or recurrence of the original disease. A particularly virulent type of rejection that is associated with damage to bile ducts, and disappearance of bile ducts may be associated with early graft loss. The survival rate at 1 year following liver transplantation ranges between 70 and 90% and is about 60% at 5 years.

Cross-matching & Immunosuppression

Decisions regarding the suitability of the donor organ for liver transplantation are currently based on ABO blood matching and organ size. HLA antigen typing is not used to match donors and recipients, although an inverse relationship between matching and survival has been reported. Many liver transplants are performed in children, so the donor liver must be of an appropriate size to fit into the child's abdominal cavity. Recently the use of livers that are made surgically smaller has drastically changed the approach to transplant in small recipients. The use of partial grafts from live donors is an extension of the work with pared-down organs from cadavers. Crossmatches are not routinely performed preoperatively but usually postoperatively. There are only a few reports of hyperacute rejection when the liver recipient has preformed antibodies against the donor. The

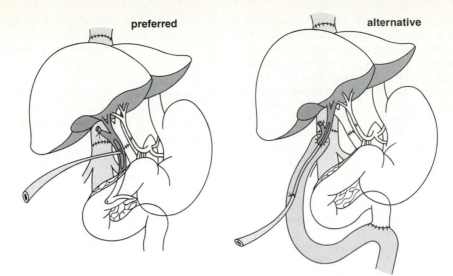

preferred alternative

Figure 60–4. Liver Transplantation. The preferred method (*A*) and the alternative technique (*B*) are shown. The donor suprahepatic vena cava, infrahepatic vena cava, portal vein, and hepatic artery are anastomosed end to end to the corresponding recipient vessels. When the recipient common duct is intact and the size matches the donor common duct, a choledochocholedochostomy (*A*) is performed. When the recipient duct is not intact (e.g. biliary atresia or sclerosing cholangitis) a choledochojejunostomy (*B*) is used.

apparent resistance of the liver to hyperacute rejection is interesting, but its cause is unknown. It has been suggested that perhaps the liver is not sensitive to preformed antibodies or that the liver mass itself results in dilution of the antibody titer to a level that is not harmful. There have been reports of combination liver and kidney transplants in recipient-donor combinations with a positive cross-match that becomes negative upon completion of the liver transplant. There has been no demonstration of increased antibody fixation to the graft. However, loss of cytotoxic antibodies could be due to the formation of soluble immune complexes. Alternatively, it may be that the blood loss associated with the liver transplant operation may dilute the antibody titers.

Rejection is readily diagnosed by percutaneous biopsy, and consensus is accumulating regarding the histologic features of acute rejection. Nonetheless, other causes of hepatic malfunction must be considered. Biliary obstruction, viral hepatitis, drug toxicity, and recurrence of the underlying disease must all be excluded. Signs and symptoms of rejection include fever, abdominal pain, ascites, hepatomegaly, and decreased appetite, all of which are nonspecific. Laboratory abnormalities do not predict for rejection but include elevation of serum bilirubin, alkaline phosphatase, and transaminases. The histopathologic features that suggest rejection include a mixed cellular portal infiltrate with bile duct epithelial damage and central vein or portal vein endothelial damage. Treatment of rejection includes the use of either methylprednisolone, antilymphoblast globulin, or

monoclonal antibody OKT 3. The use of these drugs depends on an assessment of the severity of the rejection process.

Cyclosporine has had a major impact on the results after liver transplantation. Prior to the cyclosporine era, the 1-year patient survival was in the range of 30–40%. This markedly changed with the introduction of cyclosporine after 1979. Current protocols at most centers call for cyclosporine and prednisone with or without azathioprine as prophylaxis against rejection. A few centers use antilymphocyte preparations in addition as rejection prophylaxis. Bile salts are necessary for the gastrointestinal absorption of cyclosporine, and if bile output is poor, inadequate absorption may necessitate intravenous administration of the drug. Although hepatotoxicity has been reported with cyclosporine, it is rare, and elevated postoperative liver function tests usually have another cause. The use of cyclosporine may be limited by its nephrotoxicity, which is compounded in patients with recent hepatorenal syndrome. The bone marrow suppression seen with azathioprine may be more pronounced in hypersplenic cirrhotic patients. Advances in the field of immunosuppression are eagerly awaited to avoid the complications of the currently used immunosuppressive agents.

PANCREAS TRANSPLANTATION

Unlike liver transplantation, which often is lifesaving, pancreas transplantation can be considered only life-enhancing at present. The rationale for the use of pancreas transplantation is that replacement of the ability to metabolize glucose normally will prevent the secondary sequelae of diabetes: nephropathy, neuropathy, and retinopathy. Pancreas transplantation can be effected with the whole organ, a segmental graft, or dispersed islets of Langerhans. The purpose of all three techniques is to provide biologically responsive insulin-producing tissue. Most uremic diabetic patients improve considerably with a kidney transplantation, but other long-term complications of diabetes, ie, retinopathy, angiopathy, and neuropathy do not improve. The autoimmune pathogenesis of type I insulin-dependent diabetes mellitus is evidenced by mononuclear cell infiltrate, which is seen surrounding the islets of Langerhans, and by the presence of circulatory autoantibodies directed against islet cytoplasm and cell surface antigen, which can be found in the sera of some type I diabetics (see Chapter 37). There is also a strong association of insulin-dependent diabetes mellitus with other organ-specific autoimmune endocrinopathies, and there is an association with certain HLA types of HLA-DR3 and -DR4 and -DQµ3.2 alleles. The histologic finding that the infiltrating lymphocytes are of the cytotoxic/suppressor T cell (CD8) phenotype resembles that seen in other autoimmune diseases and in allograft rejection. Therefore, distinguishing recurrent autoimmune disease from rejection in transplanted pancreatic tissue may prove difficult. More than 1500 pancreas transplants have been performed throughout the world. It may be expected that higher graft survival may be associated with transplants between HLA-identical siblings and with pancreases from donors who previously had given a kidney to the recipient. However, insulitis has occurred in a number of living-related transplants between identical twins and in a number of failed transplants from related donors. These findings have decreased the enthusiasm for the use of well-matched grafts from relatives.

Indications

Ideally, pancreas transplantation should be performed before the patient has developed any of the secondary complications of diabetes. However, not all diabetic patients suffer from secondary complications, and in fact only about 40% of individuals with type I diabetes will develop uremia. It has been difficult to balance the risk of long-term immunosuppression against the risks of developing systemic complications of diabetes. Therefore, pancreas transplantation to date has been performed on patients who were uremic and who had already received a renal transplant. However, a few centers now perform pancreas transplants in patients who have neither uremia nor kidney transplantation but have other progressive secondary complications that outweigh the risk of long-term immunosuppression. Changes

in renal glomerular basement membrane thickness before other evidence of renal malfunction may be an indication for the progression of the diabetic process.

Procedure

For the whole-organ or segmental pancreas graft, the pancreas is removed from the donor and preserved in cold storage so that it can be transported from a distant retrieval site to the facility where transplantation will take place. Preservation time in UW solution has exceeded 12 hours. Pancreas transplantation can either be done simultaneously with implantation of the kidney or sequentially in a post-kidney transplant patient with stable renal function. Simultaneous implantation of the kidney allows the use of kidney function and kidney biopsy as a marker for rejection. Various surgical techniques are used for implantation of the pancreas graft. The grafts are implanted either as a whole organ or with a small button of donor duodenum or as a distal segment of the pancreas.

Outcome

The major complications following pancreas transplantation are infection, vascular thrombosis, preservation injury, rejection, and pancreatitis. Overall graft function and patient survival rates have improved steadily since the first clinical pancreas transplant was performed in 1966. The present (1986–1988) overall graft survival at 1 year in 762 cases is 55%, and the 1-year survival rate is 88%.

Cross-matching & Immunosuppression

Pancreas transplant donors and recipients are typed and matched for ABO and HLA antigens, and a transplant is not performed in the face of a positive cross-match. The exact role of tissue typing has not been clearly defined, largely owing to small numbers of patients. In patients who have received simultaneous pancreas-kidney transplant, both organs are not uniformly rejected, but rejection of their kidney graft can frequently be used to predict ongoing rejection of the pancreas. Nonetheless, in some instances the pancreas has failed (presumably owing to rejection) while the kidney graft continues to function. The benefits of HLA-DR matching in cadaveric pancreas transplantation have been demonstrated. Zero-, one-, and 2-DR mismatches yielded 63%, 45%, and 45% 1-year graft function overall. There is 78%, 62%, and 58% 1-year graft survival in technically successful grafts with living related grafts (1984–1988). The benefit of HLA typing has been more modest: 56% of HLA-identical sibling grafts (83% of technically successful grafts), 50% of grafts from mismatched relatives (78% of technically successful grafts), and 49% of cadaveric grafts (63% of technically successful grafts) are functioning at 1 year.

Rejection of the vascularized pancreatic allograft is recognized by a loss of control over blood glucose levels. This, however, is unfortunately a relatively insensitive and late finding. Disappearance of insulin from the circulation usually parallels the plasma glucose levels and consequently cannot be used as an early indicator of rejection. Corticosteroids used for immunosuppression also tend to cause diabetogenic effects. Serum amylase levels have not been useful previously in diagnosis of rejection. However, in transplants drained into the urinary system, low levels of urinary amylase are suggestive of graft failure. This finding usually precedes changes in blood glucose levels by 24 or 48 hours, therefore allowing time for institution of antirejection therapy.

The current practice at some centers is to perform a biopsy of the graft when there is a question of rejection, even when diagnosis is not assured. The presence of vasculitis is the only certain histologic evidence for rejection because parenchymal fibrosis and inflammatory-cell infiltrate may be secondary to foreign body reaction, particularly in grafts with polymer-injected ducts or grafts associated with recurrent disease. Successful immunosuppression for pancreas transplantation appears to be more difficult than for kidney or liver transplantation. In patients who have previously received a kidney transplant and were immunosuppressed at the time of pancreas implantation and in HLA-identical sibling transplants, the use of cyclosporine and corticosteroids has been satisfactory. However, in patients who are not uremic or who are not recipients of a kidney transplant, a more potent immunosuppressive protocol involving cyclosporine, azathioprine, and prednisone has been utilized. Rejection is usually treated with intravenous bolus corticosteroids, an increase in the oral prednisone dose, or a temporary course of ALG.

Islet Cell Transplantation

A successful placement of isolated islets in nonidentical donors has been a goal for some time. Initially it was hoped that unmodified islet transplants might display the prolonged survival of other endocrine tissue. However, survival of isolated islet allografts is shorter than survival of allografts of skin, kidney, or heart regardless of placement site. Syngeneic grafts implanted in the liver, under the kidney capsule produce insulin and are able to reverse hyperglycemia, virally induced diabetes, diabetes induced by beta cell toxins, and spontaneous diabetes in BB rats and NOD mice. Since autografts cannot be used in most clinical situations, the major experimental thrust has been to perfect allograft islet transplantation.

Islet cells are obtained from either adult or fetal pancreas. The fetal pancreas contains less connective tissue, so that the relative yield of viable islets is greater but still not sufficient to render a recipient normoglycemic. The basic method for retrieving islets is via mechanical separation followed by enzymatic digestion, usually with collagenase. Secondary steps of separation are required to remove as much nonislet tissue as possible; this usually necessitates manual removal of islet tissue. The purer the islet cell separation, the longer the graft survives. Nonetheless, islets themselves contain dendritic cells and other cells capable of stimulating an immune response. A number of investigators have tried different means of reducing immunogenicity of islet tissue, such as treatment with anti-class II monoclonal antibody or irradiation. Culturing of pure islets in an oxygen-rich atmosphere has been successful in decreasing tissue immunogenicity. An alterative method that has been successful in rats and mice involves encapsulation of individual islets within a semipermeable biologic membrane across which immunocompetent cells cannot pass. All of these experiments have been performed in animal models, with prolonged reversal of the diabetic state when modified islet allografts were used. The clinical application of this work remains to be realized.

HEART TRANSPLANTATION

In 1967 the first successful human heart allograft was performed. Twenty years later, 2000 heart transplants were performed worldwide (1500 in the USA alone). Currently, the indication for cardiac allotransplantation is end-stage cardiac impairment that has been completely refractory to medical management. Absolute contraindications include severe pulmonary hypertension, infection, and cancer. Age and general medical status may be relative contraindications. Cardiac disease in most recipients is due to coronary artery disease, cardiomyopathy, rheumatic heart disease, congenital heart disease, or benign cardiac tumors.

Cardiac donors should be individuals aged 40 years or younger with established neurologic death and no preexisting cardiac disease or significant abnormalities on chest x-ray or electrocardiogram. Hydration and conservative use of vasopressor and inotropic drugs maintain optimal cardiac function and perfusion. The heart is stored by flushing the coronary circulation with mixed-electrolyte solution and preservation on ice. The heart should be implanted within 4 hours of removal from the donor. Because of a shortage of donor organs, the donor age has been raised and ischemic time extended in some institutions.

The cardiac transplantation procedure requires that the recipient be placed on cardiopulmonary bypass. Both atria of the donor heart are anastomosed to the respective atria of the recipient, and the aorta and pulmonary arteries are likewise anastomosed. Corticosteroids, cyclosporine, ALG, and OKT 3 are currently the preferred drugs for prevention of allograft rejection.

Pretransplant immunologic evaluation consists of HLA typing and screening for preformed anti-HLA antibodies. Although cardiac donors are routinely HLA typed, there is rarely an opportunity to choose among several potential recipients as there is for kidney transplantation. Hence, the potential benefits of HLA matching have not yet been realized. Nevertheless, the recipient's serum is routinely cross-matched against a random panel of lymphocytes from a number of donors. If the level of reactive antibodies is greater than 15%, a prospective cross-match between the donor and the potential recipient is necessary.

Diagnosis of allograft rejection is made on the basis of endomyocardial biopsy performed through a transvenous catheter placed in the right jugular vein. A mononuclear cell infiltrate is the characteristic hallmark of rejection. Lymphocytes, lymphoblasts, and monocytes are the predominant cell types in acute rejection. Evidence of tissue damage is found in necrosis of myocardial fibers and edema, which further impairs perfusion and function. Electrocardiographic changes of decreased voltage, sometimes associated with arrhythmias and signs of congestive heart failure, can also be demonstrated during rejection episodes. Treatment of rejection includes the use of ALG and increased levels of corticosteroids. Chronic rejection can also occur and is usually associated with atherosclerotic changes of coronary vessels. Successful retransplantation has been offered to individuals with chronic allograft rejection. Currently, graft survival at 1 year is greater than 80% in most series. In evaluating transplanted patients during the last decade survival at 5 years is approximately 70%. Patients enjoy excellent ventricular function, and more than 60% are able to return to employment or satisfactory rehabilitation.

LUNG & HEART-LUNG TRANSPLANTATION

Transplantation of one or both lungs is currently performed in a few institutions. The main problems that remain are donor supply and poor healing of the bronchial anastomosis. Heart-lung transplantation continues to be performed for both primary pulmonary failure and for cardiopulmonary failure. The procedure requires anastomosis of the trachea, right atrium, and aorta. Although the lungs remain denervated, this does not appear to contribute to ventilatory failure. Blood supply to the trachea is provided through collaterals from the coronary circulation. Currently, immunosuppression includes the use of cyclosporine, azathioprine, and ATG in the early postoperative course and corticosteroids after the establishment of tracheal healing. The diagnosis of rejection is made in the lung since rejection occurs earlier and more frequently in the lung than in the heart. The diagnosis is made by x-ray changes and changes in respiratory function and through endobronchial biopsy. Survival of heart-lung transplants is 62% after 1 year and 61% after 2 years. Patients with successful heart-lung transplantation can enjoy excellent rehabilitation.

BONE MARROW TRANSPLANTATION

Modern clinical bone marrow transplantation began in 1968, when a small number of patients with severe combined immunodeficiency disease (SCID), Wiskott-Aldrich syndrome, and advanced leukemia received infusions of marrow from HLA-identical siblings. Previous observations in animals had shown that matching the donor and recipient at the MHC loci reduced the incidence of graft-versus-host (GVH) disease and improved survival rates. Many patients have now survived for more than a decade after bone marrow transplantation for a variety of malignant and nonmalignant hematologic diseases. Laboratory and clinical advances in such areas as histocompatibility typing, prevention of GVH disease, improved supportive care, and reduced risk of relapse have made bone marrow transplantation a realistic and successful form of treatment for several usually fatal diseases (Table 60–1).

Until recently, most donors for bone marrow transplantation have been either identical twins (syngeneic) or genotypically HLA-identical individuals (allogeneic). However, only 40% of patients can be

Table 60–1. Diseases treatable by bone marrow transplantation.

Allogeneic/Syngeneic	Autologous
Aplastic anemia	Leukemia
Leukemia	AML
AML	ALL
ALL	Lymphoma
CML	Hodgkin's disease
Lymphoma	Non-Hodgkin's
Hodgkin's	High or intermediate
Non-Hodgkin's	grade
High or intermediate	T cell
grade	Burkitt's
T cell	Solid tumors
Burkitt's	Breast
Myeloma	Lung (small cell)
Immunodeficiencies	Neuroblastoma
Common variable	Ovarian
SCID	Testicular
Wiskott-Aldrich syndrome	
Agranulocytosis	
(Kostmann's syndrome)	
Osteopetrosis/genetic	
diseases	
Solid tumors	

expected to have an HLA-identical donor, and efforts to use marrow from partially matched family members or phenotypically matched unrelated donors are beginning to be successful. For diseases not involving the marrow, autologous transplantation allows the use of high-dose chemoradiotherapy and avoids the risk of GVH disease. Provocative studies using monoclonal antibodies to leukemic and other malignant cells have given credence to the idea that such marrow "purging" techniques could greatly extend the benefit of autologous transplantation to patients assumed to have indiscernible neoplastic cells remaining in the marrow.

The 5 major categories of diseases treatable by bone marrow transplantation are SCID, aplastic anemia, leukemias, lymphomas, and selected solid tumors. The cure of other genetic diseases by bone marrow transplantation is feasible (Table 60–2), but controversy remains about relative risks and benefits.

Indications & Results

A. SCID: Bone marrow transplantation is the treatment of choice for children with congenital SCID and its variants. For HLA-matched transplants, no immunosuppressive conditioning is necessary. Partially matched recipients require conditioning, usually with cyclophosphamide and busulfan rather than radiotherapy. The removal of T cells from donor marrow by lectin agglutination or monoclonal antibody and complement lysis enables parents of haploidentical children with these disorders to serve as donors.

B. Aplastic Anemia: Severe aplastic anemia has a mortality rate of 90% when treated with supportive care. Allogeneic bone marrow transplantation increases survival to 45% overall and to 70% in patients younger than 30 years. Furthermore, if patients are able to avoid pretransplantation transfusions—and hence presensitization—the overall actuarial survival at 10 years increases to 82%. Unlike the case for leukemia, rejection of the donor marrow in patients with aplastic anemia has been a major cause of failure (35% versus 10% for leukemia); this is probably due to the underlying autoimmune nature of the aplasia in some patients, to presensitization by transfusions, and to the lack of radiotherapy in the standard conditioning regimen. Irradiation is given to kill leukemic cells, but it also contributes greatly to the ablation of the immune system, which is more complete in patients treated with irradiation. Omitting irradiation results in fewer complications and lower toxicity but increases the risk of rejection. However, despite decreased risk of rejection, irradiation does not aid survival, because of increased toxicity, especially to the lungs. Newer trials of total lymphoid irradiation are encouraging because the rejection rate has been decreased to 10% without a concomitant rise in toxicity. For patients without donors and for patients older than 40 years, ATG offers a 45% chance of long-term survival without the excessive morbidity and mortality rates due to GVH disease in these groups, albeit with a greater likelihood of decreased performance status. Bone marrow transplantation should be reserved for patients not responding to ATG.

C. Acute Myelogenous Leukemia (AML): Acute myelogenous leukemia (AML) has a mortality rate of more than 90% in adults. The success of allogeneic bone marrow transplantation in the treatment of AML has been confirmed by studies worldwide, including 3 randomized trials of bone marrow transplantation versus chemotherapy. In the initial trials for relapsed AML, a long-term relapse-free survival rate of 13% was achieved in patients with no hope of survival by any other means. Now that patients receive allogeneic transplants while in remission from acute nonlymphocytic (myelogenous) leukemia, relapse rates are 15–20% and the overall survival is 40–75%, depending on the age of the recipient. Further success will depend on the improved abrogation of GVH disease and fewer infectious complications. Attempts to decrease GVH disease by T cell depletion of the donor marrow have been successful in abrogating GVH disease but, unfortunately, have been complicated by higher rates of fungal infection, a greater risk of graft rejection, and a higher risk of leukemic relapse.

Autologous transplantation for patients with AML in both first and second (or third) remission avoids the risk of GVH disease but has a potentially higher relapse rate than does allogeneic bone marrow transplantation. Preliminary results indicate that 25–40% of patients in first remission may achieve at least 1 year of disease-free survival following ablative chemotherapy and reinfusion of marrow harvested and frozen during remission. Autologous transplantation of marrow purged of residual leukemic cells with 4-hydroperoxycyclophosphamide has resulted in 35% 2-year disease-free survival for patients with AML in second or third remission.

Table 60–2. Genetic diseases treatable by bone marrow transplantation.

SCID
Wiskott-Aldrich syndrome
Fanconi's anemia
Kostmann's syndrome
Chronic granulomatous disease
Osteopetrosis
Ataxia-telangiectasia
Diamond-Blackfan syndrome
Mucocutaneous candidiasis
Chédiak-Higashi syndrome
Cartilage-hair hypoplasia
Mucopolysaccharidosis
Gaucher's disease
Thalassemia major

D. Chronic Myelogenous Leukemia (CML):
For patients with chronic myelogenous leukemia (CML) there had been no hope for cure and no improvement in survival with any form of standard therapy since splenic irradiation was first performed in the 1920s. Data now clearly show that allogeneic bone marrow transplantation will provide a 60–80% relapse-free survival in patients with CML in chronic phase. More favorable results are produced when the transplant is performed soon after diagnosis and when patients are below age 30. Especially compelling are cytogenetic analyses confirming the absence of the Philadelphia chromosome as long as 5 years after transplantation. When patients reach the accelerated phase of CML, or frank blast crisis develops, disease-free survival drops to 15%. Results of autologous transplants for CML have been uniformly poor thus far.

E. Acute Lymphoblastic Leukemia (ALL):
Allogeneic transplantation for acute lymphoblastic leukemia (ALL) has not been as successful, primarily because of a high posttransplant relapse rate (50%). Changes in the conditioning regimen may improve the outcome. A similar relapse-free survival rate of 30% in children in second remission and without HLA-matched donors has been achieved by using monoclonal anti-CALLA antibodies to deplete autologous marrow of lymphoblasts.

Procedure

Unlike other organ transplants, bone marrow aspirated from the iliac crests of a donor is entirely regenerated in 8 weeks. Since the amount harvested is only 20% of the total, the donor is not harmed immunologically or hematologically. Multiple aspirations of 5 mL each, yielding a total of 10 mL/kg of the recipient's body weight (600–1200 mL), are obtained in a single procedure under general or epidural anesthesia. The marrow is drawn through heparinized needles and placed into heparinized, buffered culture medium. This mixture is then gently filtered through fine stainless steel mesh screens to produce a single-cell suspension. Nucleated-cell counts are checked to ensure the adequacy of the withdrawn marrow. If the donor and recipient are ABO-compatible, $2–6 \times 10^8$ nucleated marrow cells/kg of the recipient's weight are infused intravenously together with erythrocytes (erythrocyte volume of 20–30%). If the donor and recipient are not ABO-compatible, either the recipient must undergo plasmapheresis to remove the anti-A or anti-B isoantibodies or the erythrocytes must be removed from the donor's marrow in vitro. Unlike the case for renal transplantation, donor-specific pretransplant transfusions do not seem to be beneficial, probably because most of the recipients have been heavily alloimmunized by prior transfusions and also because the immune system is totally ablated prior to transplantation.

Except in patients with SCID, destruction of the recipient's immune system is necessary to prevent rejection and to allow transplantation of an entirely new hematopoietic system, including new immunocompetent cells. This is usually accomplished by giving cyclophosphamide, 50–60 mg/kg for 4 or 2 days (the higher dose for patients not receiving total-body irradiation). The dose of total-body irradiation is 7.5–15 Gy, which is usually administered in fractions over 3–5 days rather than in a single dose, to avoid toxicity to the lungs and eyes. This combination of chemotherapy and radiotherapy provides a potent immunoablative and antineoplastic function for most cancer patients.

Following preparative chemoradiotherapy and infusion of the marrow, patients are extremely vulnerable to infections and bleeding. Strict isolation in rooms with laminar air flow has a significant effect on outcome only for patients with aplastic anemia. Simple precautions such as hand-washing and filtering the air to remove airborne fungi are important. The early and aggressive use of broad-spectrum antibiotics (semisynthetic penicillins or third-generation cephalosporins and aminoglycosides), as well as acyclovir and amphotericin B, is critical. Accepted practice dictates that these antibiotics not be discontinued until the absolute neutrophil count is above 500/μL following engraftment. The role of trimethoprim-sulfamethoxazole in preventing *Pneumocystis carinii* pneumonia is clearly established. The use of intravenous immunoglobulins weekly after transplantation has decreased the risks of cytomegalovirus (CMV) pneumonia and acute GVH disease. Granulocyte transfusions are not given prophylactically at most centers because of the lack of evidence that they are beneficial and because of higher risks of secondary infections, notably with CMV. Platelet transfusions, on the other hand, are given to keep the platelet count above 15,000/μL to prevent serious spontaneous hemorrhage. All blood products must be irradiated to prevent GVH disease due to viable lymphocytes in transfused cellular components or plasma.

Engraftment is heralded by a rising leukocyte count, relative monocytosis, and the appearance of circulating mature neutrophils 2–4 weeks after transplantation. Bone marrow samples at 2 and 4 weeks show increasing cellularity, and the platelet and reticulocyte counts also begin to rise. In general, all hematopoietic and immune cells of the recipient are replaced by donor cells, although there are rare examples of mixed "chimerism," most often in children who receive transplants for immunodeficiency diseases. As peripheral counts improve, antibiotics can be discontinued and transfusions become unnecessary. Patients can be discharged when they can be observed closely as outpatients, daily to twice weekly for at least the first 100 days after transplantation.

Posttransplantation Complications

The major obstacles to successful bone marrow transplantation are GVH disease, infections, interstitial pneumonia, venoocclusive liver disease, and relapse of the underlying disease. GVH disease and infections are responsible for 10–30% of morbidity and mortality in the first 30 days following transplantation.

Graft-versus-Host (GVH) Disease

The presence of immunocompetent donor cells in an immunocompromised host is a prerequisite for GVH disease. Host and donor are histoincompatible. In patients who are HLA-identical with their donors, the occurrence of GVH disease is attributed to "minor," presently undetectable differences in histocompatibility. GVH disease also can develop from lymphocytes in random blood transfusions given to neonates, patients with congenital immunodeficiencies, and cancer patients who are immunocompromised by their disease (eg, T cell leukemias, Hodgkin's disease) or by chemotherapy.

The clinical syndrome of GVH disease in humans consists of skin rash, severe diarrhea, and jaundice. Pathophysiologically, immunocompetent CD8 T cells can be found in biopsies of the skin, intestine, and liver. These tissues appear to be especially at risk because they are rich in surface DR antigens. The skin rash of acute GVH disease usually begins at the time of engraftment, 10–28 days after transplantation. It is a fine, diffuse, erythematous, macular rash often beginning on the palms, soles, or head and spreading to involve the entire trunk and sometimes the extremities. In severe GVH disease, the rash can become desquamative—the clinical equivalent of an extensive second-degree burn. Watery diarrhea is associated with malabsorption, cramps, and gastrointestinal bleeding when severe. Hyperbilirubinemia is due to GVH disease-induced inflammation of small bile ducts, and it is usually accompanied by an elevated serum alkaline phosphatase level. Elevations of alanine aminotransferase and aspartate aminotransferase are mild to moderate. A staging and grading system for GVH disease developed at the University of Washington has become standard (Table 60–3). Acute GVH disease occasionally is delayed until 30–70 days after transplantation, and then it is almost always the harbinger of chronic GVH disease.

Successful prevention of acute GVH disease began with the use of methotrexate after transplantation in outbred DLA-matched dogs. Its use in humans by the Seattle Bone Marrow Transplant Center has remained the standard by which other measures to prevent GVH disease are judged. Initial studies found that approximately 50% of patients treated with methotrexate alone developed acute GVH disease within 10–70 days after grafting, and up to half of these could die. More modern immunosuppressive

Table 60–3. Clinical staging of GVH disease by organ system.

Stage	Skin	Liver	Gastrointestinal Tract
+	Maculopapular rash < 25% body surface	Serum bilirubin 2–3 mg/dL	> 500 mL diarrhea/d
+ +	Maculopapular rash 25–50% body surface	Serum bilirubin 3–6 mg/dL	> 1000 mL diarrhea/d
+ + +	Generalized erythroderma	Serum bilirubin 6–15 mg/dL	> 1500 mL diarrhea/d
+ + + +	Generalized erythroderma with bullous formation and desquamation	Serum bilirubin > 15 mg/dL	Severe abdominal pain with or without ileus

therapy with both methotrexate and cyclosporine has reduced the risk of acute GVH disease to 25%. Cyclosporine is continued for the first 6 months after transplantation. Infusions of ATG, prednisone, and monoclonal antibodies have been used to treat established acute GVH disease with limited success. Incubating the donor marrow in vitro with anti-T cell monoclonal antibodies plus complement or similar antibodies coupled to toxins, or using a soybean lectin agglutination and sheep erythrocyte rosette-forming technique has successfully depleted the marrow of T cells and lowered the incidence of GVH disease. Interestingly, strict isolation in rooms with laminar air flow also has decreased the incidence of acute GVH disease, but only in patients with aplastic anemia. Unfortunately, studies of patients receiving T cell-depleted marrow have shown an increased risk of rejection, higher relapse rate of leukemia, increased risk of fungal infections, and risk of post-transplant Epstein-Barr virus (EBV)-related lymphoproliferative disease. These findings support the concept that donor T cells have an active graft-versus-leukemia effect and that they may also provide protection against fungi. It might be possible to selectively deplete only T cells containing specific activation antigens mediating GVH disease and not those mediating graft-versus-leukemia. A third solution might be less complete ("imperfect") T cell depletion.

Chronic GVH disease affects 25–45% of patients surviving longer than 180 days. It occurs more frequently in older patients and in those with preceding acute GVH disease. Clinically, it most closely resembles the spectrum of rheumatic or autoimmune disorders, and its main clinical effect is to produce severe immunodeficiency, leading to recurrent and life-threatening infections, much like those seen in the congenital and acquired immunodeficiency syndromes. Treatment with prednisone, alone or in combination with azathioprine, can effectively reverse many of the manifestations of chronic GVH disease in 50–75% of affected patients.

Venoocclusive Disease of the Liver

High doses of chemoradiotherapy, such as that used to condition patients prior to marrow transplantation, can cause a fibrous obliteration of small hepatic venules, known as venoocclusive disease of the liver. About 20% of patients undergoing bone marrow transplantation develop venoocclusive disease, manifested clinically as hepatomegaly, ascites, hepatocellular necrosis, and encephalopathy within 8 to 20 days after transplantation. The disease resolves in 60% of patients, persists as a major problem in 15% who die from other causes, and directly contributes to the cause of death in the rest.

The most important risk factor is the presence of hepatitis before transplantation, which, by serology and natural history, is usually non-A, non-B viral hepatitis associated with transfusions. Patients with transaminasemia before bone marrow transplantation are 3–4 times more likely to develop venoocclusive disease than are those with normal serum liver enzymes. Other risk factors include increasing age and cancers other than ALL (perhaps because ALL is also associated with younger patients).

Venoocclusive disease is the most common cause of liver dysfunction in the first 3 weeks after transplantation. Later, GVH disease of the liver, viral hepatitis (especially due to CMV), fungal liver disease, and liver injury due to drugs make the diagnosis more difficult. The timing of onset best distinguishes venoocclusive disease from GVH disease. GVH disease of the liver usually appears after day 20, and ascites from GVH disease occurs only after weeks of persistent GVH disease, whereas it is an early phenomenon in venoocclusive disease. Viral hepatitis does not usually cause ascites or encephalopathy unless there is massive liver necrosis, and neither does fatty liver with hyperbilirubinemia and elevated liver enzymes caused by total parenteral nutrition.

Infections

Infectious complications following bone marrow transplantation are from the profound lack of granulocytes and lymphocytes following ablation by the pretransplant conditioning regimen. Since full recovery of these 2 major elements of the immune system occurs separately following transplantation, it is not surprising that the risk of infection can be separated into 3 distinct phases (Table 60–4).

The first, and most dangerous, phase is the 2–4-week period prior to engraftment, when no circulating leukocytes are present. During this time, patients are at risk for both bacterial and fungal infections, which can advance extremely rapidly and cause

Table 60–4. Sequence of infections after bone marrow transplant.

Phase	Infection
I Up to engraftment	Gram-positive cocci/central lines Enterobacteriaceae Early fungi Esophagitis Fungemia
II After initial engraftment	Fungal _Aspergillus_ (less in laminar air flow) _Candida_ esophagitis Viral Correlation with GVH disease CMV Adenovirus EBV Respiratory syncytial virus, enterovirus, parainfluenza, papovaviruses
III Late	Sinopulmonary (sicca syndrome, IgA deficiency) _Streptococcus pneumoniae/ Haemophilus influenzae_ Varicella-zoster virus 85% dermatomal; ⅓ become disseminated 15% disseminated at onset Late interstitial pneumonia

death. Clinical experience and trials over the past 15 years have led to the aggressive, empirical use of broad-spectrum antibiotics (both antibacterial and antifungal). Coverage must be begun at the first sign of infection, such as fever, chills, localized pain, or change in mental status. Waiting for results of cultures may result in overwhelming and irreversible sepsis or pneumonia. The spectrum of organisms that cause infections has gradually changed. Infections due to gram-positive organisms were usually treated successfully in the early days of bone marrow transplantation. The recent increase in infections due to resistant species of staphylococci, especially _Staphylococcus epidermidis_ responsive only to vancomycin, is most probably due to the use of tunneled, central intravenous catheters in these patients. The use of these catheters has been a major factor in improved support, and there are no viable alternatives. As a result, vancomycin is empirically added to the antibiotic regimen when fever persists. Sepsis and pneumonia due to gram-negative infections have long been known to be rapidly fatal in patients with profound granulocytopenia. Marrow transplant patients are no exception. Powerful, synergistic combinations of antibiotics (semisynthetic penicillins or advanced cephalosporins and aminoglycosides) have greatly diminished the number of deaths due to these organisms. Nevertheless, there remains a high risk of death from bacterial infection—largely from gram-negative organisms—during the period of aplasia before engraftment. The overall risk is higher when acute GVH disease is present, ranging from 10% to 40% depending on age, underlying disease, and intensity of the conditioning regimen. Future efforts are focused on the use of intravenous antibiotics before infections arise, passive immunization with intravenous immunoglobulins, and modified reverse isolation techniques.

Two to 4 weeks after transplantation, the marrow begins to export granulocytes successfully to the blood; when the absolute neutrophil count reaches 500/μL and is rising, the greatest threat of bacterial infection is past. The second phase of potential infectious complications is due to the paucity and immaturity of the lymphocytes, and the greatest risk is due to fungal and viral agents during the second and third posttransplant months. An especially prominent and potent pathogen is *Aspergillus fumigatus,* which can cause vascular invasion in the lungs and brain. Although these infections can be treated with amphotericin B, they are difficult to eradicate and often are fatal. The most prominent viral pathogen is CMV: CMV pneumonia has a mortality rate of 80%. Treatment with gancyclovir and intravenous immunoglobulins has reduced the mortality rate to 40%.

Interstitial pneumonia due to nonbacterial pathogens, notably CMV, fungi, and noninfectious agents, remains a major complication of bone marrow transplantation. The incidence of interstitial pneumonia is about 35%, with a case fatality rate of 70–85% and an overall mortality rate among bone marrow transplantation patients of 24%. In about half the cases no cause can be found, and these idiopathic pneumonias are considered to be secondary to the toxicity of chemoradiotherapy. Risk factors for the development of interstitial pneumonia are (1) older recipient, (2) use of methotrexate to prevent GVH disease, (3) grade of GVH disease, (4) pretransplant performance status, (5) interval from diagnosis to transplant, and (6) dose rate of total-body irradiation.

The third phase of infectious complications occurs after the third month and lasts until the maturation of the lymphocytic arm of the immune system. This parallels the neonatal period and takes 6–18 months. During this time, there is an abnormal ratio of CD4 to CD8 T cells, T cells respond poorly to antigens, and immunoglobulin production is abnormal. This leads to a risk of infection by encapsulated bacteria such as pneumococci because of a lack of opsonic immunoglobulins. The higher risk of viral infection diminishes as T cell function gradually improves. Patients must remain relatively isolated until the immune system has fully recovered. Patients with chronic GVH disease may never recover full function of the immune system. However, the majority of surviving patients do recover full immunity and lead lives free from infection, requiring no antibiotics or other supplements. Unlike patients with solid-organ transplants, they do not need to take immunosuppressive medications to ensure engraftment, since the immune and hematopoietic systems are replaced. Once tolerance is achieved (by about 3 months after transplantation), all medications can gradually be discontinued, and patients are able to live completely normal lives.

BONE TRANSPLANTATION

Bone is more commonly transplanted than any other tissue. In general, bone-grafting operations are performed to promote healing of nonunited fractures, to restore structural integrity of the skeleton, and to facilitate cosmetic repair. Human skull defects larger than 2–3 cm are closed by neurosurgeons to protect the brain and restore bone integrity. Plastic surgeons, oral surgeons, and periodontists use fresh autografts and freeze-dried allografts in oral and maxillofacial surgery. Various bone grafts are used to promote stability of the spine and to correct spinal deformity. Autografts and allografts are used to repair the appendicular skeleton (arms and legs). When autograft sources are insufficient, allogeneic bone may be used but only in combination with an autograft, which provides a greater degree of early repair. Bone is procured for implantation by aseptic removal or by removal and subsequent sterilization by ethylene oxide or γ irradiation. Except for a fresh autograft, all other bone tissues are used after freezing because of the reduction in immunogenicity achieved by this storage technique.

Posttransplantation Course

Following grafting, one of 3 courses can occur: (1) the bone graft may become viable, acquiring the mechanical, cosmetic, and biologic characteristics of adjacent bone; (2) it may partially or completely resorb without satisfactory new-bone formation, leaving disfigurement or instability; or (3) it may become sequestrated, encapsulated, and treated by the host as a foreign body. The most likely graft to achieve optimal function in humans is the fresh autograft. However, allogeneic implants are becoming more widely used.

A bone graft transferred to a recipient undergoes several adaptive phases before ultimate incorporation into the skeletal system. Osteogenesis from surviving cells of the graft itself is characteristic only of fresh autografts. By contrast, cells from an allograft usually elicit antibody production and cell-mediated immunity and start to decay. These alloimplants slowly revascularize by invasion of capillary sprouts from the host bed during the process of resorption of the old matrix. Finally, in both autografts and allografts, osteoinduction occurs by the process of recruitment of mesenchyme-type cells into cartilage and bone under the influence of a diffusible bone morphogenetic protein derived from the bone matrix.

Bone morphogenetic protein is a recently discovered glycoprotein of MW 17,500. The target cell for its activity is an undifferentiated, perivascular mesenchymal cell whose protein synthesis is reprogrammed in favor of new-bone formation.

Temporally, healing of bone grafts follows a well-known pattern. For the initial 2 weeks, an inflammatory response occurs, associated with infiltration of the graft by vascular buds and the presence of fibrous granulation tissue, osteoclast activity, and osteocyte autolysis. There occurs a "creeping substitution" of graft bone, manifested as differentiation of mesenchymal cells into osteoblasts that deposit osteoid over devitalized trabeculae. Dead trabeculae are later remodeled internally. Thus, through appositional new-bone formation, the graft is strengthened. In contrast to cancellous bone, cortical bone grafts undergo a somewhat longer period of resorption and slower appositional phases of new-bone formation. This results in only half strength being acquired during the first 6 months and full strength 1–2 years after grafting.

Immunologic Rejection

Since bone is a composite of cells, collagen, ground substance, and inorganic minerals, all but the minerals are potentially immunogenic. Cell surface transplantation antigens associated with the MHC are the most potent immunogens within osteochondral allografts and are found on cells of osteogenic, chondrogenic, fibrous, neuronal, fatty, hematopoietic, and mesenchymal origin. Cell-rich marrow contributes significantly to immunogenicity.

Fresh allogeneic bone can sensitize the host and cause the production of circulating antibodies. Nevertheless, cellular immunity is thought to be more important than humoral antibodies in causing rejection of allogeneic bone transplants. Cartilage seems to resist destruction by antibody and cellular resorptive mechanisms, but if an immune response by the recipient develops, this protection is only relative and a low-grade, slow, immunologically mediated inflammatory response ensues, characterized by an increase in synovial fluid, leukocyte counts, antibody response, and pannus reactions.

Rejection of allogeneic bone (cortical or cancellous) elicits a response that delays healing at the site of osteosynthesis and blocks revascularization, resorption, and appositional new-bone formation. Clear-cut rejection or failure of the graft occurs in only about 10% of bone grafts.

Immunosuppression

Temporary systemic immunosuppression has been used, since MHC antigens are present in bone for only 2–3 months after transplantation. Drugs that have successfully allowed bone union include azathioprine, corticosteroids, cyclosporine, and cyclophosphamide. Because of side effects and the low rate of graft failure, these agents are no longer routinely used in human musculoskeletal transplantation. A promising new technique to diminish the antigenicity of grafts is the use of a temporary biodegradable cement that coats the donor bone and hides the bone cell antigens until these cells have died and their MHC antigens have deteriorated.

Clinical Recovery

Early ambulation and mild exercise stimulate blood flow and osteogenesis within the graft. External splinting helps to stabilize the graft. Education of the patient in proper posture, weight-bearing, turning, and exercise has been helpful in allowing sufficient time for healing.

FUTURE OF TRANSPLANTATION

The current shortage of hearts, livers, and lungs is a major impediment to offering this therapy to the growing number of eligible recipients. Stimulated by this urgent need, research into the use of xenogeneic organs (from species other than humans) is proceeding. In addition to the usual rejection problems, a more severe form of hyperacute rejection must be overcome before this approach can become a clinical reality.

Closer to implementation, however, are transplants of specific types of cells that can be utilized to replace missing genes or enzymes. One can imagine transplanting hepatic parenchymal cells for their synthesis of clotting factors, proteins, and even hematopoietic stem cells.

REFERENCES

Kidney Transplantation

Cho YW, Terasaki PI: Chap 29, p 277 in: *Long Term Survival in Clinical Transplants*. Terasaki P (editor). UCLA Tissue Typing Laboratory, 1988.

Halloran PF, Cockfield SM, Madrenas J: The molecular immunology of transplantation and graft rejection. *Immunol Allergy Clin North Am* 1989;**9**:1.

Mizel SB: The interleukins. *FASEB J* 1989;**3**:2379.

Strom TB, Kelley VE: Toward more selective therapies to block undesired immune responses. *Kidney Int* 1989;**35**:1026.

Warvariv V, Garovoy MR: Transplantation immunology. Page 752 in: *Textbook of International Medicine*. Kelley WN (editor). Lippincott, 1989.

Liver Transplantation

Caine RY (editor): *Liver Transplantation*. Grune & Stratton, 1983.

Jenkins RL et al: Liver transplantation. *Surg Clin North Am* 1985;**65**:103.

Kamada N, Caine RY: A surgical experience with five hundred-thirty liver transplants in the rat. *Surgery* 1982;**93**:64.

Shaw BW et al: Transplantation of the liver. In: *Surgical Treatment of Digestive Disease*. Moody FG, Carey LC (editors). Yearbook, 1986.

Starzl TE et al: Evolution of liver transplantation. *Hepatology* 1982;**2**:614.

Pancreas & Islet Cell Transplantation

International symposium on complications of diabetes: Current status of prevention and treatment. *Transplant Proc* (In press).

Starzl TE et al: Pancreaticoduodenal transplantation in humans. *Surg Gynecol Obstet* 1984;**159**:265.

Sutherland DER, Kendall DM: Pancreas transplantation: Registry report and a commentary. *West J Med* 1985;**143**:845.

Sutherland DER, Moundry-Munns KE: Pancreas transplants in blacks and whites. *Transplant Proc* 1989;**21**:3968.

Sutherland DER et al: One institution's experience with pancreas transplantation. *West J Med* 1985;**143**:838.

Transplantation of pancreatic islet cells. (Progress Symposium.) *World J Surg* 1984;**8**:135.

Heart & Lung Transplantation

Caves PK et al: Percutaneous transvenous endomyocardial biopsy in human heart recipients. *Ann Thorac Surg* 1973;**16**:325.

Jamieson SW: Combined heart-lung transplantation. *West J Med* 1985;**143**:829.

Jamieson SW et al: Operative technique for heart-lung transplantation. *J Thorac Cardiovasc Surg* 1984;**87**:930.

Theodore J et al: Physiologic aspects of human heart-lung transplantation: Pulmonary function status of the post-transplanted being. *Chest* 1984;**86**:349.

Bone Marrow Transplantation

Anasetti C et al: Marrow transplantation for severe aplastic anemia. *Ann Intern Med* 1986;**104**:461.

Antman K Gale RP: Advanced breast cancer: high-dose chemotherapy and bone marrow autotransplants. *Ann Intern Med* 1988;**108**:570.

Applebaum FR, Dahlberg S, Thomas ED, et al: Bone marrow transplantation or chemotherapy after remission induction for adults with acute nonlymphocytic leukemia. *Ann Intern Med* 1984;**101**:581.

Beatty PG et al: Marrow transplantation from related donors other than HLA-identical siblings. *N Eng J Med* 1985;**313**:765.

Blume KG, Petz LD (editors): *Clinical Bone Marrow Transplantation*. Churchill Livingstone, 1983.

Bone-marrow autotransplantation in man: Report of an international cooperative study. *Lancet* 1986;**2**:960.

Hobbs JR: Displacement bone marrow transplantation and immunoprophylaxis for genetic diseases. *Adv Intern Med* 1988;**33**:81.

Meyers JD: Infection in bone marrow transplant recipients. *Am J Med* 1986;**81(Suppl 1A)**:27.

Thomas ED et al: Bone marrow transplantation. (2 parts.) *N Engl J Med* 1975;**292**:832, 895.

Thomas ED et al: Marrow transplantation for the treatment of chronic myelogenous leukemia. *Ann Intern Med* 1986;**104**:155.

Bone Transplantation

Prolo DJ, Rodrigo JJ: Contemporary bone graft physiology and surgery. *Clin Orthop* 1985;**200**:322.

61

Immunosuppressive Therapy

Alan Winkelstein, MD

The growth of clinical immunology has uncovered increasing numbers of diseases that are due to aberrant immune responses. This has resulted in a search for drugs capable of inhibiting these unwanted responses. Particularly, the technical ability to successfully transplant many organs created a strong impetus for the development of safe and effective immunosuppressive regimens. Over the past 2 decades, considerable progress has been made in identifying a group of compounds capable of achieving *nonspecific* inhibition of immune response. The eventual goal in this area is to develop *specific* immunosuppression or tolerance directed only at the immune response to selected antigens. This currently remains an elusive goal.

CORTICOSTEROIDS

The glucocorticoid steroid hormones are widely and effectively used to suppress manifestations of numerous inflammatory and immune reactions. The pharmacology and anti-inflammatory effects of corticosteroids are discussed in Chapter 63. Although a clear-cut distinction between the immunosuppressive and anti-inflammatory actions of these drugs is not always possible, this section will emphasize glucocorticoid effects on the cells involved in the immune response.

Clinical research studies have often been confused by a failure to recognize that lymphocytes from different animal species vary in their susceptibility to steroid-induced lysis. In mice, rats, and rabbits, these hormones cause extensive lymphoid destruction. By contrast, normal lymphocytes from guinea pigs, monkeys, and humans are highly resistant to steroid-induced lysis. Not all human lymphocytes are resistant; steroids will effectively kill acute lymphoblastic leukemic cells and are moderately cytolytic for neoplastic B cells in chronic lymphocytic leukemia and non-Hodgkin lymphomas.

The anti-inflammatory and immunosuppressive activities of corticosteroids can be grouped conveniently into 3 general categories: the effect of these drugs on leukocyte circulation, their ability to alter specific cellular functions, and other miscellaneous anti-inflammatory activities.

Effects on Cellular Traffic

One of the most important effects of corticosteroids is to alter transiently the number of circulating leukocytes. This is illustrated in Fig 61–1, which depicts the quantitative changes in each cell type following a single intravenous injection of a glucocorticoid. There is a prompt increase in the number of neutrophils and a concomitant decrease in the total number of lymphocytes, monocytes, eosinophils, and basophils. Maximum changes are observed 4–6 hours after injection, and all counts have returned to baseline values within 24 hours.

The neutrophilia resulting from steroid administration appears to be due to at least 2 distinct activities: release of mature neutrophils from marrow reserves and reduced neutrophil egress from intravascular spaces into inflammatory exudates. As a result, the half-life of circulating neutrophils is increased.

In contrast to the neutrophilia, steroids cause a striking reduction in the number of circulating lymphocytes. This effect results from the sequestration of recirculating lymphoid cells into lymphoid tissues, including the bone marrow. The total numbers of circulating T cells are markedly decreased, B cell numbers are only modestly reduced, and numbers of null cells are unchanged. Among the T cell subsets, numbers of CD4 cells are reduced to a greater extent than are numbers of CD8 cells.

One of the important steroid-induced changes is a pronounced monocytopenia. Monocyte counts frequently decline to less than 50 cells/μl, and the reduced availability of these cells has been postulated to be of prime importance in mediating steroid-induced anti-inflammatory activities. Eosinophil and basophil numbers are also reduced in the circulation because of redistribution.

Functional Change

In addition to affecting the distribution of leukocytes, corticosteroids alter important functional activities of both lymphocytes and monocytes. Neutrophilic activities such as chemotaxis and lysosomal enzymes are not significantly impaired, but the release of nonlysosomal proteolytic enzymes such as collagenase and plasminogen activator is decreased by steroids.

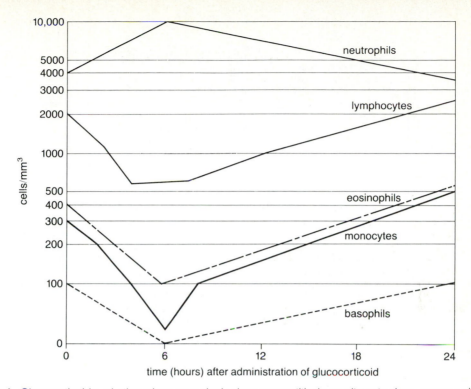

Figure 61–1. Glucocorticoids, whether given as a single dose or repetitively on alternate days, cause a decrease in lymphocyte, monocyte, basophil, and eosinophil counts and a rise in neutrophils within 4–6 hours, with a return to baseline within 24 hours. (Reproduced, with permission, from Claman HN: Glucocorticosteroids. I. Anti-inflammatory mechanisms. *Hosp Pract* 1983;**18**:123.)

T lymphocyte activities are considerably altered by corticosteroids. In vitro lymphoproliferative responses are inhibited, in part from an impairment in the synthesis and secretion of interleukin-2 (IL-2), which is essential for the clonal expansion of activated lymphocytes (Fig 61–2). The decreased availability of IL-2 is most probably an indirect result of suppressed IL-1 production by monocytes. IL-2 receptor expression is not impaired. Steroids do not alter the release of 2 other lymphokines, gamma interferon and migration inhibitory factor (MIF).

Corticosteroids can block the progression of phytohemagglutinin (PHA)-stimulated lymphocytes through the mitotic cycle (see below). They inhibit the entry of cells into the G_1 phase and arrest the progression of activated lymphocytes from the G_1 to the S phase.

Corticosteroids have less effect on B lymphocytes. Patients receiving moderate doses of prednisone are able to respond normally to test antigens. On the other hand, high-dose corticosteroid therapy modestly reduces the serum concentrations of IgG and IgA but not IgM. These changes may be observed as early as 2–3 weeks after initiation of the course of steroids. In one study using cultured spleen cells from patients with idiopathic thrombocytopenic purpura, steroids inhibited the ability of B lymphocytes to synthesize IgG. Steroid therapy does not alter the

activities of either natural killer (NK) cells or effectors of antibody-dependent cellular cytotoxicity (ADCC).

Paralleling their profound effects on the number of circulating monocytes, corticosteroids induce striking impairment in monocyte-macrophage function. They suppress the bactericidal activities of these phagocytic cells, thereby lowering resistance to infection. Steroids also interfere with the antigen-presenting function of these cells. Other effects include impaired directed migration in response to chemotactic factors, decreased response to MIF, blocking of the differentiation of monocytes to macrophages, and suppression of the capacity of monocytes to express Fc and complement receptors, which may contribute to impaired phagocytic activities.

Steroids suppress the ability of reticuloendothelial cells to phagocytose antibody-coated cells, probably by decreasing the binding of immune complexes to Fc and C3b surface membrane receptors. This impaired binding may account for their beneficial effects in diseases such as idiopathic thrombocytopenic purpura and autoimmune hemolytic anemia.

Delayed hypersensitivity skin tests are inhibited by prolonged treatment with corticosteroids. In general, these hormones must be administered for 10–14 days before skin test reactivity is impaired.

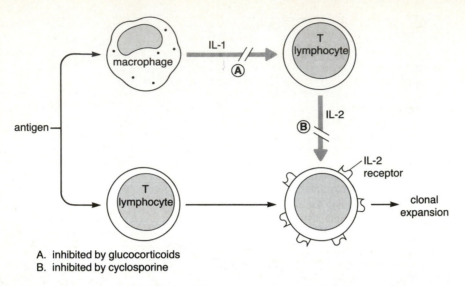

A. inhibited by glucocorticoids
B. inhibited by cyclosporine

Figure 61–2. Antigen stimulation in vivo induces monocytes to release the cytokine IL-1. This soluble mediator has numerous effects including inducing helper T cells to synthesize IL-2. Antigen stimulation also induces responsive T cells to express receptors for IL-2. When IL-2 combines with IL-2 receptor (IL-2R)-bearing lymphocytes, these cells undergo clonal expansion. Corticosteroids act primarily to inhibit IL-1 synthesis and release. Cyclosporine suppresses the release of IL-2 and inhibits IL-2R expression. The letters A and B indicate inhibition by glucocorticoids and cyclosporine, respectively.

Clinical Use

In pharmacologic quantities, these hormones are effective nonspecific inhibitors of numerous disorders of apparent immune pathogenesis. Typically, corticosteroids are most effective in suppressing acute inflammatory manifestations (see Chapter 63). By contrast, they usually do not prevent the long-term complications of the immunopathologic processes. For example, they inhibit the acute inflammatory reactions occurring in diseases such as acute rheumatic fever and rheumatoid arthritis without significantly preventing either chronic valvular heart disease or deforming arthritis.

Clinical protocols for corticosteroid administration in immunologic diseases vary with the disease; they are discussed in the relevant chapters. There are 3 general patterns to steroid therapy protocols, depending on the circumstances. The first is often used if these drugs are to be administered for extended periods. It entails the use of the smallest amount needed to partially suppress disease manifestations. An example of this is the treatment of rheumatoid arthritis with 7.5–10 mg of prednisone daily. The second approach uses larger doses in an attempt to rapidly and completely suppress manifestations of an immunologically mediated disease. Prednisone at 1–2 mg/kg is given daily, in one or divided doses. This type of therapy is often used in disorders such as autoimmune hemolytic anemia, idiopathic thrombocytopenic purpura, and various types of immune-induced glomerulonephritis. The third pattern is the pulse administration of very large doses of an intravenous corticosteroid preparation (eg, methylprednisolone at 10–30 mg/kg). These ultralarge doses are generally reserved for unusually severe or potentially life-threatening illnesses. They have also been used successfully in reversing acute allograft rejection reactions. Most studies suggest that the immunologic effects of these massive-dose steroid protocols do not differ significantly from those resulting from more conventional doses. Although the therapeutic superiority of these regimens has not been proven in controlled trials, numerous reports imply effectiveness.

Prolonged therapy with corticosteroids is not innocuous; these drugs have numerous and potentially serious side effects (see Chapter 63). It is important to recognize that chronic therapy with large doses of steroids may cause greater morbidity than does the underlying disease.

CYTOTOXIC DRUGS

Cytotoxic drugs consist of a group of chemicals with the pharmacologic property of killing cells capable of self-replication. Immunologically competent lymphocytes make up such a susceptible cell population. These drugs were originally introduced into clinical medicine for anticancer therapy; however, the initial studies revealed that many also possessed immunosuppressive activities. Thus, their use was extended to treatment of diseases caused by aberrant immune responses and to inhibition of transplant rejection reactions. There are 4 cytotoxic drugs currently in clinical use for immunosuppression: cyclophosphamide, azathioprine, methotrexate, and chlorambucil.

Although the antigen-specific cells responsible for the unwanted immune response are potentially susceptible to cytotoxic immunosuppression, it must be recognized that the immunosuppressive activities of these drugs are not limited to a single lymphocyte subset. To varying degrees, they can affect all immunologically competent cells, so that therapy leads to a generalized suppression of the immune defense system. As a result, treated patients are more susceptible to both opportunistic infections and certain neoplastic diseases.

Cytotoxic drugs are not selectively toxic for lymphocytes. They can kill nonlymphoid proliferating cells, including hematopoietic precursors, gastrointestinal mucosal cells, and germ cells in the gonads. Thus, predictable side effects of all these drugs include pancytopenia, gastrointestinal toxicities, and reduced fertility.

The lymphocytotoxic activities of different cytotoxic drugs can be related to their toxicities for cells in specific phases of the mitotic cycle (Fig 61–3). There are 4 phases in mitosis: G_1 (the pre-DNA synthetic phase), S (the DNA synthetic phase), G_2 (the premitotic phase), and M (the actual mitosis). Cells in a prolonged intermitotic period are considered to be in a G_0 phase. One group of drugs, which includes azathoprine and methotrexate, are termed "phase-specific." These drugs are cytolytic to cells as they enter a selective phase of the mitotic cycle. For example, both azathioprine and methotrexate are cytolytic for cells only when they are in the S (DNA synthetic) phase.

Cyclophosphamide and chlorambucil are classified as "cycle-specific." They are toxic for cells at all stages of the mitotic cycle, including intermitotic (G_0) lymphocytes. However, they show differential cytolytic activities; they are more toxic for actively cycling than for resting (G_0) cells. The third group, the "cycle-nonspecific" compounds, are equally cytotoxic for proliferating and intermitotic cells.

Based on animal experiments, certain principles have been formulated concerning the immunosuppressive activities of cytotoxic drugs. By extension, these principles form the basis for the use of the drugs in clinical situations. They are summarized as follows:

(1) A primary immune response is more readily inhibited than is a secondary or anamnestic reaction. Drugs that are effective in suppressing an immune response in an unsensitized animal usually show only minimal inhibitory activity in a sensitized animal. The same effect is observed in patients. For example, the primary immune response elicited by a renal transplant is readily impaired by a combination of azathioprine and corticosteroids. However, if the recipient has been presensitized to donor histocompatibility antigens, this immunosuppressive regimen is relatively ineffective in inhibiting rejection reactions.

(2) The stages of an immune response differ markedly in their susceptibility to immunosuppressants. The cellular events associated with an antigenic challenge can be subdivided into 2 phases, designated the induction phase and the established or effector phase (Fig 61–4). The former is the interval between exposure to antigen (sensitization) and the production of sensitized T cells or mature plasma cells; it is characterized by the rapid proliferative expansion of antigen-sensitive precursors. Thereafter, the reaction is considered to have entered an established phase. Most cytotoxic drugs are effective if the period of drug administration coincides with the induction phase; once the reaction has entered the established phase, they are considerably less active. Furthermore, memory lymphocytes are unresponsive to immunosuppressive drugs.

(3) The effectiveness of an immunosuppressive drug in a primary response is highly dependent on the timing of its administration relative to the initial antigenic challenge. Based on their effective interval, immunosuppressive agents are divided into 3 groups:

Group I: This group includes modes of therapy that exert their maximum immunosuppressive activity when administered just before the antigen and are considerably less effective if used after the immuno-

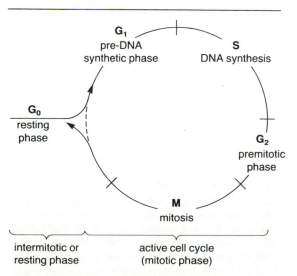

Figure 61–3. Mitotic cycles. Drugs that are selectively toxic for cells in a discrete phase of their cycle are designated phase-specific agents: most exert their toxicity for cells in the S phase. Cycle-specific agents are toxic for both intermitotic and proliferating cells but show greater toxicity for those in active cycle. Cycle-nonspecific agents show equal toxicity for all cells regardless of the mitotic activity.

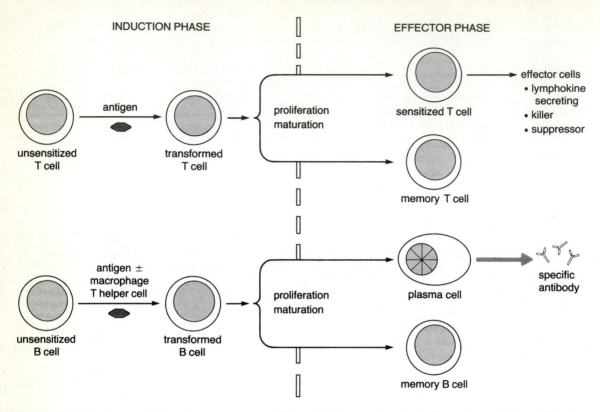

Figure 61–4. Development of an immune response. The period from antigenic challenge through the proliferative expansion of transformed lymphocytes is considered the induction phase. The period following cellular expansion is defined as the established (effector) phase.

logic challenge. Included in this group are corticosteroids, irradiation, and the cycle-nonspecific cytotoxin, nitrogen mustard.

Group II: This group includes drugs that show immunosuppressive properties only if administered in the period immediately following the antigenic challenge. They do not impair responses if used prior to the antigen. This group includes the phase-specific drugs such as azathioprine and methotrexate.

Group III: This group includes drugs that show inhibitory activity if administered either before or after antigenic stimulation, although these compounds show greater suppressive activities if used after the immune challenge. Pharmacologically, they are cycle-specific drugs; cyclophosphamide is the principal immunosuppressant in this group. The differential effects on immunity are illustrated in Fig 61–5, which shows the response to sheep erythrocytes in mice treated with an immunosuppressant either 24 hours before or 24 hours after antigenic challenge.

(4) Immunosuppressive drugs can exert differential toxicities for T and B lymphocytes. Cyclophosphamide causes a proportionately greater reduction in the number of B cells than of T cells; this correlates with its greater suppressive effects on antibody responses than on cell-mediated reactions. In clinical usage, cyclophosphamide is considered more effective in suppressing diseases of aberrant humoral immunity, such as idiopathic thrombocytopenic purpura, than in inhibiting transplant rejection reactions. By contrast, azathioprine appears more potent as an inhibitor of T cell-mediated responses.

(5) In certain circumstances, a paradoxic effect may be elicited by immunosuppressive treatment namely, augmentation of a specific response. This effect was originally noted with irradiation, which, when administered several days before an antigenic challenge, led to a greater than normal antibody response. Similar effects were then observed with 6-mercaptopurine when used before antigen challenge. With selected treatment protocols, cyclophosphamide can simultaneously suppress humoral responses and augment delayed hypersensitivity reactions to the same antigen. The heightened cellular reactions have been attributed, in part, to its toxicity for suppressor T lymphocytes.

(6) The ability to inhibit manifestations of an immune response may result from pharmacologic activ-

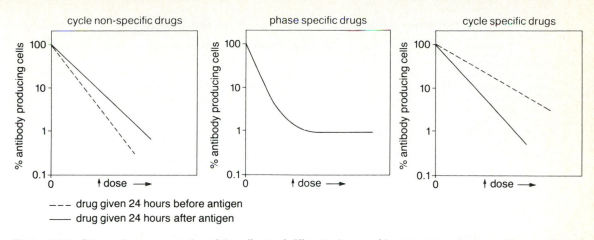

Figure 61–5. Schematic representation of the effects of different classes of immunosuppressants on the numbers of antibody-producing cells. (Reproduced, with permission, from Winkelstein A: Immune suppression resulting from various cytotoxic agents. Pages 296–316 in: *Clinics in Immunology and Allergy.* Vol 4: *Immune Suppression and Modulation.* Mitchell MS, Fahey JL (editors). Saunders, 1984.)

ities other than immunosuppression. The expression of many immune responses involves the participation of both immunologically competent cells and non-specific effector cells such as neutrophils and monocytes. The numbers or functions of these effector cells can be altered by immunosuppressive drugs, an effect that can modify or obliterate the expression of a particular response. Therefore, apparent immunosuppression can result from the anti-inflammatory properties of a specific agent. As an example, corticosteroids are potent suppressors of IgE-mediated allergic asthma and T cell-mediated allergic contact dermatitis. They inhibit inflammation in these diseases without affecting the underlying immune responses.

Clinical Use

These drugs are used to treat many autoimmune disorders. Table 61–1 is a partial list of diseases in

which cytotoxic drugs have been reported to be effective.

Despite their usage in these diseases for more than a decade, it is still difficult to ascertain their true effectiveness because there have been only a few controlled clinical trials. Controlled trials are necessary because many autoimmune diseases show unpredictable courses, with both spontaneous remissions and exacerbations. Nevertheless, cytotoxins have been widely accepted as potentially useful therapy for severe immune-related disorders.

Cytotoxic drugs have been used extensively in the treatment of rheumatic diseases. Table 61–2 compares the activities of each of the commonly used cytotoxic immunosuppressants in these diseases.

Individual Cytotoxic Drugs

A. Azathioprine: This compound is a phase-specific drug. It is a nitroimidazole derivative of the purine antagonist 6-mercaptopurine and is rapidly converted in vivo to the parent compound (6-mercaptopurine). Although there are conflicting data, most investigators believe that the addition of the imidazole side chain probably enhances its immunosuppressive potency and increases the therapeutic:toxic ratio.

Biochemically, both azathioprine and 6-mercaptopurine act by competitive enzyme inhibition to block synthesis of inosinic acid, the precursor of the purine compounds adenylic acid and guanylic acid. Therefore, the major effect is to impair DNA synthesis; this results in a decreased rate of cell replication and explains the phase-specific action of the drug. A second and less important activity is impairment of RNA synthesis.

Azathioprine appears to preferentially inhibit T cell responses compared with those resulting from

Table 61–1. Some immunologic disorders in which cytotoxic drugs are effective or probably effective.

Rheumatoid arthritis
Systemic lupus erythematosus
Systemic vasculitis
Wegener's granulomatosis
Polymyositis
Membranous glomerulonephritis
Chronic active hepatitis
Primary biliary cirrhosis
Inflammatory bowel disease
Autoimmune hemolytic anemia
Immune thrombocytopenia
Circulating anticoagulants
Multiple sclerosis
Myasthenia gravis

Table 61–2. Clinical efficacy of cytotoxic drugs in rheumatic disorders.[1]

Disease	Azathioprine	Efficacy of Chlorambucil[2]	Cyclophosphamide	Methotrexate
Rheumatoid arthritis	+ +	+	+ +	+ +
Rheumatoid vasculitis	0	+	+ +	0
Systemic lupus erythematosus	+	+	+	0
Polyarteritis nodosa	+	0	+ +	0
Polymyositis	+	0	0	+ +
Psoriatic arthritis	0	0	0	+
Wegener's granulomatosis	+	+	+ +	0
Reiter's syndrome	0	0	0	+

[1]Adapted from Nashel DJ: Mechanisms of action and clinical applications of cytotoxic drugs in rheumatic disorders. *Med Clin N Am* 1985; **69**:817.

[2]Symbols: + +, substantial evidence of effectiveness; +, benefit suggested by some studies; 0, not studied or benefit negligible.

activation of B lymphocytes. Nevertheless, both cell-mediated and humoral responses can be suppressed. In addition, azathioprine appears to effectively reduce the numbers of circulating NK and killer cells. The latter are responsible for ADCC reactions.

Before the development of cyclosporine (see below), combinations of azathioprine and corticosteroids were standard therapy for inhibition of transplant rejection reactions. These 2 agents still maintain an important role in this area. In addition, azathioprine is used to treat a spectrum of autoimmune disorders (Table 61–3). There is extensive experience with patients who have severe rheumatoid arthritis, for whom this drug is classified as a "disease-remitting" agent. Beneficial effects have also been reported in patients with other connective tissue diseases, autoimmune blood dyscrasias, and immunologically mediated neurologic diseases. This phase-specific drug may also permit the use of reduced amounts of corticosteroids in the treatment of

primary biliary cirrhosis, chronic active hepatitis, and inflammatory bowel disease. Azathioprine is administered orally, and the maximum beneficial effects generally require continuous therapy for several weeks.

The primary lymphocytotoxic effects of azathioprine are directed against actively replicating cells. Short therapeutic courses do not reduce the numbers of T or B cells in the peripheral blood, but they do decrease the number of large lymphocytes. These cells are believed to be activated lymphocytes that have entered an active proliferative cycle following exposure to appropriate antigens. Immunoglobulin levels and titers of specific antibodies are not appreciably reduced by azathioprine. The numbers of circulating neutrophils and monocytes are reduced in a dose-dependent fashion because of the drug's cytotoxicity for hematopoietic precursors.

B. Cyclophosphamide: Both experimentally and clinically, this cycle-specific drug is an extremely potent immunosuppressant with a high therapeutic:toxic ratio (Table 61–4). Because of its greater toxicity for B lymphocytes, it has more sustained suppressive activities for humoral antibody responses than for those attributed to cellular reactions. It has a variable effect on cell-mediated responses; some reactions are inhibited, whereas others are augmented. The latter phenomenon has been attributed to the toxicity of the drug for suppressor T lymphocytes.

Cyclophosphamide can be administered either orally or intravenously. The parent drug is inactive until metabolized by the liver, and the active moiety, whose structure has not yet been identified, is present in the circulation for only a few hours. The predominant cytotoxic effects are explained by its ability to cross-link DNA chains. This alkylating effect may result in the immediate death of the target cell, or the cell may incur a lethal injury that is expressed during a subsequent mitotic division. Conversely, if DNA repair can be effected, the cell will survive normally (Fig 61–6). In treated patients, cyclophosphamide causes a dose-related lymphopenia and impairs the in vitro proliferative responses of

Table 61–3. Properties and uses of azathioprine.

Trade name	Imuran
Administration	Orally, 1.25–2.5 mg/kg/d
Mechanism of action	S phase toxin (phase-specific agent) Inhibits de novo purine synthesis
Major indications	Transplant rejection reactions Chronic graft-versus-host reaction Rheumatoid arthritis ? Systemic lupus erythematosus ? Vasculitis ? Other connective tissue diseases Inflammatory bowel disease Chronic active hepatitis/primary biliary cirrhosis ? Myasthenia gravis ? Multiple sclerosis
Toxicities	Bone marrow depression Gastrointestinal irritation Hepatotoxicity (rare) Infections Cancers

Table 61–4. Properties and uses of cyclophosphamide.

Trade Name	Cytoxan
Administration	Orally 1–3 mg/kg/d Intravenously 10–20 mg/kg/every 1–3 months

Mechanism of action	Cycle-specific agent
	Binds and cross-links DNA strands
	A affects B cells more than T cells;
	   suppressor T cells more than
	   helper T cells

Major indications	Rheumatoid arthritis and vasculitis Systemic lupus erythematosus Wegener's granulomatosis Systemic vasculitis Autoimmune blood dyscrasias Immune-mediated glomerulo- nephritis

Toxicities	Bone marrow depression
	Gastrointestinal reactions
	Sterility (may be permanent)
	Alopecia
	Hemorrhagic cystitis
	Opportunistic infections
	Neoplasms (lymphoma, bladder
	   carcinoma, acute myelogenous
	   leukemia)
	Goodpasture's syndrome

residual cells. Both T and B cells are susceptible, and the selectivity of the drug for B cells appears to result from their lower recovery rate. Studies in patients with rheumatic diseases indicate that extended therapy will reduce both immunoglobulin concentrations and autoantibody titers.

Cyclophosphamide has been used successfully in the treatment of disorders believed to result from aberrant immunity. Beneficial effects have been documented in Wegener's granulomatosis, other forms of vasculitis, severe rheumatoid arthritis, the nephritis associated with systemic lupus erythematosus (SLE), autoimmune blood dyscrasias such as idiopathic thrombocytopenic purpura, autoimmune hemolytic anemia, pure erythrocyte aplasia, Goodpasture's syndrome, and immune forms of glomerulonephritis.

Although it is a potent immunosuppressant, cyclophosphamide is also toxic. The immediate side effects include a dose-dependent suppression of hematopoiesis; gastrointestinal symptoms such as abdominal pain, nausea, and vomiting; and gonadal dysfunction. In addition, this alkylating agent induces certain toxic manifestations not observed with other immunosuppressants; these include both hemorrhagic cystitis and alopecia. The delayed toxicities include an increased risk of opportunistic infections and a higher than expected occurrence of cancers, specifically non-Hodgkin lymphoma, bladder carcinoma, and acute myelogenous leukemia.

C. Methotrexate: This drug is a specific inhibitor of dihydrofolate reductase, an enzyme required for the conversion of folic acid to its active form, tetrahydrofolate (Fig 61–7). The latter compound serves as a donor of one-carbon fragments for the in vivo synthesis of thymidine. Thus, methotrexate is a potent inhibitor of DNA synthesis and is classified as a phase-specific agent.

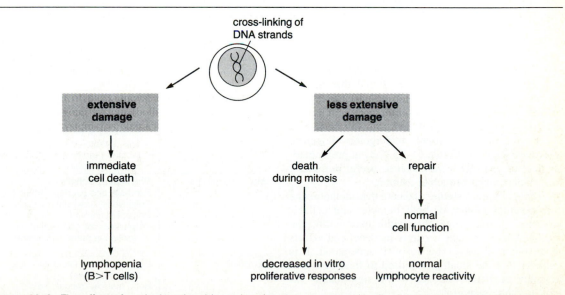

Figure 61–6. The effect of cyclophosphamide on lymphocytes appears primarily due to cross-linking DNA strands. This can result in lympholysis and decreased in vitro proliferative response. In cells that are not extensively damaged, repair can occur and the lymphocyte regains its full proliferative capacity. Because of the slow recovery of B cells, the effect is more pronounced than that on T cells.

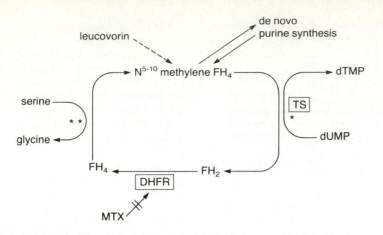

Figure 61–7. The folic acid cycle. The drug methotrexate (MTX) binds to and inhibits the enzyme dihydrofolate reductase (DHFR), thereby preventing the regeneration of tetrahydrofolate (FH_4) from dihydrofolate (FH_2). Leucovorin factor can directly antagonize the effects of methotrexate by providing a source of reduced folate. dUMP, 2-deoxyuridylate; dTMP, thymidylate; TS, thymidine synthase. *One-carbon transfer from $N^{5,10}$ methylene FH_4 to dUMP; **one-carbon transfer from serine to FH_4. (Reproduced, with permission, from Winkelstein A: Immune suppression resulting from various cytotoxic agents. Pages 296–316 in: *Clinics in Immunology and Allergy.* Vol 4: *Immune Suppression and Modulation.* Mitchell MS, Fahey JL (editors). Saunders, 1984.)

Methotrexate was one of the earliest anticancer drugs. Shortly after its introduction into clinical medicine, it was found to be effective in the treatment of psoriasis. However, the initial trials had to be terminated because of a high risk of hepatic fibrosis. Subsequently, investigators found that lower doses were equally effective in controlling psoriatic manifestations and could be administered for extended periods without inducing hepatic injury. Psoriatic patients with coexisting arthritis reported concomitant improvement in their joint disease. This led to an evaluation of methotrexate in patients with rheumatoid arthritis, and these studies showed that approximately two-thirds of the patients with severe rheumatoid arthritis achieved either partial or complete remissions. Other studies found that methotrexate effectively suppressed manifestations of polymyositis and Reiter's syndrome. It is also of considerable use in preventing graft-versus-host (GVH) reactions in patients undergoing allogeneic marrow transplants (Table 61–5). Recent preliminary studies suggest that it may also be useful in treating steroid-dependent bronchial asthma.

Athough animal studies indicate that methotrexate is a potent inhibitor of both humoral and cellular responses with a high therapeutic:toxic ratio, the mechanisms by which it exerts its beneficial effects in rheumatic diseases are not well understood. It is unlikely that the small doses used to treat immunologically mediated diseases would significantly inhibit immune responses.

A typical treatment regimen for rheumatic diseases consists of administering 2.5 mg of this drug every 12 hours for 3 doses; this course is repeated weekly. The major toxicity of methotrexate is hepatic fibrosis, which appears to be dose-related. Liver disease is rarely a problem until the total dose exceeds 1.5 g. Of particular note, hepatic fibrosis can occur with maintenance of normal liver function tests.

Other toxic manifestations include a hypersensitivity pneumonitis, mucositis, and megaloblastic anemia. With the exception of pneumonitis, these complications are rarely major problems at the doses used to treat rheumatic diseases.

Table 61–5. Properties and uses of methotrexate.

Administration	Orally 2.5–5.0 mg every 12 hours × 3 weekly
Mechanisms of action	S phase toxin (phase-specific) Competitively inhibits dihydrofolate reductase, thereby restricting synthesis of tetrahydrofolate. This is required for one-carbon transfer reactions involved in thymidine synthesis.
Major indications	Rheumatoid arthritis Psoriasis and psoriatic arthritis Polymyositis/dermatomyositis Reiter's syndrome Prophylaxis for graft-versus-host reaction in bone marrow transplants
Toxicities	Gastrointestinal (stomatitis, diarrhea, mucositis) Bone marrow (megaloblastic anemia) Hepatic fibrosis Pneumonitis Decreased fertility

D. Chlorambucil: Chlorambucil is an alkylating drug that has cytotoxic properties similar to those of cyclophosphamide. Most comparative studies suggest that it is less toxic than cyclophosphamide but not as potent an immunosuppressant.

Chlorambucil has been used extensively in Europe to treat immunologically mediated disease, and most reports suggest that it effectively responds to these disorders. These include rheumatoid arthritis, SLE, and Wegener's granulomatosis. It is the drug of choice for the treatment of idiopathic cold-agglutinin hemolytic anemia and essential cryoglobulinemia.

Chlorambucil has advantages over cyclophosphamide. It does not cause alopecia or hemorrhagic cystitis and is less irritating to the gastrointestinal tract than cyclophosphamide. Like cyclophosphamide, it will cause marrow suppression and will interfere with gonadal function. It is also a fetal toxin. It increases the risk of both opportunistic infections and certain cancers.

CYCLOSPORINE

Cyclosporine is a novel immunosuppressant with activities distinct from those of all other compounds. It is able to alter selectively the immunoregulatory activities of helper T cells without affecting suppressor T cells, B lymphocytes, granulocytes, or macrophages. Furthermore, it acts by impairing cellular functions without killing target lymphocytes. Because of its potency, it has become the standard drug for inhibition of allogeneic transplant rejection reactions; in most reports it is more effective than any other immunosuppressant. Recently, trials with cyclosporine have been initiated for the treatment of several other diseases that are presumed to be immunologically mediated.

Pharmacologically, cyclosporine is a unique cyclic undecapeptide derived from fermentation of certain soil fungi (Fig 61–8). It is not water soluble, but it can be administered either orally or intramuscularly in a lipid vehicle. Immunologically, its effects are highly selective. It specifically inhibits the activities of helper T cells while sparing suppressor T cells. Thus, it selectively blocks the immune responses, including allograft rejection, that are dependent on helper T lymphocytes.

Cyclosporine acts at an early phase of a developing immune response. In contrast to cytotoxic drugs, immunosuppression is achieved without lympholysis. Its major activity appears to be an inhibition of IL-2 synthesis and secretion (Fig 61–2). This lymphokine is required for the proliferative expansion of antigen-stimulated cells (see Chapter 7). Cyclosporine may also impair the ability of activated helper T cells to respond to IL-2, perhaps by limiting receptor expression.

Because of its ability to impair the function of helper T cells, cyclosporine can restrict the generation of antigen-specific cytotoxic and suppressor T cells. By contrast, it does not affect the activities of preformed killer or suppressor cells. T cell-dependent antibody responses are suppressed, whereas T cell-independent responses are not inhibited.

The effectiveness of this immunosuppressant may be increased by the simultaneous administration of moderate doses of corticosteroids. The 2 drugs appear to act synergistically. Cyclosporine directly inhibits IL-2 production, whereas steroids indirectly suppress the synthesis of IL-2 by blocking monocyte-macrophage release of IL-1 (Fig 61–2).

Clinically, cyclosporine has become the principal drug used to inhibit allograft rejection reactions (Table 61–6). Its development is one of the major reasons for the successful increase in transplant surgery using all types of organs, including kidney, heart, heart-lung, liver, and pancreas transplants.

Cyclosporine is also an effective means of preventing GVH reactions in major histocompatibility complex (MHC)-matched allogeneic bone marrow transplants. The drug, however, is comparatively ineffective as treatment for established GVH reactions.

Unlike cytotoxic drugs, cyclosporine is not toxic to bone marrow function. Renal failure is its major toxic effect, although this is generally reversible. It can also cause hypertension. Reversible hepatotoxicity resulting in elevations of the serum bilirubin and transaminase levels is another common side effect.

Cyclosporine has been implicated in the development of lymphomas. In particular, it appears to permit the development of B cell lymphomas, including those associated with Epstein-Barr virus (EBV). It has been postulated that this occurs because there is an escape from T cell surveillance which is normally exerted over EBV-infected B cells (see Chapter 47). Nevertheless, the overall risk of lymphoma in cyclosporine-treated transplant patients appears to be similar to that when other immunosuppressive therapy is used.

Cyclosporine treatment has additional side effects. These include gingival hyperplasia, hirsutism, and central nervous system manifestations, including seizures. In marrow transplantation patients, cyclosporine may cause potentially fatal capillary leak and a hemolytic uremic syndrome.

TOTAL LYMPHOID IRRADIATION (TLI)

Total lymphoid irradiation (TLI) is an experimental modality that offers considerable promise as a means of inducing sustained immunosuppression. Patients treated with TLI for Hodgkin's disease experience a prolonged phase of impaired immune reactivity that often persists for several years. The

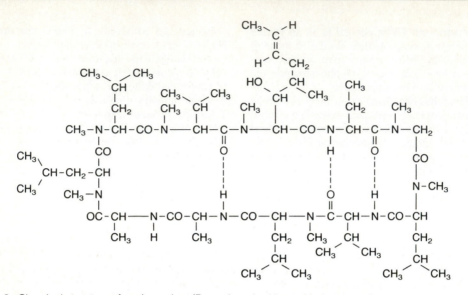

Figure 61–8. Chemical structure of cyclosporine. (Reproduced, with permission, from Cohen DJ et al: Cyclosporine: A new immunosuppressive agent for organ transplantation. *Ann Intern Med* 1984;**101:667**.)

most striking change is a decrease in the number of helper T cells.

Animal studies have confirmed the immunosuppressive effects of TLI, showing that it impairs allograft rejection and induces tolerance to MHC-mismatched marrow transplants. Furthermore, it was successful in the treatment of several experimental autoimmune diseases, including the lupuslike disorder of NZB/NZW mice.

In preliminary clinical studies, TLI suppressed manifestations of severe rheumatoid arthritis, lupus nephritis, and multiple sclerosis. Furthermore, it has been used, either alone or in combination with other agents, to inhibit transplant rejection reactions.

The mechanisms by which TLI induces long-lasting immunosuppression have not been fully defined. It produces a sustained decrease in helper T cell numbers, whereas there are only transient changes in numbers of suppressor T cells, B lymphocytes, and other lymphocytes. In vitro tests of lymphocyte function indicate that responses depending on helper T cells are suppressed and there is a prolonged phase characterized by excess suppressor T cell activity.

PLASMAPHERESIS

Diseases due to circulating autoantibodies or toxic antigen-antibody complexes could theoretically benefit from selective removal of the autoantibodies or immune complexes from the plasma. Plasma exchange (plasmapheresis) became clinically feasible with the development of automated cell separators capable of fractionating blood rapidly into its component parts. The procedure has been used experimentally to treat patients with a variety of immunologically related diseases, but there have been insufficient controlled therapeutic trials to ascertain its true effectiveness.

The technique used for plasma exchange is comparatively simple. Blood is removed, the plasma is separated by either centrifugation or membrane filtration and discarded, and the erythrocytes are reinfused into the patient. Fluid volume is maintained by administering either an albumin solution or fresh-frozen plasma. In most treatment protocols, approximately 50% of the patient's plasma is removed with each exchange procedure.

The ability of plasma exchange to remove a specific group of antibodies is dependent upon their im-

Table 61–6. Properties and uses of cyclosporine.

Administration	Orally, intravenously Variable dosage, 5–20 mg/kg/d
Mechanisms of action	Effects primarily limited to helper T cells; not cytotoxic Inhibits production of IL-2 ? Reduces expression of IL-2 receptors
Major indications	Inhibition of transplant rejection reactions
Toxicities	Nephrotoxicity Hypertension Hepatotoxicity ? Epstein-Barr virus-induced lymphomas Hirsutism, gingival hyperplasia Neurotoxicity Hemolytic uremic syndrome

munoglobin class. IgG molecules are distributed in both the intravascular and extracellular spaces, with approximately 40% contained in the vascular system. Thus, a single 50% plasma exchange can, at best, remove only 20% of a specific IgG antibody. By contrast, 85–90% of IgM antibodies are intravascular, so that a single exchange procedure can remove almost half the total quantity of pathogenic IgM antibodies. This accounts for the apparent success of plasma exchange in IgM antibody-related disorders such as idiopathic cold-agglutinin hemolytic anemia, essential cryoglobulinenemia, and the hyperviscosity syndrome associated with Waldenström's macroglobulinemia.

Plasma exchange has been most successful for 2 of the IgG antibody autoimmune diseases, myasthenia gravis and Goodpasture's syndrome. It is noteworthy that both of these diseases are characterized by the presence of highly specific tissue autoantibodies. Plasma exchange has been used, with questionable effectiveness, in intractable rheumatoid arthritis, rheumatoid vasculitis, other forms of vasculitis, lupus nephritis, posttransfusion purpura, bleeding from factor VIII antibodies, and immunologically mediated neurologic diseases such as Guillain-Barré syndrome and multiple sclerosis.

INTRAVENOUS GAMMA GLOBULIN

Replacement therapy with intravenous gamma globulin (IV-IgG) has become standard treatment for severe humoral immune deficiencies (see Chapter 25). IV-IgG has also been found to influence the course of several autoimmune diseases, particularly immune thrombocytopenia, by functioning paradoxically as an immunosuppressant or immunomodulator. It has been highly effective in treating children with the acute forms of idiopathic thrombocytopenic purpura. Although prolonged remissions in adults are rare, IV-IgG can often increase platelet counts transiently, which can be potentially life-saving in cases of bleeding diatheses resulting from severe thrombocytopenia. Although the mechanism of action in idiopathic thrombocytopenic purpura is not fully known, IV-IgG appears to act primarily by blocking FcγR on reticuloendothelial cells, thereby inhibiting the phagocytosis of antibody-coated platelets. In some cases, IV-IgG may also displace platelet-specific antibodies from the cell surface.

Based on the experience with idiopathic thrombocytopenic purpura, several other immunologically mediated diseases have been treated with IV-IgG. These include autoimmune hemolytic anemia, autoimmune neutropenia, antibody-mediated pure erythrocyte aplasia, other platelet-destructive diseases, autoantibodies against the blood-clotting factor VIII, myasthenia gravis, and Kawasaki disease. The accumulated experience to date with these conditions is

too small to determine the true effectiveness of the drug.

Several other mechanisms have been postulated to explain the immune-modulating activities. IV-IgG has been reported to nonspecifically augment suppressor T cell activities. It may also inhibit the activities of NK cells and reduce the synthesis of specific immunoglobulins. In addition, it may contain anti-idiotypic antibodies that will serve to inactivate autoantibodies.

ANTILYMPHOCYTE ANTIBODIES

The administration of heterologous antisera against lymphocyte membrane antigens is another mode of achieving nonspecific immunosuppression. Two types of antibody preparations have been used: polyclonal antibodies, which react with multiple membrane determinants, and monoclonal antibodies, which are directed at only a single antigen.

Polyclonal Antibodies

Polyclonal antibodies are generally prepared by immunizing animals with human lymphocytes. If cells from the thymus are used, the preparation is termed **antithymocyte serum (ATS)**; this is often further fractionated to obtain the globulin portion, termed **antithymocyte globulin (ATG).** Other antibodies are prepared from thoracic duct lymphocytes, splenic cells, or peripheral blood lymphocytes obtained by leukophoresis. These are referred to as either **antilymphocyte serum (ALS)** or **antilymphocyte globulin (ALG).**

Polyclonal antibodies are effective immunosuppressants in animal studies, where the primary effect is the impairment of cell-mediated responses consistent with their specificities for T lymphocytes. However, the mechanisms responsible for their immunosuppressive activities are not fully understood. They do produce lymphopenia in vivo; this is one postulated mode of action. Clinically, they are used primarily to treat organ graft rejection reactions. More recently, they have been used to treat patients with severe GVH reactions and to promote remissions in some cases of aplastic anemia.

Several major problems are associated with the use of polyclonal antibodies. (1) The preparations are not standardized, and there is no objective measure of in vivo immunosuppressive activity of a particular preparation. Thus, the amount needed to achieve a specific clinical effect cannot be predetermined. (2) These reagents are not selective for T cells. They cross-react with other types of cells, including platelets, which may lead to a destructive thrombocytopenia. (3) Heterologous antibodies are recognized as foreign proteins by the patient's immune system, thereby eliciting a humoral immune response, which may cause serum sickness (see Chapter 32).

Monoclonal Antibodies

Monoclonal antibodies, specific to lymphocyte membrane antigens, have several theoretic advantages over polyclonal antilymphocyte sera. They are highly selective in their reactivity, so they do not cross-react with nonlymphoid cells. Furthermore, the amount of a specific antibody can be accurately quantitated, allowing for more predictable dosing.

Two pan-T cell monoclonal antibodies have been used to reverse transplant rejection reactions and to treat GVH reactions in allogeneic marrow transplants. One of the antibodies used therapeutically is anti-CD3, which reacts with a determinant closely linked to the T cell antigen receptor. The other reacts with the T12 antigen, a membrane determinant on most immunologically active T lymphocytes. Initial trials suggest that each of these monoclonal antibodies has the ability to reverse some rejection reactions.

REFERENCES

General

Bach JF: *The Mode of Action of Immunosuppressive Agents.* North Holland, 1975.

Ben-Yehuda O, Tomer Y, Shoenfeld Y: Advances in therapy of autoimmune diseases. *Semin Arthritis Rheum* 1988;**17**:206.

Elion GB. Immunosuppressive agents. *Transplant Proc* 1977;**9**:975.

Fahey JL et al: Immune interventions in disease. *Ann Intern Med* 1987;**106**:257.

Hazleman B: Incidence of neoplasms in patients with rheumatoid arthritis exposed to different treatment regimens. *Am J Med* 1985;**78(Suppl 1A)**39.

Heppner GH, Calabressi P: Selective suppression of humoral immunity by antineoplastic drugs. *Annu Rev Pharmacol Toxicol* 1976;**16**:367.

Mitchell MS, Fahey JL (editors): *Immune Suppression and Modulation.* Vol 4 of: *Clinics in Immunology and Allergy* Saunders, 1984.

Penn I: The occurrence of malignant tumors in immunosuppressed states. *Prog Allergy* 1986;**37**:259.

Schein PS, Winokur SH: Immunosuppressive and cytotoxic chemotherapy: Long term complications. *Ann Intern Med* 1975;**82**:84.

Spreafico F, Tagliabue A, Vecchi A: Chemical immunodepressants. Pages 315–345 in: *Immunopharmacology.* Sirois CP, Rola-Pleszczynski M (editors). Elsevier, 1982.

Strom TB: Immunosuppressive agents in renal transplantation. *Kidney Int* 1984;**26**:353.

Tsokos GC: Immunomodulatory treatment in patients with rheumatic diseases: Mechanisms of action. *Semin Arthritis Rheum* 1987;**17**:24.

Yunus MB: Investigational therapy in rheumatoid arthritis: A critical review. *Semin Arthritis Rheum* 1988;**17**:163.

Corticosteroids

Claman HN: Glucocorticosteroids. I. Anti-inflammatory mechanisms. II. The clinical response. *Hosp Pract* 1983;**18**:123, 143.

Cupps TR, Fauci AS: Corticosteroid-mediated immunoregulation in man. *Immunol Rev* 1982;**65**:133.

Meuleman J, Katz P: The immunologic effects, kinetics and use of glucocorticosteroids. *Med Clin N Am* 1985;**69**:805.

Parrillo JE, Fauci AS: Mechanisms of glucocorticoid action on immune processes. *Annu Rev Pharmacol Toxicol* 1979;**19**:179.

Zweiman B et al: Corticosteroid effects on circulating lymphocyte subset levels in normal humans. *J Clin Immunol* 1984;**4**:151.

Cytotoxic Drugs

Ahmed AR, Hombal SM: Cyclophosphamide (cytoxan). *J Am Acad Dermatol* 1984;**11**:1115.

Austin HA et al: Therapy of lupus nephritis. *N Engl J Med* 1986;**314**:614.

Berd D et al: Augmentation of the human immune response by cyclophosphamide. *Cancer Res* 1982; **42**:4862.

Clements PJ, Davis J: Cytotoxic drugs: Their clinical application to the rheumatic diseases. *Semin Arthritis Rheum* 1986;**15**:231.

Cupps TR, Edgar LC, Fauci AS: Suppression of human B lymphocytes function by cyclophosphamide. *J Immunol* 1982;**128**:2453.

Felson DT, Anderson J: Evidence for the superiority of immunosuppressive drugs and prednisone over prednisone alone in lupus nephritis. *N Engl J Med* 1984;**311**:1528.

Nashel DJ: Mechanisms of action and clinical applications of cytotoxic drugs in rheumatic disorders. *Med Clin N Am* 1985;**69**:817.

Turk JL, Parker D: Effect of cyclophosphamide on immunological control mechanisms. *Immunol Rev* 1982;**65**:99.

Winkelstein A: Effects of cytotoxic immunosuppressants on tuberculin-sensitive lymphocytes in guinea pigs. *J Clin Invest* 1975;**56**:1587.

Winkelstein A: Effects of immunosuppressive drugs on T and B lymphocytes in guinea pigs. *Blood* 1977; **50**:81.

Cyclosporine

Bennett WM, Norman DJ: Action and toxicity of cyclosporine. *Annu Rev Med* 1986;**37**:215.

Cohen DJ et al: Cyclosporine: A new immunosuppressive agent for organ transplantation. *Ann Intern Med* 1984;**101**:667.

Total Lymphoid Irradiation

Halperin EC: Total lymphoid irradiation as an immunosuppressive agent for transplantation and the treatment of ''autoimmune'' disease: A review. *Clin Radiol* 1985;**36:**125.

Plasmapheresis

Shumak KH, Rock GA: Therapeutic plasma exchange. *N Engl J Med* 1984;**310:**762.

Antisera

Cosimi AB: Clinical development of orthoclone OKT3. *Transplant Proc* 1987;**19(Suppl 1):**7.

Goldstein G: Overview of the development of orthoclone OKT3: Monoclonal antibody for therapeutic use in transplantation. *Transplant Proc* 1987;**19 (Suppl 1):**1.

Heyworth MF: Clinical experience with antilymphocyte serum. *Immunol Rev* 1982;**65:**79.

Ortho Multicenter Transplant Study Group: A randomized clinical trial of OKT3 monoclonal antibody for acute rejection of cadaveric renal transplants. *N Engl J Med* 1985;**313:**337.

62

Immunomodulators

Howard S. Jaffe, MD, & Stephen A. Sherwin, MD

Immunomodulators are drugs that directly modify a specific immune function or have a net positive or negative effect on the activity of the immune system. The potential uses of immunomodulators in clinical medicine include the reconstitution of immune deficiency (eg, the treatment of acquired immunodeficiency syndrome [AIDS]) and the suppression of normal or excessive immune function (eg, the treatment of graft rejection or autoimmune disease). Recent advances in molecular biology have identified a growing number of substances capable of modulating immune function; these include interferons, interleukins, colony-stimulating factors, tumor necrosis factors, and monoclonal antibodies. These immunomodulators have more specific effects than do products from microorganisms such as bacillus Calmette-Guérin (BCG) and *Corynebacterium parvum,* which were used for similar purposes in the past. Experience with immunomodulators in controlled clinical trials is currently limited, but many of these may be effective for treatment of malignant, infectious, and immunologic disorders. However, since our understanding of the complex role of such agents in the immune system is still incomplete, the rational design of clinical studies remains a significant challenge. This chapter reviews the major classes of immunomodulators (cytokines, monoclonal antibodies, and nonspecific immunomodulators of microbial origin) currently being evaluated in clinical trials. A discussion of their biologic and immunologic effects is presented in Chapter 7.

CYTOKINES

Cytokines are hormonelike proteins that are produced by immune cells and other cells and that regulate the function of the immune system. They include lymphokines and monokines, which are produced by lymphocytes and monocytes, respectively. Recombinant DNA technology has provided virtually unlimited supplies of highly purified cytokines, permitting the clinical evaluation of these substances in the absence of biologically active contaminants. Most cytokines have been studied in phase I trials to determine their safety and pharmacology and in phase II trials to determine their immunomodulatory activity in specific clinical situations and to de-

fine treatment regimens. When this approach is used, it should be recognized that the maximum dose tolerated by the patient may far exceed the dose required to effect a particular desired biologic response by the immune system. The major classes of cytokines that have been evaluated clinically and are reviewed below include the interferons, interleukins, colony-stimulating factors, and tumor necrosis factors.

Interferons

The interferons are a group of proteins and glycoproteins produced by cells in response to virus, double-stranded RNA, antigen, or mitogen (see Chapter 7). They are currently classified, according to various biochemical properties, into 3 groups designated as IFN α, IFN β, and IFN γ. IFN α and IFN β (previously grouped together as type I interferons) are acid-stable and are produced primarily by leukocytes and fibroblasts in response to virus or double-stranded RNA. In contrast, IFN γ (type II interferon) is an acid-labile interferon produced primarily by T lymphocytes in response to mitogen or antigen and is often referred to as immune interferon.

A. IFN α: The major focus of recent clinical studies with human interferon has been the evaluation of recombinant or highly purified IFN α preparations in treating selected malignant and viral disorders. Table 62–1 lists tumors against which IFN α alone has clinical activity. The most impressive antitumor effects of IFN α have been noted in hairy cell leukemia and include hematologic remission, correction of pancytopenia, and significant improvement in the

Table 62–1. The antitumor effects of IFN α.

Major Activity	Minor Activity
Hairy-cell leukemia	Essential thrombocythemia
Chronic myelogenous leukemia	Kaposi's sarcoma (AIDS-related)
Basal cell carcinoma (intralesional therapy)	Multiple myeloma
Non-Hodgkin lymphoma (low grade)	Chronic lymphocytic leukemia
Cutaneous T cell lymphoma	Melanoma
Carcinoid tumor	Renal cell carcinoma
	Ovarian carcinoma (intraperitoneal therapy)
	Bladder tumors (intravesical therapy)

patient's quality of life, as evidenced by a reduction in transfusion requirements and secondary infections. Significant antitumor effects, including biopsy-proven complete responses, have also been noted in patients with advanced, heavily pretreated non-Hodgkin lymphomas and in patients with cutaneous T cell lymphomas who failed to respond to other topical and systemic therapies. Finally, IFN α has produced hematologic remissions in a majority of previously untreated patients with chronic myelogenous leukemia. More than one-third of them had a prolonged decrease in Philadelphia chromosome-positive cells on bone marrow biopsy. This effect was not seen with traditional cytotoxic chemotherapy and suggests a possible direct effect of IFN α on the expression of cells of the malignant phenotype.

It is still not yet certain that the antitumor effects seen in other cancers will result in improved survival. Moreover, the role of IFN α in combination with other agents or as an adjuvant after surgery or radiotherapy of the primary lesions has yet to be fully defined.

Extensive studies have also been carried out to evaluate the role of systemic and topical application of IFN α in the treatment of viral infections. Table 62–2 lists the viral disease that responded to IFN α in recent clinical trials. Particularly impressive results have been obtained with intensive regimens of IFN α administered intramuscularly or intralesionally to patients with papillomavirus infection of the genital tract (condyloma acuminatum). Complete responses were achieved in more than 25% of treated patients, including many who were refractory to traditional topical therapy. Because papillomavirus may be involved in the pathophysiology of dysplasia and intraepithelial neoplasia of the genital tract in women, these findings may have important implications for the prevention of cervical carcinoma.

Other studies have shown activity of IFN α in the therapy of chronic hepatitis B infection, by intranasal administration in the prophylaxis of upper respiratory tract infection, by ophthalmic application in herpes keratoconjunctivitis, and by topical application in cutaneous wart syndromes. IFN α inhibits the replication of human immunodeficiency virus (HIV) in vitro. Several clinical trials have now demonstrated that treatment of Kaposi's sarcoma with IFN α is associated with significant objective responses in patients with limited disease and less than severe immune dysfunction. Preliminary data suggest that

Table 62–2. Viral infections that respond to IFN α.

Papillomavirus
Rhinovirus
Hepatitis B virus
Human immunodeficiency virus 1
Herpesvirus

IFN α therapy can result in a reduction of HIV viremia, as measured by a decrease in p24 antigen and viral culture. However, there has not been a proven impact on long-term survival, so recent trials have focused on the combination of zidovudine (AZT) and IFN α in treating AIDS.

The administration of high doses of IFN α can result in clearly unacceptable toxicity. Most patients develop an influenzalike syndrome consisting of fever, chills, headache, and myalgia, although these symptoms tend to diminish with continued therapy and can be controlled at least partly with cyclooxygenase inhibitors and acetaminophen. Some patients develop significant fatigue and anorexia, necessitating a reduction in the dose. The most common laboratory abnormalities observed following IFN α therapy are reversible granulocytopenia and elevations of hepatic transaminase and, in some patients, antibodies to IFN α. Considerably less common problems are central nervous system toxicity, arrhythmias, and hypotension.

B. IFN β: IFN β shares antiviral, antiproliferative, and immunomodulatory properties, as well as cell surface receptors, with IFN α. However, there are differences in tumor cell sensitivities in vitro, warranting an independent clinical evaluation of IFN β. Problems in the production of IFN β have been circumvented by the production of serine-substituted recombinant IFN β. Objective evidence of antitumor effects following IFN β therapy has been seen in cancers that also respond to IFN α, including renal cell carcinoma, malignant melanoma, and hairy cell leukemia. Similarly, local administration of IFN β in the treatment of glioblastoma and cervical intraepithelial neoplasia has shown a similar efficacy to IFN α. Intravenous administration of IFN β has been associated with short-lived responses in patients with both acute and subacute adult T cell leukemias. To date, response rates and toxicity of IFN α and IFN β have been similar in cancer treatment.

C. IFN γ: While sharing many antiproliferative and antiviral effects with IFN α and IFN β, IFN γ has distinct immunomodulatory effects including macrophage activation, induction of class II histocompatibility antigens, and more pronounced synergistic interactions with other cytokines such as the interleukins and tumor necrosis factors. Therefore, the early clinical trials of IFN γ have attempted to determine treatment regimens capable of enhancing immune function in patients with both malignant and infectious diseases.

Preliminary results of IFN γ treatment in cancer patients suggest a role in combination therapy for hematologic cancers. The best results have been achieved in patients with benign-phase chronic myelogenous leukemia, who show clear objective evidence of hematologic and cytogenetic improvement with chronic IFN γ therapy. IFN γ appears to have activity in other lymphoproliferative disorders, such as Hodgkin's disease, cutaneous T cell lymphoma, chronic lymphocytic leukemia, adult T cell leukemia, and myelodysplastic syndrome, and even in some solid tumors, such as malignant melanoma and renal cell carcinoma. Although the spectrum of antitumor effects of IFN γ is similar to that of IFN α, some patients who have previously failed to respond to IFN α therapy do respond to IFN γ, and, conversely, IFN α has been active after failure of IFN γ treatment. This potential lack of cross-resistance and the demonstrated potential for these 2 interferons to act synergistically in preclinical studies have prompted the evaluation of their combined use in patients with a variety of cancers. Unfortunately, treatment-related toxicities of IFN γ and IFN α are similar.

Recent clinical trials have shown in vivo immunomodulatory effects of IFN γ. There has been clear documentation of enhancement of HLA-DR antigen and Fc receptor expression on circulating mononuclear cells, augmentation of natural killer cell function, and activation of monocyte-macrophages for both tumoricidal and antimicrobial effect. Moreover, recent studies have identified a maximal immunomodulatory treatment regimen for achieving these effects with IFN γ. Such information will be useful in future trials in patients with chronic granulomatous disease, lepromatous leprosy, and AIDS-associated toxoplasmic encephalitis. In addition, the demonstration of IFN γ inhibition of both procollagen mRNA transcription and IL-4-mediated IgE synthesis have led to the investigation of IFN γ therapy of fibrotic and allergic disorders, respectively (Table 62–3).

Interleukins

The interleukins are cytokines produced by cells of the immune system that regulate the immune response as well as hematopoiesis and metabolism (see Chapter 7). Among the interleukins, to date only interleukin-2 (IL-2) has been evaluated clinically. The observation that IL-2 can lead to the proliferation and activation of lymphokine-activated killer (LAK) cells, capable of selectively lysing tumor cells, has led to clinical trials of IL-2 alone and IL-2 plus LAK cell combination therapy of cancer. Tumor regressions in selected types of cancer have been achieved in preliminary trials. The in vivo mechanism of action of these treatment modalities has not been fully defined but is presumed to be the direct killing of tumor cells by LAK cells generated in vitro or in vivo by IL-2.

More recently, efforts to improve upon the potency and specificity of LAK cells have led to the identification of tumor-infiltrating lymphocytes. Lymphocytes extracted from freshly resected tumor tissue can be expanded in vitro by IL-2 and are capable of mediating specific lysis of autologous tumor cells.

Although high-dose IL-2 and IL-2 plus LAK cell adoptive immunotherapy can induce a significant response rate in renal cell carcinoma and melanoma, the toxicity of treatment is substantial and can include fever, chills (treated with acetaminophen and nonsteroidal and anti-inflammatory drugs), nausea, vomiting, diarrhea, marked cutaneous erythema, hypotension, fluid accumulation (up to 10% of body weight), pulmonary edema, arthritis, and hepatic, renal, and hematologic toxicity. Additionally, somnolence, confusion, and other neuropsychiatric manifestations have been observed at higher doses. The mechanism of these toxic manifestations may relate to an IL-2-induced release of secondary mediators with a consequent enhancement of vascular permeability. IL-2-related toxicity is poorly understood and represents a significant challenge to clinical use.

At present, adoptive immunotherapy with IL-2 and LAK cells or tumor-infiltrating lymphocytes may be considered an alternative but still experimental anticancer modality that can result in significant tumor regression in a minority of patients for whom no other effective therapy is available.

Colony-Stimulating Factors (CSF)

The colony-stimulating factors (CSF) are a family of glycoproteins that support hematopoietic colony formation in vitro (see Chapter 7). Five recombinant factors are currently in various stages of clinical development. There are 3 lineage-specific CSF, erythropoietin, granulocyte-colony stimulating factor (G-CSF), and monocyte-macrophage-colony stimulating factor (M-CSF), and 2 multipotential CSF, IL-3 and granulocyte-macrophage-colony stimulating factor (GM-CSF). The multipotential CSFs are capable of promoting the proliferation of earlier hematopoietic precursors (Table 62–4). These factors share many characteristics, including their ability to stimulate the function of mature cells, an overlapping effect on progenitor cells of several bone marrow lineages, and direct and indirect actions on cells outside the hematopoietic system. In addition, synergistic effects of combinations of these factors with other cytokines, eg, IL-1, IL-4, and IL-6, underscore the biologic complexity of hematopoiesis.

Table 62–3. Potential clinical applications of IFN γ.

Infectious diseases
  Chronic granulomatous disease
  Lepromatous leprosy
  Leishmaniasis
  Toxoplasmic encephalitis
Fibrotic diseases
  Scleroderma
  Keloids
IgE-mediated diseases
  Hyperimmunoglobulinemia E syndrome
  Atopic dermatitis

Table 62–4. Sources and targets of the 5 major CSF.

CSF	Major Cellular Sources	Major Target Cells
Erythropoietin	Kidneys	Erythroid
G-CSF	Monocytes, fibroblasts	Neutrophil
M-CSF	Monocytes, fibroblasts, endothelial cells	Monocyte-macrophage
IL-3	T cells	Erythroid, neutrophil, monocyte-macrophage, eosinophil, basophil, megakaryocyte
GM-CSF	T cells, fibroblasts, endothelial cells	Erythroid, neutrophil, monocyte-macrophage, eosinophil, megakaryocyte

Among the CSF, only erythropoietin appears to fit the strict definition of a hormone in that it is produced by the kidneys in response to renal delivery of oxygen and its principal site of action is the erythrocyte lineage in the bone marrow. Preliminary trials of replacement therapy in patients with end-stage renal disease have established that erythropoietin can correct anemia in these patients, but it can aggravate hypertension, cause functional iron deficiency by enhancing hematopoiesis, and complicate hemodialysis.

G-CSF administered to patients receiving cytotoxic chemotherapy for advanced cancers has resulted in a dose-dependent amelioration of neutropenia associated with chemotherapy. It has been well-tolerated and may reduce the morbidity and mortality rates associated with chemotherapy, possibly permitting higher doses and a greater antitumor response. Clinical trials of GM-CSF have documented a potential beneficial effect on bone marrow function in patients receiving high-dose chemotherapy in the setting of autologous bone marrow transplantation as well as in the treatment of advanced cancers. It has also been used in AIDS, myelodysplastic syndrome, and aplastic anemia in an attempt to stimulate bone marrow function. Preliminary results show increased bone marrow cellularity and circulating cell counts, thereby reducing transfusion requirements. However, high doses have produced marked weight gain, generalized edema, and hypotension, possibly through GM-CSF induction of other cytokines including M-CSF and tumor necrosis factor. GM-CSF also causes a dose-dependent, asymptomatic eosinophilia.

M-CSF and IL-3 have not yet undergone clinical trials. The early trials of the other CSF in patients with bone marrow failure are encouraging, but there is concern about the potential for depletion of normal hematopoietic precursor cells and possible selective enhancement of malignant clones.

Tumor Necrosis Factors (TNF)

Tumor necrosis factor (TNF) was initially defined as an antitumor activity found in the sera of animals treated with endotoxin after being primed with immunomodulators such as BCG or *C parvum* (see Chapter 7). Partially purified TNF was found to have in vitro antitumor activity apparently because of its specificity for transformed cells. This has generated considerable interest in the therapeutic potential of TNF in the treatment of cancer. Two closely related molecular species of TNF have been identified, TNF-α (identical to cachectin) and TNF-β (also called lymphotoxin).

Extensive preclinical studies have been performed to characterize the in vivo antitumor effects of TNF. Prolonged survival of patients with leukemias and regressions of established solid tumors in mice have been achieved, as well as regression of human tumor xenografts transplanted in nude mice.

The initial clinical trials of recombinant TNF-α have shown potential efficacy in gastrointestinal and bladder cancers. TNF-α can be administered safely to humans in a dose range associated with fever, chills, headaches, mild hypotension, and transient leukopenia but without severe shock or cachexia. Future studies are likely to emphasize its use locally at the tumor site and in combination with chemotherapeutic and other biologic drugs.

TNF/cachectin is released by macrophages in response to various stimuli, including endotoxin, with direct (inhibition of lipoprotein lipase) and indirect (induction of IL-1 and leukotriene release) effects. Since TNF/cachectin plays a role in septic shock, specific TNF antagonists, if discovered, could be life-saving in this condition.

MONOCLONAL ANTIBODIES

Monoclonal antibodies are produced by hybridoma technology, a procedure in which a mouse is immunized with a specific antigen and its spleen cells are then fused with a continuous B cell line, producing a hybrid antibody-secreting cell with clonal specificity for the antigen (see Chapter 18). This produces large quantities of antibodies to a single molecular epitope on the desired antigen. The early clinical trials involving cancer patients given murine monoclonal antibodies specific to human tumor antigens have identified several problems including tumor heterogeneity, limited vascular access, nonspecific antibody uptake at nontumor sites, blocking antibodies, antibody-conjugate dissociation, and the development of human antimouse antibodies. These problems have significantly limited monoclonal antibody therapy of specific cancers, particularly solid tumors. However, the use of monoclonal antibodies conjugated to radioisotopes, cellular toxins, or other drugs as a strategy for targeting the conjugated drug specifically to the neoplastic cell is currently being evaluated.

One class of monoclonal antibody has an established role in the treatment of graft rejection. The monoclonal antibody OKT 3, which has specificity for the CD3 antigen found on T cells, compares favorably with conventional high-dose corticosteroid therapy of acute renal, hepatic, and cardiac allograft rejection. There are, however, significant side effects, including influenzalike symptoms, blood pressure changes, and dyspnea (particularly following the initial dose). The development of human anti-mouse antibodies may preclude its repeated use.

NONSPECIFIC IMMUNOMODULATORS

Before the availability of highly purified compounds produced by recombinant DNA technology, a variety of nonspecific immunomodulators were used to augment host immune response in certain clinical settings. They may be divided into 3 classes: products of microbial origin, products of mammalian origin, and synthetic compounds. Table 62–5 is a partial list of such agents that have been administered to patients with selected immunodeficiencies and cancers.

Nonspecific immunomodulators of microbial origin have shown limited therapeutic benefit, low purity, and lot-to-lot product variability. The most extensively studied is BCG. When BCG is injected directly into cutaneous melanoma lesions, regression of both injected and distant, noninjected lesions can be observed, but without prolonged patient survival in prospective randomized trials. However, intravesical BCG treatment of superficial bladder carcinoma is now widely accepted in the management of such patients. BCG has also been evaluated in the active specific immunotherapy of selected cancers. This involves immunization with tumor-associated antigens plus BCG or its methanol-extracted residue. This recent approach is intended to increase host antitumor immunity as a means of preventing tumor recurrence following primary therapy.

Nonspecific immunomodulators of mammalian origin include the thymosins, hormonelike substances that are produced by the thymus gland and that have diverse biologic activities including augmentation of immune responses in both normal and thymecto-

Table 62–5. Nonspecific immunomodulators.

Products of microbial origin
  Bacillus Calmette-Guérin (BCG)
  Bestatin
  parvum
  Endotoxin
  Lentinan
  Nocardia rubra cell wall skeleton
  Picibanil (OK432)
Products of mammalian origin
  Thymosin α_1
  Thymosin fraction 5
  Thymomodulin
  Transfer factor
Synthetic compounds
  Azimexon
  Cimetidine
  Inosine pranobox
  Levamisole

mized animals. Although they are potentially useful in the treatment of selected immunodeficiency states, significant efficacy has not been demonstrated in controlled clinical trials.

Synthetic compounds such as levamisole, an antihelminthic drug capable of inhibiting suppressor T cell activity, constitute the third class of compounds. Levamisole given to patients with cancer has been associated with increases in delayed-type hypersensitivity and in increased in vitro lymphocyte proliferative and mitogenic responses. Preliminary studies of the adjuvant treatment of melanoma and colorectal cancer show promise of clinical efficacy, as measured by disease-free survival. (In this context, ''adjuvant'' refers to a therapy used following optimal local treatment of a tumor, with curative intent). However, confirmatory studies extending these observations and demonstrating an overall survival benefit have yet to be reported.

The current status of all forms of nonspecific immunomodulators for treatment of immunodeficiency diseases and cancer must be considered experimental.

FUTURE DIRECTIONS

Recent advances in molecular biology have provided insight into the complex network of interactions that occur within the immune system. The use of specific immunomodulators to strengthen a deficient immune system or bolster a normal immune system presents a unique strategy for the treatment of various disorders that will clearly affect the practice of clinical medicine for many years to come.

REFERENCES

General

Fauci AS et al: Immunomodulators in clinical medicine. *Ann Intern Med* 1987;**106:**421.

Oldham RK (editor): *Principles of Cancer Biotherapy.* Raven Press, 1987.

Cytokines

Beutler B, Cerami A: Cachectin (tumor necrosis factor): A macrophage hormone governing cellular metabolism and inflammatory response. *Endocr Rev* 1988; **9:**57.

Clark J, Longo D: Interferons in cancer therapy. In: *Cancer: Principles and Practice of Oncology.* De Vita VT, Hellmann S, Rosenberg SA (editors). Lippincott, 1987.

Clark SC, Kamen R: The human hematopoietic colony-stimulating factors. *Science* 1987;**236:**1229.

Murray HW: Interferon-gamma, the activated macrophage and host defense against microbial challenge. *Ann Intern Med* 1988;**108:**595.

Rosenberg SA et al: Use of tumor infiltrating lymphocytes and interleukin-2 in the immunotherapy of patients with metastatic melanoma. *N Engl J Med* 1988;**319:**1676.

Sieff CA: Hematopoietic growth factors. *J Clin Invest* 1987;**79:**1549.

Spiegel RJ: The alpha interferons: Clinical overview. *Semin Oncol* 1987;**14:**1.

Monoclonal Antibodies

Houghton AN, Scheinberg DA: Monoclonal antibodies: Potential applications to the treatment of cancer. *Semin Oncol* 1986;**13:**165.

Schlom J: Basic principles and applications of monoclonal antibodies in the management of carcinomas. *Cancer Res* 1986;**46:**3225.

63

Anti-Inflammatory Drugs

James S. Goodwin, MD

The distinction between immunosuppressive and anti-inflammatory drugs is not always clear, because of the extensive interaction of the biologic mechanisms of these interrelated systems. In this chapter, drugs with anti-inflammatory activity mediated at least in part by suppression of the functions of the nonspecific inflammatory cells, especially monocytes, polymorphonuclear leukocytes, and basophils, will be discussed. They are used to treat acute and chronic inflammatory process and are effective in treating inflammation whether or not the inflammation is initiated immunologically. Drugs that primarily suppress the immune response are discussed in Chapter 61.

CORTICOSTEROIDS

Glucocorticoids are the most powerful drugs currently available for the treatment of inflammatory diseases, but their use is associated with significant toxicity (also see Chapter 61). The discovery of corticosteroids was a major advance in the treatment of inflammatory diseases. Since the first successful use of hydrocortisone (Cortisol), the principal glucocorticoid of the adrenal cortex, for suppression of the clinical manifestations of rheumatoid arthritis in 1948, numerous compounds with glucocorticoid activity have been synthesized and are presently standard therapy for many immunologic and nonimmunologic inflammatory conditions.

Pharmacology & Physiology

Corticosteroids are 21-carbon steroid hormones derived from the metabolism of cholesterol. Fig 63–1 shows the structures of the commonly used synthetic corticosteroids. The activity of corticosteroids depends on the presence of a hydroxyl group on carbon-11. Two of the most commonly used corticosteroids, cortisone and prednisone, are inactive until converted in vivo to the corresponding 11-hydroxyl compounds, cortisol and prednisolone.

The clinical potency of the various synthetic steroids depends upon the rate of absorption, the concentration in target tissues, and the rate of metabolism and subsequent clearance. Table 63–1 shows the half-lives and relative potencies of the commonly used glucocorticoid preparations. Most are well absorbed after oral administration. Corticosteroid uptake is not usually affected by intrinsic intestinal diseases, and food intake does not influence absorption. Approximately 90% of endogenous circulating cortisol is bound with high affinity to the plasma protein corticosteroid-binding globulin. Another 5–8% is bound to albumin, which is a high-capacity, low-affinity reservoir for steroids. Most synthetic steroids, with the exception of prednisolone, have a low affinity for corticosteroid-binding globulin and are bound predominantly to albumin. Only the small fraction of circulating corticosteroids that are not protein-bound are free to exert a biologic action, whereas those associated with proteins are protected from metabolic degradation.

Corticosteroids are metabolized in the liver. Hydroxylation of the 4,5 double bond and ketone groups and subsequent conjugation with glucuronide or sulfate groups render steroids inactive and water soluble. The kidney excretes 95% of the conjugated metabolites, and the remainder are lost in the gut. There are individual differences in the half-lives of synthetic steroids, and patients receiving those with prolonged clearance may be at increased risk for side effects from therapy. Clearance rates of corticosteroids are also affected by other drugs and disease states. Phenytoin, phenobarbital, and rifampin can increase steroid clearance by inducing hepatic-enzyme activity. Estrogen therapy and estrogen-containing oral contraceptives impair the clearance of administered steroids and may decrease the steroid requirement. In patients with liver diseases, the metabolism of corticosteroids is not significantly altered and dose adjustments are not necessary. Dose adjustments are also generally not necessary for patients with kidney disease. Corticosteroids can lower plasma salicylate levels by enhancing their renal clearance. Patients on fixed-dose salicylate therapy may develop rapid increases to toxic levels of serum salicylate when glucocorticoids are withdrawn or tapered.

Anti-Inflammatory Effects

Administration of corticosteroids results in a complex series of changes in the actions of cells involved in inflammatory reactions. After a single dose of steroids, there is a net increase in the number of circulating neutrophils, accompanied by a decrease in the

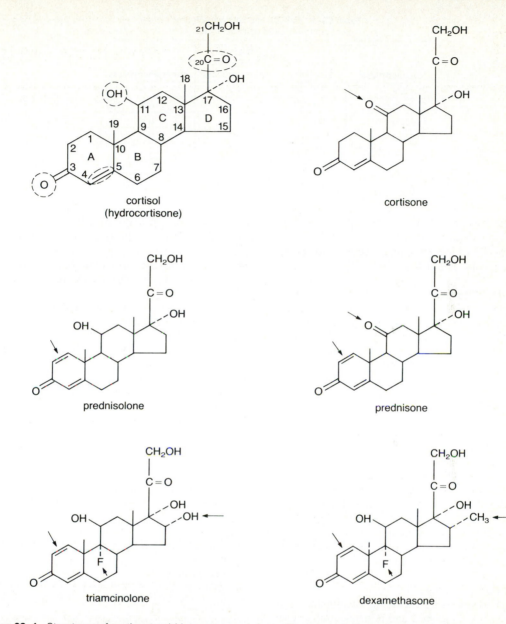

Figure 63–1. Structures of corticosteroid hormones and drugs. The arrows indicate the structural differences between cortisol and each of the other compounds.

margination, migration, and accumulation of neutrophils at sites of inflammation, which further reduces the signs of acute inflammation and also interferes with the expression of delayed-type hypersensitivity skin reactions.

Corticosteroids also directly suppress the action of cells involved in the inflammatory response, inhibiting phagocytosis by neutrophils and monocytes, the release of degradative enzymes such as collagenase and plasminogen activator by neutrophils and synovial lining cells, and the production of inflamma-

tory lymphokines and monokines such as interleukin-1 and tumor necrosis factor. Other than the clear effects found in vivo and in vitro on migration and accumulation of granulocytes and monocytes, it is difficult to know how the many other effects of corticosteroids on inflammatory cell function contribute to the anti-inflammatory effect, since this information is based largely on in vitro studies of isolated cell populations. It is assumed, however, that the so-called "lysosomal stabilizing" effects and the decreased release of inflammatory mediators and

Table 63–1. Half-life and relative potency of commonly used glucocorticoids.

Glucocorticoid	Plasma Half Life (min)	Relative Potency of Glucocorticoid	Mineralocorticoid
Cortisol	80–120	1.0	1.0
Cortisone	80–120	0.8	0.8
Prednisone	200–210	4.0	0.8
Prednisolone	120–300	5.0	0
Triamcinolone	180–240	5.0	0
Dexamethasone	150–270	30–150	0

degradative enzymes contribute to the anti-inflammatory clinical effects.

A discussion of related immunosuppressive effects of corticosteroids is in Chapter 61.

Metabolic Effects

Like other hormones, corticosteroids affect many different tissue and organ systems. At physiologic concentrations, their various metabolic effects presumably maintain normal homeostasis, but at the high concentrations used pharmacologically (or from pathologic overproduction), an accentuation of these same metabolic effects leads to target organ dysfunction.

A summary of the metabolic effects of glucocorticoids is given in Table 63–2. In general, steroids promote catabolism. They block glucose uptake by tissues, enhance protein breakdown, and decrease new protein synthesis in muscle, skin, bone, connective tissue, fat, and lymphoid tissue. DNA synthesis and cell proliferation in fibroblasts, lymphocytes, and adipocytes are inhibited. Chronic exposure to supraphysiologic levels of corticosteroids has a type of wasting effect: ie, loss of bone, connective tissue, and muscle and gain in water and fat.

Mechanism of Action

All steroid hormones including vitamin D, corticosteroids, sex hormones, and mineralocorticoid act by binding to high-affinity receptors in the cytoplasm (Fig 63–2). The steroid-receptor complex, in turn, has a high affinity for nuclear interphase chromosomes and thus binds to chromosomal DNA. This triggers DNA transcription, with the formation of messenger RNA, leading to new protein synthesis. The specific genes transcribed and proteins produced after exposure to steroid hormones vary with the different steroid hormones and also with the target cell. Specificity of cell response is manifested in at least 2 ways. (1) The steroid-receptor complex binds to specific regulatory sequences, which, in turn, leads to transcription of the particular gene containing that sequence. Presumably the steroid-receptor complex binding vitamin D attaches to regulatory sequences on different genes from those used by the complex

binding cortisol. (2) Only a small portion of the genome is capable of induction by steroid hormone because it is contained in an ''unraveled'' portion of chromatin sensitive to digestion with DNase. This unraveled portion will differ depending on the cell type.

All well-defined physiologic and pharmacologic effects of steroid hormones are thought to be mediated by the process outlined above. However, non-receptor-mediated effects of steroids, particularly at high doses, may also play an important role in their effects. One implication of this is the delay in appearance of the pharmacologic or physiologic effects after drug administration. Another implication is that glucocorticoid action is indirect; it acts by promoting the synthesis of other compounds.

Table 63–2. Metabolic effects of glucocorticoids.

Carbohydrate metabolism
  Impairs glucose uptake and utilization by peripheral tissues
  Increases gluconeogenesis and glycogen deposition in liver

Lipid metabolism
  Stimulates lipolysis and increases free fatty acid levels, an effect countered by increased insulin release and gluconeogenesis
  Increases fat deposition in truncal and facial areas

Protein metabolism
  Inhibits synthesis and enhances breakdown of proteins in many tissues, leading to negative nitrogen balance
  Increases plasma free amino acid levels

Nucleic acid metabolism
  Stimulates RNA synthesis in liver, inhibits RNA synthesis in other tissues
  Inhibits DNA synthesis in most tissues

Fluid and electrolyte metabolism
  May enhance sodium retention and potassium loss independent of mineralocorticoid action
  Increases glomerular filtration rate

Bone and calcium-metabolism
  Decreases intestinal calcium absorption
  Decreases renal reabsorption of calcium and phosphate with resulting hypercalciuria
  Inhibits osteoblast function

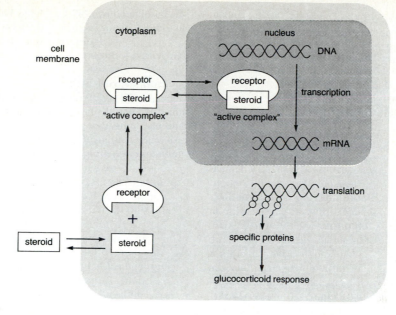

cytoplasm

nucleus

cell membrane

DNA

receptor
steroid
"active complex"

receptor
steroid
"active complex"

transcription

mRNA

receptor
+

translation

steroid — steroid

specific proteins

glucocorticoid response

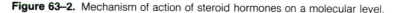

Figure 63–2. Mechanism of action of steroid hormones on a molecular level.

Cells exposed to glucocorticoids synthesize and release a phospholipase A_2-inhibitory glycoprotein, now termed lipomodulin. The inhibition of phospholipase A_2 leads, in turn, to a reduction in the release of arachidonic acid, thereby slowing production of arachidonic acid metabolites. Lipomodulin appears to be a family of molecules, one of which was recently cloned and found to have potent anti-inflammatory actions. Thus, the anti-inflammatory actions of glucocorticoids may be related, at least in part, to lipomodulin-induced reduction of arachidonic acid metabolites, the prostaglandins and leukotrienes that are generated by cyclo-oxygenase and lipoxygenase, respectively. The role of prostaglandins and leukotrienes in mediating various aspects of the inflammatory response is discussed in Chapter 14.

Toxicity

The toxicities of prolonged corticosteroid therapy are numerous and are the major limiting factor in the use of these agents. They are listed in Table 63–3. Susceptibility to side effects varies among patients; the reason for this is unknown. Some patients on prolonged, high-dose therapy appear to tolerate corticosteroids with few adverse effects, whereas others treated with small doses for brief intervals develop devastating side effects such as aseptic necrosis, osteoporosis, and vertebral collapse. In part, this differential sensitivity may be related to individual differences in plasma protein binding (with hypoalbuminemic patients at risk) and to variations in metabolism and clearance of synthetic steroids. Sensi-

Table 63–3. Side effects of glucocorticoid therapy.

Very common and should be anticipated in all patients
Negative calcium balance leading to osteoporosis
Increased appetite
Centripetal obesity
Impaired wound healing
Increased risk of infection
Suppression of hypothalamic-pituitary-adrenal axis
Growth arrest in children

Frequently seen
Myopathy
Avascular necrosis
Hypertension
Plethora
Thin, fragile skin/striae/purpura
Edema secondary to sodium and water retention
Hyperlipidemia
Psychiatric symptoms, particularly euphoria or depression
Diabetes mellitus
Posterior subcapsular cataracts

Not very common, but important to recognize early
Glaucoma
Benign intracranial hypertension
"Silent" intestinal perforation
Peptic ulcer disease (often gastric)
Hypokalemic alkalosis
Hyperosmolar nonketotic coma
Gastric hemorrhage

Rare
Pancreatitis
Hirsutism
Panniculitis
Secondary amenorrhea
Impotence
Epidural lipomatosis
Allergy to synthetic steroids

tivity to glucocorticoids in mice is closely linked to the H-2 histocompatibility region, and there is some evidence of analogous human leukocyte antigen (HLA) linkages in humans.

ASPIRIN & OTHER NONSTEROIDAL ANTI-INFLAMMATORY DRUGS (NSAID)

Each year 30 million lb of aspirin are consumed in the USA alone. Salicylates can be found in most households. Aspirin (acetylsalicylic acid) and other salicylates have been available without a physician's prescription since their introduction in the late nineteenth century. In addition to the many oral formulations, salicylates are present in most skin liniments, plasters, and ointments. The newer nonsteroidal anti-inflammatory drugs (NSAID) are also in widespread use. Hundreds have been synthesized and dozens introduced for clinical use worldwide. As a class, NSAID are the most frequently prescribed medications for patients older than 65 years. Within the last several years, ibuprofen has become available without a prescription, further contributing to the widespread consumption of NSAID.

History of NSAID

Extracts of the willow tree (Latin, salix) had been used and endorsed by Hippocrates, Pliny, Galen, and other ancient practitioners for the relief of pain and fever. Later, willow bark extract (salicylate) was substituted for the more expensive and frequently unobtainable cinchona bark extract (quinine) in the treatment of pain and fever. Salicylates achieved widespread use by the end of the nineteenth century, when simple and inexpensive ways of synthesizing the drugs were discovered. Although these drugs have been used as antipyretics and analgesics for the past century, their anti-inflammatory properties have been recognized clinically and experimentally only within the past 30 years. High-dose salicylate therapy for rheumatoid arthritis was first recommended generally in the 1950s. Since then, nonsalicylate NSAID equipotent to high-dose salicylates have steadily increased in use, being more convenient and in most cases less toxic.

Anti-Inflammatory Effects

The anti-inflammatory effects of the different NSAID are very similar in many experimental models, providing indirect support for the concept that they all share a single mechanism of action (discussed below). NSAID prevent the pain, swelling, redness, and loss of function in experimental models of inflammation as diverse as sunburn and carrageenan-induced paw edema in rats. NSAID administration decreases the rate of progressive joint destruction associated with adjuvant-induced arthritis

in rats. Clinically, NSAID have been shown to be effective in many acute and chronic inflammatory diseases, such as arthritis, tendonitis, and pericarditis.

Mechanism of Action

Since 1971 aspirin and other NSAID at therapeutic levels have been shown to inhibit the production of prostaglandins by inhibiting cyclo-oxygenase. The relative inhibiting potency in vitro of different NSAID generally parallels their anti-inflammatory potency in vivo. Cyclo-oxygenase inhibition became the in vitro screening test for new NSAID. However, the simple concept that NSAID are anti-inflammatory because they inhibit cyclo-oxygenase production of proinflammatory metabolites of arachidonic acid is not adequate to explain all their clinical effects.

Although prostaglandin E_2 causes vasodilatation and sensitizes pain receptors to agonists such as histamine, other arachidonic acid metabolites have anti-inflammatory or neutral effects. Sodium salicylate, a nonacetylated salicylate, is equally anti-inflammatory as aspirin in vivo, but has no demonstrable inhibition of cyclo-oxygenase activity in vivo or in vitro. Furthermore, aspirin ingested in low doses profoundly inhibits prostaglandin production in blood, kidneys, and vascular endothelium but has no anti-inflammatory effect, and analgesia from aspirin or other NSAID is achieved with considerably lower doses and serum concentrations than is anti-inflammatory activity. There is a dose-response relationship of analgesia and prostaglandin inhibition with all NSAID, but anti-inflammatory effects are seen only at higher doses. Analgesic-antipyretic drugs such as acetaminophen do not inhibit cyclo-oxygenase and are not anti-inflammatory. Thus, pharmacologic evidence to date links pain and fever, but not inflammation, to in vivo prostaglandin production. The effect of aspirin on prolonging the bleeding time in vivo can be prevented by prior treatment with sodium salicylate or other NSAID.

Other properties of NSAID may better explain their therapeutic anti-inflammatory effects. Inhibition of one or more lipoxygenase enzymes has been described for some NSAID in some in vitro systems. NSAID inhibit cyclic AMP-dependent protein kinase, phospholipase C, amino acid transport across cell membranes, and a variety of other membrane-associated events. The relative potency of various NSAID in inhibiting amino acid transport parallels their anti-inflammatory potency. All NSAID inhibit a variety of neutrophil and monocyte functions, such as aggregation, degranulation, and superoxide anion production.

Some other clinical effects of NSAID could be mediated by prostaglandin E inhibition. NSAID stimulates suppressor T cell activity, possibly explaining the fact that they lower rheumatoid factor levels in patients with rheumatoid arthritis. There may be a therapeutic effect attributable to the inhibition of prostaglandin E stimulation of osteoclast-activating factor production and the excretion of collagenase by monocytes.

Toxicity

Although there is still considerable question about how inhibition of cyclo-oxygenase is related to the efficacy of NSAID, there is little doubt that reduction of prostaglandin production is directly related to the important toxicities of these drugs. The major side effects are listed in Table 63–4. Between 10% and 40% of patients in controlled trials of NSAID will stop using the drug because of upper gastrointestinal symptoms such as pain, nausea, and vomiting. The newer NSAID produce fewer of these complaints than do aspirin, phenylbutazone, and indomethacin. However, in blinded, prospective, controlled clinical trials, approximately 1% of patients ingesting any of the newer NSAID develop upper gastrointestinal bleeding. The mechanism of gastrointestinal toxicity is thought to involve 3 processes, 2 of which are secondary to cyclooxygenase inhibition: (1) Prostaglandin E is a local feedback inhibitor of hydrochloric acid secretion; (2) prostaglandin E has a cytoprotective effect on gastric mucosa independent of HCl secretion; and (3) all NSAID are organic acids that can directly irritate gastric mucosa.

The major renal complication of NSAID is also related to cyclo-oxygenase inhibition. In patients with preexisting renal disease or circulatory disease resulting in decreased renal blood flow, NSAID tend to further reduce renal blood flow and glomerular filtration by eliminating prostaglandin-mediated compensatory mechanisms within the kidney. This becomes clinically important in some patients and can lead to total kidney failure, but it is almost always reversible upon cessation of the drug. The prevalence of renal complications from NSAID is difficult to estimate, because it is too rare to be detected in most prospective, controlled clinical trials. In addition, patients most likely to experience renal toxicity because of preexisting renal or heart disease are likely to be excluded from those drug trials. Renal toxicity is very rare in patients whose renal function is normal prior to the start of therapy with NSAID.

COLCHICINE

The use of colchicine for acute gouty attacks dates back to the fifth century. It is highly specific and efficacious in the treatment of acute gouty arthritis and, to a lesser extent, in the treatment of pseudogout, but it has almost no effect on other forms of arthritis or other acute inflammatory conditions. Nevertheless, colchicine has largely been replaced in the treatment of acute gouty attacks by NSAID, which work quicker, are at least as efficacious, and are less toxic. It is sometimes used as an adjunctive therapy with NSAID in chronic or polyarticular gout, and also as a prophylactic agent used in low doses (0.6 mg once or twice daily) to prevent attacks.

Recently, prophylactic chronic colchicine ingestion has been found to reduce attacks of familial Mediterranean fever and to prevent the development of amyloidosis in patients with that disease. Colchicine has been reported to slow the progression of cirrhosis in patients with alcoholic liver disease.

The mechanism of action of colchicine is not completely understood. It arrests mitosis in metaphase by inhibiting spindle formation. It binds to labile microtubules, so that disruption of neutrophil microtubules leads to decreased chemotaxis, adhesiveness, phagocytosis, and degranulation.

GOLD SALTS

Gold was introduced in 1928 as a treatment for rheumatoid arthritis because of the prevailing theory that the disease was caused by local or systemic infection. Koch and Ehrlich had shown antibacterial activity of a variety of heavy-metal salts, including gold. When the theory of the infectious origin of rheumatoid arthritis fell into disrepute in the 1950s, gold use declined, even though controlled studies demonstrated its efficacy. It was reintroduced in the 1970s and now is the leading second-line therapy for rheumatoid arthritis. Gold, penicillamine, the antimalarial hydroxychloroquine, and perhaps also the various immunosuppressive drugs (see Chapter 61) share a number of properties when used in rheumatoid arthritis and other diseases. (1) They require one to several months before any benefit is noted. (2) They can include a clinical remission wherein no

---

Table 63–4. Side effects of NSAID therapy.

Gastrointestinal
  Gastritis
  Duodenal ulcer
  Gastric ulcer

Renal
  Decreased creatinine clearance
  Acute renal failure
  Interstitial nephritis

Central nervous system
  Headache
  Confusion, memory loss, personality change, especially in the elderly

Toxicities not shared by all NSAID
  Bone marrow failure with phenylbutazone
  Rash with meclofenamate

subjective or objective evidence of continued disease activity remains. (3) They possess a narrow therapeutic spectrum. For example, gold has efficacy in rheumatoid arthritis and psoriatic arthritis but not significantly in other chronic inflammatory arthritides such as ankylosing spondylitis or systemic lupus erythematosus. (4) Many of the toxicities of the individual drugs in this class are similar. For example, gold and penicillamine can both cause rash, mouth ulcers, neutropenia, and nephritis. (5) These drugs have little or no activity in experimental animal models of arthritis. (It is ironic that the animal models now used to screen for new treatments for arthritis would not have allowed for the discovery of the most efficacious drugs!) (6) Their mechanism of action is unknown.

DRUGS THAT SUPPRESS IMMEDIATE HYPERSENSITIVITY REACTIONS

Cromolyn Sodium

Cromolyn sodium inhibits the release of mediators from mast cells, thereby blocking the tissue response and symptoms of IgE-mediated allergy. The precise mechanism of action of cromolyn sodium is unknown, but there is evidence that it interferes with calcium influx through the cell membrane. It does not interfere with the binding of IgE to mast cells, nor to the interaction of antigen with the IgE bound to mast cells. Rather, it suppresses the degranulation reaction normally triggered by the cross-linking of cell surface IgE by antigen.

Cromolyn sodium is effective only prophylactically. It is poorly absorbed after oral administration and is therefore administered by inhaler as a powder, which is effective only when administered topically to mucous membranes. It is available as a micronized powder in a metered-dose inhaler or as a powder for inhalation in a special dispenser for asthma, as a nasal aerosolized solution for allergic rhinitis, and as eye drops for allergic conjunctivitis.

The toxicity of cromolyn sodium is low and relates mostly to irritation by the inhaled powdered drug. It has no known utility in other inflammatory diseases.

Antihistamines

There are 2 classes of antihistamines, called H_1 and H_2 blockers, corresponding to the 2 types of histamine receptors found in mammalian tissues. Only H_1 blockers will be considered here because H_2 blockers do not possess noticeable anti-inflammatory activity, although they are sometimes used in allergic diseases. The pharmacologic properties of H_1-blocking antihistamines are listed in Table 63–5.

The major therapeutic role for antihistamines is in the treatment of allergic diseases involving IgE-mediated hypersensitivity reactions. They are effec-

Table 63–5. Actions of histamine at H_1 receptor sites inhibited by antihistamine.

Increased capillary permeability following histamine or antigen challenge
Smooth muscle constriction, particularly bronchial and gastrointestinal tract
Stimulation of autonomic ganglia
Secretion of exocrine glands

tive in reducing nasal and lacrimal secretions in seasonal rhinitis and conjunctivitis (hay fever). They are also effective in treating urticaria and angioedema, and they reduce pruritus associated with other dermatoses. Another major therapeutic role for antihistamines in the treatment of motion sickness and Meniere's disease.

The principal side effects of antihistamines are sedation, dryness of mucous membranes, and constipation. Recently several antihistamines have been developed that lack the sedative effect, probably because of their failure to penetrate the blood-brain barrier.

There are a large number of drugs with antihistaminic effects. The chemical classification of these drugs and representative examples are listed in Table 63–6.

Table 63–6. Commonly used antihistamines (H_1 blockers).

Classic	New Generation
Alkylamines Chlorpheniramine Dexchlorpheniramine Brompheniramine Triprolidine	Acrivastine[1,2]
Ethanolamines Diphenhydramine Dimenhydrate Clemastine Cinarrizine[2]	Ketotifen[2] Oxatomide[2]
Ethylenediamines Tripelennamine	
Piperazines Hydroxyzine Meclizine	Cetirizine[1,2,3]
Phenothiazines Promethazine	Mequitazine[1,2,3]
Piperidines Cyproheptadine Azatidine	Loratidine[1,3] Astemizole[1,3] Terfenadine[1] Azelastine[2]
Tricyclics Doxepin Amitriptyline Imipramine Desipramine	

[1]Nonsedative.
[2]Not available in the USA (as of Nov.1989).
[3]Once-a-day dosage.

Sympathomimetic (Adrenergic) Drugs

These drugs mimic the effects of sympathetic nerve stimulation. They have 2 general mechanisms of action: (1) stimulation of adrenergic receptors and (2) increase in the release of catecholamines from sympathetic nerve endings. Some drugs have both properties.

The sympathetic nervous system is not primarily involved in the pathogenesis of allergic disease, but in certain allergic reactions—particularly anaphylactic shock and acute asthma—the vascular and visceral effects will evoke a secondary sympathomimetic response to maintain homeostasis of function in the affected organs. Sympathomimetic drugs are therefore highly effective treatment in many manifestations of IgE-mediated allergy.

The diverse actions of sympathomimetic amines are explained by 2 classes of receptors, α and β, and their subclasses, α_1, α_2, β_1, and β_2 (Table 63–7).

α_1-Adrenergic agonists cause mucosal vasoconstriction and are widely used as nasal decongestants. Examples of such drugs are phenylephrine and phenylpropanolamine. For many years, epinephrine and isoproterenol were the principal sympathomimetic bronchodilators available for treatment of asthma, but their use was limited by the cardiac-stimulating properties of their α and β_1 agonist effects, respec-tively. A variety of β_2-selective bronchodilators are now available for treatment of asthma. These include metaproterenol, terbutaline, albuterol, pirbuterol, isoetharine, and procaterol. Epinephrine is the drug of choice for anaphylaxis because it has powerful α- and β-stimulating effects necessary to counteract the systemic effects of anaphylaxis.

Methylxanthines

The methylxanthines include caffeine and theophylline. Their principal use is as central nervous system stimulants and as bronchodilators. Theophylline is poorly soluble in water and may be administered as a salt, such as aminophylline or oxytriphylline. Theophylline and its salts are frequently used in treatment of chronic asthma. Side effects include nervousness, insomnia, tachycardia, ventricular arrhythmias, diuresis, anorexia, nausea, vomiting, and abdominal pain. The toxicity of theophylline is related to blood levels, which are easily obtainable in most clinical laboratories.

The mechanism of action is unknown. Methylxanthines inhibit phosphodiesterase, thereby slowing the metabolism of cyclic AMP and increasing cyclic AMP levels. However, phosphodiesterase inhibition requires a much higher theophylline concentration than is clinically effective for bronchodilatation.

Table 63–7. Tissue distribution and effects of different adrenergic receptors.

Receptor	Tissue Distribution	Action	Physiologic Effect
α_1	Vascular smooth muscle	Contraction	Vasoconstriction
	Radial muscle of pupil	Contraction	Dilates pupil
	Trigone sphincter muscle	Contraction	Inhibition of urination
	Pilomotor smooth muscle	Contraction	Erect hair
	Liver	Increase gluconeogenesis	Increase blood sugar
α_2	Central nervous system adrenergic receptors	Activation	Diverse
	Platelets	Aggregation	Aggregation
	Presynaptic peripheral adrenergic and cholinergic nerves	Inhibition of transmitter release	Diverse
	Some vascular smooth muscle	Contraction	Vasoconstriction
	Gastrointestinal smooth muscle	Relaxation	Decreased motility
β_1	Heart muscle	Increase cyclic AMP[1]	Increase heart rate, force of contraction, conduction velocity
	Coronary vessel smooth muscle	Contraction	Vasoconstriction
	Fat cells	Increase cyclic AMP	Lipolysis
β_2	Bronchial smooth muscle	Relaxation	Bronchodilation
	Liver	Increase Gluconeogenesis	Increased blood sugar
	Kidney	Increase cyclic AMP	Increased renin secretion
	Gastrointestinal smooth muscle	Relaxation	Decreased motility

[1]Activation of all β_1 or β_2 receptors results in increased cyclic AMP. A more distal action is listed, if known.

REFERENCES

General

Bray MA, Morley J: *The Pharmacology of Lymphocytes.* Springer-Verlag, 1988.

Gilman AG, Goodman LS, Gilman A: *The Pharmacologic Basis of Therapeutics.* Macmillan, 1985.

McCarty DJ (editor): *Arthritis and Allied Conditions.* Lea & Febiger, 1989.

Corticosteroids

Behrens TW, Goodwind JS: Glucocorticoids. Pages 604–621 in: *Arthritis and Allied Conditions.* McCarty DJ (editor). Lea & Febiger, 1989.

Davidson F et al: Inhibition of phospholipase A2 by "lipocortins" and calpactins. *J Biol Chem* 1987; **262:**1698.

Flower RJ, Blackwell GJ: Anti-inflammatory steroids induce biosynthesis of a phospholipase A2 inhibitor which prevents prostaglandin generation. *Nature* 1978;**278:**456.

Gustavson LE, Benet LZ: Pharmacokinetics of natural and synthetic glucocorticoids. In: *The Adrenal Cortex.* Anderson DC, Winder JSD (editors). Butterworth, 1985.

Hench PS: The reversibility of certain rheumatic and nonrheumatic conditions by the use of cortisone or of the pituitary adrenocorticotropic hormones. Le Prix Nobel en 1950. P A Norstedt Soner, 1951.

Hirata F et al: A phospholipase A2 inhibitory protein in rabbit neutrophils induced by glucocorticoids. *Proc Natl Acad Sci USA* 1980;**77:**2533.

Samulesson B: Mediators of immediate hypersensitivity reactions and inflammation. *Science* 1983;**220:**568.

NSAID

Abramson SB, Weissmann G: The mechanism of action of nonsteroidal anti-inflammatory drugs. *Arthritis Rheum* 1989;**32:**1.

Goodwin JS: Immunologic effects of nonsteroidal anti-inflammatory agents. *Med Clin North Am* 1985; **69:**793.

Goodwin JS: Toxicity of nonsteroidal anti-inflammatory drugs. *Arch Intern Med* 1987;**147:**34.

Goodwin JS, Goodwin JM: Failure to recognize efficacious treatments: A history of salicylate therapy in rheumatoid arthritis. *Perspect Biol Med* 1981;**25:**78.

Vane JR: Inhibition of prostaglandin synthesis as a mechanism of action for aspirin-like drugs. *Nature New Biol* 1971;**231:**232.

Colchicine

Goodwin JS, Goodwin JM: The tomato effect: Rejection of highly efficacious therapies. *JAMA* 1984; **251:**2387.

Reibman J et al: Colchicine inhibits inophore-induced formation of leukotriene B4 by human neutrophils: The role of microtubules. *J Immunol* 1986;**136:**1027.

Gold & Other Second-Line Agents for Rheumatoid Arthritis

Bunch TW et al: Controlled trial of hydroxychloroquine and D-penicillamine in the treatment of rheumatoid arthritis. *Arthritis Rheum* 1984;**27:**267.

Fowler PD et al: Report on chloroquine and dapsone in the treatment of rheumatoid arthritis: A 6-month comparative study. *Ann Rheum Dis* 1984;**43:**200.

Iannuzzi L et al: Does drug therapy slow radiographic deterioration in rheumatoid arthritis? *N Engl J Med* 1983;**309:**1023.

Kean WF et al: The history of gold therapy in rheumatoid arthritis. *Semin Arthritis Rheum* 1985;**14:**180.

Leibfarth JH, Persellin RH: Mechanisms of action of gold. *Agents Actions* 1981;**11:**458.

Lipsky PE, Ziff M: The mechanisms of action of gold and D-penicillamine in rheumatoid arthritis. Pages 219–235 in: *Advances in Inflammation Research.* Vol III. *Rheumatoid Arthritis.* Ziff M, Velo GP, Gorini S (editors). Raven Press, 1982.

Miller B et al: Double-blind placebo controlled crossover evaluation of levamisole in rheumatoid arthritis. *Arthritis Rheum* 1980;**23:**172.

Munthe E, Kass E, Jellum E: Evidence for enhanced radical scavenging prior to drug response in rheumatoid arthritis. Pages 211–218 in: *Advances in Inflammation Research.* Vol III. *Rheumatoid Arthritis.* Ziff M, Velo GP, Gorini S (editors). Raven Press, 1982.

Perett D: The metabolism and pharmacology of D-penicillamine in man. *J Rheumatol* 1981;**8(Suppl 7):**41.

Thompson PW, Kirwan JR, Barnes CG: Practical results of treatment with disease-modifying drugs. *Br J Rheumatol* 1985;**24:**167.

Cromolyn Sodium

Bernstein IL: Cromolyn sodium in the treatment of asthma: Coming of age in the United States. *J Allergy Clin Immunol* 1985;**76:**381.

Cockcroft DW: The bronchial late response in the pathogenesis of asthma and its modulation by therapy. *Ann Allergy* 1985;**55:**85.

Kay AB et al: Disodium cromoglycate inhibits activation of human inflammatory cells in vitro. *J Allergy Clin Immunol* 1987;**80:**1.

Antihistamines

Norman PS: Newer antihistaminic agents. *J Allergy Clin Immunol* 1985;**76:**366.

Simons FE, Simons KJ: H$_1$-receptor antagonists: Clinical pharmacology and use in allergic disease. *Pediatr Clin North Am* 1983;**30:**899.

Sympathomimetics

Fanta CH, Rossing TH, McFadden ER Jr: Treatment of acute asthma: Is combination therapy with sympathomimetics and methylxanthines indicated? *Am J Med* 1986;**80:**5.

Nelson HS: Adrenergic therapy of bronchial asthma. *J Allergy Clin Immunol* 1986;**77:**771.

Newhouse MT, Dolovich MB: Control of asthma by aerosols. *N Engl J Med* 1986;**315:**870.

Theophylline

Grant JA, Ellis EF: Update on theophylline. (Symposium.) *J Allergy Clin Immunol* 1986;**76:**669.

Weinberger M: The pharmacology and therapeutic use of theophylline. *J Allergy Clin Immunol* 1984; **73:**525.

Appendix

Glossary of Terms Commonly Used in Immunology

ABO system: A term used to designate the erythrocyte antigens used for blood typing.

Abrin: A potent toxin which is derived from the seeds of the jequirity plant and which agglutinates erythrocytes (a lectin).

Absolute catabolic rate: The mass of protein catabolized per day, which is determined by multiplying the fractional turnover rate by the volume of the plasma pool.

Accessory cells: Lymphoid cells predominantly of the monocyte and macrophage lineage that cooperate with T and B lymphocytes in the formation of antibody and in other immune reactions.

Active immunity: Protection acquired by deliberate introduction of an antigen into a responsive host.

Activated lymphocytes: Lymphocytes that have been stimulated by specific antigen or nonspecific mitogen.

Activated macrophages: Mature macrophages in a metabolic state caused by various stimuli, especially phagocytosis or lymphokine activity.

Activation: A process in which the members of the complement sequence are altered enzymatically to become functionally active.

Adaptive immunity: A series of host defenses characterized by extreme specificity and memory mediated by antibody or T cells.

Addressins: Ligands on mucosal endothelial cells for specific homing receptors on lymphocytes derived from Peyer's patches.

Adenosine deaminase: An enzyme that catalyzes the conversion of adenosine to inosine and is deficient in some patients with combined immunodeficiency syndrome.

Adjuvant: A compound capable of potentiating an immune response.

Adoptive transfer: The transfer of immunity by immunocompetent cells from one animal to another.

Adrenergic receptors: Receptors for various adrenergic agents of either the α or the β class that are present on a variety of cells and from which the action of various adrenergic drugs can be predicted.

Affinity chromatography: A technique in which a substance with a selective binding affinity is coupled to an insoluble matrix such as dextran and binds its complementary substances from a mixture in solution or suspension.

Agammaglobulinemia: See **Hypogammaglobulinemia.**

Agglutination: An antigen-antibody reaction in which a solid or particulate antigen forms a lattice with a soluble antibody. In reverse agglutination, the antibody is attached to a solid particle and is agglutinated by insoluble antigen.

Alexin (also **alexine**): A term coined by Pfeiffer to denote a thermolabile and nonspecific factor that, in concert with sensitizer, causes bacteriolysis.

Allele: One of 2 genes controlling a particular characteristic present at a locus.

Allelic exclusion: The phenotypic expression of a single allele in cells containing 2 different alleles for that genetic locus.

Allergens: Antigens that give rise to allergy.

Allergoids: Chemically modified allergens that give rise to antibody of the IgG but not IgE class, thereby reducing allergic symptoms.

Allergy (hypersensitivity): A disease or reaction caused by an immune response to one or more environmental antigens, resulting in tissue inflammation and organ dysfunction.

Allogeneic: Denotes the relationship that exists between genetically dissimilar members of the same species.

Allogeneic effect: A form of general immunopotentiation in which specific stimulation of T cells results in the release of factors active in the immune response.

Allograft (also **homograft**): A tissue or organ graft between 2 genetically dissimilar members of the same species.

Allotype: The genetically determined antigenic difference in serum proteins, varying in different members of the same species.

α/β T cells: T cells in which α and β chains of the T cell receptor are rearranged and expressed on the surface. Most T cells are of this type.

Alpha-fetoprotein (AFP): An embryonic α-globulin with immunosuppressive properties that is structurally similar to albumin.

Alternative complement pathway (also **properdin pathway**): The system of activation of the complement pathway through involvement of properdin factor D, properdin factor B, and C3b, finally activating C3 and then progressing as in the classic pathway.

Am marker: The allotypic determinant on the heavy chain of human IgA.

Amboceptor: A term coined by Ehrlich to denote a bacteriolytic substance in serum that acts together with complement or alexin, ie, antibody.

Anamnesis (also **immunologic memory**): A heightened responsiveness to the second or subsequent administration of antigen to an immune animal.

Anaphylactoid reaction: Clinical response similar to anaphylaxis but not caused by an IgE mediated allergic reaction.

Anaphylatoxin: A substance produced by complement activation that results in increased vascular permeability through the release of pharmacologically active mediators from mast cells.

Anaphylatoxin inactivator: An α-globulin with a molecular weight of 300,000 that destroys the biologic activity of C3a and C5a.

Anaphylaxis: A reaction of immediate hypersensitivity present in nearly all vertebrates that results from sensitization of tissue-fixed mast cells by cytotropic antibodies following exposure to antigen.

Anergy: A state of diminished or absent cell-mediated immunity as shown by the inability to react to a battery of common skin test antigens.

Angiogenesis factor: Released by macrophages and causes neovascularization of surrounding tissues.

Antibody: A protein which is produced as a result of the introduction of an antigen and which has the ability to combine with the antigen that stimulated its production.

Antibody-combining site: The configuration present on an antibody molecule that links with a corresponding antigenic determinant.

Antibody-dependent cell-mediated cytotoxicity (ADCC): A form of lymphocyte-mediated cytotoxicity in which an effector cell kills an antibody-coated target cell, presumably by recognition of the Fc region of the cell-bound antibody through an Fc receptor present on the effector lymphocyte.

Antigen: A substance that reacts with antibodies or T cell receptors evoked by immunogens.

Antigen-presenting cell (APC): A cell that processes a protein antigen by fragmenting it into peptides that are presented on the cell surface in concert with class II major histocompatibility molecules for interaction with the appropriate T cell receptor. B cells, T cells, dendritic cells, and macrophages can perform this function.

Antigen processing: The series of events that occurs following antigen administration and antibody production.

Antigen-binding site: The part of an immunoglobulin that binds antigen.

Antigenic competition: The suppression of the immune response to 2 closely related antigens when they are injected simultaneously.

Antigenic determinant (see **Epitope**).

Antigenic modulation: The spatial alteration of the arrangement of antigenic sites present on a cell surface brought about by the presence of bound antibody.

Antigenic shift: Periodic changes over time in the surface antigens of certain viruses. These are caused by genetic mutations.

Antiglobulin test (Coombs test): A technique for detecting cell-bound immunoglobulin. In the direct Coombs test, erythrocytes taken directly from a sensitized individual are agglutinated by antigammaglobulin antibodies. In the indirect Coombs test, a patient's serum is incubated with test erythro-

cytes and the sensitized cells are then agglutinated with an anti-immunoglobulin or with Coombs reagent.

Antilymphocyte serum: Antibodies that are directed against lymphocytes and that usually cause immunosuppression.

Antinuclear antibodies (ANA): Antibodies that are directed against nuclear constituents usually in nucleoprotein, and are present in various rheumatoid diseases, particularly systemic lupus erythematosus.

Antitoxins: Protective antibodies that inactivate soluble toxic protein products of bacteria.

Apheresis: Process of removing blood or a blood element from the body.

Armed macrophages: Macrophages capable of antigen-specific cytotoxicity as a result of cytophilic antibodies or arming factors from T cells.

Arthus phenomenon: A local necrotic lesion resulting from a local antigen-antibody reaction and produced by injecting antigen into a previously immunized animal.

Association constant (K value): The mathematical representation of the affinity of binding between antigen and antibody.

Atopy: A genetically determined state of hypersensitivity to common environmental allergens, mediated by IgE antibodies.

Attenuated: Rendered less virulent.

Autoantibody: Antibody to self antigens.

Autoantigens: Self antigens.

Autocrine: Effects of hormones on the cell that actually produces them.

Autograft: A tissue graft between genetically identical members of the same species.

Autoimmunity: Immunity to self antigens (autoantigens).

Autoradiography: A technique for detecting radioactive isotopes in which a tissue section containing radioactivity is overlaid with x-ray or photographic film on which the emissions are recorded.

B cell (also **B lymphocyte**): Strictly, a bursa-derived cell in avian species and, by analogy, a bursa-equivalent derived cell in nonavian species. B cells are the precursors of plasma cells that produce antibody.

Bacteriolysin: An antibody or other substance capable of lysing bacteria.

Bacteriolysis: The disintegration of bacteria induced by antibody and complement in the absence of cells.

Baseline cellular phagocytosis: Digestion by phagocytic cells and effector mechanisms that have developed for dealing with potential invading pathogens.

BCG (bacillus Calmette-Guérin): A viable attenuated strain of *Mycobacterium bovis* that has been obtained by progressive reduction of virulence and that confers immunity to mycobacterial infection and possibly possesses anti-cancer activity in selected diseases.

Bence Jones proteins: Monoclonal light chains present in the urine of patients with paraproteinemic disorders.

Beta lysin: A highly reactive heat-stable cationic protein that is bactericidal for gram-positive organisms.

Biosynthesis: The production of molecules by viable cells in culture.

Blast cell: A large lymphocyte or other immature cell containing a nucleus with loosely packed chromatin, a large nucleolus, and a large amount of cytoplasm with numerous polyribosomes.

Blast transformation: See **Lymphocyte activation.**

Blocking antibody: See **Blocking factors.**

Blocking factors: Substances that are present in the serum of tumor-bearing animals and are capable of blocking the ability of immune lymphocytes to kill tumor cells.

Bradykinin: A 9-amino-acid peptide that is split by the enzyme kallikrein from serum α_2-globulin precursor and that causes a slow, sustained contraction of the smooth muscles.

Bursa of Fabricius: The hindgut organ located in the cloaca of birds that controls the ontogeny of B lymphocytes.

Bursal equivalent: The hypothetical organ or organs analogous to the bursa of Fabricius in nonavian species.

C region (constant region): The carboxy-terminal portion of the H or L chain that is identical in immunoglobulin molecules of a given class and subclass apart from genetic polymorphisms.

C terminus: The carboxy-terminal end of a protein molecule.

Cachectin: A factor present in serum, which causes wasting and is identical to tumor necrosis factor alpha.

Capping: The movement of cell surface antigens toward one pole of a cell after the antigens are cross-linked by specific antibody.

Carcinoembryonic antigen (CEA): An antigen that is present on fetal endodermal tissue and is reexpressed on the surface of neoplastic cells, particularly in carcinoma of the colon.

Cardiolipin: A substance derived from beef heart, probably a component of mitochondrial membranes, that serves as an antigenic substrate for reagin or antitreponemal antibody.

Carrier: An immunogenic substance that, when coupled to a hapten, renders the hapten immunogenic.

Cationic proteins: Antimicrobial substances present within granules of phagocytic cells.

Cell-mediated immunity: Immunity in which the participation of lymphocytes and macrophages is predominant.

Cell-mediated lymphocytolysis: An in vitro assay for cellular immunity in which a standard mixed-lymphocyte reaction is followed by destruction of target cells that are used to sensitize allogeneic cells during the mixed lymphocyte reaction.

Centimorgan: A unit of physical distance on a chromosome, equivalent to a 1% frequency of recombination between closely linked genes. Also called a map unit.

Central lymphoid organs: Lymphoid organs that are essential to the development of the immune response, ie, the thymus and the bursa of Fabricius.

CH_{50} unit: The quantity or dilution of serum required to lyse 50% of the erythrocytes in a standard hemolytic complement assay.

Charcot-Leyden crystals: Hexagonal dipyramidal crystals with lysophospholipase activity derived from the eosinophil cell surface membrane.

Chase-Sulzberger phenomenon: See **Sulzberger-Chase phenomenon.**

Chemiluminescence: Release of light energy by a chemical reaction usually involving reduction of an unstable intermediate to a stable one. Used as a means of measuring respiratory burst in phagocytic cells.

Chemokinesis: Reaction by which chemical substances determine rate of cellular movement.

Chemotaxis: A process whereby phagocytic cells are attracted to the vicinity of invading pathogens.

Chromatography: A variety of techniques useful for the separation of proteins.

***cis*-pairing:** Association of two genes on the same chromosome encoding a protein.

Class I antigen: Histocompatibility antigen encoded in humans by A, B, and C loci and in mice by D and K loci.

Class II antigen: Histocompatibility antigen encoded in humans by DR, DP, and DQ loci.

Class III antigens: C4 and factor B are complement components encoded within the MHC.

Classic complement pathway: A series of enzyme-substrate and protein-protein interactions that ultimately leads to biologically active complement enzymes. It proceeds sequentially C1, 4,2,3,5,6,7,8,9.

Clonal anergy: Theory that B cell tolerance is induced by antigen-B cell contact during obligatory paralyzable phase or tolerance-sensitive phase of B cell differentiation.

Clonal deletion: A concept related to Burnet's clonal selection theory, which suggests that tolerance to self antigens results from deletion of autoreactive lymphocyte clones in embryonic life.

Clonal selection theory: The theory of antibody synthesis proposed by Burnet that predicts that the individual carries a complement of clones of lymphoid cells which are capable of reacting with all possible antigenic determinants. During fetal life, clones reacted against self antigens are eliminated on contact with antigen.

Clone: A group of cells all of which are the progeny of a single cell.

Cluster of differentiation: One or more cell surface molecules, detectable by monoclonal antibodies, that define a particular cell line or state of cellular differentiation.

***c-myc* gene:** Member of a candidate set of cancer-related genes or cellular oncogenes.

Coelomocyte: A wandering ameboid phagocyte found in all animal invertebrates containing a coelom.

Cohn fraction II: Primarily gamma globulin that is produced as the result of ethanol fractionation of serum according to the Cohn method.

Cold agglutinins: Antibodies that agglutinate bacteria or erythrocytes more efficiently at temperatures below 37 °C than at 37 °C.

Combinatorial joining: A process whereby one exon can combine alternatively with a variety of other gene segments, thereby multiplying the diversity of the gene products.

Complement: A system of serum proteins that is the primary humoral mediator of antigen-antibody reactions.

Complement fixation: A standard serologic assay used for the detection of an antigen-antibody reaction in which complement is fixed as a result of the formation of an immune complex. The subsequent failure of lysis of sensitized erythrocytes by complement that has been fixed indicates the degree of antigen-antibody reaction.

Complementarity: In genetics, the term indicates that more than one gene is required for the expression of a particular trait.

Concanavalin A (Con A): A lectin that is derived from the jack bean and stimulates predominantly the T lymphocytes.

Concomitant immunity: The ability of a tumor-bearing animal to reject a test inoculum of its tumor at a site different from the primary site of tumor growth.

Congenic (originally **congenic resistant**): Denotes a line of mice identical or nearly identical with other inbred strains except for the substitution at one histocompatibility locus of a foreign allele introduced by appropriate crosses with a second inbred strain.

Contact sensitivity: A type of delayed hypersensitivity reaction in which sensitivity to simple chemical compounds is manifested by skin reactivity.

Contrasuppression: Effects of immunoregulatory circuit that inhibit suppressor influences in a feedback loop.

Copolymer: A polymer of at least 2 different chemical moieties, eg, a polypeptide with 2 different amino acids.

Coproantibody: An antibody present in the lumen of the gastrointestinal tract.

Counterimmunoelectrophoresis: See **Electoimmunodiffusion.**
emulsified with Freund's complete adjuvant.

C-reactive protein (CRP): A β-globulin found in the serum of patients with diverse inflammatory diseases.

CREST phenomenon: A phenomenon that consists of *c*alcinosis, *R*aynaud's phenomenon, *e*sophageal dysmotility, *s*clerodactyly, and *t*elangiectasis and that occurs in patients with progressive systemic sclerosis.

Cross-matching: A laboratory test using cells from a recipient and serum from a donor to detect antibodies directed at recipient's cells.

Cross-reacting antigen: A type of tumor antigen present on all tumors induced by the same or a similar carcinogen.

Cross-reaction: The reaction of an antibody with an antigen other than the one that induced its formation.

Cryoglobulin: A protein that has the property of forming a precipitate or gel in the cold.

Cutaneous basophil hypersensitivity: An immunologically mediated inflammation in the skin with a prominent basophil infiltration occurring about 24 hours after injection of the sensitizing antigen.

Cycle-specific drugs: Cytotoxic or immunosuppressive drugs that kill both mitotic and resting cells.

Cyclo-oxygenase pathway: Enzymatic metabolism of cell membrane-derived arachidonic acid whereby prostaglandins are produced.

Cytokine: A factor such as a lymphokine or monokine produced by cells that affect other cells.

Cytotropic antibodies: Antibodies of the IgG and IgE classes that sensitize cells for subsequent anaphylaxis.

D gene region: Diversity region of genome encoding heavy chain sequences in the hypervariable region of immunoglobulin H chain.

Degranulation: A process whereby cytoplasmic granules of phagocytic cells fuse with phagosomes and discharge their contents into the phagolysosome thus formed.

Delayed hypersensitivity: A cell-mediated immune response producing a cellular infiltrate and edema that are maximal between 24 and 48 hours after antigen challenge.

Dendritic cells: Mononuclear cells that present antigens in lymphoid tissue but are distinct from the monocyte-macrophage lineage.

Desensitization: Treatment of allergic disease by repeated injections of allergen extracts. Also called "allergen immunotherapy."

Determinant groups: Individual chemical structures present on macromolecular antigens that determine antigenic specificity.

Dextrans: Polysaccharides composed of a single sugar.

Diapedesis: The outward passage of cells through intact vessel walls.

Direct agglutination: The agglutination of erythrocytes, microorganisms, or other substances directly by serum antibody.

Direct immunofluorescence: The detection of antigens by fluorescently labeled antibody.

Disulfide bonds: Chemical S–S bonds between sulfhydryl-containing amino acids that bind together H and L chains as well as portions of H–H and L–L chains.

Domains (also **homology regions**): Segments of H or L chains that are folded 3-dimensionally and stabilized with disulfide bonds.

Dysgammaglobulinemia: A term not in common use that refers to a selective immunoglobulin deficiency.

E rosette: A formation of a cluster (rosette) of cells consisting of sheep erythrocytes and human T lymphocytes.

EAC rosette: A cluster of erythrocytes sensitized with amboceptor (antibody) and complement around human B lymphocytes.

EAE (experimental allergic encephalomyelitis): An autoimmune disease in which an animal is immunized with homologous or heterologous extracts of whole brain, the basic protein of myelin, or certain polypeptide sequences within the basic protein, emulsified with Freund's complete adjuvant.

ECF-A (eosinophil chemotactic factor of anaphylaxis): An acidic peptide, molecular weight 500, that, when released, causes influx of eosinophils.

Effector cells: A term that usually denotes T cells capable of mediating cytotoxicity, suppression, or helper function.

Electroimmunodiffusion (counterimmunoelectrophoresis): An immunodiffusion technique in which antigen and antibody are driven toward each other in an electrical field and then precipitate.

Electrophoresis: The separation of molecules in an electrical field.

Encapsulation: A quasi-immunologic phenomenon in which foreign material is walled off within the tissues of invertebrates.

Endocytosis: The process whereby material external to a cell is internalized within a particular cell. It consists of pinocytosis and phagocytosis.

Endogenous pyrogen (IL-1): Factor produced by macrophages and other cells. Causes fever by reducing prostaglandins in region of hypothalamus.

Endotoxins: Lipopolysaccharides that are derived from the cell walls of gram-negative microorganisms and have toxic and pyrogenic effects when injected in vivo.

Enhancement: Improved survival of tumor cells in animals that have been previously immunized to the antigens of a given tumor.

Enterotoxin: A heat-stable toxin produced by bacteria, which produces intestinal disease.

Epitope: The simplest form of an antigenic determinant present on a complex antigenic molecule, which combines with antibody or T cell receptor.

Equilibrium dialysis: A technique for measuring the strength or affinity with which antibody binds to antigen.

Equivalence: A ratio of antigen-antibody concentration where maximal precipitation occurs.

Euglobulin: A class of globulin proteins that are insoluble in water but soluble in salt solutions.

Eukaryote: A cell or organism possessing a true nucleus containing chromosomes bounded by a nuclear membrane.

Exon: The coding segment of a DNA strand.

Exotoxins: Diffusible toxins produced by certain gram-positive and gram-negative microorganisms.

F_1 generation: The first generation of offspring after a designated mating.

F_2 generation: The second generation of offspring after a designated mating.

Fab: An antigen-binding fragment produced by enzymatic digestion of an IgG molecule with papain.

$F(ab)'_2$: A fragment obtained by pepsin digestion of immunoglobulin molecules containing the 2 H and 2 L chains linked by disulfide bonds. It contains antigen-binding activity. An $F(ab)'_2$ fragment and an Fc fragment make up an entire monomeric immunoglobulin molecule.

Fc fragment: A crystallizable fragment obtained by papain digestion of IgG molecules that consists of the C-terminal half of 2 H chains linked by disulfide bonds. It contains no antigen-binding capability but determines important biologic characteristics of the intact molecule.

Fc receptor: A receptor present on various subclasses of lymphocytes for the Fc fragment of immunoglobulins.

Felton phenomenon: Immunologic unresponsiveness or tolerance induced in mice by the injection of large quantities of pneumococcal polysaccharide.

Fetal antigen: A type of tumor-associated antigen that is normally present on embryonic but not adult tissues and that is reexpressed during the neoplastic process.

Fibronectin: A protein that has an important role in the structuring of connective tissue.

Fluorescence: The emission of light of one color while a substance is irradiated with a light of a different color.

Forbidden clone theory: The theory proposed to explain autoimmunity that postulates that lymphocytes capable of self sensitization and effector function are present in tolerant animals, since they were not eliminated during embryogenesis.

Francis skin test: An immediate hypersensitivity test for the presence of antibody on pneumococci in which pneumococcal capsular polysaccharide is injected into the skin and produces a wheal-and-flare response.

Freund's complete adjuvant: An oil-water emulsion that contains killed mycobacteria and enhances immune responses when mixed in an emulsion with antigen.

Freund's incomplete adjuvant: An emulsion that contains all of the elements of Freund's complete adjuvant with the exception of killed mycobacteria.

G cells: Gastrin-secreting cells in mucosa of the gastric antrum.

Gamma globulins: Serum proteins with gamma mobility in electrophoresis that make up the majority of immunoglobulins and antibodies.

Gammopathy: A paraprotein disorder involving abnormalities of immunoglobulins.

γ/δ T cells: T cells expressing γ and δ chains of the T cell receptor. The function of this minor T cell population is unknown.

Generalized anaphylaxis: A shocklike state that occurs within minutes following an appropriate antigen-antibody reaction resulting from the systemic release of vasoactive amines.

Genetic switch hypothesis: A hypothesis that postulates that there is a switch in the gene controlling heavy chain synthesis in plasma cells during the development of an immune response.

Genetic theory of antibody synthesis: A theory that predicts that information for synthesis of all types of antibody exists in the genome and that specific receptors are preformed on immunocompetent cells.

Germinal centers: A collection of metabolically active lymphoblasts, macrophages, and plasma cells that appears within the primary follicle of lymphoid tissues following antigenic stimulation.

Gm marker: An allotypic determinant on the heavy chain of human IgG.

Graft-versus-host (GVH) reaction: The clinical and pathologic sequelae of the reactions of immunocompetent cells in a graft against the cells of the histoincompatible and immunodeficient recipient.

Granuloma: An organized structure of mononuclear cells that is the hallmark of cell-mediated immunity.

Granulopoietin (colony-stimulating factor): A glycoprotein with a molecular weight of 45,000 derived from monocytes that controls the production of granulocytes by the bone marrow.

H chain: See **Heavy chain.**

H-2 **locus:** The major genetic histocompatibility region in the mouse.

Halogenation: A combination of a halogen molecule with a microbial cell wall that results in microbial damage.

Haplotype: The portion of the phenotype determined by closely linked genes of a single chromosome inherited from one parent.

Hapten: A substance that is not immunogenic but can react with an antibody of appropriate specificity.

Hassall's corpuscles (also **Leber's corpuscles** or **thymic corpuscles**): Whorls of thymic epithelial cells whose function is unknown.

HBcAg (also **core antigen**): The 27-nm core of hepatitis B virus, which has been identified in the nuclei of hepatocytes.

HBeAg: Low-molecular-weight component of hepatitis B nucleocapsid indicating infectious state when present in serum.

HBsAg: The coat or envelope of hepatitis B virus.

Heavy chain (H chain): One pair of identical polypeptide chains making up an immunoglobulin molecule. The heavy chain contains approximately twice the number of amino acids and is twice the molecular weight of the light chain.

Heavy chain diseases: A heterogeneous group of paraprotein disorders characterized by the presence of monoclonal but incomplete heavy chains without light chains in serum or urine.

Helper T cells: A subtype of T lymphocytes that cooperate with B cells in antibody formation.

Hemagglutination inhibtion: A technique for detecting small amounts of antigen in which the agglutination of antigen-coated erythrocytes or other particles by specific antibody is inhibited by homologous antigen.

Hematopoietic system: All tissues responsible for production of the cellular elements of peripheral blood. This term usually excludes strictly lymphocytopoietic tissue such as lymph nodes.

Hemolysin: An antibody or other substance capable of lysing erythrocytes.

Heterocytotropic antibody: An antibody that can passively sensitize tissues of species other than those in which the antibody is present.

Heterodimer: A 2-component molecule made up of different but closely joined segments, eg, T cell receptor α and β chains.

Heterologous antigen: An antigen that participates in a cross-reaction.

High dose (high zone) tolerance: Classic immunologic unresponsiveness produced by repeated injections of large amounts of antigen.

High endothelial venules: Specialized blood vessels present in lymphoid tissues with cuboidal endothelium, which allow passage of lymphocytes between cells into tissues.

Hinge region: The area of the H chains in the C region between the first and second C region domains. It is the site of enzymatic cleavage into F(ab)'$_2$ and Fc fragments.

Histamine: A bioactive amine of molecular weight 111 that causes smooth muscle contraction of human bronchioles and small blood vessels, increased permeability of capillaries, and increased secretion by nasal and bronchial mucous glands.

Histamine releasing factor: A lymphokine released from sensitized lymphocytes or antigenic stimulation that causes basophil histamine release.

Histocompatible: Sharing transplantation antigens.

HLA (human leukocyte antigen): The major histocompatibility genetic region in humans.

Homing receptors: Cell surface molecules that direct the cell to specific locations in other organs or tissues.

Homocytotropic antibody: An antibody that attaches to cells of animals of the same species.

Homologous antigen: An antigen that induces an antibody and reacts specifically with it.

Homopolymer: A molecule consisting of repeating units of a single amino acid.

Homozygous typing cells (HTC): Cells derived from an individual who is homozygous at the HLA-D locus used for MLR typing of the D locus in humans.

Horror autotoxicus: A concept introduced by Ehrlich, proposing that an individual is protected against autoimmunity or immunization against self antigens even though these antigens are immunogenic in other animals.

Hot antigen suicide: A technique in which an antigen is labeled with a high-specific-activity radioisotope (^{131}I). It is used either in vivo or in vitro to inhibit specific lymphocyte function by attachment to an antigen-binding lymphocyte, subsequently killing it by radiolysis.

Humoral: Pertaining to molecules in solution in a body fluid, particularly antibody and complement.

Hybridoma: Transformed cell line grown in vivo or in vitro that is a somatic hybrid of 2 parent cell lines and contains genetic material from both.

Hydrophilic: A hydrophilic compound is soluble in water; a hydrophilic group binds water on the exterior surfaces of proteins and cell membranes.

Hydrophobic: A hydrophobic compound is insoluble in water; a hydrophobic group is pushed to the interior of proteins or membranes, away from water.

Hyperacute rejection: An accelerated form of graft rejection that is associated with circulating antibody in the serum of the recipient and which can react with donor cells.

Hypersensitivity: See **Allergy.**

Hypervariable regions: At least 4 regions of extreme variability which occur throughout the V region of H and L chains and which determine the antibody combining site of an antibody molecule.

Hypogammaglobulinemia (agammaglobulinemia): A deficiency of all major classes of serum immunoglobulins.

Hyposensitization: See **Desensitization.**

I region: That portion of the major histocompatibility complex which contains genes that control immune responses.

Ia antigens (I region-associated antigens): Antigens that are controlled by Ir genes and are present on various tissues.

Idiotope: An epitope (antigenic determinant) on an idiotype.

Idiotype: A unique antigenic determinant present on homogeneous antibody or myeloma protein. The idiotype appears to represent the antigenicity of the antigen-binding site of an antibody and is therefore located in the V region.

IgA: The predominant immunoglobulin class present in secretions.

IgD: The predominant immunoglobulin class present on human B lymphocytes.

IgE: A reaginic antibody involved in immediate hypersensitivity reactions.

IgG: The predominant immunoglobulin class present in human serum.

IgM: A pentameric immunoglobulin comprising approximately 10% of normal human serum immunoglobulins, with a molecular weight of 900,000 and a sedimentation coefficient of 19S.

7S IgM: A monomeric IgM consisting of one monomer of 5 identical subunits.

Immediate hypersensitivity: An antibody-mediated immunologic sensitivity that manifests itself by tissue reactions occurring within minutes after the antigen combines with its appropriate antibody.

Immune adherence: An agglutination reaction between a cell bearing C$\overline{423}$ and an indicator cell, usually a human erythrocyte, which has a receptor for C3b.

Immune complexes: Antigen-antibody complexes.

Immune elimination: The enhanced clearance of an injected antigen from the circulation as a result of immunity to that antigen brought about by enhanced phagocytosis of the reticuloendothelial system.

Immune exclusion: The normal prevention of entry of antigens across mucosal membranes by secretory IgA.

Immune response genes (Ir genes): Genes that control immune responses to specific antigens.

Immune suppression: A variety of therapeutic maneuvers to depress or eliminate the immune response.

Immune surveillance: A theory that holds that the immune system destroys tumor cells, which are constantly arising during the life of the individual.

Immunization: See **Sensitization.** Natural or artificial induction of an immune response, particularly when it renders the host protected from disease.

Immunobeads: Small plastic spheres coated with antibodies or antigens, which are used to indicate immune reactions by agglutination.

Immunocytoadherence: A technique for identifying immunoglobulin-bearing cells by formation of rosettes consisting of these cells and erythrocytes or other particles containing a homologous antigen.

Immunodominant: The part of an antigenic determinant that is dominant in binding with antibody.

Immunoelectrophoresis: A technique combining an initial electrophoretic separation of proteins followed by immunodiffusion with resultant precipitation arcs.

Immunofixation electrophoresis: Technique for identification of proteins by electrophoretic separation on a gel followed by precipitation in situ with specific antibodies.

Immunofluorescence: A histo- or cytochemical technique for the detection and localization of antigens in which specific antibody is conjugated with fluorescent compounds, resulting in a sensitive tracer that can be detected by fluorometric measurements.

Immunogen: A substance that, when introduced into an animal, stimulates the immune response. The term immunogen may also denote a substance that is capable of stimulating an immune response, in contrast to a substance that can only combine with antibody, ie, an antigen.

Immunogenicity: The property of a substance making it capable of inducing a detectable immune response.

Immunoglobulin: A glycoprotein composed of H and L chains that functions as antibody. All antibodies are immunoglobulins, but it is not certain that all immunoglobulins have antibody function.

Immunoglobulin class: A subdivision of immunoglobulin molecules based on unique antigenic determinants in the Fc region of the H chains. In humans there are 5 classes of immunoglobulins designated IgG, IgA, IgM, IgD, and IgE.

Immunoglobulin class switch: The process in which a B cell precursor expressing IgM and IgG receptors differentiates into a B cell producing IgG, IgA, or IgE antibodies without change in specificity for the antigenic determinant.

Immunoglobulin subclass: A subdivision of the classes of immunoglobulins based on structural and antigenic differences in the H chains. For human IgG there are 4 subclasses: IgG1, IgG2, IgG3, and IgG4.

Immunoglobulin supergene family: A structurally related group of genes that encode immunoglobulins, T cell receptors, β_2-microglobulin, and others.

Immunomodulation: A variety of methods for therapeutic manipulation of the immune response.

Immunopathic: Referring to damage to cells, tissues, or organs from immune responses.

Immunopotency: The capacity of a region of an antigen molecule to serve as an antigenic determinant and thereby induce the formation of specific antibody.

Immunoradiometry: A technique of radioimmunoassay that employs radiolabeled antibody rather than antigen.

Immunotherapy: Either hyposensitization in allergic diseases or treatment with immunostimulants or immunosuppressive drugs or biologic products.

Indirect agglutination (also **passive agglutination**): The agglutination of particles or erythrocytes to which antigens have been coupled chemically.

Indirect immunofluorescence (also **double antibody immunofluorescence**): A technique whereby unlabeled antibody is incubated with substrate and then overlaid with fluorescently conjugated anti-immunoglobulin to form a sandwich.

Information theory of antibody synthesis: A theory that predicts that antigen dictates the specific structure of the antibody molecule.

Innate immunity: Various host defenses present from birth that do not depend on immunologic memory.

Inoculation: The introduction of an antigen or antiserum into an animal to confer immunity.

Integreins: A family of cell membrane-bound factors that promote cell adhesion.

Interferon: A heterogeneous group of low-molecular-weight proteins elaborated by infected host cells that protect noninfected cells from viral infection.

Interleukin: Chemically defined factor released from leukocytes or other cells, which has defined biologic effects.

Interleukin-1: Macrophage-derived factor (previously called LAF, or leukocyte-activating factor) that promotes short-term proliferation of T cells.

Interleukin-2: A lymphocyte-derived factor (previously called TCGF, or T cell growth factor) that promotes long-term proliferation of T cell lines in culture.

Interleukin-3: A T cell product that induces proliferation and differentiation in other lymphocytes and some hematopoietic cells.

Interleukin-4 (formerly **BCGF**): A factor that is produced by helper T cells and stimulates the growth of T and B cells.

Interleukin-5: A factor that is produced by helper T cells and stimulates B cells and eosinophils.

Interleukin-6: A factor that is produced by fibroblasts and stimulates B cell immunoglobulin production.

Interleukin-7: A factor that is produced by stromal cells and causes early T and B cell lymphopoiesis.

Interleukin-8: A factor that is produced by macrophages and chemoattracts T cells and neutrophils.

Introns: Noncoding regions of DNA interspersed among the exons.

Inv marker: See **Km marker.**

Ir genes: See **Immune response genes.**

Isoagglutinin: An agglutinating antibody capable of agglutinating cells of other individuals of the same species in which it is found.

Isoantibody: An antibody that is capable of reacting with an antigen derived from a member of the same species as that in which it is raised.

Isohemagglutinins: Antibodies to major erythrocyte antigens present in members of a given species and directed against antigenic determinants on erythrocytes from other members of the species.

Isotype: Antigenic characteristics of given class or subclass of immunoglobulin H and L chains.

Isotype switching: The process of changing synthesis of heavy-chain isotypes, eg, from μ to γ in B cells.

J chain: A glycopeptide chain that is normally found in polymeric immunoglobulins, particularly IgA and IgM.

Jarisch-Herxheimer reaction: A local or occasionally generalized inflammatory reaction that occurs following treatment of syphilis and other intracellular infections; it is presumably caused by the release of large amounts of antigenic material into the circulation.

Jones criteria: Signs and symptoms used to diagnose acute rheumatic fever.

Jones-Mote reaction: See **Cutaneous basophil hypersensitivity.**

K cell: A killer cell responsible for antibody-dependent cell-mediated cytotoxicity.

Kallikrein system: See **Kinin system.**

Kappa (κ) chains: One of 2 major types of light chains.

Kinin: A peptide that increases vascular permeability and is formed by the action of esterases on kallikreins, which then act as vasodilators.

Kinin system (also **kallikrein system**): A humoral amplification system initiated by the activation of coagulation factor XII, eventually leading to the formation of kallikrein, which acts on an α-globulin substrate, kininogen, to form a bradykinin.

Km marker (also **Inv**): An allotypic marker on the κ L chain of human immunoglobulins.

Koch phenomenon: A delayed hypersensitivity reaction by tuberculin in the skin of a guinea pig following infection with *Mycobacterium tuberculosis.*

Kupffer cells: Fixed mononuclear phagocytes of the reticuloendothelial system that are present within the sinusoids of the liver.

Kveim test: A delayed hypersensitivity test for sarcoidosis in which potent antigenic extracts of sarcoid tissue are injected intradermally and biopsied 6 weeks later in order to observe the presence of a granuloma, indicating a positive test.

L chain: See **Light chain.**

Lactoferrin: An iron-containing compound that exerts a slight antimicrobial action by binding iron necessary for microbial growth.

Lambda (λ) chain: One of 2 major types of light chains.

Langerhans cell: Bone marrow-derived macrophage with Ia cell surface antigens found in the epidermis.

Late-phase reaction: An inflammatory response that occurs about 6–8 hours after antigen exposure in IgE-mediated allergic diseases.

Latex fixation test: An agglutination reaction in which latex particles are used to passively adsorb soluble protein and polysaccharide antigens.

LE cell phenomenon: Phagocytic leukocytes that have engulfed DNA, immunoglobulin, and complement and are present as a large homogeneous mass that is extruded from a damaged lymphocyte in systemic lupus erythematosus and other rheumatoid diseases.

Lectin: A substance that is derived from a plant and has panagglutinating activity for erythrocytes. Lectins are commonly mitogens as well.

Leukocyte inhibitory factor (LIF): A lymphokine that inhibits the migration of polymorphonuclear leukocytes.

Leukotriene: A vasodilatory lipoxygenase metabolite of arachidonic acid.

Levamisole: An antihelminthic drug with possible immunostimulatory capabilities.

Ligand: Any molecule that forms a complex with another molecule, such as an antigen used in a precipitin or radioimmunoassay.

Light chain (L chain): A polypeptide chain present in all immunoglobulin molecules. Two types exist in most species and are termed kappa (κ) and lambda (λ).

Lineage infidelity: Expression following neoplastic transformation of molecules on cells that are foreign to the lineage of the cell itself.

Linkage disequilibrium: An unexpected association of linked genes in a population.

Lipopolysaccharide (also **endotoxin**): A compound derived from a variety of gram-negative enteric bacteria that have various biologic functions including mitogenic activity for B lymphocytes.

Lipoxygenase pathway: Enzymatic metabolism of cell

membrane-derived arachidonic acid whereby leukotrienes are produced.

Local anaphylaxis: An immediate hypersensitivity reaction that occurs in a specific target organ such as the gastrointestinal tract, nasal mucosa, or skin.

Locus: The specific site of a gene on a chromosome.

Low dose (low zone) tolerance: A transient and incomplete state of tolerance induced with small subimmunogenic doses of soluble antigen.

Lucio phenomenon (erythema necroticans): A variant of erythema nodosum leprosum in which necrotizing vasculitis produces crops of large polygonal lesions characterized by ulceration and sloughing of large areas of skin.

Lymphocyte: A mononuclear cell 7–12 μm in diameter containing a nucleus with densely packed chromatin and a small rim of cytoplasm.

Lymphocyte activation (also **lymphocyte stimulation, lymphocyte transformation,** or **blastogenesis**): An in vitro technique in which lymphocytes are stimulated to become metabolically active by antigen or mitogen.

Lymphocyte-defined (LD) antigens: A series of histocompatibility antigens that are present on the majority of mammalian cells and are detectable primarily by reactivity in the mixed lymphocyte reaction (MLR).

Lymphokines (also **mediators of cellular immunity**): Soluble products of lymphocytes that are responsible for the multiple effects of a cellular immune reaction.

Lymphoreticular: Referring to lymphocyte and monocyte-macrophage system and stromal elements that support its growth.

Lymphotoxin (LT): A lymphokine that results in direct cytolysis following its release from stimulated lymphocytes.

Lysosomes: Granules that contain hydrolytic enzymes and are present in the cytoplasm of many cells.

Lysozyme (also **muramidase**): The cationic low-molecular-weight enzyme present in tears, saliva, and nasal secretions that reduces the local concentration of susceptible bacteria by attacking the mucopeptides of their cell walls.

M cells: Membranous epithelial cells that overlie lymphoid tissues in the small intestine and allow limited passage of intraintestinal antigens.

M protein: Antigenic component of surface of streptococci. Cross-reacts with muscle antigens.

M protein: See **Myeloma protein.**

Macrophage chemotactic factor (MCF): A lymphokine that selectively attracts monocytes or macrophages to the area of its release.

Macrophage-activating factor (MAF): A lymphokine that will activate macrophages to become avid phagocytic cells.

Macrophages: Phagocytic mononuclear cells that derive from bone marrow monocytes and subserve accessory roles in cellular immunity.

Major basic protein: A toxic protein from the eosinophil membrane that produces tissue damage in allergic and inflammatory diseases.

Major histocompatibility complex (MHC): Genes located in close proximity that determine histocompatibility antigens of members of a species.

Mast cell: A tissue cell that has high-affinity receptors for IgE and generates inflammatory mediators in allergy.

Membrane attack complex: The terminal complement components that, when activated, cause lysis of target cells.

β_2-Microglobulin: A protein (MW 11,600) that is associated with the outer membrane of many cells, including lymphocytes, and that functions as a structural part of the histocompatibility antigens on cells.

Migration inhibitory factor (MIF): A lymphokine that is capable of inhibiting the migration of macrophages.

Mitogens (also **phytomitogens**): Substances that cause DNA synthesis, blast transformation, and ultimately division of lymphocytes.

Mixed lymphocyte culture (mixed leukocyte culture) (MLC): An in vitro test for cellular immunity in which lymphocytes or leukocytes from genetically dissimilar individuals are mixed and mutually stimulate DNA synthesis.

Mixed lymphocyte reaction (MLR): See **Mixed lymphocyte culture.**

Molecular mimicry: Immunologic cross-reactivity between determinants on an environmental antigen (such as a virus) and a self antigen, a notion that has been proposed to explain autoimmunity.

Monoclonal antibodies (Monoclonal immunoglobulin molecules): Identical copies of antibody that consist of one H chain class and one L chain type.

Monoclonal hypergammaglobulinemia: An increase in immunoglobulins produced by a single clone of cells containing one H chain class and one L chain type.

Monoclonal protein: A protein produced from the progeny of a single cell called a clone.

Monokine: Substance released from macrophage or monocyte that affects the function of another cell.

Monomer: The basic unit of an immunoglobulin molecule that is composed of 4 polypeptide chains: 2 H and 2 L.

Mononuclear phagocyte system: Mononuclear cells found primarily in the reticular connective tissue of lymphoid and other organs that are prominent in chronic inflammatory states.

Mucosal homing: The ability of immunologically competent cells that arise from mucosal follicles to traffic back to mucosal areas.

Mucosal immune system: The lymphoid tissues associated with the mucosal surfaces of the gastrointestinal, respiratory, and urogenital tracts, which produce a unique immunoglobulin (secretory IgA) and T cell immunity for these mucosal surfaces.

Multiple myeloma: A paraproteinemic disorder consisting typically of the presence of serum paraprotein, anemia, and lytic bone lesions.

Myeloma protein (M protein): Either an intact monoclonal immunoglobulin molecule or a portion of one produced by malignant plasma cells.

Myeloperoxidase: An enzyme that is present within granules of phagocytic cells and catalyzes peroxidation of a variety of microorganisms.

N terminus: The amino-terminal end of a protein molecule.

Natural antibody: Antibody present in the serum in the absence of apparent specific antigenic contact.

NBT test: A metabolic assay involving the reduction of nitro blue tetrazolium dye during activation of the hexose monophosphate shunt in phagocytic cells.

Neoantigens: Nonself antigens that arise spontaneously on cell surfaces, usually during neoplasia.

Nephelometry: The measurement of turbidity or cloudiness in a suspension or a solution.

Nephritic factor: Serum immunoglobulin with conglutinin activity that can activate the alternative complement pathway. Often present in serum of patients with membranoproliferative glomerulonephritis.

Network hypothesis: Jerne's theory of immunoregulation by a cascade of idiotype-anti-idiotype reactions involving T cell receptors and antibodies.

Neutralization: The process by which antibody or antibody in complement neutralizes the infectivity of microorganisms, particularly viruses.

Neutrophil microbicidal assay: A test for the ability of neutrophils to kill intracellular bacteria.

NK cells (natural killer cells): Cytotoxic cells belonging to the cell class responsible for cellular cytotoxicity without prior sensitization.

Nonresponder: An animal unable to respond to an antigen, usually because of genetic factors.

Northern blotting: A method for detecting RNA fragments in an RNA mixture which are separated by gel electrophoresis, blotted, and probed with labeled DNA or RNA oligmers.

Nucleoside phosphorylase: An enzyme that catalyzes the conversion of inosine to hypoxanthine and is rarely deficient in patients with immunodeficiency disorders.

Nude mouse: A hairless mouse that congenitally lacks a thymus and has a marked deficiency of thymus-derived lymphocytes.

Null cells: Cells lacking the specific identifying surface markers for either T or B lymphocytes.

NZB mouse: A genetically inbred strain of mice in which autoimmune disease resembling systemic lupus erythematosus develops spontaneously.

Oligoclonal bands: Immunoglobulins with restricted electrophoretic mobility in agarose gels found in cerebrospinal fluid of patients with multiple sclerosis and some other central nervous system diseases.

Oncofetal antigens: Antigens expressed during normal fetal development that reappear during cancer development, eg, carcinoembryonic antigen.

Oncogene: A gene of either viral or mammalian origin that causes transformation of cells in culture.

Oncogenesis: The process of producing neoplasia or malignancy.

Ontogeny: The developmental history of an individual organism within a group of animals.

Opportunistic infection: The ability of organisms of relatively low virulence to cause disease in the setting of altered immunity.

Opsonin: A substance capable of enhancing phagocytosis. Antibodies and complement are the 2 main opsonins.

Oral unresponsiveness: The process by which the mucosal immune system normally prevents immune responses to foods and intestinal bacteria while responding to potential pathogens.

Osteoclast activating factor (OAF): A lymphokine that promotes the resorption of bone.

Ouchterlony double diffusion: An immunoprecipitation technique in which antigen and antibody are allowed to diffuse toward each other and form immune complexes in agar.

Palindrome: In molecular biology, a self-complementary length of DNA which when read from the 5′ to the 3′ end displays an equivalent sequence whether read from the left or the right or forward or backward.

Paracrine: Effects of a hormone that are only local.

Paralysis: The pseudotolerant condition in which an ongoing immune response is masked by the presence of overwhelming amounts of antigen.

Paraproteinemia: A condition occurring in a heterogeneous group of diseases characterized by the presence in serum or urine of a monoclonal immunoglobulin.

Paratope: An antibody-combining site for epitope, the simplest form of an antigenic determinant.

Passive cutaneous anaphylaxis (PCA): An in vivo passive transfer test for recognizing cytotropic antibody responsible for immediate hypersensitivity reactions.

Passive immunity: Protection achieved by introduction of preformed antibody or immune cells into a nonimmune host.

Patching: The reorganization of a cell surface membrane component into discrete patches over the entire cell surface.

Peripheral lymphoid organs: Lymphoid organs not essential to the ontogeny of immune responses, ie, the spleen, lymph nodes, tonsils, and Peyer's patches.

Peritoneal exudate cells (PEC): Inflammatory cells present in the peritoneum of animals injected with an inflammatory agent.

Peyer's patches: Collections of lymphoid tissue in the submucosa of the small intestine that contain lymphocytes, plasma cells, germinal centers, and T cell-dependent areas.

Pfeiffer phenomenon: A demonstration showing that cholera vibrios introduced into the peritoneal cavity of an immune guinea pig lose their mobility and are lysed regardless of the presence of cells.

Phagocytes: Cells that are capable of ingesting particulate matter.

Phagocytosis: The engulfment of microorganisms or other particles by leukocytes.

Phagolysosome: A cellular organelle that is the product of the fusion of a phagosome and a lysosome.

Phagosome: A phagocytic vesicle bounded by inverted plasma membrane.

Phylogeny: The developmental and evolutionary history of a group of animals.

Phytohemagglutinin (PHA): A lectin that is derived from the red kidney bean (*Phaseolus vulgaris*) and that stimulates predominantly T lymphocytes.

Phytomitogens: Glycoproteins that are derived from plants and stimulate DNA synthesis and blast transformation in lymphocytes.

Pinocytosis: The ingestion of soluble materials by cells.

Plaque-forming cells: Antibody-producing cells capable of forming a hemolytic plaque in the presence of complement and antigenic erythrocytes.

Plasma cells: Fully differentiated antibody-synthesizing cells that are derived from B lymphocytes.

Plasmin: A fibrinolytic enzyme capable of proteolytically digesting C1.

Plasminogen activator: An enzyme secreted by macrophages that converts a plasma zymogen to active plasmin.

Platelet-activating factor: An inflammatory mediator that activates platelets and inflammatory cells and is considered to be important in the bronchial inflammation of asthma.

Pokeweed mitogen (PWM): A lectin that is derived from pokeweed (*Phytolacca americana*) and that stimulates both B and T lymphocytes.

Polyclonal hypergammaglobulinemia: An increase in γ-globulin of various classes containing different H and L chains.

Polyclonal mitogens: Mitogens that activate large subpopulations of lymphocytes.

Polyclonal proteins: A group of molecules derived from multiple clones of cells.

Polymerase chain reaction (PCR): A technique to amplify segments of genetic DNA or RNA of known composition with primers in sequential repeated steps.

Polymers: Immunoglobulins composed of more than a single basic monomeric unit; eg, an IgA dimer consists of 2 units.

Postcapillary venules: Specialized blood vessels lined with cuboid epithelium located in the paracortical region of lymph nodes through which lymphocytes traverse.

Prausnitz-Küstner reaction: The passive transfer by intradermal injection of serum containing IgE antibodies from an allergic subject to a nonallergic recipient.

Pre-B cells: Large immature lymphoid cells with diffuse cytoplasmic IgM that eventually develop into B cells.

Precipitation: A reaction between a soluble antigen and soluble antibody in which a complex lattice of interlocking aggregates forms.

Primary follicles: Tightly packed aggregates of lymphocytes found in the cortex of the lymph node or in the white pulp of the spleen after antigenic stimulation. Primary follicles develop into germinal centers.

Primed lymphocyte typing (PLT): A variation on the MLR in which cells are primed by allogeneic stimulation and reexposed to fresh stimulator cells. Used to type for HLA-D determinants.

Private antigen: A tumor or histocompatibility antigen restricted either to a specific chemically induced tumor or to the specific product of a given allele.

Prokaryote: An organism without a true nucleus which contain a single, linear chromosome.

Properdin system: A group of proteins involved in resistance to infection. The 2 main constitutents consist of factor A and factor B. Properdin factor A is identical with C3, a β-globulin of MW 180,000. Properdin factor B is a $β_2$-globulin of MW 95,000.

It is also called C3 proactivator, glycine-rich β-glycoprotein (GBG), or $β_2$-glycoprotein II. Properdin factor D is an α-globulin of MW 25,000 also called C3 proactivator convertase or glycine-rich β-glycoproteinase (GBGase).

Prostaglandins: A variety of naturally occurring aliphatic acids with various biologic activities, including increased vascular permeability, smooth muscle contraction, bronchial constriction, and alteration in the pain threshold.

Prothymocytes: Immature precursors of mature thymocytes that develop within the thymus gland.

Proto-oncogene: A viral oncogene present in normal mammalian DNA.

Prozone phenomenon: Suboptimal precipitation that occurs in the region of antibody excess during immunoprecipitation reactions.

Public antigen: Determinant common to several distinct or private antigens.

Pyogenic microorganisms: Microorganisms whose presence in tissues stimulates an outpouring of polymorphonuclear leukocytes.

Pyrogens: Substances that are released either endogenously from leukocytes or administered exogenously, usually from bacteria, and that produce fever in susceptible hosts.

Pyroglobulins: Monoclonal immunoglobulins that precipitate irreversibly when heated to 56°C.

Quellung: The swelling of the capsules of pneumococci when the organisms are exposed to pneumococcal antibodies.

Radioallergosorbent test (RAST): A radioimmunoassay capable of detecting IgE antibody directed at specific allergens.

Radioimmunoassay: A variety of immunologic techniques in which a radioactive isotope is used to detect antigens or antibodies in some form of immunoassay.

Radioimmunodiffusion (Rowe's method): A modification of immunodiffusion in which a radioactive antibody is incorporated in order to increase the sensitivity by means of autoradiography.

Radioimmunosorbent test (RIST): A solid-phase radioimmunoassay that can detect approximately 1 ng of IgE.

Ragocytes (RA cells): Polymorphonuclear leukocytes that have ingested characteristic dense IgG aggregates, rheumatoid factor, complement, and fibrin. They are found in the joints of patients with rheumatoid arthritis.

Raji cell test: An assay for immune complexes using the Raji lymphoblastoid cell line.

Reagin: Synonymous with IgE antibody. Also denotes a complement-fixing antibody that reacts in the Wassermann reaction with cardiolipin.

Recombinant: An animal that has experienced a recombinational event during meiosis, consisting of crossover and recombination of parts of 2 chromosomes.

Recombinatorial germ line theory: Theory proposed by Dreyer and Bennett which states that variable-region and constant-region immunoglobulin genes are separated and rejoined at DNA levels.

Rejection response: An immune response with both

humoral and cellular components directed against transplanted tissue.

Respiratory burst: The process by which neutrophils and monocytes kill certain microbial pathogens by conversion of oxygen to toxic oxygen products.

Reticuloendothelial system: See **mononuclear phagocyte system.**

Retrovirus: A virus that contains and utilizes reverse transcriptase, eg, human immunodeficiency virus or human T cell leukemia virus.

Reverse transcriptase: An enzyme present in various microorganisms that catalyzes transcription of DNA from RNA rather than in the usual direction of transcription, which occurs from DNA to RNA.

Rheumatoid factor (RF): An anti-immunoglobulin antibody directed against denatured IgG present in the serum of patients with rheumatoid arthritis and other rheumatoid diseases.

Ricin: A poisonous substance that derives from the seed of the castor oil plant and agglutinates erythrocytes (a lectin).

Rocket electrophoresis (Laurell technique): An electro-immunodiffusion technique in which antigen is electrophoresed into agar containing specific antibody and precipitates in a tapered rocket-shaped pattern. This technique is used for quantitation of antigens.

Rose-Waaler test: A type of passive hemagglutination test for the detection of rheumatoid factor that employs tanned erythrocytes coated with rabbit 7S IgG antibodies specific for sheep erythrocytes.

S region: The chromosomal region in the H-2 complex containing the gene for a serum β-globulin.

S value: Svedberg unit. Denotes the sedimentation coefficient of a protein, determined usually by analytic ultracentrifugation.

Schultz-Dale test: An in vitro assay for immediate hypersensitivity in which smooth muscle is passively sensitized by cytotropic antibody and contracts after the addition of an antigen.

Second set graft rejection: An immunologic rejection of a graft in a host that is immune to antigens contained in that graft.

Secretory IgA: A dimer of IgA molecules with a sedimentation coefficient of 11S, linked by J chain and secretory component.

Secretory immune system: A distinct immune system that is common to external secretions and consists predominantly of IgA.

Secretory component (T piece): A molecule of MW 95,000 produced in epithelial cells and associated with secretory immunoglobulins, particularly IgA and IgM.

Sensitization: See **Immunization.** Natural or artificial induction of an immune response, particularly when it causes allergy in the host.

Sensitized: Synonymous with immunized.

Sensitizer: A term introduced by Pfeiffer to denote a specific thermostable factor capable of bacterial lysis when combined with alexin.

Sequential determinants: Determinants whose specificity is dictated by the sequence of subunits within the determinant rather than by the molecular structure of the antigen molecule.

Serologically defined (SD) antigens: Antigens that are present on membranes of nearly all mammalian cells and are controlled by genes present in the major histocompatibility complex. They can be easily detected with antibodies.

Serology: Literally, the study of serum. Refers to the determination of antibodies to infectious agents important in clinical medicine.

Serotonin (5-hydroxytryptamine): A catecholamine of MW 176 that is stored in murine mast cells and human platelets and has a pharmacologic role in anaphylaxis in most species except humans.

Serum sickness: An adverse immunologic response to a foreign antigen, usually a heterologous protein.

Shwartzman phenomenon: A nonimmunologic phenomenon that results in tissue damage both at the site of injection and at widespread sites following the second of 2 injections of endotoxin.

Side chain theory: A theory of antibody synthesis proposed by Ehrlich in 1896 suggesting that specific side chains that form antigen receptors are present on the surface membranes of antibody-producing cells.

Single radial diffusion (radioimmunodiffusion): A technique for quantitating antigens by immunodiffusion in which antigen is allowed to diffuse radially into agar containing antibody. The resultant precipitation ring reflects the concentration of the antigen.

Skin-reactive factor (SRF): A lymphokine that is responsible for vasodilatation and increased vascular permeability.

Slow-reacting substances of anaphylaxis: A term used to describe the smooth muscle-constricting effect of several leukotrienes.

Slow virus: A virus that produces disease with a greatly delayed onset and protracted course.

Solid phase radioimmunoassay: A modification of radioimmunoassay in which antibody is adsorbed onto solid particles or tubes.

Southern blotting: A method for identifying DNA segments that have been digested with restriction endonucleases and electrophoresed in a gel according to size. The DNA segments are blotted onto nitrocellulose and reacted with complementary radiolabeled or enzyme-labeled probes.

Spherulin: A spherule-derived antigen from *Coccidioides immitis* used in delayed hypersensitivity skin testing for coccidioidomycosis.

Splits: Subtypes of human leukocyte antigens.

SS-A: Antibody to RNA found in Sjögren's syndrome and also associated with heart block in infants born to mothers with this antibody.

SS-B: Antibody to RNA found in Sjögren's syndrome and other rheumatic diseases.

Sulzberger-Chase phenomenon: Abrogation of dermal contact sensitivity to various chemicals produced by prior oral feeding of the specific agent.

Suppressor T cells: A subset of T lymphocytes that suppress antibody synthesis by B cells or inhibit other cellular immune reactions by effector T cells.

Surface phagocytosis: The enhancement of phagocytosis by entrapment of organisms on surfaces such as leukocytes, fibrin clots, or other tissue surfaces.

Switch: Refers to change in synthesis between heavy chains within a single immunocyte from μ to γ—eg, during differentiation. V regions are not affected by H chain switch.

Syngeneic: Denotes the relationship that exists between genetically identical members of the same species.

T antigens: Tumor antigens, probably protein products of the viral genome present only on infected neoplastic cells.

T cell (T lymphocyte): A thymus-derived cell that participates in a variety of cell-mediated immune reactions.

T cell rosette: See **E rosette.**

T piece: See **Secretory piece.**

Theliolymphocytes: Small lymphocytes that are found in contiguity with intestinal epithelial cells and whose function is unknown.

Thymopoietin (originally **thymin**): A protein of MW 7000 which is derived originally from the thymus of animals with autoimmune thymitis and myasthenia gravis and which can impair neuromuscular transmission.

Thymosin: A thymic hormone protein of MW 12,000 that can restore T cell immunity in thymectomized animals.

Thymus: The central lymphoid organ that is present in the thorax and controls the ontogeny of T lymphocytes.

Thymus-dependent antigen: Antigen that depends on T cell interaction with B cells for antibody synthesis, eg, erythrocytes, serum proteins, and hapten-carrier complexes.

Thymus-independent antigen: Antigen that can induce an immune response without the apparent participation of T lymphocytes.

Tolerance: Traditionally denotes that condition in which responsive cell clones have been eliminated or inactivated by prior contact with antigen, with the result that no immune response occurs on administration of antigen.

Toxoids: Antigenic but nontoxic derivatives of toxins.

Transcription: The synthesis of RNA molecules from a DNA template.

Transfer factor: A dialyzable extract of immune lymphocytes that is capable of transferring cell-mediated immunity in humans and possibly in other animal species.

Transgenic: Referring to an organism that contains a foreign gene.

Translation: The process of formation of a peptide chain from individual amino acids to form a protein molecule.

trans-**Pairing:** Association of two genes or opposite chromosomes encoding a protein.

Transplantation antigens: Antigens that are expressed on the surface of virtually all cells and induce rejection of tissues transplanted from one individual to a genetically disparate individual.

Trophoblast: Cell layer in placenta in contact with uterine lining. Produces various immunosuppressive substances, eg, hormones.

Tryptic peptides: Peptides produced as a result of tryptic digestion of a protein molecule.

Tuftsin: A 4-amino-acid (threonine-lysine-proline-arginine) polypeptide that enhances macrophage functions.

Tumor-specific antigens: Cell surface antigens that are expressed on malignant but not normal cells.

Tumor-specific determinants: Antigens that are found on tumor cells but are also present in different amounts or forms on normal cells.

Ultracentrifugation: A high-speed centrifugation technique that can be used for the analytic identification of proteins of various sedimentation coefficients or as a preparative technique for separating proteins of different shapes and densities.

Ultrafiltration: The filtration of solutions or suspensions through membranes of extremely small graded pore sizes.

Uropods: Long pseudopods extending from lymphocyte cytoplasm covered by cellular plasma membrane.

Urticaria (hives): Localized edematous pruritic skin plaques caused by IgE-mediated allergy.

V antigens: Virally induced antigens that are expressed on viruses and virus-infected cells.

V (variable) region: The amino-terminal portion of the H or L chain of an immunoglobulin molecule, containing considerable heterogeneity in the amino acid residues compared to the constant region.

V region subgroups: Subdivisions of V regions of kappa chains based on substantial homology in sequences of amino acids.

Vaccination: Immunization with antigens administered for the prevention of infectious diseases (term originally coined to denote immunization against vaccinia or cowpox virus).

Variolation: Inoculation with a virus of unmodified smallpox (variola).

Viropathic: Damage to host tissues that is produced directly by the presence of pathogenic viral infection.

Viscosity: The physical property of serum that is determined by the size, shape, and deformability of serum molecules. The hydrostatic state, molecular charge, and temperature sensitivity of proteins.

Von Krogh equation: An equation that relates complement to the degree of lysis of erythrocytes coated with anti-red blood cell antibodies under standard conditions. Used to determine hemolytic complement titers in serum.

Wasting disease (also **runt disease**): A chronic, ultimately fatal illness associated with lymphoid atrophy in mice who are neonatally thymectomized.

Western blotting (also **Immunoblotting**): A technique to identify particular antigens in a mixture by separation on polyacrylamide gels, blotting onto nitrocellulose, and labeling with radiolabeled or enzyme-labeled antibodies as probes.

Xenogeneic: Denotes the relationship that exists between members of genetically different species.

Xenograft: A tissue or organ graft between members of 2 distinct or different species.

Zone electrophoresis: Electrophoresis performed on paper or cellulose acetate in which proteins are separated almost exclusively on the basis of charge.

Acronyms & Abbreviations Commonly Used in Immunology

ABA	Azobenzenearsenate.
ABPA	Allergic bronchopulmonary aspergillosis.
ACTH	Adrenocorticotropic hormone.
ADA	Adenosine deaminase.
ADCC	Antibody-dependent cell-mediated cytotoxicity.
AEF	Allogeneic effect.
AFC	Antibody-forming cells.
AFP	Alpha-fetoprotein.
AGN	Acute glomerulonephritis.
AHA	Autoimmune hemolytic anemia.
AHG	Antihemophilic globulin.
AIDS	Acquired immunodeficiency syndrome.
AIHA	Autoimmune hemolytic anemia.
ALG	Antilymphocyte globulin.
ALL	Acute lymphocytic leukemia.
ALS	Antilymphocyte serum.
Am	Allotypic marker on IgA.
AMA	Antimitochondrial antibodies.
AML	Acute myelogenous leukemia.
AMP	Adenosine monophosphate.
ANA	Antinuclear antibody.
ANF	Antinuclear factor.
APC	Antigen-presenting cells.
APSGN	Acute poststreptococcal glomerulonephritis.
ARC	AIDS-related complex.
ASO	Antistreptolysin O.
ATG	Antithymocyte globulin.
ATL	Adult T cell leukemia.
B27	HLA antigen with strong disease association.
BAF	B cell-activating factor.
BAL	Dimercaprol (British anti-Lewisite).
BALT	Bronchus-associated lymphoid tissue.
BCG	Bacillus Calmette-Guérin.
BCDF	B cell differentiation factors.
BCGF	B cell growth factors.
Bf	Properdin factor B.
BFP	Biologic false-positive (tests for syphilis).
BJ	Bence Jones.
BPI	Bactericidal permeability-increasing protein.
BPO	Benzyl penicilloyl.
BSA	Bovine serum albumin.
BUDR, BUdR	5-Bromodeoxy-uridine.
C	Complement.
CAH	Chronic active hepatitis.
CALLA	Common acute lymphocytic leukemia antigen.
cAMP	Cyclic adenosine monophosphate.
CBH	Cutaneous basophil hypersensitivity.
CD	Cluster of differentiation.

CDC	Centers for Disease Control.
CD3	Antigenic marker on T cell associated with T cell receptor.
CD4	An antigenic marker of helper/inducer T cells (also designated OKT 4, T4, Leu 3).
CD8	An antigenic marker of suppressor/cytotoxic T cells (also designated OKT 8, T8, Leu 2).
cDNA	Complementary DNA.
CEA	Carcinoembryonic antigen.
CF	Complement fixation.
CFA	Colonization factor antigens (also Freund's complete adjuvant).
CFU	Colony-forming unit.
CFU-C	Colony-forming unit of cells grown in culture.
CFU-GEMM	Colony-forming unit of granulocytes erythrocytes, monocytes and megakaryocytes.
CFU-GM	Colony-stimulating factor of granulocytes and macrophages.
CFU-S	Colony-forming unit of cells grown in the spleen.
CGD	Chronic granulomatous disease.
cGMP	Cyclic guanosine monophosphate.
C_H	Constant domain of H chain.
CHS	Chédiak-Higashi syndrome.
CIg	Cytoplasmic immunoglobulin.
C_L	Constant domain of L chain.
CLL	Chronic lymphocytic leukemia.
cM	Centimorgan.
c-*myc*	An oncogene.
CMCC	Chronic mucocutaneous candidiasis.
CMI	Cell-mediated immunity.
CML	Cell-mediated lympholysis, also chronic myelogenous leukemia.
CMPGN	Chronic membranoproliferative glomerulonephritis.
CMV	Cytomegalovirus(es).
C3NeF	C3 nephritic factor.
Con A	Concanavalin A.
C3PA	C3 proactivator.
CPGN	Chronic proliferative glomerulonephritis.
CR1-CR6	Six distinct receptors for C3 fragments found on various cell types.
CREG	Cross-reactive group.
CRP	C-reactive protein.
CSA	Colony-stimulating activity.
CSF	Colony-stimulating factor.
CTL	Cytotoxic lymphocytes.
CTLL	Cloned mouse cytotoxic T lymphocytic line.

DAT	Direct antiglobulin (Coombs test); also delay-accelerating factor.
DC	Dendritic cells.
DDS	Dapsone (diaminodiphenyl-sulfone).
DEAE	Diethylaminoethyl.
DGI	Disseminated gonococcal infection.
D_H	Diversity region of immunoglobulin heavy-chain gene.
DIC	Disseminated intravascular coagulation.
D-L	Donath-Landsteiner.
DLE	Dialyzable leukocyte extracts; disseminated lupus erythematosus.
DNCB	2,4-Dinitrochlorobenzene.
DNFB	Dinitrofluorobenzene.
DNP	Dinitrophenyl.
DP	Human class II MHC allele (formerly called SB).
DPO	Dimethoxyphenylpenicilloyl.
DPT	See DTP.
DQ	Human class II MHC allele (formerly called DC, MB, and DS).
DR	D-related HLA locus in humans.
DSCG	Disodium cromoglycate.
DST	Donor-specific transfusion.
DT	Diphtheria and tetanus toxoids.
DTH	Delayed-type hypersensitivity.
DTP	Diphtheria and tetanus toxoid combined with pertussis vaccine.
EA	Early antigens (of EBV).
EA	Erythrocyte amboceptor (sensitized erythrocytes).
EAC	Erythrocyte amboceptor complement.
EAE	Experimental allergic encephalitis or encephalomyelitis.
EAN	Experimental allergic neuritis.
EB	Epstein-Barr.
EBNA	Epstein-Barr virus nuclear antigen.
EBV	Epstein-Barr virus.
ECF	Eosinophil chemotactic factor.
ECF-A	Eosinophil chemotactic factor of anaphylaxis.
ECM	Erythema chronicum migrans (in Lyme disease).
ECP	Eosinophil cationic protein.
EDTA	Ethylenediaminetetraacetate.
EFA	Enhancing factor of allergy.
EIA	Enzyme immunoassay.
ELISA	Enzyme-linked immunosorbent assay.
EMIT	Enzyme multiple immunoassay technique; a homogeneous enzyme immunoassay.
ENA	Extractable nuclear antigen.
EP	Endogenous pyrogen.
EPO	Eosinophilic peroxidase.
ER	Endoplasmic reticulum.
ESR	Erythrocyte sedimentation rate.
F_1	First generation.
F_2	Second generation.
FA	Fluorescent antibody.
FAB	French, American, British (system of leukemia classification).
Fab	Antigen-binding fragment.
FACS	Fluorescent-activated cell sorter.
Fc	Crystallizable fragment.
FCC	Follicular center cell.
FCM	Flow cytometry.

FCR	Fractional catabolic rate.
FcεR	Fc receptor specific for IgE.
FcγR	Fc receptor specific for IgG.
FcμR	Fc receptor specific for IgM.
FeLV	Feline leukemia virus.
FEV	Forced expiratory volume in 1 second.
FITC	Fluorescein isothiocyanate.
FSH	Follicle-stimulating hormone.
FTA-ABS	Fluorescent treponemal antibody absorption test.
FUDR	Fluorodeoxyuridine.
FVC	Forced vital capacity.
GALT	Gut-associated lymphoid tissue.
GBG	Glycine-rich beta-glycoprotein.
GBM	Glomerular basement membrane.
G-CSF	Granulocyte colony-stimulating factor.
GEF	Glycosylation-enhancing factor.
GFR	Glomerular filtration rate.
GGG	Glycine-rich gamma-glycoprotein.
GIF	Glycosylation inhibition factor.
GLO	Glyoxylase.
Gm	Allotypic marker on human IgG.
GM-CSF	Granulocyte-macrophage colony-stimulating factor.
GMP	Guanosine monophosphate.
gp	Glycoprotein.
gp70	Glycoprotein antigen (MW 70,000) on viral envelope of C type murine viruses.
GPA	Guinea pig albumin.
GPC	Gastric parietal cell.
G6PD	Glucose-6-phosphate dehydrogenase.
GVH	Graft-versus-host (disease).
GVHR	Graft-versus-host reaction.
HAA	Hepatitis-associated antigen.
HAE, HANE	Hereditary angioneurotic edema.
HAT	Hypoxanthine, aminopterin, and thymidine.
HAV	Hepatitis A virus.
HbA	Adult hemoglobin.
HBcAg	Low-molecular-weight nucleocapsid antigen of hepatitis B virus.
HbF	Fetal hemoglobin.
HBeAg	Protein antigen of hepatitis B.
HBIG	Hepatitis B immune globulin.
HBsAg	Hepatitis B surface antigen.
HBV	Hepatitis B virus.
HCD	Heavy chain disease.
hCG	Human chorionic gonadotropin.
HDL	High-density lipoproteins.
HDN	Hemolytic disease of newborn.
HDV	Hepatitis delta virus.
H&E	Hematoxylin and eosin (stain).
HETE	Hydroxyeicosatetraenoic acid.
HEV	High endothelial venules.
HI	Hemagglutination inhibition.
HIV	Human immunodeficiency virus.
HLA	Human leukocyte antigen.
$(H_2L_2)n$	General formula for immunoglobulin molecule.
HMP	Hexose monophosphate (shunt).
HMW-NCF	High-molecular-weight neutrophil chemotactic factor.
HPETE	Hydroperoxyeicosatetraenoic acid.
HPLC	High-performance liquid chromatography.
HRF	Homologous restriction factor.
HPRT	Hypoxanthine phosphoribosyl transferase.

HSA	Human serum albumin.
HSF	Histamine-sensitizing factor, also hepatocyte-stimulating factor.
HSV	Herpes simplex virus.
5-HT	5-Hydroxytryptamine (serotonin).
HTC	Homozygous typing cells.
HTLV	Human T cell leukemia virus.
HuFcR	Human Fc receptor.
IBL	Immunoblastic lymphodenopathy.
ICA	Islet cell antibody.
ICAM	Intracellular adhesion molecule.
ICSA	Islet cell surface antibody.
IDAT	Indirect antiglobulin (Coombs) test.
ID	Idiotype.
IDDM	Insulin-dependent diabetes mellitus.
IDU	Idoxuridine.
IEF	Isoelectric focusing.
IEL	Intraepithelial lymphocyte.
IEP	Immunoelectrophoresis.
IF	Intrinsic factor (also initiating factor).
IFA	Indirect fluorescent antibody.
IFE	Immunofixation electrophoresis.
IFN	Interferon.
IGIM	Immune globulin for intramuscular use.
IGIV	Immune globulin for intravenous use.
IL-1–IL-8	Interleukins 1–8.
INH	Isoniazid (isonicotinic acid hydrazide).
Inv	Allotypic marker on human kappa chain (κm).
Ir	Immune response (genes).
ISG	Immune serum globulin.
ITP	Idiopathic thrombocytopenic purpura.
J segment	Joining segment of DNA encoding immunoglobulins.
J_H	Joining region of immunoglobulin-bearing chains.
JRA	Juvenile rheumatoid arthritis.
K (cells)	Killer (cells).
K562	Erythroleukemic cell line.
KAF	Bovine conglutinin: conglutinin activating factor.
KLH	Keyhole limpet hemocyanin.
La	See SS-B.
LAF	Leukocyte-activating factor (see IL-1).
LAK	Lymphokine-activated killer (cells).
LAV	Lymphadenopathy-associated virus.
LCMV	Lymphocytic choriomeningitis virus.
LD	Lymphocyte-defined.
LDCC	Lectin-dependent cell-mediated cytotoxicity
LDCF	Lymphocyte-derived chemotactic factors.
LDH	Lactate dehydrogenase.
LDL	Low-density lipoproteins.
LE	Lupus erythematosus.
Lf	Limit flocculation (unit) (1/1000Lf = 0.0000003 mg).
LFA	Lymphocyte functional antigen.
LGL	Large granular lymphocytes.
LH	Luteinizing hormone.
LIF	Leukocyte inhibitory factor.
LMI	Leukocyte migration inhibition.
LPL	Lamina propria lymphocyte.
LPS	Lipopolysaccharide.
LT	Leukotriene.
LT	Lymphotoxin or lymphocytotoxin.
Lyb	Lymphocyte antigens on murine B cells.

LyNeF	Lytic nephritic factor.
Lyt	Lymphocyte antigens on murine T cells.
MAC	(Complement) membrane attack complex.
Mac-1	Macrophage-1 glycoprotein.
MAF	Macrophage-activating (-arming) factor.
MALT	Mucosa-associated lymphoid tissue.
MBP	Major basic protein.
MC(DC)	Human MHC antigen of class II type.
MCA	Methylcholanthrene.
MCF	Macrophage chemotactic factor.
MCGN	Mesangiocapillary (membranoproliferative) glomerulonephritis.
MCP	Membrane cofactor protein.
M-CSF	Monocyte-macrophage colony-stimulating factor.
MCTD	Mixed connective tissue disease.
MDP	Muramyl dipeptide.
MeBSA	Methylated bovine serum albumin.
MER	Methanol extraction residue (of phenol-treated BCG).
MF	Mitogenic factor.
MHA	Major histocompatibility antigen.
MHA-TP	Microhemagglutination test for *Treponema pallidum*.
MHC	Major histocompatibility complex.
MHD	Minimum hemolytic dilution or dose.
MIF	Migration inhibitory factor.
ML	Malignant lymphoma.
MLC	Mixed lymphocyte (leukocyte) culture.
MLD	Minimum lethal dose.
MLR	Mixed lymphocyte (or leukocyte) response or reaction.
MMI	Macrophage migration inhibition.
MMR	Measles-mumps-rubella vaccine.
6-MP	Mercaptopurine.
MPG	Methyl green pyronin.
MPO	Myeloperoxidase.
MS	Multiple sclerosis.
MTX	Methotrexate.
MuLV	Murine leukemia virus.
MW	Molecular weight.
NBT	Nitroblue tetrazolium.
NCF	Neutrophil chemotactic factor.
NF	Nephritic factor.
NK	Natural killer (cells).
NSAID	Nonsteroidal anti-inflammatory drug.
NZB	New Zealand black (mice).
NZW	New Zealand white (mice or rabbits).
OAF	Osteoclast activating factor.
OPV	Oral poliovirus.
OS	Obese strain.
OT	Old tuberculin.
PA	Pernicious anemia.
PAF	Platelet-activating factor.
PAIDS	AIDS in pediatric patients.
PAP	Peroxidase antiperoxidase.
PAS	*p-Aminosalicylic acid; periodic acid-Schiff (reaction).*
PBC	Primary biliary cirrhosis.
PCA	Passive cutaneous anaphylaxis.
PCM	Protein-calorie malnutrition.
PCP	*Pneumocystis carinii* pneumonia.
PCR	Polymerase chain reaction.
PE	Phycoerythrin.
PEC	Peritoneal exudate cells.

PFC	Plaque-forming cells.
PG	Prostaglandin.
Pg5	Urinary pepsinogen.
PGE	Prostaglandin E (PGE_1, PGE_2, $PGE_{2\alpha}$).
PGM$_3$	Phosphoglucomutase 3.
PGN	Proliferative glomerulonephritis.
PHA	Phytohemagglutinin.
PIE	Pulmonary infiltration with eosinophilia.
pIgA	Polymeric IgA.
PK (P-K)	Prausnitz-Küstner (reaction).
PLL	Poly-L-lysine.
PLT	Primed lymphocyte typing.
PMA	Phorbol myristate acetate; a tumor promotor that stimulates monocytes and lymphocytes nonspecifically.
PML	Progressive multifocal leukodystrophy.
PMN	Polymorphonuclear neutrophil.
PNA	Peanut agglutinin.
PNH	Paroxysmal nocturnal hemoglobinuria.
PPD	Purified protein derivative (tuberculin).
PRP	Polysaccharide vaccine against *Haemophilus*.
PSS	Progressive systemic sclerosis.
PTH	Post transfusion hepatitis.
PVP	Polyvinylpyrrolidone.
PWM	Pokeweed mitogen.
R	Roentgen (unit of radiation).
RA	Rheumatoid arthritis.
Ragg	Rheumatoid agglutinin.
RANA	Rheumatoid arthritis nuclear antigen.
RAST	Radioallergosorbent test.
RBC	Red blood cell (erythrocyte); red blood count.
RE	Reticuloendothelial.
RES	Reticuloendothelial system.
RF	Rheumatic fever; rheumatoid factor.
RFLP	Restriction fragment length polymorphism.
RLIg	Rh immune globulin.
RIA	Radioimmunoassay.
RIF	Receptor-inducing factor.
RIST	Radioimmunosorbent test.
RNP	Ribonucleoprotein.
Ro	See SS-A.
RPR	Rapid plasma reagin.
RSV	Respiratory syncytial virus.
S	S value or sedimentation coefficient.
SAA	Serum amyloid A.
SAC	Staphylococcal protein A of Cowan I strain.
SBE	Subacute bacterial endocarditis.
SC	Secretory component.
SCID	Severe combined immunodeficiency disease.
SCL-1	Antinuclear antibody found in scleroderma.
SD	Serologically defined.
SFA	Suppressive factor of allergy.
SIDS	Sudden infant death syndrome.
sIg	Surface immunoglobulin.
sigA	Secretory IgA.
SIRS	Soluble immune response suppressor.
SK-SD, SKSD	Streptokinase-streptodornase.
SLE	Systemic lupus erythematosus.
SMA	Smooth muscle antibody.
SMAF	Specific macrophage arming factor.
SNagg	Serum normal agglutinator.

SpA	Staphylococcal protein A.
SRBC	Sheep red blood cells.
SRF	Skin-reactive factor.
SRS-A	Slow-reacting substance of anaphylaxis.
SS	Systemic sclerosis.
SS-A	Sjögren's syndrome antibody to RNA.
SS-B	Sjögren's syndrome antibody to RNA.
SSPE	Subacute sclerosing panencephalitis.
STS	Serologic test for syphilis.
TA	Transplantation antigens.
TA1	Trophoblast antigen 1.
Tac	T cell activation receptor.
TAF	T cell-activating factor.
TATA	Tumor-associated transplantation antigen.
TBII	Thyroid-binding inhibitory immunoglobulin.
TBM	Tubular basement membrane.
T$_C$	Cytotoxic T cells.
TCGF	T cell growth factor (see IL-2).
TCR	T cell receptor.
TD	Thymus-dependent.
Td	Combined tetanus and diphtheria toxoid (adult type).
TdT	Terminal deoxynucleotidyl transferase.
TEBG	Testosterone-estrogen binding globulin.
TF	Transfer factor.
TGF	Transforming growth factor.
TGSI	Thyroid growth-stimulating immunoglobulin.
T$_H$	Helper T cells.
Thy	Thymus-derived.
TI	Thymus-independent.
TIL	Tumor-infiltrating lymphocyte.
TL	Thymic lymphocyte (antigen) on prothymocytes.
TLI	Total lymphoid irradiation.
TLX	Trophoblast lymphocyte cross-reactive antigen.
TMP	Thymocyte mitogenic protein.
TNF	Tumor necrosis factor.
TNP	Trinitrophenyl.
Tp	Precursor T cells.
TPH	Transplacental fetal hemorrhage.
TPI	*Treponema pallidum* immobilization.
TRA	Thyrotropin receptor antibody.
Ts	Suppressor T cells.
TSA	Tumor-specific antigen.
TSab	Thyroid-stimulating antibody.
TSH	Thyroid-stimulating hormone.
TSI	Thyroid-stimulating immunoglobulin.
TU	Tuberculin units.
TX	Thromboxane.
VCA	Viral capsid antigen (of EBV).
VDRL	Venereal Disease Research Laboratory.
VEA	Virus envelope antigen.
V$_H$	Variable domain of heavy chain.
VIG	Vaccinia immune globulin.
V$_L$	Variable domain of light chain.
VLDL	Very low density lipoproteins.
VSG	Variable surface glycoprotein (of trypanosomes).
VZIG	Varicella-zoster immune globulin.
WBC	White blood cell; white blood count.
Z-DNA	Methylated DNA coiled into a left-handed helix.
ZIG	Zoster immune globulin.

Glossary of Symbols Used in Illustrations

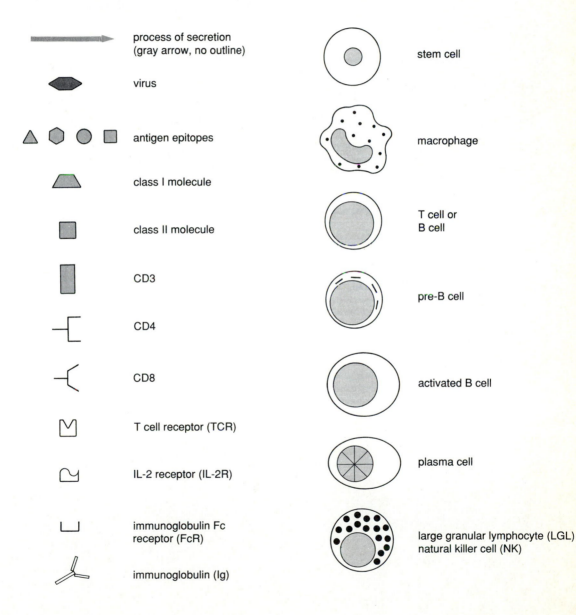

process of secretion (gray arrow, no outline)

virus

antigen epitopes

class I molecule

class II molecule

CD3

CD4

CD8

T cell receptor (TCR)

IL-2 receptor (IL-2R)

immunoglobulin Fc receptor (FcR)

immunoglobulin (Ig)

stem cell

macrophage

T cell or B cell

pre-B cell

activated B cell

plasma cell

large granular lymphocyte (LGL) natural killer cell (NK)

virus infected cell

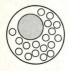 polymorphonuclear neutrophil (PMN)

eosinophil cell

mast cell

 red blood cell (RBC)

 platelets

epithelial cells

fibroblast

tumor cell

Note: Page numbers followed by a *t* or *f* indicate tables or figures, respectively.